THE

CHRONIC DISEASES,

THEIR PECULIAR NATURE

AND

THEIR HOMŒOPATHIC CURE,

BY

DR. SAMUEL HAHNEMANN.

TRANSLATED FROM THE SECOND ENLARGED GERMAN EDITION
OF 1835, BY

PROF. LOUIS H. TAFEL.

WITH ANNOTATIONS BY

RICHARD HUGHES, M. D.

EDITED BY

PEMBERTON DUDLEY, M. D.

B. Jain Publishers Pvt. Ltd.

NEW DELHI-110055

Export Edition

Reprint edition : 2001

Price Rs. 350.00 2 Vols. set

Published by :
Kuldeep Jain

For

B. Jain Publishers (P.) Ltd.
1921, Street No.10, Chuna Mandi
Paharganj, New Delhi-110 055 (INDIA)
Phones: 3670430; 3670572
FAX : 011-3610471
Email : bjain@vsnl.com
Website : www.bjainindia.com

Printed in India by:
J. J. Offset Printers
7, Wazirpur Printing Press Area,
Ring Road, Wazirpur, Delhi-110035

ISBN : 81-7021-267-7
ISBN : 81-7021-268-5
BOOK CODE : BH-2266

CONTENTS.

LIST OF MEDICINES.

CONTENTS.

TRANSLATOR'S PREFACE.

The translation here submitted to the public is the second translation of this work into English, it having before this been rendered by Dr. Charles J. Hempel and published by Wm. Radde in the years 1845-6. When it was proposed to reprint this translation, there was a strong protest made against the old version on the ground of its being to some degree inexact, and on account of its omitting not only the initials of the provers but besides this, also a great number of symptoms. These complaints have been proved well founded, especially with respect to the latter part of the work. We have taken a hundred symptoms at random here and there and compared them with the original, with the following results: in Alumina 555-655 we found only the omission of a part of symptom 556 and a partial omission and joining together of symptoms 617 and 618. So also in Graphites there is no omission except 53 (a repetition) in the first hundred, nor any other until we reach 200, 201 and 202 which are omitted. In the first hundred of Nitri acidum, however, we find 13 omissions, namely 6, 30, 32, 37, 38, 40, 43, 45, 59, 64, 65, 67 and 69. So also in Zincum from 1135 to 1235 we find 10 omissions, *i.e.*, 1136, 1138, 1152, 1170, 1187, 1197, 1207, 1220, 1222, 1225 and 1235; while 1153, 1195 and 1295 have one-half of their substance omitted. Between 1236 and 1335 there are 23 omissions, namely 1245, 1269, 1278, 1288, 1290, 1292, 1293, 1294, 1297, 1298, 1299, 1302, 1303, 1305, 1306, 1308, 1313, 1316, 1320, 1324, 1331, 1332, 1335, while one-half of the substance of symptoms 1287, 1296, 1312, 1315 and 1325 is omitted; showing the omission in this extreme case of over one-fourth. The omissions are rather impartially distributed, about one-third of the above omissions being symptoms of Hahnemann, fully one-third, those due to Nenning and the other third, distributed impartially among the various other provers.

These omissions made a new translation necessary, which was accordingly made independent of that of Dr. Hempel, though the earlier translation was consulted especially where there was any obscurity or ambiguity in the original. There is no question but that Hempel is right in what he says of the involved phraseology and the lengthy periods of Hahnemann; still we did not think it best to follow his mode of rendering, which according to his preface consists in "mastering the sense of a period, and then embodying it in a free manner in the foreign tongue." We have preferred to follow in this respect the example set by Dr. Dudgeon in his admirable translation of the *Materia Medica Pura* (London, 1880); he has faithfully rendered not only the ideas but also the expressions of Hahnemann. It is only by thus closely following the author, that we shall be sure to reproduce the ideas of the author and, indeed, in their own setting and thus in their native vigor and in the author's own original style. We have accordingly preserved the long periods of Hahnemann and his own precise, if sometimes redundant, phraseology; though, of course it was necessary to invert the periods and to arrange the phrases into the English order.

This applies chiefly to the first theoretic part of the work, and in this part we would especially acknowledge the able assistance of Dr. Pemberton Dudley, who has taken care that too close a clinging to the German original might be avoided.

We have generally endeavored to translate the same German word by the same English word, except where words have several meanings. A few particulars may here be mentioned. The frequently recurring adjective *drueckend*, which by Dr. Hempel is usually rendered with "aching" and by Dr. Dudgeon with "pressive" or with "aching," we have uniformly rendered with pressive· while we use "ache" to translate the German *weh*. There are a few words which require a varied translation according to the context: *Brust* is used both for "chest" and for "the female breast," so that *e.g. die rechte Brust* may mean either "the right breast" or "the right side of the chest;" *Hals* means either "throat" or "neck;" *Schenkel* may mean either "the thigh," "the leg" or "the whole lower limb," though for these parts usually the more specific terms *Oberschenkel*, *Unterschenkel* and *Bein* are used; *Gesicht* means either "face" or "sight." We have taken care to translate these terms according to the context in every case, though the learned reader will remember that in some of these cases there is a little ambiguity. One of the German terms which seems to have no good English equivalent is *Eingenommen* with respect to the head. It means literally "occupied" and describes the sensation produced in the head by a cold, where the parts are as it were benumbed and incapacitated from acting freely. Dr. Hempel has usually described this state of the head by "obtusion," Dr. Dudgeon usually by "confusion" or "muddled feeling." We have usually rendered it with "benumbed feeling," though as none of these terms was quite satisfactory, we have also sometimes used "muddled feeling" or obtuseness."

As was done in the *Materia Medica Pura* published in London, so we have also in this work printed the names of old school authorities cited with small capitals, while the names of other provers are in italics, so that it may be seen at a glance, whether the symptom was produced by an intentional proving (or from clinical experience), or whether it was the result of accidental poisoning or an overdose by an observer of the old school.

The Antipsoric Medicines have been annotated by Dr. Richard Hughes, of Bath, England, who in the course of his researches found occasion to rectify the numbers referring to the pages, etc. of a number of the citations. These at his suggestion were at first merely entered in the translation instead of the figures given by Hahnemann; but on second thought, it seemed more useful to give them among the other notes given by Dr. Hughes, as showing his diligence and the care given by him to these particulars.

While there seemed to be no necessity for an index to the Antipsoric Medicines, since this is furnished in the various repertories, especially in that of Bœnninghausen, it was thought useful to have an index to the first or theoretical part, and this was accordingly prepared by the translator.

L. H. TAFEL.

PREFATORY NOTE TO MATERIA MEDICA SECTION.

I have been desired, by the publishers of this new translation of Hahnemann's *Chronic Diseases*, to exercise a certain editorial superintendence over what may be called the Materia Medica section of the work. I shall do this mainly by notes appended to each pathogenesis; but in the present place I desire to state what is known in a general way about the symptom-lists in question,* and what I propose to do for them as they severally appear in the following pages.

I. In 1821 Hahnemann had been compelled to leave Leipsic, and, in difficulty where to find a place in which he could practice in freedom, had been offered an asylum in the little country town of Coethen Thither he repaired, and there he remained till his removal

* The information we have on this subject is fully given at page 31 of the later editions of my *Pharmacodynamics*. My present statement is based upon what is written there.

to Paris in 1835. He now ceased to attend acute disease, save in the family of his patron, the reigning Duke. But his fame brought him for consultation chronic sufferers from all parts; and the varied, shifting, and obstinate morbid states under which so many men and women labour were pressed closely upon his attention. The result was the theory of chronic disease which (in its latest shape) will be found in these pages, and which traces so many of its forms to a "psoric" origin. To meet the manifold disorders thus induced it seemed to him that a new set of remedies were required. Accordingly, of the three volumes of the first edition of the present work published in 1828, the two latter contained what seem to be pathogeneses of fifteen medicines hitherto strange to his *Materia Medica Pura*, and in some cases to any Materia Medica whatever. These medicines were

Ammonium carbonicum,	Magnesia muriatica,
Baryta carbonica,	Natrum carbonicum,
Calcarea carbonica,	Nitri acidum,
Graphites,	Petroleum,
Iodium,	Phosphorus,
Lycopodium,	Sepia,
Magnesia carbonica,	Silicea.

Zincum.

The pathogeneses of the foregoing (I assume them to be such from the analogy of the corresponding symptom-lists of the *Materia Medica Pura;* but they are not avowedly so) appear without a word of explanation as to how the symptoms were obtained, and without acknowledgment (as in the previous work) of fellow-observers. The absence of any co-operation on the part of others is further to be inferred from what we are told of the first announcement of the work. After six years of solitude at Coethen, Hahnemann "summoned thither his two oldest and most esteemed disciples, Drs. Stapf and Gross, and communicated to them his theory of the origin of chronic diseases, *and his discovery of a completely new series of medicaments for their cure.*" So writes Dr. Dudgeon.* This was in 1827. That he should now first reveal these new remedies, and in the following year should publish copious lists of their pathogenetic effects, confirms the inference to be drawn from his position and from his silence as to fellow-observers. He was himself between seventy and eighty years old, and it is hardly likely that he did anything at this time in the way of proving on his own person. We are compelled to the conclusion that he drew these symptoms mainly—if not entirely—

* *Lectures on Homœopathy*, p. xxx.

from the sufferers from chronic disease who flocked to his retreat to avail themselves of his treatment.

The prefatory notices to the several medicines still further substantiate this view, and throw some light on the doses with which the symptoms were obtained. He recommends all the medicines to be given in the dilutions from the 18th to the 30th (save Magnesia muriatica and Natrum carbonicum, of which he advises the 6th and 12th respectively); and repeatedly makes some such remark as this: "For a long time past I have given the 6th, 9th and 12th potencies, but found their effects too violent." Occasionally, too, he must have used the second and third triturations; as he speaks of having begun by giving a "small portion of a grain" of these, but, as this was an indefinite quantity, having subsequently dissolved and attenuated them. He mentions cases, moreover, in which he treated itch with Carbo vegetabilis and Sepia of the latter strength.

We may conclude, therefore, that it is these "violent effects" of the attenuations from the 2d to the 12th, experienced by the sufferers from chronic disease who took them, which make up the bulk—if not the whole—of the symptoms of the first issue of the *Chronic Diseases*.

In 1830 there appeared a third volume (making the fourth of the first edition) of symptom-lists, appended to two more new medicines—Kali carbonicum and Natrum muriaticum, and to five others—Carbo animalis and vegetabilis, Causticum, Conium and Sulphur—which had already found place in the *Materia Medica Pura*. Of the new ones we are told that two persons co-operated in obtaining the pathogenesis of Kali carbonicum and three in that of Natrum muriaticum—in the case of the latter the symptoms being obtained from healthy persons taking globules saturated with the 30th dilution.* Fresh associates are also acknowledged with regard to Conium. A new character is thus imprinted on the symptoms standing under the names of the several medicines, and it continues with respect to those contained in the second edition of the *Chronic Diseases*, published 1835–9, which is that here translated. Besides the twenty-two medicines of the first edition it contains twenty-five others, of which thirteen are new, and twelve had already appeared in the *Materia Medica Pura*. The new ones are:

Agaricus,
Alumina,
Ammonium muriaticum,
Anacardium,
Clematis,
Cuprum,
Euphorbium,
Mezereum,

* A specimen of these provings may be seen in the *Monthly Hom. Review* for 1889, p. 517.

Antimonium crudum,	Nitrum,
Borax,	Platina,
Sulphuris acidum.	

The old ones are:

Arsenicum,	Hepar sulphuris,
Aurum,	Manganum,
Colocynth,	Muriatis acidum,
Digitalis,	Phosphori acidum,
Dulcamara,	Sarsaparilla,
Guaiacum,	Stannum.

Those pathogeneses which had already seen the light have (generally) large additions; for all Hahnemann acknowledges contributions from fellow-observers, and for many cites symptoms from the extant literature of his day. The total number of these last is 1742.

There are, it is evident, fresh features in the pathogeneses of this second edition; and there are more than appear on the surface. Hahnemann's own additions, indeed, must be of the same character as his contributions to the first; *i. e.*, they must be collateral effects of the drugs observed on the patients to whom he gave them. They must all, moreover, be supposed to have resulted from the 30th dilution; for since 1829 he had urged the administration of all medicines at this potency. The same thing must be said of the contributions from Hahnemann's friends to this edition. They may fairly be conceived to have been provings on themselves or other healthy persons, save where, as in Wahle's symptoms of Mezereum and Hering's of Arsenic, the internal evidence is strong in the contrary direction. But they must in all cases have been evoked from the 30th dilution; for in the edition of the *Organon* published in 1833 Hahnemann recommends all provings to be made therewith, as yielding the best results. We have seen that the symptoms of Natrum muriaticum contributed by others to the fourth volume of the first edition were so obtained; and we may fairly extend the inference to all provings subsequently made. It is otherwise, however, with the provings first published in the *Materia Medica Pura*, in the present edition so largely incorporated with those of later origin. These seem, from the scanty information we have, to have been made with mother tinctures and first triturations—repeated small doses being taken until some effect was produced. Hahnemann was further able, at this time, to draw upon independent sources of drug-pathogenesy. Hartlaub and Trinks had published a Materia Medica of their own. Stapf had begun to issue his journal known as the *Archiv*, and many provings adorned its pages. Lastly, outside the Homœopathic school, Professor Joerg, of Leipsic, was following in Hahnemann's track and proving medicines on himself and his students. Of all these materials Hahnemann availed himself in the present work, which thus presents a complex whole, made up of very heterogeneous elements, and needing analysis that it may be appraised and used aright.

II. It is the giving such analysis that will constitute my editorial task. It will fall into the following categories:

1. In the preface to each medicine Hahnemann gives a list of names of "fellow-observers." To this I shall append a note, stating whether these were provers of the later or earlier times, in which case the manner of their experimentation is to be learned from what I have written above; or whether their observations already existed in print, and what information we have respecting them.

2. In the pathogeneses themselves, the first time an author is cited I shall state the nature of his contribution to the subject (supposing his work to have been accessible to me). Then—having examined his symptoms *in situ*—I shall append to each one that requires it such explanation or correction as may be necessary to set it forth in its full meaning and value.

3. The foregoing information, and any other I may be able to supply as to individual symptoms,* will be found in notes at the bottom of the page, designated by the small figures 1, 2, etc., and divided by a line from Hahnemann's own annotations, which have the usual *, †, etc. But while I have left untouched in the text the pathogenetic phenomena themselves, I have used greater freedom with the references to medical literature. These sometimes require correction, more frequently explanation—especially when transferred from the *Materia Medica Pura* or from Hartlaub and Trinks' work, in which case Hahnemann has practised omission to a very large extent, leaving those curious in the matter to refer to the previous publications. I have thought that the present volume would be more complete in itself, and more worthy of its author, were the references fully as well as rightly given; and have supplied them accordingly.

RICHARD HUGHES, M. D.

BRIGHTON, ENGLAND.

---

* See, for instance, notes to S. 114 of Colocynth and to S. 82 and 85 of Lycopodium.

EDITOR'S PREFACE.

Whatever estimate Science may finally place upon the discoveries and doctrines of Hahnemann, and whatever measure of confidence in his therapeutic belief Posterity may accord or withhold, his personality and work have achieved a position which must render them perpetually historic. His teachings have been so interwoven with the entire fabric of medical progress during the last hundred years, and are so interlaced with the formative development of the incoming century, that neither the wear and tear of time nor the dissections of criticism will ever be able to dissociate them. They are destined, inevitably, to run through the texture of every page in the future annals of medicine.

In the development of therapeutic art Hahnemann's position is more than merely transitional. He proclaims both an epoch and an era; he represents both discovery and progress. To-day, as a hundred years ago, he holds in one hand the past, in the other the future of medical achievement. The future historian, crossing the chasm between the medicine of speculative hypothesis and that based on observation of clinical and pharmaco-dynamic phenomena, will unfailingly recognize Hahnemann's agency in bringing about that remarkable transformation in medical thought and practice. And no exposition of Hahnemann's tenets, no rendition of his literary works, which fails to note and consider their historical relations and the historic individuality of their author, can be either adequate or just.

In the task of setting forth in the English tongue the works of Hahnemann, it thus becomes necessary not merely to note carefully the doctrines promulgated and the facts presented, but to exhibit also, so far as his recorded words express, and the resources of our own language enable us, the depth of the impression which his observations and discoveries must have produced upon his own mind, as well as the intensity of conviction, the earnestness of feeling, and the energy of demonstration, which characterize all his controversial writings. Long after his lineaments shall have faded from the canvas, his intellectual personality will survive in his literary creations and constitute an important feature of the medical chronicles of his time. To modify or disguise his modes of thought and expression, or to suppress the peculiarities of his literary style, would be an unpardonable distortion of the most pre-eminent figure in all medical history.

In that portion of this work in which Hahnemann considers the Nature and the Treatment of Chronic Diseases in general, and of Psora in particular, the reader will discover several peculiarities of style, some of which are not at all common to our English polemical literature. Among these we may mention: (1,) his long, and often involved, sentences; (2,) his exceedingly frequent employment of parenthetical clauses and sentences, and his not infrequent use of the parenthesis within a parenthesis; (3,) his multiplicity of iterations and reiterations—occurring twice or thrice in a single paragraph; sometimes twice in the same sentence—; (4,) his frequent interjection of words and phrases expressing anew some minor feature of the subject under discussion, but forming no part of the discussion itself; (5,) his introduction of qualifying words and phrases in certain peculiar and unusual connections, likely to escape the notice of the casual or careless reader, but evidently intended by the author to be taken at their full significance and importance and to constitute an essential element of the discussion. It may be said, in passing, that the failure to note this last-mentioned characteristic of Hahnemann's method has occasioned much misunderstanding of his doctrines.

No attempt has been made to render this work, or any portion of it, a model of concise perspicuity. On the contrary, the aim has been to retain, rather than to eliminate, the characteristic style of the original text, in order that every point in the discussion, and every shade of meaning should, if possible, be rendered exactly as the author has expressed it. The careful student, certainly the intelligent admirer, of Hahnemann could not be content with a mere transcription of his views and observations, but must insist on the opportunity to become familiar with his intellectual personality as he looks out upon the present-day world through the medium of his literary productions.

PEMBERTON DUDLEY, M. D.

PHILADELPHIA, 1896.

AUTHOR'S PREFACE.

TO THE FIRST EDITION—1828.

If I did not know for what purpose I was put here on earth—to become better myself as far as possible and to make better everything around me, that is within my power to improve—I should have to consider myself as lacking very much in worldly prudence to make known for the common good, even before my death, an art which I alone possess, and which it is within my power to make as profitable as possible by simply keeping it secret.

But in communicating to the world this great discovery, I am sorry that I must doubt whether my contemporaries will comprehend the logical sequence of these teachings of mine, and will follow them carefully and gain thereby the infinite benefits for suffering humanity which must inevitably spring from a faithful and accurate observance of the same; or whether, frightened away by the unheard of nature of many of these disclosures, they will not rather leave them untried and uninitiated and, therefore useless.

At least I cannot hope that these important communications will fare any better than the general Homœopathy which I have published hitherto. From unbelief in the efficacy of the small and attenuated doses of medicine which I made known to the medical world after a thousand warning trials, as being the most efficient, (distrusting my faithful asseverations and reasons), men prefer to endanger their patients for years longer with large and larger doses. Owing to this, they generally do not live to see the curative effects, even as was the case with myself before I attained this diminution of dose. The cause of this was, that it was overlooked that these doses by their attenuation were all the more suitable for their Homœopathic use, owing to the development of their dynamic power of operation.

What would men have risked if they had at once followed my directions in the beginning, and had made use of just these small doses from the first? Could anything worse have happened than that these doses might have proved inefficient? They surely could do no harm! But in their injudicious, self-willed application of large doses for homœopathic use they only, in fact *only* once again, went over that roundabout road so dangerous to their patients, in order to reach the truth which I myself had already successfully passed over, and indeed with trembling, so as to save them this trouble; and if they really desired to heal, they were nevertheless at last compelled to arrive at the only true goal, after having inflicted many an injury and wasted a good part of their fair life. All this I had already laid before them faithfully and frankly, and had long before given them the reasons.

May they do better with the great discovery herewith presented to them! And if they should not treat this discovery any better—well, then a more conscientious and intelligent posterity will alone have the advantage to be obtained by a faithful, punctual observance of the teachings here laid down, of being able to deliver mankind from the numberless torments which have rested upon the poor sick, owing to the numberless, tedious diseases, even as far back as history extends. This great boon had not been put within their reach by what Homœopathy had taught hitherto.

PREFACE TO THE FOURTH VOLUME.*

INQUIRY INTO THE PROCESS OF HOMŒOPATHIC HEALING.

We have no means of reaching with our senses or of gaining essential knowledge, as to the process of life in the interior of man, and it is only at times granted us to draw speculative conclusions from what is happening, as to the manner in which it may have occurred or taken place; but we are unable to furnish conclusive proofs of our explanations, from the changes which are observed in the inorganic kingdom; for the changes in living organic subjects have

* The work on the "Chronic Diseases" was originally published in five parts and every part, except the second, had its own preface, discussing some questions of general interest to Homœopathy.—*Transl.*

nothing in common with those taking place in what is inorganic, since they take place by processes entirely different.

It is, therefore, quite natural, that in presesenting the Homœopathic Therapeutics I did not venture to explain how the cure of diseases is effected by operating on the patient with substances possessing the power to excite very similar morbid symptoms in healthy persons. I furnished, indeed, a conjecture about it, but I did not desire to call it an explanation, *i. e.*, a definite explanation of the modus operandi. Nor was this at all necessary, for it is only incumbent upon us to cure similar symptoms correctly and successfully, according to a law of nature which is being constantly confirmed; but not to boast with abstract explanations, while we leave the patients uncured; for that is all which so-called physicians have hitherto accomplished.

These physicians have made many objections to the explanation I have given, and they would have preferred to reject the whole homœopathic method of curing (the only one possible), merely because they were not satisfied with my efforts at explaining the mode of procedure which takes place in the interiors of man during a homœopathic cure.

I write the present lines, not in order to satisfy those critics, but in order that I may present to myself and to my successors, the genuine practical Homœopaths, another and more probable attempt of this kind toward an explanation. This I present, because the human mind feels within it the irresistible, harmless and praiseworthy impulse, to give some account to itself as to the mode in which man accomplishes good by his actions.

As I have elsewhere shown, it is undeniable, that our vital force, without the assistance of active remedies of human art, cannot overcome even the slight acute diseases (if it does not succumb to them) and restore some sort of health, without sacrificing a part (often a large part) of the fluid and the solid parts of the organism through a so-called crisis. How our vital force effects this, will ever remain unknown to us; but so much is sure, that this force cannot overcome even these diseases in a direct manner, nor without such sacrifices. The Chronic Diseases, which spring from miasms, cannot be healed unaided, even by such sacrifices, nor can real health be restored by this force alone. But it is just as certain, that even if this force is enabled by the true (homœopathic) healing art, guided by the human understanding, to overpower and overcome (to cure) not only the quickly transient but also the chronic diseases arising from miasms in a direct manner and without such sacrifices, without loss of body and life, nevertheless, it is always this power, the vital force, which conquers. It is in this case as with the army of a country, which drives the enemy out of the country; this army ought to be called victorious, although it may not have won the victory without foreign auxiliaries. It is the organic vital force of our body which cures natural diseases of every kind directly and without any sacrifices, as soon as it is enabled by means of the correct (homœopathic) remedies to win the victory. This force would not, indeed, have been able to conquer without this assistance; for our organic vital force, taken alone, is only sufficient to maintain the unimpeded progress of life, so long as man is not morbidly affected by the hostile operation of forces causing disease.

Unassisted, the vital force is no match to these hostile powers; it hardly opposes a force equal to the hostile operation, and this, indeed, with many signs of its own sufferings (which we call morbid symptoms). By its own power, our vital force would never be able to overcome the foe of chronic disease, nor even to conquer transient diseases, without considerable losses inflicted on some parts of the organism, if it remained without external aid, without the assistance of genuine remedies. To give such support is the duty enjoined on the physician's understanding by the Preserver of life.

As I have said above, our vital force *hardly* opposes *an equal* opposition to the foe causing the disease, and yet no enemy can be overcome except by a superior force. Only homœopathic medicine can give this superior power to the invalidated vital force.

Of itself this vital principle, being only an organic vital force intended to preserve an undisturbed health, opposes only a weak resistance to the invading morbific enemy; as the disease grows and increases, it opposes a greater resistance, but at best, it is only an equal resistance; with weakly patients it is not even equal, but weaker. This force is neither capable, nor destined, nor created for an overpowering resistance, which will do no harm to itself.

But if we physicians are able to present and oppose to this instinctive vital force its morbific enemy, as it were magnified through the action of homœopathic medicines—even if it should be enlarged every time only by a little—if in this way the image of the morbific foe be magnified to the apprehension of the vital principle through homœopathic medicines, which in a delusive manner simulate the original disease, we gradually cause and compel this instinctive vital force to increase its energies by degrees, and to increase them more and more, and at last to such a degree that it becomes far more powerful than the original disease. The consequence of this is, that the vital force again becomes sovereign in its domain, can again hold and direct the reins of sanitary progress, while the apparent increase of the disease caused by homœopathic medicines, disappears of itself, as soon as we, seeing the preponderance of the restored vital force, *i. e.*, of the restored health, cease to use these remedies.

The fund or the fundamental essence of this spiritual vital principle, imparted to us men by the infinitely merciful Creator, is incredibly great, if we physicians understand how to maintain its integrity in days of health, by directing men to a healthy mode of living, and how to invoke and augment it in diseases by purely homœopathic treatment.

PREFACE TO FIFTH VOLUME.

DILUTIONS AND POTENCIES (DYNAMIZATIONS).

Dilutions, properly so-called, exist almost solely in objects of taste and of color. A solution of salty and bitter substances becomes continually more deprived of its taste the more water is added, and eventually it has hardly any taste, no matter how much it may be shaken. So, also, a solution of coloring matter, by the admixture of more and more water, becomes at last almost colorless, and any amount of shaking will not increase its color.

These are, and continue to be, real attenuations or dilutions, but no dynamizations.

Homœopathic Dynamizations are processes by which the medicinal properties, which are latent in natural substances while in their crude state, become aroused, and then become enabled to act in an almost spiritual manner on our life; *i. e.*, on our sensible and irritable fibre. This development of the properties of crude natural substances (dynamization) takes place, as I have before taught, in the case of dry substances by means of trituration in a mortar, but in the case of fluid substances, by means of shaking or succussion, which is also a trituration. These preparations cannot be simply designated as dilutions, although every preparation of this kind, in order that it may be raised to a higher potency, *i. e.*, in order that the medicinal properties still latent within it may be yet farther awakened and developed, must first undergo a further attenuation, in order that the trituration or succussion may enter still further into the very essence of the medicinal substance, and may thus also liberate and expose the more subtle part of the medicinal powers that lie hidden more deeply, which could not be effected by any amount of trituration and succussion of the substances in their concentrated form.

We frequently read in homœopathic books that, in the case of one or another person in a certain case of disease, some high (dilution) dynamization of a medicine was of no use at all, but a lower potency proved effectual, while others have seen more success from higher potencies. But no one in such cases investigates the cause of the great difference of these effects. What prevents the preparer of the medicines (and this ought to be the homœopathic physician himself; he himself ought to forge and whet the arms with which to fight the diseases)—what prevents him, in preparing a potency, from giving 10, 20, 50 and more succussive strokes against a somewhat hard, elastic body to every vial containing one drop of the lower potency with 99 drops of alcohol, so as to obtain strong potencies? This would be vastly more effective than giving only a few nerveless succussive strokes, which will produce little more than dilutions, which ought not to be the case.

The perfection of our unique art of healing and the welfare of the patients seem to make it worth while for the physician to take the trouble necessary to secure the utmost efficiency in his medicines.

Modern wiseacres have even sneered at the 30th potency, and would only use the lower, less developed and more massive preparations in larger doses, whereby they have been, however, unable to effect all that our art can accomplish. If, however, every potency is dynamized with the same number of succusive strokes, we obtain, even in the fiftieth potency, medicines of the most penetrating efficacy, so that every minute pellet moistened with it, after being dissolved in a quantity of water, can and must be taken in small parts, if we do not wish to produce too violent an action with sensitive patients, while we must remember that such a preparation contains almost all the properties latent in the drug now fully developed, and these can only then come into full activity.

PARIS, December 19th, 1838.

Nature of Chronic Diseases.

The Homœopathic healing art, as taught in my own writings and in those of my pupils, when faithfully followed, has hitherto shown its natural superiority over any allopathic treatment in a very decided and striking manner; and this not only in those diseases which suddenly attack men (the acute diseases), but also in epidemic diseases and in sporadic fevers.

Venereal diseases also have been radically healed by Homœopathy much more surely, with less trouble and without any sequelæ; for without disturbing or destroying the local manifestation it heals the internal fundamental disease from within only, through the best specific remedy. But the number of the other chronic diseases on this great earth has been immeasurably greater, and remains so.

Treatment by allopathic physicians hitherto merely served to increase the distress from this kind of disease; for this treatment consisted of a whole multitude of nauseous mixtures (compounded by the druggist from violently acting medicines in large doses, of whose separate true effects they were ignorant), together with the use of manifold baths, the sudorific and salivating remedies, the pain-killing narcotics, the injections, fomentations, fumigations, the blistering plasters, the exutories and fontanels, but especially the everlasting laxatives, leeches, cuppings and starving treatments, or whatever names may be given to all these medicinal torments, which continually varied like the fashions. By these means the disease was either aggravated and the vital force, spite of so-called tonics used at intervals, was more and more diminished; or, if any striking change was produced by them, instead of the former sufferings, there appeared a worse state—nameless diseases caused by medicine, far worse and more incurable than the original natural one—while the physician consoled the patient with the words: "The former sickness I have been fortunate enough to remove; it is a great pity that a new (?) disease has appeared, but I hope to be as successful in removing this latter as in the former." And so, while *the same disease assumed various forms*, and while new diseases were being added by the use of improper, injurious medicines, the sufferings of the patient were continually aggravated until his pitiable lamentations were hushed forever with his dying breath, and the relatives were soothed with the comforting pretense: "Everything imaginable has been used and applied in the case of the deceased."

It is not so with Homœopathy, the great gift of God!

Even in these other kinds of chronic diseases, its disciples, by following the teachings presented in my former writings and my former oral lectures, accomplished far more than all the afore-mentioned methods of curing; *i. e.*, when they found the patient not too much run down and spoiled by allopathic treatment, as was unfortunately too often the case where the patient had any money to spend.

Using the more natural treatment, Homœopathic physicians have frequently been able in a short time to remove the chronic disease which they had before them, after examining it according to all the symptoms perceptible to the senses; and the means of cure were the most suitable among the Homœopathic remedies, used in their smallest doses which had been so far proved as to their pure, true effects. And all this was done without robbing the patient of his fluids and strength, as is done by the allopathy of the common physicians; so that the patient, fully healed, could again enjoy gladsome days. These cures indeed have far excelled all that allopathists had ever—in rare cases—been able to effect by a lucky grab into their medicine chests.

The complaints yielded for the most part to very small doses of that remedy which had proved its ability to produce the same series of morbid symptoms in the healthy body; and, if the disease was not altogether too inveterate and had not been too much and in too great a degree mismanaged by allopathy, it often yielded for a considerable time, so that mankind had good reason to deem itself fortunate even for that much help, and, indeed, it often proclaimed its thankfulness. A patient thus treated might and often did consider himself in pretty good health, when he fairly judged of his present improved state and compared it with his far more painful condition before Homœopathy had afforded him its help.*

Even some gross errors of diet, taking cold, the appearance of

* Of this kind were the cures of diseases caused by a psora not yet fully developed, which had been treated by my followers with remedies which did not belong to the number of those which, later, proved to be the chief anti-psora remedies; because these remedies were not yet known. They had been merely treated with such medicines as Homœopathically best covered and temporarily removed the then apparent moderate symptoms, thus causing a kind of a cure which brought back the manifest psora into a latent condition and thus produced a kind of healthy condition, especially with young, vigorous

weather especially rough, wet and cold or stormy, or even the approach of autumn, if ever so mild, but, more yet, winter and a wintry spring, and then some violent exertion of the body or mind, but particularly some shock to the health caused by some severe external injury, or a very sad event that bowed down the soul, repeated fright, great grief, sorrow and continuous vexation, often caused in a weakened body the re-appearance of one or more of the ailments which seemed to have been already overcome; and this new condition was often aggravated by some quite new concomitants, which if not more threatening than the former ones which had been removed homœopathically were often just as troublesome and now more obstinate. This would be especially the case whenever the seemingly cured disease had for its foundation a psora which had been more fully developed. When such a relapse would take place the Homœopathic physician would give the remedy most fitting among the medicines then known, as if directed against a new disease, and this would again be attended by a pretty good success, which for the time would again bring the patient into a better state. In the former case, however, in which merely the troubles which seemed to have been removed were renewed, the remedy which had been serviceable the first time would prove less useful, and when repeated again it would help still less. Then perhaps, even under the operation of the Homœopathic remedy which seemed best adapted, and even where the mode of living had been quite correct, new symptoms of disease would be added which could be removed only inadequately and imperfectly; yea, these new symptoms were at times not at all improved, especially when some of the obstacles above mentioned hindered the recovery.

Some joyous occurrence, or an external condition of circumstances improved by fortune, a pleasant journey, a favorable season or a dry, uniform temperature, might occasionally produce a remarkable pause of shorter or longer duration in the disease of the patient, during which the Homœopath might consider him as fairly recovered; and the patient himself, if he good-naturedly overlooked some passable moderate ailments, might consider himself as healthy. Still such a favorable pause would never be of long duration, and the return and repeated returns of the complaints in the end left even the best selected Homœopathic remedies then known, and given in the most

persons, such as would appear as real health to every observer who did not examine accurately; and this state often lasted for many years. But with chronic diseases caused by a psora already fully developed, the medicines which were then known never sufficed for a complete cure, any more than these same medicines suffice at the present time.

appropriate doses, the less effective the oftener they were repeated. They served at last hardly even as weak palliatives. But usually, after repeated attempts to conquer the disease which appeared in a form always somewhat changed, residual complaints appeared which the Homœopathic medicines hitherto proved, though not few, had to leave uneradicated, yea, often undiminished. Thus there ever followed varying complaints ever more troublesome, and, as time proceeded, more threatening, and this even while the mode of living was correct and with a punctual observance of directions. The chronic disease could, despite all efforts, be but little delayed in its progress by the Homœopathic physician and grew worse from year to year.

This was, and remained, the quicker or slower process in such treatments in all non-venereal, severe chronic diseases, even when these were treated in exact accordance with the Homœopathic art as hitherto known. Their beginning was promising, the continuation less favorable, the outcome hopeless.

Nevertheless this teaching was founded upon the steadfast pillar of truth and will evermore be so. The attestation of its excellence, yea, of its infallibility (so far as this can be predicated of human affairs), it has laid before the eyes of the world through facts.

Homœopathy *alone* taught *first of all* how to heal the well-defined idiopathic diseases, the old, smooth scarlet fever of Sydenham, the more recent purples, whooping cough, croup, sycosis, and autumnal dysenteries, by means of the specifically aiding Homœopathic remedies. Even acute pleurisy, and typhous contagious epidemics must now allow themselves to be speedily turned into health by a few small doses of rightly-selected Homœopathic medicine.

Whence then this less favorable, this unfavorable, result of the continued treatment of the non-venereal chronic diseases even by Homœopathy? What was the reason of the thousands of unsuccessful endeavors to heal the other diseases of a chronic nature so that lasting health might result? Might this be caused, perhaps, by the still too small number of Homœopathic remedial means that have so far been proved as to their pure action? The followers of Homœopathy have hitherto thus consoled themselves; but this excuse, or so-called consolation, never satisfied the founder of Homœopathy—particularly because even the new additions of proved valuable medicines, increasing from year to year, have not advanced the healing of chronic (non-venereal) diseases by a single step, while acute diseases (unless these, at their commencement, threaten unavoidable death) are not only passably removed, by means of a correct application of Homœopathic remedies, but with the assistance of the never-resting, preservative vital force in our organism, find a speedy and complete cure.

Why, then, cannot this vital force, efficiently affected through Homœopathic medicine, produce any true and lasting recovery in these chronic maladies even with the aid of the Homœopathic remedies which best cover their present symptoms; while this same force which is created for the restoration of our organism is nevertheless so indefatigably and successfully active in completing the recovery even in severe acute diseases? What is there to prevent this?

The answer to this question, which is so natural, inevitably led me to the discovery of the nature of these chronic diseases.

To find out then the reason why all the medicines known to Homœopathy failed to bring a real cure in the above-mentioned diseases, and to gain an insight more nearly correct and, if possible, quite correct, into the true nature of the thousands of chronic diseases which still remain uncured, despite the incontestable truth of the Homœopathic Law of Cure, this very serious task has occupied me since the years 1816 and 1817, night and day; and behold! the Giver of all good things permitted me within this space of time to gradually solve this sublime problem through unremitting thought, indefatigable inquiry, faithful observation and the most accurate experiments made for the welfare of humanity.*

It was a continually repeated fact that the non-venereal chronic diseases, after being time and again removed homœopathically by the remedies fully proved up to the present time, always returned in a more or less varied form and with new symptoms, or reappeared annually with an increase of complaints. This fact gave me the first clew that the Homœopathic physician with such a chronic (non-venereal) case, yea in all cases of (non-venereal) chronic disease, has not only to combat the disease presented before his eyes, and must not view and treat it as if it were a well-defined disease, to be speedily and permanently destroyed and healed by ordinary homœopathic remedies, but that he has always to encounter only some separate fragment of a more deep-seated original disease.

*Yet I did not allow any of these unintermitted endeavors to become known either to the world or to my followers, not, indeed, because the ingratitude so frequently shown to me prevented me, for I heed neither ingratitude nor persecutions on my troublous path of life, which yet has not proved altogether joyless, because of the great goal toward which I have striven. No, I left it unmentioned because it is improper, yea, hurtful to speak or write of things still immature. Not until the year 1827 did I communicate the essentials of the discovery to two of my pupils, who had been of the greatest service to the art of Homœopathy, for their own benefit and that of their patients, so that the whole discovery might not be lost to the world if perchance a higher call to eternity had called me away before the completion of the book—an event not so very improbable in my seventy-third year.

The great extent of this disease is shown in the new symptoms appearing from time to time; so that the Homœopathic physician must not hope to permanently heal the separate manifestations of this kind in the presumption, hitherto entertained, that they are well-defined, separately existing diseases which can be healed permanently and completely. *He, therefore, must first find out as far as possible the whole extent of all the accidents and symptoms belonging to the unknown primitive malady* before he can hope to discover one or more medicines which may homœopathically cover the whole of the original disease by means of its peculiar symptoms. By this method he may then be able victoriously to heal and wipe out the malady in its whole extent, consequently also its separate members; that is, all the fragments of a disease appearing in so many various forms.

But that the original malady sought for must be also of a *miasmatic*, chronic nature clearly appeared to me from this circumstance, that after it has once advanced and developed to a certain degree it can never be removed by the strength of any robust constitution, it can never be overcome by the most wholesome diet and order of life, nor will it die out of itself. But it is evermore aggravated, from year to year, through a transition into other and more serious symptoms,* even till the end of man's life, like every other chronic, miasmatic sickness; *e. g.*, the venereal bubo which has not been healed from within by mercury, its specific remedy, but has passed over into venereal disease. This latter, also, never passes away of itself, but, even with the most correct mode of life and with the most robust bodily constitution, increases every year and unfolds evermore into new and worse symptoms, and this, also, to the end of man's life.

I had come thus far in my investigations and observations with such non-venereal patients, when I discovered, even in the beginning, that the obstacle to the cure of many cases which seemed delusively like specific, well-defined diseases, and yet could not be cured in a Homœopathic manner with the then proved medicines), seemed very often to lie in a former eruption of itch, which was not unfrequently confessed; and the beginning of all the subsequent sufferings usually dated from that time. So also with similar chronic patients who did not confess such an infection, or, what was probably more frequent,

---

***Not unfrequently phthisis passes over into insanity; dried-up ulcers into dropsy or apoplexy; intermittent fever into asthma; affections of the abdomen into pains in the joints or paralysis; pains in the limbs into hemorrhage, etc., and it was not difficult to discover that the later diseases must also have their foundation in the original malady and can only be a part of a far greater whole.**

who had, from inattention, not perceived it, or, at least, could not remember it. After a careful inquiry it usually turned out that little traces of it (small pustules of itch, herpes, etc.) had showed themselves with them from time to time, even if but rarely, as an indubitable sign of a former infection of this kind.

These circumstances, in connection with the fact that innumerable observations of physicians,* and not infrequently my own experience, had shown that an eruption of itch suppressed by faulty practice or one which had disappeared from the skin through other means was evidently followed, in persons otherwise healthy, by the same or similar symptoms; these circumstances, I repeat, could leave no doubt in my mind as to the internal foe which I had to combat in my medical treatment of such cases.

Gradually I discovered more effective means against this original malady that caused so many complaints; against this malady which may be called by the general name of *Psora*; *i. e.*, against the internal itch disease with or without its attendant eruption on the skin. It then became manifest to me, through the aid afforded when using these medicines in similar chronic diseases, in which the patient was unable to show a like cause, that also these cases in which the patient remembered no infection of this kind were of necessity caused by a *Psora* with which he had been infected, perhaps, even in his cradle, or in some other way that had escaped his memory; and this often received corroboration on a more careful inquiry with the parents or aged relatives.

Most painstaking observations as to the aid afforded by the antipsoric remedies which were added in the first of these eleven years have taught me evermore, how frequently not only the moderate, but also the more severe and the most severe, chronic diseases are of this origin. This observation taught me that not only most of the many cutaneous eruptions which *Willan* distinguishes with such extreme care from one another, and which have received separate names, but also almost all adventitious formations, from the common wart on the finger up to the largest sarcomatous tumor, from the malformations of the finger-nails up to the swellings of the bones and the curvature of the spine, and many other softenings and deformities of the bones, both at an early and at a more advanced age, are caused by the *Psora*. So, also, frequent epistaxis, the accumulation of blood in the veins of the rectum and the anus, discharges of blood from the same (blind or flowing piles), hemoptysis, hematemesis, hematuria, and deficient as well as too frequent menstrual discharges,

---

* So also, more lately, VON AUTENRIETH (in *Tübinger Blätter für Naturwissenschaft und Arzneikunde*, 2 vol., 2d part.)

night-sweats of several years' duration, parchment-like dryness of the skin, diarrhœa of many years' standing, as well as permanent constipation and difficult evacuation of the bowels, long-continued erratic pains, convulsions occurring repeatedly for a number of years, chronic ulcers and inflammations, sarcomatous enlargements and tumors, emaciation, excessive sensitiveness as well as deficiencies in the senses of seeing, hearing, smelling, tasting and feeling; excessive as well as extinguished sexual desire; diseases of the mind and of the soul, from imbecility up to ecstacy, from melancholy up to raging insanity; swoons and vertigo; the so-called diseases of the heart; abdominal complaints and all that is comprehended under hysteria and hypochondria—in short, thousands of tedious ailments of humanity called by pathology with various names, are, with few exceptions, true descendants of this many-formed *Psora* alone. I was thus instructed by my continued observations, comparisons and experiments in the last years, that the ailments and infirmities of body and soul which, in their manifest complaints, differ so radically and which, with different patients, appear so very unlike (if they do not belong to the two venereal diseases, *syphilis* and *sycosis*), are but partial manifestations of the ancient miasma of leprosy and itch; *i. e.*, merely descendants of one and the same vast original malady, the almost innumerable symptoms of which form but one whole and are to be regarded and to be medicinally treated as the parts of one and the same disease in the same way as in a great epidemic of typhus fever. Thus in the year 1813 one patient would be prostrated with only a few symptoms of this plague, a second patient showed only a few but different ailments, while a third, fourth, etc., would complain of still other ailments belonging to this epidemic disease, while they were, nevertheless, all sick with one and the same pestilential fever, and the entire and complete image of the typhus fever reigning at the time could only be obtained by gathering together the symptoms of all, or at least of many of these patients. Then the one or two remedies,* found to be Homœopathic, healed the whole epidemy, and therefore showed themselves specifically helpful with every patient, though the one might be suffering from symptoms differing from those of others, and almost all seemed to be suffering from different diseases.

Just so, only upon a *far larger* scale, it is with the *Psora*, this fundamental disease of so many chronic maladies, each of which seems to be essentially different from the others, but really is not; as may readily be seen from the agreement of several symptoms

*In the typhus of 1813 *bryonia* and *rhus toxicodendron* were the specific remedies for all the patients.

common to them which appear as the disease runs its course, and also from their being healed through the same remedy.

All chronic diseases of mankind, even those left to themselves, not aggravated by a perverted treatment, show, as said, such a constancy and perseverance, that as soon as they have developed and have not been thoroughly healed by the medical art, they evermore increase with the years, and during the whole of man's lifetime; and they cannot be diminished by the strength belonging even to the most robust constitution. Still less can they be overcome and extinguished. Thus they never pass away of themselves, but increase and are aggravated even till death. They must therefore all have for their origin and foundation constant chronic miasms, whereby their parasitical existence in the human organism is enabled to continually rise and grow.

In Europe and also on the other continents so far as it is known, according to all investigations, only three chronic miasms are found, the diseases caused by which manifest themselves through local symptoms, and from which most, if not all, the chronic diseases originate; namely, first, SYPHILIS, which I have also called the *venereal chancre disease;* then SYCOSIS, or *the fig-wart disease*, and finally the chronic disease which lies at the foundation of the eruption of itch; *i. e.*, the PSORA; which I shall treat of first as the most important.

PSORA is that *most ancient*, *most universal*, *most destructive*, and yet *most misapprehended* chronic miasmatic disease which for many thousands of years has disfigured and tortured mankind, and which during the last centuries has become the mother of all the thousands of incredibly various (acute and) chronic (non-venereal) diseases, by which the whole civilized human race on the inhabited globe is being more and more afflicted.

PSORA is the *oldest* miasmatic chronic disease known to us. Just as tedious as syphilis and sycosis, and therefore not to be extinguished before the last breath of the longest human life, unless it is thoroughly cured, since not even the most robust constitution is able to destroy and extinguish it by its own proper strength, *Psora*, or the Itch disease, is beside this the *oldest* and *most hydra-headed* of all the chronic miasmatic diseases.

In the many thousands of years during which it may have afflicted mankind,—for the most ancient history of the most ancient people does not reach to its origin,—it has so much increased in the extent of its pathological manifestations—an extent which may to some

† See Organon of the Healing Art, fifth edition, 1834, § 100 sqq.

degree be explained by its increased development during such an inconceivable number of years in so many millions of organisms through which it has passed,—that its secondary symptoms are hardly to be numbered. And, if we except those diseases which have been created by a perverse medical practice or by deleterious labors in quicksilver, lead, arsenic, etc., which appear in the common pathology under a hundred proper names as supposedly separate and well-defined diseases (and also those springing from *syphilis* and the still rarer ones springing from *sycosis*), all the remaining natural chronic diseases, whether with names or without them, find in PSORA their real origin, their only source.

The oldest monuments of history which we possess show the *Psora* even then in great development. Moses* 3400 years ago pointed out several varieties. At that time and later on among the Israelites the disease seems to have mostly kept the external parts of the body for its chief seat. This was also true of the malady as it prevailed in uncultivated Greece, later in Arabia and, lastly in Europe during the Middle Ages. The different names which were given by different nations to the more or less malignant varieties of leprosy, (the external symptom of *Psora*) which in many ways deformed the external parts of the body, do not concern us and do not affect the matter, since the nature of this miasmatic itching eruption always remained essentially the same.

The occidental *Psora*, which during the Middle Ages had raged in Europe for several centuries under the form of malignant erysipelas (called *St. Anthony's Fire*), reassumed the form of leprosy through the leprosy which was brought back by the returning crusaders in the thirteenth century. And though it thus spread in Europe even more than before, (for in the year 1226 there were in France alone 2,000 houses for the reception of lepers), this Psora, which now raged as a dreadful eruption, found at least an ex-

---

*In Leviticus not only in the thirteenth chapter, but also (chapt. 21, verse 20) where he speaks of the bodily defects which must not be found in a priest who is to offer sacrifice, malignant itch is designated by the word *garab*, which the Alexandrian translators (in the Septuagint) translated with *psora agria*, but the Vulgate with *scabies jugis*. The talmudic interpreter, Jonathan, explained it as *dry itch spread over the body;* while the expression, *yalephed*, is used by Moses for *lichen*, *tetter*, *herpes* (see M. Rosenmueller, *Scholia in Levit.*, p. II., *edit. sec.*, p. 124). The commentators in the so-called English Bible-work also agree with this definition, Calmet among others saying: "Leprosy is similar to an inveterate itch with violent itching." The ancients also mention the peculiar, characteristic *voluptuous* itching which attended itch then as now, while after the scratching a painful burning follows; among others Plato, who calls itch *glykypikron*, while Cicero marks the *dulcedo* of *scabies*.

ternal alleviation in the means conducive to cleanliness, which also were brought by the crusaders from the Orient; namely, the (cotton? linen?) shirts before unknown in Europe, and the more frequent use of warm baths. Through both of those means, as well as through the more exquisite diet and refinement in the mode of living introduced by increased cultivation, the external horrors of the Psora within the space of several centuries were at last so far moderated, that, at the end of the fifteenth century it appeared only in the form of the common eruption of itch, just at the time when the other miasmatic chronic disease, *syphilis*, began (in 1493) to raise its dreadful head.

Thus this eruption, externally reduced in cultivated countries to a common itch, could be much more easily removed from the skin through various means; so that with the medicinal external treatment since introduced, especially in the middle and higher classes, through baths, washes and ointments of sulphur and lead, and by preparations of copper, zinc and mercury, the external manifestations of *Psora* on the skin were often so quickly suppressed, and are so now, that in most cases either of children or of grown persons the history of itch infection may remain undiscovered.

But the state of mankind was not improved thereby; in many respects it grew far worse. For, although in ancient times the eruption of psora appearing as leprosy was very troublesome to those suffering from it, owing to the lancinating pains in, and the violent itching all around the tumors, and scabs, the rest of the body enjoyed a fair share of general health. This was owing to the obstinately persistent eruption on the skin which served as a substitute for the internal psora. And what is of more importance, the horrible and disgusting appearance of the lepers made such a terrible impression on healthy people that they dreaded even their approach; so that the seclusion of most of these patients, and their separation in leper hospitals, kept them apart from other human society and infection from them was thus limited and comparatively rare.

In consequence of the very much milder form of the *psora* during the fourteenth and fifteenth centuries, when it appeared as itch, the few pustules appearing after infection made but little show and could easily be concealed. Nevertheless they were scratched continually because of their unbearable itching, and thus the fluid was diffused around, and the psoric miasma was communicated more certainly and more easily to many other persons, the more it was concealed. For the things rendered unclean by the psoric fluid infected the persons who unwittingly touched them, and thus contaminated far more persons than the lepers, who, on account of their horrible appearance, were carefully avoided.

PSORA has thus become the *most infectious* and *most general* of all the chronic miasmas. For the miasm has usually been communicated to others before the one from whom it emanates has asked for or received any external repressive remedy against his itching eruption (lead-water, ointment of the white precipitate of mercury), and without confessing that he had an eruption of itch, often even without knowing it himself; yea, without even the physician's or surgeon's knowing the exact nature of the eruption which has been repressed by the lotion of lead, etc.

It may well be conceived that the poorer and lower classes, who allow the itch to spread on their skin for a long time, until they become an abomination to all around them and are compelled to use something to remove it, must have in the meanwhile infected many.

Mankind, therefore, is worse off from the change in the external form of the *psora*,—from leprosy down to the eruption of itch—not only because this is less visible and more secret and therefore more frequently infectious, but also especially because the *psora*, now mitigated externally into a mere itch, and on that account more generally spread, nevertheless still retains unchanged its original dreadful nature. Now, after being more easily repressed, the disease grows all the more unperceived within, and so, in the last three centuries, after the destruction* of its chief symptom (the external skin-eruption) it plays the sad rôle of causing innumerable secondary symptoms; *i. e.*, it originates a legion of chronic diseases, the source of which physicians neither surmise nor unravel, and which, therefore, they can no more cure than they could cure the original disease when accompanied by its cutaneous eruption; but these chronic diseases, as daily experience shows, were necessarily aggravated by the multitude of their faulty remedies.

So great a flood of numberless nervous troubles, painful ailments, spasms, ulcers (cancers), adventitious formations, dyscrasias, paralyses, consumptions and cripplings of soul, mind and body were never seen in ancient times when the *psora* mostly confined

* The external eruption of itch may not only be driven away by the faulty practices of physicians and quacks, but unfortunately it not unfrequently of its own accord withdraws from the skin (see below, *e. g.*, in the observation of the older physicians, Nos. 9, 17, 26, 36, 50, 58, 61, 64, 65). *Syphilis* and *sycosis* both have an advantage over the itch disease, in this, that the chancre (or bubo) in the one and the fig-wart in the other never leave the external parts until they have been either mischievously destroyed through external repressive remedies or have been in a rational manner removed through the simultaneous internal cure of the whole disease. The venereal disease cannot, therefore, break out so long as the chancre is not artificially destroyed by external applications, nor can the secondary ailments of sycosis break out so long as the

itself to its dreadful cutaneous symptom, leprosy. Only during the last few centuries has mankind been flooded with these infirmities, owing to the causes just mentioned.*

It was thus that PSORA became the *most universal* mother of chronic diseases.

The *psora*, which is now so easily and so rashly robbed of its

fig-wart has not been destroyed by faulty practice; for these local symptoms, which act as substitutes for the internal disease, remain standing even until the end of man's life, and prevent the breaking out of the internal disease. It is, therefore, just as easy to heal them then, even in their whole extent; *i. e.*, thoroughly, through their specific internal medicines, which need only to be continued until these local symptoms (chancre and fig-wart) which are in their nature *unchangeable* except through artificial external application, are thoroughly healed. Then we may be quite certain that we have thoroughly cured the internal disease; *i. e.*, *syphilis* and *sycosis*.

This good feature *psora* has lost in the present more and more mitigated nature of its chief symptom, which has changed from leprosy to itch in the last three centuries. The eruption of itch by no means remains as persistently in its place on the skin as the chancre and the fig-wart. Even if the eruption of itch has not (as is nearly always the case) been driven away from the skin through the faulty practices of physicians and quacks by means of desiccating washes, sulphur ointments, drastic purgatives or cupping, it frequently disappears, as we say, *of itself*; *i. e.*, through causes which are not noticed. It often disappears through some unlucky physical or psychical occurrence, through a violent fright, through continual vexations, deeply-affecting grief, through catching a severe cold, or through a cold temperature (see below, observation 67); through cold, lukewarm and warm river baths or mineral baths, by a fever arising from any cause, or through a different acute disease (*e. g.*, smallpox; see below, observation 39); through persistent diarrhœa, sometimes also perhaps through a peculiar want of activity in the skin, and the results in such a case are just as mischievous as if the eruption had been driven away externally by the irrational practice of a physician. The secondary ailments of the internal *psora* and any one of the innumerable chronic diseases flowing from this origin will then break out sooner or later.

But let no one think that the *psora* which has been thus mitigated in its local symptom, its cutaneous eruption, differs materially from ancient leprosy. Even leprosy, when not inveterate, could in ancient times not seldom be driven from the skin by cold baths or by repeated dipping in a river and through warm mineral baths (see below, No. 35); but also then the evil effects resulting were as little regarded as the more modern physicians regard the acute diseases and the insidious maladies which do not fail to develop sooner or later from the indwelling *psora* when an eruption of the present itch disease has disappeared of itself or has been violently driven away.

*That the drinking of warm coffee and Chinese tea which has spread so generally in the last two centuries, and which has so largely increased the irritability of the muscular fibre as well as the excessive excitability of the nerves, has further augmented the tendency of this period to a multitude of chronic diseases, and has thus aided the *psora*, I least of all *can doubt*, as I have made prominent, perhaps too prominent, the part which coffee takes with re-

ameliorating cutaneous symptom, the eruption of itch, which acts vicariously for the internal disease, has been producing within the last three hundred years more and more secondary symptoms, and indeed so many that at least *seven-eighths* of all the chronic maladies spring from it as their only source, while the *remaining eighth* springs from *syphilis* and *sycosis* or from a complication of two of these three miasmatic chronic diseases, or (which is rare) from a complication of all three of them. Even *syphilis*, which on account of its easy curability yields to the smallest dose of the best preparation of mercury, and *sycosis*, which on account of the slight difficulty in its cure through a few doses of thuja and nitric acid in alternation, only pass into a tedious malady difficult to cure when they are complicated with psora. Thus PSORA *is among all diseases the one which is most misapprehended, and, therefore, has been medically treated in the worst and most injurious manner.*

It is incredible to what an extent modern physicians of the common school have sinned against the welfare of humanity; since, with scarcely an exception, teachers of medicine and the more prominent modern physicians and medical writers have laid down the rule and taught it as an infallible theorem that: "Every eruption of itch is merely a local ailment of the skin, in which ailment the remaining organism takes no part at all, so that it may and must be driven away from the skin at any time and without any scruple, through local applications of sulphur ointment or of the yet more active ointment of Jasser, through sulphur fumigations, by solutions of lead and zinc, but most quickly by the precipitates of mercury. If the eruption is once removed from the skin everything is well and the person is restored and the whole disease removed. Of course, if the eruption is neglected and allowed to spread upon the skin, then it may eventually turn out that the malignant matter may find opportunity to insinuate itself through the absorbent vessels into the mass of humors, and thus to corrupt the blood, the humors and the health. Then, indeed, man may finally be afflicted with ailments from these malignant humors, though these might soon again be removed from the body by purgatives and abluents; but through prompt removal of the eruption

spect to the bodily and mental sufferings of humanity, in my little work on "The Effects of Coffee" (*Die Wirkungen des Kaffee's.* Leipzig, 1803). This, perhaps undue, prominence given was owing to the fact that I had not then as yet discovered the chief source of chronic diseases in the *psora.* Only in connection with the excessive use of coffee and tea, which both offer palliatives for several symptoms of *psora*, could *psora* spread such innumerable, such obstinate chronic sufferings among mankind; for psora alone could not have produced this effect.

from the skin all sequelæ are prevented, and the internal body remains entirely healthy."

These horrible untruths have not only been, and are still being taught, but they are also carried out in practice. The consequence is that at the present day the patients in all the most celebrated hospitals, even in those countries and cities that seem most enlightened, as well as the private itch-patients of the lower and higher classes, the patients in all the penitentiaries and orphan asylums, in other civil and military hospitals, wherever such eruptions are found—in short, the innumerable multitude of patients, without exception, are treated, not only by physicians unknown to fame, but by all, even those *most celebrated*, with the above mentioned external remedies,* using perhaps at the same time large doses of flowers of sulphur, and strong purgatives (to cleanse the body, as they say). These physicians think that the more quickly these eruptions are driven from the skin the better. Then they dismiss the patients from their treatment as cured, with brazen assurance and the declaration that everything is now all right,† without regarding or being willing to notice the ailments which sooner or later are sure to follow; *i. e.*, the

* Then, as these gentlemen dream in their perverted minds, in which they have disposed of the nature of this most important disease in their arbitrary way and without consulting nature, then these frivolous gentlemen assure us, the matter of the itch has not yet had time to penetrate inwardly and to be received by the absorbent vessels to the detriment of the whole mass of humors: But how then, O conscientious men! if even the first little pustule of itch with its unbearable voluptuous itching, forcing a man irresistibly to scratch, and with the following burning pain, is *in every case and every time* the proof of a universal itch-disease which has been previously developed in the interior of the whole organism, as we shall see below? How then, if in accordance with this fact any external repression of the itch-eruption can not only do nothing toward alleviating the internal general disease, but rather as thousands of facts go to prove, compel it to develop and break forth quickly into innumerable, different, acute sufferings, or gradually into chronic sufferings, which make mankind so helpless and miserable? Can you then heal these? Experience says no; you cannot do it.

† In some vigorous itch patients the vital force, following the law of nature on which it rests (her instinct showing more wisdom than the intelligence of her destroyers), after some weeks, drives back to the skin the eruption seemingly destroyed by itch ointments and purgatives; the patient returns to the hospital and the mischievous destruction of the eruption, by means of ointments and lotions of solutions of lead and zinc, is renewed. I have seen in military hospitals this eruption thus destroyed in an irrational and cruel manner three times in succession within a few months, while the quack who applied the ointment pretended that the patient must have been infected anew with itch three times in this short period, which was really impossible.

Psora which shows itself from within in a thousand different diseases.* If the deceived wretches then sooner or later return with the malady following *unavoidably* on such a treatment; *e. g.*, with swellings, obstinate pains in one part or another, with hypochondriac or hysterical troubles, gout, consumption, tubercular phthisis, continual or spasmodic asthma, blindness, deafness, paralysis, caries of the bones, ulcers (cancer), spasms, hemorrhages, diseases of the mind and soul, etc., the physicians imagine that they have before them something entirely new and treat it again and again according to the old routine of their therapeutics in a useless and hurtful manner, directing their medicines against phantom diseases; *i. e.*, against causes invented by them for the ailments as they appear, until the patient, after many years' suffering continually aggravated, is at last freed from their hands by death, the end of all earthly maladies.†

The older physicians were more conscientious in this matter and observed with less prejudice. They saw clearly and became convinced that innumerable ailments and the most severe chronic diseases follow the destruction of the itch-eruption from the skin. And since this experience compelled them to assume the existence of an internal disease, in every case of itch they endeavored to extirpate this internal malady by means of a multitude of internal remedies, as good as their therapeutics afforded. It was, indeed, but a useless endeavor, because the true method of healing, which it could only be the prerogative of Homœopathy to discover, was unknown to them. Nevertheless this sincere endeavor was praiseworthy, since it was founded on an appreciation of the great internal disease present together with the eruption of itch, which internal disease it was necessary to remove. This prevented their reliance on the mere local destruction of the itch from the skin, as practiced by modern physicians, who think that they cannot quickly enough drive it away—as if it were a mere external disease of the skin—without regarding

* I wrote this six years ago, but even at this day the physicians of the old school continue to act and teach with the same criminal negligence. In this most important medical affair they have up to this day not become the least bit wiser or more humane.

† By accident (for they cannot give any but a feigned reason for their action) they found out a refuge which temporarily often alleviates the sufferings of their patients when they can not do anything at home with their prescriptions against the unknown disease; that is, they send him to some sulphur bath or other, where the patients often get rid of a small part of their *Psora*, and thus are also at the first use of the baths for a time relieved of their chronic disease; but afterwards they fall back into the same or a kindred ailment, and the repetition of the bath then avails little or nothing, because the cure of a developed *Psora* requires a far more adequate treatment than the impetuous use of such baths.

the great injuries attending such a course. The older physicians, on the other hand, have warningly laid these injuries before our eyes in their writings, giving thousands of examples.

The observations of those honest men are too startling to be rejected contemptuously, or ignored by conscientious men.

I shall here adduce some of these numerous observations handed down to us, which I might increase by an equal number of my own if the former were not already abundantly sufficient to show with what fury the internal *Psora* manifests itself when the external local symptom which serves to assuage the internal malady is hastily removed. They also show that it must be a matter of conscience for the physician who loves his fellow-man to direct all his endeavors to cure, first of all, the internal malady, whereby the cutaneous eruption will at the same time be removed and destroyed and all the subsequent innumerable lifelong chronic sufferings springing from the *Psora* be prevented or, if they are already embittering the life of the patient, be cured.

The diseases, partly acute but chiefly chronic, springing from such a one-sided destruction of the chief skin-symptom (eruption and itching) which acts vicariously and assuages the internal *Psora* (which destruction is erroneously called "*Driving the itch into the body*") are innumerable; as manifold as the peculiarities of bodily constitutions and of the outer world which modifies them.

A brief survey of the manifold misfortunes resulting thence is given by the experienced and honest LUDWIG CHRISTIAN JUNCKER in his *Dissertatio de Damno ex Scabie Repulsa*, *Halle*, 1750, p. 15–18. He observed that with young people of a sanguine temperament the suppression of itch is followed by phthisis, and with persons in general who are of a sanguine temperament it is followed by piles, hemorrhoidal colic and renal gravel; with persons of sanguino-choleric temperament by swellings of the inguinal glands, stiffening of the joints and malignant ulcers (called in German *Todenbrüche*); with fat persons by a suffocating catarrh and mucous consumption; also by inflammatory fever, acute pleurisy and inflammation of the lungs. He further states that in autopsies the lungs have been found indurated and full of cysts containing pus; also other indurations, swellings of the bones and ulcers have been seen to follow the suppression of an eruption. Phlegmatic persons in consequence of such suppressions suffered chiefly from dropsy; the menses were delayed, and when the itch was driven away during their flow, they were changed into a monthly hemoptysis. Persons inclined to melancholy were sometimes made insane by such repression; if they were pregnant the fœtus was usually killed. Sometimes the suppression of the itch causes sterility,* in nursing women the milk is generally lacking, the menses disappear prematurely; in older women the uterus becomes ulcerated, attended with deep, burning pains, with wasting away (cancer of the womb).

His experiences were frequently confirmed by the observations † of others, as *e. g.* with reference to

Asthma, Lentilius *Miscell. med. pract.* Tom. I., p. 176. **Fr. Hoffmann** *Abhandlung v. d. Kinderkrankheiten*, Frft.,1741, p. 104. **Detharding** in *Append. ad Ephem. Nat. Cur. Dec.* III., *ann 5 et, 6 et in obs. parallel. ad obs. 58.* **Binninger,** *Obs. Cent.* V., *obs. 88.* **Morgagni,** *de sedibus et. caus. morb. Epist.* XIV., 35. *Acta Nat. Cur. Tom.* V *obs.* 47. **J. Juncker,** *Consp. ther. spec. tab.* 31. **F. H. L. Muzell,** *Wahrnehm. Samml.* II. *Cas. 8.*[1] **J. Fr. Gmelin** in

*A pregnant Jewess had the itch on her hands and drove it away in the eighth month of her pregnancy so that it might not be seen during the period of her delivery. Three days afterwards she was delivered and the lochial discharge did not appear and she was seized with a high fever; since that time for seven years she had been sterile and had suffered from leucorrhœa. Then she became poor and had to walk a great distance barefooted; hereupon the itch again appeared and she thus lost her leucorrhœa and her other hysteric affections; she became again pregnant and was safely delivered. (*Juncker*, ibid.)

† When writing the first edition of the Chronic Diseases, I was not as yet acquainted with **Autenrieth's** *Versuche fuer die prakt. Heilkunde aus den Klinishen Anstalten von Tübingen*, 1808. But I saw on examining the work, that what he says about diseases following the driving away of itch through local applications, is only a confirmation of what I had already found with the other hundred writers. He also had observed that the external driving away of itch was followed by ulcers on the feet, pulmonary consumption, hysterical chlorosis, with various menstrual irregularities; white swelling of the knee, dropsy of the joints, epilepsy, amaurosis, with obscured cornea ; glaucoma, with complete amaurosis ; mental derangement, paralysis, apoplexy and curvature of the neck ; these he erroneously attributed to the ointments alone. But his own slow local driving away of the eruption by means of sulphuret of potash and soft soap, which he in vain calls *healing* it, is in no way better. Just as if his treatment were anything else than a local driving away of the eruption from the skin! Of any true cure he knows just as little as the other Allopaths, for he writes: "It is, of course, absurd to endeavor to cure itch (scab) by internal remedies." No! it is not only absurd, but even wretched to undertake to cure an internal itch-disease which cannot be cured by any *local* application, through any but *internal* means, which alone can cure the disease *thoroughly and with certainty.*

[1] A man 30 to 40 years of age had been afflicted with the itch a long time before, and it had been driven away by ointments ; from which time he had become more and more asthmatic. His respiration became at last, even when not in motion, very short and extremely labored, emitting at the same time a continuous hissing sound, but attended with only little coughing. He was ordered an injection of one drachm of squills, and to take internally 3 grains of squills. But by mistake he took the drachm of squills internally. He was near

Gesner's *Samml. v. Beob. V.* S. 21.[2] **Hundertmark.-Zieger** *Dissert. de scabie artificiale, Lips.* 1758, p. 32.[3] **Beireis—Stammen.** *Diss. de causis cur imprimis plebs scabie laboret.* Helmst., 1792, p. 26.[4] **Pelargus** (*Storch*) *Obs. clin. Jahrg.*, 1722, p. 435 *n* 438.[5] *Breslauer Sammlung v. Jahre* 1727, p. 293.[6] **Riedlin,** the father, *Obs. Cent.* II., *obs.* 90. Augsburg, 1691.[7]

Suffocating Catarrh, Ehrenfr. Hagendorn, *hist. med. phys. Cent.* I., *hist* 8, 9.[8] **Pelargus**, *Obs. clin. Jahrg.*, 1723, p. 15.[9]

---

losing his life with an indescribable nausea and retching. Soon after this the itch appeared again on his hands, his feet and his whole body in great abundance, and by this means the asthma was at once removed.

[2] The violent asthma was combined with general swelling and fever.

[3] A man of 32 years had the itch driven away by sulphur ointment, and he suffered for eleven months from the most violent asthma until by drinking birch-juice the eruption was brought back on the twenty-third day.

[4] A student was seized with the itch just as he was going to dance, on which account he had it driven out by a practitioner with sulphur ointment, But soon after, he was attacked by such a severe asthma that he could only draw breath by throwing his head back, and was almost suffocated during the attacks. After thus wrestling with death for an hour, he would cough up little cartilaginous pieces which would ease him for a very short time. Having returned home to Osterode he suffered continually for two years of this disease, being attacked about ten times a day, which could not even be mitigated through the help of his physician, **Beireis**

[5] A boy of 13 years having suffered from his childhood with *tinea capitis* had his mother remove it for him, but he became very sick within eight or ten days, suffering with asthma, violent pains in the limbs, back and knee, which were not relieved until an eruption of itch broke out over his whole body a month later,

[6] *Tinea capitis* in a little girl was driven away by purgatives and other medicines, but the child was attacked with oppression of the chest, cough and great lassitude. It was not until she stopped taking the medicines, and the *tinea* broke out again, that she recovered her cheerfulness and this, indeed, quickly.

[7] A boy of 5 years suffered for a long time from itch, and when this was driven away by a salve it left behind a severe melancholy with a cough.

[8] Owing to *tinea capitis*, which had been driven off by rubbing with almond oil, there arose an excessive lassitude of all the limbs, headache on one side, loss of appetite, asthma, waking up at night with suffocating catarrh, with severe rattling and whistling on the chest and convulsive twisting of the limbs, as if about to die, and hematuria. When the tinea broke out again, he recovered from all these ailments.

A 3-year-old girl had the itch, for several weeks; when this was driven out by an ointment she was seized the next day by a suffocating catarrh with snoring, and with numbness and coldness of the whole body, from which she did not recover until the itch re-appeared.

[9] A girl of twelve years had the itch with which she had frequently suffered, driven away from the skin by an ointment, when she was seized with an acute fever with suffocative catarrh, asthma and swelling, and afterward with pleurisy. Six days afterward, having taken an internal medicine containing sulphur, the

Suffocations from Asthma, Joh. Phil. Brendel, *Consilia med.*, *Frft.*, 1615, *Cons.*, 73. *Ephem. Nat. Cur.*, Ann. II., obs. 313. **Wilh. Fabr. V. Hilden,** *Obs. Cent.* III., *Obs.* 39.[10] **Ph. R. Vicat.** *Obs. Pract.*, *obs.* 35, *Vitoduri*, 1780.[11] **J. J. Waldschmid,** *Opera*, p. 244.[12]

Asthma with General Swelling. Waldschmid, ibid. **Hoechstetter,** *Obs. Dec.* III., *obs.* 7 Frft. et Lips, 1674, p. 248. **Pelargus,** *Obs. Clin. Jahrg.*, 1723, p. 504.[13] **Riedlin,** the father, *Obs. Cent.* II., *obs.* 91.[14]

Asthma with Dropsy of the Chest. Storch *in Act. Nat. Cur. Tom.* V., *obs.* 147. **Morgagni,** *de sed. et causis morb.* XVI., Art. 34.[15] **Richard,** *Recueil d'observ. de Méd. Tom.* III., p. 308, à Paris, 1772. **Hagendorn,** as above, Cent. II., hist. 15.[16]

Pleurisy and Inflammation in the Chest, Pelargus, as above, p. 10.[17] **Hagendorn,** as above, *Cent.* III., *hist.* 58. **Giseke,** *Hamb.*

---

itch again appeared and all the ailments, excepting the swelling, disappeared; but after twenty-four days the itch again dried up, which was followed by a new inflammation in the chest with pleurisy and vomiting.

[10] The dyspnœa of a youth, 20 years, caused by the driving away of itch was so great that he could not get any breath, and his pulse was hardly perceptible, in consequence of which he suffocated.

[11] A moist herpes on the left upper arm of a youth of 19 years was finally locally removed by many external applications. But soon after, there ensued a periodical asthma which was suddenly increased by a lengthy foot-tour in the heat of summer, even to suffocation, with a puffed up bluish-red face and quick, weak, uneven pulse.

[12] The dyspnœa from the driven out itch came on very suddenly, and the patient was suffocated.

[13] A 5-year-old girl had had for some time large itch vesicles on the hands, which dried up of themselves. Shortly after, she became sleepy and tired and was seized with dyspnœa. The following day the asthma continued and her abdomen became distended.

[14] A 50 year old farmer, who had been long tortured with the itch, while he was driving it out by external applications, was seized with a dyspnœa, a loss of appetite and a swelling of the whole body.

[15] A girl in Bologna drove away the itch with an ointment and was seized with the most severe asthma without fever. After two blood-lettings her strength decreased so much and the asthma was so much augmented that she died on the following day. The whole chest was filled with bluish water, also the pericardium.

[16] A girl of 9 years with the *tinea capitis* had it driven away, when she was seized with a lingering fever, a general swelling and dyspnœa; when the *tinea* broke out again she recovered.

[17] A man of 46 drove out his itch with a sulphur ointment. Thereupon he was seized with inflammation in the chest with bloody expectoration, dyspnœa and great anguish. The following day the heat and the anguish became almost unbearable and the pains in the chest increased on the third day. Then sweat broke out. After fourteen days the itch broke out again and he felt better. But he had a relapse, the itch dried up again and he died on the 13th day after the relapse.

Abhandl., p. 310. **Richard**, as above. **Pelargus**, as above. *Jahrg.*, 1721, p. 23 and 114,[18] and *Jahrg.*, 1723, p. 29,[19] also in *Jahrg.*, 1722, p. 459.[20] **Sennert** *praxis med. lib.* II., *P.* III., *Cap.* 6, p. 380. **Jerzembsky,** *Diss. Scabies salubris in hydrope*, Halae, 1777.[21] **Karl Wenzel,** *Die Nachkrankheiten von zurückgetretener Krätze*, Bamb., 1826, p. 49.[22]

Pleurisy and Cough, Pelargus, as above, Jahrg., 1722, p, 79.[23]

Severe Cough, Richard, as above. **Juncker,** *Conspect. med. theor. et pract. tab.*, 76. **Hundertmark,** as above, p. 23.[23*]

Hemoptysis, Phil. Georg. Schroeder, *Opusc.* II., p. 322. **Richard,** as above. **Binninger,** Obs. Cent. V., obs. 88.

Hemoptysis and Consumption. Chn. Max Spener, *Diss. de ægro febri maligni, phthisi complicata laborante*, Giess, 1699.[24] **Baglio,** *Opera*, p. 215. **Sicelius** *Praxis casual. Exerc.* III., *Cas.* I., Frft et Lips, 1743.[25] **Morgagni,** as above, XXI., *Art.* 32.[26] **Unzers** *Arzt* C C C., p. 508.[27] **Karl Wenzel,** as above, p. 32.

---

18 A thin man died of inflammation in the chest and other ailments twenty days after driving out the itch.

19 A boy of 7 years whose *tinea capitis* and itch dried up, died after four days from an acute fever and asthma accompanied with expectoration.

20 A youth who removed his itch with a lead ointment, died four days afterward of a disease of the chest.

21 A general dropsy was quickly cured by a return of the itch, but when this was suppressed by a severe cold, pleurisy supervened and death ensued in three days.

22 A young peasant was attacked with acute fever with pleurisy and dyspnœa, six days after driving out an eruption of itch with sulphur ointment.

23 A school boy of 13 years was seized with cough and stitches in the chest, when his itch dried up. These ailments disappeared when the itch broke out again.

23 *A man of 36 years had the itch removed sixteen months ago by an ointment of lead and mercury; he suffered since from a whooping cough accompanied with great anguish.

24 A youth of 18 years had the itch, which he finally drove away with a black looking lotion. A few days after, he was seized with chills and heat, lassitude, oppression of the heart, headache, nausea, violent thirst, cough and difficulty in breathing; he expectorated blood, commenced to speak deliriously, his face was deadly pale and sunken, the urine was deep red without sediment.

25 An eruption of itch in a youth of 18 years driven out by a mercurial plaster.

26 Itch which disappeared from the skin of itself, was followed by a lingering fever and fatal expectoration of pus; at the autopsy the left lung was found full of pus.

27 A robust looking candidate for the ministry who was about to preach in a few days and therefore wished to free himself from his old itch, rubbed himself one day with itch ointment, and in a few hours, soon after noon he passed away with anxiety, dyspnœa and tenesmus; the autopsy showed that the whole of the lungs was filled with liquid pus.

Collection of Pus in the Chest. F. A. Waitz, *Medic. Chirurg. Aufsätze Th.* I., p. 114, 115.[28] **Preval,** in the *Journal de Médec.*, LXI., p. 491.

Cysts of Pus in the Intestines, Krause. Schubert, *Diss. de scabie humana.* Lips, 1779, p. 23.[29]

Great Degeneration of a Great Part of the Intestines. J. H. Schulze, in *Act. Nat. Cur. Tom.*, 1 *obs.*, 231.[30]

Degeneration of the Brain. Dimenbrock, *Obs. et Curat. med.*, *obs.* 60. **Bonet,** *Sepulchretum anat.*, *Sect.* IV., *obs.* 1, § 1[31] and § 2.[32] **J. H. Schulze, as above.**

Hydrocephalus, *Acta helvet.*, V., p. 190.

Ulcers in the Stomach. L. Chn. Juncker, *Diss. de scabie repulsa*, Halle, 1750, p. 16.[33]

Sphacelus of the Stomach and Duodenum. Hundertmark, as above, p. 29.[34]

General Dropsical Swelling.[35]

Dropsy of the Chest. Hessler in Karl Wenzel, as above, p. 100 and 102.

---

[28] Empyema followed the driving away, through external means, of an eruption of itch which had come out a few years before, and appeared especially in March and April.

[29] A young man who had been warned by (the good physician and) Prof. Krause against the use of sulphur ointment for the re-appearing itch did not follow his advice, but rubbed himself with it, when he died of constipation. In his body, at the autopsy, were found sacs of pus in his abdominal viscera.

[30] Also the diaphragm and the liver were diseased.

[31] A little prince of two years had his *tinea capitis* driven away; in consequence, after his death, much bloody water was found under his skull,

[32] In a woman who had driven out the *tinea* by a lotion, one-half of the brain was found putrefied and filled with yellow humor.

[33] A man of rank, of a cholerico-sanguine temperament, was afflicted with gouty pains of the abdomen and pains as from gravel. After the removal of the gout through varions remedies the itch broke out, which he drove out through a desiccating bath of tan-bark; an ulcer formed on his stomach, which, as the autopsy showed, hastened his death.

[34] A boy of 7 weeks and a youth of 18 years died very suddenly from an itch driven out through a sulphur ointment. At the autopsy in the case of the infant the upper part of the stomach immediately below the orifice was found destroyed by gangrene, and in the second case that part of the duodenum into which the biliary duct and the pancreatic duct empty was found similarly diseased. A similar fatal inflammation of the stomach from driven out itch, in *Morgagni*, as above, LV., art. 11.

[35] Of this, innumerable cases are found in a number of writers of which I only desire to mention the one reported in **J. D. Fick**, *Exercitatio med. de scabie retropulsa*, Halle, 1710, § 6, where an eruption of itch driven out by application of mercury, left behind it general dropsy, which was only mitigated by the re-appearance of the eruption.

Dropsy of the Abdomen, Richard, as above, and with several other observers.

Swelling of the Scrotum (in boys). **Fr. Hoffmann**, *Med. rat. syst.*, III., p. 175.

Red Swelling of the Whole Body. Lentilius, *Misc. med. pract.*, Part I., p. 176.

Jaundice. Baldinger, *Krankheiten ein. Armee*, p. 226. **Joh. Rud. Camerarius**, *Memorab. Cent.*, X., § 65.

Swelling of the Parotid Glands. Barette, in the *Journal de Méd.*, XVIII., p. 169.

Swelling of the Cervical Glands, Pelargus, as above, **Jahrg.**, 1723, p. 593.[36] **Unzer**, *Arzt.* Part VI., *St.* 301.[37]

Obscuration of the Eyes and Presbyopia, Fr. Hoffman, *Consult. med.*, 1 Cas. 50.[38]

Inflammation of the Eyes, G. W. Wedel. Snetter, *Diss.* **de Ophthalmia**, Jen., 1710. **Hallmann**, in *Kœnigl. Vetenskaps Handl.* f. A. X., p. 210.[39] **G. Chph. Schiller**, *de Scabie humida*, p. 42, Erford. 1747.

The author of the book *Epidemion lib.* 5, No. 4, who gives his name as **Hippocrates**, first mentions the sad result of such a case, where an Athenian was seized by a violently itching eruption, spread over the whole body and especially over the genital organs; he expelled it by the use of the warm baths on the island of Melos, but died of the resulting dropsy.

[36]A boy of 8 or 9 years, who had been shortly before healed of *tinea* showed many swellings of the glands of the neck by which his neck was drawn crooked and stiff.

[37]A youth of 14 years had the itch in June, 1761. He rubbed with a gray ointment and the itch passed away. Upon this the glands behind both of his ears swelled up; the swelling on the left ear passed away of itself, but the right one in five months became monstrously enlarged and about August began to pain him. All the glands of the neck were swollen. On the outside the large gland was full of hard knots and without sensitiveness, but internally there was an obtuse pain, especially at night; at the same time he suffered from dyspnœa and obstructed deglutition. All means used to produce suppuration were in vain; it became so large that the patient was suffocated in the year 1762.

[38]A girl of 13 years was seized with the itch, especially on the limbs, in the face and on the pudenda; this was finally driven away by ointments of zinc and sulphur, whereupon she gradually became weak of sight. Little dark bodies floated before her eyes, and these could also be seen from without floating in the aqueous humor of the anterior chamber of the eye. At the same time she could not recognize small bodies except with spectacles. The pupils were dilated.

[39]A girl had a violent eruption of itch on the legs, with large ulcers in the bend of the knee. Being attacked with smallpox the itch was suppressed. This induced a humid inflammation of the white of the eye and of the eyelids, with itching and suppuration of the same, and the vision of dark bodies floating before her eyes; this lasted for two years. Then for three days she put on the

Cataract, Chn. Gottlieb Ludwig, *Advers. med.* II., p. 157.[40]

Amaurosis, Northof, *Diss. de scabie,* Gotting., 1792, p. 10.[41] **Chn. G. Ludwig,** as above.[42] **Sennert,** *prax. lib.* III., *Sect.* 2, *Cap.* 44. **Trecourt,** *chirurg. Wahrnehmungen,* p. 173. Leipz. 1777. **Fabricius ab Hilden.** *Cent.* II., *obs.* 39.[43]

Deafness. **Thore** in *Capelle, Journal de santé,* Tom. I. **Daniel,** *Syst. aegritud.* II., p. 228. **Ludwig,** as above.

Inflammation of the Bowels, Hundertmark, *Diss. de scabie artificiali, Lips.* 1758, p. 29.

Piles, Hemorrhoids, *Acta helvet.* V., p. 192.[44] **Daniel,** *Syst. aegritud.* II., p. 245.[45]

Abdominal Complaints, Fr. Hoffmann, *Med. rat. syst.* III., p. 177.[46]

Diabetes (Mellitaria), *Comment. Lips.* XIV., p. 365. *Eph. Nat. Cur. Dec.* II., *ann.* 10, p. 162. **C. Weber,** *Obs.* f. I., p. 26.

Suppression of Urine, Sennert, Prax. lib. 3, p. 8. **Morgagni,** as above, XLI., *art.* 2.[47]

Erysipelas, Unzer *Artz, Th.* V., St. 301.[48]

---

stockings of a child afflicted with the itch. On the last day a fever broke out with dry cough, tension in the chest, with inclination to vomit. On the following day the fever and the tension of the chest diminished and a sweat broke out, which increased until erysipelas broke out on both legs, and on the following day these passed over into the real itch. The eyes then improved.

[40] A man whose itch had been driven off, but who was of robust constitution, was seized with cataract.

[41] From itch expelled by external application there arose amaurosis, which passed away when the eruption re-appeared on the skin.

[42] A vigorous man, when the itch had been expelled from the skin, was seized with amaurosis and remained blind to an advanced age.

[43] Amaurosis from the same cause, with terrible headache.

[44] Bleeding piles returned every month.

[45] In consequence of itch driven off by external applications, loss of blood up to eight pounds within a few hours, colic, fever, etc.

[46] After the expulsion of itch a most violent colic, pain in the region of the left lower ribs, restlessness, lingering fever, anxiety and obstinate constipation.

[47] A young peasant had driven off the itch with ointment, and shortly after he suffered from suppression of urine, vomiting and at times from a pain in the left loin. Still he, after awhile, passed urine a few times, but only a little, of dark color and attended with pains. In vain the attempt was made to empty it with a catheter. At last the whole body swelled up, difficult and slow respiration ensued, and he died on about the twenty-first day after the suppression of the itch. The bladder contained two pounds of urine just as dark, but the abdominal cavity, water, which being held for awhile over the fire thickened into a sort of albumen.

[48] A man rubbed himself with mercurial ointment against the itch, when

Discharges of acrid humors. Fr. Hoffman, *Consult. Tom.* II., *Cas.* 125.

Ulcers, Unzer *Arzt, Th.* V., St. 301.[49] **Pelargus**, as above, *Jahrg.*, 1723, p. 673.[50] *Breslauer Samm.*, 1727, p. 107.[51] **Muzell**, *Wahrnehm.* II., *Cas.* 6.[52] **Riedlin**, the son, *Cent. obs.* 38.[53] **Alberti–Gorn**, *Diss. de scabi.*, p. 24. Halle, 1718.

Caries. Richard, as above.

Swelling of the Bones of the Knee. Valsalva in Morgagni, *de sede et caus. morb.* I. art. 13.

Pain in the bones, *Hamburger Magaz.*, XVIII., p. 3, 253.

Rachitis and Marasmus in Children, Fr. Hoffman. *Kinderkrankh. Leipz.*, 1741, p. 132.

Fever, B. V. Faventinus, *Medicina empir.*, p. 260. **Ramazzini**, *Constit. epid. urbis.* II. No. 32, 1691.[54] **J. C. Carl** in *Act. Nat. Cur.* VI., *obs.* 16.[55]

Fever. Reil, *Memorab. Fasc.* III., p. 169.[56] **Pelargus**, as above; Jahrg., 1721, p. 276,[57] and *ibid. Jahrg.*, 1723.[58] **Amatus**,

---

there followed an erysipelatous inflammation in the neck, of which he died after five weeks.

[49] A woman, after using a mercurial ointment against itch, had a putrescent eruption all over her body, so that whole pieces of flesh rotted away; she died in a few days with the greatest pains.

[50] A youth of 16 years had the itch for some time; when this passed away ulcers broke out on the legs.

[51] After rubbing with an ointment against the itch there followed with a man of 50 years tearing pains in the left shoulder for five weeks, when several ulcers broke out in the arm-pit.

[52] A quack gave a student an ointment for the itch, from which it disappeared indeed, but instead of it an incurable ulcer broke out in the mouth.

[53] A student who had been for a long time afflicted with the itch drove it off with an ointment, and instead of this there broke out ulcers on his arms and legs, and glandular swellings in the arm-pits. These ulcers were finally cured by external applications, when he was seized with dyspnœa and then with dropsy, and from these he died.

[54] Many observations are found there respecting cases where the itch, being driven off by ointments, there followed fever and blackish urine, and where, when the itch was brought back to the skin, the fever disappeared and the urine became like that of a healthy person.

[55] A man and a woman had an eruption of itch on the hand, of many years' standing, and as often as it dried up fever always ensued, and as soon as this came to an end the eruption of itch again returned; and yet this itch extended but to a small part of the body and was not driven off by external applications.

[56] Itch was suppressed by a fever that set in; when the fever was removed it returned.

[57] A mother put ointment on the *tinea* of a boy of 9 years; it passed away, but there followed a violent fever.

[58] A child, 1 year old, had had for some time *tinea capitis* and an eruption in the face; both these had shortly before dried up, when there followed heat, cough and diarrhœa. A return of the eruption on the head gave alleviation.

Lusit. Cent. II., Cor. 33. **Schiller** *Diss. de scabie humida*, Erford, 1747, p. 44.[59] **J. J. Fick**, *Exercitatio med. de scabie retropulsa*, Halle, 1710, § 2.[60] **Pelargus**, as above, *Jahrg.*, 1722, p. 122.[61] Also *Jahrg.*, 1723, p. 10, p. 14[62] and p. 291. **C. G. Ludwig**, *Advers. med.* II., pp. 157–160.[63] **Morgagni**, as ab. X., *art.* 9;[64] XXI., art. 31;[65] XXXVIII., *art.* 22;[66] LV., *art.* 3.[67]

Fever. **Lanzonus**, in *Eph. Nat. Cur.*, *Dec.* III., *ann.* 9 and 10, *obs.* 16 and 113. **Hoechstetter**, *Obs. med.*, *Dec.* VIII.,

---

[59] A woman of 43 years, long afflicted with dry itch, rubbed her joints with an ointment of sulphur and mercury, and thus drove it off; this was followed by pains under the right ribs, lassitude in all the limbs, heat and feverish irritation. After using sudorific remedies for six days, large vesicles of itch broke out all over the body.

[60] Two youths, brothers, drove off the itch by one and the same remedy, but they lost all appetite, a dry cough and a lingering fever set in, they became emaciated and fell into a slumbrous stupor, so that they would have died if the eruption had not luckily re-appeared on the skin.

[61] With a three-year old child when *tinea capitis* had disappeared of itself, there arose a violent fever on the chest, cough and weariness, and it only recovered when the eruption re-appeared on the head.

[62] A journeyman purse-maker, who had to make some embroidery, drove off his frequent itch with lead-ointment. Scarcely was the itch drying off in consequence, when he was seized with chills, heat, dyspnœa and a rattling cough, of which he suffocated on the fourth day.

[63] A vigorous, healthy man of 30 years was taken with the itch and drove the eruption from the skin, but was then seized with a catarrhal fever with an uncontrollable perspiration; he was slowly recovering from it when he was seized without any further cause by another fever. The attacks began with anxiety and headache, and increased with heat, a quick pulse and morning sweats. There was added an unusual sinking of the strength, and delirious speech, anxious tossing about, a sobbing respiration with suffocation—a disease which despite all medicines ended with death.

[64] With a boy the itch passed away of itself; this was followed by fever. The itch now appeared more violent and the fever passed away, but the child grew thin, and when the itch again dried up there followed diarrhœa, convulsions and soon afterwards death.

[65] Itch disappeared from the skin of itself, on which lingering fever, expectoration of pus and lastly death followed, and at the autopsy the left lungs were found full of pus.

[66] A woman of 30 years had for a long time pain in the limbs and a strong eruption of itch, which she drove off with ointment, when she was attacked by fever with violent heat, thirst and raging headache, which was accompanied with delirious speech, uncontrollable dyspnœa, tumefaction of the body and great distension of the abdomen. She died on the sixth day of the fever. The abdomen contained much air, and especially the stomach was distended with air, filling half of the abdomen.

[67] A man whose *tinea capitis* had passed off from intense cold, was seized after eight days with a malignant fever, with vomiting, accompanied at last with hiccough; he died in consequence on the ninth day.

Cas. 8.[68] **Triller.** **Wehle,** *Diss. nullam medicinam interdum esse optimam*, Witemb., 1754.[69] **Fick,** as ab., § 1.[70] **Waldschmidt,** *Opera.*, p. 241. **Gerbizius,** in *Eph. Nat. Cur., Dec.* III., *ann.* 2, *obs.* 167. **Amatus,** *Lusit.*, Cent. II., Curat. 33.[71] **Fr. Hoffmann,** *Med. rat. system*, T. III., p. 175.[72]

Tertian Intermittent Fever. **Pelargus,** as ab., Jahrg., 1722, p. 103, cfr. with p. 79.[73] **Juncker,** as ab., *tab.* 79; *Eph. Nat. Cur., Dec.* I., *ann.* 4. **Welsch,** *Obs.* 15. **Sauvages,** *Spec.* 11. **De Hautesierk,** *Obs., Tom.* II., p. 300; *Comment. Lipsienses* XIX., p. 297.

Quartan Fever, Thom. Bartholinus, *Cap.* 4, *hist.* 35. **Sennert,** *Paralip.*, p. 116. **Fr. Hoffman,** *Med. rat. system* III., p. 175.[74]

Vertigo and a Total Sinking of the Strength, Gabelchofer, *Obs. Med. Cent.* II., *obs.* 42.

Vertigo Like Epilepsy, Fr. Hoffmann, *Consult. Med.* I., *Cas.* 12.[75]

In the same article **Morgagni** mentions the case of a man who, having scabs from itch on the arms and on other parts, drove off nearly the whole eruption by a sulphurated shirt, but was seized at once with drawing pains on the whole body combined with fever, so that he could neither rest at night nor move about in the daytime; also the tongue and the fauces were thus attacked. With much trouble the eruption was brought out again on the skin, and thus his health was restored.

[68] A malignant fever with opisthotonus from driving off the itch.

[69] A young merchant had driven off the itch with ointment, when he was suddenly seized with such hoarseness that he could not speak a loud word; then followed dry asthma, loathing of food, severe cough, troublesome especially at night and robbing him of sleep, violent ill-smelling night-sweats, and, despite of all medical treatment, death.

[70] A burgomaster, 60 years of age, was infected with the itch, and suffered unspeakably from it through the nights; he used many medicines in vain, and at last was taught by a beggar a so-called infallible remedy, composed of *oleum laurinum*, flowers of sulphur and lard. Having rubbed with this several times he was, indeed, freed from the eruption, but soon after he was seized with a violent chill, followed by an excessive heat all over the body, vehement thirst, a gasping asthma, sleeplessness, violent trembling all over the body and great lassitude, so that on the fourth day he expired.

[71] From the same cause a fever combined with insanity, precipitating death.

[72] After driving off itch, most frequently acute fevers with a great sinking of the strength follow. In one such case the fever lasted seven days, when the eruption of itch re-appeared and stopped the fever.

[73] A boy of 15 years for a long time had *tinea capitis* and had received from *Pelargus* a strong purgative to cure it; he was seized with pain in the back, cutting pains during micturition, followed by tertian fever.

[74] Old people have especially dry itch, and if this is driven off by external applications usually quartan fever ensues, which vanishes as soon as the itch re-appears on the skin.

[75] A count, 57 years old, had suffered for three years with dry itch. It was

Epilepsy Like Vertigo, Fr. Hoffmann, as ab., p. 30.[76]

Convulsions, Juncker, as ab. tab. 53. **Hoechstetter**, *Eph. Nat. Cur. Dec.* 8, *Cas.* 3. *Eph. nat. cur. dec.* 2, *ann. obs.* 35, and *ann.* 5, *obs.* 224. **D. W. Triller. Welle**, *Diss. nullam medicinam interdum esse optimam*, Viteb., 1754, § 13, 14.[77] **Sicelius**,

---

driven off, and he enjoyed for two years an apparently good health only he had during this time two attacks of vertigo, which gradually so increased that once after finishing his meal he was seized with such vertigo that he would have fallen to the floor if he had not been supported. He was covered with an icy perspiration, his limbs trembled, all the parts of his body were as dead, and he repeatedly vomited up a sour substance. A similar attack followed six weeks later, then once a month for three months. He indeed retained consciousness, but there always followed heaviness of the head and a drunken stupor. At last these attacks came daily, though in a milder form. He could not read nor think nor turn around quickly nor stoop down. This was attended with sadness, sorrowful, anxious thoughts and sighs.

[76] A woman of 36 years had the itch driven from the skin a few years before with mercurial remedies. Her menses became irregular, and were often interrupted for ten or even fifteen weeks; she was at the same time constipated. Four years ago during pregnancy she was seized with vertigo, and she would suddenly fall down while standing or walking. While sitting she would retain her senses during the vertigo and could speak, eat and drink. At her first attack she felt in her left foot, as it were, a crawling sensation and formication, which terminated in a violent jerking up and down of the feet. In time these attacks took away consciousness, and afterwards in traveling in a carriage there came an attack of real epilepsy which returned thrice in the following winter. During these attacks she could not speak; she did not indeed turn her thumbs inward, but yet there was foam at her mouth. The sensation of formication in the left foot announced the attack, and when this sensation reached the pit of the stomach it suddenly brought on the fit. This epilepsy was removed by a woman with five powders, but instead of it her vertigo reappeared, but much more violently than before. It also commenced with a crawling sensation in the left foot, which rose up to the heart; this was attended with great anxiety and fear, as if she were falling down from a height, and while supposing that she had fallen she lost consciousness and speech; at the same time her limbs moved convulsively. But also outside of these attacks the least touch of her feet caused her the most intense pain as if from a boil. This was attended with severe pains and heat in the head and with loss of memory.

[77] After an itch driven away by ointment there followed with a girl a most profound swoon, and soon after the most terrible convulsions and death.

[78] A girl of 17, in consequence of *tinea capitis* which disappeared of itself, was seized with continual heat in the head and attacks of headache. She sometimes suddenly started up as if from fright, and while awake she was seized with convulsive motions of the limbs, especially of the arms and hands, as also with oppression in the pit of the stomach as if her breast was laced together; with moaning; then her limbs would jerk convulsively and she would start up.

Decas Casuum I., *Cas.* 5.[78] **Pelargus**, as ab., *Jahrg.*, 1723, p. 545.[79]

Epileptic Convulsions and

Epilepsy, J. C. Carl in *Act. Nat. Cur.* VI., obs. 16.[80] **E. Hagendorn**, as above, *hist.* 9.[81] **Fr. Hoffmann**, *Consult. med.* I., *Cas.* 31.[82]; *ibid. med. rat. syst. T.* IV., P. III., *Cap.* I., and in *Kinderkrankheiten*, p. 108. **Sauvages**, *Nosol. spec.* 11. **de Hautesierk**, *obs. T.* II., p. 300. **Sennert**, *prax.* III., *Cap.* 44. *Eph. Nat. Cur. Dec.* III., *ann.* 2, *obs.* 29. **Gruling**, *obs. Med. Cent.* III., *obs.* 73. **Th. Bartolin**, *Cent.* III., *hist.* 20. **Fabr. de Hilden**, *Cent.* III., *obs.* 10.[83] **Riedlin**, *lin. med. ann.*, 1696, *Maj. obs.* 1.[84] **Lentilius**, *Miscell. med. pr.*, P. I., p. 32. **G. W. Wedel**, *Diss. de aegro epileptico, Jen.*, 1673.[85] **Herrm. Grube**, *de arcanis medicorum non arcanis, Hafn.*, 1673, p. 165.[86] **Tulpius**, *obs. lib.* I., *Cap.* 8.[87] **Th. Thompson**, *Medic. Rathpflege, Leipzig*, 1779, pp. 107, 108.[88]

---

[79] A full-grown man who had been for some time affected with tremor of the hands had his *tinea* dry up. He was thereupon seized with great lassitude and red patches without heat broke out on his body. The tremor passed over into convulsive shaking, bloody matter was discharged from his nose and his ears, he also coughed up blood, and he died on the 23d day amidst convulsions.

[80] A man who had driven off a frequently occurring eruption of itch with an ointment fell into epileptic convulsions, which disappeared again when the eruption reappeared on the skin.

[81] A youth of 18 years drove off the itch with a mercurial ointment and two months after he was unexpectedly seized with convulsions, which attacked all the limbs of the body, now this, now that; with painful constriction of the breast and the neck, coldness of the limbs and great weakness. The fourth day he was seized with epilepsy, foaming at the mouth, while the limbs were strangely contorted. The epilepsy only yielded when the eruption returned.

[82] With a boy, whose tinea had been driven off by rubbing it with almond oil.

[83] With children, combined with suffocating catarrh.

[84] A servant girl after twice rubbing her itch with ointment had an attack of epilepsy.

[85] A youth of 18, who had driven out itch with mercurial remedies, was seized a few weeks later with epilepsy, which returned after four weeks with the new moon.

[86] A boy of 7 months was seized with epilepsy, while the parents were unwilling to acknowledge that he had had the itch. But when the physician enquired more particularly, the mother confessed that the little boy had some vesicles of itch on the sole of the foot, which had soon yielded to lead ointment; the child, as she said, had no other sign of the itch. The physician correctly recognized in this the only cause of the epilepsy.

[87] Two children were freed from epilepsy by the breaking out of humid tinea, but the epilepsy returned when the tinea was incautiously driven off.

[88] Five-year-old itch passed away and this, after several years, produced epilepsy.

Hundertmark, as ab., p. 32.[89] **Fr. Hoffmann**, *Consult. med.* I., Cas. 28, p. 141.[90]

Apoplexy. Cummius in *Eph. Nat. Cur. Dec.* I., *ann.* 1, *obs.* 58. **Mobius,** *Institut. med.*, p. 65. **J. J. Wepfer**, *Histor. Apoplect. Amstel.*, 1724, p. 457.

Paralysis, **Hoechstetter**. *Obs. med. Dec.* VIII., *obs.* 8, p. 245. *Journal de Méd.*, 1760, Sept., p. 211. **Unzer**, *Arzt* VI., *St.* 301.[91] **Hundertmark**, as above, p. 33.[92] **Krause**. **Schubert**, *Diss. de scabie humani corp.*, *Lips.*, 1779, p. 23.[93] **Karl Wenzel**, as above, p. 174.

Melancholy, **Reil**, *Memorab. Fasc.*, III., p. 177.[94]

Insanity, **Landais** in **Roux**, *Journ. de Médecine*, Tom. 41. **Amat. Lusitanus**, *Curat. med. Cent.* II., *Cur.* 74. **J. H. Schulze**,

---

[89] The itch in a youth of 20 years was suppressed by a purgative which was allowed to act violently for several days, after which he for two years suffered daily the most violent convulsions, until, through the use of birch-juice, the itch was brought back to the skin.

[90] A young man of 17 years, of vigorous constitution and good intelligence, was attacked three years ago, after itch had been driven out, first by hemoptysis and then by epilepsy, which grew worse through medicines until the fits came on every two hours. Another surgeon, through frequent blood-lettings and many medicines, effected that he remained free from epilepsy for four weeks, but soon afterwards the epilepsy returned while he was taking his noonday nap, and the patient had two or three fits in the nights; at the same time he was attacked with a very severe cough and suffocating catarrh, especially during the nights, when he expectorated a very fetid fluid. He was confined to his bed. At last, after much medicine, the disease increased so much that he had ten fits at night and eight during the day. Nevertheless he never in these fits either clenched his thumbs or had foam at his mouth. His memory is weakened. The attacks come at the approach of meal-time, but more frequently after meals. During his nightly attacks he remains in the deepest sleep without awaking, but in the morning he feels as if bruised all over. The only warning of a fit consists in his rubbing his nose and drawing up his left foot, but then he suddenly falls down.

[91] A woman, after having the itch driven out, had paralysis of one leg and remained lame.

[92] After driving oft the itch with sulphur ointment, a man of 53 years had hemiplegia.

[93] A minister who for a long time had in vain used internal remedies against the itch finally grew tired of it and drove it off with ointment, when his upper extremities were, in a measure, paralyzed and a hard, thick skin formed in the palms of the hands, full of bloody chaps and insufferable itching.

In the same place the author mentions also a woman whose fingers contracted from an itch driven out by external means; she suffered of them a long time.

[94] He found an idiotic melancholy arise in consequence of suppressed itch; when the itch broke out again the melancholy disappeared.

Brune, *Diss. Casus aliquot mente alienatorum*, Halle, 1707. Cas. 1, p. 5.[95] **F. H. Waitz**, *medic.-chirurg. Aufsätze*, *Th.* 1, p. 130.[96] *Altenburg*, 1791. **Richter** in *Hufel. Journal*, XV., II. **Grossmann** in **Baldinger's** *neuem Magaz.*, XI., I.[97]

Who, after meditating on even these few examples which might be much increased from the writings of the physicians of that time and from my experience,* would remain so thoughtless as to ignore the great evil hidden within, the *Psora*, of which evil the eruption of itch and its other forms, the *tinea capitis*, milk crust, tetter, etc., are only indications announcing the internal, monstrous disease of the whole organism, only local external symptoms which act vicariously and mitigatingly for the internal disease? Who, after reading even the few cases described, would hesitate to acknowledge that the *Psora*, as already stated, is the *most destructive* of all chronic miasmas? Who would be so stolid as to declare, with the later allopathic physicians, that the itch-eruption, tinea and tetters

---

[95] A student, 20 years old, had the humid itch, which so covered his hands that he became incapable of attending to his work. It was driven off by sulphur ointment. But shortly after it appeared how much his health had suffered from it. He became insane, sang or laughed where it was unbecoming, and ran until he sank to the ground from exhaustion. From day to day he became more sick in soul and in body, until at last hemiplegy came on and he died. The intestines were found grown together into a firm mass, studded with little ulcers full of protruberances, some of the size of walnuts, which were filled with a substance resembling gypsum.

[96] The same story.

[97] A man of 50 years with whom, after driving away the itch by ointments, general dropsy had set in; when the itch re-appeared and drove away the swelling he drove it away again, when he fell into raving madness, while head and neck swelled up to suffocation; at last blindness and complete suppression of urine were added. Artificial irritants applied to the skin and a strong emetic brought back the itch again; when the eruption extended over the whole body all the former accidents disappeared.

* An opponent, of the old school, has reproached me that I have not adduced my own experience to prove that the chronic maladies, when they are not of syphilitic or sycotic origin, spring from the miasma of itch, as such proofs from experience would have been convincing. Oho! If the examples here adduced by me from both the older and from modern non-Homœopathic writings have not yet enough convincing proof, I should like to know what other examples (even my own not excepted) could be conceived of as more striking proofs? How often (and I might say almost always) have opponents of the old school refused all credence to the observations of honorable Homœopathic physicians, because they were not made before their own eyes and because the names of the patients were only indicated with a letter; as if private patients would allow their names to be used! Why should I endure the like? And do I not prove my point in a manner most indubitable and most free from partisanship through the experience of so many other honest practitioners?

are only situated superficially upon the skin and may, therefore, without fear, be driven out through external means since the internal of the body has no part in it and retains its health?

Surely, among all the crimes which the modern physicians of the old school are guilty of, this is the most hurtful, shameful and unpardonable!

The man who, from the examples given and from innumerable others of a like nature, is not willing to see the exact opposite of that assertion blinds himself on purpose and works intentionally for the destruction of mankind.

Or are they so little instructed as to the nature of all the miasmatic maladies connected with diseases of the skin that they do not know that they all take a similar course in their origin? And that all such miasmas become first internal maladies of the whole system before their external assuaging symptom appears on the skin?

We shall more closely elucidate this process, and in consequence we shall see that all miasmatic maladies which show peculiar local ailments on the skin are always present as internal maladies in the system *before* they show their local symptom externally upon the skin; but that only in acute diseases, after taking their course through a certain number of days, the local symptom, together with the internal disease, is wont to disappear, which then leaves the body free from both. In chronic miasmas, however, the outer loca symptom may either be driven from the skin or may disappear of itself, while the internal disease, if uncured, neither wholly nor in part ever leaves the system; on the contrary, it continually increases with the years, unless healed by art.

I must here dwell the more circumstantially on this process of nature, because the common physicians, especially of modern days, are so deficient in vision; or, more correctly stated, so blind that although they could, as it were, handle and feel this process in the origin and development of acute miasmatic eruptional diseases, they nevertheless neither surmised nor observed the like process in chronic diseases, and therefore declared their local symptoms as secondary growths and impurities existing merely externally on the skin, without any internal fundamental disease, and this as well with the chancre and the fig-wart as with the eruption of itch, and therefore—since they overlooked the chief disease or perhaps even boldly denied it—by a mere external treatment and destruction of these local ailments they have brought unspeakable misfortunes on suffering humanity.

With respect to the origin of these three chronic maladies, as in the acute, miasmatic eruptional diseases, three different important moments are to be more attentively considered than has hitherto been done: *First*, the time of infection; *secondly*, the period of time during which the whole organism is being penetrated by the disease infused, until it has developed within; and *thirdly*, the breaking out of the external ailment, whereby nature externally demonstrates the completion of the internal development of the miasmatic malady throughout the whole organism.

The infection with miasmas, as well of the acute as of the above-mentioned chronic diseases, takes place, without doubt, in *one single moment*, and that moment, the one most favorable for infection.

When the smallpox or the cowpox catches, this happens in the moment when in vaccination the morbid fluid in the bloody scratch of the skin comes in contact with the exposed nerve, which then, irrevocably, dynamically communicates the disease to the vital force (to the whole nervous system) in the same moment. After this moment of infection no ablution, cauterizing or burning, not even the cutting off of the part which has caught and received the infection, can again destroy or undo the development of the disease within. Smallpox, cowpox, measles, etc., nevertheless will complete their course within, and the fever peculiar to each will break out with its smallpox, cowpox, measles,* etc., *after a few days*, when the internal disease has developed and completed itself.

The same is the case, not to mention several other acute miasmas, also when the skin of man is contaminated with the blood of cattle

* We may justly ask: Is there in any probability any miasma in the world, which, when it has infected from without, does not first make the whole organism sick before the signs of it externally manifest themselves? We can only answer this question with, *no*, there is none!

Does it not take three, four or five days after vaccination is effected, before the vaccinated spot becomes inflamed? Does not the sort of fever developed—the sign of the completion of the disease—appear even later, when the protecting pock has been fully formed; *i. e.*, on the seventh or eighth day?

Does it not take ten to twelve days after infection with smallpox, before the inflammatory fever and the outbreak of the smallpox on the skin take place?

What has nature been doing with the infection received in these ten or twelve days? Was it not necessary to first embody the disease in the whole organism before nature was enabled to kindle the fever, and to bring out the eruption on the skin?

Measles also require ten or twelve days after infection or inoculation before this eruption with its fever appears. After infection with scarlet fever seven days usually pass before the scarlet fever, with the redness of the skin, breaks out.

What then did nature do with the received miasma during the intervening days? What else but to incorporate the whole disease of measles or scarlet fever in the entire living organism before she had completed the work, so as to be enabled to produce the measles and the scarlet fever with their eruption.

affected with anthrax. If, as is frequently the case, the anthrax has infected and caught on, all ablutions of the skin are in vain; the black or gangrenous blister, nearly always fatal, nevertheless, always comes out after four or five days (usually in the affected spot); *i. e.*, as soon as the whole living organism has transformed itself to this terrible disease.

(It is just so with the infection of half-acute miasmas without eruption. Among many persons bitten by mad dogs—thanks to the benign ruler of the world—only few are infected, rarely the twelfth; often, as I myself have observed, only one out of twenty or thirty persons bitten. The others, even if ever so badly mangled by the mad dog, usually all recover, even if they are not treated by a physician or surgeon.*) But with whomsoever the poison acts, it has taken effect in the moment when the person was bitten, and the poison has then communicated itself to the nearest nerves and, therefore, without contradiction, to the whole system of the nerves, and as soon as the malady has been developed in the whole organism (for this development and completion of the disease nature requires at least several days, often many weeks), the madness breaks out as an acute, quickly fatal disease. Now if the venomous spittle of the mad dog has really taken effect, the infection usually has taken place irrevocably in the moment of contagion, for experience shows that even the immediate excision† and amputation of the infected part does not protect from the progression of the disease within, nor from the breaking out of the hydrophobia—therefore, also, the many hundreds of other much lauded external means for cleansing, cauterizing and suppurating the wound of the bite can protect just as little from the breaking out of the hydrophobia.

From the progress of all these miasmatic diseases we may plainly see that, after the contagion from without, the malady connected with it in the interiors of the whole man must first be developed; *i. e.*, the whole interior man must first have become thoroughly sick of small-pox, measles or scarlet fever, before these various eruptions can appear on the skin.

---

* We are indebted especially to the careful English and American physicians for these comforting experiences—to HUNTER and HOULSTON (in *London Med. Journal*, Vol. I.), and to VAUGHAN, SHADWELL and PERCIVAL, whose observations are recorded in Jam. Mease's "*On the Hydrophobia, Philadelphia*, 1793."

† An eight-year-old girl, in Glasgow, was bitten by a mad dog on the 21st of March, 1792. A surgeon *immediately exsected the wound altogether*, kept it suppurating and gave mercury until it produced a mild salivation, which was kept up for two weeks; nevertheless hydrophobia broke out on the 27th of April and the patient died on the 29th of April. M. DUNCAN'S *Med. Comment, Dec.* II., *Vol.* VII., *Edinb.* 1793, and *The New London Med. Journ.*, II.

For all these *acute* miasmatic diseases the human constitution possesses that process which, as a rule, is so beneficent: to wipe them out (*i. e.*, the specific fever together with the specific eruption) in the course of from two to three weeks, and of itself to extinguish them again, through a kind of decision (*crisis*), from the organism, so that man then is wont to be entirely healed of them and, indeed, in a short time, unless he be killed by them.*

In the chronic miasmatic diseases nature observes *the same course* with respect to the mode of contagion and the antecedent formation of the internal disease, before the external declarative symptoms of its internal completion manifests itself on the surface of the body; but then that great remarkable difference from the acute diseases shows itself, that in the chronic miasmata the entire internal disease, as we have mentioned before, remains in the organism during the whole life, yea, it increases with every year, if it is not exterminated and thoroughly cured *by art.*

Of these chronic miasmata I shall for this purpose only adduce those two, which we know somewhat more exactly; namely, the *venereal chancre* and the *itch.*

In impure coition there arises, most probably at the very moment in the spot which is touched and rubbed, the specific contagion.

If this contagion has taken effect, then the whole living body is in consequence seized with it. Immediately after the moment of contagion the formation of the venereal disease in the whole of the interior begins.

In that part of the sexual organs where the infection has taken place, nothing unnatural is noticed in the first days, nothing diseased, inflamed or corroded; *so also all washing and cleansing of the parts immediately after the impure coition is in vain.* The spot remains healthy according to appearance, only the internal organism is

* Or have these various, acute, half-spiritual miasmas the peculiar characteristic that—after they have penetrated the vital force in the first moment of the contagion (and each one in its own way has produced disease) and then, like parasites, have quickly grown up within it and have usually developed themselves by their peculiar fever, after producing their fruit (the mature cutaneous eruption which is again capable of producing its miasma)—they again die out and leave the living organism again free to recover?

On the other hand, are not the chronic miasmas disease-parasites which continue to live as long as the man seized by them is alive, and which have their fruit in the eruption originally produced by them (the itch-pustule, the chancre and the figwart, which in turn are capable of infecting others) and which do not die off of themselves like the acute miasmas, but can only be exterminated and annihilated by a *counter-infection*, by means of the potency of a medicinal disease quite similar to it and stronger than it (the anti-psoric), so that the patient is delivered from them and recovers his health?

called into activity by the infection (which occurs usually in a moment), so as to incorporate the venereal miasma and to become thoroughly diseased with the venereal malady.

Only when this penetration of all the organs by the disease caught has been effected, only when the whole being has been changed into a man entirely venereal, *i. e.*, when the development of the venereal disease has been completed, only then diseased nature endeavors to mitigate the internal evil and to soothe it, by producing a local symptom which first shows itself as a vesicle (usually in the spot originally infected), and later breaks out into a painful ulcer called the chancre; this does not appear before five, seven or fourteen days, sometimes, though rarely, not before three, four or five weeks after the infection. This is therefore manifestly a chancre ulcer which acts vicariously for the internal malady, and which has been produced from within by the organism after it has become venereal through and through, and is able through its touch to communicate also to other men the same miasma; *i. e.*, the venereal disease.

Now, if the entire disease thus arising is again extinguished through the internally given specific remedy, then the chancre also is healed and the man recovers.

But if the chancre is destroyed through local applications* before the internal disease is healed,—and this is still a daily practice with physicians of the old school,—the miasmatic chronic venereal disease remains in the organism as syphilis, and it is aggravated, if not then cured internally, from year to year until the end of man's life, even the most robust constitution being unable to annihilate it within itself.

Only through the cure of the venereal disease, which pervades the whole internal of the body (as I have taught and practiced for many years), the chancre, its local symptom, will also simultane-

*The venereal disease not only breaks out through the removal of the chancre by the cautery,—in which case some wretched casuists have considered syphilis as resulting from the driving back of the poison out of the chancre into the interior of the body, which up to this time is supposed by them to have been healthy,—no, even after the quick removal of the chancre without any external stimulants, the venereal disease breaks out, which gives additional confirmation, if this were needed, of the indubitable pre-existence of syphilis in the system. "*Petit* cut off a part of the *labia minora*, in which for some days a venereal chancre had appeared; the wound healed, indeed, but the venereal disease broke out notwithstanding." M. s. *Fabre*, *Lettres*, *supplément à son traité des maladies vénériennes*, *Paris*, 1786. Of course! because the venereal disease was present in the whole interior of the body even before the outbreak of the chancre.

ously be cured in the most effective manner; and this is best effected without the use of any external application for its removal—while the merely local destruction of the chancre, without any previous general cure and deliverance of man from the internal disease, is followed by the most certain outbreak of syphilis with its sufferings.

Psora (itch disease), like *syphilis*, is a miasmatic chronic disease, and its original development is similar.

The itch disease is, however, also the *most contagious* of all chronic miasmata, far more infectious than the other two chronic miasmata, the venereal chancre disease and the figwart disease. To effect the infection with the latter there is required a certain amount of friction in the most tender parts of the body, which are the most rich in nerves and covered with the thinnest cuticle, as in the genital organs, unless the miasma should touch a wounded spot. But *the miasma of the itch needs only to touch the general skin*, especially with tender children. The disposition of being affected with the miasma of itch is found with almost everyone and under almost all circumstances, which is not the case with the other two miasmata.

No other chronic miasma infects more generally, more surely, more easily and more absolutely than the miasma of itch; as already stated, it is the most contagious of all. It is communicated so easily, that even the physician, hurrying from one patient to another, in feeling the pulse has unconsciously * inoculated other patients with it; wash which is washed with wash infected with the itch; † new gloves which had been tried on by an itch patient, a strange lodging place, a strange towel used for drying oneself have communicated this tinder of contagion; yea, often a babe, when being born, is infected while passing through the organs of the mother, who may be infected (as is not infrequently the case) with this disease; or the babe receives this unlucky infection through the hand of the midwife, which has been infected by another parturient woman (or previously); or, again, a suckling may be infected by its nurse, or, while on her arm, by her caresses or the caresses of a strange person with unclean hands; not to mention the thousands of other possible ways in which things polluted with this invisible miasma may touch a man in the course of his life, and which often can in no way be anticipated or guarded against, so that men who have never been infected by the *psora* are the exception. We need not to hunt for the causes of infection in crowded hospitals, factories, prisons, cr in orphan houses, or in the filthy huts of paupers; even in active life, in retirement, and in the

*CAR. MUSITANI, *Opera de tumoribus, Cap.* 20.

†As WILLIS has noticed in TURNER, *des maladies de la peau, traduit de l'anglois, à Paris,* 1783, *Tom.* II., *Cap.* 3, p. 77.

rich classes, the itch creeps in. The hermit on Montserrat escapes it as rarely in his rocky cell, as the little prince in his swaddling clothes of cambric.

As soon as the miasma of itch, *e. g.*, touches the hand, in the moment when it has taken effect, it no more remains local. Henceforth all washing and cleansing of the spot avail nothing. Nothing is seen on the skin during the first days; it remains unchanged, and, according to appearance, healthy. There is no eruption or itching to be noticed on the body during these days, not even on the spot infected. The nerve which was first affected by the miasma has already communicated it in an invisible dynamic manner to the nerves of the rest of the body, and the living organism has at once, all unperceived, been so penetrated by this specific excitation, that it has been compelled to appropriate this miasma gradually to itself until the change of the whole being to a man thoroughly psoric, and thus the internal development of the *psora*, has reached completion.

Only when the whole organism feels itself transformed by this peculiar chronic-miasmatic disease, the diseased vital force endeavors to alleviate and to soothe the internal malady through the establishment of a suitable local symptom on the skin, the itch-vesicles. So long as this eruption continues in its normal form, the internal *psora*, with its secondary ailments, cannot break forth, but must remain covered, slumbering, latent and bound.

Usually it takes six, seven or ten, perhaps even fourteen days from the moment of infection before the transformation of the entire internal organism into *psora* has been effected. Then only, there follows after a slight or more severe chill in the evening and a general heat, followed by perspiration in the following night, (a little fever which by many persons is ascribed to a cold and therefore disregarded), the outbreak of the vesicles of itch, at first fine as if from miliary fever, but afterwards enlarging on the skin*—first in the region of the spot first infected, and, indeed, accompanied with a *voluptuously tickling itching* which may be called *unbearably agreeable* (*Grimmen*), which compels the patient so irresistibly to rub and to scratch the vesicles of itch, that, if a person restrains himself forcibly from rubbing or scratching, a shudder passes over the skin of the whole body. This *rubbing* and *scratching* indeed satisfies somewhat for a few moments, but there then *follows immediately a long-*

* Far from being an independent, merely local, cutaneous disease, the vesicles or pustules of itch are the reliable proof that the completion of the internal *psora* has already been effected, and the eruption is merely an integrating factor of the same; for this peculiar eruption and this peculiar itching make a part of the essence of the whole disease in its natural, least dangerous state.

continued burning of the part affected. Late in the evening and before midnight this itching is most frequent and most unbearable.

The vesicles of itch contain in the first hours of their formation a lymph clear as water, but this quickly changes into pus, which fills the tip of the vesicle.

The itching not only compels the patient to rub, but on account of its violence, as before mentioned, to rub and scratch open the vesicles; and the humor pressed out furnishes abundant material for infecting the surroundings of the patient and also other persons not yet infected. The extremities defiled even to an imperceptible degree with this lymph, so also the wash, the clothes and the utensils of all kinds, when touched, propagate the disease.

Only this skin symptom of the *psora* which has permeated the whole organism (and which as more manifestly falling under the cognizance of the senses has the name of *itch*), only this eruption, as well as the sores which later arise from it and are attended on their borders with the itching peculiar to *psora*, as also the herpes which has this peculiar itching and which becomes humid when rubbed (the tetter), as also the *tinea capitis*—these alone can propagate this disease to other persons, because they alone contain the communicable miasma of the *psora*. But the remaining secondary symptoms of the *psora*, which in time manifest themselves after the disappearance or the artificial expulsion of the eruption, *i. e.*, the general psoric ailments, cannot at all communicate this disease to others. They are, so far as we know, just as little able to transfer the *psora* to others, as the secondary symptoms of the venereal disease are able to infect other men (as first observed and taught by J. HUNTER) with syphilis.

When the itch-eruption has only lately broken out and is not yet widely spread on the skin, nothing of the general internal malady of the *psora* is as yet to be noticed in the state of the patient. The eruptional symptom acts as a substitute for the internal malady and keeps the *psora* with its secondary ailments as it were latent and confined.*

In this state, the disease is most easily cured through specific remedies internally administered.

But if the disease is allowed to advance in its peculiar course

* As also the chancre, when not expelled, acts vicariously and soothingly for the syphilis within, and does not permit the venereal disease to break out, so long as it remains undisturbed in its place. I examined a woman who was free from all the secondary symptoms of the venereal disease; with her a chancre had remained in its place untreated for two years, and had gradually acquired the size of almost an inch in diameter. The best preparation of *Mercury*, internally administered, soon and entirely healed, not only the internal malady, but also the chancre.

without the use of an internal curative remedy or an external application to drive away the eruption, the whole disease within *rapidly* increases, and this increase of the internal malady makes necessary a corresponding increase of the skin-symptom. The itch-eruption, therefore, in order to be able to soothe and to keep latent the increased internal malady, has to spread and must finally cover the whole surface of the body.

Yet even at this acme of the disease the patient still appears healthy in every other respect; all the symptoms of the internal *Psora*, now so much increased, still remain covered and assuaged through the skin-symptom augmented in the same proportion. But so great a torture, as is caused by so unbearable an itching spread over the whole body, even the most robust man cannot continue to bear. He endeavors to free himself from these torments at any price, and, as there is no thorough help for him with the physicians of the old school, he endeavors to secure deliverance at least from this eruption, which itches so unbearably, even if it should cost his life; and the means are soon furnished him, either by other ignorant persons, or by Allopathic physicians and surgeons. He seeks deliverance from his external tortures, without suspecting the greater misfortune which unavoidably follows, and is bound to follow, on the expulsion of the external skin-symptom (which hitherto has acted vicariously for the internal enlarged psora-disease), as has been sufficiently proved by the observations mentioned before. But when he thus drives away such an eruption of itch by external applications, he exposes himself to a similar misfortune, and acts just as unreasonably, as a person who in order to be quickly delivered from poverty, and thus as he supposes to make himself happy, steals a great sum of money, and is, therefore, sent to the dungeon and the gallows.

The longer the itch-disease has already lasted, whether the eruption, as is usually the case, has spread over the greater part of the skin, or whether, owing to a peculiar lack of activity in the skin, (as in some cases) the eruption has been confined to a few vesicles of itch*—in both cases, supposing only that the *Psora* together with its skin-sympton has grown old, the expulsion of the eruption of itch, whether greater or smaller or even as small as you please, is attended with the most destructive consequences on account of the internal itch-disease (*psora*) with its unspeakable sufferings, which, through its long continuance, has increased to a high degree and then unavoidably breaks forth.

But the ignorance of the uninstructed layman may be pardoned if

*See the observation to No. 86, p. 29.

he drives out the itch-eruption and the troublesome itching by a cold shower-bath, by rolling in snow, by cupping, or by rubbing the whole skin, or only the skin around the joints, with sulphur mixed with lard; for he does not know to what dangerous accidents and outbreaks of the Psora-disease, that lurks within, he thereby opens the door and ingress. But who will pardon the men whose office and duty it is to know the extent of the inevitably following, illimitable misfortune, resulting from the external expulsion of the itch-eruption, owing to the *Psora* which is then aroused from the whole organism, and who ought to have guarded against it in every way by a thorough internal cure of the whole of this disease,* when we

* For even when the itch-disease has reached this high degree, the eruption, together with the internal malady, in one word, the whole *psora*, may still be healed by the internal, specific Homœopathic remedies, with greater difficulty, indeed, than in the beginning, immediately after its origin, but still *far more easily and certainly* than after a complete expulsion of the eruption by mere external applications, when we must cure the internal *psora* as it brings forth its secondary symptoms and develops into nameless chronic diseases. The itch-disease, though it may have advanced so far, may nevertheless in its *entire* state be most easily, certainly and thoroughly cured, together with its external eruption, through the suitable internal remedies, without the least local application, just as the venereal chancre disease may *most surely and easily* be thoroughly cured often by the least, single dose of the best preparation of mercury internally administered—when the chancre, without calling in the aid of the least external remedy, quickly becomes a mild ulcer, and in a few days heals of itself, so that no trace of secondary symptoms (venereal disease) then ever appears or can appear, since the internal symptom has been cured together with the local symptom, as I have taught for many years orally and in my writings, and have proved by my cures of this kind.

How can we excuse the whole host of physicians, who, hitherto, after treating this generally spread venereal disease for more than three hundred years, nevertheless remain so ignorant in recognizing its nature, that in looking at a chancre they even to this day acknowledge nothing diseased in the infected patient, but this same chancre, and do not see the syphilis, which was already present within and had been developed in the whole organism, even before the breaking out of the chancre; and so they blindly suppose, that the chancre is the only venereal evil which is to be extirpated, and that this needs but to be destroyed by external applications, in order to be able to declare the man cured; and this without being instructed, by the many thousand cases in their experience, that by the local extermination of the chancre they have never done anything but injury, as they have only deprived the syphilis pre-existing within of its diverting local symptom, and have thereby compelled the internal malady to break out only the more certainly and dreadfully (and a manner more difficult of cure), as venereal disease. How can such a universal, pernicious obliquity of vision be excused?

Or why did these physicians never reflect on the origin of the figwarts? Why did they always overlook the internal universal malady, which is the cause of these excrescences? It is only when this is recognized, that it can

see them treat the itch patients all in the same erroneous manner; yea, with even more violent internal and external remedies, with sharp purgatives, with the Jasser ointment, with lotions of acetate of lead, with the sublimate of mercury or sulphate of zinc, but especially with an ointment prepared of fat with flowers of sulphur or with a preparation of mercury; with which they lightly and carelessly destroy the eruption, declaring "this is merely an impurity located in the skin, and must be driven out; then everything will be well and the man will be healthy and free from every ailment." Who can pardon them if they are not willing to learn from the many warning examples recorded by the older, more conscientious observers, nor by the many thousands of other examples, which frequently,

---

be thoroughly cured by its Homœopathic remedies, which then cause the fig-warts to be healed, without the application of any external means of destruction.

But even if a shadow of an excuse might be offered for this sad negligence and ignorance, and if anyone would claim that these physicians have only had three and one-half centuries, in which to discern clearly the true nature of *syphilis*, and that they might have learned this truth after a still more extended practice (still I have endeavored, though in vain, to convince them of their error a number of years ago and since then from time to time), nevertheless, that general negligence of previous physicians and, I may well say, their obstinate *blindness*, are quite without excuse, in that they did not recognize the internal pre-existing malady, the *psora*, which lies at the bottom of the itch-disease, which has infected men for several thousands of years, and that they ignored in their proud levity all the facts which point to it, so that they might continue the delusion and leave the world in its destructive infatuation that: *the unbearably itching pustules are only a mere superficial ailment of the skin, and by their local destruction man is delivered from the whole disease, and has fully recovered.*

Not perchance mere medical scribblers, no, the greatest and most celebrated physicians of modern and most modern days have made themselves guilty of this grievous error (or shall I say of this intentional crime), from von Helmont even to the latest advocates of the Allopathic medical practice.

By the use of the above mentioned remedies, they indeed usually reached their aim; *i. e.*, the driving away of the eruption and of the itching from the skin, and they supposed in the intoxication of their spirit (or at least they pretended), they had destroyed the disease itself and, indeed, totally, and they sent away the patients, thus abused, assuring them that they were again healthy.

All the sufferings, which follow the one-sided destruction of the cutaneous eruption, which belongs to the natural form of the *psora*, they passed off as a newly arisen disease, owing to quite another origin. In their narrowness of mind, they never regarded the innumerable, plain testimonies of honest observers of earlier days, which record the sad consequences of the local expulsion of the itch-eruption, which often followed so closely, that a man would have to deny his reason, or else acknowledge them as the immediate result of the indwelling severe malady (the *psora*), which had been deprived of the local symptom (the cutaneous eruption), destined by nature to alleviate the internal malady, whence the uncured internal disease has been compelled to a manifest outbreak of its secondary symptoms.

yea, almost daily, come before their eyes? Yet they cannot see nor be convinced as to the certain, quickly fatal or lifelong insidious misfortune they bring upon the itch-patient through the destruction of his eruption, as they thus merely unfetter the internal malady (psora), which is laden with innumerable ailments. This disease is neither destroyed nor cured; and so this thousand-headed monster, instead of being conquered, is inexorably let loose against the deceived patient to his destruction, by tearing down the barriers that shut it in.

It may easily be imagined, as experience also teaches, that the more months a neglected itch-eruption has flourished on the skin, the more surely has internal *psora*, which underlies it, been able to reach, in even a moderate space of time, a great—and finally its greatest—degree, which dreadful increase it also then proves through the more dangerous consequences, which the expulsion of so inveterate an eruption unavoidably draws after it in every case.

On the other hand, it is just as certain that the eruption of a few vesicles of itch which has broken out only a few days before, in consequence of a recent infection, may be expelled with less *immediate* danger; as the internal *psora* that has sprung up in the whole organism has not yet had time to grow up to a high degree, and we must confess that the expulsion of a few vesicles of itch, that have just arisen, often shows no *immediate*, manifestly strong, evil consequences. Wherefore with delicate and aristocratic persons, or their children, it usually remains unknown, that a single vesicle or a few vesicles itching violently, which showed only a few days and were at once treated by the careful physician with lead ointment or a lotion of lead, and which disappeared the following day, had itch for their foundation.

However small the internal *psora* may be at the time of the quick suppression of an itch-eruption, which has only developed a few vesicles and which is then followed by only moderate ailments and complaints (which are then usually, from ignorance, ascribed by the domestic physician to other causes of little import): the internal malady of *psora*, although as yet of slight degree, remains in its character and in its chronic nature the same general psoric disease of the whole organism; *i. e., without the aid of art it is ineradicable, and cannot be extirpated by the strength of even the best and most robust bodily constitution, and it will increase even to the end of the patient's life.* It is usually the case, indeed, that this disease, deprived as early as possible of the first traces of its cutaneous symptom by local applications, will grow but slowly in the beginning and will make but slow progress in the organism—much slower progress than where the eruption has been allowed to remain for a long time on the skin; for in the latter case the progress of the internal *psora* is of immense rapidity; but the disease, nevertheless, increases unceasingly, and even in the best cases and under the most favorable external circumstances, quietly and often for years unperceived by the eyes; so that anyone, who does not know the signs of its latent presence, would suppose and declare such persons to be healthy and free from any internal malady. Often for years it does not manifest itself in prominent symptoms, which might be called manifest diseases.

Many hundred observations have gradually acquainted me* with the signs, by which the internally slumbering,† hitherto latent *psora* (itch-malady) may be recognized even in those cases where it has not yet manifested itself in any startling disease, so that I am able to root out and to thoroughly cure this malady with its roots, more easily before the internal *psora* has risen to a manifest (chronic) disease, and has developed to such a fearful height that the dangerous conditions make the cure difficult and in some cases impossible.

There are many signs of the *psora* which is gradually increasing within, but is as yet slumbering, and has not yet come to the full outbreak of a manifest disease; but no one person has all these symp-

* It was more easy to me, than to many hundreds of others, to find out and to recognize the signs of the Psora as well when latent and as yet slumbering within, as when it has grown to considerable chronic diseases, by an accurate comparison of the state of health of all such persons with myself, who, as is seldom the case, have never been afflicted with the *psora*, and have, therefore, from my birth even until now in my eightieth year, been entirely free from the (smaller and greater) ailments enumerated here and further below, although I have been, on the whole, very apt to catch acute epidemic diseases, and have been exposed to many mental exertions and thousand fold vexations of spirit.

† Allopathy has also assumed *hidden* (*latent*) conditions of disease in patients, in order to explain, or, at least, to excuse its blind inroads with violent medicines, blood-lettiug, anodynes, etc. These so-called *qualitates occultæ Fernelii* are, however, wholly suppositious and imaginary, as (according to the statement of this same physician) they are supposed not to be recognizable by any manifestations and symptoms. But whatever does not make known its hidden, imaginary existence by any sign does not exist for us men, who are limited by our Creator in our cognizance of things to observations—it is consequently a phantom of a roving fancy. It is quite different with the various forces *slumbering* (*latent*) in nature; despite their ordinary occultness, they, nevertheless, show themselves when the requisite circumstances and conditions appear; *e. g.*, latent heat, even in metals that feel cold, is manifested when they are rubbed, just as the Psora manifests itself; *e. g.*, as a drawing pain in the sheaths of the muscles, when the person infected with Psora has been exposed to a draught, etc.

toms; the one has more of them, the other a smaller number; the one has at present only one of them, but in the course of time he will also have others; he may be free from some, according to the peculiar disposition of his body or according to the external circumstances of different persons.

SYMPTOMS OF LATENT PSORA.

Mostly with children: frequent discharge of ascarides and other worms; unsufferable itching caused by the latter in the rectum.

The abdomen often distended.

Now insatiable hunger, then again want of appetite.

Paleness of the face and relaxation of the muscles.

Frequent inflammations of the eyes.

Swellings of the cervical glands (scrōfula).

Perspiration on the head, in the evening after going to sleep.

Epistaxis with girls and youths (more rarely with older persons), often very severe.

Usually cold hands or perspiration on the palms, (burning in the palms).

Cold, dry, or ill-smelling sweaty feet, (burning in the soles of the feet).

The arms or hands, the legs or feet, are benumbed by a slight cause.

Frequent cramps in the calves (the muscles of the arms and hands).

Painless subsultus of various portions of the muscles here and there on the body.

Frequent or tedious dry or fluent coryza or catarrh,* or impossibility of catching a cold even from the most severe exposure, even while otherwise having continually ailments of this kind.

Long continued obstruction of one or both nostrils.

Ulcerated nostrils (sore nose).

Disagreeable sensation of dryness in the nose.

Frequent inflammation of the throat, frequent hoarseness.

Short tussiculation in the morning.

Frequent attacks of dyspnœa.

Predisposition to catching cold (either in the whole body or only in the head, the throat, the breast, the abdomen, the feet; *e. g.*, in a draught,† (usually when these parts are inclined to perspiration), and many other, sometimes long continuing ailments arising therefrom.

---

* The epidemic catarrhal fevers and catarrhs which seize almost everyone, even the healthiest persons (Grippe, Influenza), do not belong to this category.

† Persons not afflicted with *psora*, though draughts and damp cold air may not be agreeable to them, do not suffer any colds or evil after-effects therefrom.

Predisposition to strains, even from carrying or lifting a slight weight, often caused even by stretching upward and reaching out the arms for objects which are hung high (so also a multitude of complaints resulting from a moderate stretching of the muscles: headache, nausea, prostration, tensive pain in the muscles of the neck and back, etc.)

Frequent one-sided headache or toothache, even from moderate emotional disturbances.

Frequent flushes of heat and redness of the face, not unfrequently with anxiety.

Frequent falling out of hair of the head, dryness of the same, many scales upon the scalp.

Predisposition to erysipelas now and then.

Amenorrhœa, irregularities in the menses, too copious, too scanty, too early (too late), of too long duration, too watery, connected with various bodily ailments.

Twitching of the limbs on going to sleep.

Weariness early on awaking; unrefreshing sleep.

Perspiration in the morning in bed.

Perspiration breaks out too easily during the daytime, even with little movement (or inability to bring out perspiration).

White, or at least very pale tongue; still more frequently cracked tongue.

Much phlegm in the throat.

smell from the mouth, frequently or almost constantly, especially early in the morning and during the menses, and this is perceived either as insipid, or as slightly sour, or as if from a stomach out of order, or as mouldy, also as putrid.

Sour taste in the mouth.

Nausea, in the morning.

Sensation of emptiness in the stomach.

Repugnance to cooked, warm food, especially to meat (principally with children).

Repugnance to milk.

At night or in the morning, dryness in the mouth.

Cutting pains in the abdomen, frequently or daily (especially with children), more frequently in the morning.

Hard stools, delaying usually more than a day, clotted, often covered with mucus (or nearly always soft, fermenting stools, like diarrhœa).

Venous knots on the anus; passage of blood with the stools.

Passing of mucus from the anus, with or without fæces.

Itching on the anus.

Dark urine.

Swollen, enlarged veins on the legs (swollen veins, varices).

Chilblains and pains as from chilblains, even outside of the severe cold of winter; even, also, in summer.

Pains as of corns, without any external pinching of the shoes.

Disposition to crack, strain or wrench one joint or another.

Cracking of one or more joints on moving.

Drawing, tensive pains in the neck, the back, the limbs, especially, also, in the teeth (in damp, stormy weather, in northwest and northeast winds, after colds, overlifting, disagreeable emotions, etc.).

Renewal of pains and complaints while at rest, and disappearance of the same while in motion.

Most of the ailments come on at night, and are increased with a low barometer, with north and northeast* winds, in winter and towards spring.

Uneasy, frightful, or at least too vivid, dreams.

Unhealthy skin; every little lesion passes into sores; cracked skin of the hands and of the lower lips.

Frequent boils, frequent felons (whitlows).

Dry skin on the limbs; on the arms, the thighs, and also at times on the cheeks.

Here or there a rough, scaling spot on the skin, which causes at times a voluptuous itching and, after the rubbing, a burning sensation.

Here or there at times, though seldom, a single insufferably pleasant, but unbearably itching vesicle, at its point sometimes filled with pus, and causing a burning sensation after rubbing, on a finger, on the wrist or in some other place.

Suffering from several or from a greater number of these ailments (even at various times and frequently), a person will still consider himself as healthy, and is supposed to be so by others. He may also lead a quite endurable life in such a state, and without much hindrance, attend to his business as long as he is young or still in his vigorous years, and so long as he does not suffer any particular mishap from without, has a satisfactory income, does not live in vexation or grief, does not overexert himself; but especially if he is of quite a cheerful, equable, patient, contented, disposition. With such persons the *psora* (internal itch malady), which may be recognized by a connoisseur by means of a few or by more of the above symptoms, may slumber on for many years within, without causing any continuing chronic disease.

---

*In Europe northeast winds are cold, sharp and dry, corresponding to our west winds.—*Transl.*

But still, even in such favorable external relations, as soon as these persons advance in age, even moderate causes (a slight vexation, or a cold, or an error in diet, etc.), may produce *a violent attack of (however only a brief) disease:* a violent attack of colic, inflammation of the chest or the throat, erysipelas, fever and the like, and the violence of these attacks seems to be out of proportion to its moderate cause. This is mostly wont to happen in fall or winter, but often also by preference in springtime.

But even where a person, whether a child or an adult, who has the *psora* slumbering within him, shows much semblance of health, but happens upon the opposite of the above-described favorable conditions of life, when his health and whole organism have been very much weakened and shaken by a prevalent epidemic fever or an infectious acute disease,* smallpox, measles, whooping cough, scarlet fever, purple rash, etc , or through an external severe lesion, a shock, a fall, a wound, a considerable burn, the breaking of an arm or a leg, a hard labor, the confinement due to a disease (*usually helped on by the incorrect and weakening Allopathic treatment*), confinement at a sedentary occupation in a gloomy, close room, weakening the vital force; the sad losses of beloved relatives bending down the soul with grief, or daily vexation and annoyance which embitter the life; deterioration of the food or an entire want of what is necessary and indispensable, exposure and inferior food beating down man's courage and strength; then the *psora*, which has hitherto slumbered, awakes and shows itself in the heightened and augmented symptoms enumerated below, in its transition to the formation of severe maladies; one or another of the nameless (psoric) chronic diseases† breaks out and *most of all*

* At the termination of an acute fever there often follows, as if incited by such a fever, an appearance of an old *psora* residing in the body, as an eruption of itch. This the physicians explain as a new generation of itch in this individual body replete with bad humors (*scilicet*), since they know nothing of a *psora* in man which may be quiescent for a long period. But the itch-disease cannot now be generated or arise or be created anew of itself, just as no smallpox or cow-pox, no measles, no venereal chancre disease, etc., can now make its appearance with any man without previous infection.

† The one or the other disease, according to the original bodily constitution, a peculiar mode of living, a peculiar disposition of the mind often arising from the individual education or a more receptive or more weakened condition of some part of the body, gives a peculiar direction to the disease, and thus causes the itch disease to lead to the origin of the one or the other disease, so as to show itself preferably in that one direction and develop itself in that particular modification. A passionate, peevish disposition gives an extraordinary predisposition to the development of the *psora;* so also previous exhaustion through frequent pregnancies, excessive nursing of infants, extraordinary hardships, *exhaust-*

through weakening and exhausting improper treatment by allopathic physicians, they are aggravate dfrom time to time without intermis-

---

ing erroneous medical treatment, debauchery, and a profligate mode of living. The internal itch-disease is, as before mentioned, of such a peculiar nature that it may remain, as it were, tied down and covered up for a long time through external favorable surroundings, so that a man may seem to the superficial observer healthy for years, even for many years, until circumstances unfavorable to the body or the soul, or to both, may arise, and serve as a hostile impulse to awaken the disease slumbering within and thus develop its germs. His acquaintances and his physician, yea, the patient himself, can not then comprehend how his health could so suddenly fall into a decline. To bring some examples for explanation from my own experience: After a simple fracture of a limb attended with confinement to bed for five or six weeks, there may follow diseased conditions of another kind, the cause of which cannot be guessed, which diseased condition, even when measurably removed, nevertheless returns, and which even without any error in diet nevertheless at their return show aggravation. This is mostly the case in fall (winter) and spring and becomes a tedious ailment increasing from year to year, a lasting cure for which, without the substitution of a still worse disease for it by an allopathic cure, has been hitherto vainly sought for in the councils of former physicians and also in visits to mineral springs. There are in man's life innumerable stumbling-blocks or unfavorable occurrences of this kind which serve to awaken the *psora* (the internal itch-disease) which till then has been slumbering (perhaps for a long time previously) and which cause its germs to develop. They are often of such a nature that the grave evils which gradually follow on them are out of all proportion to them, so that no rational man can consider those occurrences as sufficient causes for the chronic diseases which follow and which are often of a fearful character. But such a man is compelled to acknowledge a deeper seated hostile cause of these appearances, which cause has only now developed itself.

For example, a young married woman who, viewed superficially and according to the common standard, was healthy, but who had in her childhood been infected with *psora*, had the misfortune to be thrown out of her carriage while in the third month of her pregnancy, from which she suffered not only slight injury and the fright, but also a miscarriage, and the attending loss of blood gave her a considerable set-back. In a few weeks, however, her youthful constitution had pretty well recovered, and she might have been assured of a speedy return to lasting good health, when the announcement of the dangerous illness of a beloved sister, living at a distance, threw her back and augmented her former ailments, which had not yet been quite removed, by the addition of a multitude of nervous disorders and convulsions, thus turning them into a serious illness. Better news from her sister, indeed, follow, and at last good news. At last her sister, entirely restored herself, pays her a visit. But the sick young wife still remains sick, and even if she seems to recover for a week or two, her ailments nevertheless return without any apparent cause. Every succeeding confinement, even when quite easy, every hard winter, adds new ailments to the old, or the former disorders change into others still more troublesome, so that at last there ensues a serious chronic illness, though no one can see why the full vigor of youth, attended by happy external surroundings, should not have soon wiped out the consequence of that

sion, often to a fearful height, if external circumstances favorable for the patient do not interpose, and cause a moderation in the process of the malady.

---

one miscarriage; still less can it be explained why the unfortunate impression of those sad tidings should not have disappeared, on hearing of the recovery of her sister, or at least on the actual presence of her sister fully restored.

If the cause must at all times be proportionate to its effect and consequence, as is the case in nature, no one can see how, after the removal of the causes assailing her health, the resulting ailments could not only continue, but even increase from year to year, if their cause were not in something else, something deeper, so that those unhappy occurrences (the miscarriage and the sad tidings), since they both disappeared of themselves and therefore could not possibly yield a sufficient ground for the ensuing chronic disease, can only be regarded as the occasion, but not the efficient cause, of the development of a hostile power of greater importance, pre-existent in the internal organism but hitherto quiescent.

In a similar manner, a robust merchant, apparently healthy, despite some traces of internal *psora*, perceptible only to the professional examiner, may in consequence of unlucky commercial conjunctures become involved in his finances, even so as to approach bankruptcy, and at the same time he will fall gradually into various ailments and finally into serious illness. The death of a rich kinsman, however, and the gaining of a great prize in a lottery, abundantly cover his commercial losses; he becomes a man of means—but his illness, nevertheless, not only continues but increases from year to year, despite all medical prescriptions, in spite of his visiting the most famous baths, or rather, perhaps, with the assistance of these two causes.

A modest girl, who, excepting some signs of internal *psora*, was accounted quite healthy, was compelled into a marriage which made her unhappy of soul, and in the same degree her bodily health declined, without any trace of venereal infection. No allopathic medicine alleviates her sad ailments, which continually grow more threatening. But in the midst of this aggravation, after one year's suffering, the cause of her unhappiness, her hated husband, is taken from her by death, and she seems to revive, in the conviction, that she is now delivered from every occasion of mental or bodily illness, and hopes for a speedy recovery; all her friends hope the same for her, as the exciting cause of her illness lies in the grave. She also improves speedily, but unexpectedly she still remained an invalid, despite the vigor of her youth; yea, her ailments but seldom leave her, and are renewed from time to time without any external cause, and they are even aggravated from year to year in the rough months.

A person who had been unjustly suspected and become involved in a serious criminal suit, and who had before seemed healthy, with the exception of the marks of latent *psora* mentioned above, during these harassing months fell into various diseased states. But finally the innocence of the accused is acknowledged, and an honorable acquittal followed. We might suppose that such a happy, gratifying event would necessarily give new life to the accused and remove all bodily complaints. But this does not take place, the person still at times suffers from these ailments, and they are even renewed with longer or briefer intermissions, and are aggravated with the passing years, especially in the wintry seasons.

How shall we explain this? If that disagreeable event had been the cause, the *sufficient* cause, of these ailments, ought not the effect; *i. e.*, the disease, to

But even if favorable external conditions should again check the rapid development of a disease that has broken out, true health can not be lastingly restored by any of the modes of treatment hitherto known, and the customary allopathic treatments, with their aggressive, inappropriate remedies—such as baths, mercury, prussic acid, iodine, digitalis, quinine, starvation and other fashionable remedies included—only hasten death, the end of all those maladies which the physician cannot heal.

When once, under the above-mentioned unfavorable outward surroundings, the transition of the *psora* from its slumbering and bound condition to its awakening and outbreak has taken place, and the patient leaves himself to the injurious activity of the usual allopathic physician, who deems it appropriate to his office and his income to mercilessly assault the organism of the patient (as we are sorry to witness every day) with the battering-rams of his violent, inappropriate remedies and weakening treatments;—in such a case, the external circumstances of the patient and his situation with respect to his surroundings may have changed ever so favorably, but the aggravation of the disease nevertheless proceeds under such hands without any escape.

The awakening of the internal *psora* which has hitherto slumbered and been latent, and, as it were, kept bound by a good bodily constitution and favorable external circumstances, as well as its breaking out into more serious ailments and maladies, is announced by the increase of the symptoms given above as indicating the slumbering *psora*, and also by a numberless multitude of various other signs and complaints. These are varied according to the difference in the bodily constitution of a man, his hereditary disposition, the various errors in his education and habits, his manner of living and diet, his employments, his turn of mind, his morality, etc.

Then when the itch-malady develops into a manifest secondary disease there appear the following symptoms, which I have derived and observed altogether from accounts of diseases which I myself have treated successfully and which confessedly originated from the contagion of itch, and were mixed neither with syphilis nor sycosis.

---

have entirely ceased of necessity, after the removal of the cause? But these ailments do not cease, they are in time renewed and even gradually aggravated, and it becomes evident that those disagreeable events could not have been the sufficient cause of the present ailments and complaints—it is seen that they *only served as an occasion and impetus toward the development of a malady, which till then only slumbered within.*

The recognition of this old internal foe, which is so frequently present, and the science which is able to overcome it, make it manifest, that generally an indwelling itch disease (*psora*) was the ground of all these ailments, which can not be overcome even by the vigor of the best constitution, but only through art.

I am quite willing to believe that many more symptoms may have occurred in the experience of others.

I would only add further, that among the symptoms adduced there are also such as are entirely opposed to each other, the reason of which may be found in the varying bodily constitutions existing at the time—when the outbreak of the internal *psora* occurred. Yet the one variety of symptoms is found more rarely than the other and it offers no particular obstruction to a cure:

Vertigo; reeling while walking.

Vertigo; when closing the eyes, everything seems to turn around with him; he is at the same time seized with nausea.

Vertigo; on turning around briskly, he almost falls over.

Vertigo, as if there was a jerk in the head, which causes a momentary loss of consciousness.

Vertigo with frequent eructations.

Vertigo even when only looking down on the level ground, or when looking upward.

Vertigo while walking on a road not enclosed on either side, in an open plain.

Vertigo; she seems to herself now too large, now too small, or other objects have this appearance to her.

Vertigo, resembling a swoon.

Vertigo, passing over into unconsciousness.

Dizziness; inability to think or to perform mental labor.

Her thoughts are not under her control.

She is at times quite without thought (sits lost in thought).

The open air causes dizziness and drowsiness in the head.

Everything at times seems dark and black before his eyes, while walking or stooping, or when raising himself from a stooping posture.

Rush of blood to the head.[1]

Heat in the head (and in the face).[2]

A cold pressure on the top of the head.[3]

Headache, a dull pain in the morning immediately on waking up, or in the afternoon when walking rapidly or speaking loudly.

Headache on one side, with a certain periodicity (after 28, 14 or a less number of days), more frequently during full moon, or during the new moon, or after mental excitement, after a cold, etc.; a pressure or other pain on top of the head or inside of it, or a boring pain over one of the eyes.[4]

---

[1] While the mind is uneasy, with anxiety and disinclination to work.

[2] Not unfrequently accompanied with coldness of the hands and feet.

[3] Usually accompanied with anxiety.

[4] At the same time a great internal disquiet and anxiety, especially in the

Headache daily at certain hours; *e. g.*, a stitching in the temples.[1]

Attacks of throbbing headache (*e. g.*, in the forehead) with violent nausea as if about to sink down, or, also, vomiting; starting early in the evenings, repeated every fortnight, or sooner or later.

Headache as if the skull were about to burst open.[2]

Headache, drawing pains.[3]

Headache, stitches in the head (passing out at the ears).[4]

Roaring noise in the brain, singing, buzzing, humming, thundering, etc.

The scalp full of drandruff, with or without itching.

Eruption on the head, tinea capitis, malignant tinea with crusts of greater or less thickness, with sensitive stitches when one of the places becomes moist; when it becomes moist a violent itching; the whole crown of the head painfully sensitive to the open air; with it hard swellings of the glands in the neck.

The hair of the head as if parched.

The hair of the head frequently falls out, most in front, on the crown and top of the head; bald spots or beginning baldness of certain spots.

Under the skin are formed painful lumps, which come and pass away, like bumps and round tumors.[5]

Feeling of contraction in the skin of the scalp and the face.

Paleness of the face during the first sleep, with blue rings around the eyes.

Frequent redness of the face, and heat.[6]

---

abdomen; a lack of stools, or frequent, scanty evacuations attended with anxiety; heaviness in the limbs, quivering in the whole body, tension of all the nerves with great irritability and sensitiveness; the eye can not bear any light, lachrymation, sometimes with swelling of the eyes; the feet are cold; at times attended with dry coryza; often chills, then again a flying heat; conjoined with this, continuous nausea, also at times, retching and vomiting; she lies either as if stunned, or throws herself anxiously from side to side, the attacks lasting from twelve to twenty-four and more hours. After these attacks either great weariness with sadness, or a feeling of tension all over the body. Before these attacks there are frequently jerks of the limbs during sleep and starting up from sleep, anxious dreams, gnashing of the teeth in sleep and tendency to start at any sudden noise.

[1] Which also swell at times, with lachrymation of the one eye.

[2] In some cases a drawing pain from the nape of the neck toward the occiput, at times also over the whole head and face, which is often bloated from it, while the head aches when touched, not infrequently attended with nausea.

[3] Usually while walking, especially while walking and moving after meals.

[4] At the same time everything frequently appears dark before her face.

[5] Which also in rare cases pass over into suppuration.

[6] He at times also becomes quite weak and weary from it or anxious, and he perspires on the upper part of the body; his eyes at times become dim;

Yellowish, yellow color of the face.

Sallow yellowish complexion.

Erysipelas on the face.[1]

Pressive pain on the eyes, especially late in the evening; he must shut them.

He cannot look long at anything, else everything flickers before him; objects seem to move.

The eyelids, especially in the morning, are as if closed; he cannot open them (for minutes; yea, even for hours); the eye-lids are heavy as if paralyzed or convulsively closed.

The eyes are most sensitive to daylight; they are pained by it and close involuntarily.[2]

Sensation of cold in the eyes.

The canthi are full of pus-like mucus (eye-gum).

The edges of the eyelids full of dry mucus.

On the edges of the eyelids, inflammation of single Meibomian glands or of several of them.

Inflammations of the eyes, of various kinds.[3]

Yellowness around the eyes.

Yellowness of the white of the eye.[4]

Dim, opaque spots on the cornea.[5]

Dropsy of the eye.

Obscuration of the crystalline lens, cataract.

Squinting.

Far-sightedness; he sees far in the distance, but cannot clearly distinguish small objects held close.

Short-sightedness; he can see even small objects by holding them close to the eye, but the more distant the object is, the more indistinct it appears, and at a great distance he does not see it.

False vision; he sees objects double, or manifold, or only the one-half of them.

Before his eyes there are floating as it were flies, or black points, or dark streaks, or networks, especially when looking into bright daylight.

The eyes seem to look through a veil or a mist; the sight becomes dim at certain times.

---

everything becomes black before his eyes, his mind is sad; his head also feels as if too full, with burning in the temples.

[1] In some cases with much fever, also at times with burning, itching, stinging watery blisters in the face, which turn into scabs (Erysipelas bullosum.)

[2] Usually with more or less inflammation.

[3] The *fistula lachrymalis* has probably never any other cause than the itch-disease.

[4] Or gray color of the same.

[5] Even without having had any previous inflammation of the eyes.

Night-blindness; he sees well in daytime, but, in the twilight he cannot see at all.

Blindness by day; he can only see well during the twilight.

Amaurosis; uninterrupted dimness of vision[1] increased finally even to blindness.

Painfulness of various spots in the face, the cheeks, the cheekbones, the lower jaw, etc., when touched; while chewing, as if festering inwardly; also like stitches and jerks; especially in chewing there are jerks, stitches and a tension so that he cannot eat.[2]

The hearing is excessively irritateb and sensitive; she cannot bear to hear a bell ring without trembling; he is thrown into convulsions by the beating of the drum, etc.; many sounds cause pains in the ear.

There are stitches in the ear, outwardly.[3]

Crawling sensation and itching in the ear.

Dryness in the ear; dry scabs within, without any ear-wax.

Running from the ear of thin, usually ill-smelling pus.

Pulsation in the ear.

Various sounds and noises in the ear.[4]

Deafness of various degrees even up to total deafness, with or without noise in the ear; occasionally worse, according to the weather.

Swelling of the parotid glands.[5]

Epistaxis, more or less profusely, more or less frequently.

The nostrils as it were stopped up.[6]

Sensation of dryness in the nose, troublesome even when the air passes freely.

Polypi of the nose (usually with the loss of the power of smelling); these may extend also through the nasal passages into the fauces.

Sense of smell, weak, lost.

---

[1] More frequently without opacity of the crystalline lens than with it.

[2] During chewing or speaking there is at times also a similar twitching on the sides of the head, where protuberances like painful bumps often arise. When the pain is still more unbearable and at times combined with a burning pain, it is called Fothergill's pain in the face.

[3] Especially while walking in the open air.

[4] Such as clinking, rushing, seething, roaring, humming, chirping, ringing, drumming, thundering, whizzing, fluttering, murmuring, etc.

[5] Often with stinging pains in the glands.

[6] Either one or both, or alternately, first one, then the other; often there is only the sensation of being stopped up, while the air can be freely drawn in through it.

Sense of smell perverted.[1]

Too violent sensation of smell, higher and highest sensitiveness for even imperceptible odors.

Scabs in the nose; discharge of pus or hardened clots of mucus.[2]

Fetid smell in the nose.

Nostrils frequently ulcerated, surrounded with pimples and scabs.

Swelling and redness of the nose or the tip of the nose, frequent or continual.

Under the nose, or on the upper lip, long-lasting scabs or itching pimples.

The red of the lips is quite pale.

The red of the lips is dry, scabby, peeling off; it chaps.

Swelling of the lips, especially of the upper lip.[3]

The inside of the lips is lined with little sores or blisters.[4]

Cutaneous eruption of the beard and of the roots of the hairs of the beard, with itching.

Eruptions of the face of innumerable kinds.[5]

Glands of the lower jaw swollen, sometimes passing over into chronic suppuration.

Glandular swellings down the sides of the neck.

Gums bleeding at a slight touch.

Gums, the external or the internal, painful, as if from wounds.

Gums, with erosive itching.

Gums, whitish, swollen, painful on touching.

Gums, recession, leaving the front teeth and their roots bare.

Gnashing of the teeth during sleep.

Looseness of the teeth, and many kinds of deterioration of the teeth, even without toothache.

Toothache of innumerable varieties, with varying causes of excitation.

She cannot remain in bed at night, owing to toothache

On the tongue, painful blisters and sore places.

Tongue white, coated white or furred white.

Tongue pale, bluish-white.

Tongue full of deep furrows; here and there, as if torn above.

Tongue dry.

Sensation of dryness on the tongue, even while it is properly moist.

---

[1] *E. g.*, the smell of manure or some other peculiar smell is in the nose.

[2] Sometimes also a discharge of acrid mucus from the nose.

[3] At times with a burning, biting pain.

[4] Often very painful, coming and passing away.

[5] Milk-crust, pimples, blotches, herpes and carcinomatous ulcers of the nose, lips and face (also called *cancer*), with burning and stinging pain.

Stuttering, stammering; also at times sudden attacks of inability to speak.

On the inside of the cheeks painful blisters or sores.

Flow of blood from the mouth; often severe.

Sensation of dryness of the whole internal mouth, or merely in spots, or deep down in the throat.[1]

Fetid smell from the mouth.

Burning in the throat.

Constant flow of saliva, especially while speaking, particularly in the morning.

Continual spitting of saliva.

Frequent mucus deep down in the throat (the fauces), which he has to hawk up and expectorate frequently during the day, especially in the morning.

Frequently inflammation of the throat, and swelling of the parts used in swallowing.

Insipid, slimy taste in the mouth.

Intolerably sweet taste in the mouth, almost constantly.

Bitter taste in the mouth, mostly in the morning.[2]

Sourish and sour taste in the mouth, especially after eating, though the food tasted all right.[3]

Putrid and fetid taste in the mouth.

Bad smell in the mouth, sometimes mouldy, sometimes putrid like old cheese, or like fetid foot-sweat, or like rotten sour krout.

Eructations, with the taste of the food, several hours after eating.

Eructations, empty, loud, of mere air, uncontrollable, often for hours, not infrequently at night.

Incomplete eructation, which causes merely convulsive shocks in the fauces, without coming out of the mouth.

Eructation, sour, either fasting or after food, especially after milk.

Eructation, which excites to vomiting.

Eructation, rancid (especially after eating fat things).

Eructation, putrid or mouldy, early in the morning.

Frequent eructations before meals, with a sort of rabid hunger.

Heart-burn, more or less frequent; there is a burning along

---

[1] Chiefly on waking up at night or in the morning, with or without thirst; with a great deal of dryness in the throat, often a pricking pain in swallowing.

[2] Not rarely, this is constant.

[3] Rarely an offensively sweet taste in the mouth, even without eating or drinking.

the chest, especially after breakfast, or while moving the body.

Water-brash, a gushing discharge of a sort of salivary fluid from the stomach, preceded by writhing pains in the stomach (the pancreas), with a sensation of weakness (shakiness), nausea causing as it were a swoon, and gathering of the saliva in the mouth, even at night.[1]

The ruling complaints in any part of the body are excited after eating fresh fruit, especially if this is acidulous, also after acetic acid (in salads, etc.).

Nausea early in the morning.[2]

Nausea even to vomiting, in the morning immediately after rising from bed, decreasing from motion.

Nausea always after eating fatty things or milk.

Vomiting of blood.

Hiccough after eating or drinking.

Swallowing impeded by spasms, even causing a man to die of hunger.

Spasmodic, involuntary swallowing.

Frequent sensation of fasting and of emptiness in the stomach (or abdomen), not unfrequently with much saliva in the mouth.

Ravenous hunger (canine hunger), especially early in the morning; he has to eat at once else he grows faint, exhausted and shaky, (or if he is in the open air he has to lie straight down).

Ravenous hunger with rumbling and grumbling in the abdomen.

Appetite without hunger; she has a desire to swallow down in haste various things without there being any craving therefor in the stomach.

A sort of hunger; but when she then eats ever so little, she feels at once satiated and full.

When she wants to eat, she feels full in the chest and her throat feels as if full of mucus.

Want of appetite; only a sort of gnawing, turning and writhing in the stomach urges her to eat.

Repugnance to cooked, warm food, especially to boiled meat,

---

[1] This also at times turns into vomiting of water, mucus, or a gush of acrid acid—more frequently after eating flour dumplings, vegetables causing flatulence, baked prunes, etc.

[2] Often coming very suddenly.

and hardly any longing for anything but rye-bread (with butter), or for potatoes.[1]

In the morning, at once, thirst; constant thirst.

In the pit of the stomach there is a sensation of swelling painful to the touch.

Sensation of coldness in the pit of the stomach.

Pressure in the stomach or in the pit of the stomach, as from a stone, or a constricting pain (cramp).[2]

In the stomach, beating and pulsation, even when fasting.

Spasm in the stomach; pain in the pit of the stomach as if drawn together.[3]

Griping in the stomach; a painful griping in the stomach;[4] it suddenly constricts the stomach, especially after cold drinking.

Pain in the stomach, as if sore, when eating even the most harmless kinds of foods.

Pressure in the stomach, even when fasting, but more from every kind of food, or from particular dishes, fruit, green vegetables, rye-bread, food containing vinegar, etc.[5]

During eating, feels dizzy and giddy, threatening to fall to one side.

After the slightest supper, nocturnal heat in bed; in the morning, constipation and exceeding lassitude.

After meals, anxiety and cold perspiration with anxiety.[6]

During eating, perspiration.

Immediately after eating, vomiting.

After meals, pressure and burning in the stomach, or in the epigastrium, almost like heartburn.

After eating, burning in œsophagus from below upward.

After meals, distension of the abdomen.[7]

---

[1] Especially in youth and childhood.

[2] In some cases even while fasting, and causing him to wake up out of sleep at night, sometimes oppressing the breathing.

[3] Usually a short time after eating.

[4] Not infrequently with vomiting of mucus and water, without which in such a case the griping is not alleviated.

[5] Even after partaking of the slightest quantity of such things, there may also ensue colic, pain or numbness of the jaws, tearing pain in the teeth, copious accumulation of mucus in the throat, etc.

[6] There may also be pains, renewed now and then; *e. g.*, stitches in the lips, griping and digging in the abdomen, pressure in the chest, heaviness in the back and the small of the back, even to nausea; when nothing but an artificially excited vomiting will give relief. With some the anguish is aggravated after eating, even to an impulse to destroy themselves by strangulation.

[7] With this, at times, weariness in the arms and legs.

After meals, very tired and sleepy.[1]

After meals, as if intoxicated.

After meals, headache.

After meals, palpitation of the heart.

Alleviation of several, even remote, complaints from eating.

The flatus does not pass off, but moves about, causing many ailments of body and of spirit.[2]

The abdomen is distended by flatus,[3] the abdomen feels full, especially after a meal.

Sensation as if the flatus ascended; followed by eructations—then often a sensation of burning in the throat, or vomiting by day and by night.

Pain in the hypochondria when touched, and in motion, or also during rest.

Constricting pain in the epigastrium, immediately under the ribs.

Cutting pains in the abdomen, as if from obstructed flatus; there is a constant sensation of fulness in the abdomen—the flatus rises upwards.

Cutting pains in the abdomen almost daily, especially with children, oftener in the morning than in other parts of the day, sometimes day and night, without diarrhœa.

Cutting pains in the abdomen, especially on the one side of the abdomen, or the groin.[4]

In the abdomen, qualmishness, a sensation of voidness, disagreeable emptiness,[5] even immediately after eating, he felt as if he had not eaten anything.

From the small of the back, around the abdomen, especially below the stomach, a sensation of constriction as from a bandage, after she had had no stool for several days.

Pain in the liver, when touching the right side of the abdomen.

Pain in the liver, a pressure and tension—a tension below the ribs on the right side.

Below the last ribs (in the hypochondria), a tension and pressure all over, which checks the breathing and makes the mind anxious and sad.

---

[1] Often until the patient lies down and sleeps.

[2] At times drawing pains in the limbs, especially in the lower limbs, or stitches in the pit of the stomach, or in the side of the abdomen, etc.

[3] The flatus often ascends; less frequently a great quantity of flatus is discharged, especially in the morning, without smell and without alleviating the other ailments; in other cases flatulence, with a great quantity of excessively fetid flatus passing off.

[4] The cutting pain also at times passes down into the rectum and down the high.

[5] In some cases alternating with a contractive pain in the abdomen.

Pain in the liver, stitches—mostly when stooping quickly.

Inflammation of the liver.

Pressure in the abdomen as from a stone.[1]

Hardness of the abdomen.

Crampy colic, a grasping pain in the bowels.

In colic, coldness on one side of the abdomen.

A clucking, croaking and audible rumbling and grumbling in the abdomen.[2]

So-called uterine spasms, like labor pains, grasping pains often compelling the patient to lie down, frequently quickly distending the abdomen without flatulence.

In the lower abdomen, pains pressing down toward the genitals.[3]

Inguinal hernias, often painful while speaking and singing.[4]

Swellings of the inguinal glands, which sometimes turn into suppuration.

Constipation; delayed stools sometimes for several days, not infrequently with repeated ineffectual urging to stool.

Stools hard, as if burnt, in small knots, like sheep-dung, often covered with mucus, sometimes also enveloped by veinlets of blood.

Stools of mere mucus (mucous piles).

Passage of round worms from the anus.

Discharge of pieces of tape-worm.

Stools, in the beginning very hard and troublesome, followed by diarrhœa.

Very pale, whitish stool.

Gray stools.

Green stools.

Clay-colored stools.

Stools with putrid, sour smell.

At the stools, cutting pains in the rectum.

Stools show diarrhœa for several weeks, months, years.[5]

Frequently repeated diarrhœa, with cutting pains in the abdomen, lasting several days.

---

[1] Which often rises to the pit of the stomach, digging and causing vomiting.

[2] At times only in the left side of the abdomen, passing upwards with the inspiration and downward with the expiration.

[3] Pressing down as if to cause a prolapsus, and when it is passed she feels heavy in all her limbs, the limbs go to sleep; she must stretch and extend her limbs.

[4] Inguinal hernias rise as a rule only from internal psora, excepting the few cases, when these parts are injured by great external violence, or when the hernia arises from superhuman exertions of the body through lifting or pushing quickly, while in a great fright.

[5] Usually preceded by rumbling or fermentation in the abdomen; chiefly in the morning.

After a stool, especially after a softer, more copious evacuation, great and sudden prostration.[1]

Diarrhœa, soon so weakening, that she cannot walk alone.

Painless and painful hemorrhoidal varices[2] on the anus, in the rectum (blind piles).

Bleeding hemorrhoidal varices on the anus or in the rectum[3] (running piles), especially during stools, after which the hemorrhoids often pain violently for a long time.

With bloody discharges in the anus or in the rectum, ebullition of blood through the body and short breathing.

Formication and itching formication in the rectum, with or without the discharge of ascarides.

Itching and erosion in the anus and the perinæum.

Polypi in the rectum.

During micturition, anxiety, also at times prostration.

At times too much urine is discharged, succeeded by great weariness.[4]

Painful retention of urine (with children and old people).

When he is chilled (feels cold through and through), he cannot urinate.

At times owing to flatulence, she cannot urinate.

The urethra is constricted in parts, especially in the morning.[5]

Pressure on the bladder, as if from an urging to urinate, immediately after drinking.

He cannot hold the urine for any length of time, it presses on the bladder, and passes off while he walks, sneezes, coughs or laughs.

Frequent micturition at night; he has to get up frequently at night for that purpose.

Urine passes off in sleep involuntarily.

---

[1] Especially, weakness in the pit of the stomach, anxiety, restlessness, also at times chills in the abdomen or the small of the back, etc.

[2] Which not infrequently have a slimy fluid oozing from them.

[3] *Fistulæ in ano* have probably never any other cause than this malady, especially when to this there are added a stimulating diet, an excess in spirituous liquors, frequent laxatives, a sedentary occupation and abuse of the sexual instinct.

[4] *Diabetes*, which with Allopathic remedies is usually so fatal, has probably never any other origin than this malady.

[5] The urine frequently passes off as thin as a thread, or the stream spreads out; the urine is only discharged in jerks at long intervals; these interruptions are frequently caused by a spasm in the neck of the bladder which antagonizes the action of the bladder and springs from the same psoric malady. So also inflammation of the bladder from strictures of the urethra, and the *fistula in vesica* are always of psoric origin, though in rare cases *sycosis* may be complicated with the *psora*.

After urinating, the urine continues to drip out for a long time.

Whitish urine, with a sweetish smell and taste, passes off in excessive abundance, with prostration, emaciation and inextinguishable thirst (diabetes).

During urination, burning, also lancinating pains in the urethra and the neck of the bladder.

Urine of penetrating, sharp odor.

The urine quickly deposits a sediment.

The urine discharged is at once turbid like whey.

With the urine there is discharged from time to time a red sand (kidney grits).

Dark-yellow urine.

Brown urine.

Blackish urine.

Urine with blood particles, also at times complete hematuria.

Discharge of prostatic fluid after urination, but especially after a difficult stool (also almost constant dripping of the same).[1]

Nocturnal passage of semen, too frequent, one, two or three times a week, or even every night.[2]

Nightly discharge of the genital fluid in a women, with voluptuous dreams.

Nocturnal pollutions, even if not frequent, yet immediately attended by evil consequences.[3]

Semen passes off almost involuntarily in daytime, with little excitation, often even without erection.

Erections very frequent, long continuing, very painful without pollutions.

The semen is not discharged, even during a long-continued coition and with a proper erection,[4] but it passes off afterward in nocturnal pollutions or with the urine.

Accumulation of water in the tunica vaginalis of the testicle (hydrocele).

There is never a complete erection, even with the most voluptuous excitement.

---

[1] Sometimes also consumption from the constant oozing out of the prostatic fluid.

[2] With healthy chaste young men, pollutions naturally only take place every twelve or fourteen days, without any attending troubles, and they are followed by cheerfulness and a feeling of strength and serenity.

[3] Gloominess, obtuseness, dimness of the thinking powers, diminished vividness of the imagination, want of memory, depression, melancholy; the vision is weakened, as well as the digestion and the appetite; stools are retained, a rush of blood to the head ensues, also toward the anus, etc.

[4] The testicles in such a case are never drawn up to the body, but hang down more or less.

Painful twitches in the muscles of the penis.

Itching of the scrotum, which is sometimes beset with pimples and scabs.

One or both of the testicles chronically swollen, or showing a knotty induration (*Sarcocele*).

Dwindling, diminution, disappearance of one or both testicles.

Induration and enlargement of the prostatic gland.

Drawing pain in the testicle and the spermatic chord.

Pain as from contusion in the testicle.

Lack of the sexual desire in both sexes, either frequent or constant.[1]

Uncontrollable insatiable lasciviousness,[2] with a cachectic complexion and sickly body.

Sterility, impotence, without any original organic defect in the sexual parts.[3]

Disorders of the menstrual function; the menses do not appear regularly on the twenty-eighth day after their last appearance, they do not come on without other ailments and not at once, and do not continue steadily for three or four days with a moderate quantity of healthy-colored, mild blood, until on the fourth day it imperceptibly comes to an end without any disturbance of the general health of body and spirit; nor are the menses continued to the forty-eighth or fiftieth year, nor do they cease gradually and without any troubles.

The menses are slow in setting in after the fifteenth year and later, or after appearing one or more times, they cease for several months and for years.[4]

The menses do not keep their regular periods, they either come

---

[1] Often for years, yea, for many years. The male and the female genital parts cannot then be excited to any agreeable or voluptuous sensation—the body of the male penis hangs down relaxed, is thinner than the glans penis, which feels cold and is of a bluish or white color; in the female parts the labia are not excitable, they are relaxed and small; the vagina almost numb and insensible, and usually dry; sometimes there is a falling out of the hair of the pudenda, or entire bareness of the female genital parts.

[2] Metromania and Nymphomania are of the same origin.

[3] Too frequent coition from impotent lasciviousness, with too sudden a passing off of immature, watery semen, or lack of erection, or lack of the issue of semen, or lack of sexual desire—menses too copious, or a constant flow of blood; watery, scanty or deficient menses; copious discharge of mucus from the vagina (leucorrhœa), indurated ovaries, the breasts have either dwindled down or become knotty; insensibility, or merely painful sensibility of the genital organs, are merely the proximate usual symptoms of sterility or impotence with the one sex or the other.

[4] Consequent sallow paleness and tumefaction of the face, heaviness of the limbs, swelling of the feet, chilliness, weariness, asthma (chlorosis), etc.

several days too early, sometimes every three weeks, or even every fortnight.[1]

The menses flow only one day, only a few hours, or in imperceptibly small quantities.

The menses flow for five, six, eight and more days, but only intermittently, a little flow every six, twelve, twenty-four hours, and then they cease for half or whole days, before more is discharged.

The menses flow too strongly, for weeks, or return almost daily (bloody flux).[2]

Menses of watery blood or of brown clots of blood.

Menses of very fetid blood.

Menses accompanied with many ailments, swoons or (mostly stitching) headaches, or contractive, spasmodic, cutting pains in the abdomen and in the small of the back; she is obliged to lie down, vomit, etc.

Polypi in the vagina.

Leucorrhœa from the vagina, one or several days before, or soon after, the monthly flow of blood, or during the whole time from the one menstrual discharge to the other, with a diminution of the menses, or continuing solely instead of the menses; the flow is like milk, or like white, or yellow mucus, or like acrid, or sometimes like fetid, water.[3]

Premature births.

---

[1] The menses rarely come several days too late, and flow then in too great abundance, with prostrating weariness and many other ailments.

[2] Often followed by swelling of the face, of the hands and feet, painful spasms in the breast and the abdomen, innumerable ailments from nervous debility, excessive sensitiveness, as well in general, as of particular sensory organs, etc., and before the appearance of the flow, anxious dreams, frequent awakenings with a rush of blood to the head, palpitation, restlessness, etc. With a more violent flow of blood from the uterus, there are often cutting pains in the one side of the abdomen and in the groin; the cutting pain sometimes descends into the rectum and into the thigh; then she frequently cannot urinate, or sit down, on account of her pains; after these pains the abdomen aches as if it were festering.

[3] Leucorrhœa, especially the more malignant kind, is accompanied by an innumerable multitude of ailments. Not to mention the lesser ones (such as the itching of the pudenda and the vagina, with excoriation on the outside of the pudenda and the adjacent part of the thigh, especially in walking), hysterical states of all kinds follow the more severe cases of this troublesome flux, as also disturbances of the mind and spirit, melancholy, insanity, epilepsy, etc. Often it comes in the form of an attack, and then it is preceded by a digging in the one side of the abdomen, or by burning in the stomach, in the lower abdomen, in the vagina, or stitches in the vagina and in the mouth of the uterus, or a constrictive pain in the uterus and pressure toward the vagina as if everything were about to fall out, also at times most keen pains in the small of the back; the flatus is obstructed, causing pain, etc. Has the so-called uterine cancer any other origin than this (psora) malady?

During pregnancies great weariness, nausea, frequent vomiting, swoons, painful varicose veins on the thighs and the legs, and also at times on the labia, hysteric ailments of various kinds, etc.

Coryza at once, whenever she comes into the open air; then usually a stuffed coryza while in her room.

Dry coryza and a stuffed nose often, or almost constantly, also sometimes with intermissions.

Fluent coryza at the least taking of cold, therefore mostly in the inclement season and when it is wet.

Fluent coryza, very often, or almost constantly, also in some cases uninterruptedly.

He cannot take cold, even though there have been strong premonitory symptoms of it, simultaneously with other great ailments from the itch malady.

Hoarseness, after the least amount of speaking; she must vomit in order to clear her voice.

Hoarseness, also sometimes aphony (she cannot speak loud but must whisper), after a slight cold.

Constant hoarseness and aphony for years; he cannot speak a loud word.

Suppuration of the larynx and the bronchia (laryngo-bronchial phthisis).[1]

Hoarseness and catarrh very often, or almost constantly; his chest is continually affected.

Cough; frequent irritation and crawling in the throat; the cough torments him, until perspiration breaks out on his face (and on his hands).

Cough, which does not abate until there is retching and vomiting, mostly in the morning or in the evening.

Cough, which terminates every time with sneezing.

Cough mostly in the evening after lying down and whenever the head lies low.

Cough, waking the patient up after the first brief sleep.

Cough, especially in the night.

Cough, worst after awaking in the morning.

Cough, worst after eating.

Cough, at once with every deep breath.

Cough, causing a sensation of soreness in the chest, or at times stitches in the side of the chest or the abdomen.

Dry cough.

---

[1] Inflammation of the larynx (croup) cannot take place with any child that is free from latent psora or has been made free from it by treatment.

Cough, with yellow expectoration resembling pus, with or without spitting of blood.[1]

Cough, with excessive expectoration of mucus and sinking of the strength (mucous phthisis).

Attacks of whooping cough.[2]

Violent, at times unbearable stitches in the chest at every breath; cough impossible for pain; without inflammatory fever (spurious pleurisy).

Pain in the chest on walking, as if the chest was about to burst.

Pressive pain in the chest, at deep breathing or at sneezing.

Often a slightly constrictive pain in the chest, which, when it does not quickly pass, causes the deepest dejection.[3]

Burning pain in the chest.

Frequent stitches in the chest, with or without cough.

Violent stitches in the side; with great heat of the body, it is almost impossible to breathe, on account of stitches in the chest with hemoptysis and headache; he is confined to his bed.

Night-mare; he usually suddenly awakes at night from a frightful dream, but cannot move, nor call, nor speak, and when he endeavors to move, he suffers intolerable pains, as if he were being torn to pieces.[4]

Obstruction of the breath, with stitching pains in the chest at the slightest amount of walking;[5] he cannot go a step farther (angina pectoris).

Asthma, merely when moving the arms, not while walking.

Attacks of suffocation especially after midnight; the patient has to sit up, sometimes he has to leave his bed, stand stooping forward, leaning on his hands; he has to open the windows, or go out into the open air, etc.; he has palpitations; these are followed by eructations or yawning, and the spasm terminates with or without coughing and expectoration.

---

[1] Suppurative pulmonary phthisis has probably seldom any other cause than this malady, even when it seems as if the fumes of quicksilver or arsenic had caused it; at least most of these cases of suppurative phthisis originate in pneumonias mismanaged with blood-letting, and this disease may always be considered as the manifestation of latent Psora.

[2] She is suddenly compelled to cough, but cannot do so, as her breath fails her, even to suffocation, with a dark-red, bloated face; usually the œsophagus is then also constricted, so that not a drop of water will pass; after eight or ten minutes, there follow eructations from the stomach, and the spasm terminates.

[3] Usually the attacks last from evening to morning, the whole night.

[4] Such attacks, in some cases, also occur several times in one night, especially when he has not been out in the open air during the day.

[5] Especially when ascending a height.

Palpitation with anxiety, especially at night.

Asthma, loud, difficult, at times also sibilant respiration.

Shortness of breath.

Asthma, on moving, with or without cough.

Asthma, mostly while sitting down.

Asthma, spasmodic; when she comes into the open air it takes her breath.

Asthma, in attacks, lasting several weeks.

Dwindling of the breasts, or excessive enlargement of the same, with retroceding nipples.

Erysipelas on one of the breasts (especially while nursing).

A hard, enlarging and indurating gland with lancinating pains in one of the mammæ.[1]

Itching, also moist and scaly eruptions around the nipples.

In the small of the back, in the back and in the nape of the neck, drawing (tearing), tensive pains.

Lancinating, cutting, painful stiffness of the nape of the neck; of the small of the back.

Pressive pain between the shoulder-blades.

Sensation of pressure upon the shoulders.

In the limbs, drawing (tearing), tensive pains, partly in the muscles and partly in the joints (rheumatism).

In the periosteum, here and there, especially in the periosteum of the long bones, pressive and pressive-drawing pains.[2]

Stitching pains in the fingers or toes.[3]

Stitches in the heels and soles of the feet while standing.

Burning in the soles of the feet.[4]

In the joints a sort of tearing, like scraping on the bone, with a red, hot swelling which is painfully sensitive to the touch and to the air, with unbearably sensitive, peevish disposition (gout, podagra, chiragra, gout in the knees, etc.).[5]

The joints of the fingers, swollen with pressive pains, painful when touching and bending them.

---

[1] Is it probable that the different varieties of cancer of the breast have any other origin than this psora malady?

[2] These spots then also pain on being touched, as if they were bruised or sore.

[3] In worse, chronic cases, this is aggravated into a cutting pain.

[4] Especially at night under a feather bed.

[5] The pains are either worse in daytime, or at night. After every attack, and when the inflammation is past, the joints of the hand are painful, as also those of the knee, the foot, those of the big toe when moved, when he stands up, etc., they feel intolerably benumbed and the limb is weakened.

Thickening of the joints; they remain hard swollen, and there is pain on bending them.

The joints, as it were, stiff, with painful, difficult motion, the ligaments seem too short.[1]

Joints, painful on motion.[2]

Joints crack on moving, or they make a snapping noise.

The joints are easily sprained or strained.[3]

Increasing disposition to *strains* and to *overlift* oneself even at a very slight exertion of the muscles, even in slight mechanical work, in reaching out or stretching for something high up, in lifting things that are not heavy, in quick turns of the body, pushing, etc. Such a tension or stretching of the muscles often then occasions long confinement to the bed, swoons, all grades of hysterical troubles,[4] fever, hemoptysis, etc., while persons who are not psoric lift such burdens as their muscles are able to, without the slightest after effects.[5]

The joints are easily sprained at any false movement.[6]

In the joint, of the foot there is pain on treading, as if it would break.

Softening of the bones, curvature of the spine (deformity, hunchback), curvature of the long bones of the thighs and legs (*morbus anglicus*, rickets).

Fragility of the bones.

Painful sensitiveness of the skin, the muscles and of the periosteum on a moderate pressure.[7]

---

[1] *E. g.*, the *tendo Achillis* on standing erect, stiffness of the tarsus, of the knees, either transient (after sitting, when rising), or permanent (contraction.)

[2] *E. g.*, the shoulder-joint on raising the arm; the tarsus pains on treading as if it was about to break.

[3] *E. g.*, the tarsus, the wrist-joint, the joint of the thumb.

[4] Often also, at once severe headache in the crown of the head, which is then also painful externally when touched, or suddenly a pain in the small of the back, or pain in the uterus, not unfrequently stitches in the side of the breast, or between the shoulder blades, which check the respiration, or painful stiffness of the neck or spine, frequent audible eructations, etc.

[5] The common people, especially in the country, seek alleviation through a sort of mesmeric stroking, but without lasting effects; the tendency to overlifting nevertheless remains. It is usually a woman (called a *stroking woman*) who makes with the tips of her thumbs passes over the shoulder blades toward the shoulders or along the spine, sometimes also from the pit of the stomach along below the ribs, only they usually exert too strong a pressure while stroking.

[6] *E. g.*. the ankle at a false step, so also the shoulder-joint. Of this kind is also the gradual luxation of the hip-joint (*i.*, *e.* of the head of the femur from the *acetabulum*, when the leg then becomes too long, or too short, causing limping).

[7] As when he moderately strikes against something, it becomes very painful

Intolerable[1] pain in the skin (or in the muscles, or in the periosteum) of some part of the body from a slight movement of the same or of a more distant part; *e. g.*, from writing there arises a pain in the shoulder or in the side of the neck, etc., while sawing or performing other hard labor with the same hand causes no pain; a similar pain in the adjacent parts, from speaking and moving the mouth; pain in the lips and in the back at a slight touch.

Numbness of the skin or of the muscles of certain parts and limbs.[2]

Dying off of certain fingers or of the hands or feet.[3]

Crawling or also prickling formication (as from the limbs going to sleep) in the arms, in the legs and in other parts (even in the finger-tips).

A crawling, or whirling, or an internally itching *restlessness*, especially in the lower limbs (in the evening in bed or early on awaking); they must be brought into another position every moment.

Painful sensation of cold in various parts.

Burning pains in various parts (frequently without any change in the usual external bodily temperature).

Coldness, repeated or constant of the whole body, or of the one side of the body; so also of single parts, cold hands, cold feet which frequently will not get warm in bed.

Chilliness, constant, even without any change in the external bodily temperature.

Frequent flushes of heat, especially in the face, more frequently with redness than without; sudden, violent sensation of heat during rest, or in slight motion, sometimes even from speaking, with or without perspiration breaking out.

Warm air in the room or at church is exceedingly repugnant to

---

and for a long time; the parts on which he lies in bed are very painful, wherefore he frequently turns over at night; the posterior muscles of the thigh and the bone on which she sits are quite sore; a slight stroke with the hand on the thighs causes great pain. A slight knock against a hard object leaves blue marks, suffusion of blood.

[1] Of incredible variety. Often burning, jerking, lancinating, but often also indescribable, are these pains which communicate a similar intolerable excessive sensitiveness to the mind. These pains thus affect chiefly the upper parts of the body, or the face (*tic douloureux*), or the skin of the neck, etc., at even a gentle touch, in speaking and chewing,—in the shoulder at a slight pressure, or movement of the finger.

[2] The sense of touch is lacking; the parts feel hard and tumid, either periodically or permanently (constant insensibility).

[3] The limb then becomes white, bloodless, without feeling and quite cold, often for hours, especially while it is cool (stroking with a piece of zinc toward the tips of the fingers or the toes usually drives it away quickly, but only as a palliative).

her, makes her restless, causes her to move about (at times with a pressure in the head, over the eyes, not infrequently alleviated by epistaxis).

Rushes of blood, also at times a sensation of throbbing in all the arteries (while he often looks quite pale, with a feeling of prostration throughout the body).

Rush of blood to the head.

Rush of blood to the chest.

Varices, varicose veins in the lower limbs (varices on the pudenda), also on the arms (even with men), often with tearing pains in them (during storms), or with itching in the varices.[1]

Erysipelas, partly in the face (with fever), partly on the limbs, on the breast while nursing, especially in a sore place (with a prickling and burning pain).

Whitlow, paronychia (sore finger with festering skin).

Chilblains (even when it is not winter) on the toes and fingers, itching, burning and lancinating pains.

Corns, which even without external pressure cause burning, lancinating pains.

Boils (furuncles), returning from time to time, especially on the nates, the thighs, the upper arms and the body. Touching them causes fine stitches in them.

Ulcers on the thighs, especially, also upon the ankles and above them and on the lower part of the calves, with itching, gnawing, tickling around the borders, and a gnawing pain as from salt on the base of the ulcer itself; the parts surrounding are of brown and bluish color, with varices near the ulcers, which, during storms and rains, often cause tearing pains, especially at night, often accompanied with erysipelas after vexation or fright, or attended with cramps in the calves.

Tumefaction and suppuration of the humerus, the femur, the patella, also of the bones of the fingers and toes (*spina ventosa*).

Thickening and stiffening of the joints.

Eruptions, either arising from time to time and passing away again; some voluptuously itching pustules, especially on the fingers or other parts, which, after scratching, burn and have the greatest similarity to the original itch-eruption;

or *nettle-rash*, like stings and water-blisters, mostly with burning pain;

or *pimples* without pain in the face, the chest, the back, the arms and the thighs;

---

[1] The swellings of the arteries (aneurismata) seem to have no other origin than the *psora*.

or *herpes* in fine miliary grains, closely pressed together into round, larger or smaller spots of mostly reddish color, sometimes dry, sometimes moist, with itching, similar to the eruption of itch and with burning after rubbing them. They continually extend further to the circumference with redness, while the middle seems to become free from the eruption and covered with smooth, shining skin (*herpes circinatus*). The moist herpes on the legs are called salt-rheum;

or *crusts* raised above the surrounding skin, round in form, with deep-red, painless borders, with frequent violent stitches on the parts of the skin not yet affected;

or *small, round spots* on the skin, covered with bran-like, dry scales, which often peel off and are again renewed without sensation;

or *red spots of the skin*, which feel dry, with burning pain; somewhat raised above the rest of the skin.

Freckles, small and round, brown or brownish spots in the face, on the hands and on the chest, without sensation.

Liver spots, large brownish spots which often cover whole limbs, the arms, the neck, the chest, etc., without sensation or with itching.

Yellowness of the skin, yellow spots of a like nature around the eyes, the mouth, on the neck, etc., without sensibility.[1]

Warts on the face, the lower arm, the hands, etc.[2]

Encysted tumors in the skin, the cellular tissue beneath it, or in the *bursæ mucosæ* of the tendons (exostosis), of various forms and sizes, cold without sensibility.[3]

Glandular swellings around the neck, in the groin, in the bend of the joints, the bend of the elbow, of the knee, in the axillæ,[4] also in the breasts.

Dryness of the (scarf) skin either on the whole body with inability to perspire through motion and heat, or only in some parts.[5]

---

[1] After riding in a carriage, yellowness of the skin comes on most quickly, if it is not yet constant but only occasional.

[2] Especially in youth. Many remain only a short time and pass away to give place to another symptom of psora.

[3] The fungus hematodes, which has lately become such a dreadful plague, has, according to the conclusions I am compelled to draw from several cases, no other source than psora.

[4] At times they pass over, after lancinating pains, into a sort of chronic suppuration, in which, however, instead of pus, only a colorless mucus is secreted.

[5] Especially on the hands, the outer side of the arms and legs, and even in the face; the skin is dry, rough, parched, feels chapped, and often has scales like bran.

Disagreeable sensation of dryness over the whole body (also in the face, around and in the mouth, in the throat, or in the nose, although the breath passes freely through it).

Perspiration comes too easily from slight motion; even while sitting, he is attacked with perspiration all over, or merely on some parts; *e. g.*, almost constant perspiration of the hands and feet,[1] so also strong perspiration in the axillæ[2] and around the pudenda.

Daily morning sweats, often causing the patient to drip, this for many years, often with sour or pungent-sour smell.[3]

One-sided perspiration, only on one side of the body, or only on the upper part of the body, or only on the lower part.

Increasing susceptibility to colds, either of the whole body (often even from repeatedly wetting the hands, now with warm water, then with cold, as in washing clothes), or only susceptibility of certain parts of the body, of the head, the neck, the chest, the abdomen, the feet, etc., often in a moderate or slight draught, or after slightly moistening these parts;[4] even from being in a cooler room, in a rainy atmosphere, or with a low barometer.

So-called *weather prophets; i. e.*, renewed severe pains in parts of the body which were formerly injured, wounded, or broken, though they have since been healed and cicatrized; this renewed pain sets in, when great changes of the weather, great cold, or a storm are imminent, or when a thunderstorm is in the air.

Watery swelling, either of the feet alone, or in one foot, or in the hands, or the face, or the abdomen, or the scrotum, etc., alone, or again cutaneous swelling over the whole body (dropsies).

Attacks of sudden heaviness of the arms or legs.

Attacks of paralytic weakness and paralytic lassitude of the one arm, the one hand, the one leg, without pain, either arising suddenly and passing quickly, or commencing gradually and constantly increasing.

---

[1] The latter is usually very fetid and so abundant that, after even a short walk, the soles of the feet, the heels and toes are soaked and sore.

[2] Not infrequently of red color or of a rank smell like that of he goats or that of garlic.

[3] Here belongs the perspiration of psoric children on their head after going to sleep in the evening.

[4] The ailments following from it, immediately afterwards, are then considerable and manifold: Pains in the limbs, headaches, catarrh, sore throat, and inflammation of the throat, coryza, swelling of the glands of the neck, hoarseness, cough, dyspnœa, stitches in the chest, fever, troubles of digestion, colic, vomiting, diarrhœa, stomachache, rising of water from the stomach, also stitches in the face and other parts, jaundice-like color of the skin, etc. No person who is not psoric ever suffers the least after-effects from such causes.

Sudden bending of the knees.

Children fall easily, without any visible cause. Also similar attacks of weakness, with adults, in the legs, so that in walking one foot glides this way and the other that way, etc.

While walking in the open air sudden attacks of faintness, especially in the legs.[1]

While sitting, the patient feels intolerably weary, but stronger while walking.

The predisposition to spraining and straining the joints at a mis-step, or a wrong grasp, increases at times even to dislocation; *e. g.*, in the tarsus, the shoulder-joint, etc.

The snapping and cracking of the joints at any motion of the limb increases with a disagreeable sensation.

The going to sleep of the limbs increases and follows on slight causes; *e. g.*, in supporting the head with the arm, crossing the legs while sitting, etc.

The painful cramps in some of the muscles increase and come on without appreciable cause.

Slow, spasmodic straining of the flexor muscles of the limbs.

Sudden jerks of some muscles and limbs even while waking; *e. g.*, of the tongue, the lips, the muscles of the face, of the pharynx, of the eyes, of the jaws, of the hands and of the feet.

Tonic shortening of the flexor muscles (tetanus).

Involuntary turning and twisting of the head, or the limbs, with full consciousness (St. Vitus' dance).

Sudden fainting spells and sinking of the strength, with loss of consciousness.

Attacks of tremor in the limbs, without anxiety. Continuous, constant trembling, also in some cases beating with the hands, the arms, the legs.

Attacks of loss of consciousness, lasting a moment or a minute, with an inclination of the head to the one shoulder, with or without jerks of one part or the other.

Epilepsies of various kinds.

Almost constant yawning, stretching and straining of the limbs.

Sleepiness during the day, often immediately after sitting down, especially after meals.

Difficulty in falling asleep, when abed in the evening; he often lies awake for hours.

---

[1] At times the feeling of faintnees seems to rise up even to the scrobiculus cordis, where it turns into a ravenous hunger, which suddenly deprives him of all strength; he is attacked with tremor and has immediately to lie down for a while.

He passes the nights in a mere slumber.

Sleeplessness, from anxious heat, every night, an anxiety which sometimes rises so high, that he must get up from his bed and walk about.

After three o'clock in the morning, no sleep, or at least no sound sleep.

As soon as he closes his eyes, all manner of phantastic appearances and distorted faces appear.

In going to sleep, she is disquieted by strange, anxious fancies; she has to get up and walk about.

Very vivid dreams, as if awake; or sad, frightful, anxious, vexing, lascivious dreams.

Loud talking, screaming, during sleep.

Somnambulism; he rises up at night, while sleeping with closed eyes, and attends to various duties; he performs even dangerous feats with ease, without knowing anything about them when awake.

Attacks of suffocation while sleeping (nightmare).

Various sorts of severe pains at night, or nocturnal thirst, dryness of the throat, of the mouth, or frequent urinating at night.

Early on awaking, dizzy, indolent, unfreshed, as if he had not done sleeping and more tired than in the evening, when he lay down; it takes him several hours (and only after rising) before he can recover from this weariness.

After a very restless night, he often has more strength in the morning, than after a quiet, sound sleep.

Intermittent fever, even when there are no cases about, either sporadic or epidemic,[1] or endemic; the form, duration and type of the fever are very various; quotidian, tertian, quartan, quintan or every seven days.

Every evening, chills with blue nails.

Every evening, single chills.

Every evening, heat, with a rush of blood to the head, with red cheeks, also at times an intervening chill.

Intermittent fever of several weeks' duration, followed by a moist itching eruption lasting several weeks, but which is healed again during a like period of intermittent fever, and alternating thus for years.

Disturbances of the mind and spirit of all kinds.[2]

---

[1] Epidemic intermittent fevers probably never seize a man who is free from psora, so that wherever there is a susceptibility to them, it is to be accounted a symptom of psora.

[2] I have never either in my practice, nor in any insane asylum, seen a patient suffering from melancholy, insanity, or frenzy whose disease did not have

Melancholy by itself, or with insanity, also at times alternating with frenzy and hours of rationality.

Anxious oppression, early on awaking.

Anxious oppression in the evening after going to bed.[1]

Anxiety, several times a day (with and without pains), or at certain hours of the day or of the night; usually the patient then finds no rest, but has to run hither and thither, and often falls into perspiration.

Melancholy, palpitation and anxiousness causes her at night to wake up from sleep (mostly just before the beginning of the menses).

Mania of self-destruction [2] (spleen?).

A weeping mood; they often weep for hours without knowing a cause for it.[3]

Attacks of fear; *e.g.*, fear of fire, of being alone, of apoplexy, of becoming insane, etc.

Psora as its foundation, complicated at times, however, though rarely, with syphilis.

[1] This causes some patients to break out into a strong perspiration; others feel from it merely flushes of blood and throbbing in all the arteries; with others, the anxious oppression tends to constrict the throat, threatening suffocation, while others have a sensation, as if all the blood in their arteries were standing still, causing anguish. With others, this oppression is associated with anxious images and thoughts, and seems to rise from them, while with others, there is oppression without anxious ideas and thoughts.

[2] This kind of disease of the mind or spirit, which is also merely psoric, seems not to have been taken into consideration. Without feeling any anxiety, or anxious thoughts, therefore also, without any one's perceiving such anxiety in them, apparently in the full exercise of their reason, they are impelled, urged, yea, compelled by a certain feeling of necessity, to self-destruction. They are only healed by a cure of the *Psora*, if their utterances are noticed *in time*. I say *in time*, for in the last stages of this kind of insanity it is peculiarly characteristic of this disease, not to utter anything about such a determination to anyone. This frenzy manifests itself in fits of one-half or of whole hours, usually in the end daily, often at certain times of the day. But besides these fits of destructive mania, such persons have usually also fits of anxious oppression, which seem, however, to be independent of the former fits, and come at other hours, accompanied partly with pulsation in the pit of the stomach, but during these they are not tormented with the desire of taking their own life. These attacks of anxiety which seem to be more of a bodily nature, and are not connected with the other train of thoughts, may also be lacking, while the fits of suicidal mania rule in a high degree; they may also return, when that mania is in a great part extinguished through the anti-psoric remedies, so that the two seem to be independent of one another, though they have the same original malady for their foundation.

[3] This is a symptom, however, which seems to be caused by the diseased state, especially of the female sex, in order to soothe temporarily more and greater nervous disorders.

Attacks of passion, resembling frenzy.

Fright caused by the merest trifles; this often causes perspiration and trembling.

Disinclination to work, in persons who else are most industrious; no impulse to occupy himself, but rather the most decided repugnance thereto.[1]

Excessive sensitiveness.[2]

Irritability from weakness.[2]

Quick change of moods; often very merry and exuberantly so, often again and, indeed, very suddenly, dejection; *e. g.*, on account of his disease, or from other trifling causes. Sudden transition from cheerfulness to sadness, or vexation without a cause.

These are some of the leading symptoms observed by me, which, if they are often repeated, or become constant, show that the internal *Psora* is coming forth from its latent state. They are at the same time the elements, from which (under unfavorable external conditions) the itch-malady, as it manifests itself, composes the illimitable number of chronic diseases, and with one man assumes the one form, with another another, according to the bodily constitution, defects in the education, habits, employment and external circumstances, as also modified by the various psychical and physical impressions. It thus unfolds into manifold forms of disease, with so many varieties, that they are by no means exhausted by the disease-symptoms enumerated in the pathology of the old school, and erroneously designated there as well-defined, constant and peculiar diseases.*

---

[1] Such a person, when she desired to begin one of her domestic occupations, was seized with anxiety and oppression; her limbs trembled, and she became suddenly so weary, she had to lie down.

[2] All physical and psychical impressions, even the weaker and the weakest, cause a morbid excitement, often in a high degree. Occurrences affecting the mind, not only such as are of a sad and vexatious kind, but also those of a joyous kind, cause surprising ailments and disorders; touching tales, yea, even thinking of them and recalling them, cause a tumultuous excitement of the nerves, and drive the anxiety into the head, etc. Even a little reading about indifferent things, or looking attentively at an object; *e. g.*, while sewing, attentively listening even to indifferent things, too bright a light, the loud talking of several people at the same time, even single tones on a musical instrument, the ringing of bells, etc., cause harmful impressions: trembling, weariness, headache, chills, etc. Often the senses of smell and of taste are immoderately sensitive. In many cases even moderate bodily motion, or speaking, also moderate warmth, cold, open air, wetting the skin with water, etc. Not a few suffer even in their room from a sudden change of the weather, while most of these patients complain during stormy and wet weather, few of dry weather with a clear sky. The full moon also with some persons, and the new moon with other, has an unfavorable effect.

***They** bear the following names: Scrofula, rickets, spina ventosa, atrophy,

These are the characteristic secondary symptoms* of the long-unacknowledged, thousand-headed monster, pregnant with disease, the *Psora*, the original miasmatic malady which now makes its manifest appearance.†

---

marasmus, consumption, pulmonary consumption, asthma, tabes mucosa, laryngeal phthisis, chronic catarrh, constant coryza, difficult dentition, worms and consequent diseases, dyspepsia, abdominal cramps, hypochondria, hysteria, dropsy, dropsy of the abdomen, dropsy of the ovaries, of the uterus, hydrocele, hydrocephalus, amenorrhœa, dysmenorrhœa, uterine hemorrhages, hematemesis, hemoptysis and hemorrhages, vaginal hemorrhages, dysuria, ischuria, enuresis, diabetes, catarrh of the bladder, hematuria, nephralgia, gravel of the kidneys, stricture of the urethra, stricture of the intestines, blind and running piles, fistula of the rectum, difficult stools, constipation, chronic diarrhœa, induration of the liver, jaundice, cyanosis, heart diseases, palpitation, spasms of the chest, dropsy of the chest, abortion, sterility, metromania, impotence, induration of the testicles, dwindling of the testicles, prolapsus uteri, inversion of the womb, inguinal, femoral and umbilical hernias, dislocations of the joints from an internal cause, curvature of the spine, chronic inflammations of the eyes, fistula lachrymalis, short-sightedness and long-sightedness, day blindness and night blindness, obscuration of the cornea, cataracts, glaucoma, amaurosis, deafness, deficient smell or taste, chronic one-sided headache, megrim, tic douloureaux, tinea capitis, scab, crusta lactea, tetters (herpes), pimples, nettle-rash, encysted tumors, goitre, varices, aneurism, erysipelas, sarcomas, osteosarcoma, scirrhus, cancer of the lips, cheeks, breast, uterus, fungus hematodes, rheumatism, gout in the hips, knotty gout, podagra, apoplectic fits, swoons, vertigo, paralysis, contractions, tetanus, convulsions, epilepsy, St. Vitus' dance, melancholy, insanity, imbecility, nervous debility, etc.

* The supreme royal councillor *Kopp*, an Allopath, who is unwillingly and only half and half approaching Homœopathy, pretends to have seen chronic diseases disappear of themselves—he may have seen some particular symptoms disappear, which symptoms the old school, in its shortsighted fashion, considered with him as so many entire diseases!

† I will grant that the doctrine, that "all chronic non-venereal diseases which are not extinguishable by the vital force, in an orderly course of life, while external circumstances are favorable, but which even increase with the years, are of psoric origin," is for all who have not fully weighed my reasons and for all narrow-minded people, too great, too overwhelming. But it is none the less true. Or should we regard such a chronic disease as not being psoric, because the patient cannot remember, that he at sometime, all the way back to his birth, has had several or more (intolerably voluptuously) itching pustules of itch on his skin, or (since the itch-disease is considered as something disgraceful) is not willing to acknowledge it? His non-acknowledgment here proves nothing to the contrary.

Since at all times, all the innumerable chronic diseases resulting from an acknowledged preceding itch (when this has not been cured) are ineradicable through the vital force, and advance in their equable course as psoric ailments, and are continually aggravated: so long as the doubters of the psora doctrine cannot show me *any other source* which is at least as probable for a (non-veneric) ailment, which, despite of favorable external conditions, correct diet, good morality and vigorous bodily constitution, nevertheless increases every year, without any preceding infection from itch so far as memory goes: so long I have on my side an overpowering analogous probability, *i. e.*, 100 to 1, that also the individual cases of chronic disease, which show *a like progression*, probably also are, yea, must also be of a psoric nature, although the patient cannot or will not remember a preceding infection.

It is easy to doubt matters which cannot be laid before our ocular vision, but in itself this doubt proves nothing at all, for according to the old rule of logic: *negantis est probare.*

To prove the psoric nature of these chronic diseases without acknowledged infection, we do not even need the fact that the anti-psoric remedies prove effectual therein; this serves only like the proof to a correctly solved mathematical problem.

Now since, in addition, the other remedies, although also selected according to the similarity of their symptoms, do not by far yield so durable and thorough a cure in such chronic diseases, as those which are recognized as anti-psoric, and which are selected in as Homœopathic a manner, because these more than the others are adequate to the whole extent of the endless number of symptoms of the great psora malady: I do not see why men will deny to the latter the title of the especially *anti-psoric* remedies, unless this springs from dogmatism.

And just as little is there any good reason for contradicting me, when I (*Organon*, § 73,) explain the acute diseases which return from time to time; *e. g.*, inflammations of the throat, of the chest, etc., as flaming up from a latent *psora*, simply because their inflammatory state, as they say, is mostly to be combatted by means of the anti-phlogistic remedies, which are not anti-psoric; *i. e.*, Aconite, Belladonna, Mercury and the like. These, nevertheless, have their source in a latent psora, because their customary return cannot be prevented by anything but a final cure with anti-psoric remedies.

vent without any preceding infection from such sources [illegible] there [illegible] psoric [illegible] the [illegible] of chronic diseases [illegible] also are [illegible] of a psoric nature, although [illegible] of [illegible].

It is easy [illegible] but in itself this [illegible] of [illegible] nature.

To prove the psoric nature of these chronic diseases without [illegible] and [illegible] the fact that the anti-psoric remedies [illegible] [illegible] only [illegible] psoric [illegible] problem.

[illegible] other remedies, although [illegible] in the [illegible] of their symptoms, [illegible] pure [illegible] diseases [illegible] and which are [illegible] the [illegible] extent of [illegible] of the [illegible] remedies [illegible]

[illegible] and [illegible] the acute diseases [illegible] inflammation [illegible] of the [illegible] [illegible] combated by means of the antipsoric remedies, which are not anti-psoric.

Acute [illegible], [illegible] and the like [illegible] their source [illegible] cannot be [illegible] by anything but a [illegible] cure with anti-psoric remedies.

Cure of the Chronic Diseases.

CURE.

We now proceed to the medical Homœopathic treatment of the illimitably large number of chronic diseases, which, after the above gained knowledge of their threefold nature, has not, indeed, become easy, but—what without this knowledge was before impossible—has at last become *possible*, since the homœopathically specific remedies for each one of these three different miasmata have in great part been discovered.

The first two miasmata, which cause by far the smaller part of the chronic diseases, the *venereal chancre-disease* (*syphilis*) and the *figwart-disease* (sycosis), with their sequelæ, we will treat first, in order that we may have a free path to the therapeutics of the immeasurably greater number of the various chronic diseases which spring from *Psora*.

SYPHILIS.

The second chronic miasma, which is more widely spread than the figwart-disease, and which for three and a half [now four] centuries has been the source of many other chronic ailments, is the miasm of the venereal disease proper, the chancre-disease (syphilis). This disease only causes difficulties in its cure, if it is entangled (complicated) with a psora that has been already far developed—with sycosis it is complicated but rarely, but then usually at the same time with psora.

In the cure of the venereal disease, three states are to be distinguished:

1. When syphilis is still alone and attended with its associated local symptom, the *chancre*, or at least if this has been removed by external applications, it is still associated with the other local symptom, which in a similar manner acts vicariously for the internal disorder, the bubo.*

2. When it is alone, indeed, *i. e.*, without any complication with a second or third miasma, but has already been deprived of the vicarious local symptom, the chancre (and the bubo).

3. When it is already complicated with another chronic disease, *i. e.*, with a psora already developed, while the local symptom may either be yet present, or may have been removed by local applications.

The chancre appears, after an impure coition, usually between the seventh and fourteenth days, rarely sooner or later, mostly on the member infected with the miasma, first as a little pustule, which changes into an impure ulcer with raised borders and stinging pains, which if not cured remains standing on the same place during man's lifetime, only increasing with the years, while the secondary symptoms of the venereal disease, syphilis, cannot break out as long as it exists.

In order to help in such a case, the Allopathic physician destroys this chancre, by means of corroding, cauterizing and desiccating substances, wrongly conceiving it to be a sore arising merely from without through a local infection, thus holding it to be a merely

* Very rarely the impure coition is at once followed by the bubo alone without any preceding chancre; usually the bubo only comes after the destruction of the chancre by local applications, and is a very troublesome substitute for the same.

ways, in secondary ailments; for the figwart-miasm, which rules in the whole organism, has been in no way diminished, either by the external destruction of the above-mentioned excrescences, or by the mercury which has been used internally, and which is in no way appropriate to sycosis. Besides the undermining of the general health by mercury, which in this disease can only do injury, and which is given mostly in very large doses and in the most active preparations, similar excrescences then break out in other parts of the body, either whitish, spongy, sensitive, flat elevations, in the cavity of the mouth, on the tongue, the palate and the lips, or as large, raised, brown and dry tubercles in the axillæ, on the neck, on the scalp, etc., or there arise other ailments of the body, of which I shall only mention the contraction of the tendons of the flexor muscles, especially of the fingers.

The gonorrhœa dependent on the figwart-miasma, as well as the above-mentioned excrescences (*i. e.*, the whole sycosis), are cured most surely and most thoroughly through the internal use of Thuja,* which, in this case, is Homœopathic, in a dose of a few pillets as large as poppy seeds, moistened with the dilution potentized to the decillionth† degree, and when these have exhausted their action after fifteen, twenty, thirty, forty days, alternating with just as small a dose of nitric acid, diluted to the decillionth degree, which must be allowed to act as long a time, in order to remove the gonorrhœa and the excrescenses; *i. e.*, the whole sycosis. It is not necessary to use any external application, except in *the most inveterate and difficult* cases, when the larger figwarts may be moistened every day with the mild, pure juice pressed from the green leaves of Thuja, mixed with an equal quantity of alcohol.

But if the patient was at the same time affected with another chronic ailment, as is usual after the violent treatment of figwarts by Allopathic physicians, then we often find developed psora ‡ com-

---

patient, has been developed by means of a strongly affecting, irritating or weakening treatment by Allopathic physicians. In such a case frequently secondary gonorrhœas remain, which can only be cured by an anti-psoric treatment.

* Materia Medica Pura, Part V.

† If further doses of Thuja are required, they are used most efficiently from other potencies (viii., vi., iv., ii.), a change of the modification of the remedy, which facilitates and strengthens its ability of affecting the vital force.

‡ This psora is hardly ever found in its developed state (and thus capable of entering into complication with other miasmata) with young people who have just been infected and seized by the figwart-disease, and who have not had to pass through the usual mercurial treatment, which never runs its course without the most violent assaults on the constitution; by this pernicious derangement of the whole organism, the psora, even if slumbering ever so soundly, will be awakened, if, as is often the case, it was present within.

plicated with sycosis, when the psora, as is often the case, was latent before in the patient. At times, when a badly treated case of venereal chancre disease had preceded, both these miasmata are conjoined in a threefold complication with syphilis. Then it is necessary first to come to the assistance of the most afflicted part, the *psora*, with the specific anti-psoric remedies given below, and then to make use of the remedies for sycosis, before the proper dose of the best preparation of mercury, as will be described below, is given against the syphilis; the same alternating treatment may be continued, until a complete cure is effected. Only, each one of these three kinds of medicine must be given the proper time to complete its action.

In this reliable cure of sycosis from within, no external remedy (except the juice of Thuja in inveterate bad cases) must be applied or laid on the figwarts, only clean, dry lint, if they are of the moist variety.

SYCOSIS.

First, then, concerning sycosis, as being that miasma which has produced by far the fewest chronic diseases, and has only been dominant from time to time. This *figwart-disease*, which in later times, especially during the French war, in the years 1809–1814, was so widely spread, but which has since showed itself more and more rarely, was treated almost always, in an inefficient and injurious manner, internally with mercury, because it was considered homogeneous with the venereal chancre-disease; but the excrescences on the genitals were treated by Allopathic physicians always in the most violent external way by cauterizing, burning and cutting, or by ligatures. These excrescences usually first manifest themselves on the genitals, and appear usually, but not always, attended with a sort of gonorrhœa* from the urethra, several days or several weeks, even many weeks after infection through coition; more rarely they appear dry and like warts, more frequently soft, spongy, emitting a specifically fetid fluid (sweetish and almost like herring-brine), bleeding easily, and in the form of a coxcomb or a cauliflower (*brassica botrytes*). These, with males, sprout forth on the glans and on, or below, the prepuce, but with women, on the parts surrounding the pudenda; and the pudenda themselves, which are then swollen, are covered often by a great number of them. When these are violently removed, the natural, proximate effect is, that they will usually come forth again, usually to be subjected again, in vain, to a similar, painful, cruel treatment. But even if they could be rooted out in this way, it would merely have the consequence, that the figwart-disease, after having been deprived of the local symptom which acts vicariously for the internal ailment, would appear† in other and much worse

* Usually in gonorrhœa of this kind, the discharge is from the beginning thickish, like pus; micturition is less difficult, but the body of the penis swollen somewhat hard; the penis is also in some cases covered on the back with glandular tubercles, and very painful to the touch.

† The miasm of the other common gonorrhœas seems not to penetrate the whole organism, but only to locally stimulate the urinary organs. They yield either to a dose of one drop of fresh parsley-juice, when this is indicated by a frequent urgency to urinate, or a small dose of cannabis, of cantharides, or of the copaiva balm, according to their different constitution and the other ailments attending it. These should, however, be always used in the higher and highest dynamizations (potencies), unless a psora, slumbering in the body of the

local ulcer, such also it is declared to be in their writings. They falsely suppose, that when it appears, no internal venereal disease is as yet to be thought of, so that when locally exterminating the chancre, they suppose that they remove all the venereal disease from the patient at once, if only he will not permit this ulcer to remain too long in its place, so that the absorbent vessels do not get time to transfer the poison into the internal organism, and so cause by delay a general infection of the system with syphilis. They evidently do not know, that the venereal infection of the whole body commenced with the very moment of the impure coition, and was already completed before the appearance of the chancre. The Allopathic doctor destroys in his blindness, through local applications, the vicarious external symptom (the chancre ulcer), which kind nature intended for the alleviation of the internal extensive venereal general disease; and so he inexorably compels the organism to replace the destroyed first substitute of the internal venereal malady (the chancre) by a far more painful substitute, the bubo, which hastens onward to suppuration; and when the Allopath, as is usually the case, also drives out this bubo through his injurious treatment, then nature finds itself compelled to develop the internal malady through far more troublesome secondary ailments, through the outbreak of the whole chronic syphilis, and nature accomplishes this, though slowly, (frequently not before several months have elapsed), but with *unfailing certainty*. Instead of assisting, therefore, the Allopath does injury.

John Hunter says:* "Not one patient out of fifteen will escape syphilis, if the chancre is destroyed by mere external applications," and in another passage in his book† he says: "The result of destroying the chancre ever so early, and even on the first day of its appearance, if this is effected by local applications was always the consequent outbreak of syphilis."

Just as emphatically Fabre declares:‡ "Syphilis always follows on the destruction of the chancre by local applications. He relates that *Petit* cut off a part of the labia of a woman, who had thereon for a few days a venereal chancre; the wound healed, but syphilis, nevertheless, broke out."

How, then, could physicians, despite of all these facts and testimonies, close their eyes and ears to the truth: that the whole vener-

* *Abhandl. über die vener. Krankheit* (Treatise on the Venereal Disease), Leipsic, 1787, p. 531.

† *Abhandl. über die vener. Krankheit*, Leipsic, 1787, pp. 551–553.

‡ *Fabre*, *Lettres*, *Supplément à son traité des maladies* vénériennes. *Paris*, 1786

eal disease (syphilis) was already developed within, before the chancre could appear, and that it was a most unpardonable mistake to forward the certain outbreak of the syphilis, already present within, into the venereal disease, by driving away and destroying the chancre by external means, and thereby destroying the fair opportunity afforded of curing this disease in the easiest and most convincing manner, through the internal specific remedy, while the chancre was yet fully present! The disease is not cured except when through the effect of the internal remedy alone, the chancre is cured; but it is fully extinguished, as soon as through the action of the internally operating medicine alone (without the addition of any external remedy) the chancre is completely cured, without leaving any trace of its former presence.

I have never, in my practice of more than fifty years, seen any trace of the venereal disease break out, so long as the chancre remained untouched in its place, even if this were a space of several years (for it never passes away of itself), and even when it had largely increased in its place, as is natural in time with the internal augmentation of the venereal disorder, which increase takes place in time in every chronic miasma.

But whenever anyone is so imprudent, as to destroy this vicarious local symptom, the organism is ready to cause the internal syphilis to break out into the venereal disease, since the general venereal disease dwells in the body from the first moment of infection.

For in the spot, into which at the impure coition the syphilitic miasma had been first rubbed in and had been caught, it is, in the same moment, no more local: the whole living body has already received (perceived) its presence, the miasma has already become the property of the whole organism. All wiping off and washing off, however speedy, and with whatever fluid this be done (and as we have seen, even the exsection of the part affected), is too late—is in vain. There is not to be perceived, indeed, any morbid transmutation in that spot during the first days, but the specific venereal transformation takes place in the internal of the body irresistibly, from the first moment of infection until syphilis has developed itself throughout the whole body, and only then (not before), nature, loaded down by the internal malady, brings forth the local symptom peculiar to this malady, the chancre, usually in the place first infected; and this symptom is intended by nature to soothe the internal completed malady.

Therefore also, the cure of the venereal disease is effected most easily and in the most convincing manner, so long as the chancre (the bubo) has not yet been driven out by local applications, so long as the chancre (the bubo) still remains unchanged, as a vicarious symptom of the internal syphilis. In this state, and especially when it is not yet complicated with psora, it may be asserted from manifold experience and with good reason, *that there is on earth no chronic miasma, no chronic disease springing from a miasma, which is more curable and more easily curable than this.*

In this *first* simple state and simple cure, when the chancre (or the bubo) is still present, and there is no complication with a developed psora, no prominent chronic ailment from a psoric origin (usually there is none such with young, lively persons), and with latent psora syphilis combines as little as sycosis—in this *first* state it needs only one little dose of the best mercurial remedy, in order to cure thoroughly and forever the whole syphilis with its chancre, within fourteen days. In a few days after taking such a dose of mercury, the chancre (without any external application) becomes a clean sore with a little mild pus, and heals of itself—as a convincing proof, that the venereal malady is also fully extinguished within; and it does not leave behind the least scar, or the least spot, showing any other color than the other healthy skin. But the chancre, which is not treated with external application, would never heal, if the internal syphilis had not been already annihilated and extinguished by the dose of mercury; for so long as it exists in its place, it is the natural and unmistakable proof of even the least remainder of an existing syphilis.

I have, indeed, in the second edition of the first part of *Materia Medica Pura* (Dresden, 1822), described the preparation of the pure semi-oxide of mercury, and I still consider this to be one of the most excellent anti-syphilitic medicines; but it is difficult to prepare it in sufficient purity. In order, therefore, to reach this wished for goal in a still simpler manner, free from all detours, and yet just as perfectly (for in the preparation of medicines we cannot proceed in too simple a manner), it is best to proceed in the way given below, so that one grain of quite pure running quick-silver is triturated three times, with 100 grains of sugar of milk each time, up to the millionth attenuation, in three hours, and one grain of this third trituration is dissolved, and then potentized through twenty-seven diluting phials up to (x) the decillionth degree, as is taught at the end of this volume, with respect to the dynamization of the other dry medicines.

I formerly used the billionth dynamization (ii) of this preparation in 1, 2 or 3 fine pellets moistened with this dilution, as a dose, and this was done successfully for such cures; although the preparation of the higher potencies (iv, vi, viii), and finally the decillionth potency (x), show some advantages, in their quick, penetrating and yet mild action for this purpose; but in cases where a second or third dose (however seldom needed) should be found necessary, a lower potency may then be taken.

Just as the continued presence of the chancre (or the bubo) during the cure shows the continued presence of syphilis, so when the chancre (and the bubo) heal merely from the internally applied mercury, without any addition of a remedy used for the local symptom, and yet this disappears without leaving any trace of its former presence; it is incontrovertibly sure, that also every trace of the internal syphilis was extinguised at the moment of the completion of the cure of the chancre or the bubo.

But just as incontrovertibly does it follow that every disappearance of the chancre (or the bubo) owing to a mere local destruction, since it was no real cure founded on the extirpation of the internal venereal disease through the internally given appropriate mercury medicine, leaves to us the certainty that the syphilis remains behind; and every one who supposes himself healed by any such merely local, pretended cure, is to be considered as much venereally diseased as he was before the destruction of the chancre.

The *second* state in which, as mentioned above, syphilis may have to be treated, is the rare case when an otherwise healthy person, affected with no other chronic disease (and thus without any developed psora), has experienced this injudicious driving away of the chancre through local applications, effected by an ordinary physician in a short time and without attacking the organism overmuch with internal and external remedies. Even in such a case,—as we have not as yet to combat any complication with psora—all outbreaks of the secondary venereal disease may be avoided, and the man may be freed from every trace of the venereal miasma through the before-mentioned simple internal cure effected by a like dose of the above mentioned mercurial medicine—although the certainty of his cure can no more be so manifestly proved as if the chancre had still been in existence during this internal cure, and as if it had become a mild ulcer simply through this internal remedy, and had been thus manifestly cured of itself.

But here also there may be found a sign of the non-completed as well as of the completed cure of the internal syphilis which has not yet broken out into the venereal disease; but this sign will only manifest itself to an exact observer. In case the chancre has been driven out through local application, even if the remedies used had not been very acrid, there will always remain in the place where it stood, as a sign of the unextinguished internal syphilis, a discolored, reddish, red or blue scar; while on the contrary when the cure of the whole venereal disease has been effected by the internal remedy, and if thus the chancre heals of itself without the action of an external application, and when it disappears because it is no more needed as a substitute and alleviator of an internal venereal disorder which now has ceased, then the spot of the former chancre can no more be recognized, for the skin covering that place will be just as smooth and of the same color as the rest, so that no trace can be discerned of the spot where the chancre had stood.

Now if the Homœopathic physician has carefully taken cognizance of the presence of the discolored scar remaining after the quick, merely local expulsion of the venereal local symptom, as a sign of the unextinguished internal syphilis, and if the person to be healed is otherwise in good health, and consequently his venereal disorder is not yet complicated with psora, he will also, even now, be able to free him from every remainder of the venereal miasma by one dose of the best preparation of mercury as above described, and he will be convinced that the cure is completed, from the fact that during the time of the activity of the specific remedy the scar will again assume the healthy color of the other skin and all discoloration of that spot will disappear.

Even when, after the expulsion of the chancre by local applications, the bubo has already broken out but the patient is not yet seized with any other chronic disease, and consequently the internal syphilis is not yet complicated with a developed psora (which is nevertheless a rare case), the same treatment will also here, while the bubo is only developing, produce a cure ; and its completion will be recognized by the same signs.

In both cases, if they have been rightly treated, the cure is a complete one, and no outbreak of the venereal disease need any more be apprehended.

The most difficult of all these cases, the *third*, is still to be treated: when the man at the time of the syphilitic infection was already laboring under a chronic disease, so that his syphilis was complicated with psora, even while the chancre yet existed, or when, even while there was no chronic disease in the body at the outbreak of the chancre, and the indwelling psora could only be recognized by its tokens, an allopathic physician has, nevertheless, destroyed the local symptom, not only slowly and with very painful external applications, but has also subjected him for a long time to an internal treatment, weakening and strongly affecting him, so that the general health has been undermined and the psora which had as yet been latent within him has been brought to its development and has broken out into chronic ailments, and these irrepressibly combine with the internal syphilis, the local symptom of which had been at the same time destroyed in such an irrational manner. Psora can only be complicated with the venereal disease when it has been developed and when it has ultimated itself in a manifest chronic disease; but not when it is as yet latent and slumbering. By the latter the cure of syphilis is not obstructed, but *when complicated with developed psora, it is impossible to cure the venereal disease alone.*

Only too often, I should say, do we find the syphilis which has remained uncured after the merely local destruction of the chancre, complicated with awakened psora, not always because the psora was already developed before the venereal infection—for this is rarely the case with young people—but because it is violently awakened and brought to its outbreak by the usual treatment of the venereal disease. By means of friction with mercury, large doses of calomel, corrosive sublimate and similar acrid mercurial remedies, (which originate fever, dysenteric abdominal ailments, chronic exhausting salivation, pains in the limbs, sleeplessness, etc., without possessing sufficient anti-syphilitic power to cure the chancre-miasma mildly, quickly and perfectly,) they assault the venereal patient often for many months, with the intermediate use of many weakening warm baths and purgatives; so that the internal slumbering psora (whose nature causes it to break forth in all great convulsions and in the weakening of the general health) is awakened before the syphilis can be cured by such an injudicious treatment, and thus becomes associated and complicated therewith.

There arises in this manner and through this combination what is called a *masked*, *spurious syphilis*, and in England *pseudo syphilis*, a monster of a double disease,* which no physician hitherto has been able to cure, because no physican hitherto has been acquainted with the psora in its great extent and its nature, neither in its latent nor its developed state; and no one suspected this dreadful combination with syphilis, much less perceived it. No one, therefore, could heal the developed psora, the only cause of the uncurableness of this bastard syphilis,—nor could they in consequence free the syphilis from this horrible combination so as to make it curable, just as the psora remains incurable if the syphilis has not been extirpated.

In order to reach this so-called masked venereal disease successfully, the following rule must serve the homœopathic physician:

* Yea, after such a treatment it is even more than a double disease; the sharp mercurial medicines, in large and frequent doses, have also added their medicinal disease, which when we consider in addition the debility caused by such treatment, must place the patient in a most sad state. In such a case hepar sulphuris is probably to be preferred to the pure sulphur.

After removing all hurtful influences that affect the patients from without and after settling on a light and yet nourishing and strengthening diet for the patient, let him first give the anti-psoric medicine which is homœopathically the best fitting to the then prevailing state of disease, as will be shown below; and when this medicine has completed its action, also probably a second, most suitable to the still prominent psora symptoms, and these should be allowed to act against the psora, until they have effected all that can be at present done against it—then should be given the dose above described of the best mercurial preparation to act against the venereal disease for three, five to seven weeks; *i. e.*, so long as it will continue to produce an improvement in the venereal symptoms.

In inveterate and difficult cases, however, this first course will hardly accomplish all that is desired. There usually still remain some ailments and disorders, which cannot be definitely classed as purely psoric, and others which cannot be classed as definitely syphilitic, and these require yet some additional aid. A repetition of a similar process of cure is here required; *i. e.*, first another application of one or more of the antipsoric remedies that have not yet been used, and which are homœopathically the most appropriate, until whatever seems still unsyphilitically morbid—*i. e.*, psoric—may disappear, when the before mentioned dose of the mercurial remedy, but in another potency, should be given again and allowed to complete its action, until the manifest venereal symptoms (the pricking, painful ulcer of the tonsils, the round copper-colored spots that shimmer through the epidermis, the eruptive pimples which do not itch and are found chiefly in the face upon a bluish-red foundation, the painless cutaneous ulcers on the scalp and the penis, which are smooth, pale, clean, merely covered with mucus, and almost level with the healthy skin, etc., and the boring, nightly pains in the exostoses) have entirely passed away. But since these secondary venereal symptoms are so changeable that their temporary disappearance gives no certainty of their complete extinction, we must also wait for that more conclusive sign of the complete extirpation of the venereal miasm afforded by the return of the healthy color and the entire disappearance of the discoloration found in the scar which remains after the extirpation of the chancre by local, corrosive applications.

I have, in my practice, found only two cases* of the threefold

*A master tiler from the Saxon-Erz Mountains, whose dissolute wife had infected him with a venereal disease in his genitals, concerning which it was not apparent from his description whether it was a chancre or a figwart, had been so maltreated by violent mercurial remedies that he had lost his uvula, and his nose was so affected that the fleshy parts had mostly been eaten away,

complication of the three chronic miasms, the figwart disease with the venereal chancre miasm and at the same time a developed psora, and these cases were cured according to the same method; *i. e.*, the psora was treated first, then the one of the other two chronic miasmata, the symptoms of which were at the time the most prominent, and then the last one. The remaining psoric symptoms had then still to be combatted with suitable remedies, and then lastly what there yet remained of sycosis or syphilis, by means of the remedies given above. I would also remark that the complete cure of sycosis which has taken possession of the whole organism before the outbreak of its local symptom, is demonstrated, like that of the chancre miasma, by the complete disappearance of the discoloration on the spot of the skin, which discoloration remains after every merely local destruction of the figwart as a sign of the unextirpated sycosis.

---

and the remaining part was swollen and inflamed and pierced like a honeycomb with ulcers. This was attended with great pain and an intolerably fetid smell. In addition he had a psoric ulcer on the leg. The anti-psoric remedies improved the ulcers up to a certain degree: they healed the ulcer on the leg, they took away the burning pain and most of the fetid smell of the nose; also the remedies given to cure the sycosis caused some improvement—but as to the sum total nothing further was effected until he received a small dose of protoxide of mercury, after which everything was fully healed and he was restored to full health, excepting the irreparable loss of his nose.

complications of the same chronic miasms, the [illegible] disease will [illegible] [illegible] at the same time a [illegible] and these cases [illegible] according to the same method [illegible] the [illegible] first, then the one of the other two [illegible] [illegible] the symptoms of which at that time [illegible] the most prominent [illegible] [illegible] remaining [illegible] symptoms, but [illegible] still to be [illegible] with suitable remedies [illegible] [illegible] [illegible] by means of the [illegible] [illegible] [illegible] [illegible] then [illegible] the whole [illegible] [illegible] [illegible] [illegible] [illegible] the [illegible] of the [illegible] spot of the skin [illegible] [illegible] [illegible] [illegible] [illegible] of the [illegible]

and the [illegible] [illegible] [illegible] [illegible] [illegible] [illegible] [illegible] [illegible] [illegible] the [illegible] [illegible] the [illegible] [illegible] they took [illegible] the [illegible] [illegible] [illegible] also the [illegible] [illegible] [illegible] [illegible] [illegible] [illegible] of [illegible] every [illegible] healed and he was [illegible] health [illegible] the [illegible]

PSORA.

I think it necessary before proceeding to the doctrine of the *third* chronic miasma, the most important of all, psora, to premise the following general remark:

For the infection with the only three known chronic miasmatic diseases there is usually needed but one moment; but the development of this tinder of infection, so that it becomes a general disease of the entire organism, needs a longer time. Not until a certain number of days have elapsed, when the miasmatic disease has received its complete internal development in the whole man—not until then, from the fulness of internal suffering, the local symptom breaks forth, destined by a kind nature to take upon itself in a certain sense the internal disease, and in so far to divert it in a palliative manner and to soothe it, so that it may not be able to injure and endanger the vital economy too much. The local symptom has its place on the least dangerous part of the body, the external skin, and, indeed, on that part of the skin where, during the infection, the miasma had touched the nearest nerves.

This process of nature, which repeats itself continually and evermore in the same manner in chronic miasmata, aye,—even in those which are acute and constant,—ought not to have escaped the penetration of physicians, at least not in venereal diseases, to the treatment of which they have applied themselves now for more than three hundred years; and then they could not have avoided drawing a conclusion as to the process of nature in the other two chronic miasmata. It was, therefore, irrational and unpardonably thoughtless of them to suppose that every chancre evolved by the organism after several days, often after quite a number of days, as the result of the completed internal malady, was a thing merely adventitious from without and situated on the skin without any internal connection, so that it might be simply removed by cauterizing, "so as to prevent the poison from the chancre (*scilicet*) from being absorbed into the internal parts, and thus from causing man to be afflicted with the venereal disease." Irrational and unpardonably thoughtless was this false idea of the origin of the venereal chancre, which caused the injurious practice of the external cauterization of the chancre, producing as its unavoidable, shameful effect, the breaking out of the venereal disease from the internal which has continued in its diseased state. This has been the case in several hundred thousands of cases these last three centuries. Just as irrational and thoughtless is the notion of physicians of the old school, even of the most modern times, that itch is *merely a disease of the skin*, in which the internal portion of the body takes no part. According to this groundless supposition, therefore, nothing better can be done than to remove this ailment from the surface of the skin, although the extirpation of the internal psora disease which causes the cutaneous eruption is necessary as an aid, and when this is cured also the cutaneous ailment, being the necessary consequence of the internal disease, will naturally disappear—*cessante causa, cessat effectus.*

For in its complete state, *i. e.*, so long as the original eruption is still present on the skin so as to assuage the internal malady, the entire disease of the psora may be cured most easily, quickly and surely.

But when by the destruction of this original cutaneous eruption, which acts vicariously for the internal malady, it has been robbed then the psora is put in the unnatural position of dominating in a merely one-sided manner the internal finer parts of the whole organism, and thus of being compelled to develop its secondary symptoms.

How important and necessary the cutaneous eruption is for the original psora, and how carefully in the only thorough cure of itch, that is, the internal cure, every external removal of the eruption must be avoided, we may see from the fact that the most severe chronic ailments have followed as secondary symptoms of the internal psora after the original itch-eruption has been driven out, and that when, in consequence of a great revolution in the organism, this itching eruption re appears on the skin, the secondary symptoms are so suddenly removed, that these grievous ailments, often of many years' standing, are wont to disappear, at least temporarily, as if by a miracle. See the before quoted observations of older physicians, Nos. 1, 3, 5, 6, 8, (9), 16, (17), (21), 23, 33, 35, 39, 41, 54, 58, 60 72, 81, 87, 89, 94.

But let no one suppose that an internal psora, which, after the external destruction of the original cutaneous eruption, has broken out into secondary chronic ailments, can, through the re-appearance of such an itch-like eruption on the skin, come into just as normal a state as before, or that it can be cured just as easily as if it were still the original eruption and as if this had not been as yet removed.

This is not at all the case. Even the eruption following immediately after the infection has no such unchanging constancy and pertinacity on the skin as the chancre and the figwarts show on the spots where they first appear,* but not infrequently disappears from the skin also from other causes † than from artificial remedies used purposely for its destruction, and so also from other causes unknown.‡

So that the physician must not waste any time even in the original eruption, if he would complete the cure while the itch-disease is still entire, by the use of internal anti-psoric remedies. Such a respite can be expected still less in this secondary eruption, which has been brought out on the skin by any cause after the local extirpation of the eruption; for the second eruption is wont to be far more inconstant and changeable, so that it often passes away on much slighter provocation in a few days—a proof that it lacks much of the complete quality of the primitive itch-eruption, so that the physician cannot count on it in the thorough cure of the psora.

This proneness to change, in the itch-like eruption which has been called a second time to the skin, seems evidently to be caused by the fact that the internal psora, after the destruction of the original itch-eruption is unable to give to the secondary eruption the full qualities belonging to the primary eruption, and is already much more inclined to unfold itself in a variety of other chronic diseases; wherefore a thorough cure is now much more difficult, and is simply to be conducted as if directed against the internal psora.

The cure is not, therefore, advanced by producing such a secondary eruption through internal remedies, as has sometimes been effectually attempted (see Nos. 3, 9, 59, 89); or by its re-appearance through other unknown causes (see Nos. 1, 5, 6, 8, 16, 23, 28, 29, 33, 35, 39, 41, 54, 58, 60, 72, 80, 81, 87, 89, 94) or, especially, through the help of a fever (see No. 64, also 55, 56, 74). Such a secondary eruption is always very transitory, and so unreliable and rare that we cannot build our hope of cure on it, nor expect from it the advancement of any thorough cure.

But even if, by any means, such a secondary eruption might, after a fashion, be produced, and even were it in our power to retain

* Neither of these ever passes away of itself, unless destroyed externally on purpose, or the entire disease is healed internally.

† *E. g.* through cold, see No. 67 of the above-mentioned observations; through small-pox, No. 39; through warm baths, No. 35.

‡ See Nos. 9, 17, 26 (36), 50, 58, 61, 64, 65, in which observations it may be seen at the same time that after such disappearances of the original itch-eruption without appreciable cause just as many ill effects are wont to follow as when it has been driven away artificially through local applications.

it on the skin for a longer period, we cannot at all count on it for an assistance in the cure of the whole psoric malady.*

It remains, therefore, an established truth, that the cure of the entire destructive Psora through antipsoric remedies is effected most easily only while the original eruption of itch is still present. From this it again appears how unconscionable it is of the allopathic physicians, to destroy the primitive itch eruption through local applications instead of completely eradicating this grave disease from the whole living organism by a cure from within, which at that stage is

* There was a time when, not yet fully convinced of this fact, I thought that the cure of the entire psora might be rendered easier by an artificial renewal of the cutaneous eruption effected through a sort of checking of the perspiratory function of the skin, so as to excite it homœopathically to the reproduction of the eruption. For this purpose I found most serviceable the wearing of a plaster mostly on the back (but where practicable also on other portions of the skin); the plaster was prepared by *gently* heating six ounces of Burgundy pitch, into which, after removing it from the fire, an ounce of turpentine produced from the larch-tree (called Venetian turpentine) was stirred until it was perfectly mixed. A portion of this was spread on a chamois skin (as being the softest), and laid on while still warm. Instead of this, there might also be used so-called tree-wax (made of yellow wax and common turpentine), or also taffeta covered with elastic resin; showing that the itching eruption evolved is not due to any irritation caused by the substance applied; nor does the plaster first mentioned cause either eruption or itching on the skin of a person who is not psoric. I discovered that this method is the most effective to cause such an activity of the skin. Yet despite of all the patience of the sick persons (no matter how much they might internally be affected with the psora), I never could evolve a complete eruption of itch, least of all one that would remain for a time on the skin. What could be effected was only that some itching pustules appeared, which soon vanished again, when the plaster was left off. More frequently there ensued a moist soreness of the skin, or at best a more or less violent itching of the skin, which in rare cases extended also to the other parts not covered by the plaster. This, indeed, would cause for a time a striking alleviation of even the most severe chronic diseases flowing from a psoric source; *e. g.*, suppuration of the lungs. But this much could not be attained on the skin of many patients (frequently all that could be attained was a moderate or small amount of itching), or again, if I could produce a violent itching, this frequently became too unbearable for the patient to sustain it for a time sufficient to produce an internal cure. When the plaster then was removed in order to relieve him, even the most violent itching, together with the eruption present, disappeared very soon, and the cure had not been essentially advanced by it; this confirms the observation made above, that the eruption if evolved a second time (and so also the itching reproduced) had not by any means the full characteristics of the eruption of the itch which had originally been repressed, and was therefore of little assistance in the real advancement of a thorough cure of the psora through internal remedies, while the little aid afforded loses all value owing to the often unbearable infliction of the artificially produced eruption and itching of the skin, and the weakening of the whole body which is inseparable from the titillating pain.

as yet very easy, and by thus choking off in advance all the wretched consequences that we must expect from this malady if uncured; *i. e.*, all the secondary, chronic, nameless sufferings which follow it.

The excuse of the private physician (for the physician at the hospital has no excuse at all) amounts to nothing. He will say, indeed: "If it is not known—and hardly ever does it become demonstrably known—where, when, at what occasion and from what person avowedly suffering from itch the infection has been derived, then he could not discover from the present, and often insignificant little eruption whether it was real itch; so he was not to be blamed for the evil consequences, if he supposed it to be something else and endeavored to remove it from the skin as soon as possible by a lotion of lead solution, or an ointment of cadmia, or white percipitate of mercury, according to the wishes of the aristocratic parents."

This excuse, as above said, amounts to nothing. For, *first* of all, ***no cutaneous eruption of whatever kind it may be***, ought to be expelled through external means by any physician who wishes to act conscientiously and rationally.* The human skin does not evolve of itself, without the co-operation of the rest of the living whole, any eruption, nor does it become sick in any way, without being induced and compelled to it by the general diseased state, by the lack of normality in the whole organism. In every case there is at the bottom a disorderly state of the whole internal living organism, which state must first be considered; and therefore the eruption is only to be removed by internal healing and curative remedies which change the state of the whole; then also the eruption which is based on the internal disease will be cured and healed of itself, without the help of any external remedy, and frequently more quickly than it could be done by external remedies.

Secondly, even if the physician should not have presented to him the original, undestroyed form of the eruption,—*i. e.*, the pustule of itch which in the beginning is transparent, then quickly filled with pus, with a narrow red margin all around it,—even if the eruption should consist only of small granules like the miliary eruption, or appear like scattered little pimples or little scabs, still he cannot for a moment be in doubt as to whether the eruption is itch, if the child or even the suckling only a few days old, uninterruptedly rubs and scratches the spot, or, if it is an adult, when he complains of the titillation of a voluptuously itching eruption (or even only a few pimples) which is unbearable without scratching, especially in the evening and at night, and when this is followed by a burning pain. In such a case we can never doubt as to the infection with itch,

*See "Organon of the Healing Art," fifth edition, § 187–203.

though in genteel and wealthy families we can seldom secure the information and the certainty as to how, where and from whom the infection has been derived; for there are innumerable imperceptible occasions whereby this infection may be received, as taught above.

Now when the family physician notices this in time, then without any external application, the simple dose of one or two pills as large as poppy-seeds, moistened with the potentized sulphur in alcohol, as described below, will fully and abundantly suffice to cure a child and to deliver it from the entire disease of itch, both the eruption and the internal itch malady (psora).

The homœopathic physician in his private practice seldom gets to see and to treat an eruption of itch spread over a considerable part of the skin and coming from a fresh infection. The patients on account of the intolerable itching either apply to some old woman, or to the druggist or the barber, who, one and all, come to their aid with a remedy which, as they suppose, is immediately effective (*e.g.*, lard mixed with flowers of sulphur). Only in the practice of the barracks, of prisons, hospitals, penitentiaries and orphan asylums those infected have to apply to the resident physician, if the surgeon of the house does not anticipate him.

Even in the most ancient times when itch occurred, for it did not everywhere degenerate into leprosy, it was acknowledged that there was a sort of specific virtue against itch in *sulphur;* but they knew of no other way of applying it, but to destroy the itch through an external application of it, even as is done now by the greater part of the modern physicians of the old school. A. C. Celsus has several ointments and salves (V. 28) some of which consist merely of sulphur mixed with tar, while others contain also compounds of copper and other substances; these he prescribes for the expulsion of itch, and this he supposes to be its cure. So also the most ancient physicians, like the moderns, prescribed for their itch patients baths of warm sulphurous mineral water. Such patients are usually also delivered from their eruption by these external sulphur remedies. But that their patients were not really cured thereby, became manifest, even to them, from the more severe ailments that followed, such as general dropsy, with which an Athenian was afflicted when he drove out his severe eruption of itch by bathing in the warm sulphur baths of the island of Melos (now called Milo), and of which he died. This is recorded by the author of Book V. Epidemion, which has been received among the writings of Hippocrates (some three hundred years before Celsus).

Internally the ancient physicians gave no sulphur in itch, because they, like the moderns, did not see that this miasmatic disease was, at the same time *and especially*, an internal disease.

Modern physicians have never given sulphur *only*, and internally, to cure the itch, because they have never recognized the itch-disease as being also an internal *and*, indeed, *chiefly* internal disease. They only gave it in connection with the external means of driving away the itch, and, indeed, in doses which would act as purgatives,—ten, twenty and thirty grains at a dose, frequently repeated,—so that it never became manifest how useful or how injurious this internal application of such large doses, in connection with the external application, had been; *at least* the whole itch-disease (psora) *could never* be thoroughly healed thereby. The external driving out of the eruption was simply advanced by it as by any other purgative, and with the same injurious effects as if no sulphur at all had been used internally. For even if sulphur is used only internally, but in the above described large doses, without any external destructive means, it can never thoroughly heal a psora; partly because in order to cure as an antipsoric and homœopathic medicine, it must be given only in the smallest doses of a potentized preparation, while in larger and more frequent doses the crude sulphur* in some cases increases the malady or at least adds a new malady; partly because the vital force expels it as a violently aggressive remedy through purging stools or by means of vomiting, without having put its healing power to any use.

Now if, as experience teaches, not even the fresh itch-disease which

* Here it is proper to subjoin the words of an impartial and even practical connoisseur of Homœopathy, the deep-thinking, many-sided scholar and indefatigable investigator of truth, Count Buquoy, in his *Anregungen für ph. w. Forschungen* (Leipzig, 1825, p. 386 sgg.). After assuming that a drug, which in a normal state of health causes the symptoms *a*, *b*, *g*,—in analogy with other physiological phenomena, produces the symptoms *x*, *y*, *z*, which appear in an abnormal state of health—can act upon this abnormal state in such a way that the disease-symptoms *x*, *y*, *z*, are transformed into the drug symptoms *a*, *b*, *g*, which latter have the peculiar characteristic of temporariness or transitoriness; he then continues: "This transitory character belongs to the group of symptoms of the medicine *a*, *b*, *g*, which is substituted for the group of symptoms belonging to the disease, merely because the medicine is used in an *extraordinarily small* dose. Should the homœopathic physician give the patient *too large* a dose of the homœopathic remedy indicated, the disease *x*, *y*, *z* may indeed be transformed into the other, *i. e.*, into *a*, *b*, *g* but the new disease *now sits just as firmly fixed* as the former *x*, *y*, *z;* so that the organism *can just as little free itself from the disease a*, *b*, *g*, as it was able to throw off the original disease *x*, *y*, *z*. If a *very large* dose is given, then *a new*, often *very dangerous disease* is produced, or the organism does its utmost to free itself very quickly from the poison (through diarrhœa, vomiting, etc.)."

is the most easy to cure of all, *i. e.*, the internal, recently formed psora together with the external, recent eruption, can be thoroughly healed by external applications accompanied with large quantities of flowers of sulphur, it may easily be seen, that the psora, after it has been deprived of its eruption and has become merely internal and inveterate, having developed secondary ailments and thus having changed into chronic diseases of various kinds, for the same reason can be just as little cured by a quantity of sulphur flowers, or by a number of baths in sulphurous mineral waters, or on the other hand by simultaneously drinking the same or a similar water; in a word, it cannot be cured by a superabundance and frequent repetition of this remedy, although it is of itself antipsoric.* It is true that many such chronic patients by the first treatment at the baths seem to get rid for some time of the symptoms of their disease (therefore we see an incredible throng of many thousands, suffering from innumerable different chronic ailments at Teplitz, Baden, Aix-la-Chapelle, Neundorf, Warmbrunn, etc.); yet they are not on that account restored to health, but instead of the original chronic (psoric) disease, they have for a time come under the dominion of a sulphur-disease (another, perhaps more bearable, malady). This in time passes away, when the psora again lifts its head, either with the same morbid symptoms as before, or with others similar but gradually more troublesome than the first, or with symptoms developing in nobler parts of the organism. Ignorant persons will rejoice in the latter case, that their former disease at least has passed away, and they hope that the new disease also may be removed by another journey to the same baths. They do not know, that their changed morbid state is merely a transformation of the same psora; but they always find out by experience, that their second tour to the baths causes even less alleviation, or, indeed, if the sulphur-baths are used in still greater number, that the second trial causes aggravation.

Thus we see that either the excessive use of sulphur in all its forms, or the frequent repetition of its use by allopathic physicians in the treatment of a multitude of chronic diseases (the secondary psoric ailments) have taken away from it all value and use; and we

* Used in small doses, sulphur as one of the antipsoric remedies will not fail to make a brief beginning of a cure of the chronic (non-venereal and therefore psoric) diseases. I know a physician in Saxony who gained a great reputation by merely adding to his prescriptions in nearly all chronic diseases flowers of sulphur, and this without knowing a reason for it. This *in the beginning* of such treatments is wont to produce a strikingly beneficent effect, but of course *only* in the beginning, and therefore after that his help was at an end.

may well assert that, to this day, hardly anything but injury has been done by allopathic physicians through the use of sulphur.

But even supposing that anyone should desire to make the only correct use of sulphur in this kind of disease, it will seldom be possible to do this with the same desired success as where the homœopathic physician finds a recent case of the itch-disease with its still existing eruption. Even when, owing to its undeniable anti-psoric effects, sulphur may be able of itself to make the beginning of a cure, after the external expulsion of the eruption, either with the still hidden and latent psora or when this has more or less developed and broken out into its varied chronic diseases, it can nevertheless be but rarely made use of for this purpose, because its powers have usually been already exhausted, because it has been given to the patient already before by allopathic physicians for one purpose or another, perhaps has been given already repeatedly; but sulphur, like most of the antipsoric remedies in the treatment of a developed psora that has become chronic, can hardly be used three or four times (even after the intervening use of other antipsoric remedies) without causing the cure to retrograde.

The cure of an old psora that has been deprived of its eruption, whether it may be latent and quiescent, or already broken out into chronic diseases, can never be accomplished with sulphur alone, nor with sulphur-baths either natural or artificial.

Here I may mention the curious circumstance that in general—with the exception of the recent itch-disease still attended with its unrepressed cutaneous eruption, and which is so easily cured from within*—every other psoric diathesis, *i. e.*, the psora that is still latent within, as well as the psora that has developed into one of the innumerable chronic diseases springing from it, is very seldom cured by any single anti-psoric remedy, but requires the use of several of these remedies—in the worst cases the use of quite a number of them—one after the other, for its perfect cure.

This circumstance need not astonish us when we consider that the psora is a chronic miasma of quite peculiar and especial character which in several thousands of years has passed through several millions of human organisms, and must have assumed such a vast extension of varied symptoms,—the elements of those innumerable,

---

*Recent itch-disease with its still present cutaneous eruption has been cured at times without any external remedy by even *one* very small dose of a properly potentized preparation of sulphur and thus within two, three or four weeks; once a dose of ½ grain of carbo vegetabilis potentized a million fold sufficed for a family of seven persons, and three times a like dose of as highly potentized sepia was sufficient.

chronic, non-venereal ailments, under which mankind now groans,—and could transmute itself into such an indefinite multitude of forms differing from one another as it gradually ultimated itself in the various bodily constitutions of individual men who differed from one another in their domiciles, their climatic peculiarities, their education, habits, occupations,* modes of life and of diet, and was moulded by varying bodily and psychic relations. It is, therefore, not strange, that one single and only medicine is insufficient to heal the entire psora and all its forms, and that it requires several medicines in order to respond, by the artificial morbid effects peculiar to each, to the unnumbered host of psora symptoms, and thus to those of all chronic (non venereal) diseases, and to the entire psora, and to do this in a curative homœopathic manner.†

It is only, therefore, as already mentioned, when the eruption of itch is still in its prime and the infection is in consequence still recent, that the complete cure can be effected by sulphur alone, and then at times with but a single dose. I leave it undecided, whether this can be done in every case of itch still in full eruption on the skin, because the ages of the eruption of itch infecting patients is quite various. For if the eruption has been on the skin for some time (although it may not have been treated with external repressive remedies) it will of itself begin to recede gradually from the skin. Then the internal psora has already in part gained the upper hand; the cutaneous eruption is then no more so completely vicarious, and ailments of another kind appear, partly as the signs of a latent psora, partly as chronic diseases developed from the internal psora. In such a case sulphur alone (as little as any other single antipsoric remedy) is usually no longer sufficient to produce a complete cure, and the other antipsoric remedies, one or another according to the remaining symptoms, must be called upon to give their homœopathic aid.

The homœopathic medical treatment of the countless chronic diseases (non-venereal and therefore of psoric origin) agrees essentially in its general features with the homœopathic treatment of human diseases as taught in the *Organon of the Art of Healing;* I shall

---

* *I. e.*, occupations which called more fully into play one or another organ of the body, one or another function of the spirit and mind.

† I refrain from hinting through what exertions and through how many careful observations, investigations, reflections and varied experiments I have finally succeeded after eleven years in filling up the great chasm in the edifice of the homœopathic healing art, the cure of the innumerable chronic diseases, and thus in completing as far as possible the blessings which this art has in store for suffering humanity.

now indicate what is especially to be considered in the treatment of chronic diseases.

As to the *diet and mode of living* of patients of this kind I shall only make some general remarks, leaving the special application in any particular case to the judgment of the homœopathic practitioner. Of course everything that would hinder the cure must also in these cases be removed. But since we have here to treat lingering, sometimes very tedious diseases which cannot be quickly removed, and since we often have cases of persons in middle life and also in old age, in various relations of life which can seldom be totally changed, either in the case of rich people or in the case of persons of small means, or even with the poor, therefore limitations and modifications of the strict mode of life as regularly prescribed by Homœopathy must be allowed, in order to make possible the cure of such tedious diseases with individuals so very different. A strict, homœopathic diet and mode of living does not *cure* chronic patients as our opponents pretend in order to diminish the merits of Homœopathy, but the main cause is the medical treatment. This may be seen in the case of the many patients who trusting these false allegations have for years observed the most strict homœopathic diet without being able thereby to diminish appreciably their chronic disease; this rather increasing in spite of the diet, as all diseases of a chronic miasmatic nature do from their nature.

Owing to these causes, therefore, and in order to make the cure possible, the homœopathic practitioner must yield to circumstances in his prescriptions as to *diet* and *mode of living*, and in so doing he will much more surely, and therefore more completely, reach the aim of healing, than by an obstinate insistence on strict rules which in many cases cannot be obeyed.

The daily laborer, if his strength allows, should continue his labor; the artisan his handiwork; the farmer, so far as he is able, his field work; the mother of the family her domestic occupations according to her strength; only labors that would interfere with the health of healthy persons should be interdicted. This must be left to the intelligence of the rational physician.

The class of men who are usually occupied, not with bodily labor, but with fine work in their rooms, usually with sedentary work, should be directed during their cure to walk more in the open air, without, on that account, setting their work altogether aside.

Persons belonging to the higher classes should also be urged to take walks more than is their custom. The physician may allow this class the innocent amusement of moderate and becoming dancing amusements in the country that are reconcilable with a strict diet, also social meetings with acquaintances, where conversation is the chief amusement ; he will not keep them from enjoying harmless music or from listening to lectures which are not too fatiguing ; he can permit the theatre only exceptionally, but he can never allow the playing of cards. The physician will moderate too frequent riding and driving, and should know how to banish intercourse which should prove to be morally and psychically injurious, as this is also physically injurious. The flirtations and empty excitations of sensuality between the sexes, the reading of indelicate novels and poems of a like character, as well as superstitious and enthusiastic books, are to be altogether interdicted.*

Scholars ought also to be induced to (moderately) exercise in the open air, and in bad weather to do some light mechanical work in doors; but during the medical treatment mental occupation should be limited to work from memory, since straining the head by reading is hardly ever to be allowed, or at least only with great limitation and a strict definition as to the quantity and quality of what is read, *i. e.*, in treating any of the more severe chronic diseases. In mental disorders it can never be allowed.

All classes of chronic patients must be forbidden the use of any domestic remedies or the use of any medicines on their own account. With the higher classes, perfumeries, scented waters, tooth-powders and other medicines for the teeth must also be forbidden. If the patient has been accustomed for a long time to woolen under-clothing, the homœopathic physician cannot suddenly make a change; but as the disease diminishes the woollen under-garments may in warm weather be first changed to cotton and then, in warm weather, the patient can pass to linen. Fontanels can be stopped, in chronic diseases of any moment, only when the internal cure has already made progress, especially with patients of advanced age.

The physician cannot yield to the request of patients for the continuation of their customary home-baths; but a quick ablution, as

---

* Physicians frequently wish to assume importance by forbidding without exception all sexual intercourse to chronic patients who are married. But if both parties are able and disposed to it, such an interdict is, to say the least, ridiculous, as it neither can nor will be obeyed (without causing a greater misfortune in the family). No legislature should give laws that cannot be kept nor controlled, or which would cause even greater mischief if kept. If one party is incapable of sexual intercourse this of itself will stop such intercourse. But of all functions in marriage such intercourse is what may least be commanded or forbidden. Homœopathy only interferes in this matter through medicines, so as to make the party that is incapable of sexual intercourse capable of it, through antipsoric (or anti-syphilitic) remedies, or on the other hand to reduce an excitable consort's morbidity to its natural tone.

much as cleanliness may demand from time to time, may be allowed; nor can he permit any venesection or cupping, however much the patient may declare that he has become accustomed thereto.

As to *diet*, all classes of men who wish to be cured of a lingering disease, can suffer some limitation, if the chronic disease does not consist of an ailment of the abdomen; with the lower classes there need to be no very strict limitations, especially if the patient is able to remain at work in his trade, thus giving motion to the body. The poor man can recover health even with a diet of salt and bread, and neither the moderate use of potatoes, flour-porridge nor fresh cheese will hinder his recovery; only let him limit the condiments of onions and pepper with his meagre diet.

He who cares for his recovery can find dishes, even at the king's table, which answer all the requirements of a natural diet.

Most difficult for a homœopathic physician is the decision as to drinks. Coffee has in great part the injurious effects on the health of body and soul which I have described in my little book (*Wirkungen des Kaffees* [Effects of Coffee], Leipzig, 1803); but it has become so much of a habit and a necessity to the greater part of the so-called enlightened nations that it will be as difficult to extirpate as prejudice and superstition, unless the homœopathic physician in the cure of chronic diseases insists on a general, absolute interdict. Only young people up to the twentieth year, or at most up to the thirtieth, can be suddenly deprived of it without any particular disadvantage; but with persons over thirty and forty years, if they have used coffee from their childhood, it is better to propose to discontinue it gradually and every day to drink somewhat less; when lo and behold! most of them leave it off at once, and they will do so without any peculiar trouble (except, perhaps, for a few days at the commencement). As late as six years ago I still supposed that older persons who are unwilling to do without it, might be allowed to use it in a small quantity. But I have since then become convinced that even a long-continued habit cannot make it harmless, and as the physician can only permit what is best for his patient, it must remain as an established rule that chronic patients must altogether give up this part of their diet, which is insidiously injurious; and this the patients, high or low, who have the proper confidence in their physician, when it is properly represented to them, almost without exception, do willingly and gladly, to the great improvement of their health. Rye or wheat, roasted like coffee in a drum and then boiled and prepared like coffee, has both in smell and in taste much resemblance to coffee; and rich and poor are using this substitute willingly in several countries.

The like may be said concerning the expensive and so-called fine sorts, as well as concerning the cheap sorts of Chinese, tea which so flatteringly allures the nerves and so secretly and inevitably infests and weakens them. Even when made very weak and when only a little is drank only once a day it is never harmless, neither with younger persons nor with older ones who have used it since their childhood; and they must instead of it use some harmless warm drink. Patients, according to my extensive experience, are also willing to follow the advice of their faithful adviser, the physician in whom they have confidence, when this advice is fortified with reasons.

With respect to the limitation in wine the practitioner can be far more lenient, since with chronic patients it will be hardly ever necessary to altogether forbid it. Patients who from their youth up have been accustomed to a plentiful use of pure * wine cannot give it up at once or entirely, and this the less the older they are. To do so would produce a sudden sinking of their strength and an obstruction to their cure, and might even endanger their life. But they will be satisfied to drink it during the first weeks mixed with equal parts of water, and later, gradually wine mixed with two, three and four and finally with five and six parts of water and a little sugar. The latter mixtures may be allowed all chronic patients as their usual beverage.

More absolutely necessary in the cure of the chronic diseases is the giving up of whisky or brandy. This will require, however, as much consideration in diminishing the quantity used, as firmness in executing it. Where the strength appreciably diminishes at giving it up totally, a small portion of good, pure wine must be used instead of it for a little while, but later, wine mixed with several parts of water, according to circumstances.

Since, according to an inviolable law of nature, our vital force always produces in the human organism the opposite of the impressions caused by physical and medicinal potencies in all the cases in which there are such opposites, it may easily be understood, as accurate observation also testifies, that spirituous liquors, after having simulated refreshment and heightened vital warmth immediately after partaking them, must have just the opposite after-effects, owing to this opposite reaction of the vital force of the organism. Weakness

* Even for men in quite good health it is improper and in many ways injurious to drink pure wine as a customary beverage, and morality only permits its use in small quantities at festive occasions. A youth cannot keep his sexual desires under control up to his marriage unless he altogether avoids banquets. Gonorrhœa and chancre are due to such excesses.

and a diminution of the vital warmth are the inevitable consequences of their use—states which ought to be removed as far as possible from the chronic patient by every true physician. Only an allopath who has never accustomed himself to observation and to reflection, and who is unwilling to acknowledge the injurious effects of his palliatives, can advise his chronic patients to daily drink strong, pure wine to strengthen themselves; a genuine Homœopath will never do this (*sed ex ungue leonem!*).

The permission of beer is quite questionable! Since the artifices of brewers in modern times seem to intend, by their addition of vegetable substances to the extract of malt, not only to prevent it from souring, but also and especially to tickle the palate and to cause intoxication, without any regard to the injurious qualities of these malignant additions which often deeply undermine the health when daily used, and which cannot be discovered by any inspection, the honest physician cannot allow his patient to drink whatsoever is called *beer;* for even in the white beer (thin beer) and the porter, which on account of their lack of bitterness seem so harmless, not infrequently have narcotic ingredients added to give them the much-liked intoxicating quality in spite of their diminished quantity of malt.

Among the articles of diet which are generally injurious to chronic patients are also all dishes containing vinegar or citric acid. These are especially apt to cause disagreeable sensations and troubles in those afflicted with nervous and abdominal ailments. They also either antagonize or excessively increase the effects of several medicines. For such patients also very acid fruit (as sour cherries, unripe gooseberries and currants) are to be allowed only in very small quantities, and sweet fruits only in moderate quantity; so also baked prunes as a palliative are not to be advised to those inclined to constipation. To the latter, as also to those suffering from weak digestion, veal which is too young is not serviceable. Those whose sexual powers are low should limit themselves in eating young chickens and eggs, and should avoid the irritating spice of vanilla, also truffles and caviare, which as palliatives hinder a cure. Ladies with scanty menses must avoid the use of saffron and cinnamon for the same reason; persons with weak stomachs should avoid cinnamon, cloves, amomum, pepper, ginger and bitter substances, which, being palliatives, are also injurious while under homœopathic treatment. Vegetables causing flatulency should be forbidden in all abdominal troubles and where there is an inclination to constipation and costiveness. Beef and good wheat-bread or rye-bread, together with cow's milk and a moderate use of fresh butter, seem to be the most natural and harmless food for men, and also for chronic patients; only little salt should be used. Next to beef in wholesomeness are mutton, venison, grown chickens and young pigeons. The flesh and fat of geese and ducks are even less to be permitted to chronic patients than pork. Pickled and smoked meats should be rarely used and only in small quantities.

Sprinkling chopped raw herbs on soups, putting pot-herbs into vegetables, and eating old, rancid cheese must be avoided.

In using the better quality of fish their preparation should be especially looked to; they had best be prepared by boiling and used sparingly with sauces not much spiced; but no fish dried in the air or smoked; salt fish (herrings and sardines) only rarely and sparingly.

Moderation in all things, even in harmless ones, is the chief duty of chronic patients.

In considering diet, the use of tobacco should also be carefully considered. Smoking in some cases of chronic diseases may be permitted, when the patient had been accustomed to an uninterrupted use of it, and if he does not expectorate; but smoking should always be limited, and more so if the mental activity, sleep, digestion or the evacuations are defective. If evacuations regularly only take place after smoking, the use of this palliative must be all the more circumscribed, and the same result must be obtained in a lasting manner through the appropriate antipsoric remedies. More objectionable yet, however, is the using of snuff, which is wont to be abused as a palliative against rheum and obstruction of the nose and insidious inflammation of the eyes, and which being a palliative, is a great hindrance in the cure of chronic diseases; it can, therefore, not be allowed with such patients, but must be diminished every day and at last stopped. An especial reason for this is also that in snuff the medicinal liquors (sauces) with which almost all snuff is medicated touches with its substance the nerves of the inner nose and injures just as if a foreign medicine were taken, which is less the case with the burning, smoking tobacco in which the strength is disintegrated by the heat.

I now pass to the other hinderances to the cure of chronic diseases which must be avoided as far as possible.

All those events in human life which can bring the psora latent and slumbering within, which has hitherto manifested itself only by some of the signs mentioned above, wherein the patient varies from a state of health, so as to break out into open chronic diseases, these same events if they occur to a person already a chronic patient may not only augment his disease and increase the difficulty of curing it, but, if they break in on him violently, may make his disease incurable, if the untoward circumstances are not suddenly changed for the better.

Such events are, however, of very various nature, and therefore of different degrees of injurious influence.

Excessive hardships, laboring in swamps, great bodily injuries and wounds, excess of cold or heat, and even the unsatisfied hunger of poverty and its unwholesome foods, etc., are not by any means very powerful in causing the fearful malady of psora which lies in ambush, lurking in secret to break forth into serious chronic diseases, nor of great consequence in aggravating a chronic disease already present; yea, an innocent man can, with less injury to his life, pass ten years in bodily torments in the bastile or on the galleys rather than pass some months in all bodily comfort in an unhappy marriage or with a remorseful conscience. A psora slumbering within, which still allows the favorite of a prince to live with the appearance of almost blooming health unfolds quickly into a chronic ailment of the body, or distracts his mental organs into insanity, when by a change of fortune he is hurled from his brilliant pinnacle and is exposed to contempt and poverty. The sudden death of a son causes the tender mother, already in ill health an incurable suppuration of the lungs or a cancer of the breast. A young, affectionate maiden, already hysterical, is thrown into melancholy by a disappointment in love.

How difficult it is, and how seldom will the best antipsoric treatment do anything to relieve such unfortunates!

By far the most frequent excitement of the slumbering psora into chronic disease, and the most frequent aggravation of chronic ailments already existing, are caused by grief and vexation.

Uninterrupted grief and vexation very soon increase even the smallest traces of a slumbering psora into more severe symptoms, and they then develop these into an outbreak of all imaginable chronic sufferings more certainly and more frequently than all other injurious influences operating on the human organism in an average human life; while these two agencies just as surely and frequently augment ailments already existing.

As the good physician will be pleased when he can enliven and keep from ennui the mind of a patient, in order to advance a cure which is not encumbered with such obstructions, he will in such a case feel more than ever the duty incumbent upon him to do all within the power of his influence on the patient and on his relatives and surroundings, in order to relieve him of grief and vexation. This will and must be a chief end of his care and neighborly love.

But if the relations of the patient cannot be improved in this respect, and if he has not sufficient philosophy, religion and power over himself to bear patiently and with equanimity all the sufferings and afflictions for which he is not to blame, and which it is not in his power to change; if grief and vexation continually beat in upon him, and it is out of the power of the physician to effect a lasting removal of these most active destroyers of life, he had better give up the treatment* and leave the patient to his fate, for even the most masterly management of the case with the remedies that are the most exquisite and the best adapted to the bodily ailment will avail nothing, nothing at all, with a chronic patient thus exposed to continual sorrow and vexation, and in whom the vital economy is being destroyed by continuous assaults on the mind. The continuation of the fairest edifice is foolish, when the foundation is being daily undermined, even if but gradually, by the play of the waves.

Almost as near, and often nearer yet, to incurability are the chronic diseases, especially with great and rich men, who for some years, besides the use of mineral baths,† have passed through the hands of various, often of *many*, allopathic physicians, who have tried on them one after another all the fashionable modes of cure, the remedies which are so boastingly lauded in England, France and Italy,—all strongly acting mixtures. By so many unsuitable medicines, which are injurious by their violence and their frequent repetition in large doses, the psora which always lies within, even if not combined with syphilis, becomes every year more incurable, as do also the chronic ailments springing from it; and after the continuation of such irrational medical assaults on the organism for several years it becomes almost quite incurable. It cannot well be decided, since these things take place in the dark, whether these heroic unhomœopathic doses have added, as may be suspected, new ailments to the original disease, which ailments through the largeness of the doses and their frequent repetition have now become lasting and as it were chronic, or whether through abuse there has resulted a crippling of the different faculties of the organism, *i. e.*,

---

* Unless the patient should have little or no cause for his grief and sorrow, or hardly any incitement from without to vexation, and in consequence would need more particularly to be treated with respect to his mental disorder, by means of the antipsoric remedies, which are at the same time suited to the rest of his chronic disease. Such cases are not only curable, but often even easily curable.

† Every time the baths are used, even when the water is not in itself unsuitable to the ailment, they are to be considered as the use of large doses often repeated of one and the same violently acting medicine, the violent operation of which can seldom be salutary, and must often result in the aggravation of the morbid state, yea, even to the patient's utter destruction.

those of irritability, of sensation and of reproduction, and so (probably from both causes) there has arisen the monster of various ailments, fused into one another, which can no longer be rationally viewed as a simple natural ailment. In short, this many-sided disharmony and perversion of parts and of forces most indispensable to life present a chaos of ailments which the homœopathic physician should not lightly declare curable.

By such treatments, which are incapable of curing the original disease, but are exhausting and debilitating, the aggravation of the psora is not only hastened from within, but new artificial and threatening ailments are generated by such delusive allopathic cures, so that the vital force, thus attacked from two sides, often is unable to escape.

If in such cases the sad consequences of these indirect assaults of the old methods of cure were dynamic disturbances only, they would surely either disappear of themselves when the treatment is discontinued, or they ought at least to be extinguished again effectively through homœopathic medicines. But this is not at all the case; they do not yield. Very likely by these indirect, continuous and repeated assaults on the sensitive, irritable fiber by such injudicious medicinal disease-potencies, which are given in large doses frequently repeated, the vital force is obliged to meet this attack and to endeavor either to dynamically change these tender internal organs which are assaulted so mercilessly, or to reconstruct them materially so as to make them unassailable to such violent attacks, and thus to protect and shield the organism from general destruction. Thus, *e. g.*, this force, which instinctively preserves life, beneficially shields the fine sensitive skin of the hand with a callous covering of hard, horny skin in persons with whom the skin is exposed to frequent injuries during hard labor whereby the skin is injured by hard, scratching materials or by corroding substances. So also in a long continued allopathic treatment, which has no true healing power with respect to the disease, no direct pathic (homœopathic) relation to the parts and processes concerned in the chronic disease, but internally assaults other delicate parts and organs of the body, in such cases the vital force, in order to protect the whole from destruction, dynamically and organically transmutes these fine organs; *i. e.*, either makes them inactive or paralyzes them, or dulls their sensitiveness, or makes them altogether callous. On the one side the most tender fiber is abnormally thickened or hardened, and the more vigorous fibers consumed or annihilated—thus there arise artificially, adventitious organisms, malformations and degenerations, which at post-mortem examinations are cunningly ascribed to the malignancy of the original disease. Such an internal state is not infrequent, and is in many cases incurable. Only where there are still sufficient vital powers in a body not too much bowed down by age (but where under an allopathic régime do we not find the powers wasted?) under favorable external circumstances, the vital force dynamically freed from its original disease by the careful homœopathic (antipsoric) treatment of a practiced physician, may succeed in gradually reasserting itself, and in gradually absorbing and transforming those (often numerous) adventitions secondary formations which it was compelled to form. Such a transformation is, however, only possible to a still energetic vital force, which has been in great part set free from its psora. Only however, under favorable external circumstances, and after the lapse of a considerable time and usually in only an imperfect manner, does the vital force succeed in this almost creative endeavor. Experience proves daily that the more zealously the allopath puts into practice in chronic diseases his perverse destructive art (often with great care, industry and persistence), the more he ruins his patients in health and life.

How can perversions, introduced into patients in this manner frequently for years, be transformed in a short time into health even by the best, *i. e.*, the true method of cure, which has never assumed to itself the power of *directly* influencing organic defects?

The physician has to meet in such cases no natural, simple psoric disease. He can therefore promise an improvement only after a long period of time, but never a full restoration, even if the vital powers are not (as is so frequently the case) altogether wasted; for where this is the case, he would feel compelled to desist from treatment even at the first glance. First the many chronic medicinal diseases which pass over the fluctuating state of health must gradually be removed (perhaps during a several months' stay in the country almost without medicine); or they must depart as of themselves through the activity of the vital force, when the antipsoric treatment has to some degree begun, with an improved manner of living and a regulated diet. For who could find remedies for all these ailments artificially produced by a confused mass of strong unsuitable medicines? The vital force must first absorb and reform what it has compulsorily deformed, before the true healer will in time see again before him a partially cleared malady similar to the original one, and which he will then be able to combat.*

*On the other hand, the most dreadful diseases of every kind which have not been spoiled by any medical fatuity, in the families of farm laborers and other day laborers, on whom of course no ordinary physician presses his services, are *quite commonly*, almost as if by a miracle, cured by the antipsoric remedies in a short time, and are transformed into lasting good health.

Woe to the young homœopathic physician who has to found his fame upon the cure of those diseases, of rich and prominent persons, which by a mass of allopathic evil arts have degenerated into such monstrosities! With all his care he will end in failure!

A similar great hindrance to a cure of far-advanced chronic diseases is often found in the debility and weakness into which youths fall who are spoiled by rich parents, being carried away by their superabundance and wantonness, and seduced by wicked companions through destructive passions and excesses, through revelings, abuse of the sexual instinct, gambling, etc. Without the least regard for life and for conscience, bodies originally robust are debilitated by such vices into mere semblances of humanity, and are besides ruined by perverse treatment of their venereal diseases, so that the psora, which frequently lurks within, grows up into the most pitiable chronic diseases, which, even if the morality of the patient should have improved, on account of the depressing remorse, and the little remnant of their wasted vital powers, accept antipsoric relief only with the greatest difficulty. Such cases should be undertaken by homœopathic physicians as curable only with the greatest caution and reserve.

But where the above-mentioned often almost insurmountable obstacles to the cure of these innumerable chronic diseases are not present,* there is nevertheless found at times, especially with the lower classes of patients, a peculiar obstruction to the cure, which lies in the source of the malady itself, where the psora, after repeated infections and a repeated external repression of the resulting eruption, had developed gradually from its internal state into one or more severe chronic ailments. A cure will, indeed, also be certainly effected here, if the above-mentioned obstacles do not prevent, by a judicious use of the antipsoric remedies, but only with much patience and considerable time, and only with patients who observe the directions and who are not too aged nor too much debilitated.

But in these difficult cases also the wise arrangement of nature is

* One additional obstacle to the homœopathic cure of chronic diseases, and one which is not very rare but is still usually disregarded, is: *The suppressed sexual instinct* with marriageable persons of either sex, either from non-marriage owing to various causes not removable by a physician, or where in married persons sexual intercourse of an infirm wife with a vigorous husband, or of the infirm husband with a vigorous wife has been absolutely and forever interdicted by an injudicious physician, as is not infrequently the case. In such cases a more intelligent physician, recognizing the circumstances and the natural impulse implanted by the Creator, will give his permission and thus not infrequently render curable a multitude of hysterical and hypochondriac states, yea, often even melancholy and insanity.

manifested in aid of our efforts, if we only make a good use of the favorable moment offering. For experience informs us that in a case of itch arising from a new infection, even when, after several preceding infections and repressions of the eruption, the psora has made considerable progress in the production of chronic diseases of many kinds, the itch which has last arisen, if it has only still kept its full primitive eruption unhindered on the skin, may be cured almost as easily as if it were the first and the only one, *i. e.*, usually by merely one or a few doses of the appropriate antipsoric medicine, and that by such a cure the whole psora of all the preceding infections, together with its outbreaks into chronic ailments, is cured.*

Nevertheless it is not advisable to intentionally cause a new artificial infection with itch, even if the patient felt no repugnance to it (as is nevertheless, frequently the case) merely on account of the easier cure in that case of the old psora which had been several times renewed; because in severe chronic diseases of a non-venereal and therefore psoric origin,—as *e. g.* suppuration of the lungs, a complete paralyzation of one or another part of the body, etc.,—the itch miasma rarely retains its hold, and, as far as experience shows, it clings less when caused by an artificial inoculation than when it originates from an accidental, unintentional infection.

I have little further to say to the physician already skilled in the homœopathic art as to how he is to operate in the cure of chronic diseases, except to direct him to the antipsoric remedies appended to this work; for he will know how to use these remedies for this noble end successfully. I have only to add a few *cautions*.

First of all, the great truth is established that all chronic ailments, all great, and the greatest, long continuing diseases (excepting the few venereal ones) spring from psora alone and only find their thorough cure in the cure of the psora; they are, consequently, to be healed mostly only by antipsoric remedies, *i. e.*, by those remedies which in their provings as to their pure action on the healthy human body manifest most of the symptoms which are most frequently perceived in latent as well as in developed psora.

The homœopathic physician, therefore, in curing a chronic (non-

*The same is the case, according to the merciful arrangement of nature, with syphilis, where, after a local destruction of the chancre or the bubo and after a consequent breaking out of the venereal disease, a new infection takes place. The new infection, while the chancre remains undisturbed, may be cured, together with the venereal disease sprung from the former infection, just as easily by a single dose of the best mercurial preparation, as if the first chancre were still present,—provided that no complication with either of the other two chronic miasmata, especially the psoric, has taken place; for in such a case, as has been mentioned above, the psora must first be removed.

venereal) disease, and in all and in every symptom, ailment and disorder arising in this disease, no matter what seductive name these may have in common life or in pathology, will usually and especially look to the use of an antipsoric medicine selected according to strictly homœopathic rules, in order to surely attain his end.

Let him not think, while a well-chosen antipsoric medicine is acting and the patient some day feels a moderate headache, or else a moderate ailment, that he must give the patient at once some other medicine, whether an antipsoric or another remedy; or if perchance a sore throat should arise, that he must give another remedy, or another on account of diarrhœa, or another on account of some moderate pain in one part or another, etc.

No! the homœopathic antipsoric medicine having been chosen as well as possible to suit the morbid symptoms, and given in the appropriate potency and in the proper dose, the physician should *as a rule* allow it to finish its action without disturbing it by an intervening remedy.

For if the symptoms occurring during the action of the remedy have also occurred, if not in the last few weeks, at least now and then some weeks before, or some months before in a similar manner, then such occurrences are merely a homœopathic excitation, through the medicine, of some symptom not quite unusual to this disease, of something which had perhaps been more frequently troublesome before, and they are a sign that this medicine acts deeply into the very essence of this disease, and that consequently it will be more effective in the future. The medicine, therefore, should be allowed to continue and exhaust its action undisturbed, without giving the least medicinal substance between its doses.

But if the symptoms are different and had never before occurred, or never in this way, and, therefore, are peculiar to this medicine and not to be expected in the process of the disease, but trifling, the action of the medicine ought not for the present to be interrupted. Such symptoms frequently pass off without interrupting the helpful activity of the remedy; but if they are of a burdensome intensity, they are not to be endured; in such a case they are a sign that the antipsoric medicine was not selected in the correct homœopathic manner. Its action must then be checked by an antidote, or when no antidote to it is known, another antipsoric medicine more accurately answering its symptoms must be given in its place; in this case these false symptoms may continue a few more days, or they may return, but they will soon come to a final end and be replaced by a better help.

Least of all, need we to be concerned when the usual customary symptoms are aggravated and show most prominently on the first days, and again on some of the following days, but gradually less and less. This so-called homœopathic aggravation is a sign of an incipient cure (of the symptoms thus aggravated at present), which may be expected with certainty.

But if these aggravated original symptoms appear on subsequent days still of the same strength as at the beginning, or even with an increased severity, it is a sign that the dose of this antipsoric remedy, although properly selected according to homœopathic principles, was too large, and it is to be apprehended that no cure will be effected by it; because the medicine in so large a dose is able to establish a disease, which in some respects, indeed, is similar to it; with respect to the fact, however, that the medicine in its present intensity unfolds also its other symptoms which annul the similarity, it produces a dissimilar chronic disease instead of the former, and, indeed, a more severe and troublesome one, without thereby extinguishing the old original one.

This will be decided in the first sixteen, eighteen or twenty days of the action of the medicine which has been given in too large a dose, and it must then be checked, either by prescribing its antidote, or, if this is not as yet known, by giving another antipsoric medicine fitting as well as possible, and indeed in *a very moderate dose*, and if this does not suffice to extinguish this injurious medicinal disease, another still should be given as homœopathically suitable as possible.*

Now when the stormy assault caused by too large a dose of medicine, although homœopathically selected, has been assuaged through an antidote or the later use of some other antipsoric remedies, then, later on, the same antipsoric remedy—which had been hurtful only because of its over-large dose—can be used again, and, indeed, as soon as it is homœopathically indicated, with the greatest success, only in a *far* smaller dose and in a *much* more highly potentized attenuation, *i. e.*, in a milder quality.

The physician can, indeed, make no worse mistake than *first*, to consider as too small the doses which I (forced by experience) have reduced after manifold trials and which are indicated with every antipsoric remedy and *secondly*, the wrong choice of a remedy, and

*I have myself experienced this accident, which is very obstructive to a cure and cannot be avoided too carefully. Still ignorant of the strength of its medicinal power, I gave *sepia* in too large a dose. This trouble was still more manifest when I gave *lycopodium* and *silicea*, potentized to the one-billionth degree, giving four to six pellets, though only as large as poppy seeds. *Discite moniti!*

thirdly, the hastiness which does not allow each dose to act its full time.

The first error I have already spoken of, and would only add that nothing is lost if the dose is given even smaller than I have prescribed. *It can hardly be given too small*, if only everything in the diet and the remaining mode of life of the patient which would obstruct or counteract the action of the medicine is avoided. The medicine will still produce all the good effects which can at all be expected from a medicine, if only the antipsoric was homœopathically, correctly, selected according to the carefully investigated symptoms of the disease, and if the patient does not disturb its effects by his violation of the rules. If ever it should happen that the choice has not been correctly made, *the great advantage remains, that the incorrectly selected medicine in this smallest dose may in the manner indicated above be counteracted more easily*, whereupon the cure may be continued without delay with a more suitable antipsoric.

As to the *second* chief error in the cure of chronic diseases (*the unhomœopathic choice of the medicine*) the homœopathic beginner (many, I am sorry to say, remain such beginners their life long) sins chiefly through inexactness, lack of earnestness and through love of ease.

With the great conscientiousness which should be shown in the restoration of a human life endangered by sickness more than in anything else, the Homœopath, if he would act in a manner worthy of his calling, should investigate first the whole state of the patient, the internal cause as far as it is remembered, and the cause of the continuance of the ailment, his mode of life, his quality as to mind, soul and body, together with all his symptoms (see directions in *Organon*), and then he should carefully find out in the work on Chronic Diseases as well as in the work on Materia Medica Pura a remedy covering in similarity, as far as possible, all the moments, or at least the most striking and peculiar ones, with its own peculiar symptoms; and for this purpose he should not be satisfied with any of the existing repertories,—a carelessness only too frequent; for these books are only intended to give light hints as to one or another remedy that might be selected, but they can never dispense him from making the research at the first fountain heads. He who does not take the trouble of treading this path in all critical and complicated diseases, and, indeed, with all patience and intelligence, but contents himself with the vague hints of the repertories in the choice of a remedy, and who thus quickly dispatches one patient after the other, does not deserve the honorable title of a genuine Homœopath, but is rather to be called a bungler, who on that account has continually to change his remedies until the patient loses patience; and as his ailments have of course only been aggravated he must leave this aggravator of diseases, whereby the art itself suffers discredit instead of the unworthy disciple of art.

This disgraceful love of ease (in the calling which demands the most conscientious care) often induces such would-be Homœopaths to give their medicines merely from the (often problematic) statement of their use (*ab usu in morbis*) which are enumerated in the introductions to the medicines, a method which is altogether faulty and strongly savors of allopathy, as these statements usually only give a few symptoms. They should only serve as a confirmation of a choice made according to the pure actions of the medicines; but never to determine the selection of a remedy which can cure only when used according to the exact similitude of its homœopathic symptoms. There are, we are sorry to say, even authors who advise following this empiric pathway of error!

The *third* leading mistake which the homœopathic physician cannot too carefully nor too steadfastly avoid while treating chronic diseases, is in hastily and thoughtlessly—when a properly moderate dose of a well selected antipsoric medicine has been serviceable for several days,—giving some other medicine in the mistaken supposition that so small a dose could not possibly operate and be of use more than eight or ten days. This notion is sought to be supported by the statement that on some day or other, while allowed to continue its action, the morbid symptoms which were to be eradicated, had shown themselves somewhat from time to time.

But if once a medicine, because it was selected in a correct homœopathic manner, is acting well and usefully, which is seen by the eighth or tenth day, then an hour or even half a day may come when a moderate homœopathic aggravation again takes place. The good results will not fail to appear but may, in very tedious ailments, not show themselves in their best light before the twenty-fourth or thirtieth day. The dose will then probably have exhausted its favorable action about the fortieth or fiftieth day, and before that time it would be injudicious, and an obstruction to the progress of the cure, to give any other medicine. Let it not be thought, however, that we should scarcely wait for the time assigned as the probable duration of action to elapse, before giving another antipsoric medicine: *that we should hasten to change to a new medicine in order to finish the cure more quickly.* Experience contradicts this notion entirely, and teaches on the contrary, that a cure cannot be accomplished more quickly and surely than by allowing the suitable antipsoric to continue its actions *so long as the improvement con-*

tinues, even if this should be several, yea, *many** days beyond the assigned, supposed time of its duration, so as to delay as long as practicable the giving of a new medicine.

Whoever can restrain his impatience as to this point, will reach his object the more surely and the more certainly. Only when the old symptoms, which had been eradicated or very much diminished by the last and the preceding medicines commence to rise again for a few days, or to be again perceptibly aggravated, then the time has most surely come when a dose of the medicine most homœopathically fitting should be given. Experience and careful observation alone can decide; and it always has decided in my manifold, exact observations, so as to leave no doubt remaining.

Now if we consider the great changes which must be effected by the medicine in the many, variously composite and incredibly delicate parts of our living organism, before a chronic miasm so deeply inrooted and, as it were, parasitically interwoven with the economy of our life as psora is, can be eradicated and health be thus restored: then it may well be seen how natural it is, that during the long-continued action of a dose of antipsoric medicine selected homœopathically, assaults may be made by it at various periods on the organism, as it were in undulating fluctuations during this long-continued disease. Experience shows that when for several days there has been an improvement, half hours or whole hours or several hours will again appear when the case seems to become worse; but these periods, so long as only the original ailments are renewed and no new, severe symptoms present themselves, only show a continuing improvement, being homœopathic aggravations which do not hinder but advance the cure, as they are only renewed beneficent assaults† on the disease, though they are wont to appear at times sixteen, twenty or twenty-four days after taking a dose of antipsoric medicine.

---

* In a case where *sepia* had showed itself completely homœopathically antipsoric for a peculiar headache that appeared in repeated attacks, and where the ailment had been diminished both as to intensity and duration, while the pauses between the attacks had also been much lengthened, when the attacks re-appeared I repeated the dose, which then caused the attacks to cease for one hundred days (consequently its action continued that long), when it reappeared to some degree, which necessitated another dose, after which no other attack took place for, now, seven years, while the health was also otherwise perfect.

† These attacks, however, if the antipsoric remedy was selected fittingly and homœopathically and the dose was a moderate one, during its continued action take place, ever more and more rarely and more feebly, but if the doses were too strong they come more frequently and more strongly, to the detriment of the patient.

As a rule, therefore, the antipsoric medicine in chronic diseases continue their action the longer, the more tedious the diseases are. But *vice versa* also those medicines which in the healthy body show a long period of action act only a short time and quickly in acute diseases which speedily run their course (*e. g.* belladonna, sulphur, arsenic, etc.) and their periods of action are shorter, the more acute the diseases. The physician must, therefore, in chronic diseases, allow all antipsoric remedies to act thirty, forty or even fifty and more days *by themselves*, so long as they continue to improve the diseased state perceptibly to the acute observer, even though gradually; for so long the good effects continue with the indicated doses and these must not be disturbed and checked by any new remedy.*

---

* The importance of avoiding the above-described two errors will hardly be realized by physicians. These great, pure truths will be questioned yet for years even by most of the homœopathic physicians, and will not, therefore, be practiced, on account of the theoretical reflection and the reigning thought: "It requires quite an effort to believe that so little a thing, so prodigiously small a dose of medicine, could effect the least thing in the human body, especially in coping with such enormously great, tedious diseases; but that the physician must cease to reason, if he should believe that these prodigiously small doses can act not only two or three days, but even twenty, thirty and forty days and longer yet, and cause, even to the last day of their operation, important, beneficent effects otherwise unattainable." Nevertheless this true theorem is not to be reckoned among those which should be comprehended, nor among those for which I ask a blind faith. I demand no faith at all, and do not demand that anybody should comprehend it. Neither do I comprehend it; it is enough, that it is a fact and nothing else. Experience alone declares it, and I believe more in experience than in my own intelligence. But who will arrogate to himself the power of weighing the invisible forces that have hitherto been concealed in the inner bosom of nature, when they are brought out of the crude state of apparently dead matter through a new, hitherto undiscovered agency, such as is potentizing by long continued trituration and succussion. But he who will not allow himself to be convinced of this and who will not, therefore, imitate what I now teach after many years' trial and experience (and what does the physician risk, if he imitates it exactly?), *he who is not willing to imitate it exactly*, can leave this greatest problem of our art unsolved, *he can also leave the most important chronic diseases uncured*, as they have remained unhealed; indeed, up to the time of my teaching. I have no more to say about this. It seemed to me my duty to publish the great truths to the world that needs them, untroubled as to whether people can compel themselves to follow them exactly or not. If it is not done with exactness, let no one boast to have imitated me, nor expect a good result.

Do we refuse to imitate any operation until the wonderful forces of nature on which the result is based are clearly brought before our eyes and made comprehensible even to a child? Would it not be silly to refuse to strike sparks from the stone and flint, because we cannot comprehend how so much combined caloric can be in these bodies, or how this can be drawn out by rubbing or striking, so that the particles of steel which are rubbed off

But if these appropriately selected antipsoric medicines are not allowed to act their full time, when they are acting well, the whole treatment will amount to nothing. Another antipsoric remedy which may be ever so useful, but is prescribed too early and before the cessation of the action of the present remedy, or a new dose of the same remedy which is still usefully acting, can in no case replace the good effect which has been lost through the interruption of the complete action of the preceding remedy, which was acting usefully, and which can hardly be again replaced.

It is a *fundamental rule* in the treatment of chronic diseases: *To let the action of the remedy, selected in a mode homœopathically appropriate to the case of disease which has been carefully investigated as to its symptoms, come to an undisturbed conclusion, so long as it visibly advances the cure and the while improvement still perceptibly progresses.* This method forbids any new prescription, any interruption by another medicine and forbids as well *the immediate repetition of the same remedy*. Nor can there be anything more desirable for the physician than to see the improvement of the patient proceed to its completion unhindered and perceptibly. There are not a few cases, where the practiced careful Homœopath sees a single dose of his remedy, selected so as to be perfectly homœopathic, even in a very severe chronic disease, continue uninterruptedly to diminish the ailment for several weeks, yea, months, up to recovery; a thing which could not have been expected better in any other way, and could not have been effected by treating with several doses or with several medicines. To make the possibility of this process in some way intelligible, we may assume, what is not very unlikely, that an antipsoric remedy selected most accurately according to homœopathic principles, even in the smallest dose of a high or the highest potency can manifest so long-continued a curative force, and at last cure, probably, only *by means of a certain infection* with a very similar medicinal disease which overpowers the original disease, by the process of nature

---

by the stroke of the hard stone are melted, and, as glowing little balls, cause the tinder to catch fire? And yet we strike fire with it, without understanding or comprehending this miracle of the inexhaustible caloric hidden in the cold steel, or the possibility of calling it out with a frictional stroke. Again, it would be just as silly as if we should refuse to learn to write, because we cannot comprehend how one man can communicate his thought to another through pen, ink and paper—and yet we communicate our thoughts to a friend in a letter without either being able or desirous of comprehending this psychico-physical miracle! Why, then, should we hesitate to conquer and heal the bitterest foes of the life of our fellow-men, the chronic diseases, in the stated way, which, punctually followed, is the best possible method, because we do not see how these cures are effected?

itself, according to which (*Organon*, § 45, Fifth Edition,) two diseases which are different, indeed, in their kind but very similar in their manifestations and effects, as also in the ailments and symptoms caused by it, when they meet together in the organism, the stronger disease (which is always the one caused by the medicine, § 33, ibid.) destroys the weaker (the natural one). In this case every new medicine and also a new dose of the same medicine, would interrupt the work of improvement and cause new ailments, an interference which often cannot be repaired for a long time.

But if any unfavorable effects are evolved by the present dose of medicine, *i. e.*, troublesome symptoms which do not belong to this disease, and if the mind of the patient becomes depressed, if only a little at first, still increasingly, then the next dose of the same medicine, given immediately after the former, cannot but become injurious to the patient. Yet when a sudden great and striking improvement of a tedious great ailment follows immediately on the first dose of a medicine, there justly arises much suspicion that the remedy has only acted palliatively, and therefore must never be given again, even after the intervention of several others remedies.

Nevertheless there are cases which make an *exception* to the rule, but which not every beginner should risk finding out.*

The only allowable *exception* for an *immediate repetition of the same medicine* is when the dose of a well-selected and in every way suitable and beneficial remedy has made some beginning toward an improvement, but its action ceases too quickly, its power is too soon exhausted, and the cure does not proceed any further. This is rare in chronic diseases, but in acute diseases and in chronic diseases that rise into an acute state it is frequently the case. It is only then,—as a practiced observer may recognize—*when the peculiar symptoms of the disease to be treated, after fourteen, ten, seven, and even fewer days, visibly cease to diminish, so that the improvement manifestly has come*

* Still there has been of late much abuse of this immediate repetition of doses of the same medicine, because young Homœopaths thought it more convenient to repeat, without examination, a medicine which in the beginning had been found to be homœopathically suitable, and which had therefore in the beginning proved serviceable, and even to repeat it frequently without examination, so as to heal more quickly.

We may declare at once, that the practice of late, which has even been recommended in public journals of giving the patient several doses of the same medicine to take with him, so that he may take them himself at certain intervals, without considering whether this repetition may affect him injuriously, seems to show a negligent empiricism, and to be unworthy of a homœopathic physician, who should not allow a new dose of a medicine to be taken or given without convincing himself in every case beforehand as to its usefulness.

to a stop, without any disturbance of the mind and without the appearance of any new troublesome symptoms, so that the former medicine would still be perfectly homœopathically suitable, only then, I say, is it useful, and probably necessary to give a dose of the same medicine of a similarly small amount, but most safely in a different degree of dynamic potency.* When the remedy is thus modified, the vital force of the patient will allow itself more easily to be further affected by the same medicine, so as to effect by it everything that may be expected of this medicine and in this ailment.†

To adduce an example: a freshly arisen eruption of itch belongs to those diseases which might soonest permit the repetition of the dose (sulphur), and which does permit it the more frequently, the sooner after the infection the itch is received for treatment, as it then approaches the nature of an acute disorder, and demands its remedies in more frequent doses than when it has been standing on the skin for some time. But this repetition should be permitted only when the preceding dose has largely exhausted its action (after six, eight or ten days), and the dose should be just as small as the preceding one, and be given in a different potency. Nevertheless it is in such a case often serviceable, in answer to a slight change of symptoms, to interpose between the doses of pure sulphur, a small dose of *Hepar sulphuris calcareum*. This also should be given in various potencies, if several doses should be needed from time to time. Often also, according to circumstances, a dose of Nux vomica (x) or one of mercury (x)‡ may be used between.

If I except sulphur, Hepar sulphuris and in some cases Sepia, the other antipsoric remedies can seldom be usefully given in imme-

---

* If it, *e. g.*, has first been given in the 30th potency, it will now be given in perhaps the 18th, and if a repetition should be again found serviceable and necessary, it might afterwards be given in the 24th, and later perhaps also in the 12th and 6th, etc., if, *e. g.*, the chronic disease should have taken on itself an acute character. A dose of medicine may also have been suddenly counteracted and annihilated by a grave error in the regimen of the patient, when perhaps a dose of the former serviceable medicine might again be given with the modification mentioned above.

† In cases where the physician is certain as to the homœopathic specific to be used, the first attenuated dose may also be dissolved in about four ounces of water by stirring it, and one-third may be drunk at once, and the second and third portions on the following days; but it should each time be again stirred so as to increase the potency and thus to change it. Thereby the remedy seems to take a deeper hold on the organism and hasten the restoration in patients who are vigorous and not too sensitive.

‡ That the itch-patient during such a treatment must avoid every external application, however harmless it may appear, *e. g.*, the washing with black soap, is not necessary to emphasize.

diately repeated doses. Indeed it is hardly ever needed in chronic diseases, as we have a goodly supply of antipsoric remedies at our disposal, so that as soon as one well-selected remedy has completed its action, and a change of symptoms, *i. e.*, a change in the total image of the disease, appears, another antipsoric remedy homœopathically appropriate to the altered case may be chosen to greater advantage and with a more sure prospect of hastening the cure, than if we take the risk of prescribing the former medicine which now is no longer altogether adequate. Nevertheless in very tedious and complex cases, which are mostly such as have been mismanaged by allopathic treatment, it is nearly always necessary to give again from time to time during the treatment, a dose of Sulphur or of Hepar (according to the symptoms), even to the patients who have been before dosed with large allopathic doses of Sulphur and with sulphur-baths; but then only after a previous dose of Mercury (x).

Where, as is usually the case in chronic diseases, various antipsoric remedies are necessary, the more frequent sudden change of them is a sign that the physician has selected neither the one nor the other in an appropriately homœopathic manner, and had not properly investigated the leading symptoms of the case before prescribing a new remedy. This is a frequent fault into which the homœopathic physician falls in urgent cases of chronic diseases, but oftener still in acute diseases from overhaste, especially when the patient is a person very dear to his heart. I cannot too urgently warn against this fault.

Then the patient naturally falls into such an irritated state that, as we say, no medicine acts, or shows its effect,* yea, so that the power of response in the patient is in danger of flaring up and expiring at the least further dose of medicine. In such a case no further benefit can be had through medicine, but there may be in use a calming mesmeric stroke made from the crown of the head (on which both the extended hands should rest for about a minute) slowly down over the body, passing over the throat, shoulders, arms, hands, knees and legs down over the feet and toes. This may be repeated if necessary.

A dose of homœopathic medicine may also be moderated and softened by allowing the patient to smell† a small pellet moistened

* That a homœopathically potentized dose of medicine should ever fail of having an effect in a treatment conducted *with care*, I think impossible; I have never experienced it.

† Even persons born without the sense of smell or who have lost it through disease, may expect equally efficient help from drawing in the imperceptible vapor (proceeding from the medicine and contained in the vial) through one

with the selected remedy in a high potency, and placed in a vial the mouth of which is held to the nostril of the patient, who draws in only a momentary little whiff of it. By such an inhalation the powers of any potentized medicine may be communicated to the patient in any degree of strength. One or more such medicated pellets, and even those of a larger size may be in the smelling-bottle, and by allowing the patient to take longer or stronger whiffs, the dose may be increased a hundred fold as compared with the smallest first mentioned. The period of action of the power of a potentized medicine taken in by such inhalation and spread over so large a surface (as that of the nostrils and of the lungs) lasts as long as that of a small massive dose taken through the mouth and the fauces.

Such medicated pellets kept in a stoppered vial retain their medicinal power quite undiminished, even if the vial be opened a number of times in many years for the purpose of inhalation; *i. e.*, if the vial be preserved from sunshine and heat. This method of allowing the patient to be acted upon by smelling the potentized medicine has great advantages in the manifold mishaps which often obstruct and interrupt the treatment of chronic diseases. The antidote to remove these mishaps as quickly as possible the patient may also best receive in greater or less strength through inhalation, which acts most quickly on the nerves and so also affords the most prompt assistance, by which also the continuation of the treatment of the chronic disease is least delayed. When the mishap has thus been obviated most speedily, the antipsoric medicine before taken frequently continues its interrupted action for some time. But the dose of the inhaled medicine must be so apportioned to the morbid interruption that its effect just suffices to extinguish the disadvantage arising from the mishap, without going any deeper or being able to continue its operation any further.

If a homœopathic physician, scrupulous at the wrong occasion, should ask me how he might fill up the many days after giving a dose, so that it may continue its action undisturbed during the above-mentioned long time, and so satisfy, without injuring, the patient who every day* asks for his medicine, I reply with two

nostril or the other, as those do who are gifted with the sense of smell. From this it follows that the nerves possessing merely the sense of touch receive the salutary impression and communicate it unfailingly to the whole nervous system.

*No old established custom among the people, be it ever so hurtful, can be suddenly changed. So also the homœopathic physician cannot avoid allowing a new chronic patient to take at least one little powder a day; the difference between this and the many medicinal doses of allopaths is still very

words, that he should be given every day at the usual time for medicine a dose of sugar of milk, about three grains, which shall be marked as usual with continuous numbers.* I remark here, that I consider the sugar of milk thus used as an invaluable gift of God.†

We cannot flatter ourselves that the antipsoric medicine given was rightly selected, or that it will forward the cure of a chronic disease, if it quickly and entirely destroys as if by a stroke of magic the most troublesome symptoms, old, great, continuous pains, tonic

---

great. During this daily taking of a powder, following the numbers, it will be a great benefit to the poor patient who is often intimidated by slanderers of the better medical art, if he does not know whether there is a dose of medicine in every powder, nor again, in which one of them? If he knew the latter, and should know, that to-day's number contains the medicine of which he expects so much, his fancy would often play him an evil trick, and he would imagine that he feels sensations and changes in his body, which do not exist; he would note imaginary symptoms and live in a continual inquietude of mind; but if he daily takes a dose, and daily notices no evil assault on his health, he becomes more equable in disposition (being taught by experience), expects no ill effects, and will then quietly note the changes in his state which are actually present, and therefore can only report the truth to his physician. On this account it is best that he should daily take his powder, without knowing whether there is medicine in all or in a certain powder; thus he will not expect more from to-day's powder than from yesterday's or that of the day before.

* Chronic patients who firmly trust in the honesty and skill of their physician will be satisfied, without any after thoughts, to receive such a dose of sugar of milk every two, four or seven days, according to the disposition of each, and nevertheless retain a firm confidence, as, indeed, is only just and reasonable.

† There were some anxious purists, who were afraid that even the pure sugar of milk, either in itself or changed by long trituration, might have medicinal effects. But this is a vain, utterly unfounded fear, as I have determined by very exact experiments. We may use the crude, pure sugar of milk as a food, and partake of considerable quantities of it, without any change in the health, and so also the triturated sugar. But to destroy at the same time the fear to which utterance has been given by some hypochondriacs, that through a long trituration of the sugar of milk alone, or in the potentizing of medicines, something might rub off from the porcelain mortar (silica), which being potentized by this same trituration would be bound to become strongly acting Silicea($_1$), I took a new porcelain triturating bowl in which the glazing had been rubbed off, with a new porcelain pestle, and had one hundred grains of pure sugar of milk, divided into portions of thirty-three grains, triturated eighteen times for six minutes at a time and as frequently scraped for four minutes with a porcelain spatula, in order to develop by this three hours' strong trituration a medicinal power either of the sugar of milk or of the silica or of both; but my preparation remained as indifferent and unmedicinal as the crude, merely nutritive sugar of milk, of which I convinced myself by experiments on very sensitive persons.

or clonic spasms, etc., so that the patient almost immediately after taking the medicine, fancies himself as much freed from sufferings as if he were already restored, and as if in heaven. This deceptive effect shows that the medicine here acts enantiopathically as an opposite or palliative, and that in the days following we cannot expect anything from this remedy but an aggravation of the original disease. As soon then as this deceptive improvement within a few days begins again to turn to aggravation, it is high time to give either the antidote to this medicine, or, when this cannot be had, a medicine which is homœopathically more appropriate. Very rarely will such an enantiopathic remedy do any good in the future. If the medicine which is thus antipathic at once in the beginning, *i. e.*, which seemed so to alleviate, is inclined to reciprocal action, it is possible that when the aggravation from this dose takes place, a second dose of the same remedy may produce the contrary, and thus bring about a lasting improvement, as I have at least perceived in Ignatia.

In such cases we may also successfully use, for the ailments following after a few days from such an antipathic remedy, one of the remaining medicines from the considerable store laid down in *Materia Medica Pura*, in the "*Archiv der homœopathischen Heilkunst*" or in the "*Annalen.*" This may be done for a few days until the Psora-disease returns to its customary routine course, when a homœopathically selected antipsoric medicine is to be given to continue the cure.

Among the mishaps which disturb the treatment only in a temporary way, I enumerate: overloading the stomach (this may be remedied by hunger, *i. e.*, by only taking a little thin soup instead of the meal and a little coffee); disorder of the stomach from fat meat, especially from eating pork (to be cured by fasting and *pulsatilla*); a disorder of the stomach which causes rising from the stomach after eating and especially nausea and inclination to vomit (by highly potentized *antimonium crudum*); taking cold in the stomach by eating fruit (by smelling of *arsenicum*); troubles from spirituous liquors (*nux vomica*); disorder of the stomach with gastric fever, chilliness and cold (*bryonia alba*); fright (when the medicine can be given at once, and especially when the fright causes timidity, by *poppy-juice* (*opium*); but if aid can only be rendered later, or when vexation is joined with the fright, by *aconite;* but if sadness is caused by the fright, *ignatia seeds*); vexation which causes anger, violence, heat, irritation, by *chamomilla*, (but if beside the vexation there is chilliness and coldness of the body, by *bryonia*); vexation with indignation, deep internal mortification (attended with throwing away what was held in the hand, by *staphisagria*); indignation with silent internal mortification (by *colocynthis*); unsuccessful love with quiet grief (by *ignatia*); unhappy love with jealousy (by *hyoscyamus*); a severe cold (next to keeping the house or the bed) by *nux vomica;* when diarrhœa resulted, by *dulcamara;* or if followed by pains, *coffea cruda;* or if followed by fever and heat, by *aconite;* a cold which is followed by suffocative fits, (by *ipecacuanha*); colds followed by pains and an inclination to weep, (by *coffea cruda*); cold with consequent coryza and loss of the sense of smell and of taste, (by *pulsatilla*); over-lifting or strains (sometimes by *arnica*, but most certainly by *rhus toxicodendron*); contusions and wounds inflicted by blunt instruments, (by *arnica*); burning of the skin (by compresses of water mixed with a dilution of highly potentized *arsenicum*, or uninterruped application for hours of alcohol heated by means of very hot water); weakness from loss of fluids and blood, (by china); homesickness with redness of the cheeks, (by *capsicum*).

But during the treatment of chronic diseases by antipsoric remedies we often need the other non-antipsoric store of medicines in cases where epidemic diseases or intermediate diseases (*morbi intercurrentes*) arising usually from meteoric and telluric causes attack our chronic patients, and so not only temporarily disturb the treatment, but even *interrupt* it for a longer time. Here the other homœopathic remedies will have to be used, wherefore I shall not enter upon this here, except to say that the antipsoric treatment will have for the time to be totally discontinued, so long as the treatment of the epidemic disease which has also seized our (chronic) patient may last, even if a few weeks in the worst cases may thus be lost. But here also, if the disease is not too severe, the above mentioned method of applying the medicine by smelling a moistened pellet is often sufficient to help, and the cure of the acute disease may thus be extraordinarily shortened.

The intelligent homœopathic physician will soon note the point of time when his remedies have completed the cure of the epidemic intermediate disease* and when the peculiar course of the chronic (psoric) malady is continued.

* Usually these epidemic intermediate diseases appear in the form of a fever (if they are not the permanent miasms, small-pox, measles, dysentery, whooping cough, etc.). There are fevers of various kinds, a continuous acute fever, or a slow remittent, or an intermittent fever. Intermittent fevers appear almost every year in a somewhat changed form. Since I have learned to cure chronic diseases and maladies by a homœopathic extirpation of their psoric source, I have found the epidemically current intermittent fevers almost every year different in their character and in their symptoms, and they therefore require almost every year a different medicine for their specific cure. One year they require arsenicum, another belladonna, another antimonium crudum, or spigelia, aconite, with ipecacuanha, alternating with nux vomica, sal ammoniacum,

The symptoms of the original chronic disease will, however, always be found somewhat varied after the cure of such a prevailing intermediate disease. Also another part of the body will be found suffering, so that the homœopathic physician will choose his antipsoric remedy according to the totality of the remaining symptoms, and not simply give the one he intended to give before the intermediate disease appeared.

When the physician is called to treat such a prevalent disease in a patient whom he had not before attended as a chronic patient he will not unfrequently find, especially if the fever was considerable, that after overcoming it by the remedies which had been homœopathically specific with other patients of this kind, the full restoration to health does not follow even with good diet and mode of living: but incidents of another kind will show themselves (usually called after-pains or secondary diseases) and these will gradually be aggravated and threaten to become chronic. Here the homœopathic physician will nearly always have to meet a psora which is developing into a chronic disease, and this will have to be cured according to the principles here laid down.

Here is a fitting opportunity to note that the great epidemic diseases: smallpox, measles, purple rash, scarlet fever, whooping cough, fall dysentery and typhoid, when they complete their course

---

natrum muriaticum, opium, cina, alone or in alternation with capsicum, or capsicum alone, menyanthes trifoliata, calcarea carbonica, pulsatilla, one of the two carbos, arnica, alone or in alternation with ipecacuanha, and with these they were cured in a few days. I would not, indeed, except any one of the non-antipsoric medicines, if they are only homœopathic to the whole complex of the symptoms of the prevailing fever, in its attack as well as in its apyrexia (see *von Bœnninghausen*, Versuch e. hom. Therapie d. Wechselfiebers, 1833, Muenster), but I would almost always except cinchona; for this can only *suppress its type* in many large doses in a concentrated form (as quinine), and then it changes it into a cachexy of quinine, which it is difficult to cure. (*China* is only appropriate to the *endemic* intermittent fever in marshy regions, and even this can only be rightly cured by it in connection with antipsoric remedies.) Even at the beginning of the treatment of an *epidemic* intermittent fever, the homœopathic physician is most safe in giving every time an attenuated dose of sulphur or in appropriate cases, hepar sulphuris in a fine little pellet or by means of smelling, and in waiting its effects for a few days, until the improvement resulting from it ceases, and then only he will give, in one or two attenuated doses, the non-antipsoric medicine which has been found homœopathically appropriate to the epidemy of this year. These doses should however only be given at the end of an attack. *With all patients in intermittent fever, psora is essentially involved in every epidemy*, therefore an attenuated dose of sulphur or of hepar sulphuris is necessary at the beginning of every treatment of epidemic intermittent fever, and makes the restoration of the patient more sure and easy.

especially without a judicious homœopathic treatment, leave th organism so shaken and irritated, that with many who seem restored the psora which was before slumbering and latent now awake quickly, either into itch-like eruptions * or into other chronic dis- orders, which then reach a high degree in a short time, if they ar not treated properly in an antipsoric manner. This is due to th great exhaustion of the organism which still prevails. The allo- pathic physician, when such a patient, as is frequently the case dies after all his unsuitable treatment, declares that he has died fro the *sequelæ* of whooping cough, measles, etc.

These *sequelæ* are, however, the innumerable chronic diseases i numberless forms of developed psora which have hitherto bee unknown as to their origin and consequently remained uncured.

Epidemic and sporadic fevers, therefore, as well as the miasmati acute diseases, if they do not soon terminate and pass directl over into good health, (even when the epidemic and acute mias matic part has found a homœopathic specific which has been rightl used against them), often need an antipsoric assistance, which I hav usually found in sulphur, if the patient had not used shortly befor a medicine containing sulphur, in which case another antipsori suitable to this particular case will have to be used.

Endemic diseases, with their striking pertinacity, depend almos wholly on a psoric complication, or on psora modified by the peculi arity of the nature of the locality (and the especial mode of life c the inhabitants), so that, *e. g.*, in intermittent fever originating in marshy region, the patients, even after removal into a dry region often remain uncured despite of all their use of china, unless th antipsoric treatment is especially used. The exhalation fro swamps seems to be one of the strongest physical causes of the devel opment of the psora latent within with so many persons † and thi

---

* When such an eruption appears in any quantity, it is called by write *scabies spontanea* (spontaneous itch)—a mere chimera and nonentity, for as fa as history goes, no itch has arisen except from infection, and it cannot no arise again of itself without infection with the miasma of itch. But this phe nomenon after acute fever is nothing else than the secondary eruption so ofte mentioned above springing from the slumbering and latent psora remainin within after the repression (or more rarely the gradual disappearance) from th skin of the original eruption of itch. This eruption frequently leaves the ski of itself and it has never been proved that it infected any other person with th itch.

† Presumably these exhalations possess a quality which as it were paralyze the vital force of the organism (which in an ordinary state of health is able t keep down the internal psora which always endeavors to manifest itself) an thus predisposes to putrid and nervous fevers.

most of all in hot countries. Without an almost regular use of the best antipsoric method of cure, we shall never succeed in removing the murderous qualities of humid climates and changing them into passably healthy, habitable regions. Man may accustom himself to the extreme degrees of atmospheric heat, as well as to the most violent cold, and can live joyous and healthy in both extremes, Why should he not be able to accustom himself to marshy regions just as well as to the driest mountain regions, if there were not a hitherto undiscovered and unconquered enemy of vigorous life and lasting health, lying in ambush in marshy regions, *i. e.*, psora? Wherever psora lies latent within (and how frequently is this the case?) it is developed into chronic diseases of every kind, especially those in which the liver is most affected, through stagnant water and the gases that emanate from damp soil and from swamps; and this is effected *more surely*, yea, *unavoidably* by these causes than by any other physical power injurious to health.

The latest symptoms that have been added to a chronic disease which has been left to itself (and thus has not been aggravated by medical mismanagement) are always the first to yield in an antipsoric treatment; but the oldest ailments and those which have been most constant and unchanged, among which are the constant local ailments, are the last to give way; and this is only effected, when all the remaining disorders have disappeared and the health has been in all other respects almost totally restored. In the general maladies which come in repeated attacks, *e. g.* the periodic kinds of hysteria, and different kinds of epilepsy, etc., the attacks may quickly be made to cease by a suitable antipsoric; but to make this cessation reliable and lasting, the whole indwelling psora must be completely cured.

The frequent request of a patient to have one symptom, which above others is troublesome to him, removed first of all, is impracticable, but the ignorant patient should be excused for his request.

In the daily written report during the use of an antipsoric medicine, the patient who lives *at a distance* should underscore once, for the information of the physician, those incident symptoms during the day, which after a considerable time or a long time he has now felt again for the first time; but those which he never had before and which he first felt on that day, he should *underscore twice*. The former symptoms indicate that the antipsoric has taken hold of the root of the evil, and will do much for its thorough cure, but the latter, if they appear more frequently and more strongly, give the physician a hint that the antipsoric was not selected quite homœopathically, and should be interrupted in time and replaced by a more appropriate one.

When the treatment is about half completed, the diminished disease commences to return into the state of a latent psora; the symptoms grow weaker and weaker, and at last the attentive physician will only find traces of it; but he must follow these to their complete disappearance, for the smallest remnant retains a germ for a renewal of the old ailment.* If the physician should here give up the treatment and suppose what the common man (and also the higher class of the non-medical public) is apt to say: "It will now likely get right of itself," a great mistake would be made; for in time there would develop, (especially when any important untoward events take place), out of this little remnant of this only diminished psora, a new chronic disease which gradually would increase unavoidably, according to the nature of diseases springing from unextinguished chronic miasms as shown above.

The *cito, tuto et jucunde* (quickly, safely and pleasantly) of Celsus, the patient may reasonably ask from his physician, and from the homœopath he can rightly *expect* this in acute diseases springing from occasional causes, as well as in the well-defined intermediate diseases prevalent at times (the so-called intercurrent diseases).

But with especial regard to the "Cito" (quickly), *i. e.*, the hastening of the cure, the nature of the case forbids it, at least in inveterate chronic ailments.†

The cure of great chronic diseases of ten, twenty, thirty and more years' standing (*if they have not been mismanaged by an excess of allopathic treatments, or indeed, as is often the case, mismanaged into incurableness*) may be said to be quickly annihilated if this is done in one or two years. If with younger, robust persons this takes place in one-half the time, then on the other hand in advanced age, even with the best treatment on the part of the physician and the most punctual observance of rules on the part of the patient and his attendants, considerable time must be added to the usual period of the cure. It will also be found intelligible that such a long-continued

*So from the water-polypus which has several of its branches lopped off, in time new branches will shoot forth.

†Only an ordinary ignorant practitioner can lightly promise to cure a severe inveterate disease in four to six weeks. He need not, indeed, keep his promise! What does he risk, if as a matter of course, his treatment only aggravates the disease? Can he lose anything? Any honor? No; for his colleagues, who are like him do no better. Can he lose in self-respect? Should he yet have any to lose?

(psoric) chronic disease, the original miasm of which has had so much time and opportunity in a long life to insert its parasitical roots as it were, into all the joints of the tender edifice of life, is at last so intimately interwoven with the organism that even with the most appropriate medical treatment, careful mode of life and observance of rules on the part of the patient, great patience and sufficient time will be required to destroy this many armed polypus in all its parts, while sparing the independence of the organism and its powers.

The strength of a patient under an antipsoric treatment, even if it should be continued ever so long, ought continually to increase from the very commencement of the correct treatment even to the restoration of health and of the normal state. The strength increases during the whole of the cure without the use of the so-called tonics, and the patients joyously rise up again of themselves in proportion as their life is delivered from its corroding enemy.*

The best time for taking a dose of antipsoric medicine seems to be, not an hour before going to bed but, rather, early in the morning while fasting. The medicine in the numbered paper † (as also all that succeed) if it is desired that it should act but feebly, should be taken dry and allowed to dissolve on the tongue, or be moistened with two or three drops of water on a spoon, and by itself, without in either case drinking anything after it or eating anything within half an hour or a whole hour.‡

After taking the medicine the patient should keep perfectly quiet at least a full hour, but without going to sleep (sleep delays the be-

* It is inconceivable how allopathic physicians could think of curing chronic diseases through a continuance of exhausting and debilitating treatments, without being restrained by their lack of success from repeating continually their perverse treatment. The *amara* which they give between, together with the quinine, without being able to supply the strength lost, only add new evils.

† Numbering the powders continuously has the convenience that the physician when the patients render their daily report (especially those living at a distance) putting first the date and the number of the powder taken that day, can recognize the day when the patient took his medicine, and can judge of the progress of its action according to the report of the following day.

‡ If the medicine is to act more strongly it must be stirred in a little more water until dissolved before taking it, and in still more water if it is to act still more strongly, and the physician should order the solution taken a portion at a time. If he orders the solution taken in one or three days it must be stirred up not only the first time, but also the other two times, by which every part thus stirred acquires another somewhat higher degree of potency, and so is received more willingly by the vital force. To direct the use of the same solution for a greater number of days is not advisable, as the water, kept longer, would begin to putrefy. How a dose for smelling may be adapted to all degrees of strength, I have mentioned above.

ginning of the action of the medicine). He must avoid during this hour, as indeed throughout the treatment, all disagreeable excitement, nor should he strain his mind immediately after taking the dose, in any way, either by reading or computing, by writing, or by conversations requiring meditation.

The dose of antipsoric medicine must not be taken by females shortly before their menses are expected, nor during their flow; but the dose can be given, if necessary, four days, *i. e.*, about ninety-six hours after the menses have set in. But in case the menses previously have been premature or too profuse, or two long-lasting, it is often necessary to give on this fourth day a small dose of *nux vomica* (one very small pellet, moistened with a high dynamization) to be smelled, and then, on the fourth or sixth day following, the antipsoric. But if the female is very sensitive and nervous, she ought, until she comes near her full restoration, to smell such a pellet once about every time seventy-two hours after the beginning of her menses, notwithstanding her continued antipsoric treatment.*

Pregnancy in all its stages offers so little obstruction to the antipsoric treatment, that this treatment is often most necessary and useful in that condition.† *Most necessary*, because the chronic ailments then are more developed. In this state of woman, which is quite a natural one, the symptoms of the internal psora are often manifested most plainly ‡ on account of the increased sensitiveness of the female

---

* In such a morbid state of the menses nothing can be done in the cure of chronic diseases without the intermediate use of Nux vomica, which here specifically reduces to order the disharmony arising in the functions of the nerves from so disorderly a flow of the menses, and so quiets this excessive sensitiveness and irritability, which put an insurmountable obstacle in the way of the curative action of the antipsoric remedies.

† In what more certain way could, *e. g.*, the return of miscarriage, which is almost exclusively due to psora, be prevented, and, indeed, be lastingly prevented, than through a judicious antipsoric treatment before or at least during pregnancy? In what more reliable way could the states of the womb, which are not infrequently dangerous, and sometimss fatal even in a proper presentation of the fœtus and in a natural labor, be removed in advance than by a timely antipsoric treatment during pregnancy? Even the improper presentation of the child has, if not always, still very often its only cause in the psoric sickliness of the mother, and the hydrocephalus and other bodily defects of the child have surely this cause! Only the antipsoric treatment of the sickly wife if not before, at least during pregnancy, can remove in advance the mother's inability for suckling, as also in suckling prevent the frequent sore breasts, the soreness of the nipples, the frequent inclination to erysipelatous inflammations of the breasts and their abscesses, as well the hemorrhages of the uterus during suckling.

‡ Nevertheless, the entire opposite frequently takes place, so that the wife who before pregnancy was always sickly, and uninterruptedly complaining,

body and spirit while in this state; the antipsoric medicine therefore acts more definitely and perceptibly during pregnancy, which gives the hint to the physician to make the doses in these cases as small and in as highly potentized attenuations as possible, and to make his selections in the most homœopathic manner.

Sucklings never receive medicine; the mother or wet-nurse receives the remedy instead, and through their milk it acts on the child very quickly, mildly and beneficially.

The corporeal nature (called the life-preserving principle or vital force) when left to itself, since it is without reason, cannot provide anything better than palliatives in chronic diseases and in the acute diseases springing thence which cause sudden danger to life, owing to the indwelling psora. These are the causes of the more frequent secretions and excretions of various kinds taking place of themselves now and then in chronic (psoric) diseases, as *e. g.*, diarrhœas, vomiting, perspiration, suppurations, hemorrhages, etc. All these are attended with only temporary alleviations of the chronic original malady, which owing to the losses of humors and of strength thereby only becomes more and more aggravated.

Allopathy has, so far, not been able to do any more than this toward a genuine cure of the chronic diseases; it could only imitate the unreason in corporeal nature in its palliatives (usually without an equal alleviation and with a greater sacrifice of strength). It caused therefore, more than the other, a hastening of the general ruin, without being able to contribute anything to the extinction of the original malady. To this class belong all the many, indescribable purgatives, the so-called dissolvents, the venesection, cupping, the applying of leeches now so insanely frequent, the sudorifics, the artificial sores, setons, fontanels, exutories, etc.

God be praised, the homœopathic physician who is acquainted with the means of a radical cure, and who thus through the antipsoric treatment can destroy the chronic disease itself, has so little need of the above mentioned applications, which only hasten dissolution, that he has on the contrary to use all care that the patient may not secretly use some of these appliances, following the old routine, diffused over the whole earth by allopathy. He can never yield to the request of the patient, *e. g.*, that he has become accustomed to being bled so and so many times a year, or to be cupped,

---

feels in unusual good health during every pregnancy and only during this state. And with such cases this time of pregnancy may very well be made use of for antipsoric treatment, which in such a case is directed against the symptoms of the morbid state before pregnancy, so far as this can be remembered.

or to use purgatives or warm baths, and that he therefore needs them. Such things cannot be permitted.

The homœopathic physician who is a master of his art, and God be praised! there is now a not inconsiderable number of such masters in homœopathy, never allows a drop of blood to be drawn from his patient; he never needs any such or similar means of weakening the body, for such a course evermore remains the negation of curing. Only journeymen, half homœopaths still, I am sorry to say, use such a *contradictio in adjecto* (*weakening while desiring to cure*).*

Only in the one case, where, as in many chronic diseases, the delay in passing evacuations causes great trouble, he will permit (*in the beginning of the treatment* before the antipsoric medicine has had the time [in its after-effects] to produce improvement in this point) if the stool is not passed for three or four days, a clyster of clean, lukewarm water without the least admixture, also perhaps a second, if an evacuation does not result within a quarter of an hour. Rarely a third injection will be needed, after waiting a third quarter of an hour. This help which acts chiefly mechanically by expanding the rectum, is harmless when repeated after three or four days if it is necessary, and, as before mentioned, only at the beginning of the treatment—for the antipsoric medicines, among which in this respect lycopodium next to sulphur has the pre-eminence, usually soon remove this difficulty.

The inexcusable wasting fontanels the homœopathic physician must not at once suppress, if the patient has had them for some time (often for many years), nor before the antipsoric treatment has already made perceptible progress, but if they can be diminished without totally stopping them, this may safely be done even in the beginning of the treatment.

So also the physician should not at once discontinue the woolen underclothing, which is said to prevent the taking of cold and the recommendation of which is carried very far by the ordinary physicians in default of any real assistance. Though they are a burden to the patient, we should wait until there is a visible improvement

*This may well be pardoned with journeymen and beginners; but when they assume to boast of this noviceship and declare in public journals and books that the incidental use of blood-letting and leeches is indispensable, yea, that it is more essentially homœopathic, they become ridiculous and are to be pitied as tyros and as laboring under delusion; and their patients also are to be pitied. Is it laziness or a haughty preference for their old (although ruinous) allopathic routine, or is it lack of love for their fellowmen which prevents a deeper entering into true, beneficent Homœopathy and an elevation into the troublesome but correct and useful selection of the remedy homœopathically specific in every case, and into that mastery of Homœopathy now no more rare?

effected by the antipsorics which remove the tendency to taking cold, and until the warmer season comes. With patients who are very weakly, he should in the beginning change to cotton shirts which rub and heat the skin less, before requiring patients to put linen underclothing on their skin.

For many easily perceived reasons, but especially in order that his delicate doses of medicine may not be interfered with in their action, the homœopathic physician can not in his antipsoric treatment allow the intermediate use of any hitherto customary domestic remedy, no perfumery of any kind, no fragrant extracts, no smelling-salts, no Baldwin tea, or any other herb teas, no peppermint confection, no spiced confections or anise-sugar or stomach drops, or liqueurs, no Iceland-moss, or spiced chocolate, no spice-drops, tooth-tinctures or tooth-powders of the ordinary kinds, nor any of the other articles of luxury.

So-called warm and hot baths for the sake of cleanliness, to which spoiled patients are usually very much attached, are not to be allowed, as they never fail to disturb the health; nor are they needed, as a quick washing of a part or of the whole of the body with lukewarm soap-water fully serves the purpose without doing any injury.

At the end of these directions for treating chronic diseases, I recommended, in the first edition, the lightest electric sparks as an adjuvant for quickening parts that have been for a long time paralyzed and without sensation, these to be used besides the antipsoric treatment. I am sorry for this advice, and take it back, as experience has taught me, that this prescription has nowhere been followed strictly, but that larger electric sparks have always been used to the detriment of patients; and yet these larger sparks have been asserted to be very small. I, therefore, now advise against this so easily abused remedy, especially, as we can easily remove this appearance of enantiopathic assistance; for there is an efficient *homœopathic* local assistance for paralyzed parts or such as are without sensation. This is found in cold water* locally applied (at 54° Fahrenheit) from mountain-springs and deep wells; either by pouring on these parts for one, two or three minutes, or by douche-baths over the whole body of one to five minutes duration, more rarely or more frequently, even daily or oftener according to the circumstances, together with the appropriate, internal, antipsoric treatment, sufficient exercise in the open air, and judicious diet.

* Water of this and a lower temperature has the primary power of depriving the parts of the living body partly of sensation and partly of motion, in such cases it therefore gives local homœopathic assistance.

THE MEDICINES.

The medicines which have been found most suitable and excellent in chronic diseases so far, I shall present in the following part according to their pure action on the human body, as well those used in the treatment of the diseases of psoric origin, as those used in syphilis and in the figwart-disease.

That we need far fewer remedies to combat the latter than the psora can not with any thinking man form an argument against the chronic miasmatic nature of the latter and still less against the fact that it is the common source of the other chronic diseases.

The psora, a most ancient miasmatic disease, in propagating itself for many thousands of years through several millions of human organisms, of which each one had its own peculiar constitution and was exposed to very varied influences, was able to modify itself to such a degree as to cause that incredible variety of ailments which we see in the innumerable chronic patients, with whom the external symptom (which acts vicariously for the internal malady), *i. e.* the more or less extensive eruption of itch, has been driven away from the skin by a fatal art, or in whom it has disappeared of itself from the skin through some other violent incident.

Hence it seems to have come to pass that this half-spiritual miasma, which like a parasite seeks to inroot its hostile life in the human organism and to continue its life there, could develop itself in so many ways in the many thousands of years, so that it has even caused to spring forth and has born modified offshoots with characteristic properties, which do not indeed deny their descent from their stock (the common psora) but, nevertheless, differ from one another considerably by some peculiarities. These changes are due in some part to the varying physical peculiarities and climatic differences of the dwelling-places of men afflicted with the psora,* and in part are moulded by their varying modes of life, *e. g.* children in

* E. g. the *Sibbens* or *Rade-Syge* commonly found in Norway and in the northwest of Scotland; the *Pellagra* in Lombardy; the *plica polonica* (Koltun, Trichiasis) in Poland and Carinthia, the tumorous leprosy in Surinam; the raspberry-like excrescences (Frambösia) in Guinea called *yaws* and in America *pian;* the exhaustive fever in Hungary called *Tsömör*, the exhausting malady of Virginia (*asthenia Virginensium*), the human degeneration in the deep Alpine villages called *cretin*, the *goitre* in the deep valleys and at their entrances, etc.

the corrupt city air develop rhachitis, *spina ventosa*, *softening of the bones. curvatures. cancer of the bones. tinea capitis*, scrofula, ringworm; adults exhibit nervous debility, nervous irritability, gout of the joints, etc. And so also the other great varieties in the mode of ilving and in the occupations of men with their inherited bodily constitutions give to the psoric diseases so many modifications, that it may easily be understood, that more numerous and more varied remedies are needed for the extirpation of all these modifications of the psora (antipsoric remedies).

I have often been asked by what signs a substance may beforehand be recognized as antipsoric? But there can be no such external visible marks in them; nevertheless while proving several powerful substances as to their pure effects on the healthy body, several of them by the complaints they caused showed me their extraordinary and manifest suitableness for homœopathic aid in the symptoms of clearly defined psoric diseases. Some traces of their qualities leading in this direction gave me in advance some hint as to their probable usefulness; *e. g.* the efficacy of the herb *Lycopodium*, much praised in Poland for the *plica polonica* pointed me to the use of the pollen of lycopodium in similar psoric ailments. The circumstance that some hemorrhages have been arrested by large doses of salt was another hint. So was the usefulness of Guaiacum, Sarsaparilla and Mezereum, even in ancient times where venereal diseases could not be healed by any amount of mercury unless one or the other of these herbs had first removed the psora complicated with it.

As a rule it was developed from their pure symptoms, that most of the earths, alkalies and acids, as well as the neutral salts composed of them, together with several of the metals cannot be dispensed with in curing the almost innumerable symptoms of psora. The similarity in nature of the leading antipsoric, sulphur, to phosphorus and other combustible substances from the vegetable and the mineral kingdoms led to the use of the latter, and some animal substances naturally followed them by analogy, in agreement with experience.

Still only those remedies have been acknowledged as antipsoric whose pure effects on the human health gave a clear indication of their homœopathic use in diseases manifestly psoric, confessedly due to infection; so that, with an enlargement of our knowledge of their proper, pure medicinal effects, in time it may be found necessary to include some of our other medicines among the antipsoric remedies; although even now we can with certainty cure, with the antipsorics now recognized, nearly all non-venereal (psoric) chronic diseases, if the patients have not been loaded down and spoiled through allopathic mismanagement with severe medicine-diseases, and when their vital force has not been depressed too low, or very unfavorable external circumstances make the cure impossible. Nevertheless, it need not be specially stated that the other proved, homœopathic medicines, not excepting *mercury*, cannot be dispensed with in certain states of the psoric diseases.

Homœopathy, by a certain treatment of the crude medicinal substances, which had not been invented before its foundation and development, advances them into the state of progressive and high development of their indwelling forces, in order that it may then use them in curing in the most perfect manner. Some of these medicines in their crude state seem to have a very imperfect, insignificant medicinal action (*e. g.* common salt and the pollen of lycopodium). Others (*e. g.* gold, quartz, alumina) seem to have none at all, but all of them become highly curative by the preparation peculiar to Homœopathy. Other substances, on the other hand, in their crude state are, even in the smallest quantities, so violent in their effects that if they touch the animal fibre, they act upon it in a corroding and destructive manner (*e. g.* arsenic and corrosive sublimate) and these medicines are rendered by the same preparation peculiar to Homœopathy not only mild in their effects, but also incredibly developed in their medicinal powers.

The changes which take place in material substances, especially in medicinal ones, through long-continued trituration with a non-medicinal powder, or when dissolved, through a long-continued shaking with a non-medicinal fluid, are so incredible, that they approach the miraculous, and it is a cause of joy that the discovery of these wonderful changes belongs to Homœopathy.

Not only, as shown elsewhere, do these medicinal substances thereby develop their powers in a prodigious degree, but they also change their physico-chemical demeanor in such a way, that if no one before could ever perceive in their crude form any solubility in alcohol or water, after this peculiar transmutation they become wholly soluble in water as well as in alcohol—a discovery invaluable to the healing art.

The brown-black juice of the marine animal *Sepia*, which was formerly only used for drawing and painting, is in its crude state soluble only in water, not in alcohol; but by such a trituration it becomes soluble also in alcohol.

The yellow Petroleum only allows something to be extracted from it through alcohol when it is adulterated with ethereal vegetable oil; but in its pure state while crude it is soluble neither in water nor in alcohol (nor in ether). By trituration it becomes soluble in both substances.

So also the *pollen of lycopodium* floats on alcohol and on water, without either of them showing any action upon it—the crude lycopodium is tasteless and inactive when it enters the human stomach; but when changed in a similar manner through trituration it is not only perfectly soluble in either fluid, but has also developed such extraordinary medicinal powers, that great care must be taken in its medicinal use.

Who ever found marble or oyster-shells soluble in pure water or in alcohol? But this mild *lime* becomes perfectly soluble in either, by means of this mode of preparation; the same is the case with *baryta* and *magnesia* and these substances then exhibit astonishing medicinal powers.

Least of all will anyone ascribe solubility in water and alcohol to quartz, to rock-crystal (many crystals of which have contained enclosed in them drops of water for thousands of years unchanged), or to sand; nor would any one ascribe to them medicinal power, and yet by the dynamization (potentizing)* peculiar to Homœopathy, by melting silica with an alkaline salt, and then precipitating it from this glass, it not only becomes soluble without any residuum in water and in alcohol, but also then shows prodigious medicinal powers.

What can I say of the pure metals and of their sulphurets, but that all of them, without any exception become by this treatment equally soluble in water and in alcohol, and every one of them develops the medicinal virtue peculiar to it in the purest, simplest manner and in an incredibly high degree?

But the chemical medicinal substances thus prepared now also stand above the *chemical* laws.

A dose of phosphorus, potentized highly in a similar manner, may lie in its paper envelope in the desk, and, nevertheless, when taken after a whole year's interval, it will still show its full medicinal power; not that of phosphoric acid, but that of the unchanged, uncombined phosphorus itself. So that no neutralization takes place in this its elevated, and as it were, glorified state.

The medicinal effects of natrum carbonicum, of ammonium car-

---

*In its crude condition and without this preparation quartz and pebbles do not seem to allow a development of their medicinal powers by trituration and therefore it is that the triturating of various medicines with the indifferent sugar of milk in the porcelain triturating bowl seems to impart to them no admixture of *silicea* as some anxious purists have vainly feared.

bonicum, of baryta, of lime, and of magnesia, in this highly potentized state, when a dose of one of them has been taken, is not neutralized like basic substances taken in a crude form by a drop of vinegar taken afterwards; their medicinal effect being neither changed nor destroyed.

Nitric acid when thus given in its highly potentized state in which it is serviceable for homœopathic medicinal use, is not changed by a little crude lime or crude soda given after it, as to its strong well defined medicinal action; therefore it is not neutralized.

In this *preparation*, peculiar to Homœopathy, we take one grain in powder of any of the substances treated of in the six volumes of Materia Medica Pura,* and especially those of the antipsoric substances † following below, *i. e.*, of silica, carbonate of baryta, carbonate of lime, carbonate of soda and sal ammoniac, carbonate of magnesia, vegetable charcoal, animal charcoal, graphites, sulphur, crude antimony, metallic antimony, gold, platina, iron, zinc, copper, silver, tin. The lumps of the metals which have not yet been beaten out into foil, are rubbed off on a fine, hard whetstone under water, some of them, as iron, under alcohol; of mercury in the liquid form one grain is taken, of petroleum one drop instead of a grain, etc. This is first put on about one-third of 100 grains of pulverized sugar of milk, and

* Vegetable substances which can only be procured dry, *e. g.*, cinchona bark, ipecacuanha, etc., are prepared by the same kind of trituration and will completely dissolve when potentized a million fold, not less, with their peculiar powers, in water and alcohol, and may then be preserved as medicines far more easily than the easily spoiled alcoholic tinctures. Of the juiceless vegetable substances, such as oleander, thuja, the bark of mezereum, etc., we may, without making a mistake, take of each about one and a half grains of the fresh leaves, bark, root, etc., without any further preparation, and triturate the same three times with 100 grains of sugar of milk to the millionfold powder trituration. A grain of this dissolved in alcohol and water may be developed in the diluting vials with alcohol to the necessary degree of potency of their powers by giving for each potency two succussive strokes. Also with the freshly expressed juices of the herbs it is best to at once put one drop of the same with as much sugar of milk as is taken for the preparation of the other medicines, so as to triturate it to the millionfold powder attenuation, and then a grain of this attenuation is dissolved in equal parts of water and alcohol, and must be potentized to a further dynamization through the twenty-seven diluting vials by means of two succussive strokes. The fresh juices thus seem to acquire more of dynamization, as experience teaches me, than when the juice without any preparation by triturating is merely diluted in thirty vials of alcohol and potentized each time with two succussive strokes.

† Even phosphorus which is so easily oxidized by exposure to the air is potentized in a similar manner, and thus rendered soluble in these two liquids, and is thus prepared as a homœopathic medicine; but in this case some precautions are used, which will be found below.

placed in an unglazed porcelain mortar, or in one from which the glaze has been first rubbed off with wet sand; the medicine and the sugar of milk are then mixed for a moment with a porcelain spatula, and the mixture is triturated with some force for six minutes, the triturated substance is then for four minutes scraped from the mortar and from the porcelain pestle,* which is also unglazed, or has had its glazing rubbed off with wet sand, so that the trituration may be homogeniously mixed. After this has been thus scraped together, it is triturated again without any addition for another six minutes with equal force. After scraping together again from the bottom and the sides for four minutes this triturate (for which the first third of the 100 grains had been used), the second third of the sugar of milk is now added, both are mixed together with the spatula for a moment, triturated again with like force for six minutes; then having again scraped the triturate for four minutes, it is triturated a second time (without addition) for six minutes more, and after scraping it together for another four minutes it is mixed with the last third of the powdered sugar of milk by stirring it around with the spatula, and then the whole mixture is again triturated for six minutes, scraped for four minutes, and a second and last time triturated for six minutes; then it is all scraped together and the powder is preserved in a well-stoppered bottle with the name of the substance and the signature 100 because it is potentized one hundred fold.†

* That after the completion of every three hours' trituration of a medicinal substance, the mortar, pestle and spatula are to be several times scalded with boiling water, being after every scalding wiped quite dry and clean, I presuppose as indispensable, so that no idea of spoiling any medicine that may be triturated in it in future may be entertained. If the further precaution is used of exposing mortar, pestle and spatula to a heat approaching red heat, this will dissipate every thought that any least rest of the medicine last triturated can cling to them, and thus even the most scrupulous mind will be satisfied.

† Only phosphorus needs some modification in the preparation of the first attenuation to the 100th degree. Here the hundred grains of sugar of milk are at once put into the triturating bowl and, with about twelve drops of water they are stirred by means of the wet pestle into a thickish pap; one grain of phosphorus is then cut into numerous pieces, say twelve, and kneaded in with the moist pestle and rather stamped than rubbed into it, while the mass which often clings to the pestle is as often scraped into the mortar. Thus the little crumbs of phosphorus are rubbed to little invisible dust particles in the thick pap of sugar of milk even in the first two periods of six minutes each, without the appearance of the least spark. During the third period of six minutes the stamping may pass over into rubbing, because the mass is then approaching the form of powder. During the succeeding three periods of six minutes each the trituration is carried on only with a moderate force, and after every six minutes the powder is scraped from the mortar and the pestle for several minutes, which is done easily, as this powder does not adhere tenaciously. After the sixth period

To potentize the substance to the ten thousandth attenuation, one grain of the powder last mentioned as being the one hundredth is taken with one-third of 100 grains of fresh sugar of milk, stirred in the mortar with a spatula and treated as above, so that every third is triturated twice for six minutes at a time, and after every trituration is scraped together (for about four minutes), before the second third of the sugar of milk is added and after this has been similarly treated the last third of sugar of milk is stirred into it and again similarly triturated twice for six minutes at a time, when it is scraped together, put in a stoppered vial with the signature $\frac{}{10000}$ as it contains the medicine potentized to the ten thousandth attenuation.*

The same is done with one grain of this powder (marked $\frac{}{10000}$) in order to bring it to I, and thus to attenuate it to the millionfold potency.

In order to produce a homogeneity in the preparation of the homœopathic and especially the antipsoric remedies, at least in the form of powders, I advise the reducing of medicines only to this millionth potency, no more and no less and to prepare from this the solutions and the necessary potencies of these solutions; this has been my own custom.

The trituration should be done with force, yet only with so much force that the sugar of milk may not be pressed too firmly to the mortar, but may be scraped up in four minutes.

Now in preparing the solutions † from this, and in bringing the medicines thus potentized one millionfold, into the fluid form, (so that their dynamization may be still further continued), we are aided by the property of *all* medicinal substances, that, when brought to the potency I, they are soluble in water and alcohol; this property is still unknown to chemistry.

---

of trituration the powder, when standing exposed to the air in the dark, is only feebly luminous, and has but a slight odor. It is put into a well-stoppered vial and marked phosphorus $\frac{}{100}$, the other two triturations $\frac{}{10000}$, and $\frac{1}{\text{mill.}}$ are prepared like those from other dry medicinal substances.

* Thus it will be seen that every attenuation (that to $\frac{}{100}$, that to $\frac{}{10000}$, and also the third to $\frac{}{1000000}$ or I) is prepared by six times triturating for six minutes and six times scraping together for four minutes each time. Thus each one requires one hour.

† In the beginning I used to give a small part of a grain of the powders potentized to the $\frac{}{10000}$ or the I degree by trituration, as a dose. But since *a small part of a grain* is too indefinite a quantity, and since Homœopathy must avoid all indefiniteness and inexactness as much as possible, the discovery that all medicines may be changed from potentized medicinal powders into fluids with which a definite number of pellets may be moistened for a dose, was of great value to me From liquids the higher potencies may also be easily prepared.

The first solution cannot be made in pure alcohol, because sugar of milk will not dissolve in alcohol. The first solution is therefore made in a mixture of half water and half alcohol.

To one grain of the medicinal powder triturated to the millionfold potency I, fifty drops of distilled water are dropped in and by turning the vial a few times round on its axis it is easily dissolved, when fifty drops of good alcohol* are added, and the vial, which ought only to be filled to two-thirds of its capacity by the mixture, ought to be stoppered and shaken twice (*i. e.* with two down-strokes of the arm). It is marked with the name of the medicine and $\overline{100\ \text{I}}$.† One drop of this is added to ninety-nine or one hundred drops of pure alcohol, the stoppered vial is then shaken with two strokes of the arm and marked with the name of the medicine and designated $\overline{10000\ \text{I}}$. One drop of this is added to ninety-nine or one hundred drops of pure alcohol, the corked vial is then shaken with two strokes of the arm and marked with the name of the medicine and $_{\text{II}}$. The preparation of the higher potencies is then continued with two strokes of the arm‡ every time to the $\overline{100\ \text{II}}$, $\overline{10000\ \text{II}}$, $_{\text{III}}$, etc., but to attain a simple uniformity in practice only the vials with the full numbers $_{\text{II, III, IV, V,}}$‖ etc., are used in practice, but the intermediate

---

* For the fifty drops of water as well as for the fifty drops of alcohol a vial containing just that quantity may be used, so that we need not then count the drops, especially as drops of water are not easily counted when it flows from a vial, the mouth of which is not roughened by rubbing with sand.

† It will be well to mark on the label that it has been shaken twice, together with the date.

‡ After many experiments and searching comparisons with the patients I have for several years preferred from conviction to give to the medicinal fluids which are to be elevated to higher potencies and at the same time to be rendered milder, only two shakes (with two strokes of the arm) instead of the ten shakes given by others, because the potentizing in the latter case by the repeated shaking passes far beyond the attenuation at every step (though this is one hundred fold); while yet the end striven for is to develop the medicinal powers only in the degree that the attenuation may reach the end aimed for: to moderate in some degree the strength of the medicine while its power of penetration is increased. The double shake also increases the quantity of the medicinal forces developed, like the tenfold shake, but not in as high a degree as the latter, so that its strength may, nevertheless, be kept down by the one hundred fold attenuation effected, and we thus obtain every time a weaker though somewhat more highly potentized and more penetrating medicine.

‖ Instead of the fractional numbers $\frac{1}{1000000}$ $(\frac{1}{\text{I}})$, $\frac{1}{1000000000000}$ $(\frac{1}{\text{II}})$, etc., these degrees of dynamization are frequently so expressed that only the exponent showing how often one hundred has been multiplied into itself is expressed, thus instead of ^{1}, $_{100}(^{3})$: instead of $\frac{1}{\text{II}}$, $_{100}(^{6})$; instead of ^{1}, $_{100}(^{9})$; instead of $\frac{1}{100}\text{III}$ $_{100}(^{10})$; instead of $\frac{1}{10000}\text{IX}$, $_{100}(^{29})$ and instead of decillion $\frac{1}{\text{X}}$, $_{100}(^{30})$, thus only the exponents as to the third, sixth, ninth, tenth, twenty-ninth and thirtieth potency, etc.

numbers are preserved in boxes or cases with their labels. Thus they will be protected from the effect of daylight.

As the shaking is *only* to take place through *moderate* strokes of the arm, the hand of which holds the vial, it is best to choose the vials just so large that they will be two-thirds filled with 100 drops of the attenuated medicine.

Vials that have contained a remedy must never be used for the reception of any other medicine, though they be rinsed ever so often, but new vials must be taken every time.

The pellets which are to be moistened with the medicine should also be selected of the same size, hardly as large as poppy-seeds, made by the confectioner, partly so that the dose may be made small enough, and partly that homœopathic physicians in the preparation of medicines, as also in the giving of doses, may act alike, and thus be able to compare the result of their practice with that of other Homœopaths in the most certain manner.

The moistening of pellets is best done with a quantity, so that a drachm or several drachms of pellets are put into a little dish of stoneware, porcelain or glass; this dish should be more deep than wide, in the form of a large thimble; several drops of the spirituous medicinal fluid should be dropped into it (rather a few drops too many), so that they may penetrate to the bottom and will have moistened all the pellets within a minute. Then the dish is turned over and emptied on a piece of clean double blotting paper, so that the superfluous fluid may be absorbed by it, and when this is done, the pellets are spread on the paper so as to dry quickly. When dry, the pellets are filled in a vial, marked as to its contents, and well stoppered.

All pellets moistened with the spirituous liquid have when dry a dull appearance; the crude, unmoistened pellets look whiter and more shining.

To prepare the pellets to give to patients, one or a couple of such little pellets are put into the open end of a paper capsule containing two or three grains of powdered sugar of milk; this is then stroked with a spatula or the nail of the thumb with some degree of pressure until it is felt, that the pellet or pellets are crushed and broken, then the pellets will easily dissolve if put into water.

Wherever I mention pellets in giving medicine, I always mean the finest, of the size of poppy-seeds, of which about 200 (more or less) weigh a grain.

The antipsoric medicines treated of in what follows contain no so-called *idiopathic* medicines, since their pure effects, even those of the potentized miasma of itch (*Psorin*) have not been proved enough, by far, that a safe homœopathic use might be made of it. I say *homœopathic* use, for it does not remain *idem* (the same); even if the prepared itch substance should be given to the same patient from whom it was taken, it would not remain *idem* (the same), as it could only be useful to him in a potentized state, since crude itch substance which he has already in his body as an *idem* is without effect on him. But the dynamization or potentizing changes it and modifies it; just as gold leaf after potentizing is no more crude gold leaf inert in the human body, but in every stage of dynamization it is more and more modified and changed.

Thus potentized and modified also, the itch substance (*Psorin*) when taken is no more an *idem* (same) with the crude original itch substance, but only a *simillimum* (thing most similar). *For between* IDEM *and* SIMILLIMUM *there is no intermediate for any one that can think;* or in other words between *idem* and *simile* only *simillimum* can be intermediate. Isopathic and *æquale* are equivocal expressions, which if they should signify anything reliable can only signify *simillimum*, because they are not *idem* (ταυτον).

SECOND PART.

ANTIPSORIC MEDICINES.

PREFACE

CONCERNING THE TECHNICAL PART OF HOMŒOPATHY.[1]

Since I last* addressed the public concerning our healing art, I have had among other things also the opportunity to gain experience as to the best possible mode of administering the doses of the medicines to the patients, and I herewith communicate what I have found best in this respect.

A small pellet of one of the highest dynamizations of a medicine laid dry upon the tongue, or the moderate smelling of an opened vial wherein one or more such pellets are contained, proves itself the smallest and weakest dose with the shortest period of duration in its effects. Still there are numerous patients of so excitable a nature, that they are sufficiently affected by such a dose in slight acute ailments to be cured by it if the remedy is homœopathically selected. Nevertheless the incredible variety among patients as to their irritability, their age, their spiritual and bodily development, their vital power and especially as to the nature of their disease, necessitates a great variety in their treatment, and also in the administration to them of the doses of medicines. For their diseases may be of various kinds: either a natural and simple one but lately arisen, or it may be a natural and simple one but an old case, or it may be a complicated one (a combination of several miasmata), or again what is the most frequent and worst case, it may have been spoiled by a perverse medical treatment, and loaded down with medicinal diseases.

I can here limit myself only to this latter case, as the other cases cannot be arranged in tabular form for the weak and negligent, but must be left to the accuracy, the industry and the intelligence of able men, who are masters of their art.

Experience has shown me, as it has no doubt also shown to most of my followers, that it is most useful in diseases of any magnitude (not excepting even the most acute, and still more so in the half-

---

[1] This preface was prefixed to Vol. III. of the "Chronic Diseases," published in the year 1837.—*Tr.*

* In the beginning of the year 1834 I wrote the first two parts of this work and although they together contain only thirty-six sheets, my former publisher, Mr. Arnold, in Dresden, took two years to publish these thirty-six sheets. By whom was he thus delayed? My acquaintances can guess that.

acute, in the tedious and most tedious) to give to the patient the powerful homœopathic pellet or pellets only in solution, and this solution in divided doses. In this way we give the medicine, dissolved in seven to twenty tablespoonfuls of water without any addition, in acute and very acute diseases every six, four or two hours; where the danger is urgent, even every hour or every half-hour, a tablespoonful at a time; with weak persons or children, only a small part of a tablespoonful (one or two teaspoonfuls or coffeespoonfuls) may be given as a dose.

In chronic diseases I have found it best to give a dose (*e. g.*, a spoonful) of a solution of the suitable medicine at least every two days, more usually every day.

But since water (even distilled water) commences after a few days to be spoil, whereby the power of the small quantity of medicine contained is destroyed, the addition of a little alcohol is necessary, or where this is not practicable, or if the patient cannot bear it, I add a few small pieces of hard charcoal to the watery solution. This answers the purpose, except that in the latter case the fluid in a few days receives a blackish tint. This is caused by shaking the liquid, as is necessary every time before giving a dose of medicine, as may be seen below.

Before proceeding, it is important to observe, that our vital principle cannot well bear that the same unchanged dose of medicine be given even twice in succession, much less more frequently to a patient. For by this the good effect of the former dose of medicine is either neutralized in part, or new symptoms proper to the medicine, symptoms which have not before been present in the disease, appear, impeding the cure. Thus even a well selected homœopathic medicine produces ill effects and attains its purpose imperfectly or not at all. Thence come the many contradictions of homœopathic physicians with respect to the repetition of doses.

But in taking one and the same medicine repeatedly (which is *indispensable* to secure the cure of a serious, chronic disease), if the dose is in every case varied and modified only a little in its degree of dynamization, then the vital force of the patient will calmly, and as it were willingly receive *the same* medicine even at brief intervals very many times in succession with the best results, every time increasing the well-being of the patient.

This slight change in the degree of dynamization is even effected, if the bottle which contains the solution of one or more pellets is merely well shaken five or six times, every time before taking it.

Now when the physician has in this way used up the solution of the medicine that had been prepared, if the medicine continues useful, he will take one or two pellets of the same medicine in a lower potency (*e. g.* if before he had used the thirtieth dilution, he will now take one or two pellets of the twenty-fourth), and will make a solution in about as many spoonfuls of water, shaking up the bottle, and adding a little alcohol or a few pieces of charcoal. This last solution may then be taken in the same manner, or at longer intervals, perhaps also less of the solution at a time; but every time the solution must be shaken up five or six times. This will be continued so long as the remedy still produces improvement and until new ailments (such as have never yet occurred with other patients in this disease), appear; for in such a case a new remedy will have to be used. On any day when the remedy has produced too strong an action, the dose should be omitted for a day. If the symptoms of the disease alone appear, but are considerably aggravated even during the more moderate use of the medicine, then the time has come to break off in the use of the medicine for one or two weeks, and to await a considerable improvement.*

When the medicine has been consumed and it is found necessary to continue the same remedy, if the physician should desire to prepare a new portion of medicine from the same degree of potency, it will be necessary to give to the new solution as many shakes, as the number of shakes given to the last portion amount to when summed up together, and then a few more, before the patient is given the first dose; but after that, with the subsequent doses, the solution is to be shaken up only five or six times.

In this manner the homœopathic physician will derive all the benefit from a well selected remedy, which can be obtained in any special case of chronic disease by doses given through the mouth.

But if the diseased organism is affected by the physician through

* In treating acute cases of disease the homœopathic physician will proceed in a similar manner. He will dissolve one (two) pellet of the highly potentized, well selected medicine in seven, ten or fifteen tablespoonfuls of water (without addition) by shaking the bottle. He will then, according as the disease is more or less acute, and more or less dangerous, give the patient every half hour, or every hour, every two, three, four, six hours (after again well shaking the bottle) a whole or a half tablespoonful of the solution, or, in the case of a child, even less. If the physician sees no new symptoms develop, he will continue at these intervals, until the symptoms present at first begin to be aggravated; then he will give it at longer intervals and less at a time.

As is well known, in cholera the suitable medicine has often to be given at far shorter intervals.

Children are always given these solutions from their usual drinking vessels; a teaspoon for drinking is to them unusal and suspicious, and they will refuse the tasteless liquid at once on that account. A little sugar may be added for their sake.

this same appropriate remedy at the same time in sensitive spots other than the nerves of the mouth and the alimentary canal, *i. e.* if this same remedy that has been found useful is at the same time in its watery solution rubbed in (even in small quantities) into one or more parts of the body which are most free from the morbid ailments (*e. g.* on an arm, or on the thigh or leg, which have neither cutaneous eruptions, nor pains, nor cramps)—then the curative effects are *much* in creased. The limbs which are thus rubbed with the solution may also be varied, first one, then another. Thus the physician will receive a greater action from the medicine homœopathically suitable to the chronic patient, and can cure him more quickly, than by merely internally administering the remedy.

This mode of procedure has been frequently proved by myself and found extraordinarily curative; yea, attended by the most startling good effects; the medicine taken internally being at the same time rubbed on the skin externally. This procedure will also explain the wonderful cures, of rare occurrence indeed, where chronic crippled patients *with sound skin* recovered quickly and permanently by a few baths in a mineral water, the medicinal constituents of which were to a great degree homœopathic to their chronic disease.*

The limb, therefore, on which the solution is to be rubbed in, must be *free from cutaneous ailments.* In order to introduce also here change and variation, when several of the limbs are free from cutaneous ailments, one limb after the other should be used, in alternation, on different days, (best on days when the medicine is not taken internally). A small quantity of the solution should be rubbed in with the hand, until the limb is dry. Also for this purpose, the bottle should be shaken five or six times.

Convenient as the mode of administering the medicine above described may be, and much as it surely advances the cure of chronic diseases, nevertheless, the greater quantity of alcohol or whiskey or

---

*On the other hand such baths have also inflicted a proportionally greater injury with patients who suffered from ulcers and cutaneous eruptions; for these were driven by them from the skin, as may be done by other external means, when after a short period of health, the vital force of the patient transferred the internal uncured disease to another part of the body, and one much more important to life and health. Thus *e. g.* may be produced the obscuration of the crystalline lens, the paralysis of the optic nerve, the destruction of the sense of hearing; pains also of innumerable kinds in consequence torture the patient, his mental organs suffer, his mind becomes obscured, spasmodic asthma threatens to suffocate him, or an apoplectic stroke carries him off, or some other dangerous or unbearable disease takes the place of the former ailment. Therefore the homœopathic remedy given internally must never be rubbed in on parts which suffer from external ailments.

the several lumps of charcoal which have to be added in warmer weather to preserve the watery solution were still objectionable to me with many patients.

I have, therefore, lately found the following mode of administration preferable with careful patients. From a mixture of about five tablespoonfuls of pure water and five tablespoonfuls of French brandy—which is kept on hand in a bottle, 200, 300 or 400 drops (according as the solution is to be weaker or stronger) are dropped into a little vial, which may be half-filled with it, and in which the medicinal powder or the pellet or pellets of the medicine have been placed. This vial is stoppered and shaken until the medicine is dissolved. From this solution one, two, three or several drops, according to the irritability and the vital force of the patient, are dropped into a cup, containing a spoonful of water; this is then well stirred and given to the patient, and where more especial care is necessary, only the half of it may be given; half a spoonful of this mixture may also well be used for the above mentioned external rubbing.

On days, when only the latter is administered, as also when it is taken internally, the little vial containing the drops must every time be briskly shaken five or six times; so also the drop or drops of medicine with the tablespoonful of water must be well stirred in the cup.

It would be still better if instead of the cup a vial should be used, into which a tablespoonful of water is put, which can then be shaken five or six times and then wholly or half emptied for a dose.

Frequently it is useful in treating chronic diseases to take the medicine, or to rub it in in the evening, shortly before going to sleep, because we have then less disturbance to fear from without, than when it is done earlier.

When I was still giving the medicines in undivided portions, each with some water at a time, I often found that the potentizing in the attenuating glasses effected by ten shakes was too strong (*i. e.*, the medicinal action too strongly developed) and I, therefore, advised only two succussions. But during the last years, since I have been giving every dose of medicine in an incorruptible solution, divided over fifteen, twenty or thirty days and even more, no potentizing in an attenuating vial is found too strong, and I again use ten strokes with each. So I herewith take back what I wrote on this subject three years ago in the first volume of this book on page 149.

In cases where a great irritability of the patient is combined with extreme debility, and the medicine can only be administered by allowing the patient to smell a few small pellets contained in a vial, when the medicine is to be used for several days, I allow the patient to smell daily of a different vial, containing the same medicine, indeed, but every time of a lower potency, once or twice with each nostril according as I wish him to be affected more or less.

ANTIPSORIC MEDICINES.

AGARICUS MUSCARIUS.*

(TOAD-STOOL.)

Agaricus is the fetid toad-stool with scarlet-red top, which is studded with whitish warts and has a white border. Of the toad-stool carefully dried take one grain, or two grains of the fresh plant, and triturate it like any of the other medicines with sugar of milk for three hours; this preparation is afterwards dissolved, attenuated and potentized by two successive strokes for every potency until we reach the thirtieth potency (or x).

Apelt found it useful in pains of the upper jaw-bone and of the teeth, as well as in pains of the bones of the lower limbs (seemingly in the marrow) and finally in itching eruptions as large as millet seeds, set closely together; as also in lassitude following coition.

Whistling cured with it convulsions and trembling, and *J. C. Bernhard* cured with it even several varieties of epilepsy.

Dr. Woost saw the effects of agaricus in large does extend for seven or eight weeks.

Camphor is the chief antidote in ailments due to toad-stool even when they become chronic.

The abbreviations of the names of my fellow-provers are as follows:

Ap., Apelt; Gr., Dr. Gross; Fr. H., Dr. Frederick Hahnemann,

---

* Agaricus appears for the first time in this second edition, but Hahnemann acknowledges that his fellow observers and he himself also had already published their observations—Hahnemann with his son and Langhammer in Vol. IX., Apelt in Vol. X., of the *Archiv;* Gross Schreter and Stapf in the *Prakt. Mitth. d. cen. Gesell. hom. Aerzte* for 1828, Ng., Seidel, Sch., and Woost in Hartlaub and Trink's *Arzneimittellehre*, Vol. III., 1831. Apelt proved a tincture of the fresh fungus, beginning with six to eight drops of the tincture and going on to the twelfth and thirtieth potencies; he gives his symptoms in schema form only, and does not indicate how each one was obtained. Of the doses taken by Gross we have no record, and the same may be said of the remaining observers; but from the dates of their publications it may fairly be inferred that their provings were made after the earlier rather than the later manner. For the same reasons Hahnemann's own symptoms--to which no addition has here been made --may be accounted as derived from provings on the healthy and not from observations on the sick. Triturations of the dried fungus seem to have been used by all but Apelt. (Concerning Ng. see note on preface to Alumina.)--*Hughes.*

Lgh., *Dr. Langhammer; Ng.*, an anonymous contributor; *Sdl.*, *Seidel; St.*, *Medicinalrath Dr. Stapf; Schrt.*, *Schréter; Sch.*, another anonymous contributor; and *Wst.*, *Dr. Woost*, in Oschatz*

AGARICUS MUSCARIUS.

Dejection of mind. [*Ap.*]

Despondency. [*Ap.*]

Anxious forebodings, as if she were about to experience something disagreeable. [*Ap.*]

Unsteadiness and restlessness of spirit and of body (after ½ hour.) [*Schrt.*]

5. The mind is restless and troubled; he was always solely occupied with his present and his future condition. [*Lgh.*]

Disinclination to speak, without being ill-humored. [*Ap.*]

He compels himself to speak, but answers in few words, though otherwise cheerful. [*Ap.*]

It seems as if he could not find the words to express himself. [*Ap.*]

Disinclination to speak with fretfulness, peevishness and disinclination to work. [*Lgh.*]

10. Fretful mood. [*Wst.*]

Very peevish and irritable. [*Ap.*]

Ill-humored and indifferent. [*Sdl.*]

While at other times full of great solicitude, she is now altogether indifferent. [*Ap.*]

Indifferent, self-absorbed mood with aversion to all occupation. [*Sdl.*]

15. **Disinclination to all work.** [*Ap.—Gr.*]

He trifles with all manner of things, merely to avoid working. [*Schrt.*]

Disgust for all work which occupies the mind, and if he nevertheless undertakes it, there arise a rush of blood to the head, throbbing in the arteries, flushes in the face, and the thinking faculty is disturbed. [*Sdl.*]

Forgetful; he finds it difficult to recall what he has before heard and thought. [*Schrt.*]

Loss of consciousness. [LERGER, *Memorabilien* vol. iii, p. 334.]

20. Drunken fearless frenzy with bold, vengeful determinations. [*Voigtel* A. M. L. vol. ii, part ii, p. 352.]

Shy insanity. [MURRAY, *Apparatus Medicam*. v, 557.

---

*Throughout the work the symptoms without a name or mark are contributed by myself. With respect to the symptoms of other contributors, I have sometimes found it necessary for the convenience of my readers to abbreviate phrases unnecessarily extended, sometimes also to substitute more intelligible expressions in the place of obscure or idiomatic ones. I have not knowingly omitted anything essential.—*Sam. Hahnemann.*

Frenzy. [VOIGTEL ibid.]

Fearless, threatening, destructive frenzy, also such as turns against itself and injures itself, combined with great exertion of strength. [MURRAY ibid.]

Causes cheerfulness. [*Pharmakol. Lex.* vol. i, p. 74.]

25. Cheerful, careless mood. [*Wst.*]

Cheerful mood but without any impulse toward conversation. [*Ap.*]

Extravagant fancy, rapture, prophesying, making verses. [*Murray* ibid.]

Quiet, equable, sociable, active, and glad of having done his duty (curative action). [*Lgh.*]

Muddled feeling in the head. [*Ap.*]

30. Muddled feeling in the head with dull pains (aft. 2 h.). [*Schrt.*]

Muddled feeling and heaviness in the head (aft. 5 h.). [*Sch.*]

Continued heaviness in the head (aft. 5 h.). [*Sch.*]

Painful heaviness in the forehead (on 5th d.). [*Ng.*]

Sensation of a tugging down heaviness in the two temples, reaching to the middle of the ears, as if there were a heavy load hanging on both sides of the head, more during the day than in the morning, and worse when touched. [*Fr. H.*]

35. Heaviness of the head as after intoxication (aft. ½ h.). [*Schrt.*]

In the morning heaviness and chaotic sensation in the head, as if he had been on a spree the day before; this lasts for six days. [*Sch.*]

Dulness, imbecility (after-effects in old age). [*Murray, App. Med.* v, p. 557.]

Dizziness, stupefaction.

Dizziness as from intoxication. [VOIGTEL, ibid.]

40. Pleasant intoxication. [MURRAY, ibid.]

Drunkenness. [*Pharmakol. Lex.* ibid.]

Reeling and sinking down (on 2d d.). [LERGER, ibid].

Reeling when walking in the open air (aft. 1 h.) [*Ap.*]

Reeling as from spirituous liquors; in walking in the open air he staggers about. [*Lgh.*]

45. Vertigo.

Vertigo and stupidity in the morning (aft. 3 h.). [*Fr. H.*]

Vertigo in the morning as after a spree (aft. ¼ h.) [*Ap.*]

Vertigo coming on especially in the morning and lasting for 1-8 minutes, returning after short intervals several times during the day. [*Ap.*]

Strong sun-light in the morning causes a momentary vertigo, even to falling down. [*Wst.*]

50. Attacks of vertigo with a tottering gait and obscuration of the vision even as to near objects, coming and going at intervals of five minutes; this can only be entirely removed by the reception of different ideas. [*Ap.*]

Vertigo while meditating while walking in the open air (aft. 8 d.) [*Ap.*]

Attacks of vertigo in the open, air which passed away in the room, for several days. [*Sch.*]

Vertigo in the room while turning around. [*Ap.*]

Vertigo which passes away for a length of time by quickly turning about or by turning the head. [*Ap.*]

55. Headache early in bed. [*Ap.*]

Headaches of various kinds in the left half of the occipital bone, *while sitting*. [*Ap.*]

Dull headache in the right temple. [*Ap.*]

Dull headache especially **in the forehead**, during which he has to move his head to and fro; this causes the eyes to close as if for sleep. [*Ap.*]

Dull, stupefying headache with thirst and heat especially in the face (at once). [*Schrt.*]

60. Dull pressive headache which passes away after a copious stool, with flushes of heat. [*Wst.*]

Pressive headache in fits and starts, before going to bed.

Pressure in the frontal sinuses. [*Ap.*]

Violent pressive pain in the forehead with vertigo, while sitting down. [*Ap.*]

Pressure from the forehead down on the upper half of the eyeballs (aft. 1½ h.). [*Wst.*]

65. Violent pressure in the right temple or the temporal bone. [*Gr.*]

Pressure on the upper part of the left temporal bone just above the auricle, extending deep into the brain, increased by pressure or by touching the hair, attended with complete despondency. [*Ap.*]

Painful pressure in the zygomatic process of the left temporal bone. [*Gr.*]

Pressure in the occiput (on 1st d.). [*Sdl.*]

Violent pressive headache, especially in the occiput; after dinner (on 9th d.). [*Sdl.*]

70. Pressure with stitches in the forehead above the eyes. [*Ap.*]

Painful drawing pressure from the left side of the forehead to the right, while sitting down (aft. ½ h.) [*Lgh.*]

Drawing pains in the head, early on awaking, with pressure on the eye-balls. [*Sdl.*]

Drawing pain in the forehead. [*Ap.*]

Drawing from both sides of the frontal bone to the root of the nose. [*Gr.*]

75. Very painful drawing through the temples, forehead or eyeballs. [*Sdl.*]

Drawing in the head in all directions with a sensation as if becoming unconscious. [*Gr.*]

Drawing pain in the occiput, in the afternoon. [*Ap.*]

Drawing headache in the occiput early in bed, as if the result of lying in a wrong position, increased by extending the arms and stretching while holding the breath. [*Wst.*]

Drawing cutting pain in the forehead while standing; when sitting down this becomes a pressive stupefaction of the head (aft. 1½ h.). [*Lgh.*]

80. Intermittent drawing and tearing pain in the forehead (aft. 33 h.). [*Lgh.*]

Tearing in the forehead, just above the root of the nose. [*Ap.*]

Tearing in the region of the right temple. [*Gr.*]

Tearing in the left side of the occiput, returning at short intervals. [*Ap.*]

Jerking tearing in the head, terminating behind the right ear where it is most painful.

85. Headache as if the brain were being torn.

Tearing with pressure in the whole left circumference of the brain, strongest in the left orbit and zygoma with a muddled feeling in the head (aft. 8 h.). [*Gr.*]

Tearing stitches in the occiput from one side to the other, early in the morning (on the 2d d.). [*Wst.*]

Violent lancinating tearing from the crown to the left ear (aft. 6 h.). [*Wst.*]

Fine stitches in the right temple (aft. ½ h.). [*Schrt.*]

90. Burrowing pain in the head, lasting only a few minutes, but returning very frequently. [*Ap.*]

Violent burrowing pain in the left frontal eminence (aft. 3 h.). [*Ap.*]

Boring pains deep in the brain at the crown of the head. [*Ap.*]

Pain as from a nail in the right side of the head. [*Gr.*]

Throbbing in the crown of the head with a desperation bordering on frenzy.

95. Tearing drawing pains externally in the integuments of the head (the skin and bones), increased by pressure, especially in a little spot on the crown, which pains as if it were internally festering, at night (aft. 18 d.). [*Sdl.*]

Sensitiveness of the skin of the head as if ulcerating.

Twitches in the skin of the forehead over the right eye. [*Ap.*]

Repeated painless twitches on the right temple, beside the eye (the 7th d.). [*Ng.*]

Cramplike pain in the left temple (aft. 37 h.). [*Lgh.*]

100. Sensation of cold as of ice on the right frontal bone which is covered with hair, while externally it feels warm. [*Ap.*]

After a preceding itching and scratching, icy cold in the region of the coronal suture frequently returning, and progressively more in front until it comes into the part of the forehead not covered with hair. [*Ap.*]

Itching of the hairy scalp. [*Ap.*]

Itching of the whole hairy scalp, as if it were healing; this provokes scratching. [*Lgh.*]

Troublesome itching of the hairy scalp, especially early after rising; it passes away by scratching with a sharp comb. [*Wst.*]

105. Pimples on the hairy scalp. [*Ap.*]

In the eyebrows, itching. [*Ap.*]

Falling out of the hair of the eyebrows. [*Ap.*]

Pressure in the eyes. [*Fr. H.*]

Pressure in the left eyeball (aft. 10 h.). [*Wst.*]

110. Pressure in the eyes and inclination to close them, without sleepiness, after dinner. [*Ap.*]

Pressure in the eyes and upon the forehead, as if something were pressing inwardly (aft. 10 min.). [*Schrt.*]

Pressure in the corner of the left eye, as if from the presence of a foreign body. [*Ap.*]

Pressure and drawing in the eyeballs, especially on the left, reaching into the forehead (on 4th d.). [*Sdl.*]

Very painful drawing in the eyeballs (on 3d and 4th d.) [*Sdl.*]

115. Spasmodic pain under the curve of the right eyebrow, which renders the opening of the eyes difficult (aft. 5 h.). [*Lgh.*]

Itching and tickling in the right eye (aft. 1 h.). [*Schrt.*]

Tickling itching in the left eye, which necessitates rubbing (aft. 3 h.). [*Lgh.*]

Itching and quivering of the left lower eyelid, necessitating rubbing. [*Ap.*]

Itching and pressing in the right eye, which only ceases for a short time on rubbing it. [*Schrt.*]

120. **Burning of the eyes** with a sensation of contraction, in the evening (on 1st d.). [*Ng.*]

Burning of the inner canthi of the eyes, as though they were inflamed, with increased painfulness on being touched. [*Gr.*]

Burning in the inner canthi when he compresses the lids. [*Gr.*]

Burning pressive pains over the right eye with lachrymation (aft. 1½ h.). [*Sch.*]

Redness of the white of the eye. [*Fr. H.*]

125. Yellow color of the white of the eyes (on 3d d.). [*Sdl.*]

Swelling of the lids of the left eye toward the inner canthus, whereby the eye is somewhat diminished in size. [*Ap.*]

Contraction of the eyelids (aft. 2 h.). [*Schrt.*]

Contraction and narrowing of the inner canthus of the left eye. [*Ap.*]

Sensation of contraction of the right eye with increased brightness of vision, followed by itching in the eyeball and lachrymation, and finally twitching in the left eye such as had previously occurred in the right eye; wine at once did away with this symptom [*Ap.*][1]

130. **Contraction of the open space between the eyelids for several days** without swelling and often with twitching and quivering of the eyelids. [*Ap.*]

The open space between the eyelids is narrower than usual, and can only be enlarged by exertion. [*Schrt.*]

Twitching in the eyeballs often, first in one and then in the other, in the left eye it is sometimes accompanied with lachrymation. [*Ap.*]

Frequent twitching and pressure in the left eyeball while reading. [*Ap.*]

---

[1] 129. This symptom with 5, 327, 506, 582, 692, 694 and 708 on a second application occurred in a patient affected with involuntary twitching of the right eyelid, for which he held to the open eye for a few moments a vial of the thirtieth dilution.

Twitching with pressive pain in the left eyeball at any time of the day and under any circumstances; it necessitates wiping the eyes, but this does not cause it to cease. [*Ap.*]

135. Frequent quivering in the eyelids, mostly in only a small portion of them and extending more towards one canthus. [*Ap.*]

Quivering of the right lower eyelid, with pulsation of an artery to the left and at the back of the nose, and twitching in the skin on the left side of the nose. [*Ap.*]

Dryness of the eyes. [*Ap.*]

The lachrymal caruncle of the left eye is enlarged for several days. [*Ap.*]

Lachrymation of the right eye (on 1st and 2d d.). [*Ng.*]

140. Lachrymation of the right eye (aft. 3 h.). [*Schrt.*]

Sensation in the eyes as if they ought to be constantly wiped. [*Fr. H.*]

The eyelids are joined together as if by mucous threads, and this only passes away temporarily by wiping them.

Gum in the canthi of the eyes (aft. 6 h.). [*Lgh. Schrt.*]

Viscous yellow humor (at first white) **which glues the eyelids together**; this exudes continually, even during the day; but most in the mornings and evenings in the inner canthi. [*Gr.*]

145. The pupils are first dilated (aft. ¾ h.) then contracted (aft. 25 h.). [*Lgh.*]

Gradual diminution of the vision while walking in the open air (aft. 7 h.). [*Ap.*]

Great weariness (weakness) of the eyes, things grow pale if she looks for some time at any object. [*Ap.*]

Short-sightedness and dimness of vision of both eyes. [*Ap.*]

Very indistinct vision; objects must be quite near to his eyes in order that he may properly distinguish them. [*Ap.*]

150. He is obliged in reading to bring the letters more and more closely to his eyes, in order to distinguish them clearly, then he must at once remove them to a greater distance, as else the vision becomes dim again. [*Ap.*]

Dimness before the eyes, with sleepiness. [*Wst.*]

Dimness of vision, everything appears obscured as if seen through turbid water, so that he must make a great effort to recognize objects. [*Ap.*]

All objects appear enveloped in a fog and thus obscured. [*Ap.*]

Whatever comes before his eyes is as it were covered with a cobweb and obscured. [*Ap.*]

155. A black fly floats before his left eye at the distance of half a yard and when winking it flits to and fro. [*Fr. H.*]

In rainy weather a brown fly flits before the left eye toward the inner canthus. [*Ap.*]

In closing the right eye, there appears before the left a small somewhat elongated dark-brown spot, which flits about pretty near to the eye, mostly in an oblique direction toward the inner corner of the eye. [*Ap.*]

He imagines that he sees things double. [*Wst.*]
Photophobia. [*Ap.*]

160. Earache, a tearing in the auditory meatus of the right ear, which is excited and increased by cold air penetrating into the ear, extends to the upper jaw and continues several days. [*Ap.*]

Stitches in the left mastoid process. [*Wst.*]

Itching in and behind the ears. [*Ap.*]

Itching in the external meatus of the right ear. [*Ap.*]

Itching with tickling in the right ear, inciting to scratching (aft. 29 h.). [*Lgh.*]

165. Itching, mostly in the left ear, which induces boring with the finger. [*Ap.*]

Itching on the lobules of the ears. [*Ap.*]

Itching on the external ear compelling him to rub; this causes redness and soreness, without stopping the itching. [*Ap.*]

Itching, redness and burning of the ears, as if they had been frozen. [*Gr.*]

Itching and pimples on the posterior surface of the external ear. [*Ap.*]

170. Sensation in the ears as if ear-wax was running out. [*Ap.*]

Buzzing in the ears.

Ringing in the right ear while walking in the open air (aft. 4 h.). [*Lgh.*]

On the nose: a sudden pressure on the upper part of the dorsum of the nose. [*Ap.*]

Sharp stitches in the left side of the root of the nose. [*Gr.*]

175. Great sensitiveness of the inner walls of the nose. [*Ap.*]

Itching on the outer surface of the nose. [*Ap.*]

Violent itching on the alæ of the nose, compelling him to rub. [*Ap.*]

Pricking in the right nostril and eye, as from an incitation to sneezing. [*Ap.*]

Tickling itching in the left nostril, that compels rubbing (aft. 14 h.). [*Lgh.*]

180. Burning pain in the nose and the eyes (from the vapor).

Soreness and inflammation of the internal paries of the nose. [*Ap.*]

Blowing of blood from the nose in the morning immediately after rising from bed, followed by violent bleeding from the nose (aft. 33 h.). [*Gr.*]

Epistaxis. [*Sch.*]

Increased acuteness of olfaction. [*Ap.*]

185. In the face, in the left cheek, stitches extending upward from the lower jaw (aft. 1 h.). [*Wst.*]

Obtuse stitches in the right cheek-bone. [*Schrt.*]

Lancinating, drawing pain in the right cheek (aft. 2h.). [*Sch.*]

Quick throbbing of an artery in the left cheek with shooting stitches from the left eye to the upper jaw. [*Ap.*]

Quivering, like pulsation, in the right cheek (aft. 8 d.). [*Ap.*]

190. Burning of the cheeks. [*Wst.*]

Burning in the cheeks (aft. 1 or 2 h.). [*Sdl.*]

Redness of the face without any perceptible heat. [*Sdl.*]

Redness of the face with itching and burning, as after freezing the parts. [*Gr.*]

Itching in the face. [*Ap.*]

195. Itching in the whiskers. [*Ap.*]

Itching on the forehead, inducing scratching and pimples there. [*Ap.*]

An itching pimple by the side of the mouth.

On the lips and in the throat a tearing pain (from the vapor)

Dryness and burning of the lips (on 1st d.). [*Ng.*]

200. Burning chaps on the upper lip (on 4th d.). [*Ng.*]

Bluish lips (1st and 2d d.). [*Sdl.*]

On the right side of the chin, a painful pressure. [*Gr.*]

Stitches, fine and sharp, on a small spot of the chin, just under the upper lip. [*Gr.*]

Stitches in the chin as from needles (immediately). [*Schrt.*]

205. Spasmodic drawing in the chin and lower jaw (aft. 2 h.). [*Sdl.*]

In the articulation of the lower jaw, violent pricking as from needles. [*Schrt.*]

Severe tearing pain in the lower jaw on the right side. [*Gr.*]

Toothache, tearing pain in the teeth of the lower jaw, increased by cold. [*Ap.*]

Pulsating, tearing pain in the upper back molars on the left side; in the afternoon. [*Ap.*]

210. Gnawing pain in the molars of the upper jaw, then itching in the left ear, immediately after which the toothache starts again, in the afternoon. [*Ap.*]

Dull (incipient) toothache on the left side of the upper jaw. [*Ap.*]

Drawing pain in the lower incisors. [*Wst.*]

Drawing stitches in the lower incisors which draw toward the left angle of the lower jaw (aft. 1 h.). [*Schrt.*]

Dulness of the incisors of the lower jaw, [*Wst.*]

215. The front teeth feel too long and very sensitive in the evening (on 3d d.). [*Ng.*]

The gums are painful and the saliva tastes acrid (the first 10 d.). [*Ng.*].

Painfulness and bleeding of the gums. [*Ap.*]

Swelling of the gums, with pains. [*Ap.*]

Bad smell from the mouth. [*Ap.*]

220. Bad smell from the mouth early in the morning, attended with a fetid taste in the mouth. [*Fr. H.*]

Morbidly putrid smell from the mouth (on the 8th–10th d.). [*Sdl.*]

Acrid smell from the mouth as after horse-radish, but he does not perceive it himself. [*Ap.*]

Soreness in the whole of the inner mouth, especially in the palate (on 5th d.). [*Ng.*]

The palate feels sore, as though the skin had been pulled off, and is very sensitive (on 1st d.). [*Ng.*]

225. The tongue is sore. [*Ap.*]

A small, painful ulcer by the side of the frænum of the tongue (on 9th d.). [*Sdl.*]

Whitish tongue set at its point with dirty yellow aphthæ, with a sensation as if the skin would peel off, immediately after a meal (aft. 4 h.). [*Gr.*]

The tongue coated white. [*Lgh.—Schrt.*]

Very pale tongue, thinly coated with white mucus. [*Ap.*]

230. Yellow coating of the tongue on its back part (on 7th–10th d.). [*Sdl.*]

Slimy tongue. [*Ap.*]

Fine stitches in the tip of the tongue (aft. 4 h.). [*Schrt.*]

Foam at the mouth. [*Lerger, Memorab.* vol. iii, 334.]

Water gathers in the mouth (with pains in the abdomen) (on 2d d.). [*Ng.*]

235 Flow of saliva from the mouth.

Sometimes especially when raising, the head fluid saliva runs into his bronchia, causing violent vomiting. [*Wst.*]

The saliva tastes very acrid (on first 10 d.). [*Ng.*]

Disagreeable taste in the mouth, with yellow-coated tongue (on 7th–10th d.). [*Sdl.*]

Insipid taste in the mouth. [*Schrt.*]

240. Bitter taste in the mouth (on 12th d.). [*Sdl.*]

Lack of thirst, absence of thirst. [*Sdl.*]

Thirst, in the afternoon (on 2d d.). [*Ng.*]

Want of appetite. [*Ap.*]

No appetite for eating, but for drinking. [*Ap*].

245. No taste for bread. [*Ap.*]

Great hunger but no appetite, also in the morning. [*Ap.*]

Great desire for food, often bordering on a ravenous appetite (4th–8th d.). [*Sdl.*]

For several days he suddenly gets hungry, when he swallows his food hastily and with great eagerness. [*Ap.*]

Increased appetite toward evening, he feels as if he could not be satiated; and he swallows his food hastily and eagerly, as if ravenous (aft. 8 h.). [*Lgh.*]

250. Toward evening he is suddenly seized with a ravenous hunger, with perspiration over the whole body, great weariness and trembling of the limbs. [*Ap.*]

After eating retching in the œsophagus and pressure in the stomach. [*Ap.*]

After dinner, pressure in the pit of the stomach with painful drawing and pressure in the eyeballs, distaste for work and indolent disposition (on 10th d.). [*Sdl.*]

After supper, feverish shuddering. [*Ap.*]

Frequent eructation of mere air, as if from a deranged stomach (aft. ½ h.). [*Lgh.*]

255. Empty eructation. [*Ap.*]

Frequent empty eructations alternating with hiccup during the (customary) smoking (aft. 1 h.). [*Lgh.*]

Eructation with qualmishness in the stomach (aft. 3 h.). [*Schrt.*]

Eructation with the taste of the ingesta. [*Ap.*]

Eructation with the taste of the ingesta, early in the morning. [*Fr. H.*]

260. Heartburn.

Hiccup, immediately after taking the medicine. [*Ap.*]

Hiccup, in the afternoon. [*Ap.*]

Frequent hiccups (aft. 26 h.). [*Lgh.*]

A sense of nausea, rising even into the mouth.

265. Nausea soon after taking the medicine. [*Sdl.*]

Nausea with colicky pains. [*Ap.*]

Nausea and inclination to vomit (aft. 2 h.). [*Schrt.*]

Nausea immediately after a meal, alleviated by eructations. [*Wst.*]

Pressure in the stomach with inclination for stool. [*Ap.*]

270. Pressure at the cardiac orifice. [*Wst.*]

Pressive pain in the region of the upper left border of the stomach, both while standing and walking (aft. 2 h.). [*Ap.*]

Oppressive heaviness in the stomach. [*Ap.*]

Pressure in the scrobiculus cordis (1st and 9th d.). [*Sdl.*]

Pressure in the scrobiculus cordis, extending to the sternum.

275. After breakfast, pressure in the pit of the stomach, which in the afternoon passes over into a burrowing in the epigastrium, which in the evening passes off with the discharge of flatus (on 16th d.). [*Sdl.*]

Tensive pain in the stomach, extending to the left clavicle when respiring deeply, toward evening (on 9th d.). [*Sdl.*]

Spasmodic drawing in the region of the scrobiculus cordis, extending to the chest, toward evening (on 9th d.). [*Sdl.*]

Spasmodic colicky cutting in the abdomen like cramps of the stomach, immediately under the diaphragm back toward the spine, while sitting (aft. 1½ h.). [*Wst.*]

Pain in the region of the hypochondria and of the scrobiculus cordis as if the viscera of the chest were being pressed in, more violent after meals. [*Gr.*]

280. In the hypochondria on the left side of the last true rib, a pressive pain returning momentarily with a sensation on the corresponding spot on the right side as if there were a pain from an old gun-shot wound (aft. 2 h.). [*Wst.*]

Acute throbbing pain under the left hypochondria, which often extends up to the third and fourth rib, in the afternoon (on 8th d.). [*Sdl.*]

Dull pressure in the spleen in the evening in bed while lying, on the left side, diminished by turning on the right side. [*Wst.*]

Stitches under the short ribs on the left side during inspiration and especially while bending forward in sitting. [*Gr.*]

In the region of the liver, sharp stitches as from needles. [*Gr.*]

285. Dull stitches in the liver during inspiration. [*Gr.*]

Violent pain in the abdomen (aft. 4 h.). [LERGER, l. c.]

Painful pressure in the lumbar region (aft. 2 h.). [*Wst.*]

Violently pressive pain in the region of the left kidney, at night, disturbing the sleep (on 12th d.). [*Sdl.*]

Pressure and fulness of the abdomen, after moderately eating of light food. [*Ap.*]

290. Troublesome fulness of the whole abdomen, making sitting and breathing difficult. [*Wst.*]

Inflated abdomen. [LERGER, l. c.]

Inflated abdomen. [*Ap.*]

Sensation of writhing in the abdomen.

Writhing pain in the abdomen. [*Ap.*]

295. Pinching in the abdomen. [*Ap.*]

Pinching under the navel with distention of the abdomen. [*Ap.*]

Violent pinching of the abdomen with diarrhœa-like stools. [*Ap.*]

Pinching and cutting in the epigastrium, in the evening (on 9th d.). [*Sdl.*]

Cutting in the umbilical region (aft. 2 h.). [*Wst.*]

300. Cutting pains in the abdomen, without stools. [*Ap.*]

Cutting in the abdomen, as from incipient diarrhœa, in the evening. [*Wst.*]

Cutting, with flatus moving about in the bowels and distention of the abdomen, only for a short time alleviated by eructations and the discharge of flatus (aft. 1 h.). [*Wst.*]

Cutting in the abdomen as after a purgative, followed by a fluid stool with diminution of the pains (on 2d d.). [*Ng.*]

Sensation in the abdomen as if diarrhœa were setting in.

305. Dull and very painful stitches at the superior anterior process of the iliac bones. [*Gr.*]

A stitch on the right side next to the spine in the region of the right kidney (aft. ½ h.). [*Wst.*]

Simple pains in the inguinal region. [*Wst.*]

Pain as from a sprain on the left side of the groin, only while walking (aft. 4½ h.). [*Lgh.*]

Troublesome itching of the hypogastrium with goose-skin, it lasts almost the whole night and only ceases in the morning after perspiration. [*Wst.*]

310. Flatus moves audibly to and fro in the abdomen. [*Ap.*]

Growling, rumbling and rolling about in the abdomen. [*Schrt.*]

Loud growling in the abdomen early in the morning (on 2d d.). [*Ap.*]

Loud rumbling in the belly (aft. ½ h.). [*Fr. H.*]

Clucking in the epigastrium. [*Gr.*]

315. Loud gurgling in the bowels, deep down. [*Ap.*]

Loud painless din, like far off thunder, in the belly, with a sensation as if a stool were coming, in the evening. [*Ap.*]

Restlessness in the abdomen as if urging to stool, with the passage of frequent flatus with hardly any smell.

Passage of much flatus. [*Fr. H. and Lgh.*]

Passage of flatus with sensation as in diarrhœa. [*Ap.*]

320. Frequent passage of fetid flatus. [*Ap.*]

Flatus smelling of garlic. [*Ap.*]

When flatus passes, itching in the rectum (on 6th d.). [*Sdl.*]

The whole day a constant sensation in the bowels as if there should be a stool, which having been passed copiously in the morning only ensues again late in the evening. [*Ap.*]

Constipation for two days. [*Sdl.*]

325. After several days' constipation, a solid stool. [*Ap.*]

Stools are passed every other day and are solid. [*Ap.*]

The stool, which before that came daily, is lacking for three days and then is solid. [*Ap.*]

Stool of very hard fæces. [*Ap.*]

Hard dark-colored evacuations (on 3d d.). [*Sdl.*]

330. Knotty stool at night after violent colicky pains, with subsequent severe tenesmus and urging to stool without effect (on 3d d.). [*Ap.*]

First a knotty stool and after a quarter of an hour a watery stool with violent colicky pains, fermentation in the abdomen and great nausea. [*Ap*]

First a solid stool, then a pappy stool and a short time after a diarrhœa-like evacuation. [*Ap.*]

Colic followed by a knotty stool, then diarrhœic, early in the morning (on 2d d.). [*Ap.*]

Soft stools, after the previous usual morning stool had properly been passed [*Schrt.*]

335. Soft, pap-like stool, every day. [*Ap.*]

The evacuations become pappy (on 6th d.). [*Sdl.*]

Passage of a large quantity of pappy stool (aft. 12–38 h.). [*Lgh.*]

Watery stool with violent colic and urging, early in the morning (on 3d d.). [*Ap.*]

340. **Diarrhœic stools with violent pinching in the abdomen,** early in the morning (on 2d d.). [*Ap.*]

Five consecutive passages of fluid, yellow fæces with pinching in the hypogastrium and passage of flatus without smell. [*Ng.*]

Stools of diarrhœa with passage of much flatus (aft. 6 h.). [*Ap.*]

Slimy diarrhœa with much flatus. [*Fr. H.*]

Passage of mucus in the stool with flatus. [*Fr. H.*]

345. Before and during the stool, violent pinching and cutting in the abdomen. [*Ap.*]

During the diarrhœic stool, painful drawing inward of the stomach and belly. [*Ng.*]

During and after the stool, itching in the anus (on 3d and 4th d.). [*Sdl.*]

After the stool, belly-ache, as from poison, early in the morning (on 7th, 9th d.). [*Ap*]

After the stool, gurgling in the belly. [*Ap.*]

350. In the anus tickling itching, compelling scratching (aft. ¾ h.). [*Lgh.*]

Itching and creeping in the anus. [*Wst.*]

Creeping in the anus (aft. 3 h.). [*Schrt.*]

Prickling in the anus, as from worms. [*Sdl.*]

Urging to urinate, with very little discharge of urine (aft. ¾ h.) [*Lgh.*]

355. Repeated urging to urinate, with copious discharge of urine, while the penis is completely relaxed (aft. 4 h.). [*Lgh.*]

Frequent micturition. [*Ap.*]

Frequent micturition, though she had drunk but little (on 4th d.). [*Ng.*]

Scanty emission of urine, without increase in quantity. [*Ap.*]

Diminution of the urine and rare emission of the same. [*Ap.*]

360. The urine is discharged slowly with a feeble stream, at times only drop by drop; he often has to bear down to hasten the flow. [*Ap.*]

The urine sometimes stops for a few moments and then sets in again. [*Ap.*]

Retention of the urine. [*Ap.*]

Scanty, reddish urine (on 1st, 2d d.). [*Sdl.*]

Clear, lemon-yellow urine. [*Ap.*]

365. In urinating, a spasmodic drawing in the left inguinal region (aft. 3 d.) [*Wst.*]

In the orifice of the urethra, creeping and itching (aft. 2 h.). [*Schrt.*]

A stitch in the urethra, as if a red-hot steel was pushed through (aft. 3 h.). [*Wst.*]

Sensation in the urethra as if he had not finished urinating. [*Wst.*]

Sensation in the urethra as if a drop of cold urine was passing through. [*Wst.*]

370. **Discharge of viscid, glutinous mucus from the urethra.** [*Schrt.*]

Itching in the hairs of the pudenda. [*Ap.*]

In the penis a quickly passing, voluptuous itching. [*Wst.*]

Tickling itching of the border of the prepuce, compelling him to rub it (aft. 5 h.). [*Lgh.*]

Tickling itching of the scrotum compelling him to rub it, while sitting (aft. 12 h.) [*Lgh.*]

375. Drawing in the testicles with discomfort, awkwardness and sleepiness, in the evening.

Spasmodic drawing in the left testicle and spermatic cord. [*Wst.*]

Long continued erections (1st night). [*Sdl.*]

Stiffness of the penis, early in the morning. [*Schrt.*]

Frequent ercetions, also in the night. [*Ap.*]

380. Pollutions (1st night). [*Sdl.*]

Nocturnal effusion of seed without lascivious dreams. [*Lgh.*]

Great dislike of all sexual intercourse. [*Schrt.*]

Excitement of the sexual instinct. [*Ap.*]

After the siesta, uncontrollable desire in the sexual organs for seminal emission, and after the emission, pressive tension under the ribs without any indications of flatulence.

385 **Great inclination for coition, while the penis is relaxed.** [*Ap.*]

When desiring coition in the evening, he could, in spite of all exertions, produce no erection and had to desist; in the night following, a copious pollution. [*Schrt.*]

In spite of strong excitation, no voluptuous sensation during coition. [*Ap.*]

During coition, a copious emission of semen followed by a very long sleep. [*Ap.*]

Very tardy emission of seed during coition. [*Ap.*]

390. Deficient emission of seed during coition, with subsequent exhaustion of the body. [*Ap.*]

After every coition great weariness for several days. [*Ap.*]

Strong nocturnal perspiration after every act of coition, with general exhaustion of the body for several days. [*Ap.*]

After coition he is so much affected that he perspired violently for two nights, with burning itching of the skin, first on the upper part of the chest and the shoulders, then also on the abdomen and the arms. [*Ap.*]

Tickling itching on the female pudenda. [*Ap.*]

395. Stronger flow of the menses. [*Fr. H.*]

Sneezing without catarrh. [*Ap.*]

Frequent sneezing without coryza (aft. 12, 22 h.). [*Lgh.*]

Frequent sneezing, always twice in succession (on 1st d.). [*Ng.*]

Repeated sneezing immediately after taking the medicine. [*Ap.*]

400. Early in the morning repeated severe sneezing while in bed. [*Ap.*]

Dryness of the nose. [*Ap.*]

Dryness of the nose, with sensation of coryza. [*Ap.*]

Constant dryness of the nose only once or twice a day two or three drops of water flow down. [*Ap.*]

Frequent dropping of clear water from the nose, without coryza. [*Ap.*]

405. While stooping down, clear water drops from the nose. [*Ap.*]

After snuffing a little tobacco, there immediately follows a copious flow of viscid mucus from the nose. [*Ap.*]

Copious discharge of thick mucus from the nose on blowing it (aft. 5 d.). [*Ap.*]

Dry white mucus in small quantities in the nose, with a frequent sensation as if it contained much mucus. [*Ap.*]

Coryza, in the afternoon. [*Wst.*]

410. Sudden coryza with sneezing. [*Wst.*]

Coryza with stopping of the nose, especially while stooping down (on 7th d.). [*Ng.*]

Dry coryza. [*Schrt.*]

Fluent coryza. [*Ap.*]

Hoarseness and roughness of the throat. [*Schrt.*]

415. Upon slightly hawking, small balls of mucus are detached. [*Ap.*]

Expectoration of small flakes of mucus or firm pellets of mucus, almost without any cough. [*Ap.*]

Irritation to cough [*Ap.*]

Often returning tickling irritation in the bronchia, causing a slight cough. [*Ap.*]

Frequent cough after meals, without expectoration. [*Ap.*]

420. A dry cough after dinner, while sitting down, disturbs his after-dinner nap. [*Ap.*]

Breath very short.

Very short breath and asthma, while walking slowly. [*Ap.*]

She must often stop in walking in order to take breath. [*Ap.*]

Difficult breathing (aft. 8 d.) [*Ap.*]

425. Difficult breathing as if the cavity of the thorax were surcharged with blood (aft. 4 h.). [*Gr.*]

Tightness of the chest. [*Ap*].

Severe constriction of the chest. [*Ap.*]

Her chest feels so constricted that she must stop quickly when she tries to take a slow and deep breath. [*Ap.*]

Constriction which draws her chest together tightly; she must take breath often and deeply, which renders walking difficult for her. [*Ap.*]

430. Constriction of the chest in the region of the diaphragm, attended with a painful drawing (aft. ½ h.). [*Wst.*]

Constriction of the chest, with strong throbbing of the blood-vessels for 1 or 2 days. [*Sdl.*]

Sensation of constriction in the region of the heart, as if the cavity of the thorax was contracted. [*Gr.*]

Tightness of the chest. [*Ap.*]

Pains in the lower part of the chest, especially in the region of the scrobiculus cordis, as if the viscera of the chest were being pressed together, aggravated after meals. [*Gr.*]

435. Painful pressure on the middle of sternum, worse while inspiring (aft. 2½ h.). [*Gr.*]

Tension in the lower part of the chest, while moving and while sitting, so that it takes the breath away. [*Ap.*]

Stitches in the region of the lungs, soon passing away. [*Ap.*]

Stitching pain in the middle of the chest. [*Wst.*]

Stiches in the chest below the paps (aft. 14 and 30 h.). [*Gr.*]

440. Fine stitches in the left side of the chest where the ribs cease, while sitting with the chest bent forward. [*Gr.*]

Stitches, while inspiring, in the left side of the chest where the ribs cease. [*Gr.*]

Pinching pain in the left part of the chest obliquely downward to the navel. [*Fr. H.*]

Pain as from a sprain in the interior of the chest, which increases especially while taking a deep breath; in the evening (on 9th d.). [*Sdl.*]

Burning pain in the left half of the chest (on 3d d.). [*Sdl.*]

445. Fine burning and prickling on various parts of the chest, especially on the sternum (aft. 1 h.). [*Gr.*]

Palpitation while standing, very painful. [*Wst.*]

Pulsating sore pain in particular small spots on the chest, especially on the right half; at night and also in daytime (aft. 14 d.). [*Sdl.*]

Itching, externally on the chest, passing over into burning. [*Ap*].

Burning itching on the chest (and in the back). [*Ap.*]

450. On the nipples, violent itching. [*Ap.*]

Burning itching and pimples on the left nipple. [*Ap.*]

Copious perspiration on the chest at night. [*Ap.*]

On the left side of the coccyx, an itching corrosion. [*Gr.*]

Itching inciting, to scratching, on the left tuberosity of the ischium. [*Gr.*]

455. When he sits down, the parts on which he sits feel as if bruised or as if he had been sitting on them a long time. [*Gr.*]

In the left, nates violent tearing pain with sensation of coldness, very severe while sitting, less severe when rising and walking (for 8 days). [*Ap.*]

Drawing tearing in the left nates; it wakes him in bed at night out of his sleep. [*Ap.*]

Carbuncle on the right part of the nates. [*Schrt.*]

In the small of the back, when rising after having been sitting, a violent pain which hinders him in rising and also impedes the motion of the thighs. [*Ap.*]

460. Violent pain in the small of the back while sitting and lying, alleviated by motion (on 1st and 3d d.). [*Sdl.*]

He feels bruised in the small of the back, especially while standing. [*Wst.*]

Pain as from a sprain in the region of the small of the back on the left side (on 6th and 8th d.). [*Sdl.*]

Violent jerking pain in the small of the back, in raising the thigh while sitting. [*Ap.*]

Pain in the back as after long continued stooping. [*Wst.*]

465. When rising from sitting, and straightening the body, stiffness in the back with violent pain in the left loin, which prevents his straightening himself; while sitting he feels no pain, and can turn himself to every side without pain. [*Ap.*]

Spasmodically pressive, drawing pain, lasting for several hours, starting from the back, seemingly in the middle of the chest in the œsophagus; in the afternoon (on 5th and 7th d.). [*Sdl.*]

Pressive boring pain, in the middle of the back (on 2d d.). [*Sdl.*]

Spasmodic painful jerks in the left side of the back. [*Wst.*]

Tearing pain now on the right side, now on the left of the lumbar vertebræ, while walking. [*Ap.*]

470. Tearing between the shoulders, frequent (on 4th d.). [*Ng.*]

Lancinating pain between the shoulders (on 2d d.) [*Ng.*]

Bruised feeling in the muscles of the back. [*Wst.*]

Bruised feeling in the muscles of the back, they feel too short when he bends forward; in the morning after a good night's sleep, as well while lying in bed as also later while sitting down, two days in succession. [*Wst.*]

Bruised feeling in the region of the loins, especially while lying and sitting. [*Sdl.*]

475. Pain as from a bruise or a sprain in the whole back, with an inclination to stretch it (on 3d and 4th d.). [*Sdl.*]

Weakness of the muscles of the back; he finds it difficult to sit straight without leaning against something. [*Gr.*]

In bending the spine aches as if it were too weak to support the weight of the body. [*Gr.*]

Paralytic pain as from weakness back in the loins, aggravated by walking and standing (aft. 12 h.). [*Gr.*]

Sensation of paralysis along the lumbar vertebræ, immediately above the border of the os ilium; this hinders him in walking when he has risen. [*Ap.*]

480. Quivering in the muscles of the right lumbar region, in the evening (on 9th d.). [*Sdl.*]

Tickling itching on the back. [*Ap.*]

Burning itching on the back. [*Ap.*]

In the muscles of the nape of the neck pain, as from a sprain, as if from lying on the back (aft. 32 h.). [*Lgh.*]

Bruised feeling in the muscles of the nape; they feel too short when bending forward; early in the morning while lying abed and later while sitting. [*Wst.*]

485. Stiffness in the neck (aft. 2 h.). [*Sdl.*]

Between the neck and the shoulders, suddenly a violent pressure. [*Gr.*]

In the shoulder-joint, rheumatic drawing with weakness of the whole arm (on 15th d.). [*Sdl.*]

The arms feel bruised. [*Ap.*]

No strength in the arms. [*Ap.*]

490. Painful weariness of the arms. [*Ap.*]

He has often to change the position of his arms to relieve the pains in them. [*Ap.*]

Itching on the arms. [*Ap.*]

Pimples with burning itching, of the size of millet, on the arms. [*Ap.*]

The upper arms are painful to the touch. [*Ap.*]

495. Tearing on the left upper arm. [*Ap.*]

Fine sharp stitches in front on the head of the right humerus. [*Gr.*]

Burning on the upper arm, above the left elbow. [*Gr.*]

The upper arm feels lame from much writing. [*Gr.*]

Tickling itching, urging him to scratch, on the point of the left elbow (aft. 3 h.). [*Lgh.*]

500. In the fore-arm a dull but very severe pain. [*Ap.*]

Violent rheumatic pains in the whole left fore-arm, extending into the thumb while resting; in the afternoon. [*Ap.*]

Tearing in the right fore-arm. [*Ap.*]

Tearing in the left fore-arm, in the bone of the elbow, while at rest. [*Ap.*]

Twitching and quivering on the upper surface of the right fore-arm, extending to the ball of the thumb. [*Ng.*]

505. Burning pain on the front side of the left fore-arm, near to the wrist, as if from a burn. [*Gr.*]

Burning itching on the right fore-arm, compelling him to scratch; after scratching, there appear white lumps as large as millet, while the skin scales off like bran. [*Ap.*][1]

In the hand, dull pain in the metacarpal bone of the left middle finger. [*Ap.*]

Drawing pains in the metacarpal bones of the left hand. [*Ap.*]

Tearing in the carpus of the left hand. [*Ap.*]

510. The left hand goes to sleep at night even up to the middle of the fore-arm (on 5th d.). [*Ng.*]

Trembling of the hands. [*Ap.*]

Trembling of the hands as if from old age, when he moves the hands or when he holds something in them (aft. 1½ h.). [*Lgh.*]

Tickling itching on the right carpus, compelling him to scratch (aft. 1½ h.)]*Lgh.*]

Tickling itching compelling him to scratch, in the right palm (aft. 7 h.). [*Lgh.*]

515. **Itching, redness and burning on the hands as if they were frozen.** [*Gr.*]

Inflamed pimples of the size of a grain of millet on the back of the left hand. [*Ap.*]

In the index-finger of the right hand, drawing. [*Ap.*]

Tearing between the thumb and index finger of the right hand. [*Gr.*]

Violent tearing in the right middle finger (aft. 23 h.). [*Gr.*]

520. Tearing in the lower joints of the fingers of the left hand, where they join with the metacarpal bones, without any reference to motion (aft. 1 h.). [*Gr.*]

Jerking tearing in the last two fingers of the right hand. [*Gr.*]

Cramp-like pain in the ball of the right thumb while writing (aft. 1–8 h.). [*Lgh.*]

Cramp-like pain in the ball of the left thumb; while standing and walking, disappearing in sitting (aft. 6 h.). [*Lgh.*]

Burning and formication in the index of the right hand as if a paronychia were forming, after some days this is followed by frequent numbness of the finger and great long-continued sensitiveness of the same to cold. [*Wst.*]

525. Titillating itching, inciting him to scratch, on the ball of the right thumb (aft. 8 h.). [*Lgh.*]

Titillating itching as from freezing on the inner border of the right index (aft. 5 h.). [*Lgh.*]

Itching, redness and burning of the fingers as after freezing. [*Gr.*]

Pain in the hips for twenty-four hours; this is not felt painfully while sitting, but very much so in walking. [*Wst.*]

Pains in the legs (of almost all kinds), **arising nearly al-**

---

[1] See note to symptom 129. These pimples only lasted an hour.—*Hughes.*

ways while sitting and standing, more seldom while walking; they diminish and pass off through motion. [*Ap.*]

530. Tearing in the legs, constant while sitting, improved by motion. [*Ap.*]

Great weariness of the legs, he knows not how to rest them. [*Ap.*]

Weakness of the (feet) **legs;** they are so weak while standing, that the body is constantly in a wavering motion. [*Gr.*]

He can hardly lift his legs for weariness and heaviness. [*Ap.*]

Great heaviness in the legs. [*Ap.*]

535. Heaviness in the legs, as if tired out and broken down. [*Schrt.*]

The legs go to sleep as soon as he crosses them. [*Ap.*]

In the thighs, violent pain while crossing them. [*Ap.*]

Pressive pain as from a peg driven in on the exterior side of the thigh above the knee. [*Gr.*]

Painful pressure in the left thigh. [*Wst.*]

540. Rheumatic drawing in the external side of both thighs, in walking after sitting. [*Wst.*]

Constant paralytic drawing in the left thigh down to the knee, both in rest and in motion; in the afternoon. [*Wst.*]

Drawing tearing in the right thigh while crossing it over the left; this passes away again while stretching it (aft. 1 h.). [*Lgh.*]

Tearing at the head of the left femur, which disturbs the night's rest. [*Ap.*]

Tearing just below the lesser condyle of the femur. [*Ap.*]

545. Tearing in the right thigh, in walking and sitting. [*Ap.*]

Tearing with sensation of coldness on the posterior side of the left thigh. [*Ap.*]

Tearing which excites a feeling of numbness in the whole thigh, from the joint of the left thigh down to the knee. [*Ap.*]

Painful weariness of the thigh. [*Ap.*]

The thighs are painful as after great foot-tours. [*Ap.*]

550. Painful lameness of the left thigh. [*Wst.*]

Paralytic pain in the right thigh, especially while walking; the thigh feels as if too heavy and as if a load lay upon it (aft. 8 h.). [*Gr.*]

Corrosive itching on the anterior side of the left thigh. [*Gr.*]

Itching pimple on the thigh above the left knee, with violent burning while scratching it. [*Wst.*]

The knee-joints pain early in the morning after rising from bed, while sitting down. [*Ap.*]

555. The pain in the knees increases while sitting and diminishes and passes away while walking. [*Ap.*]

Drawing in the left knee. [*Ap.*]

Drawing in both knee-joints at the same time. [*Ap.*]

Tearing in the right knee-joint while standing and sitting. [*Ap.*]

Constant boring, tearing in the right knee while sitting. [*Ap.*]

560. Jerking on the inner side of the right knee. [*Ap.*]

Stitches as from needles above the left hough (aft. 36. h.). [*Gr.*]

Sudden giving way of the left knee while walking; in the afternoon. [*Wst.*]

Pain as from a sprain in the left knee while walking. [*Ap.*]

Painful lameness in the left hough. [*Wst.*]

565. In the legs the pain increases while standing, so that he is soon compelled to walk or to sit down, and this pain begins when he has only stood a minute. [*Ap.*]

The pain in the tibia increases and is constant while sitting, but passes off while walking. [*Ap.*]

Pressure as from a bruise on the inner side of the muscles of the calves while sitting; somewhat alleviated by standing and by touching these parts, but the pain becomes more severe again after sitting down (aft. 2 h.). [*Lgh.*]

Drawing pain in the leg, from the right knee to the toes while sitting. [*Ap.*]

Painful drawing on the posterior side of the left leg, down from the calf, passing off while walking; in the afternoon. [*Wst.*]

570. Drawing, tearing in the right tibia. [*Ap.*]

Tearing in the leg, down to the lower point of the tibia. [*Ap.*]

Tearing in the left tibia. [*Ap.*]

Tearing in the exterior surface of the right calf, while sitting down (on 1st d.). [*Ng.*]

Violent stitch on the exterior side of the calf (aft. 2 h.). [*Lgh.*]

575. Fine stitches on the inside of the right leg and toward the tibia. [*Gr.*]

Bruised pain in the legs. [*Ap.*]

Pains in the legs as if from exhaustion, after passing through typhoid fevers. [*Ap.*]

Heaviness in the calves.

Burning with pressure, on the upper part of the tibia below the knee. [*Gr.*]

580. Sensation on the upper part of the tibia and on the head of the fibula as if a warm hand was laid upon them. [*Gr.*]

Burning itching on the legs in the evening, while undressing, with a desire to scratch, and increased burning afterwards; the skin becomes dry and cracks easily for five weeks and after that time it peels off. [*Wst.*]

Burning itching, inciting to scratch, on the left leg, with little white knots as large as millet grains after scratching; these scale off like bran. [*Ap.*][1]

On the left foot a tearing pressure on the inner side of the ankle, while sitting (aft. 35 h.) [*Lgh.*]

Tearing in the hollow of the right foot, while sitting. [*Ap.*]

585. Tearing in the soles of the feet, while walking. [*Ap.*]

Lancinating pain on the outside of the left ankle (while sitting) (aft. 5 h.). [*Lgh.*]

Fine stitches in the dorsum of the right foot. [*Gr.*]

---

[1] As in symptom 506.

Stitches in the lower surface of the heel, while sitting. [*Ap.*]

Violent stitches in the middle of the left foot, beginning at the ankles, while resting. [*Ap.*]

590. Stitches in the lower surface of the first and second metatarsus. [*Ap.*]

Cramp in the sole of the foot, at night. [*Ap.*]

Pain in the heels as if bruised, while standing. [*Gr.*]

Heaviness and relaxed state of the feet. [*Wst.*]

Corrosive itching on the dorsum of the right foot. [*Gr.*]

595. Corrosive itching on the interior side of the left ankle. [*Gr.*]

Drawing in the toes of the left foot. [*Ap.*]

Drawing tearing on the lower side of the big toe of the right foot, while sitting. [*Ap.*]

Tearing in the ball of the big toe of the left foot, frequent (aft. 2d d.). [*Ng.*]

Twitching in the ball of the big toe of the left foot (on 1st d.). [*Ng.*]

600. Painful jerking in the left big toe. [*Ap.*]

Stitches in the toes while resting. [*Ap.*]

Sharp stitches in the toes of the left foot, while standing (aft. ¼ h.). [*Lgh.*]

Stitches, where there was formerly a corn.

Painful, dull stitches in the last three toes of the right foot (aft. 20 h). [*Gr.*]

605. Burrowing pain in the toes of the right foot. [*Ap.*]

Soreness of the little right toe as if from tight shoes (aft. 6. h.). [*Lgh.*]

Soreness on the corn of the second toe of the left foot, as if from a tight shoe (aft. 3 h.). [*Lgh.*]

Tickling itching inciting to scratch, on the toes, as if they were frozen (aft. 11 h.). [*Lgh.*]

Itching, burning and redness of the toes, as if they had been frozen. [*Gr.*]

610. The skin of the whole body itches. [*Ap.*]

The herpes extends. [*Ap.*]

All parts of the body are painfully sensitive; if any part is only lightly pressed, it pains for a long time. [*Gr.*]

Spasmodic pains in the muscles of the whole body, here and there, now in the upper, then in the lower limbs, while sitting. [*Lgh.*]

Tearing of different long bones, especially at their extremities. [*Gr.*]

615. Stitches as of needles in various parts of the body (aft. ½ h.). [*Gr.*]

Fine pricking and burning in various parts of the body (aft. 1 h.). [*Gr.*]

Drawing pain, now in the right upper arm, then in the left knee-joint; now in the right, then in the left thigh. [*Ap.*]

The ailments are wont to appear simultaneously in various parts, especially on both halves of the body above the small of the back. [*Ap.*]

While sitting down, pains of various kinds simultaneously in all parts of the body. [*Ap.*]

620. While sitting, boring pains in the whole head, the thighs, and the tibial and tarsal bones, with sleepiness and relaxed state of the whole body. [*Ap.*]

He feels most comfortable while walking very slowly. [*Ap.*]

Convulsions. [VOIGTEL, A. M. L. vol. ii, part 2, p. 352.]

Several spasms quickly following each other in the back part of the chest right across, then in the epigastrium and afterward in the hypogastrium, especially on the right side, with a sensation as if there was a shaking through the whole body; while standing in the evening. [*Ap.*]

Concussion of the nerves. [*Pharmakol. Lex.*, vol. i, p. 74.]

625. Convulsions. [MURRAY, *Apparat. Medic.*, v, 557.]

Epilepsy. [MURRAY, ibid.]

The epileptic attacks become more violent and follow in shorter intervals, with an epileptic patient.[1] [*Ap.*]

With two epileptic patients the attacks become more violent and return at shorter intervals, but soon the intervals are lengthened and the attacks become extremely mild.[1] [*Ap.*]

Uncomfortable feeling of disease in the whole body. [*Ap.*]

630. Weakness and painful sensitiveness in all the limbs, with pains in the heels when standing. [*Gr.*]

Lack of strength of all parts. [*Fr. H.*]

Marked lack of strength. [*Ap.*]

Great lassitude and staggering gait (shortly). [*Sdl.*]

Sensation of trembling in the whole body (aft. 1 h.). [*Sdl.*]

635. **Trembling.** [VOIGTEL, ibid., *Pharmakol. Lex.*, ibid.]

Anxious trembling with weariness. [*Ap.*]

Lassitude (aft. 12–16 h.). [MURRAY, ibid.]

Lassitude and heaviness in the limbs. [*Fr. H.*]

Heaviness in the whole body, especially in the calves.

640. Painful weariness in the arms and legs. [*Ap.*]

After a short walk his arms feel as if bruised next day. [*Ap.*]

The long bones of the upper and lower limbs, as also all the joints, feel as if bruised after any exercise, with painfulness of the muscles when touched. [*Ap.*]

After a short, brisk walk, great weariness. [*Ap.*]

When ascending a little eminence, he feels faint, with copious perspiration. [*Ap.*]

645. In bed, he knows not what position to take, for sheer weariness. [*Ap.*]

In the morning, weariness. [*Ap.*]

Frequent yawning. [*Ap.*]

Yawning, stretching and extending the limbs (aft. 1 h.). [*Schrt.*]

Frequent yawning, as if he had not done sleeping (aft. 7½ h.). [*Lgh.*]

650. Frequently repeated yawning, so violent as to make him

[1] 627, 628, from the 12th and 30th potency, respectively.—*Hughes.*

giddy, in the morning, while walking in the open air (at once). [*Ap.*]

Frequent yawning with sleepiness, so that he can hardly keep from falling asleep; in the forenoon. [*Ap.*]

Sleepy and tired, the whole day. [*Ap.*]

Irresistible sleepiness, compelling him to lie down. [*Wst.*]

Sleepiness with heaviness of the head (at once). [*Schrt.*]

655. Sleepiness, at once in the morning, one hour after rising. [*Schrt.*]

In the forenoon, while reading, he could not keep from going to sleep. [*Ap.*]

After dinner irresistible sleepiness. [*Ap.*]

Despite of great sleepiness in the forenoon, he cannot go to sleep. [*Ap.*]

With great and tired somnolence, he could not sleep during the day on account of the abundance of ideas. [*Ap.*]

660. **After dinner sleep oppressed his eyes, and yet the pain and uneasiness in his legs would not allow him to go to sleep.** [*Ap.*]

So sleepy at 8 o'clock in the evening that he had to go to bed, while a peculiar apprehension that some one might disturb him did not allow him to go to sleep for a whole hour, after which he slept almost till morning. [*Schrt.*]

When he went to bed in the evening, being very sleepy, he yet could not go to sleep on account of uneasiness in his body and weariness in his legs; so again later, after having been waked up by a dream. [*Ap.*]

After a good sleep, he yet was not refreshed, and rose without desiring to do so. [*Ap.*]

He had to compel himself to rise in the morning. [*Ap.*]

665. After a two hours' nap after dinner. he could not become wide awake. [*Ap.*]

Uneasy sleep (the 1st–3d nights). [*Sdl.*]

Uneasy sleep, broken by awaking several times. [*Wst.*]

Frequent waking up at night (on 5th d.). [*Ng.*]

He often awakes at night, becomes wide awake, but falls asleep again after a while. [*Ap.*]

670. Frequently waking up at night, as if he had done sleeping. [*Lgh.*]

Frequent, anxious awaking at night. [*Sdl.*]

Waking up at night, with violent urging to urinate, with copious micturition (aft. 19 h.). [*Lgh.*]

She is waked up soon after going to sleep by a spasmodic cough lasting 10 minutes, with a painful tickling in the larynx and down the throat. [*Wst.*]

He wakes up in the night from a feeling of coldness in the whole of the left leg. [*Wst.*]

675. Light sleep with many dreams and ever changing images. [*Wst.*]

Sleep interrupted by anxious dreams. [*Ap.*]

Internal disquiet in bad dreams which he cannot recollect,

without any movement of the body; on awaking all unrest had disappeared.

Frequent awaking through vexatious dreams. [*Ap.*]

Dreams of a disagreeable nature often wake him at night from sleep. [*Ap.*]

680. Vivid dreams partly pleasant, partly disagreeable. [*Lgh.*]

Chilly shivers through the whole night. [*Ap.*]

Shivers over the whole body (aft. 10 min.). [*Gr.*]

A shiver runs through the body from above downwards. [*Gr.*]

Very sensitive to cool air. [*Ap.*]

685. The least sensation of cool air causes goose-skin. [*Ap.*]

Much inclined to chilliness. [*Ap.*]

As soon as he comes into the open air or raises the cover of his bed at night he is chilly. [*Ap.*]

Great internal chilliness. [*Ap.*]

Almost constant chilliness, he cannot get warm, especially in the morning in his room. [*Wst.*]

690. A chill runs over him, down his left leg to the foot. [*Wst.*]

Chill in the back, as if cold water were running down, when he leans his back against his chair. [*Ap.*]

Very chilly in the evening.[1] [*Ap.*]

In evening when lying down, shaking chill for ten minutes. [*Wst.*]

In the evening, a long-continued chill which increases to shaking.[2] [*Ap.*]

695. Every evening a feverish chill without thirst and without subsequent heat. [*Ap.*]

Shaking chill, when he lifts his bed-covers. [*Ap.*]

Shaking chill with yawning. [*Ap.*]

Chill, while the face, hands and feet are warm. [*Ap.*]

Violent chills, with shaking of the whole body and trembling of the hands while writing, while the hands are cold, but the face properly warm, without thirst or subsequent heat. [*Lgh.*]

700. Warmth in the face and the whole upper body, in frequent flushes of 5–10 minutes.

Increased warmth in the body at night. [*Ap.*]

Violent attack of heat in the evening, so that the cheeks glow, while the hands are cold, with subsequent long-continued thirst without following perspiration (aft. 12 h.). [*Lgh.*]

Heat at night, but as soon as she turns over or lifts the bed-cover she is chilled. [*Ap.*]

At night, continual heat, then perspiration. [*Lgh.*]

705. Heat with perspiration, in repeated attacks the whole afternoon, with a dull headache without thirst; when putting on his hat in the evening, the heat and perspiration increase, with hurried respiration and great prostration. [*Schrt.*]

Perspiration after only moderate bodily exertion. [*Ap.*]

Perspiration while walking. [*Ap.*]

---

[1] See note to symptom 129, with sleepiness.—*Hughes.*

[2] See note to symptom 129, followed by symptom 708.—*Hughes.*

Night-sweat during uneasy sleep.[1] [*Ap.*]

Small quick pulse of 80 beats, early in the morning. [*Wst.*]

710. **The pulse grows slower** (aft. 2 h.). [*Ap.*]

The pulse, at other times strong and full, becomes small, weak and hardly perceptible. [*Ap.*]

Weak, unequal, intermittent pulse. [*Ap.*]

The pulse is less intermittent in the morning. [*Ap.*]

After drinking coffee, the pulse became less intermittent and rose from 50 up to 60 beats. [*Ap.*]

715. Undulating, weak, slow pulse. [*Ap.*]

ALUMINA.

(OXIDE OF ALUMINUM.)

To secure quite pure clay, a matter of some difficulty, we may use the following process: Pure muriate of lime which has been thoroughly dried by heating in a porcelain bowl is pulverized while still hot, and dissolved in as much alcohol as is required. Half an ounce of white Roman alum from Solfatara is dissolved in five parts of distilled water and to remove any adherent earth is filtered. The sulphuric acid contained in it is precipitated in the form of gypsum, by dropping in the alcoholic solution of muriate of lime until the solution of alum is no longer rendered turbid thereby. The clear watery fluid on top then contains muriate of alumina, from which this earth is precipitated by means of alcoholic spirits of ammonia. It is then well washed and then thoroughly heated in order to completely remove the ammonia. The powder is then, while warm, preserved in a well-stoppered glass vial, and is pure alumina. One grain of this is then triturated in the well-known manner with thrice one hundred grains of sugar of milk. Through solution and further dilution with alcohol, it is then brought to the decillionth potency, in the manner directed at the conclusion of the first volume with respect to dry medicinal substances. Alumina has proved itself an important antipsoric.

It proved itself excellent when it was otherwise homœopathically suitable to the case, when one or several of the following states were present:*

---

[1] See note to symptom 129, profuse and oily, not offensive, preceded by sympt. 694.—*Hughes.*

* I am sorry to say the significance of the use of medicines as given in the preface to most of the remedies, and which have often been unreliably reported,

Moroseness; *anxiety;* solicitude; timidity; dislike to work; difficulty in recollecting and reflecting; *vertigo;* headache as if the hair was pulled out, with nausea; pressure on the forehead; rush of blood to the eyes and nose, with epistaxis; itching of the forehead; heaviness of the face, (*Hg.*) tumor-like swellings in the face, (*Hg.*) sensation of coldness in the eyes, while walking in the open air; pressure, every evening, in the corner of the eye as from a grain of sand; closing of the eyes from pus, and lachrymation; buzzing before the ear; redness of the nose; tearing, lancinating pain in the cheek-bone; dryness in the mouth; *eructation;* many years' tendency to rising from the stomach; acid risings; disordered appetite, now strong, now wanting; *frequent nausea*; pains in the scrobiculus cordis and the hypochondria while stooping; colic in the morning; inactivity of the rectum; *itching of the anus;* urinating at night; discharge of prostatic juice during difficult stools; excessive sexual desire; scanty menses; pains during the menses; *leucorrhœa;* proneness to frequent colds of many years' standing; coryza and cough; rawness in the throat; catarrh of the throat and of the chest; dyspnœa; asthma; cough; itching in the breasts; pain in the thyroid cartilage on touching it; palpitation of the heart; shocks of the heart; *pains in the small of the back*, while at rest; paralytic *heaviness in the arm;* pains in the arms, while they are hanging down or while they are stretched out in bed; stitches in the wrist while working; chapping and excoriation of the hands; paronychia; at night the legs go to sleep, are stiff and numb; painful weariness of the articulations of the feet while sitting; cold feet; burning sensation in the toes; twitching and trembling in the limbs; frequent stretching and extension of the limbs while sitting; disagreeable lack of vital warmth; ill effects of vexation; falling asleep late; the sleep is too light; dreamy sleep; stupor, unrefreshing sleep; chilliness in the evening; fever and ague, the chills appearing immediately after the warm soup at dinner-time. (*Bte.*)

According to *Bute*, Bryonia is an antidote to the excessive fever-

---

has been now and then misunderstood, having been regarded as determining the choice of remedies in the treatment of diseases (as *indications*); this they cannot and should not be; they are not names of diseases healed, but only of separate symptoms which, in treating a disease with the specified medicine, were either diminished or removed—*ab usu*. To use them otherwise is a deceptive procedure which we leave now as before to our allopathic step-brothers. They are, on the contrary, only to serve to furnish occasionally a little confirmation of the correct choice of the homœopathic remedy, already found out from their pure peculiar medicinal effects, as *indicated* according to the similarity of the symptoms of disease of the special case under consideration.

effects of alumina. Others mention Chamomilla and Ipecacuanha as antidotes.

The abbreviations of the names of my fellow-provers are *Hb., Dr. Hartlaub, Sen.; Ng.;* S., Dr. Schréter; Tr., Dr. Trinks; Bte., Dr. H. G. Bute, of Philadelphia.*[1]

ALUMINA.

Dejected and joyless; he only desires to be left alone, forenoon (on 8th d.). [*Ng.*]

(He is exuberantly merry.)

Great changableness in his mental moods.

Dejected as to his disease.

5. He thinks that he cannot get well again. [*S.*]

* By these two letters merely (a real anonymity) *Hartlaub* and *Dr. Trinks* designate a man who furnished the greatest number of symptoms in the provings of medicines for their "*Annalen,*" which often appear in very negligent, diffuse and vague expressions. I could merely extract therefrom what was useful under the supposition that he has acted as an honest, careful man. But it is hardly to be excused that the Homœopathic public should be expected to give absolute credit to an unknown person designated merely with the two letters N-g in this most important and serious work which requires circumspection, acuteness of the senses, subtle gift of observation and strict criticism of one's own sensations and perceptions, as well as a correct choice of expression, in prosecuting a work which is an indispensable foundation of our healing art.[2]

[1]The pathogenesis of Alumina resembles that of Agaricus, in appearing for the first time in the second edition, but being made up almost entirely of already published provings. Hahnemann's own symptoms may be included in this description; for Hering writes (*Guiding Symptoms* sub voce): Hahnemann had proved the pure earth when Hartlaub and Trinks edited a collection of 975 symptoms, obtained from four provers,"--the Hartlaub, Ng., Schreter and Trinks of the above list--"in their *Arzneimittellehre* in 1829. The year after, Hahnemann published his own observations in Stapf's *Archiv;* viz. 215 symptoms obtained from a much better preparation. Hartlaub simply purified his preparation by washing it, which never can suffice, but Hahnemann subjected his to a red heat." No information is given as to the subjects and doses of his provings (if provings they were); but with Hartlaub and Trinks the 1st trituration and 9th dilution were employed. Of the source of Bute's symptoms we have no information.--*Hughes.*

[2] This note of Hahnemann has led to a good deal of mistrust of the symptoms of the anonymous observer in question, which has been iucreased by their exeessive number. Dr. Roth having counted more thau eleven thousand in the several contributions to our Materia Medica made by him between 1828 and 1836. The same critic also says, that he has found great sameness in his pathogenetic lists. Dr. Hering, however (Allen's Encyclopædia III, 640) has explained why "Ng."--the surgeon Cajatan Nenning--had to keep his name concealed; and has shown that his symptoms were obtained by genuine provings on healthy subjects. Nenning himself has given in the *Allg. hom. Zeitung* for 1839 a similar account to explain the copiousness of his symptom lists. "A number of persons in part related to me and in part friendly (they were millinery pupils of his wife's) were gathered together by me, and in consideration of board and payment, made experiments. Along with them were also my two daughters; and with complete reliance on the honesty of them all, I gave one medioine to one and another to another, writing down all that they reported. It was a matter of conscience on my part not to omit the smallest particular, and that thereby frequent repetitions have arisen, I grant readily, but I thought that just in that way the sphere of action of the medicine could be best recognized."--*Hughes.*

Fancy paints to itself nothing but disagreeable, sad pictures (on 1st d.). [*Tr.*]

Sad thoughts constantly enter her mind, which compel her to weep, with restlessness and anxiety as if something bad would happen to her; whatever she looks at, fills her with sadness (on 11th d.). [*Ng.*]

Involuntary moaning and groaning as if in great pain, without his knowing it. [*Bte.*]

In the morning when awaking, as if depressed by sorrow, without clear consciousness.

10. She looks at everything in the worst light, and weeps and cries for hours (on 2d d.).

The boy falls into continuous weeping against his wish, lasting ½ an hour.

Anxiety with much restlessness, the whole day (on 2d. d.). [*Ng.*]

Serious, anxious mood.

Anxious, introverted, vexed mood. [*Tr.*]

15. Anxiety with stupid obtuseness in the head and pressure on the forehead (aft. 12 h.). [*Hb.*]

Anxiety with external heat and **restlessness, as if she had done something wicked.**

Anxiety and fearfulness, as if he had committed a crime (on 5th d.). [*Ng.*]

Restlessness in the evening, **as if evil was imminent.**

Anxiety with palpitation of the heart and pulsation in various parts of the chest and the abdomen (on 4th d.). [*Tr.*]

20. In the morning, anxiety as if he were to have an attack of epilepsy in a few hours.

Apprehension of losing his thoughts, his reason.

She cannot see blood nor a knife without horrible thoughts pressing in upon her, as if she should, *e. g.*, commit suicide; though she has the greatest horror of it.

Excited, over-worked, and yet discontented, because not enough had been done.

Very timid, is startled at hearing the least thing fall.

25. Varying moods through the day, now confidence, then again faint-heartedness.

Discontented with everything, and as it were desperate.

Cross and **peevish**; she mutters continually. [*S.*]

Ill-humored, nothing pleases him. [*Ng.*]

Cross and ill-humored, of which she is herself conscious; at 1 P. M. (on 1st d.). [*Ng.*]

30. Peevish mood (on 1st d.). [*Tr.*]

Peevish and inclined to weep, with hot lobules of the ears (aft. 2 d.).

Extremely peevish and self-willed.

She does not wish to do what others wish.

She is extremely peevish, and everything is offensive to her; she only wishes to scold and to raise a fuss, in the afternoon (on 5th d.). [*Ng.*]

35. He laughs contemptuously at everything.

Indisposition to every kind of occupation, and ennui, in the forenoon.

Dislike to every occupation (on 1st d.). [*Tr.*]

Indifference, distraction and peevishness. [*Tr.*]

Great absent-mindedness and irresolution (2d d.). [*Tr.*]

40. Inattention to what is read, the thoughts will not remain concentrated on any subject (1st d.). [*Tr.*]

The thoughts are occupied with various subjects, without any of them remaining so as to be clearly recognized (4th d.). [*Tr.*]

He constantly makes slips of the tongue and uses other words than he desires.

Lack of power of recollection and great weakness of memory.

Striking forgetfulness. [*Bte.*]

45. Continuous great weakness of memory.

Lack of memory for many weeks. [*Bte.*]

Great forgetfulness. [*Tr.*]

Inability to think connectedly.

Dulness of mind.

50. Inability and dislike to mental work. [*Bte.*]

Unbearable *ennui*, one hour seems to him as half a day. [*Bte.*]

Everything is easy to him, the powers of his understanding and of his body seem excited (1st d.). [*Ng.*]

Great liveliness of spirit, alternating with absence of mind, while thought, vision and hearing seem indistinct and to have almost vanished.

Numb feeling in the head, with a fear that he would become unconscious.

55. A numb feeling in the head as if his consciousness was outside of his body; when he says anything, he feels as if another person had said it; and when he sees anything, as if another person had seen it, or as if he could transfer himself into another, and only then could see.

In the morning, the head feels obtuse and silly, which passes after rising (3d d.). [*Ng.*]

In the morning, his head feels muddled and hot.

Numb feeling in the head, with heat in the face. [*Tr.*]

From time to time, weakness in the head.

60. Great **stupefaction**, with apprehension of falling forward.

Violent vertigo while walking and sitting, as if about to fall over, often for several days, with straining in the nape toward the head.

Vertigo even to falling, *the whole room turns with her;* she has to sit down at once, in the afternoon at 4 (3d day). [*S.*]

Vertigo, everthing turns around with him; with nausea.

Everything turns around with him before his eyes.

65. Vertigo in the morning, as if she should turn about, with a fainting sort of nausea; after breakfasting on rolls the nausea ceased, but there was acidity in the mouth (11th d.). [*S.*]

Vertigo in the morning.

Staggering while walking, as if from drunkenness. [*Bte.*]

Quickly-passing vertigo in the morning. [*S.*]

Vertigo increased by stooping. [*S.*]

70. Vertigo even to falling over while walking; she had to hold herself up by the wall (24th d.). [*S.*]

The whole day giddiness, even to falling down; to moderate the giddiness she has to wipe her eyes (11th d.). [*S.*]

Giddiness almost continuous for several days, somewhat like a light intoxication from beer. (31st d.). [*S.*]

The head is always giddy, as soon as she opens her eyes (16th d.). [*S.*]

The head feels as if in a fog and intoxicated; she feels as if she ought to turn around, for 9 days; this symptom alternated with a pain in the kidneys, so that as this pain increased the giddy feeling diminished, and *vice versa* (aft. 30 d.). [*S.*]

75. He becomes intoxicated even by the weakest spirituous drink.

Headache, increasing by walking in the open air.

Pains in the head and in the nape of the neck, beginning when going to bed and diminishing only in the morning after rising.

Headache, obliging the person to lie down, with dry heat and coughing during sleep, the whole afternoon.

Headache on the left side (aft. 18 h.). [*Hb.*]

80. Dull pain in the occiput for a short time (aft. ½ h.). [*Tr.*]

Headache in the occiput as if bruised, passing off on lying down.

The head feels heavy and hot in the morning.

Great heaviness of the head, with paleness and weariness.

Heaviness of the head, with a sensation as if he would fall over while sitting up straight, but worse when stooping, at 1 P. M. (5th d.). [*Ng.*]

85. Heaviness of the head, with a muddled feeling in the forehead and sensitiveness to the touch in the crown of the head at 4 P. M. (2d d.). [*Ng.*]

Sharp, pressive pain in the head over the eyes.

Pressing out at the forehead, after dinner (5th d.). [*Ng.*]

Inward pressure in the forehead. [*Ng.*]

Inward pressure on the right temple, after dinner. [*Ng.*]

90. Screwing pressure on the head.

Pressive headache above the eyes from both temples, during the evening; and at night in bed, heat and afterwards perspiration (aft. 2 h.).

Compressive (pinching) headache in the forehead over the eyes, as if coming from the temples (aft. 3–12 h.).

Headache, tearing and pressing together from both sides, in the evening (aft. 2½ h.), with a shaking chill, many evenings in succession.

Sensation as if the right side of the head were being pressed or screwed toward the other, and as if a heavy weight were lying on the crown of the head, 8½ A. M. (2d d.). [*Ng.*]

95. Pains as if the inside of the head were being screwed together, with stitches in the forehead and such violent heaviness in the

crown of the head, that on stooping, the head threatens to tumble off while standing at 2 P. M. (2d. d.). [*Ng*].

Sensation of constriction around the forehead, attended with pain (aft. ¼ h.). [*Ng.*]

Obtuse, pressive headache, aggravated by walking (1st d.). [*Tr.*]

Burning, **pressive pain with warmth in the fore part of the head, after dinner, both while standing** and sitting; relieved in the open air and does not return in the room. [*Ng.*]

Headache as if from being bruised, with some redness of the cheeks. [*Bte.*]

100. Peculiarly malignant headache, as if the brain was shattered, as in putrid fever. [*Bte.*]

Benumbing tension of a small spot of the right temple, which passes off when it is pressed upon, but immediately returns when the pressure is remitted, in the forenoon (2d d.). [*Ng.*]

Drawing and pulsating tension in the right occiput, in the forenoon (1st d.). [*Ng.*]

Headache, a painful drawing in the right side of the head.

Boring drawing pain in the left temporal region, in the evening (3d d.). [*Tr.*]

105. Tearing headache in the forehead, which is alleviated in the open air, in the evening (3d d.). [*Ng.*]

Tearing in the whole head, in the forenoon (1st d.). [*Ng.*]

Tearing in the right temple (the spot burns on being rubbed) (aft. ½–2h.). [*Ng.*]

Tearing and shooting in the right side of the head in the forenoon, also in the left frontal protuberance, in the evening (1st d.). [*Ng.*]

Tearing in the forehead, in the forenoon, turning into shooting pains in the afternoon (2d d.). [*Ng.*]

110. Tearing pain extending up the left temple, with subsequent stitches in the right temple (aft. 2 h.). [*Ng.*]

Headache, like tearing and also stitches in the ears, somewhat relieved by pressing upon it with the hand, for 4 days toward evening (aft. 6d.). [*S.*]

Headache, violent stitching pain in the brain with nausea.

Stabs as from a knife, darting through the head from time to time.

Stitches darting through the head at every step.

115. A stitch in the head, as if passing all around the head.

Sharp stitches in the right side of the head, while stooping in working (28th d.). [*Ng.*]

A stitch in the right temple, as with a large dull instrument, leaving behind it pain as from a wound, lasting a short time (aft. 13th d.). [*S.*]

Stitches in the temple while singing, ceasing as soon as she stopped singing (aft. 33 d.). [*S.*]

Stitches in particular spots in the head. [*Tr.*, *Ng.*]

120. Stitches in the head toward the crown (2d and 3d. d.). [*Hb.*]

Stitches in the forehead, with muddled and heavy sensation in the head, in the afternoon (3d d.). [*Ng.*]

Stitches in the forehead while going to sleep (10th d.). [*S.*]

Stitches in the fore and back parts of the head after eating, worse toward evening (aft. 37 d.). [*S.*]

Stitches from within outward, in the afternoon (8th d.). [*Ng.*]

125. Painful boring into the right temple, in the evening (5th d.). [N*g.*]

Constant boring and tearing in both temples, in the forenoon (4th d.). [*Ng.*]

Pulsating headache in the crown above the right temporal region, on awaking in the morning.

Throbbing and stitches in the forehead and the right side of the head, in the afternoon (2d d.). [*Ng.*]

Throbbing and pressure in the right temple, like a strong pulsation, with pressure on the crown as from a heavy weight, in the afternoon (2d d.). [*Ng.*]

130. Pulsating headache on going upstairs, after dinner (2d d.). [*Tr.*]

Beating and raging in the crown of the head, forenoon (2d d.). [*Ng.*]

Beating and tearing on the upper part of the right side of the head, 1 P. M. [*Ng.*]

Rythmic beating in the whole head, in the afternoon while walking and in bed in the morning (aft. 3d d.). [*Ng.*]

While stooping, a rushing in the head in the rythm of the pulsation, relieved somewhat on rising up; after dinner. [*Ng.*]

135. **The headache is relieved, when the person quietly lays his head on the bed.** [*Bte.*]

After dinner, heat in the head, with a sensation while stooping, as if the whole brain was about to fall forward; this passes when he rises (1st d.). [*Ng.*]

Feeling of internal warmth in the forehead, while none is felt externally, with muddled feeling for ½ hour. [*Ng.*]

She feels heat rising from the stomach into the head, in the forenoon. [*Ng.*]

Headache, with a sensation as if a worm were crawling under the cranium, also like cutting and gnawing.

140. Sensation as if something were crawling (between the skin and the flesh) from both the temples toward the forehead, where it presses outward, as if about to press through there. [*Bte.*]

A sensation spreads over the head externally, as if the skin were going to sleep (3d. d.). [*Hb.*]

Pressure externally on the occiput and the forehead, **as if from a tight hat.**

On the upper part of the forehead, a small spot painful to the touch, in the morning (10th, 11th d.). [*Tr.*]

External tearing in the right temple, with subsequent constant boring and beating internally (2d d.). [*Ng.*]

145. External stitching as from an awl in a small spot on the left side of the head, near the crown. [*S.*]

External pinching and griping on the head, with a chilly sen sation toward the occiput, worse while stooping, in the evening. [*S.*]

Pain in the left region of the vertex, as if some one were pulling her upward by a lock of her hair (1st d.).

The hair of the head pains when touched, as if the place were sore.

Falling out of the hair (aft. 8 d.). [*S.*]

150. Dryness of the hair of the head.

Itching (formication and crawling sensation), here and there on the head. [*Ng.*]

Unbearable itching on the head; he has to scratch until it bleeds, and after scratching the skin feels sore. [*Hb.*]

The hairy scalp itches, and is full of white scales. [*Hb.*]

Dryness and parched feeling of the hair of the head.

155. A cluster of pimples on the hairy scalp behind the right ear, with tensive pain. [*Ng.*]

Eruptional pimples on the forehead and on the neck.

Quivering sensation of the eyebrows. [*Bte.*]

Pressure on the eyes, she could not open them.

Pressure in the eyes and sensitiveness to the light. [*Hb.*]

160. Pressure in the right eye in the evening, while writing or reading. [*Tr.*]

Pressure in the left eye, as if something had fallen into it, just below the upper eyelid, during the whole day (5th d.). [*S.*]

Pressure on the left eyeball (aft. ½ h.). [*Tr.*]

Alternating pressure in the eyelids (1st d.). [*Tr.*]

Tension about the left eye (2d d.). [*Ng.*]

165. Tearing in the right upper eyelid while looking down; when looking upward, a sensation as if the upper lid was longer and was hanging down; then stitches in the right side of the head (2d d.). [*Ng.*]

Tearing in the upper border of the orbit.

A burning stinging smarting, as from some acid in a corner of the eye.

Stitching in the canthi. [*Ng.*]

Stitching in the lower eyelid. [*Hb.*]

170. Frequent violent itching in the eyes.

Itching in the canthi and the lids. [*Ng.*]

Excoriations in the interior of the eyes, in the evening; the eyelids then close irresistibly.

Sensation of excoriation and dryness in the inner canthi. [*Hb.*]

Smarting in the left eye as from soap, in the evening.

175. Tearing smarting pain in the eye.

Smarting, burning pain in the eyes in the morning (2d d.). [*Tr.*]

Burning of the eyes, early on awaking. [*Ng.*]

Burning in the eyes, especially when he looks upward.

Burning and pressure in the eyes.

180. Burning and pressure in the eyes and in the nose, as if she were catching a cold in the nose. [*S.*]

Burning in the canthi (2d, 3d d.). [*Tr.*]

Burning and increased secretion of mucus in the eyes, at night and sometimes in the morning, with itching. [*Tr.*]

Every evening, burning and dryness of the eyelids, with pain in the inner left canthus, and with a secretion of dry gum, every morning for more than a week. [*Hb.*]

Redness of the eyes, with excoriations in the canthi and dulness of vision; in the evening while reading, he sees a halo around the light; he has to wipe his eyes frequently, and they become closed at night from suppuration; this lasts a long time. [*Hb.*]

185. Redness of the right eye, with sensation of soreness and lachrymation (3d and 4th d.). [*Hb.*]

Inflammation of the conjunctiva of the right eye, without any severe pains, in the evening (1st d.). [*Tr.*]

On the left lower eyelid, a pimple with stinging pain.

Repeated commencement of a stye on the upper eyelid. [*Hb.*]

The eyelashes fall out.

190. Weakness of the eyelids, they are continually tending to close, without any sleepiness, in the afternoon. [*Ng.*]

He cannot easily open the left eye, because it seems to him as if the upper eyelid was hanging down too far, wherefore he frequently wipes his eyes, so as to see better (5th d.). [*Ng.*]

The upper eyelid feels as if it were paralyzed, hangs down and only half covers the eye (29th d.).

When he has lightly closed his eyes in bed, they often contract spasmodically and painfully with a jerk, and if he wishes to open his eyes at night, even in the dark, they ache violently, with pressive pains as if from a most bright sunlight suddenly admitted, and they contract again; he can get but little sleep at night, and during the day there is frequent quivering in the right upper eyelid. [*Hb.*]

Tremor of the left eye, as if it would leap out, worse toward evening and while looking down; alleviated by closing the eyes or by looking up or when she holds it with her hand; at the same time the eye is sensitive to the light, so that she had to close it frequently, for 3 days (aft. 47 d.). [*S.*]

195. Lachrymation of the eyes in the open air.

Frequent lachrymation of the eyes, without pains. [*S.*, *Ng.*]

Lachrymation of the eyes, early on awaking. [*Hb.*, *Ng.*]

Running of the eyes and burning, with a sensation as if the face was swollen (1st d.). [*Ng.*]

A mucous humor is continually secreted in the right eye (gum).

200. The eyes secrete much mucus during the night, for several days successively. [*S.*]

Early on awaking, much dry eye-gum.

The eyes, early on awaking, are glued together and burn when opened, with photophobia. [*Ng.*, *Hb.*]

Nightly agglutination of the eyes for several weeks, with inflamed conjunctiva and with secretion of gum during the day;

in the light, especially in the evening, he feels as if there was a gauze before his eyes, compelling him to wipe them, though it does not thereby pass off, and he sees a halo around the light (aft. 10 d.). [*Hb.*]

The eyes, which are agglutinated in the morning, smart and are dim, which passes away after washing (2d d.). [*Ng.*]

205. **Dimness of vision, as if looking through a mist.**

Dimness of vision, at times in the open air, and disappearing in the room. [*Tr.*, *Ng.*]

Dimness of vision as through a fog, in the evening (1st, 30th d.). [*Ng.*, *Tr.*]

Dimness of vision, compelling him to continually wipe his eyes; this alleviates the dimness; with a sensation in the eyes as if they were about to be agglutinated in the canthi (11th d.). [*Ng.*, *Tr.*]

The right eye is dim-sighted, as if a feather or a hair were before it, which she thinks she must remove (6th and 7th d.). [*S.*]

210. She can neither read nor sew at night, on account of the dulness and dryness of the eyes; also during the day her eye-sight is dull (while her sight was at other times acute).

After long looking, there is weakness of the eyes (4th d.). [*Ng.*]

Squinting of both eyes. [*Tr.*]

Flickering and mist before the eyes. [*Tr.*]

Short flickering and as it were spots before the eyes, a kind of vertigo.

215. After blowing the nose, little white stars glimmer before the eyes (4th d.). [*Ng.*]

He sees a light before his eyes, even when closing them.

Whatever she looks at, appears to her yellow (34th, 35th d.). [*Ng.*]

Tension in the ears (2d, 3d d.). [*Tr.*]

Tearing in, behind and under the ears. [*Ng.*]

220. **Stitches in the ears**, especially in the evening (aft. 30 d.) [*Hb.*]

Stitches in the left ear (7th d.). [*S.*]

Stitches from within outward through the ear. (aft. 4 h.). [*Tr.*]

Stitches into the ears. [*Ng.*]

At night short stitches deep in the right ear (aft. 4 h.). [*Ng.*]

225. Frequent stitches into the hollow of the ear as with a knife. [*Ng.*]

Boring in the ear in the morning, in the afternoon in the hollow of the ear, which also pains when pressed upon (4th d.). [*Ng.*]

Throbbing in the ear.

Violent itching in both ears, increased by rubbing with the finger (aft. 50 h.).

Itching and formication in the interior meatus auditorius. [*Ng.*, *Tr.*]

230. On the right ear a watery, transparent vesicle without any pain. [*Bte.*]

Itching before and behind the ears and on the lobules. [*Ng.*]

Itching burning on the anterior border of the right ear (1st d.). [*Ng.*]

For many evenings a hot, red ear.

Discharge of pus from the right ear (aft. 11 d.). [*Hb.*]

235. It seems to her as if something lay outside before the ear.

On blowing her nose the ear is obstructed, but when she swallows, it opens again.

Humming of the ears, in the evening

Humming of the ears in the morning; the stools at the same time are harder than usual. [*S.*]

Buzzing before the ears, as from bells, early on rising from bed.

240. Hissing in the ear.

Loud whistling in the ear.

While swallowing there is a crackling sound in the ear.

Especially in chewing there is a crackling sound of the tympanum.

His voice sounds changed to him for one hour in his right ear (4th d.). [*Ng.*]

245. Intermittent burning pain in the right nostril, in the evening (1st d.). [*Tr.*]

Tearing in and near the right nasal cavity, which passes away only for a short time when pressed upon (2d d.). [*Ng.*]

Itching on the dorsum, the side and around the orifice of the nose. [*Ng.*]

Violent itching of one ala of the nose for 1 hour.

Ulcerated nostrils.

250. Soreness with scabs in the right nostril; with a discharge of much thick, yellowish mucus from the nose (the first 4 weeks). [*Ng.*]

On the right side of the nose two pimples with burning, stinging pain.

A furuncle on the nose.

Bleeding of the nose. [*Ng.*]

In blowing his nose, pure blood is discharged.

255. The septum of the nose is swollen, red and painful to the touch; in the evening the pains are aggravated with stitches in the forehead (1st d.). [*S.*]

Swelling and induration of the left nostril, which is painful to the touch (8th d.). [*S.*]

Sour smell in the nose, in the morning (3d d.). [*Ng.*]

Excessively acute sense of smell.

Weakness of olfaction.

260. Lowering, ill-humored expression of countenance. [*Ng.*]

Quickly alternating paleness and redness of the face.

Tearing in the sides of the face, especially in the right side, in the zygoma, where it passes away on rubbing, or with tearing in the teeth on this side. [*Ng.*]

The cheeks are of a coppery red, as with brandy-drinkers. [*Bte.*]

Heat and tension in the left side of the face, in the evening (1st d.). [*Tr.*]

265. Tension and drawing in the jaws and cheeks, with increased secretion of saliva (2d d.). [*Tr.*]

Drawing and tearing in the left cheek and gums, in the afternoon (aft. 30th d.). [*S.*]

Formication in the right side of the face as from ants with, stitches in the hollow of the ear and tearing in the right knee. [*Ng.*]

The skin of the face is tense, even around the eyes, as if the white of an egg was drying upon it, after dinner (while walking in the open air) (5th d.). [*Ng.*]

His face appears to him to be larger or swollen and the eyes smaller, so that it impedes his vision, after dinner (1st d.). [*Ng.*]

270. Paleness of the face.

Daily flushes of heat in his face.

A red spot which pains on his right cheek.

The skin of the face rough, especially on the forehead.

Sensation on the chin as if cobwebs enclosed it.

275. Violent itching in the face.

Itching on the forehead, the cheeks, around the eyes, and the chin. [*Ng.*]

Itching of the cheek with burning after scratching. [*Ng.*]

Itching formication as from an insect on the right side of the lower jaw. [*Ng.*]

Itching with a violent impulse to scratch, in the face and below the chin, on which small pimples like rash arise (4th d.). [*Ng.*]

280. Itching pimples on the forehead, the right side of the nose, and the left angle of the mouth (on being pressed upon these coalesce) (6th to 9th d.). [*Ng.*]

A pimple on the right cheek which pains as if sore when touched.

Small red pimples on the right cheek; they are rough to the touch and painless (12th d.). [*S.*]

The vermillion of the lips is bluish (during and after the fever). [*Bte.*]

Small pimples on the chin which pass away on the following morning (aft. 8th and 13th d.). [*Ng.*]

285. Eruptive granules on the left cheek and on the forehead (10th d.). [*Ng.*]

One furuncle after the other on the left cheek.

Itching on a crust, already dry, of an unhealed little furuncle on the forehead, which passes away on scratching. [*Ng.*]

Firm closure of the jaws (1st h.). [*Tr.*]

Tensive pain in the articulations of the jaws, in chewing or opening the mouth.

290. The jaw is swollen, that he cannot open his mouth without pain; stitches ran up to the cheek-bone and to the temple.

Both the lips seem to him to be larger and swollen. [*Ng.*]

Swelling of the lower lip.

Swelling of the lips with vesicles on them.

Tickling of the left angle of the mouth and the right zygoma, which passes away by scratching. [*Ng.*]

295. On the inner surface of the lip a clear looking vesicle as large as a pea (2d d.). [*Tr.*]

Eruption on the lower lip, like a crust.

The lips peel off (4th d.). [*Ng.*]

Chapped, dry **lips**. [*Ng.*, *Tr.*, *S.*]

Considerable retraction of the lower jaw; the upper teeth extend far over the lower for 3 days. [*Bte.*]

300. Drawing pain in the gums as if sore.

Swelling of the gums.

Bleeding of the gums (4th d.). [*Hb.*]

Ulceration of the roots of all the teeth. [*Bte.*]

An ulcer forms on the gums of the lower row on the left side; this breaks open at once and discharges blood which has a salty taste (4th d.). [*Ng.*]

305. Drawing pain from a tooth even to the ear, into the side of the head.

The toothache extends down to the larynx with a nervous excitement, as it does often after taking cold or after the use of chamomile. [*Bte.*]

Drawing pains in the row of teeth of the right side, in the evening; passing away after going to bed. [*Ng.*]

Jerking pain in one of the first molars of the left upper row (1st d.). [*Ng.*]

Jerking and tearing toothache wakes her up after midnight and passes away when she rises (5th d.). [*Ng.*]

310. Drawing tearing pain in the anterior lower teeth, extending to the zygoma and the temple.

Tearing in the molars at various times of the day, at times extending to the temples. [*Ng.*]

Gnawing pain in an anterior molar of the lower jaw with tearing behind the ear and a sensation as if it would tear it out; worst at 9 P. M., then slowly decreasing, somewhat alleviated by sitting up in bed, and after midnight there is merely a gnawing pain in the tooth. The pain is unchanged under all circumstances, during the day it merely mutters. [*Ng.*]

In the evening boring (tearing, digging) in the teeth (aft. 1 h.).

Boring in various hollow teeth.

315. Cutting toothache in the open air and while lying down, in the evening in bed (aft. 2–3 h.).

Tickling in the teeth and at their roots, immediately after dinner (4th, 5th d.). [*Ng.*]

Sensation of coldness in the teeth, with great sensitiveness of the same. [*Ng.*]

The hollow teeth ache severely when any food gets into them.

Pressive pain in an incisor while chewing and also otherwise.

320. The teeth pain severely while chewing, she does not dare to press them together (aft. 2 d.).

The worst toothache is felt, at the least chewing, the roots of the teeth then ache as if they were ulcerated.

On chewing, one of the stumps pains as if it were being violently pushed into the socket.

On pressing the teeth together there is toothache, as if the teeth were loose.

Bruised pain in a molar of the right upper row, alleviated by pressing upon the tooth, which appears loose (11th d.). [*Ng.*]

325. An upper molar is painful to the touch.

Two rotten molar teeth (above and below) interfere with one another on opening the mouth. [*Bte.*]

The teeth feel as if they were too long (1st d.). [*Tr.*]

Thick, ill-smelling mucus on the teeth (5th d.). [*Ng.*]

Continuous sensation in the mouth as if it had been burned (after dinner) (aft. 48 h.). [*Ng.*]

330. Formication on the inner surface of the cheeks (aft. 3 h.). [*Tr.*]

Painfulness of the inner mouth, palate, tongue and of the gums, as if sore, so that he can hardly eat for it.

Numerous little ulcers in the mouth.

On awaking, the mouth is parched and the tongue cleaves to the palate.

Water gathers in the mouth. [*Bte.*]

335. In the morning much expectoration of saliva and mucus. [*Bte.*]

Thick mucus runs into the mouth from the posterior nares.

Musty, rotten smell from the mouth.

(Transient stinging) formication in the tongue (1st h.). [*Tr.*]

Itching of the tip of the tongue, so that he would like to scratch it to pieces (aft. 5th, 7th d.). [*Ng.*]

340. Sensation of roughness on the tongue (aft. ¾ h.). [*Ng.*]

Tongue coated white, with a clean taste. [*S.*]

Tongue coated yellowish-white, with a bitter taste. [*S.*]

Pressive pain in the left tonsil during swallowing, and otherwise (1st d.). [*Tr.*]

Obtuse stitches in the right tonsil in the morning (4th d.). [*Tr.*]

345. Swollen tonsils (6th d.). [*Tr.*]

On both sides of the neck a sensation as of an external swelling with shooting pains.

Sore throat while swallowing. [*S.*]

Sore throat, pressive pain in the throat, even when not swallowing, with hands internally hot (aft. 2 h.).

Pressive pain in the throat as if from a tumor there, with feeling of soreness, hoarseness and dryness of the throat.

350. Violently pressive pain in the throat even when only swallowing saliva, in the evening, for several days in succession, caused by a swelling of the throat (4th d.). [*Tr.*]

Vehemently pressive pain as if a spot in the œsophagus was

constricted or pressed together in the middle of the chest, especially while swallowing, but also at other times, with alternating oppression of the chest and palpitation of the heart, especially after meals (8th, 9th d.). [*Tr.*]

Spasmodic pressive pain in the middle of the chest, while swallowing food and drinks. [*Tr.*]

Sensation of constriction from the gullet down to the stomach with every morsel swallowed.

Constriction of the œsophagus, as well as inactivity of the same, early on awaking.

355. At night impeded swallowing as if from a spasmodic constriction of the throat (1st d.). [*Tr.*]

Constrictive (pressive) pain in the fauces and in the inner throat (in the pharynx with much mucus in the mouth) in the evening (1st and 2d d.). [*Tr.*]

Pressive tensive pain in the inner right side of the throat even to the ear (1st d.). [*Tr.*]

Drawing tensive pains on the right side of the throat, especially when moving the tongue (9th d.). [*Tr.*]

At night a spasmodic drawing pain in the side of the throat and the ear, disturbing the sleep, and increased by swallowing (9th d.). [*Tr.*]

360. Transient stitches, darting hither and thither in the throat, and at times, while swallowing a sensation as if something pointed were sticking in it (in the evening) (2d and 4th d.). [*Tr.*]

Stitching in the throat, during (empty) deglutition. [*Hb. Ng.*]

Hoarseness, in the evening (and at night) which compels hawking, and accumulation of mucus in the throat several days in succession. [*Tr. Ng.*]

Sensation of scraping in the throat, as from swallowing pepper (aft. 3 h.). [*Tr.*]

Constant griping scraping in the throat, lasting for a long time (5th d.). [*Ng.*]

365. Scratching above in the throat.

After eructation, scratching in the neck, compelling him to hawk (2d d.). [*Ng.*]

(Burning) pain as of soreness in the throat (during and) even when not swallowing, in the evening, several days in succession (4th d.). [*Tr.*]

Burning in the throat, in the evening (3d d.). [*Tr.*]

Burning in the throat, like heartburn and hoarseness (5th d.). [*Ng.*]

370. Inflammation of the fauces, which is distinctly terminated by a livid color in the bucal cavity for several days (aft. 2 d.). [*Tr.*]

Inflammatory redness in the back part of the throat (9th d.). [*Tr.*]

Great dryness in the throat, the mouth and the lips, as if these parts were parched with heat, attended with a tormenting thirst.

Dryness in the throat and mouth (soon after taking the medicine). [*Tr.*]

In the evening, dryness in the throat which forces him to hawk (3d d.). [*Tr.*]

375. Dryness, with a sensation of scraping in the throat (1st d.). [*Ng.*]

The ailments of the throat are most violent in the evening and at night; least in the forenoon, and are alleviated by eating and drinking warm things. [*Tr.*]

Increased secretion of saliva in the mouth, with a sensation of contraction there or with constant formication in the surfaces of the cheeks (aft. ½ h.). [*Tr.*]

In the evening in bed, much saliva collects in the mouth (3d d.). [*Tr.*]

Frequent gathering of watery saliva in the mouth, which he has to spit out all the day, most of all in the afternoon, not at all at night (aft. 10 min. and 2d.). [*Ng.*]

380. The secretion of saliva becomes a real ptyalism. [*Tr.*]

Increased secretion of mucus (and saliva) (1st and 2d d.). [*Tr. Ng.*]

Collection of much mucus in the mouth, which being spit out is continually renewed again, with dryness in the throat (1st d.). [*Tr.*]

Especially in the evening and early on awaking, there is a collection of thick, viscid mucus in the throat, which increases the soreness of the throat, compels frequent hawking, and can only be ejected with difficulty, in little lumps (1st d.). [*Tr.*]

Thick, viscid mucus flows into the throat from the posterior nares.

385. After hawking up phlegm with much difficulty, the throat becomes very sensitive. [*Ng.*]

He cannot hawk up the phlegm from his throat, because it is too far down. [*Ng.*]

A piece of phlegm comes into his throat, which threatens to choke him until he swallows it down (aft. 10 min.). [*Ng.*]

Hawking up of (salty) phlegm, after dinner (2d d.). [*Ng.*]

Constant collection of (sweetish or acidulous) water in the mouth (5th, 8th d.). [*Ng.*]

390. Dryness of the mouth, though saliva is not deficient, which frequently causes painful deglutition. [*Tr.*]

Bloody taste in the mouth for ½ hour (7th d.). [*Ng.*]

Sweet taste in the throat with vertigo, then expectoration of mucus mixed with blood, early in the morning (28th d.). [*Ng.*]

Astringent acrid taste on the tongue, as from eating sloes (1st, 8th d.). [*Ng.*, *Tr.*]

Bitter taste in the evening, after eating apples.

395. Bitter taste in the mouth (soon after taking the medicine). [*Ng.*]

Bitter and phlegmy taste in the mouth, early on arising (5th d.). [*Ng.*]

Bitterish insipid taste in the mouth. [*Hb.*]

Everything tastes disagreeable. [*Bte.*]

Disagreeable metallic taste in the mouth in the morning (4th, 5th d.). [*Tr.*]

400. A sourish taste arises in his throat all at once, without eructation, in the forenoon (4th d.). [*Ng.*]

An acid fluid rises into his mouth.

Sourish taste in his throat, then a bitter retching up, soon after eating his milk-soup in the evening (4th d.). [*Ng.*]

Sourish, salty taste (1st d.). [*Tr.*]

Rancid taste in the throat and hoarseness, compelling him to hawk (4th d.). [*Ng.*]

405. All food especially in the evening appears to her as tasteless and unseasoned, bread tastes like sponge (1st and 2d d.). [*Ng.*]

Meat, especially, seems to her to have no taste.

Beer tastes to her bitter and nauseous, causing her to retc (12th d.). [*Ng.*]

No desire to eat, no appetite, no hunger; food has, indeed, no bad taste, rather none at all; everthing tastes like straw or shavings.

She has no aversion to food, but no desire to eat at all, and when she sees food, she has at once enough, and could go the whole day without eating; this for many days.

410. Little hunger and no appetite for many days (even when he does not eat any dinner) (1st d., 15th d.). [*Ng.*]

Diminished appetite with fullness of the abdomen. [*Tr.*]

He has no appetite and eats with aversion. [*S.*]

Aversion to meat.

He abominates meat, it even causes vomiting for three days (aft. 6 d.). [*Ng.*]

415. Aversion to his customary smoking of tobacco.

Disagreeable feeling of hunger and emptiness in the stomach, and yet but little appetite.

She has hunger, and yet she does not enjoy her food. [*Ng.*]

Almost constant hunger; he could eat all the time.

Very violent hunger. [*Hb.*]

420. Voracious hunger; he is all in a tremble for his meals and can hardly wait for them. [*S.*]

Strong appetite for vegetables, fruit and soft food.

Smoking of tobacco causes ailments.

Smoking of tobacco does not give him any pleasure and makes him dizzy, for four days. [*Ng.*]

After eating potatoes, stomach-ache, sick feeling, nausea, and then colicky pains. [*Ng.*]

425. After eating at noon and in the evening, hiccough.

As soon as she has eaten anything, she feels a pressure in her stomach; she nevertheless enjoys her food. [*S.*]

Soon after eating, a sharp, pressive pain in the left hypogastrium.

After every meal, at noon and in the evening, pinching in the abdomen (aft. 29 d.). [*Ng.*]

After meals in the evening, violent nausea and tremulousness.

430. After supper, nausea, loathing and weariness, for several evenings,

After dinner, a drawing sensation in the stomach, which causes a feeling of tension in the whole body, making her so tired, she had to lie down.

Much thirst the whole day, also at dinner. [*Ng.*]

Hiccough after dinner, and also after eructations following the soup at breakfast (1st and 2d d.). [*Ng.*]

Heartburn after supper.

435. Heartburn after drinking water.

Heartburn, with a copious flow of water from the mouth. [*Hb.*]

Waterbrash. [*S.*]

Frequent empty eructations (aft. 2 h.).

Empty eructations after supper (2d d.). [*Ng.*]

440. Eructations with pressive pain on the chest during meals (aft. ¾ h.). [*Ng.*]

Frequent eructations with the taste of the milk-soup eaten, from supper-time till going to bed. [*Ng.*]

Bitter eructations after eating potatoes, so that he shook for loathing, in the evening (5th d.). [*Ng.*]

Rancid eructations, which leave behind a long continued burning in the throat (1st d.). [*Tr.*]

Rancid eructation, especially after dinner (10th–13th d.). [*Tr.*]

445. Rancid eructation after the soup at breakfast. [*Ng.*]

Sharp, corrosive eructations.

Sour eructation in the evening in bed.

Sour eructation with burning in the throat, like heartburn (1st d.). [*Ng.*]

In the forenoon, acidity rises into his mouth; this is long continued and attended with a sensation of heat in the mouth.

450. Belching up of sour mucus, then burning in the throat like heartburn, frequently, especially after soup at breakfast.

Sweetish risings from the stomach, with a sweetish taste of the mucus hawked up, long continued, in the morning (3d d.). [*Ng.*]

Sensation of loathing and qualmishness in the fauces (1st d.).

Qualmishness in the stomach with a fainting sort of nausea and vertigo, in which the room turns round with her, with subsequent muddled feeling in the head (10th d.). [*S.*]

Frequent nausea (especially during the chills). [*Bte.*]

455. Nausea with risings of air. [*S.*]

Nausea and chilliness the whole day. [*S.*]

Attack of nausea with headache, paleness of the face, loss of appetite, repeated evacuations, loathing, followed by nausea and chills running over him; after a walk he has to lie down (11th d.). [*Hb.*]

Nausea-like fainting in the morning; better after breakfast (9th d.). [*S.*]

Nausea early on awaking, qualmishness in the stomach with weariness, with stitches over the eyes and pains in the kidneys on moving (9th d.). [*S.*]

460. While standing she feels sick with nausea.

Nausea even to fainting, depriving her of her breath, at night.

Nausea, early in the morning at 4 o'clock.

Frequent nausea as if he should vomit, and yet he has a tolerable appetite.

Inclination to vomit, in the morning. [*S.*]

465. In the morning, retching as if about to vomit.

Inclination to vomit, after eructations of air, with chilliness of the body, which passes from the feet into the body. [*S.*]

Nausea with inclination to vomit and retching, so that she had to put her finger down her throat, when she vomited mucus and water; but the breakfast eaten two hours before remained (14th d.). [*S.*]

Violent stomach-ache with external sensitiveness of the stomach to pressure, in the evening (6th d.). [*Ng.*]

Pressure in the stomach up to the throat, after eating potatoes, alleviated by eructations, in the morning (8th d.). [*Ng.*]

470. Pressure in the stomach as from a stone, after eating milk-soup, relieved by eructations, in the evening (4th d.). [*Ng.*]

Pressure in the stomach, toward noon or evening. [*Hb.*, *Ng.*]

Violent pressure in the scrobiculus cordis and thence great oppression on the chest, she had to stand still every few moments, and could not go on. [*S.*]

Stomach-ache, it feels full or bloated, with external sensitiveness to pressure, empty eructation and fermentation; or loud grumbling and rumbling in the abdomen, as if something was working there, after dinner (1st, 5th d.). [*Ng.*]

Twisting together and constriction in the region of the stomach, extending to the chest and throat, with labored breathing. [*Hb. Ng.*]

475. Pressure and constriction in the region of the stomach (31st d.). [*Hb.*]

Pressive contractive sensation in the scrobiculus cordis, extending into the chest and between the shoulder-blades (13th d.). [*Hb.*]

Sensation like cutting, in the region of the stomach which is also sensitive to pressure, in the afternoon (2d d.). [*Ng.*]

Stitches in the pit of the stomach and up into the chest.

After dinner till evening, stitches in the stomach and in the chest, out at the shoulders, with short breath and great oppression, several days (aft. 12th d.). [*Ng.*]

480. Some time after meals, gnawing in the region of the stomach 2d, 3d d.). [*Tr.*]

Griping sensation in the stomach, in the afternoon (1st d.). [*Ng.*]

Drawing pain in the stomach.

Drawing pain from the pit of the stomach to the fauces, with difficult breathing.

Pressive aching pain over the stomach and in the epigastrium, transversely, in the afternoon.

485. Pain as from a sore, festering in the scrobiculus cordis, early on turning in bed.

Tearing pain as from a sore, from the scrobiculus cordis into the abdomen, as if everything was being torn out.

Pressive formication in the scrobiculus cordis, as from a worm (aft. 2 h.). [*Ng.*]

Sensation of coldness in the stomach, as if she had drunk cold water, in the evening, also in the forenoon after eructations, and during constant sour eructations, which cease in the afternoon (2d, 5th d.). [*Ng.*]

In stooping, the liver is continually sensitive and painful.

490. Tearings in the liver.

Tearing from the region of the right hypochondrium into the hip, in the forenoon (1st d.). [*Ng.*]

On rising up from stooping, violent stitches in the right side of the abdomen, as if in the liver; they check breathing. (11th d.).

Stitches in the region of the right hypochondrium while standing, passing away on sitting down. [*Ng.*]

In the evening continual shooting pain under the left lower ribs, up into the scrobiculus cordis (5th d.).

495. Dull stitches alternately under the left short ribs and in the right side of the abdomen (4th d.). [*Tr.*]

Stitches in both hypochondriac regions. [*Ng.*]

Sensation as if the two hypochondriac regions were forcibly pressed or screwed together, in the forenoon (1st d.). [*Ng.*]

Long continued burning and stitching in the region of the right hypochondria as if it was deeply cut into by a bandage, in the afternoon (1st d.). [*Ng.*]

Frequently a momentary drawing pain under the right ribs, both while sitting and walking.

500. Pressure from both sides of the epigastrium toward one another, with painfulness of the spot on pressure from without (aft. 2 h.). [*Ng.*]

Constant pressure and burning in the abdomen.

Pressure and stitches in the abdomen after meals (5th d.). [*Hb.*]

Pressing inwardly into the region of the navel, with stitches, in the afternoon, while standing. [*Ng.*]

Pressure and heaviness in the abdomen.

505. The abdomen seems to him to hang down heavy, for 2 hours in the afternoon while walking. [*Ng.*]

Early before eating, a spasmodic pain from the bladder to the chest, disappearing after breakfast. [*S.*]

Violent griping in the abdomen every time she takes cold, or as often as she goes out into the cold. [*Ng.*]

Griping and twisting in the abdomen (aft. 1 h.).

In the evening, griping about the navel (1st d.). [*Tr.*]

510. At the usual breakfast, griping below the navel, with fulness and distention of the abdomen (1st d.). [*Tr.*]

Sudden griping here and there in the abdomen, which then passes into the small of the back, where it gnaws painfully for a long time in the afternoon (16th d.). [*Ng.*]

Griping in the abdomen with heat in the stomach (aft. 1 h.). [*Ng.*]

Griping in the abdomen, in the bed in the evening; this ceases after saliva gathers in the mouth (2d and 3d d.). [*Tr.*]

On awaking, griping in the abdomen and tenesmus, she could scarcely reach the water-closet, where she, fainting, leaned against the wall; there was no evacuation, but after much urging all in vain, the colicky pains ceased (12th d.). [*S.*]

515. In the afternoon and at night, griping, stitching, tearing pain in the left side of the abdomen to the hypochondria and up into the sternum (7th d.).

Towards evening a colicky griping and tearing in the abdomen, with chilliness of the body; alleviated by applying warm cloths. [*S.*]

Flatulent colic.

Violent attacks of colic after dinner, during the afternoon, improved by a short nap, but soon returning, as it seemed, through motion with violent tenesmus and frequent passage of excrements until the evening, so that the anus pains with stitches as if sore, and he cannot sit down without pains; on the following day involuntary discharge of fluid mucus from the anus (aft. 14 d.). [*Hb.*]

Soon after rising, tearing sensation in the abdomen.

520. During bodily exertions, pain in both sides of the abdomen as if something in it was about to tear; this pain extends down to the thighs.

Frequent cutting pain in the abdomen, without distension or stool (2d d.). [*Ng.*]

While sitting bent over, sharp cutting pains, transversely over the abdomen (aft. 5 h.). [*Tr.*]

Violent cutting and gurgling sounds in the whole abdomen, whence the pain passes as a violent contortion into the stomach, this is followed by a violent pressive pain in the chest, with arrest of breathing; from 4 P. M. to 11 P. M. [*Ng.*]

Drawing pains in the abdomen.

525. Stitches darting about in the abdomen and in the hypochondria, as if something were about to fall out (7th d.). [*Hb.*]

Digging about the navel, as after a cold, in the afternoon (2d d.). [*Ng.*]

Rolling about and painless digging in the abdomen (aft. ½ h.). [*Ng.*]

Aching in the abdomen as after a copious stool, after which an urging remains (aft. 10 d.). [*S.*]

Aching in the epigastrium, like an inclination to diarrhœa; then a soft stool without diminution of the colic (11th d.). [*S.*]

530. After diarrhœic stools following a colic, there remained a violent ache in the abdomen, especially in a spot, where when a girl she had an internal ulcer which opened. The pain was as if from a violent blow, she had to stroke place, bending her body, hold her hand upon it, which somewhat alleviated the pain, but it continued uniformly the whole day, whether sitting or standing (17th d.). [*S.*]

Violent colicky pains in the left side of the abdomen, as if an ulcer was forming, with nausea (34th d.). [*S.*]

The pains in the abdomen are diminished by warmth. [*Ng.*]

Sensation of cold in the abdomen, in the afternoon. [*Ng.*]

Sudden burning in the stomach in the afternoon. [*Ng.*]

535. Pains in the region of the kidneys.

Pain in the region of both the kidneys, above the small of the back, as if bruised, or as if after driving on rough roads, worse on stooping or turning around; as it were pressing inward, so that she cries out; it is almost constant for several days (4th d.). [*S.*]

Pain in the loins, especially in walking and stooping (10th d.). [*S.*]

In the morning, pain in the kidneys, better in the afternoon. [*S.*]

(Griping and) stitches in the flanks and the inguinal regions (on ascending the stairs). [*Ng.*]

540. Severe cutting and burning in the inguinal region the whole forenoon, till evening. [*S.*]

Pulsating pain in the left side of the hypogastrium, about the abdominal ring while sitting (4th d.).

Pressure in both inguinal regions toward the sexual organs in the evening (3d d.). [*Ng.*]

Lancinating, pressive pain in the region of the abdominal ring, as if a hernia would press out, with tension into the side of the abdomen; on the painful spot a knot may be felt like a strangulated hernia.

Inguinal hernia protrudes violently (aft. ½ h.).

545. The hernia did not protrude during the first days, then every day till the 12th day; the 30th day it seemed about to become strangulated, then it protruded every day till the 50th day, but continually less, and finally it did not protrude at all for months. [*S.*]

The hernia protrudes a good deal toward evening, becomes constricted in the inguinal region, and could not be reduced, with the most violent pains, which compelled her to bend double and prevented her from walking, until it was at last reduced of itself after quietly sitting for half an hour (30th d.). [*S.*]

In the abdominal muscles above the left inguinal region a drawing pain for a quarter of an hour, when she dances or walks quickly.

Jerking on the left side of the abdomen, frightening her (2d d.). [*Ng.*]

Tension of the abdominal muscles from reaching high.

550. Sensation of flatulence, as if the abdomen was continually becoming fuller after supper (5th d.). [*Ng.*]

Fulness of the abdomen with rushes of blood toward the chest after meals, for several days (aft. 3 d.). [*Tr.*]

Great distension of the abdomen with empty risings and two diarrhœic stools without alleviation (18th d.). [*Ng.*]

After meals much distension with strong ineffectual tenesmus, followed afterwards by the passage of two hard balls of excrement; then she took a walk, the tension of the abdomen continuing despite the frequent passage of flatus; only when after her walk a copious evacuation followed, was she relieved (9th d.). [*S.*]

At night painful distention of the hypogastrium, which does not allow her to sleep, with constipation (11th d.). [*Ng.*]

555. The abdomen is tense and quite hard, without any painful sensation. [*Hb.*]

There is a rumbling motion in the abdomen, like an anxious unrest, without the passing of any flatus; a small evacuation gives no relief (aft. 1 h.).

Distension and grumbling in the abdomen without the passage of flatus (1st d.). [*Ng.*]

Loud rumbling and noise in the abdomen without pain.

Much grumbling flatus in the abdomen; but the flatus passes freely with a feeling of weakness of the sphincter of the anus. [*Bte.*]

560. Much audible rumbling and moving about in the abdomen. [*Ng.*]

Loud rumbling in the abdomen, also after meals. [*Tr.*]

Rumbling and grumbling in the abdomen, afterwards eructations. [*S.*]

Frequent urging to pass flatus. [*Ng.*]

Passage of flatus with relief of the fulness of the stomach, in the evening (5th d.). [*Ng.*]

565. Loud passage of flatus.

Much fetid flatus (passing off quietly), at night and also after dinner (1st, 7th d.). [*Ng.*]

Urging to stool without evacuation (3d d.).

Tenesmus (1st d.). [*Ng.*]

Constipation (8th, 11th d.). [*Ng.*]

570. No stools during the first days. [*S.*]

Stools only every two days and solid, at times mixed with blood. [*S.*]

After a troublesome pressure in the hypogastrium and long continued urging, the stool ensues slowly and only by straining the abdominal muscles; all the bowels seem inactive from lack of the peristaltic motion; stool not hard (aft. 2 d.).

The rectum is inactive, as if it lacked the power to evacuate the fæces, and lacked the peristaltic motion; the stool is soft and of thin formation, and can only be evacuated by a great exertion of the abdominal muscles (aft. 16 h.).

The rectum is as if paralyzed (2d d.).

375. Hard stool, passed with difficulty, with pain in the anus. [*Hb.*]

While bearing down for the stool, which is laborious, urine passes involuntarily (2d d.).

Pressing and bearing down during the stool, which is very firm, knotty and scanty, after previous urging to stool (2d d.). [*Ng*]

Firm, hard and scanty stool, with pressure and pain in the anus and difficult discharge (the first days). [*Ng.*]

Only a very small quantity of hard fæces are discharged, with pressure and excoriation in the rectum.

580. **Stools far too scanty.** [*Hb.*]

(Firm) stool covered with whitish mucus, after pressure in

the region of the stomach, which ceases immediately after the stool (aft. 30 d.). [*Hb.*]

Light colored stool.

The first part of her stool is liquid and squirts out forcibly, but the latter portion appears burned (5th d.). [*Ng.*]

The stool which previously came always in the evening, comes in the morning. [*S.*]

385. The stool comes 3 or 4 times, but is otherwise as usual without any trouble, for some time. [*Hb.*]

Soft (almost fluid) stool with burning in the anus; also in the evening after previous urging, which returns at night (2d, 5th d.). [*Ng.*]

Attacks of little stools of diarrhœa with colic, of 2 or 3 days duration.

Diarrhœa after previous colic. [*S.*]

Diarrhœa after 6 days of constipation; also 6 evacuations a day with previous colic, which sometimes even continues after the stool. [*S.*]

590. Liquid stools with colicky pains before, or cutting pains during, their discharge (3d, 5th d.). [*Ng.*]

In the evening two diarrhœic stools, the last part of which is lumpy (2d d.). [*Ng.*]

Diarrhœa with tenesmus in the rectum. [*S.*]

Tenesmus of the rectum and bladder, which ceases after an evacuation. [*S.*]

Before the stool, disagreeable pressure in the region of the stomach (9th d.). [*Hb.*]

595. Before the stool, which now is solid, now soft, but always scanty, there is griping in the abdomen. [*S.*]

Much tenesmus before there is an evacuation.

After the stool much ineffectual urging in the epigastrium and the sides of the abdomen without any urging to stool in the rectum or anus (without tenesmus).

At the evacuation he felt as if the rectum was dried up and contracted, yet the stool itself was normal. [*S.*]

In the evening during the stool a chill over the whole body (5th d.). [*Ng.*]

600. After the stool, throbbing in the small of the back.

After the stool, while digestion is going on, he has a sensation of scraping in the stomach and in the mouth.

After a difficult evacuation, pricking as of needles in the anus.

After a stool, which is difficult from the sensation of constriction of the rectum and contraction of the anus, there is a pain in the anus as if excoriated.

After a difficult discharge of hard stool like laurel-berries, with cutting pains in the anus as if this was too narrow, there is a discharge of blood in a jet with subsequent smarting pains as of soreness in the anus and up the rectum (aft. 17 d.).

605. During a stool blood drops from the rectum.

Passage of blood with a firm stool (9th and 30th d.). [*Hb.*]

Passage of bloody mucus, during and outside of the stools.

While walking, dark blood is discharged from her anus.

Protrusion of a varix from the rectum, which enlarges while walking; diminished by the night's rest.

610. Varices of the rectum always enlarge in the evening, with burning pain, and humid.

Humidity of the varices and stitches therein.

Severe itching in the fold between the nates and in the anus, increased by rubbing.

Itching on the anus, aggravated by scratching (1st–2d d.). [*Ng.*]

Itching on the anus for a considerable time (aft. 30 d.). [*Hb.*]

615. Itching *burning in the anus.*

Itching, with burning and stitching in the rectum. [*S.*]

Itching in the anus, with a sensation as if it would pulsate. [*S.*]

Tickling in the rectum as from worms. [*S.*]

Pressure in the anus (3d d.). [*Tr.*]

620. Painful pressure in the perinæum, but quickly passing away. [*S.*]

Momentary pressure in the perinæum on blowing the nose. [S.]

Pain in the perinæum when touched, as if it were bruised. [*S.*]

Stitches in the perinæum. [*S.*]

[Soreness in the perinæum, during gonorrhœa (aft. 4 w.).] [*Hb.*]

625. Sensation as if the parts between the scrotum and the anus were inflamed. [*S.*]

Sweating of the perinæum, with unbearable itching, aggravated by rubbing, when it pains. [*Hb.*]

Pressure and drawing in the region of the bladder, especially at its neck (4th and 5th d.). [*Tr.*]

While walking in the open air, tearing, jerking stitches in the urethra, up towards the hypogastrium.

Itching burning in the urethra.

630. In the urethra and between the scrotum a pleasant, voluptuous itching. [*S.*]

Sensation of dryness in front in the urethra, as if the skin there were without sensation, especially in the morning. [*S.*]

Sensation of heat in the urethra which passes off by lying still. [*S.*]

Feeling of weakness in the bladder and the sexual organs, in the evening; he is afraid of wetting his bed. [*Bte.*]

Strong urging to urinate. [*S.*, *Ng.*]

635. Pressure and urging to urinate, without increased discharge (soon after taking the medicine). [*Tr.*]

Early on waking, an urging to urinate, with difficult and delayed passage of the urine, which issues in a thin jet from the female urethra (7th d.).

He has to rise several times at night to urinate (1st and 4th d.). [*Ng.*]

Much water-colored urine.

Increased secretion of urine for several days. [*Tr.*, *Ng.*]

640. Frequent emission of (copious) pale urine (after burning in the urethra). [*Ng.*]

Increased quantity of pale (hot) urine with burning. [*Tr.*, *Ng.*]

Emission of a quantity of straw-yellow, clear urine (4th, 5th d.). [*Tr.*, *Ng.*]

Rare but copious micturition (6th d.). [*Ng.*]

Frequent micturition with scanty emission, in the evening (1st d.). [*Ng.*]

645. Diminished urine (in the morning), with cutting anteriorly in the urethra (4th, 5th, 6th d.). [*Ng.*]

A whole day without micturition or stool. [*Ng.*]

No urine in the forenoon, but in the afternoon frequent emission of an increased quantity of reddish urine, which becomes turbid over night and leaves a sediment (1st d.). [*Ng.*]

She emits very little urine, which leaves, as sediment, a red sand.

The urine, of a deep yellow color, soon deposits a large loose cloud (1st and 5th d.). [*Ng.*]

650. The urine, on standing, leaves a thick white sediment. [*Hb.*]

Pale urine with turbid sediment. [*Ng.*]

White, turbid urine, as if chalk had been stirred into it. [*S.*]

The stream of urine is twisted. [*S.*]

(A sort of fright when about to urinate.) [*S.*]

655. While urinating, a burning sensation, like fire, much worse in the evening (1st d.). [*S.*, *Ng.*]

(After sitting for some time, he feels no discomfort while urinating, but when he takes some exercise the urine burns him.) [*S.*]

(Cutting anteriorly in the urethra, while urinating and also for some time afterward, as if the urine ran over an inflamed spot (aft. 18 d.). [*Hb.*]

After micturition, the urethra becomes hot, then he has a burning sensation, and he has tenesmus of the bladder and rectum. [*S.*]

(After micturition, there is a long continued burning, which makes him ill-humored and discouraged.) [*S.*]

660. (Involuntary micturition, almost twenty times a day, only a little being emitted at a time, with gonorrhœa) (aft. 4 w.). [*Hb.*]

Pressure on the sexual organs.

Tickling of the sexual organs and the thighs.

Formication on the glans. [*S.*]

Itching on the glans (4th d.) [*Tr.*]

665. Drawing from the glans through the urethra (aft. 5d.). [*Tr.*]

(When stroking the penis there is felt a drawing, pinching pain extending to the glans; attended with a poor appetite.) [*S.*]

Sensation as if the glans were squeezed together, for two minutes. [*S.*]

(Gonorrhœa over six weeks (aft. 14 d.) with a severe and painful swelling of the inguinal glands, cutting pain during micturition and pain in the perinæum, especially violent at the end of the second week; the pain in the perinæum is particularly severe while standing, rising and sitting down.) [*Hb.*]

Secretion of much smegma behind the glans.

670. Soreness on the inner surface of the foreskin.

Contractive pain in the right spermatic cord, when the right testicle is drawn up and is also sensitive and painful (2d d.). [*Tr.*]

The left testicle is hard and when touched there is an indescribable aching. [*S.*]

Itching on the scrotum, passing off by scratching (2d d.). [*Ng.*]

It seems to lessen the sexual impulse and to increase the erections in the beginning, while in its after effects the inclination for coition is increased, but the erections are lacking.

675. Lack of the sexual instinct (at once, for several days).

Indifference to sexual intercourse. [*S.*]

During the first weeks increased sexual instinct, but after that, it is lessened and quieted.

Many erections in the evening and night while lying down, and in the afternoon while sitting down (1st, 3d d.). [*Tr.*]

In the night priapism. [*S.*]

680. (In the night while waking, almost continuous painful erections, which are imperfect, but cause a sensation as if the member were festering, with short, fine, piercing stitches in the whole member, like jerks) (aft. 4 w.). [*Hb.*]

Frequent and violent erections and pollutions (aft. 3 and 33 d.). [*Hb.*, *Tr.*]

Pollutions two nights in succession (aft. 15 d.).

The first four nights in succession, pollutions with voluptuous dreams.

Almost every other night, pollution with voluptuous dreams.

685. Pollution during the noon siesta.

After a pollution, all the former ailments are renewed and much aggravated (2d d.).

At the beginning of coition as well as during erections, a violent pressure on the perinæum. [*S.*]

During coition, pressure in the perinæum. [*S.*]

(The seed emitted in coition is thick and lumpy like jelly.) [*S.*]

690. Jerking stitches on the left side of the pudenda up into the breast.

On the left side of the vagina, a ticking pain as from a watch, with a pulsation as when pus is gathering in an ulcer, for 2 days, unchanged by any circumstances; but nothing could be felt or seen (36th d.). [*S.*]

Menses very scanty and only 3 days. [*Ng.*]

Menses in diminished quantity and very pale (aft. 3d d.).

Menses too early (by 3, 11 days), also too short and scanty. [*Ng.*]

695. The menses ought to have appeared 10 days before, but did not appear; only one day (aft. 52 d.) during a walk, when there was an urging to urinate, a little dark-colored bloody water passed, then nothing more; the menses only appeared in the 3d month (with a woman of 48 years).

The menses which had gradually ceased, reappear (aft. 17 d.).

The menses (aft. 9 d.) in diminished quantity; but 4 weeks later (aft. 37 d.) in great abundance.

The menses appeared 5 days earlier, very strong on the 2d day, and lasted as usual for 8 days; preceded by colic; on the 6th day diarrhœa. [*S.*]

Before the appearance of the menses, disturbed sleep, many dreams, and when she wakes from them, she has rushes of blood, heat in the face, headache and palpitations.

700. Six days before the menses appeared, there was a strong flow of mucus from the vagina, with tremulousness, weariness and a sensation as if everything were falling out of her.

Several days before the appearance of the menses, colic during stools, as if preceding diarrhœa, also griping, twisting and pressure, as if from labor-pains.

During the menses, colic and greater weariness than usual.

During the menses distention of the abdomen and excessive flow of blood.

The menses having appeared on the 6th day without any trouble, there came on the second day a flowing coryza with pain in the nose, the head and the forehead, increased by blowing the nose; during the last days diarrhœa and colic were added (aft. 2 d.). [*S.*]

705. During the menses she was obliged to urinate frequently, which corroded the genital organs (6th d.). [*S.*]

Violent headache before the menses, which set in 4 days too early, the headache ceased when the menses appeared, but it reappeared after they had flowed for one day, and continued during the whole period; the flow was weaker than usual and lasted 5 days (aft. 22 d.). [*S.*]

The menses leave behind, after their course, considerable prostration of mind and body; a little work and a moderate walk exhaust her and she feels low-spirited.

Leucorrhœa. [*Ng.*]

The leucorrhœa (which had been flowing before) ceased. [*Hb.*]

710. Leucorrhœa after the menses, painless, lasting 3 days (aft. 27 d.). [*S.*]

Frequent acrid leucorrhœa.

Acrid leucorrhœa with burning in the genital organs and still more in the rectum; these parts were, as it were, inflamed and excoriated, so that she found walking difficult, relieved by washing with cold water; the leucorrhœa was frequent and almost flowed over her feet; at the same time appeared blood like bloody water 3 days after the catamenia had ceased (22d d.). [*S.*]

Leucorrhœa like bloody water in the afternoon, while walking in the open air (and while sitting down), and also at night. [*Ng.*]

Severe leucorrhœa of transparent mucus, but only during the daytime, without pain and without colic.

715. Leucorrhœa, quite transparent and clear like water, and like transparent mucus, stiffening the shift (aft. 8 d.). [*S.*]

Yellow mucus flows from the vagina (aft. several d.).

Itching in the pudenda during the leucorrhœa. [*Ng.*]

* * * * * * *

Frequent sneezing (and hiccough) without coryza (1st, 2d, 7th d.). [*Ng.*]

The nose is stopped up (1st d.).

720. The left nostril is stopped up (10th d.). [*Tr.*]

Indisposition as from coryza, which cannot develop itself.

A sensation in the nose as if a cold in the head were coming on in the evening, for several days (4th d.). [*Tr.*]

Catarrh with sneezing and obstruction of the nose, the whole day (3d d.). [*Ng.*]

Dry coryza (9th d.). [*Ng.*]

725. Severe dry coryza, especially at night, with great dryness of the mouth.

Sudden violent fluent coryza from the left nostril, while the right is entirely obstructed.

First fluent coryza, then a severe dry coryza, so that he cannot breathe through either nostril.

Secretion of much thick and viscid mucus from the nose. [*Hb.*]

Water runs from the right nostril without coryza. [*Ng.*]

730. Running coryza (with obscured voice), afternoon and morning (4th, 6th d.). [*Ng.*]

Running coryza with frequent sneezing and lachrymation. [*S.*]

Snoring during the siesta (6th d.). [*Ng.*]

Rattling and whistling through the nose with obscured voice, afternoon (3d d.). [*Ng.*]

Rattling in the chest, from mucus (5th d.). [*Ng.*]

735. Sibilus in the bronchia and sensation of smothering in the chest, while breathing.

Constantly adhering mucus in the bronchia, which compels hawking, without detaching much mucus. [*Hb.*]

In the morning on awaking, the throat feels raw and the chest coated with mucus; he cannot hawk up anything, and has to sneeze frequently (aft. 12 h.).

Feeling of dryness in both sides of the chest (15th d.).

Hoarseness, early in the morning (16th d).

740. Frequently quite hoarse, so that her voice fails her, not relieved by hawking, mostly in the afternoon and evening.

Hoarse and raw feeling in the throat, the whole afternoon (aft. 5 d.). [*Ng.*]

Scraping and raw sensation in the throat, urging to cough (evening, 4th d.). [*Ng.*, *Tr.*]

Strong tickling in the throat, frequently exciting cough (4th d.). [*Tr.*]

Irritation to cough, in the larynx. [*S.*]

745. Irritation to cough, with frequent spitting out of saliva. [*Tr.*]

Cough, with scratching in the throat. [*Ng.*]

Cough which makes the chest feel sore, in the forenoon (3d d.). [*Ng.*]

Cough with pressive pain in the occiput.

Frequent (short and dry) cough, forenoon and evening. [*Ng.*, *Tr.*]

750. Short fits of cough, causing a tearing, shooting pain in the right temple and the vertex.

Violent, dry, short, continuous cough with sneezing, with a shooting, tearing and pinching pain in the nape of the neck to the right shoulder.

Dry cough at night, with dryness in the throat (aft. 24 h.). [*Ng.*]

Dry cough coming in the morning and suddenly, quickly passing away, or continuing in the open air and then also in the room (1st, 6th d.). [*Ng.*]

Constant dry cough causing vomiting with interception of breath and lancinating pain in the left hypogastrium up to the hypochondria and the scrobiculus cordis.

755. Severe dry cough during the day, every fit is of long continuance, only after 2 days these fits become rare and loose.

Violent dry cough early on arising, followed later by some expectoration (4th, 6th d.). [*Ng.*]

Cough with much expectoration, especially in the morning.

(The cough, with expectoration in the morning, ceases, (curative effect) (5th d.). [*S.*]

(Cough with expectoration, with raw and hoarse throat, with fluent coryza.) [*S.*]

760. Cough with slight rattling of phlegm; curative effect. [*S.*]

Sudden violent, though short cough, when with much exertion he expectorates a lump of mucus mixed with blood, in the afternoon (5th d.). [*Ng.*]

Difficult breathing, forenoon. [*S.*]

His chest is oppressed.

Oppression of the chest (1st d.). [*Tr*].

765. Sensation in the throat as if it were constricted and the air cut off, as in a violent sore throat, but lasting only a few minutes at a time (the first 7 d.). [*Hb.*]

Oppression of the chest.

Pressure, rush of blood and pulsation in the chest (aft. 2 h.). [*Ng.*, *Tr.*]

The chest feels as it were contracted, with anguish (11th d.). [*Ng.*]

Sensation of constriction about the chest, while sitting bent together, passing away when he rises up, in the afternoon (1st d.). [*Ng.*]

770. In stooping at her work, her chest feels constricted, so she could scarcely breathe, as if she was laced too tightly; passing away when walking in the open air (9th d.). [*S.*]

In a strong exertion, lifting, carrying, etc., pain in the chest on the left side of the sternum, with soreness ot the spot to the touch (aft. 10 d.). [*Hb.*]

Sensation of soreness within the ches, to nmoving or turning the body. [*S.*]

Sensation of soreness as if from enlargement of the chest (1st, 9th d.). [*Hb.*]

Weight in the chest with short breath, without cough, only in the afternoon (18th d.). [*Ng.*]

775. Pressive pain and tightness of the chest.

Pressure on the chest. [*S.*]

Pressure on the chest, on sitting bent forward while writing.

Dry pressure anteriorly under the sternum. [*S.*]

Pressure on the sternum, aggravated on walking in the evening. [*S.*]

780. Sensation as of a heavy pressure, above on both sides of the chest, on strong exertion, less while sitting, none at all while lying down; no change by touching it.

Pressure here and there in the chest. [*Ng.*]

Pressure in the chest, followed by empty eructations without alleviation, at times passing through to the back and worse in walking in the forenoon (1st and 20th d.). [*Ng.*]

Pressure on the chest, with short breath and inclination to cough, often ceasing and then again returning. [*Ng.*]

Pressure on the chest during a (pre-existent) cough and after it, during which suddenly a paralyzing pain passes through the fore-arm, so that this becomes weary and powerless (aft. ½ h.). [*Ng.*]

785. Pressive pain in the middle of the chest, alternating with a sensation of tightness and violent palpitation, especially after meals (8th, 9th d.). [*Tr.*]

At night, severe pressive pain in the chest, which disturbs the sleep which is otherwise calm; the pain is not increased by breathing, but by bending the head forward; for several days (aft. 5 d.). [Tr.]

At night while lying on the back, pressure in the chest with short breath; passing off when lying on the side (2d d.). [*Ng.*]

Disagreeable contractive sensation on a small spot below the left chest (aft. 2 h.). [*Ng.*]

Pinching pain in the upper part of the chest, in the evening while sitting down (1st d.). [*Tr.*]

790. Pain in the chest as if cut to pieces or sore, after dinner till 10 P. M.; better on going to bed, but returning the following morning (with the early cough with a sensation of exhaustion in the chest,) with empty eructations and short breath, 7th d., [*Ng.*]

While walking fast, sensation as if cut to pieces in the chest with pressure; relieved by sitting, for fourteen days (20 d.). [*Ng.*]

Pain below in the sternum, as if from excoriation, extending to the stomach, followed by hoarseness.

Sensation of soreness in the chest and in the scrobiculus cordis with fatiguing cough, lachrymation and tenaciously adhering expectoration. [*S.*]

Stitches in the chest here and there, sometimes aggravated by inspiration, sometimes burning. [*Ng.*]

795. Tearing stitch like a lightning-flash from the right loins to the left part of the chest, through the scrobiculus cordis, while catching breath.

In stooping, a stitch from the left side of the abdomen out into the middle of the chest, at every breath; then also while standing upright.

Stitches above on both sides of the chest during, active motion; no stitches while sitting and walking; then it only presses with taking away of the breath.

Stitches under the sternum, increased by talking, at the same time a pressing together of the chest as from a tight corset (35th d.). [*S.*]

Sharp stitches in the upper part of the chest (3 d.). [*Tr.*]

800. Boring pain now in the middle, now in the sides of the chest, aggravated on inspiration, at times in the evening and then relieved by rising up and walking. [*Ng.*]

Chill in the interior of the sternum.

Continuous warmth in the middle of the chest (aft. 5 min.). [*Ng.*]

Heat anteriorly in the chest; she feels the heat while breathing.

Burning in the whole right side of the chest, with stitches and straining in a false rib on the right side,in the afternoon (1st d.). [*Ng.*]

805. Daily palpitation of the heart, early on awaking.

Frequent palpitation of the heart; several irregular beats, short and long ones intermixed.

Fine stitches in the left breast at 9 A. M. (2d d.). [*Ng.*]

External pressure on the lower part of the chest, (somewhat diminished by rubbing). [*Ng.*]

Itching on the sternum, passing off on scratching (15th d.). [*Hb.*]

810. Crawling as of insects on the left clavicle (and over the right side of the chest with itching smarting); after scratching, the spot itches and burning blisters appear (16th d.). [*Ng.*]

Blister on the right side of the chest and on the neck, with burning pain; at the same time glowing of the face and chilliness in the rest of the body, but the sleep is sound and dreamless. [*S.*]

Itching on the coccyx.

At the point of the coccyx painful twitches in the forenoon (2d d.). [*Ng.*]

Sensation of screwing together in the right ilium (1st d.). [*Ng.*]

815. Gnawing pain in the coccyx, unchanged by walking, but alleviated by stretching (1st d., evening). [*Ng.*]

Violent pain in the small of the back, like gnawing, drawing up between the shoulders, where it becomes so violent that she feels like weeping (relieved by chamomile) (32d d.). [*Ng.*]

Tearing stitching pain in the small of the back, in the evening before going to sleep, in bed.

Jerking tearing in the small of the back, especially on moving.

Pain in the small of the back while walking.

820. Violent pain as from a bruise in the small of the back and (in the morning) in the coccyx when touched (4th, 7th d.). [*Ng.*]

Pain in the sacrum and in the back as if from a bruise.

Eruptive pimples on the back.

Burning itching, like a flea-bite, in the region of the left loins so that he shudders; it lasted a long time and only passed off after long continued scratching. [*Ng.*]

Itching on and between the shoulder blades. [*Ng.*]

825. Itching, crawling and smarting in the whole back, the small of the back, followed by a rumbling pain. [*Ng.*]

Strong pressure in the back, before the protusion of a varix from the rectum.

Tearing pain in the left shoulder-blade (aft. 34 d.).

Violent pain along the whole of the back, stitches and twitches, so that she cannot stoop nor pick up anything with her hand; increased on inspiration (3d d.). [*Hb.*]

Fine stitches from the back to the region of the ribs (aft. 2 h.). [*Ng.*]

830. From time to time, a severe stitch in the middle of the back.

Pain in the back, as if a red hot iron was thrust through the lowest vertebræ.

Burning on the upper end of the left shoulder-blade, somewhat diminished by rubbing. [*Ng.*]

Two days in succession, stitches and cutting in the shoulder-blades with chilliness therein.

Gnawing and stitches in the shoulder-blades (2d d.). [*Ng.*]

835. Stitches between the shoulder-blades.

Stitches between (and in) the shoulder-blades, with arrest of breathing (1st, 2d d.). [*Ng.*]

Painful stiffness between the shoulder-blades, later drawing into the region of the ribs and the kidneys. [*Bte.*]

Painful tension between the shoulder-blades in the forenoon (2d d.). [*Ng.*]

Painful drawing in the muscles of the neck, not changed by rubbing and moving of the head, in the forenoon (1st d.). [*Ng.*]

840. Violent tension in the nape of the neck for 1 hour in the afternoon (1st d.). [*Ng.*]

In the morning stiffness of the neck and the upper part of the back, with drawing pains, passing off through motion (4th d.). [*Tr.*]

Stitches in the nape of the neck.

Stitches in the nape and the right side of the neck, only passing off on long continued rubbing. [*Ng.*]

The neck pains on moving the head.

845. **Itching in the nape and in the throat** (aft. 18 d.). [*S.*, *Ng.*]

Violent itching on the throat and chest, as if from flea-bites (aft. 10 d.). [*S.*]

Violent itching on the throat, neck and chest, without any visible eruption; only on touching it, there is felt here and there a hard granule (14th d.). [*S.*]

Little blisters on the right side of the throat (8th d.). [*Ng.*]

Stitches in the glands on the right side and a drawing pressure in those of the left side of the neck (aft. ½ h.). [*Tr.*]

850. Stitches in the neck externally on the left side, alleviated by pressing upon it; at the same time, tearing in the head and stitches in the ears (aft. 12 d.). [*S.*]

Pressing and drawing in gland, on the left side of the neck.

Swelling on the glands of the side of the neck.

Stiffness of the muscles of the neck, so that she cannot turn her head to the left.

Pain as from a sprain in the shoulder-joint, especially on raising up the arms.

855. Frequently intermittent tearing in both axillæ, in the afternoon (4th d.). [*Ng.*]

Sudden jerk or shake in the right shoulder (aft. 2 h.). [*Ng.*]

Eruption across the shoulders of little reddish granules with a pointed pustule in the middle, which only cause some burning in the evening (aft. 6 and 14 d.). [*Tr.*]

Stitches in the axillæ, the shoulders, and the arms, also at night. [*Ng.*]

Tearing pains at various times in the arms and in all parts of the same, in the shoulders, the axillæ, upper arms, elbows, fore-arms, etc. [*Ng.*]

860. Tearing in the arms, from the upper arms to the fingers, and from the fingers and wrists into the shoulders. [*Ng.*]

Paralytic bruised pains, in the arms, at times in the small of the back, from the right upper arm to the left fore-arm and vice versa. [*Ng.*]

Great weariness in the arms, which he can hardly raise up (3d d.). [*Tr.*]

Weariness of the arms.

Great tiredness in one arm.

865. Sensation of tightness in the arm as from cold.

From time to time heat in the right arm, sensible even externally.

Burning (with tension) in the arms (the upper arms) and the fingers, and in the left elbow, as from a red-hot iron. [*Ng.*]

Swelling (soft, red) on the arm, and violent stitches therein.

Itching on all parts of the arms, passing off through scratching. [*Ng.*]

870. Pain as if from a sprain, in the upper arm.

Drawing pain in the left humerus (2d d.). [*Tr.*]

Tearing pain at the back part of the upper arm extending into the shoulder-blades, while sneezing and coughing.

Stitches in the muscles of the left upper arm (after several h.).

(Lancinating) **tearing** in the upper arm and **in the elbow,** as if in the bone, in the forenoon. [*Ng.*]

Lancinating pain in the elbow and wrist, as if from a sprain.

Almost constant boring pain in the point of the elbow.

Pain above the point of the elbow, especially on leaning upon it, as from a sharp pressure in the upper arm.

In the fore-arm an aching drawing pain, while at rest.

Drawing, tearing pain in the fore-arm even to the hand, in the morning on awaking.

880. Painful tearing in the fore-arm, as if in the bone, for one minute, thrice.

Tearing in the fore-arms into the wrists and the fingers. [*Ng.*]

Constant visible twitching or quivering on the right fore-arm and on the posterior joint of the left thumb. [*Ng*]

Extraordinary heaviness in the fore-arms and hands, while her arms seem to her to be shorter. [*Ng.*]

His left fore-arm goes to sleep every day; there is a pricking sensation in it from the hand to the elbow.

885. On waking up, the right hand is asleep.

The left wrist is sensitive, so that he cannot lift up anything without the greatest pains. [*Hb.*]

Distended veins on the hands, in the afternoon and evening. [*Ng.*]

Itching on the palms and the back of the hands and between the fingers, passing away on scratching. [*Ng.*]

After violent itching of the hands, the skin peels off like bran, on the 3d day; at the same time there appears behind the left thumb and index-finger a little red spot which burns violently, but only for one day. [*Ng.*]

890. Continual disagreeable coldness of the hands.

Rough, chapped hands, bleeding easily. [*Hb.*]

On the right index-finger a sensation, as if sprained. [*S.*]

The middle fingers pain on being moved.

Drawing pain in the thumb and index.

895. Tearing in and between the fingers. [*Ng.*]

The left thumb went to sleep twice in the afternoon, and then for a long time there was a crawling sensation in it. [*Ng.*]

Formication in the fingers of the right hand, with burning stitches as from ants, in the evening (6th d.). [*Ng.*]

Gnawing under the nails of the fingers, with formication up the arms, up to the clavicle. [*Ng.*]

Swelling of the fingers.

900. Itching on and between the fingers, passing off by scratching. [*Ng.*]

Itching on the fingers of the right hand, aggravated by scratching and rubbing.

Itching about the posterior joints of the fingers, aggravated by rubbing, which causes an unbearable pain in the bones of the fingers.

Formicating burning itching between the index and middle finger of the left hand. [*Ng.*]

Inclination to festering in the tips of the fingers; there appears there a white suppurating spot with lancinating pains, which, however, also passes away again without breaking open. [*Hb.*]

905. A scar on the finger, caused by a cut 9 years ago at a dissection, begins to itch (9th–12th d.). [*Tr.*]

Extreme brittleness of the finger nails; they break off when about to be cut. [*Bte.*]

Pain in the right hip-joint.

Tearing pain above both the hips and on the upper border of the pelvis.

Tearing in the hip-bone. [*Ng.*]

910. Stitches in the right region of the pelvis. [*Ng.*]

Stitches in the left hip, which branch off into the small of the back and into the flanks, and return at the inspiration. [*Ng.*]

Cutting as with a knife across the right nates, in the forenoon (2d d.). [*Ng.*]

In sitting, the nates go to sleep.

Pain in the left hip as if bruised, aggravated by pressure, in the morning (4th d.). [*Ng.*]

915. Tearing and stitches in the hip-joint and immediately above the knee, in paroxysms. [*Bte.*]

Furuncle on the right hip, terminating in suppuration. [*Ng.*]

Pain in the legs and loins while moving.

After walking, pain in the legs and loins, preventing her from sleeping.

Drawing in the legs.

920. **Tearing in the legs**, both the thighs and the legs, while sitting and lying down, especially at night. [*Ng.*]

In the thighs and the legs long continued straining downwards, almost like cramp; lasting only a few minutes, but returning frequently.

Gnawing pain in the legs. [*Bte.*]

For several evenings, about 7 o'clock, restlessness in the legs foı ½ hour, before she went to sleep.

Heaviness in the legs, so that she can scarcely lift them.

925. Great weight in the lower limbs, so that he can hardly drag them along; he staggers in walking, and has to sit down; in the evening (5th d.). [*Ng.*]

Great weariness of the legs, while sitting down. [*Ng.*]

Burning and smarting itching, passing off by scratching, on the thighs. [*Ng.*]

Itching (and a fine eruption) on the inside of the right thigh. [*Ng.*]

Pain in the left hough, the boy cannot stand well upon his foot.

930. At night, violent pain in the hough down to the heel.

A sensation of pressure into the left hough, while walking, after rising from being seated. [*Ng.*]

Drawing pain in the houghs while ascending the stairs, but not while descending.

Drawing pain in both knees on ascending the stairs, but not while merely bending or touching them.

Pain in the patella, but only when pressing upon it with the hand and when flexing the knee-joint.

935. Jerking, sharp pressure from without inward on the patella.

Tearing in the knees and patellæ. [*Ng.*]

In the evening before going to sleep, a lancinating, tearing pain in the knee.

Dull tearing on the inside of the left knee, in the evening (19th d.).

Violent tearing from the knees downward out at the toes, with a sensation of swelling at the knee; in the afternoon till evening (relieved by walking) (21st d.). [*Ng.*]

940. Stitches in the left knee, only while sitting, passing away when walking in the open air. [*Ng.*]

Stitches and tearing in the right knee, in the evening (1st d.). [*Ng.*]

Painful boring in the right knee (aft. 2 h.). [*Ng.*]

Cracking of the right knee in walking.

Trembling of the knees.

945. The knees appear to her larger during the pains. [*Ng.*]

Weariness of the legs, especially in the middle of the tibiæ, as if bruised; while standing and walking, when it is worst, she feels like sinking down; (diminished while sitting and lying down), especially in the evening. [*Ng.*]

Pain as from bruises on the right tibia, especially during motion.

In the evening in bed, stitches in the right tibia [*Ng.*]

Lancinating, cramp-like pain in the right leg, with a feeling of numbness during the siesta while sitting, and also after awaking.

950. Tearing in the legs at various times. [*Ng.*]

Tearing drawing in the leg, extending from the external ankle.

In the evening, tearing in the tendo Achillis of both legs (5th d.). [*Ng.*]

Keen, drawing pain in the tendo Achillis while at rest, not while walking.

Painless drawing down in both calves (aft. 2 h.). [*Ng.*]

955. Tearing in the calves.

In walking, the muscles of the calves seem too short, they feel strained (aft. 20 h.).

Tensive pain on the inside of the calves, while walking.

Tension (and burning) on the outside of the right calf, in the evening (2d d.). [*Ng.*]

The (previously existing) tension in the calves (the soles of the feet and the toes, in cramps and paralysis of the legs) is much increased and includes the knee, so that he cannot keep erect; then a burning, lancinating and sometimes also a cutting pain in the calves and the soles (1st d.). [*Hb.*]

960. Repeated cramp of the calves.

When she puts one foot across the other, or steps upon her toes, she is every time immediately seized with painful cramps of the calves.

Cramps in the calves, as if the tendons were too short after rising from his seat; passing off when walking, before that his legs suddenly became so weary that he was afraid to rise, in the afternoon (2d d.). [*Ng.*]

Painless beating or throbbing in the left calf, like a pulsation, in the morning (4th d.). [*Ng.*]

Violent formication in both calves, as from ants, after supper (5th d.). [*Ng.*]

965. Itching of the calves. [*Ng.*]

Sensation in the left heel as if it were being pressed together from both sides (2d d.). [*Ng.*]

Tearing in the feet and ankles at various times. [*Ng.*]

Heaviness in the feet, with tearing. [*S.*]

Heaviness in the feet, with great weariness in the legs (3 d.) [*Ng.*]

970. The right foot goes to sleep, with formication. [*Ng.*]

Painful drawing below the ankles (10th d.). [*Hb.*]

Pain in the bones on the dorsum of the foot, on touching, with itching of those parts (1st d.). [*Hb.*]

On trying to step upon the foot, intense stitches in the ankle of the right foot and violent cutting from the left big toe into the heel, so that he is unable to step on his foot (2d d.). [*Hb.*]

Numbness of the heel on stepping on his foot.

975. Stitching (tickling) and pricking sensation in the soles of the feet. [*Hb.*, *Ng.*]

Itching in the sole of the foot.

Tickling itching in the sole of the foot. [*Bte.*]

Burning stitches in the sole of the right foot, in the evening and morning, passing off after rubbing. [*Ng.*]

Tension in the sole of the foot, in the forenoon (2d d.). [*Ng.*]

980. Painful sensitiveness of the sole of the right foot.

Pain in the sole of the foot, when stepping on it, as if it were too soft and swollen.

The hard skin of the sole of the foot is very sensitive to the touch and causes, even of itself, violent pressive pain.

The old, hard skin on the feet becomes very sensitive. [*Hb.*]

Excoriating **stitches in the corns.**

985 An ulcer on the sole of the foot, which had almost healed, causes a lancinating pain on stepping on it in the room, after walking in the open air. [*Ng.*]

Lancinating pain in the ball of the great toe. [*Hb.*]

Burning lancinations in the left big toe, near the nail, at night. [*Hb.*]

Cutting in the right big toe, as if he were walking on knives, in the morning while walking (4th d.). [*Ng.*]

Formication in the big toe, as if it had been frozen (2d d.). [*Ng.*]

990. Itching of the toes after staying in the cold air. [*Hb.*]

Itching of the toes and feet when getting warm in walking; this ceases immediately after the walk (aft. 30 d.). [*Hb.*]

Itching, with shining redness of the big toes; painful on ex ternal pressure (aft. 4 d.). [*Hb.*]

Itching of the toes, with redness as if they had been frozen, worse after scratching, in the evening (3d, 4th, 16th d.). [*Ng.*]

Tetters between the toes.

995. Corns are very painful. [*Bte.*]

Drawing in the limbs.

Tension in the dorsum of the feet and hands, like burning, as if from a swelling.

Continual burning and stitches in the anus, with stiffness of the back, so that she cannot move well.

(Dull, pressive pains in the bones, especially of the legs, the chest and the back.)

1000. Tearing in the left shoulder-blade, in the arms, the hands and the legs, especially in the evening (3d d.).

Pains darting quick as lightning in the right shoulder, the small of the back and the abdomen; then as if bruised (2d d.). [*Ng.*]

Pain as from a bruise in the loins, above the hips, and in the muscles of the calves in walking.

Pain as from a bruise in the back and all the limbs as in fever and ague. [*Bte.*]

On entering the room after walking in the open air, there is oppression and nausea during speaking.

1005. After walking in the open air, excessive cheerfulness and a staring look; then, with every motion, a cold shudder and perspiration with chilliness about the head; when going to bed the head, the hands and feet are hot.

During bodily exertions a rush of heat over the whole body, then shaking and chilly shuddering, with a burning sensation in the abdomen.

During bodily labor, a cramp-like sensation like numbness up the whole of the left leg, so also in the left arm, with a reeling stupefaction of the head, in intermittent attacks (14th d.).

All the muscles feel as if paralyzed. [*Bte.*]

In the morning, paralytic weakness in all the limbs, with stupefaction of the head in paroxysms of several minutes (10th d.).

1010. Rigidity in the hands and feet, as if they were asleep, early on awaking; after rising and walking about, it passed away.

The ring finger and the little finger, also the knee and lastly the heel, go to sleep after sitting.

Slow, tottering gait, as after a severe illness. [*Bte.*]

An attack in the evening: she feels sick and things turn around with her, with constant palpitation and severe anxiety, lasting the whole night till the next forenoon.

On entering the room after walking in the open air, anxiety and nausea during speaking ensues.

1015. An attack in the evening; violent pain in the small of the back and vertigo, then urging to stool with a discharge of mere blood; she felt as if paralyzed in the small of the back; it gave her no support in sitting up straight.

An attack: rush of blood to the head, black before the eyes, vertigo, ringing before the ears and sleepiness.

An attack: first he sat still without answering, then anxious groaning for 5 minutes, then for 10 minutes severe convulsive laughter, then again weeping; then alternately laughter and weeping.

In the evening in bed, inclination to convulsive laughter (th5 d.).

Tremulous excitement of the whole nervous system. [*Bte.*]

1020. Shaking pulsation through the whole body. [*Bte.*]

Sensation of contraction in the right index finger and the foot, as if the tendons were too short; if he touches anything with the finger, he feels as if electrified. [*S.*]

During the siesta, when he is about to go to sleep while sitting, a jerk through head and limbs, like an electric shock, with stupefaction.

His arm and also his head are jerked backwards several times, with anxiety.

In the evening, twitches in both legs at once, especially in the legs and feet, then an inclination in the arms to turn about and to stretch upward.

1025. Involuntary twitches now and then, and movements of one foot, of the fingers, etc.

Involuntary movements of the head and of other members.

Twitchings in all the limbs.

Tortures in the limbs as if the bones were compressed, with pressure in the joints.

Restlessness, obliged always to move the feet and to walk about.

1030. Restlessness, both while sitting and lying down, she has to move the hands and the feet, now here, now there.

Most of the troubles seem to come while sitting and to be alleviated by walking. [*Ng.*]

All the symptoms are aggravated immediately after dinner. [*Bte.*]

Most of the troubles appear soon after dinner and in the evening. [*Ng.*]

Many of the troubles come after dinner and last till evening, while they vanish in the forenoon and at night. [*Ng.*]

1035. Potatoes seem to aggravate or to again call forth the symptoms. [*Ng.*]

He feels best after meals. [*S.*]

He feels somewhat better every other day. [*S.*]

He feels pretty well during the day; most of the troubles come on in the morning and evening. [*S.*]

The patient appears better in the open air and in the evening. [*Ng.*]

1040. **Disposition to colds**; even in the room she becomes hoarse; improved by walking in the open air.

Perspiration at every motion and afterwards shuddering from chilliness, as if the person had taken cold.

Sensation in the limbs, as if cold had been taken; during the day frequent chilliness and in the evening heat in the face.

Unbearable itching of the whole body, especially on getting warm, and in bed; he has to scratch until he bleeds and after scratching the skin is painful. [*Hb.*]

Itching on the whole of the body, especially in the face (7th d.).

1045. Itching here and there in small spots of the body, mostly in the evening; does not disappear from scratching. [*Ng.*]

Violent itching of the whole body, as if an eruption would break out (5th d.). [*Hb.*]

Severe itching and fretting of the skin of the whole body, relieved but little by scratching.

Stinging itching of the back and also of the side of the abdomen (2d d.).

Stinging, now here, now there, on the whole body, especially in the evening. [*Ng.*]

1050. The tetters (small, white, itching pimples in groups) multiply. [*Hb.*]

Itching of the tetters, *especially towards evening*. [*Hb.*]

Violently itching miliary eruption on the arms and legs without redness, with bleeding of serum after scratching. [*Bte.*]

Itching stinging in the tetters. [*Hb.*]

Little injuries of the skin become excoriated and inflamed.

1055. **Great lassitude of the body,** especially after walking in the open air, with yawning, stretching and extension of the limbs, sleepiness and *inclination to lie down*, which however increases the weariness (1st and 3d d.). [*Tr.*]

Lassitude throughout the whole body, with dullness of the thinking faculty, flying heat in the face and anxiety (4th d.).

A little talking and a little walk fatigues him.

Especially much wearied by talking.

Excessively **tired and weary**; he must sit down.

1060. Tremulous weariness.

Weariness in the forenoon and severe chilliness; in the afternoon she shook from cold in the back. [*S.*]

Very weary in the whole body, with chilliness and headache (33d d.). [*Ng.*]

Weary, dizzy in the head, the pulse often feverish, and in disposed to work, for several days; also little appetite; after dinner sleepy; heaviness in the body, frequent inclination to eructation, which however does not take place at all or only imperfectly (aft. 4 w.). [*Hb.*]

Fatigued, weary, so that she can hardly lift her feet, at the same time sleepy and lazy (22d d.). [*S.*]

1065. Irresistible inclination to lie down (aft. 3 h.).

Weary and sleepy.

Much yawning, with sleepiness (only passing away in the open air). [*Ng.*]

Constant yawning, also before dinner, without sleepiness. [*Tr.*, *Ng.*]

Sleepiness during the day.

1070. With great weariness, she is irresistibly overcome in the forenoon by sleep; she lies down and sleeps soundly for 1 hour, when the weariness has disappeared and she feels very well. [*Ng.*]

Great drowsiness in the evening, even while standing.

Great drowsiness in the evening, as early as 6 o'clock. [*Ng.*]

She goes to sleep early in the evening. [*S.*]

In the morning when rising, she feels as if she had not slept enough; weary, with yawning.

1075. In the morning after a restless sleep, he is still tired and does not want to rise. [*Hb.*]

He always desires to sleep late in the morning. [*S.*]

He always has to sleep longer in the morning than usual, and can not rouse himself; on the other hand, he can not at once go to sleep in the evening. [*S.*]

In the evening, he is late in getting to sleep on account of frequent fantastic imaginings (2d d.). [*Tr.*]

Can not go to sleep for a whole hour in the evening, but afterwards he sleeps well. [*Ng.*]

1080. He can not go to sleep before midnight, hindered as it were by a heavy feeling in his arms.

He can not go to sleep before midnight, and throws himself from one side to the other (2d d.). [*Ng.*]

At night, restless in all the limbs, this prevents his going to sleep.

She can not find rest at night anywhere, she throws herself about and everything hurts her, for several nights (aft. 15 d.). [*Ng.*]

Restless sleep: he throws himself about in the bed; he feels hot and anxious; at the same time twitches of the limbs and starting before going to sleep. [*S.*]

1085. During the first nights, a very restless sleep. [*S.*]

Restless sleep; she often turned over; **she felt hot**, she mostly lay uncovered; her sleep was only a slumber without refreshing her, with many dreams and **frequent awaking** (7th d.). [*S.*]

Restless sleep, with toothache. [*Bte.*]

Frequent awaking at night, for 8 days (12th d.). [*Ng.*]

Awaking before midnight from a dry cough, first with chilliness, and later with a dry heat. [*Ng.*]

1090. After midnight a restless sleep, he awakes often and tosses about in his bed. [*Hb.*]

At night in bed, beating at the roots of his teeth like pulsation. [*Bte.*]

At 12 at night, he awakes from violent griping and rumbling in the abdomen, which passes away toward morning (aft. 12 d.). [*Ng.*]

At night in bed, headache.

In the evening in bed, griping in the scrobiculus cordis.

1095. Violent pains at night, in the hough and down to the heel.

He awakes at night with cramps and tightness of the chest (after a long walk on the day before).

Early about 4 o'clock, waking up from chilliness of the whole body, with violent contraction in the stomach, constant empty eructation which relieves; then four fluid stools in succession, with continual chilliness and with subsequent burning in the anus; the chilliness lasts till evening (32d d.). [*Ng.*]

At night on awaking, anxiety, oppressed breathing and copious perspiration.

Is waked up about 4 or 5 in the morning by anguish in his heart, as if perspiration would break out, which does not appear; on rising, the anguish immediately disappears.

1100. Awaking toward morning, he is tormented with thoughts of anguish of death, on account of imaginary pains while sleeping.

Awaking **in the morning with depression as from sorrow,** without clear consciousness.

Awaking early, with nausea and qualmishness in the stomach, and fatigued as if the sleep had in no way refreshed her; at the same time a quick feverish pulse with internal heat (3d d). [*S.*]

Early in bed on awaking, a drawing, smarting sensation in the urethra.

Starting up after midnight from an anxious dream (that a horse pursued him and wanted to bite him) (10th d.). [*Ng.*]

1105. Violent starting from sleep, before midnight, and a complete awaking (7th d.). [*Ng.*]

She talked aloud in her sleep, laughed and wept.

Much talking in sleep, as if he had anxious dreams.

Before midnight great restlessness during sleep with violent weeping and disconsolate grief, without any proper consciousness, for some minutes.

She moans and groans at night as if she were weeping, but she is unconscious of it, soon after going to sleep (7th d.).

1110. He rises at night unconsciously from his bed and with his eyes firmly closed, he walks anxiously from one room into the other, rubbing his eyes; being brought again to bed, the boy went straight to sleep again.

The sleep is too sound, she has to be waked up.

Sound (dreamy) sleep with erections. [*Tr.*]

The sleep is deep toward morning, with dreams that tire the head (aft. 10 h.).

Good sleep with many (agreeable) dreams. [*S.*]

1115. Agreeable dreams about receiving money and the like. [*Ng.*]

Confused dreams. [*S.*]

Shameful dream. [*Ng.*]

Many dreams, but all of a disagreeable kind. [*S.*]

Dreams of quarrels and vexation. [*Ng.*]

1120. Dreams of falling stars, of a conflagration, of marriages. [*Ng.*]

Dreams of thieves, with anxious awaking.

Dreams of committing a theft or that she had fallen among robbers. [*Ng.*]

Dreams of death and burial. [*Ng.*]

Tormenting dreams, which on awaking leave behind them a deadly fear.

1125. **Distressing dreams** with restless sleep.

Anxious dreams towards morning, the sleep being otherwise good (aft. 12 d.). [*S.*]

Frightfully anxious dreams and nightmare.

Anxious dreams, *e. g.*, the flayer forces dog's meat into his mouth. [*S.*]

In his dream he has to descend from a height, and thinks that he must fall.

1130. A dream, that she is in a ferry-boat sinking in the river, with anxious awaking. [*Ng.*]

A dream that he is going about in a river, in which he sees snakes and other animals of which he is afraid. [*Ng.*]

He dreams of ghosts, and makes a noise in the night, so that he wakens. [*S.*]

The whole night, chilliness and restless sleep (33 d.). [*Ng.*]

Chilly, shudders by the warm stove (15th d.).

1135. In the evening from 7 to 8, a chill, so that she has to go to bed from cold, but can not for a long time get warm even in bed (5th d.). [*Ng.*]

Very sensitive to cold air, especially in the feet. [*Bte.*]

Internal chill and shuddering, with a desire for the warm stove, and extending and stretching the limbs, worse *after warm drinks.*

Chilly feeling in the open air.

Chilly over the whole body; the feet are like ice the whole day, with heat in the head, also in the room (1st d.). [*Ng.*]

1140. With an internal chill, external warmth, especially in the cheeks, with dark redness of the same as with brandy drinkers. [*Bte.*]

With an external chill, hot cheeks and cold hands. [*Bte.*]*

Chills running over the body, without thirst and without subsequent heat or perspiration, from 4 to 6 in the afternoon, with beating pains in the forehead and in the occiput, relieved by pressing upon it with the hand (9th d.). [*S.*]

Chilliness, constant eructations, bitter taste in the mouth, frequent gathering of saliva, great lassitude and headache as if the head would split, especially above in the vertex, with vertigo (alleviated by a dose of Ipecac) (34th d.). [*Ng.*]

Shudderings one after another, in the evening (2d d.). [*Hb.*]

1145. Every other day, feverish shudderings over the whole body, toward evening, without thirst, with lack of appetite, sleeplessness and restless tossing in bed. [*S.*]

In the evening, feverish movements, shuddering and chilliness, aggravated by the least movement, and only now and then a transient flush of the face (1st d.). [*Tr.*]

Evening fever; severe chill about 5 o'clock, especially in the back and the feet, so that she could not get warm by the warm

* Bryonia is an antidote to fevers caused by Alumina. [*Bte.*]

stove; after ½ hour, perspiration without thirst (6th, 7th d.). [*Ng*].

Evening fever, chill and heat, frequently alternating, with a hot face and chills and shuddering in the rest of the body.

Internal chilliness, with hot hands and hot lobes of the ear (aft. 2 h.).

1150. After ½ hour's chilliness, heat of the body and perspiration of the face. [*Tr.*]

Pleasant, transient warmth in the right side of the face, in the afternoon (5th d.). [*Ng.*]

Sudden flush of the face, with redness, but only transient (5th d.). [*Ng.*]

Sensation in the body as after having been violently heated, while sitting (the first days). [*Tr.*]

In the evening, heat in the whole body for 2 hours; it seems to start from the head (5th d.). [*Ng.*]

1155. Feverish weariness, with internal heat.

Towards evening, heat in the whole body, especially in the feet, then a shaking chill, so that she had to go to bed, where she soon went to sleep; neither in the heat nor in the chill, any thirst or other trouble (11th d.). [*S.*]

Heat before midnight, keeping him from going to sleep. [*Ng.*]

Distressing heat at night and perspiration.

Sudden heat, with perspiration and distressing palpitation.

1160. In the morning, if she remains in bed after 6 o'clock, she begins to perspire, for several mornings (aft. 9 d.) [*S.*]

Rushes of blood, with increased pulse, and trembling of the hands while writing; also after meals, with heat of the whole body and perspiration of the face (1st d.). [*Tr.*]

AMMONIUM CARBONICUM, CARBONATE OF AMMONIA.

SAL VOLATILE.

(The salt obtained from equal parts of sal-ammoniac and crystalline carbonate of soda, triturated together and sublimated at a moderate heat.*)

* Instead of procuring this salt from chemical laboratories, as our druggists do of late, and then, in order to free it from any contents of lead which may be suspected, subliming it again, (G. Pharm. boruss. P. 134,) (what a round about course!) we need only to put an ounce of the above-mentioned mixture into a good sized medicine bottle which is loosely corked, place this bottle in an iron pan filled with sand, immersing the bottle as deeply as the mixture extends, sublimate the ammonia by fire into the upper part of the bottle and then break this off in order to secure the contents.

Of this salt one grain is triturated for 1 hour with 100 grains of sugar of milk, as I have described in the first part, in the *directions* for preparing antipsoric remedies, and we thus get the first one hundredfold, potentized powder-attenuation ($\frac{1}{100}$). One grain of this powder, again, is triturated with 100 grains of fresh sugar of milk in a similar manner to $\frac{1}{10000}$, and one grain of this is triturated with another 100 grains of sugar of milk to the millionfold potentized powder-attenuation (I). One grain of this (as given in the directions) is dissolved in 100 drops of alcohol mixed with water, and shaken twice, forming a liquid ($\frac{1}{100}$ I) which is then potentized through 27 additional vials, each containing 100 drops of good alcohol, up to the decillionth attenuation (X) by two strokes of the arm. With this 1, 2 or 3 of the finest pellets are moistened for a dose, which, when homœopathically selected, at times operates for more than 36 days.

This medicine serves in its way very well for curative antipsoric purposes in chronic diseases, especially in cases where the following symptoms prevail or are present among others:

Timidity; disobedience; obstinacy; loathing of life; uneasiness in the evening; distress; anxiety with weakness; diminished faculty of thinking; vertigo while sitting and reading; *long continued headache;* headache as if it would burst out at the forehead; headache with nausea; hammering headache; falling out of the hair; dry pus on the eyelids; burning and sensation of cold in the eyes; obscuration of vision, with a glimmer before the eyes; black dots and streaks of light, hovering before the eyes; cataract (aft. 32 d.); short-sightedness; hardness of hearing, with suppuration and itching of the ear; humming and ringing before the ears; itching of the nose; suppurating pustules in the nose; bleeding of the nose, in the morning while washing; freckles; chaps from the left upper lip across the cheek to the ear; cracking in the articulation of the jaw, while chewing; long-continued looseness of the teeth; sore throat as if raw; pain as of soreness in the throat; swelling of the interior of the mouth; after eructations, taste of the food and drinks partaken of; bitter taste in the mouth, especially after eating; scraping and burning, up the œsophagus, after a meal; headache, after a meal; nausea after a meal; during a meal, a dizzy vertigo; irresistible inclination to eat sugar; *thirst;* lack of appetite in the morning; sour eructations; heartburn; eructation and vomiting; stomachache; spasms of the stomach; contractive pain in the scrobiculus cordis, while stretching; burning pain in the liver; boring stitches in the liver, in the evening while sitting; restlessness in the abdomen; concussive pain in the hypogastrium when setting the foot down; constipation; difficult evacuations; colic with diarrhœa; blood with the stools; discharge of blood from the anus (flowing piles); *itching of the anus; varices of the anus;* nightly micturition; pollutions; (lack of sexual instinct;) *menses too scanty;* sterility with too scanty menses; catamenia too short and too scanty; menses too early; with the catamenia, pressure on the genitals, cutting in the abdomen, tearing in the back and in the genital organs, compelling her to lie down; watery discharge from the uterus; *leucorrhœa;* copious, excoriating, acrid leucorrhœa; long-continued dryness of the nose; chronic *coryza; dry coryza;* dyspnœa; *asthma; cough;* cough with hoarseness, while the body is warm; cough from tickling in the throat, with expectoration; cough during the day; cough at night; stitches in the small of the back, while coughing; burning in the chest from below upward; tearing from the upper left side of the chest to the shoulder-joint; stitches in the fleshy part of the chest; goitre; swelling of the cervical glands, with an itching eruption of the face and body; pain in nape of the neck; rigidity of the arms and fingers and numbness of the same at night, in the morning and while grasping something; *pain in the wrist-joint, sprained some time previous*; swelling of the fingers, while the arms hang down; the fingers go to sleep; great weariness of the legs; drawing pain in the legs, while sitting; stitches in the heel; perspiration of the feet; swelling of the feet; cramp in the sole of the foot; pain of a sprain in the ball of the big toe, at night in bed; burning in the hands and feet; feeling of weakness in the limbs, while walking in the open air; dislike to taking walks; drawing and tension in the small of the back and the joints; curvature of the bones; warts; burning, stitches and tearing pains in the corns; drowsiness during the day; sleeplessness at night; nightmare, when going to sleep; fever-heat in the head, with cold feet; chilliness in the evening; perspiration.

This medicine may be advantageously repeated after some intermediate remedies. Smelling of a solution of camphor moderates its excessive action.

The abbreviations of my fellow provers are: *Hb.*, *Dr. Hartlaub; Ng.* Gr.*, *Dr. Gross; Stf.*, medical councillor *Dr Stapf, Tr.*, *Dr. Trinks; S.*, *Dr. Schreter.*[1]

*See note under Alumina.

[1] Ammonium carbonicum had already appeared in the first edition of the *Chronic Diseases* and the new symptoms from Hahnemann published in the second, must be of the same origin as those of the first. The greater number of the additions is from "*Ng.*," published with a few from Hartlaub and Trinks in vol. II, of their *Arzneimittellehre*. The nature of the observations of *Ng.* has already been stated under Alumina. Schreter's pathogenesis (without information as to its mode of production, appears in vol. III of the same work. The symptoms of Gross and Stapf—four only in all: Sympt. 656, 669, 670 and 675—are of unknown origin.—*Hughes.*

AMMONIUM CARBONICUM.

Serious mood.

Gloomy, almost tearful humor, towards evening (2d d.). [*Ng.*]

Very lugubrious, with thoughts of death.

Grieving and sorrowful.

5. Thoughts of previous annoyances torment him.

Anxious and distressed about her diseased condition.

Sad, dejected, feeling as if a misfortune was imminent, with sensation of coldness in the forenoon. [*Ng.*]

Every afternoon between 5 and 6 o'clock she is seized with anguish, as if she had committed the greatest crime; this passes off in the evening.

Many afternoons she is seized with weakness and timidity, so that she cannot control herself and knew not what to do; in the evening this state passes off.

10. Severe compression of the heart, he knows not how to help himself.

The mind is restless and feels uncanny (2d d.). [*S.*]

She finds no rest, and prospers in nothing (4th d.). [*Ng.*]

Sighs. [*S.*]

Not disposed to anything. [*S.*]

15. Indisposed to work.

Cloudy weather makes her excessively ill-humored.

Peevish in the morning.

Ill and peevish humor, sometimes with headache in the forenoon. [*Ng.*]

Very unamiable, irritated, ill-humored, she answers only reluctantly (on the 2d day of her menses). [*Ng.*]

20. Nothing pleased her.

She could not bear any noise.

The child is very self-willed. [*Gr.*]

Can bear no contradiction.

Very peevish and passionate.

25. Peevish, passionate, abusive, in the evening (6th d.). [*Ng.*]

In the evening after supper the mood improves (with the cessation of headache and of the pains in the stomach). [*Ng.*]

Very easily frightened.

Excessive and nervous exaltion.

Sometimes extravagantly merry.

30. He often laughs immoderately at a trifle (aft. 38 d.). [*Ng.*]

He seems as if beside himself.

His head is very thoughtless.

Very forgetful, and there is headache when he reflects. [*Ng.*]

Very forgetful, distracted, cannot recollect (9th d.).

35. Very distracted and easily loses himself when telling a tale, passing from his train of thoughts into other thoughts and expressions which he did not wish to utter (8th d.).

Anxious distraction, so that in speaking he does not at last know how to finish his speech.

She can not well arrange her ideas.

He speaks incorrectly, makes mistakes in speaking, and uses one word for another in telling a tale.

He easily makes slips in writing and reckoning (9th d.).

40. **Numb and muddled feeling of the head** (aft. ¼ h.).

Stupefaction of the head. [*S.*]

After sitting a while (toward evening) dizziness as from intoxication.

When turning the body, everything turns with him and his head is dizzy.

Vertigo, and staggering of the feet, he must hold himself to avoid falling, for several days (aft. 3 d.). [*Ng.*]

45. Vertigo, at night and in the morning (aft. 2d.).

In the morning, vertigo with glimmering before his eyes, he has to sit down.

Frequent vertigo, early on arising and lasting the whole day, worse in the evening, he feels as if the objects whirled around with him, also at night when he moves his head. [*Ng.*]

At once in the morning, dizzy, sick at stomach and without appetite.

Vertigo, with sickness at the stomach in the morning, soon passing off in walking (4th d.). [*Ng.*]

50. Headache, early in bed, with nausea rising up into the throat, as if she would vomit, passing off after 2, 3 hours.

Headache and pains in the stomach, with ill humor the whole day (3d d.). [*Ng.*]

Headache after dinner (5th d.). [*Ng.*]

Headache with heaviness in the forehead in the morning, but worse in the afternoon (8th d.). [*Ng.*]

Pressure on the head above, for ½ h (aft. 6 d.).

55. After being heated, pressure over the whole head (aft. 10 d.).

Headache, now here now there in the brain; a pressure with stitches over one eye-brow.

The head feels very heavy.

Heaviness and beating in the forehead, after dinner. [*Ng.*]

Heaviness in the left side of the head, becoming worse in bed (46th d.). [*Ng.*]

60. The right side of the head seems to her heavier, and as if the head were about to fall over to that side (1st d.) [*Ng.*]

Pressive sensation of fulness in the forehead as from coal-gas.

Straining fulness in the vertex and the forehead, as if the head would burst there.

In stooping, there is a tension in the nape of the neck, and in front, the head feels as if it would burst open with pain.

Headache, throbbing in the forehead as if it would burst open.

65. Raging in the right frontal protuberance, as if everything were coming out there (2d d.). [*Ng.*]

Compressive pain in the head as from a vice.

A drawing pain in the periosteum of the forehead awakens her early from her sleep, for several mornings; it passes away after rising.

Drawing and tearing in the whole head, soon after rising, and during the whole day (23d d.). [*Ng.*]

Tearing in the temples, in the morning and evening. [*Ng.*]

70. Tearing, upward behind the left ear, up into the crown, with a sensation, as if the head were split open. [*Ng.*]

Lancinating headache all the day.

Lancinations here and there in the head, and especially on the right side, deep in the brain, passing away in the open air (4th, 42d d.). [*Ng.*]

Lancinations in the left temple, increased while chewing.

Stitches in the left temple, as from a dull instrument. [*S.*]

75. Stitches as from a needle, above the right eye. [*S.*]

Stitches over the left eye, so violent that it often contracts the eyes, after meals (4th d.). [*Tr.*]

Boring stitches behind the right frontal protuberance, deep in the brain, at dinner (2d d.). [*Ng.*]

Headache, like a sharp knocking or chopping; she could not move for pain, and had to lie still.

Painful throbbing and beating in the temple, the left side of the head and the left occiput, at times with yawning. [*Ng.*]

80. On moving the head, and on pressing upon the head, pain as of ulceration in the whole head, especially in the occiput and in a gland situated there, for some time. [*Ng.*]

On moving the head, a sensation as if the brain fell hither and thither, toward the side to which he stoops, sometimes with lancinating pains; a symptom which leaves him no rest at night, for several weeks. [*Ng.*]

Headache, as if water or something else were in the head.

Sensation as if the brain were loose in the head.

The head easily catches cold.

85. Itching of the head, with great sensitiveness of the integuments of the head, when scratching (10th d.). [*Ng.*]

Severe **itching on the hairy scalp**, especially of the occiput.

Sensation as if the hairs would stand on end, with formication on the whole head, and a feeling of cold there; after coming into the room from the open air. [*Ng.*]

The hairs are painful to the touch.

The skin of the head and the hairs are keenly sensitive when stroked with the hand; the movement made him shudder (the first evening).

90. The eyes are weak; the child winks continually. [*Gr.*]

On awaking, and when about to go to sleep, there is a pressure upon the eyelids so that he can not open them, although internally he is awake.

Pressure in the eyes. [*S.*]

Pressure and cutting in the eyes (4th d.).

Pressure and fine stitches in the eyes (2d d.).

95. Stitches as from needles and pressure in the eyes. [*S.*]

Smarting in the eyes, and itching of the edges of the lids.

Itching and smarting of the eyes, which passes off by rubbing (in the morning) (1st, 4th, 12th d.). [*Ng.*]

Burning of the eyes the whole day, especially early on awaking, with photophobia, and in the evening, when going to sleep. [*Ng.*]

In the right upper eyelid, a stye is becoming inflamed, with a sensation of tension (2d d.).

100. Inflammation of the right inner canthus, painless (26th d.)

Eyes inflamed and dim of vision.

The right eye somewhat inflamed and dim of vision. [*S.*]

The eyes are closed with gum in the morning.

The eyes, after a good sleep, are agglutinated in the morning; she can not open them for a time. [*Ng.*]

105. The eyes are glued together in the morning, during the day they run. [*S.*]

During reading, his eyes run.

Watery eye; the white of the eye is full of red veins, as in an incipient inflammation of the eyes.

The right eye is watery, and the vessels in the cornea are plainly visible. [*S.*]

Severe lachrymation, especially of the right eye, both in the open air and in the room. [*Ng.*]

110. In sneezing, white stars glimmer before the eyes. [*Ng.*]

A large black spot floats before the eyes, after she has been sewing.

In the distance, and also when straining her sight on near objects, objects appear double to her. [*Ng.*]

Frequent painful stitches in the right ear. [*Ng.*]

Stitches in the left ear (2d d.).

115. At night, beating in the left ear, while lying on it, but passing off on turning over (6th d.). [*Ng.*]

Twitching and pinching in the internal ear.

Twitching tension about the left ear, as also in the cheek-bone and in the temple, with swelling of the cervical glands.

Tension behind the right ear. [*Ng.*]

Tearing below and behind the ears, at times extending to the crown, the occiput and the nape of the neck, as well as towards the shoulders (aggravated by moving the head), after dinner. [*Ng.*]

120. Hard swelling of the glands of the ear.

In the morning, an itching above the ears, which extends over the whole body (3d d.).

Formication and digging in the left ear, passing afterwards into the lower jaw (10th d.). [*Ng.*]

A sound in the ears as from a distant shot, 5 or 6 times an hour.

Buzzing before the left ear. [*Ng.*]

125. Illusion of hearing; he thinks that a bell is ringing. [*Ng.*]

In the night, buzzing in the left ear (2d d.).

Daily after midnight, a rustling in the (right) ear, on which he is lying in bed. [*Ng.*]

Humming before the ears, as if they were hard of hearing and as if something were lying before them (aft. 17 d.).

The hearing is diminished.

130. Painful sensitiveness of a deaf ear to a loud sound; her whole body shakes from it.

Tearing in the left nostril, and at the same time in the left elbow, in the bone and extending toward the hand. [*Ng.*]

A quivering on the left side of the nose, which seemed to draw up the ala of the nose.

Sensation in the point of the nose while stooping, as if the blood were accummulating in it. [*Ng.*]

His nose pains when he draws in the air through it.

135. Swelling, feeling of soreness and itching in the right nostril, and formication in it as from coryza; the nose is running (aft. 3d.).

A pustule on the tip of the nose.

A suppurating pustule on the side of the nose.

A little blister in front, on the septum of the nose. [*Ng.*]

A furuncle with pus on the tip of the nose. [*Ng.*]

140. An acrid fluid flows from the nose.

Water runs from the nose on stooping.

Pus drops from one of the nostrils, on blowing the nose in the morning (5th d.).

Bloody mucus blown out of the nose, frequently.

Blood comes from the left nostril, on blowing his nose (2d d.). [*Ng.*]

145. **Bleeding of the nose** (8th d.).

Bleeding of the nose after meals (2d d.).

Violent pain on the right side of the face.

Painful tension and tearing in the right side of the face (2d d.). [*Ng.*]

Pressive pain in the zygoma.

150. Drawing pain in the cheek-bone.

Contraction of the skin of the forehead and in the face.

Sensation as of stretching in the face, she has to rub her eyes and face, as in drowsiness. [*Ng.*]

Heat in the face, during mental exertion.

Heat in the head and face, with red cheeks. [*Ng.*]

155. Redness of the left cheek. [*Ng.*]

Paleness of the face, with nausea, and mental and bodily fatigue.

Wretched appearance. [*Gr.*]

Paleness of the face, with headache and stomachache and very ill humor (4th d.). [*Ng.*]

Pale, bloated face, for a long time (aft. 30 d.). [*Ng.*]

160. In the morning on awaking, tension of the skin of the face (on the nose and both lips), as if the face were swollen.

Hard swelling of the cheek, as well as of the glands of the ears and neck.

On the cheek, white spots, as large as lentils, like herpes, which continually exfoliate.

Furuncle on the cheek and around the ear.

Little furuncle and nodules, discharging blood and water, on the cheek, the corner of the mouth and on the chin. [*Ng.*]

165. Eruption, like little furuncles, on the forehead.

Eruption of pimples and vesicles on the forehead.

Pustules on the forehead and the tip of the nose. [*S.*]

Miliary eruption about the chin, painless.

Pustule on the forehead, the temple, the cheek and the chin. [*Ng.*]

170. Pustules on the cheeks, during the menses. [*Ng.*]

Itching on the mouth; both lips itch.

A pimple on the upper lip, with burning pain.

Burning vesicles on the vermilion of both lips. [*Ng.*]

Vesicles on the right corner of the mouth and the upper lip. [*Ng.*]

175. Eruption on the mouth.

Scaly eruption, like herpes, around the mouth.

Scaly skin on the chin, with severe itching, not passing off by scratching. [*Ng.*]

The upper lip pains as if chapped.

The lower lip is cracked open in the middle, with burning pain and bleeding.

180. Chapped lips and sore corners of the mouth.

Dry, cracked, chapped lips, with burning and a sensation as if full of vesicles. [*Ng.*]

Pain and swelling of the glands under the chin, with tension of the same on moving the mouth. [*Ng.*]

Under the gums, on the jaw, a swelling as large as a pigeon's egg, which pains violently simply from the motion of the jaw in chewing.

The gums are so sensitive that she dares not touch them with the tongue (41st d.). [*Ng.*]

185. Stitches on the inner, upper gums on the right side. [*Ng.*]

Itching of the gums, which bleed after scratching. [*Ng.*]

The gums are inclined to bleed.

Sensation of swelling, and actual swelling and inflammation of the gums. [*Ng.*]

Swelling of the gums, with swelling of the cheek.

190. Abscess on the gums, with discharge of pus.

Pain in two of the molars, as when sweets get into a hollow tooth. [*S.*]

Violent toothache, with heat in the same side of the head (aft. 12 d.).

Violent toothache in the evening, as soon as she gets to bed, through the whole night, not alleviated by any change of position. [*Ng.*]

At night, toothache, and the following day, a swollen cheek; then a swollen nose, and red spots in the face and on the neck.

195. When a warm fluid gets into the mouth, it darts painfully through the teeth and the lower jaw of one side for 5 or 10 minutes.

Pain in almost all the teeth, especially while chewing; he

can not speak for pain, and admitted no air into the mouth, as it makes the pain unbearable.

The teeth ache, when brought together in biting.

A lower anterior incisor becomes very painful, when biting on it, on the 3d day of the menses. [*Ng.*]

Toothache, day and night, especially during (and after) eating, alleviated by applying warm cloths and pressure, during the menses. [*Ng.*]

200. Drawing **toothache, also during the menses.** [*Ng.*]

Drawing toothache during the menses, relieved by eating (aft. 6 h.).

Drawing toothache as if in the jaws, extending to the ears and the cheeks, only when eating and biting on the teeth. [*Ng.*]

Twitching in an infected molar after dinner, ceasing on picking with a tooth-pick. [*Ng.*]

Tearing pains in the upper row of teeth.

205. Drawing tearing in a molar, after a journey in wet cold weather (aft. 23d d.). [*Ng.*]

Tearing, jerking, griping in the teeth, extending to the ears, also at **night** in a hollow molar; alleviated by smelling of hepar **sulphuris.** [*Ng.*]

Before midnight, tearing in the teeth and jaws, extending into the ears; **she has** to roll around continually, and the teeth are **also sensitive when** she bites on them, on the 3d day of her menses. [*Ng.*]

Tearing in the upper molars of the left side, with frequent gathering of water in the mouth, and gnawing in the left shoulder (10th d.). [*Ng.*]

Tearing toothache in the left upper row, as if in the roots, as if an ulcer were forming there (36th d.). [*Ng.*]

210. Sensation as if there were an abscess at the roots of the teeth, which was about to break open from the access of air or from pressure on the tooth.

Stitches in a sound molar, in the open air. [*S.*]

Lancinating toothache, uninterrupted for 8 days.

Lancinating pain in the molars on biting, he could only chew with the incisors (at once and on 2d d.).

A severe shooting pain in an upper hollow tooth, on touching it with the tongue.

215. Pain as from soreness in a hollow molar (aft. ½ h.). [*Hb.*]

Throbbing and pressive toothache (aft. 3 d.).

In the evening pain in the teeth as if they were pinched in a vice.

Sensation in the teeth as if there were no strength in them to bite. [*S.*]

The teeth become very dull.

220. Dulness of the molars, and on biting on them, they seem loose.

The teeth feel dull and too long. [*S.*]

Teeth often seem too long, as if from acids.

A tooth which before has often been painful, seems to be longer and becomes painful (2d d.). [*Ng.*]

On sucking a molar, blood comes out. [*Ng.*]

225. The decay of the teeth progresses rapidly. [*Ng.*]

The teeth fall out, even sound ones.

Burning vesicles on the inner side of the lower lip. [*Ng.*]

On the inner side of the lower lip, a painful white vesicle.

The mouth on the inside becomes full of painless vesicles. [*Ng.*]

230. **Vesicles on the tongue,** especially on its border.

Vesicles on the tip of the tongue, hindering both speaking and eating, with a burning pain.

Pustules on the tongue, with burning, stinging pain, especially on the border and under the tongue.

Little ulcer on the tip of the tongue, painful as if sore, at every movement of the tongue. [*S.*]

Pain as from an ulcer on the palate, on touching it with the tongue; the part pells on the following day. [*Ng.*]

235. The anterior half of the tongue is as it were stiff and hard in the morning (4th d.). [*Ng.*]

Burning on the tip of the tongue, worse when touched. [*Ng.*]

Redness and inflammation in the interior of the mouth and throat; all of it pains as if sore and raw.

Sensation in the mouth as if it were swollen. [*S.*]

The cavity of the mouth seems to her so narrow, that she hardly dares open her mouth and move her tongue, because she is afraid of striking against the parts with the tongue (40th d.). [*Ng.*]

240. Speaking often becomes difficult for her, as if from weakness of the organs of speech and as if from a pain similar to stomach-ache (aft. 3d d.).

Sore throat towards evening. [*S.*]

In swallowing, the throat hurts as if the right tonsil was swollen.

Swelling of the tonsils, with impeded deglutition, especially in the morning and evening.

Sensation **as if something stuck in the throat which impeded swallowing,** with a choking pressure in the morning and evening. [*S.*, *Ng.*]

245. It seems to her as if something stuck in the throat on the right side, impeding the swallowing (aft. 6 min.).

Sore throat, with a sensation of scraping.

Rawness and scraping in the throat. [*Ng.*]

Soreness in the throat.

Burning in the throat down the œsophagus, as if from alcohol. [*Ng.*]

250. Severe sore throat, like stitches and drawing or tearing, more painful in talking. (3d d.).

Pressure in the throat, with external swelling of the same on both sides.

In the evening, dryness of the mouth, not relieved by drinking; the mouth in the morning feels as if parched.

Great dryness and heat in the mouth, at night (aft. 12 d.).

Dryness in the mouth and throat.

255. Early on awaking, dryness of the mouth and throat. [*Ng.*]

In the afternoon and evening, dryness in the mouth and throat, with thirst. [*Ng.*]

The lips are always dry, and stick together (15th d.). [*Ng.*]

Gathering of salty water in the mouth. [*Ng.*]

She has to spit out much saliva, for several days.

260. Frequent collection of watery saliva in the mouth; she has to spit out continually. [*Ng.*]

Bad smell in the mouth, which he perceives himself, for a long time. [*Ng.*].

Sweet taste in the mouth, with bloody saliva (5th d.). [*Ng.*]

Bloody taste in the mouth, during the whole time of proving. [*Ng.*]

In the morning, bad taste and smell in the mouth.

265. In the morning, bitter taste in the mouth, and the whole day sick at the stomach (aft. 10 d.).

Early on awaking, bitter taste in the mouth (2d d.). [*Ng.*]

Nasty, sourish taste in the mouth.

After drinking milk, a sour taste.

Taste of foods, sourish and metallic.

270. Constant eructations.

Frequent **suppressed eructations.**

Much empty eructation, especially the first day.

Frequent eructations of air, in the evening and after dinner (5th d.). [*Ng.*]

Eructation with the taste of ingesta.

275. During and after supper, eructation with taste of the food eaten (10th d.). [*Ng.*]

Sour eructation.

Frequent heartburn.

Early (after the chill) hiccup (2d d.). [*Ng.*]

In the morning nausea and coated tongue (aft. 8 d.).

280 Early after rising, nausea, till the afternoon, with chill in the whole body, followed by vomiting of some water; during the menses (aft. 55 d.). [*Ng.*]

In walking, loathing and nausea in the stomach, as if about to vomit (4th d.). [*Ng.*]

Constant adipsia, during the whole time of proving. [*Ng.*]

Constant thirst.

The whole afternoon, constant thirst (6th d.). [*Ng.*]

285. No appetite, but constant thirst.

She cannot eat at noon, without drinking (aft. 10 d.).

Little hunger and appetite (though he relishes his meals) (2d, 8th d.). [*Ng.*]

Lack of appetite, in the morning.

Milk is repugnant to her.

290. No appetite for meat and cooked dishes, only for bread and cold dishes; for several days (during her menses). [*Ng.*]
Hunger and appetite is increased (1st, 2d d.). [*Ng.*]
Very strong hunger and appetite (aft. 18 d.).
Rabid hunger (aft. 2 h.).
At noon increased hunger, and yet *she is sated with little food* (4th, 6th d.). [*Ng.*]
295. **At dinner, heat in the face**, also after dinner.
At dinner, tearing in the right temple.
During and after dinner she feels sick and fatigued (during the menses) (9th d.). [*Ng.*]
During supper, loathing of it and stomachache (8th d.). [*Ng.*]
After supper, stitches in the chest.
300. **After meals, sickness at the stomach.**
Every day, immediately after dinner, qualmishness and nausea, for an hour.
Immediately after dinner, discomfort, with pressure in the stomach and in the forehead, for several hours (aft. 4 h.).
After meals, oppression and pressure in the stomach.
After eating, severe pressure in the scrobiculus cordis, then nausea, and vomiting of all that has been eaten; afterward sour taste in the mouth; for five days (aft. 16 d.).
305. After dinner it is very difficult for her to speak.
Feeling as if the stomach were overloaded, until 3 hours after dinner.
The stomach feels full, tremulous (during the menses). [*Ng.*]
Feeling of emptiness in the stomach. [*S.*]
Stomachache, with tendency to watery risings (6th d.). [*Ng.*]
310. Painfulness of the stomach, also when touched (4th d.) [*Ng.*]
Pressure of the clothes on the stomach.
Pressure in the stomach.
Pressure in the stomach after meals.
Pressure in the stomach after supper (aft. 12 h.).
315. Pressive heaviness in the scrobiculus cordis.
Pressure in the stomach, with qualmishness and sensitiveness in the scrobiculus cordis.
Pressure and contraction of the stomach (and of the chest), with loathing and qualmishness (4th d.). [*Ng.*]
Pressure in the stomach, early in the morning, passing over into qualmishness and nausea.
Griping, rolling and gurgling in the stomach. [*Ng.*]
320. Gnawing in the right side of the stomach.
Tearing, boring pain in the region of the stomach, up to the upper lumbar vertebræ.
Feeling of coldness in the region of the stomach.
Burning in the region of the stomach.
Burning heat, first in the stomach, then also in the abdomen soon after taking the medicine). [*Ng.*, *S.*]
325. Heat in the stomach, spreading thence into the bowels, as from drinking strong wine (aft. ¼ h.).

Pressive pain under the right ribs, in the region of the liver.

Pain as from soreness in the liver.

Stitches below the left ribs, in the evening. [*Ng.*]

Pressure over the navel as from a button.

330. Early (at 3 o'clock) awaking from a violent pain in the abdomen, two days before her menses (41st d.). [*Ng.*]

Pressure in the hypogastrium for 3 h., also during dinner (aft. 2 h.).

Pressive pain in the left side of the abdomen, in the morning (aft. 12 h.).

Painful compression on both sides of the hypogastrium, only while sitting, alleviated by motion and by stretching (5th d.). [*Ng.*]

Sudden, painful contraction of the bowels up to the region of the stomach, relieved by compressing the abdomen with the hands, and passing off after going to bed (33d d.). [*Ng.*]

335. Colic, consisting of contraction and griping, first in the epigastrium, then in the hypogastrium, in the morning, so violent that qualmishness and collection of water in the mouth ensued, even to a swoon, with chilliness, 12 h. before the menses set in (aft. 9 d.).

At dinner, griping in the left side of the abdomen, passing away later on by emission of flatus. [*Ng.*]

In the forenoon, violent griping, contraction and rolling about in the abdomen, arising during a walk in the open air and only relieved by warmed cloths and lying on the stomach, appearing again in the evening, and also in the following morning in the cold, after which it improves in the room (17th d.). [*Ng.*]

Contractive cramps deep in the hypogastrium, and in stooping, also in the small of the back (38th d.).

Tightness and obstruction of the abdomen.

340. Cutting pain in the hypogastrium, while the abdomen is very small (16th d.). [*Ng.*]

Early (at 7 o'clock) violent colic (aft. 48 h.).

Cutting and smarting in the abdomen, as from worms, with contractive pain in the stomach and chills and sweat; this does not allow him to go to sleep before morning, and the pain returns early on awaking. [*Ng.*]

Stitches in the abdomen, impeding him in walking.

In the evening, while stooping, stitches in the left side of the abdomen.

345. Stitches passing transversely deep in the hypogastrium, while standing.

Burning, deep within, in the left side of the abdomen (2d d.). [*Ng.*]

(Griping and) sharp stitches in the right flanks, while stretching (20th d.). [*Ng.*]

Heaviness in the abdomen.

In the groin and the hough, painful pressure.

350. Sensation of fulness and bloatedness in the left flank. [*Ng.*]

An elastic swelling, as large as the fist, in the left flank, in the evening after lying down, with bruised pain in this spot, which does not allow her to lie on that side, and is also sensitive when pressing upon it; on waking up, the swelling and pain have disappeared (9th d.). [*Ng.*]

In the left groin a hernia appears (2d d.).

Extraordinary distension of the abdomen.

Bloatedness of the abdomen, with retention of stools. [*Ng.*]

355. Croaking, clucking and movements in the abdomen, as from flatus. [*Ng.*]

Clucking in the stomach, as in cramps or while fasting, after every deglutition, for several days (aft. 16 d.). [*Ng.*]

Rumbling and aching in the abdomen. [*S.*]

Accumulation of flatus, with griping of the abdomen. [*Ng.*]

Tendency to painful, flatulent colic.

350. Passage of much flatus.

Frequent discharge of flatus, in the afternoon, evening and night, with the customary stools (4th d.). [*Ng.*]

Retention of urine during the first days, followed by soft stools; with all provers. [*Ng.*]

Constipation (the first 4 d.). [*Tr.*]

Delayed, hard, solid stool, consisting of lumps which can be discharged by her only with difficulty. [*Ng.*]

365. Hard, painful evacuation, with pricking as of needles in the anus. [*Ng.*]

Hard stool, surrounded, as it were, with bloody streaks (aft. 22 h.).

Very soft stool, twice daily (3d and 4th d.). [*S.*, *Ng.*]

Early in the morning, diarrhœa with colic. [*S.*]

Diarrhœa of fæces and mucus, with cutting in the abdomen before and during the same (8th d.). [*Ng.*]

370. Stool largely mixed with mucus.

Evacuations by stools always connected with much urging.

With normal stools violent cutting in the rectum.

During the evacuation, a *griping pain in the abdomen*, drawing across the abdomen to the small of the back and the rectum, relieved by bending the body, and ceasing entirely after the stool (28th d.). [*Tr.*]

Before and after the soft stool, colic.

375. After the stool, first scraping in the anus, then burning.

After a copious stool, discharge of a milky prostatic fluid.

During and after stool, discharge of blood.

The varices of the rectum protrude much during the evacuation, and they **are painful** for a long while after, so that she cannot walk at all (aft. 7 d.).

The varices of the rectum protrude also when there is no evacuation, but recede when lying down.

380. There appear varices of the anus, with pains as from excoriation, and moist.

He cannot sleep at night, on account of the burning in the anus; he had to get up from bed on this account, and because of strong urging to stool.

Itching of the anus.

The child becomes sore between the legs.

Strong **pressure of the urine on the bladder**, with cutting in it.

385. Continual urging to micturition, also at night, with diminished emission (with burning). [*Ng.*]

She has to get up at night to urinate.

Nocturnal repeated micturition, at times quite copious. [*Ng.*]

The boy emits his urine at night (toward morning) **involuntarily while sleeping** (1st and 2d night, and aft. 16 d.).

Very frequent micturition, especially the first day.

390. Frequent, copious micturition, especially in the evening. [*Ng.*]

Increased, turbid urine. [*Ng.*]

The urine at noon is very pale yellow, and is the first after the previous evening. [*Ng.*]

White, **sandy urine**, for several days (aft. 9 d.).

The urine after dinner is reddish, like water mixed with blood.

395. Blood comes from the urethra.

After micturition, strong drawing anteriorly in the urethra (in the evening, on going to bed).

Much itching on the genitals.

Itching of the scrotum.

Perspiration of the scrotum.

400. Frequent relaxation of the testicles.

Drawing pain in the testicles.

At times, drawing in the testicles, relieved by tying them up.

Increased weight of the testicles; he had to use a suspensory.

Choking pain in the testicles and spermatic cords, with sensitiveness of the testicles to the touch; caused mostly by involuntary erections.

405. Continual **involuntary erections,** in the morning (13th d.).

Stiffness of the penis, without any impulse to coition (6th d.).

The sexual instinct quiescent for some time (aft. 7 d.).

(Total lack of sexual impulse).

Aversion to the other sex.

410. Violent excitation to coition, without any special voluptuous thoughts and almost without erections (aft. 5 d.).

Violent voluptuous desire with trembling of the body, almost without erection.

Pollutions almost every night.

Pollution two days after coition.

(After coition strong circulation of the blood and palpitation).

415. Violent itching of the pudenda.

Excoriation of the pudenda and anus, especially painful during micturition.

Swelling, itching and burning of the female pudenda (aft. 12 d.).

Constant itching of the mons veneris, which always returns after scratching. [*Ng.*]

The menses appear three to five days too late and once they are omitted altogether. [*Ng.*]

420. It brings the menses six days too soon.

The catamenia, always else quite regular, appear a day too soon. [*Tr.*]

The menses appear (after a long drive in the cold air) four days too soon and are very copious especially at night, as also in sitting and driving; preceded by griping pains in the abdomen with lack of appetite. [*Ng.*]

Menses on the 18th day (aft. 7 d.).

The menses flow more copiously owing to it (at once).

425. The blood of the catamenia is blackish, often in whole lumps, with spasmodic pains in the abdomen and hard stools, discharged after urging; the flow very strong. [*Ng.*]

The blood of the catamenia is colored very little.

The menstrual blood is acrid, so as to make the thigh sore, causing a burning pain. [*Ng.*]

Before the menses, pains in the abdomen and the small of the back. [*Ng.*]

Before and during the menses paleness of the face.

430. During the menses unconquerable sadness.

Toothache during the menses. [*Ng.*]

During the menses violent colic, with griping, pressure and tension between the shoulder-blades.

Violent tearing in the abdomen during the menses which set in one day too soon. [*S.*]

During the menses severe pain in the small of the back.

435. During the period violent coryza (9th d.).

During the menses great lassitude of the whole body, especially of the thighs, with yawning, toothache, pains in the small of the back and chilliness. [*Ng.*]

Severe **leucorrhœa** (aft. 2, 7, 8, 9 d.).

Watery, burning leucorrhœa (13th, 14th d.). [*Ng.*]

Frequent sneezing in the morning in bed.

440. Frequent violent sneezing (5th d.). [*Ng.*]

Nose obstructed. [*S.*]

The nose is very much obstructed without a cold.

At night the nose is so much obstructed that she has always to breathe through the mouth (aft. 4 d.).

After a sound nap in the forenoon, she wakes up at 1 o'clock with anxiety as if she were suffocating, because her nose was entirely obstructed and she could only breathe with difficulty with her mouth open, so that her chest pained her from the difficult breathing (aft 12 d.).

445. Coryza with rattling in the nose and obstruction of the same with husky voice. [*Ng.*]

Coryza with stoppage of the left nostril. [*Ng.*]

Dry coryza preventing the least passage of air through the nose, especially at night.

Fluent coryza (4th d.).

Severe fluent coryza with tearing in the left cheek. [*Ng.*]

450. Most violent fluent coryza with cough.

Dropping of water from the nose without coryza. [*Ng.*]

There is a continual discharge of acrid water burning the upper lip during the menses (43d d.). [*Ng.*]

Constriction of the larynx from both sides of the neck.

Drawing, stinging, itching, in the larynx.

455. Hoarseness and sensation of rawness in the throat. [*Ng.*]

Hoarseness, he can only talk with difficulty, as this increases the hoarseness (2d d.).

Severe and frequent **hoarseness.**

Hoarseness so that she cannot speak aloud (aft. 16 d.).

His chest is oppressed, so that he can hardly speak, with coryza and much expectoration of mucus, especially in the morning.

460. The chest feels raw; when he calls loudly he is hoarse.

Catarrh with difficult hearing and burning in the region of the stomach.

Frequent hawking on account of the collection of mucus in the throat. [*Ng.*]

Rattling in the bronchia, as from mucus, for several days. [*Ng.*]

He has to cough for a quarter of an hour in the evening, in bed.

465. **Cough at night.**

The child coughs very violently every morning about 3 or 4 o'clock.

In the middle of the night, violent, dry cough.

Cough with asthma (6th d.). [*Ng.*]

Cough with asthma in the evening in bed for half an hour.

470. Cough with the greatest violence from the depth of the chest.

Cough which draws the chest together.

Cough, while the chest under the sternum pains as if raw and sore.

The cough causes pain in the jaws, which is not perceived on touching them.

Cough with pain below in the sternum.

475. Cough with stitches in the sternum (1st d.).

Cough with a stitch in the scrobiculus cordis every time.

Cough with heat in the head. [*Ng.*]

Short, subdued cough, from an irritation of the larynx with a painful sensation of spasmodic asthma. Soon after irritation to coryza in the nose and scraping and scratching soreness in the throat, with difficult expectoration of a little mucus (aft. ½ h.). [*Hb.*]

Dry cough, especially at night, as from feathery dust in the throat. [*Ng.*]

480. Cough with expectoration of mucus and soreness of the throat. [*Ng.*]

Cough the whole day and early in the morning, with much expectoration of mucus. Early in bed, constant cough with expectoration of mucus affecting the chest and head.

Cough with expectoration of mucus with little specks of blood (aft. 8 d.).

Cough with expectoration of bloody mucus, heaviness

on the chest and short breath, especially in ascending a mountain (6th, 18th d.). [*Ng.*]

485. Bloody expectoration, when hawking up.

After rawness and taste of blood in the mouth, cough with expectoration of bright red blood, with burning and heaviness of chest, heat and redness in the face and trembling in the whole body (4th d.). [*Ng.*]

Difficult breathing, it made him retch (short cough).

At night very difficult respiration; the coverlet must not touch his mouth, else he is afraid of suffocating (7th d.). [*Ng.*]

After every exertion he is asthmatic, with palpitation. [*Ng.*]

490. Tightness in the middle of the chest when breathing and also when not; the spot pains, when pressing upon it, as after a blow. [*Ng.*]

A paroxysm of asthma, lasting eight days; he could only with the greatest effort mount a few steps, could only draw breath with the greatest exertion, and only in the open air; he could not come into a heated room; he would there become deadly pale, and could do nothing but sit still (aft. 21 d.).

Short breath, with stitches in the chest. [*Ng.*]

Short breath, especially on going up stairs. [*Ng.*]

In breathing, frequent stitches in the hands and the fingers.

495. In expiration something seems to draw down into the chest, which keeps the breath from being expelled (7th d.). [*Ng.*]

The chest is as it were faint.

Long-continued weakness of the chest and catarrh (aft. 4 w.). [*Ng.*]

Heaviness of the chest, as if from accumulation of blood (4th, 5th, 7th d.) [*Ng.*]

Heaviness and tightness of the chest, when walking in the open air. [*Ng.*]

500. She feels as it were a hundred weight upon her chest, with pains; she only wishes to be able to cough, so as to be relieved (7th d.). [*Ng.*]

Rush of blood to the chest (after writing).

Heat in the chest.

Great oppression of the chest.

While standing, a sensation in the chest, as if the lungs were being drawn down (6th d.). [*Ng.*]

505. Bruised pain in the middle of the chest, in the morning (4th d.). [*Ng.*]

Painful pressure on the chest, especially while lying abed.

Compressive pressure on the chest.

Stitches in the chest near the last true rib, while breathing and singing.

Stitches in the sternum, on the right side of the chest and under the left breast, where it pains as if bruised when touched. [*Ng.*]

510. When stooping, stitches in the chest, alleviated by straightening up (16th d.). [*Ng.*]

Stitches in the right breast when stooping.

While walking, stitches in the right side of the chest. [*S.*]

Under the right breast, at the lowest rib, early when raising himself in bed, twenty to thirty stitches in succession, also when not breathing; also at other times of the day.

Stitches in the left breast, through a great part of the night, preventing her from lying on the left side.

515. Severe stitches in the left side of the chest, beginning in the region of the heart and drawing down to the side, and afterward more to the back (aft. 11 d.).

Frequently a stitch in the heart.

Frequent palpitation of the heart, with a drawing in of the epigastrium and a feeling of weakness in the scrobiculus cordis.

Audible palpitation of the heart and quickened heart-beat; on pressing on it with the hand, the blood seemed to rise up to the throat, with dyspnœa (while resting).

The cartilage of the sternum cracks on bending back the chest, with a pressure in the middle of the chest.

520. The right breast is painful to the touch (3d d.).

Red miliary eruption on the chest.

A small red furuncle over the right breast, which is only painful when touched. [*Ng*]

On the coccyx stitches, where before there was itching.

Pain in the small of the back, aggravated by motion and by walking.

525. When stooping, pain in the small of the back; she feels as if the muscles were not strong enough to support the body, which always tends to fall forward; better on rising up (2d d.). [*Ng.*]

Pain, as from a bruise, in the small of the back (on the 2d day of the menses). [*Ng.*]

When walking in the open air a pain darted suddenly into the small of the back (crick in the back), most painful on rising after long-continued sitting.

Twitching pain in the small of the back.

Drawing pain from the small of the back into the legs.

530. In the small of the back and the loins, a pressive drawing pain, only while resting (sitting, standing and lying down) in day-time; disappearing in walking.

In the small of the back and the loins a violently beating pain, while at rest, not changing when touched.

Gnawing pain in the small of the back and the hips, going thence to the abdomen and back again, both in rest and in motion (16th d.). [*Ng.*]

Sudden stitches in the right loin.

Pain in the back, on motion. [*S.*]

535. A jerk in the back, at night, while sleeping (7th d.). [*Ng.*]

Pressure in the back.

Burning on the back, especially on the small of the back, several times a day.

With stitches, as from fleas, a vesicle forms on the left shoulder-blade. [*Ng.*]

In the neck, severe burning pain, in the morning (10th d.). [*Ng.*]

540. Drawing from the neck down the back (6th d.). [*Ng.*]

Stiff neck on turning the head.

Drawing pain in the nape of the neck, with stitches in the head, over the temple, with bloated face.

Pressure on the left shoulder.

The knot of glands in the axilla becomes painful and swells.

545. In the right shoulder-joint a drawing pain (aft. 14 d.)

Twitching tearing in the right shoulder-joint, at rest and in motion (37th d.). [*Ng.*]

Tearing in the joints of the upper limbs.

Tearing in the shoulders. [*Ng.*]

Several tears in the left shoulder, towards the chest. [*Ng.*]

550. Pain, as from a bruise, in the left shoulder, at rest and in motion. [*Ng.*]

Pain as of a bruise in the left shoulder-joint and elbow-joint (in the evening).

A small furuncle on the left shoulder. [*Ng.*]

Burning on a little spot of the upper arm and the fore-arm (11th d.). [*Ng.*]

In the arms and hands, a drawing pain.

555. Paralytic drawing in the left arm, from the axilla into the wrist.

Sensation of paralysis in the right arm (14th d.). [*Hb.*]

Sensation of paralysis and heaviness of the right arm; she has no strength in it and must let it hang down; the hand at the same time is swollen and cold for half an hour (aft. 2 h.).

The right arm seems to weigh a hundred weight, and to be powerless.

The right arm for many days becomes quite weak and cold, appearing to be asleep and lifeless; this was again followed by a tingling sensation.

560. In the night (3 to 4 o'clock) she involuntarily stretches her arm out of the bed and awakes from the pain in it, as it is cold, stiff, and in the elbow-joint heavy like lead; she has to use the other hand to bring it back into bed, because it is too stiff, and when moved and in bed there is a tearing pain in the joints of the shoulder, the elbow and the wrists.

Cramp in the right arm, which pulled the arm backward three times in succession; then heat of the body and turbid white urine.

Twitching and quivering in the right upper arm (4th d.). [*Ng.*]

Cracking in the elbow-joint when in motion.

Groaning pain in the elbow-joint in straightening the arm in front of him.

565. Stiffness of the elbow-joint.

Boring pain in the elbow-joint in the fossa which receives the process.

Sharp stitches in the elbow.

Tearing in the elbow (in the bone) extending forward into the little finger (4th, 5th d.). [*Ng.*]

In the left fore-arm, in the middle, a violent pain, in the evening in bed with a sensation as if the bones there would forcibly bend inward and break of (2d d.). [*Ng.*]

570. Itching of the inside of the right fore-arm, with burning after scratching, and the appearance of small red pimples, spots and granules, which do not cease to itch after scratching, until they become deep red on the following day (4th, 5th d.). [*Ng.*]

In the wrist, tension while at rest, aggravated by motion; he feels as if he could not move his hand (2d d.). [*Ng.*]

Tearing in the wrist extending into the fingers, ceasing when she gets warm in bed.

Painful tearing in the left wrist, as if in the marrow, toward the little finger (6th d.). [*Ng.*]

Frequent going to sleep of the (right) hand, on which she lies at night (4th d.). [*Ng.*]

575. Trembling of the hands (aft. 7 d.).

Distended veins and blueness of the hands, after washing them in cold water. [*Ng.*]

The skin of the hands in a child becomes quite hard, and chaps in deep fissures.

Peeling off of the skin of the palms of the hands (aft. 4 d.).

In the fingers a pinching pain on stretching them apart.

580. Cramp in the posterior joint of a finger, so that he cannot extend it, with a stinging pain; from morning to evening, while staying in the cold (2d d.). [*Ng.*]

Drawing pain from the tips of the fingers down into the hand, as if from constant mesmerizing (1st d.).

Tearing in the fingers and in the thumb-joint. [*Ng.*]

Pain as from a bruise in the left thumb, in the cold (2d d.). [*Ng.*]

Twitching, griping in the left thumb, as if in the bone, with yawning (11th d.). [*Ng.*]

585. Visible twitching and quivering in the left thumb. [*Ng.*]

Swelling of the middle joint of the right middle finger, with painfulness while touching or bending it.

On the nates, a burning, itching.

In the hip-joint a severe pain while walking.

Every morning in bed, a severe pain in the hip-joint, as if it was rotten and beaten in two, so that he can not turn over while lying down; after rising and more yet after walking, the pain decreases, and in the afternoon passes away entirely; for 4 weeks.

590. Drawing pain down from the left hip.

His legs are contracted.

The tendons in the leg feel as if too short.

Pain like a sprain in the left leg, while walking.

Restlessness in the legs.

595. Twitches in the leg, toward evening.

Heaviness in the legs so that he can hardly lift them, in the evening (8th d.). [*Ng.*]

Suddenly great weakness in the lower limbs, so that she has trouble in getting along, after dinner (2d d.). [*Ng.*]

Great weariness in the thighs and legs. [*Ng.*]

In the evening, while lying down, jerking scraping on th bones of the thighs and legs, so that she has to jerk up her leg momentarily, and cannot lie still, but is obliged to walk about.

600. In the right thigh, a severe pain, as if the inmost marrow wa shaken up, aggravated by lying and sitting for a quarter of a hour (aft. some h.).

Great wearisome pain in the thighs, as if they would fall off or as if the tendons would tear off; alternating with pains in th small of the back; she knows not what to do for pains (on the 3 day of her menses). [*Ng.*]

Bruised pain in the thighs.

Bruised pain in the middle point of the thighs in rest and motion (during the menses.) [*Ng.*]

Pain in the thigh as if beaten blue, impeding her walk, (bu only while walking and in being pressed upon in touching.)

605. Pain as if crushed, passing away by rubbing, in the righ thigh, immediately above the knee (11th d.). [*Ng.*]

Pain as from a sprain in the left thigh, with a feeling of weak ness and of sudden collapse of the legs in walking.

Stiffness in the thighs, in walking.

Pain as if the tendons were too short, in a spot of the lef thigh, above the knee; only when pressing upon it or sitting, bu not else (3d d.). [*Ng.*]

A blue spot, as large as a child's hand, above the knee, wher it burns exceedingly.

610. After itching, a deep-seated burning furuncle on the knee [*Ng.*]

A knot over the right knee, deep in the skin, only painful o pressure. [*Ng.*]

A small furuncle, only painful on being pressed upon, in th left knee. [*Ng.*]

Tearing in the knees and knee-joints. [*Ng.*]

Boring pain in and upon the patella.

615. Boring and drawing in the knee, and thence restlessness i the legs, so she has to move them continually, without alleviatin the restlessness.

Twitching in both patellæ, in the evening, several times i succession (5th d.). [*Ng.*]

Twitches in both knees and legs.

In moving the knee, a grating sound.

On sitting down and in turning the leg, a pain in the kne as if sprained.

620. Burning redness like scarlatina, in the right knee and down t leg; putting the cold hand upon it increases the pain (20th, 21 d.). [*Ng.*]

In the legs a paralytic pain, as if they were going to slee alleviated by walking (7th d.). [*Ng.*]

Frequent going to sleep of the legs, while sitting and stan ing, and at night, when lying upon them. [*Ng.*]

Tearing below the knee and on the left tibia (11th d.). [*Ng.*]

Cramp in the legs, frequently, especially in the muscles of the tibiæ and the feet.

625. While lying down, cramp in the leg, which became, however, unbearable on rising, compelling him to lie down.

In the calf, severe cramp, on walking in the open air, so that he had suddenly to stand still.

Straining in the calf (from a cold?).

Violent stitches deep in the calves (14th d.). [*Hb.*]

Above the right heel, stitches.

630. In the heel, early, on awaking, a keen pain, as if the bones were festered through.

Formication in the left heel, and sensation as if festering, when touched (aft. 5 d.). [*Ng.*]

Twitching tearing in the right heel (37th d.). [*Ng.*]

In the joints of the feet and the ankles, a tearing which draws down into the toes, and ceases when she becomes warm in bed.

Drawing pain at the external ankle (4th d.). [*Ng.*]

635. Cold feet.

In the evening chilliness in the feet, especially on going to bed.

Rapid swelling of the feet up to the calves.

Great weariness in the feet as if fatigued (2d d.). [*Ng.*]

Trembling in both feet (aft. 9 h.).

640. Formication in the dorsum of the left foot as from going to sleep (11th d.). [*Ng.*]

Violent formication and itching in the sole of the foot, so that it can hardly be borne, so that she feels like scratching the skin off; after scratching, the spot burns, in the evening (after lying down). [*Ng.*]

Tearing in the soles of both feet (11th d.). [*Ng.*]

Sharp stitches on the ball of right foot.

Stinging, tearing and twitching in the big toe.

645. Frequent painful twitching in the ball of the great toe (which had been frozen when she was a child).

Several days, especially in the evening, when going to sleep she had attacks of severe stinging and drawing in the balls of both the big toes as if they had been frozen.

Itching formication in the ball of the right great toe as from a chilblain. [*Ng.*]

The left big toe is hot to the touch and pains with a burning sensation as if he had burned himself, especially from the pressure of boots and in damp weather; when taking off the boot and when resting the foot on something and in walking the pain is alleviated (14th to 36th d.).

The big toe becomes red, thick and painful, especially in the evening in bed, and the whole foot swells up.

650. In walking the ball of the big toe pains as if festering.

On the skin of the whole body much itching.

Itching of the whole body in the morning for three hours.

Itching here and there, in many parts of the body, mostly passing away on scratching, or burning painfully. [*Ng.*]

Violent itching of the whole body, here and there, and, after scratching, burning vesicles and pimples or hard granules. [*Ng.*]

655. Burning pimples, like millet seed, on the neck and the fore-arm. [*Ng.*]

Every evening about 7 o'clock a strange uneasiness which wakes the child from its rest; it tosses about restlessly and cries until about 10 o'clock it falls into a sound sleep lasting the whole night; during its restlessness the head is, as it were, bloated and glowing hot; next morning the face is spotted as if scarlatina was coming on. [*Gr.*]

The whole upper part of the body is red as if covered with scarlatina.

Miliary eruption on the right side of the neck and the left fore-arm.

Around the elbow small red tubercles and about the neck large ones, with cutting pain; only a few of them suppurate.

660. The warts become inflamed.

A mild tetter becomes red, with itching and burning, and disappears after some days.

The humor in an ulcer becomes fetid.

Unusual sensitiveness to cold in the skin.

Chilliness while undressing.

665. A cold causes coryza and hoarseness.

She cannot bear the evening air; her feet become heavy; the air is unpleasant to her and every part of her body hurts.

She is very much fatigued by walking in the open air.

Very much fatigued by walking in the open air. [*Ng.*]

Extreme sensitiveness to the open air. [*Gr.*]

670. While walking in the open air he is easily heated. [*Stf.*]

After walking in the open air violent headache, which lasts during the evening.

Several ailments seem to appear and to be aggravated in the open air. [*Ng.*]

Cracking in the joints, while walking.

Tearing pain in the whole body and especially in the thighs.

675. Violent rheumatic drawing pain through all the limbs, hands, feet, head, neck, etc. [*Stf.*]

Stinging drawing, now in the right arm, now in the legs.

Fine stitches in the head, in the finger tips and toes.

Pain in the occiput, in the chest and from the two shoulder-blades down to the ribs.

Feeling of numbness in the (right) side on which she lies in bed, passing away on turning over (2d d.). [*Ng.*]

680. Going to sleep of the hands and feet while sitting, passing away by motion. [*Ng.*]

Cold hands and feet even when well wrapped up and in the warm room.

In the forenoon and night all her limbs ache, with a gnawing pain in the small of the back, more while at rest than in motion (41st d.). [*Ng.*]

The right side of the body seems more affected than the left. [*Ng.*]

Visible emaciation of the whole body. [*Ng.*]

685. Paroxysm: Toward noon everything turned black before her eyes; the letters seemed to move; the breath was checked with previous lassitude; on quickly rising from his seat, he became, as it were, rigid all over the body, his arms and legs extended outwardly, while the fingers were clenched; he had to forcibly stretch them out which made them movable again (4th d.).

Toward evening she became suddenly unwell, so that she thought she would faint; alleviated by walking up and down in the open air, though there was yet an occasional stitch in the right side (aft. 10 d.).

She is very much incommoded from much speaking and hearing people talk, her hands and feet grow cold from it.

The whole day, a slight perspiration, as if from exhaustion.

The whole day weary and fatigued, without being either sad or cheerful (aft. 24 h.).

690. Extremely weary.

She often cannot stand, when she first leaves her bed, from weariness (aft. 48 h.).

Indescribably great exhaustion; she often cannot sit, but has to lie down from asthenia for hours (aft. 24 h.).

She lies down as if exhausted and stupefied for several hours.

While walking in the open air, exhaustion and ill-humor; he, as it were, trembled for weakness.

695. While walking, her whole body trembles.

She staggers when rising.

Great exhaustion in the limbs, and total indisposition for work.

In the forenoon and morning great exhaustion and lassitude of body, as if he had worked too much, alleviated by walking in the open air. [*Ng.*]

Broken-down feeling of the whole body, lack of tone and weeping mood early in the morning on rising.

700. Sensation in the limbs as if broken down, also in the evening.

Especially in the evening hours great fatigue and weakness in the limbs, especially in the knees and legs, so that he has to lie down (1st and 2d d.). [*Hb.*]

Great exhaustion, inviting to sleep, in the forenoon for an hour.

Frequent extending and stretching ofthe body, in the morning, as if he had not done sleeping (2d d.).

Disposition to stretch arms and legs.

705. Much yawning, with collection of water in the mouth, weariness, uneasiness and chilliness. [*Ng.*]

In the evening severe, spasmodic yawning.

Drowsiness in daytime; he has to sit down and sleep in the afternoon, else his eyes ache.

Drowsiness by day; he has to lie down in the forenoon and afternoon.

When she is unoccupied as, *e. g.*, at meals, she becomes very very sleepy; but when she is at work the drowsiness passes away.

710. Sleepy during the day, with yawning (1st, 4th d.). [*Ng.*]

After supper invincible sleepiness, and yet on lying down he **does** not sleep soundly during the night.

He soon becomes sleepy in the evening, but his sleep is uneasy for several weeks. [*Ng.*]

Late in going to sleep (the 1st night).

He cannot go to sleep in the evening, for a long time, without any particular reason; but he afterwards sleeps soundly (2d d.). [*Ng.*]

715. (Nightmare when going to sleep.)

The earlier she goes to sleep, the better is her sleep; the later she goes to bed the less she can sleep.

He often, when in bed at night, cannot go to sleep for two, three or four hours from restlessness, dry heat and sometimes from burning in the stomach.

On account of itching and stinging of the skin he cannot go to sleep at night.

He does not go to sleep till about 4 o'clock in the morning, when he falls into a dull sleep, perspiring, till 7 A. M.

720. Very light sleep at night; she awakes at every slight sound. [*Ng.*]

Uneasy, unrefreshing sleep every night; he tosses about.

His sleep is restless and broken; he sleeps little and wakes up frequently.

Restless sleep, with frequent awakening, several nights, especially during the menses. [*Ng.*]

Frequent awakening at night, with chilliness (1st d.) [*Ng.*]

725. She awakes at night, every half hour, and is then tired in the morning.

He wakes up at night, between 1 and 2 o'clock, and cannot again go to sleep for two hours (2d d.).

After midnight she wakes up with stomachache and cannot again go to sleep till 4 o'clock.

Frequent awaking, with moaning and groaning, for several weeks. [*Ng.*]

Awaking in a fright, several times, after midnight, when he cannot again go to sleep; many nights. [*Ng.*]

730. Frequent violent starting up terrified from sleep at night, with great timidity afterwards. [*Ng.*]

Sleep full of dreams (aft. 2 d.)

He dreams, waking, during the night.

Vivid dreams, with one who never before dreamed.

Sleep full of varied dreams.

735. She dreams whole stories.

Romantic dreams.

Lacivious dreams, three nights in succession, about practising coition, and on awaking a sensation as of emission of seed, which yet was not true.

Confused dreams.

Anxious dreams.

740. Dreams every night, with an anxious ending, from which he waked up early (at 3 A. M.).

Distressing dreams of danger and hardship. [*Ng.*]
Distressing dreams about ghosts; he cried out in his sleep.
Dreams of death and of dying.
Dreams of dying and corpses. [*Ng.*]
745. Disgusting dreams about lice (aft. 18 d.). [*Ng.*]
Dreams of quarrels (3d and 7th d.) [*Ng.*]
She tells in her dreams what she thought of while waking.
In the evening in bed, anguish, she cannot lie still.
At night an attack of great anguish, as if she had to die, with cold sweat, audible palpitation and involuntary flow of tears; she could not move her eyes nor speak, with audible dyspnœa and trembling of the hands (aft. 19 d.).
750. Vertigo at night, everything turned with her; she had to sit up in bed.
Rush of blood to the head, at night, and on awaking, heat in the face.
At night, boring, lancinating headache.
Before her eyes sparks, when she awakes at night.
In the teeth, drawing, at night and on awaking.
755. Qualmishness, the whole night, so that she could not sleep (aft. 8 h.).
Pressure in the stomach, at night.
Violent colic, two nights in succession, which only ceased on the passage of copious flatus.
He wakes up at night for micturition.
Dry coryza and stopped nose, in the evening and at night, while in bed.
760. Much hawking and expectoration of salty mucus, at night.
Heaviness and pressure in the sternum, at night.
Great pain in an excrescence (*ganglium*) on the hand, so that she wakes up, at night.
In the ball of the big toe, in the evening, in bed, a piercing pain.
Perspiration on the legs at night.
765. At night, about 3 o'clock, his upper body and arms were jerked, with a tearing pain for ten minutes, while he was in full consciousness, causing great exhaustion.
All her lower limbs pain at night, with gnawing pains in the small of the back (41st d.). [*Ng.*]
He can only turn over slowly in bed, because the motion causes him pain. [*Ng.*]
He can lie with more ease on his left side than on his right. [*Ng.*]
Extraordinary rush of blood at night; it seems as if the blood would burst his arteries and his heart.
770. At night, he often feels a chill in his sleep, but on awakening he quickly becomes warm again.
Chill and cold at night, so that he cannot get warm again, especially in his feet, and he cannot go to sleep. [*Ng.*]
Chilly sensation, frequently towards evening and until he goes to bed.

In the evening, often a feverish chill.

Shaking chill before going to sleep.

775. Chill and coldness in the open air, or when he comes into a room from the open air. [*Ng.*]

Evening attacks of chills, often with the hair standing on end, blue hands and blue nails, chattering of the teeth and shaking; at times with a nightly heat following, and perspiration in the morning. [*Ng.*]

In the evening, in bed, from 9 to 12 o'clock, a chilly shivering alternating with heat and much restlessness (aft. 10 d.).

Several days chills and heat, mostly shaking chills and subsequently a general dry heat; some perspiration, only in the morning.

Alternately chill and heat, with sensitiveness to cold; nausea, thirst, pressure on the chest, with stitches in the left side of the chest, tearing in the forehead and muddled feeling of the head, alternate redness and paleness of the cheeks, pressure in the stomach, with tendency to eructation, attended with severe catarrh and sleeplessness; for several days (during the menses). [*Ng.*]

780. Feverish heat, many evenings in succession, for 1½ hours, with headache.

Heat at night (19th d.). [*Ng.*]

Heat in the whole body, especially in the abdomen, in the forenoon (11th d.). [*Ng.*]

Continually warm and anxious, in the forenoon (before the menses) (42 d.). [*Ng.*]

Feverish heat in the head, with cold feet.

785. Constant night-sweats.

He perspires almost every night, and is quite hot in the morning.

Morning-sweats.

Perspiration toward morning (1st d.). [*Ng.*]

Morning-sweat in the joints (aft. 16 d.).

AMMONIUM MURIATICUM, CHLORIDE OF AMMONIUM, SAL AMMONIAC.

We take one drachm of sal ammoniac in lumps, as being the purest. This is dissolved in 1½ drachms of boiling distilled water, filtered through white printing paper and then set in the cellar to quietly crystallize. Of the crystallized and dried salt* one grain is then triturated three times with one hundred grains of sugar of milk within three hours to the millionfold powder-attenuation, and then in

* *Sal ammoniacum depuratum.*

Ammonium muriaticum, first appearing here, has its pathogenesis mainly made up from one published in 1833, in Hartlaub and Trinks' *Annalen*, Vol. iv. It is a joint one as will be seen by the names of Hartlaub and Nenning always standing in a pair after the symptoms. Hahnemann's own observation will have been on patients, as shown in the preface; Rummel's are probably from provings with the 30th dilution.—*Hughes.*

dilution it is diluted and potentized to the 30th development of power, as has been taught concerning the other dry drugs at the end of the first volume.

This natural salt, which has been abused by allopathy so frequently and in such large doses, in diseases of every kind, shows itself in homœopathic practice as an excellent anti-psoric, even in a dose of one or two of the smallest pellets moistened with a potency of high degree, and administered in dilution of more or less water (according as it is desired to act more or less strongly), or also by smelling of such a larger or smaller pellet.

This salt deserves in a high degree further provings as to its pure effects.

This medicine has proved itself particularly efficacious where one or more of the following symptoms appeared:

Lugubrious, peevish, indifferent mood; *flying spots and points before the vision*, in day-time and in the evening at candle-light; (hard hearing); Ringing and buzzing in the ears; ulcerated corners of the mouth; tensive pains in the articulations of the jaws, during chewing and opening the mouth; empty eructation; lancinating pains in the left hypochondrium, early on awaking in bed, with dyspnœa compelling the person to sit up; the groin, on being touched, feels as if it were festered and swollen; tendency to constipation; discharge of blood during stool; pain as of soreness in the rectum and passing upwards in sitting; during the menses vomiting and diarrhœa; pressive and contractive *pain in* the abdomen and *the* back during the menses; during the menses, pain in the small of the back; tearing in the feet during the menses; while sneezing, tearing stitches in the nape of the neck into the shoulders; severe cough; tightness in the chest during manual labor; stiffness in the small of the back; stitches in the right shoulder-blade in respiring; tearing stitching pain as of spraining in the left hip; *cold feet;* paralytic weakness in the limbs, with dizziness; drowsiness in the day-time, with indolence and indisposition to work; night-sweats.

The abbreviations of the names of my fellow provers are *Ng.*; *Hb.*, *Dr. Hartlaub; Rl.*, *Dr. Rummel.*

AMMONIUM MURIATICUM.

Great seriousness.

Anxious and melancholy, as if internal grief or sorrow were gnawing in her heart. [*Ng.*, *Hb.*]

She does not know what to do for anguish, she would like to weep, and does weep at times (1st d.). [*Ng.*, *Hb.*]

During this anguish, bitter taste and nauseous, bitter eructation. [*Ng.*, *Hb.*]

5. She sits ill-humored, lost in thoughts, and it is difficult to make her speak, in the evening (15th d.). [*Ng.*, *Hb.*]

Very peevish, as if from internal vexation, in the morning, and dazed, as if she had not done sleeping (3d d.). [*Ng.*, *Hb.*]

Irritable and peevish, in the forenoon; after dinner her mood improves (8th d.). [*Ng.*, *Hb.*]

Very irritable, peevish and timid. [*Rl.*]

In speaking about an important matter, he becomes excessively excited.

10. Involuntary, strong aversion to certain persons.

Gloomy in the head, as after a spree (14th d.). [*Ng.*, *Hb.*]

Dizzy and numbed in the head, in the room; this passes off when in the air, in the morning (4th d.). [*Ng.*, *Hb.*]

Vertigo, as if about to fall to one side; worse on motion, passing away when in the air; frequently (3d d.). [*Ng.*, *Hb.*)

Vertigo and **fullness in the head, so that it seems too heavy** (1st and 25th d.). [*Ng.*, *Hb.*]

15. Feeling of heaviness in the head, almost daily, on rising. [*Ng.*, *Hb.*]

Heaviness in the forehead, frequently during day (with internal sensation of heat and some perspiration). [*Ng.*, *Hb.*]

Headache, extremely violent for several days. [*Rl.*]

Headache in the crown, as if the head were broken in two (4th d.). [*Ng.*, *Hb.*]

Pressure in the forehead, with feeling of heat there, early, after an uneasy night. [*Ng.*, *Hb.*]

20. Pressing down into the forehead, toward the root of the nose, with a sensation as if the brain was torn in pieces, early on rising (25th d.). [*Ng.*, *Hb.*]

The occiput feels as if compressed in a vice, later also on both sides of the head, with great ill-humor (17th d.). [*Ng.*, *Hb.*]

Pinching pain in the occiput in a small spot (11th d.). [*Ng.*, *Hb.*]

Painful twitching up into the left temple (3d d.). [*Ng.*, *Hb.*]

Tearing in the head, mostly in the right temple, whence it also passes into the side of the face (also during the menses, and in the forehead and the right side of the head in sitting) (6th, 7th, 15th, 17th d.). [*Ng.*, *Hb.*]

25. Stitches in the left temple, forehead and side of the head, also in the crown, when stooping, with a feeling there as if the head had burst (2d to 5th d.). [*Ng.*, *Hb.*]

Stitches and pressure in the head, especially on the left side, in the room (2d d.). [*Ng.*, *Hb.*]

Boring in front in the forehead, early on rising, and almost the whole day (5th d.). [*Ng.*, *Hb.*]

Glowing heat in the right side of the head, every evening.

Frequent rushes of heat in the head (25th d.). [*Ng.*, *Hb.*]

30. Feeling of heat and fullness in the head, early on rising. [*Hb.*, *Ng.*]

Burning pain, and at times stitches in the left temple, of itself, as also while chewing and sneezing; not **aggravated by external touch.**

Itching of the hairy scalp, urging to constant scratching (3d d.). [*Ng.*, *Hb.*]

Itching pimples on the right side of the occiput, in the evening, passing away at night (aft 19 d.). [*Hb.*, *Ng.*]

In the eyes, pains.

35. Over the border of the right orbit, hammering or knocking, as from a large body (15th d.). [*Ng.*, *Hb.*]

Tearing in the upper border of the right eye, first aggravated, then improved by pressing upon it (15th d.). [*Ng.*, *Hb.*.]

Tearing in the external canthus.

Tearing in the eyeballs.

Burning in the eyes, especially in the corners, also early on rising, so that she can not look into the light; this passes off on washing (3d and 4th d.). [*Ng.*, *Hb.*]

40. For several evenings, the eyes burn only during the twilight; as soon as light comes into the room, it ceases. [*Hb.*, *Ng.*]

In the evening, burning and closing of the eyes, as from drowsiness, which passed off when light was brought in (15th d.). [*Ng.*, *Hb.*]

At night, the eyes burn, with profuse lachrymation.

Twitching and quivering of the eyes, passing away by rubbing (4th and 14th d.). [*Ng.*, *Hb.*]

Quivering in the lower eyelids, especially in the left one, during the whole time of proving. [*Hb.*, *Ng.*]

45. Lachrymation of the eyes, early on rising (3d d.). [*Ng.*, *Hb.*]

Agglutinated eyes, early on awaking, with burning in the canthi, on washing (2d d.). [*Ng.*, *Hb.*]

Redness of the white of the eyes, with itching of the eyes.

A vesicle in the white of the eye.

A mist before the eyes, which prevents her from seeing clearly, either in the air or the brightest sunshine, either what is close or what is distant; but she sees better in the room. [*Ng.*, *Hb.*]

50. Early, for several mornings, dimness of the eyes, as if foggy, passing away on washing. [*Hb.*, *Ng.*]

Sensation, in the left eye, as if a body was rising up which prevented her from seeing, in the forenoon (14th and 15th d.). [*Ng.*, *Hb.*]

Yellow spots before the eyes, while sewing, and when she looks down through the window into the garden (2d d.). [*Ng.*, *Hb.*]

Lancinating pains in the ears, passing inwards and outwards, also with boring and burning, most when walking in the air. [*Ng.*, *Hb.*]

Digging and tearing in the right ear, also at night when lying on it, a digging and rolling as if something wanted to come out. [*Ng.*, *Hb.*]

55. Twitching (with boring) in the ears, also behind the left ear, around a humid tetter. [*Hb.*, *Ng.*]

Tickling in the right ear. [*Hb.*, *Ng.*]

Itching in both ears, not passing away by scratching, with running out of fluid wax for several days (aft. 5 d.). [*Hb.*, *Ng.*]

Painful pimple on the anthelix of the right ear.

Itching pimples in the right external concha, urging to constant scratching. [*Hb.*, *Ng.*]

60. Growling and thundering in the right ear, while sitting, also at night, with rhythmic or pulse-like strokes (6th d.). [*Hb.*, *Ng.*]

Sore nose, within and on the borders of the nostrils.

Pain as of ulceration in the left nasal passage, with sensitiveness to external touch, returning often (aft. 3 d.). [*Hb.*, *Ng.*]

External swelling of the left side of the nose, with formation of bloody crusts in the nose (3d d.). [*Hb.*, *Ng.*]

Bleeding of the nose from the left nostril, after previous itching (3d d.). [*Ng.*, *Hb.*]

65. Color of the face very pale. [*Rl.*]

Twitching pain in the right upper side of the face in a small spot, ceasing when pressing upon it, but returning at once (15th d.). [*Ng.*]

Tearing in the bones of the face, especially in the zygoma and the lower jaw, also in the evening. [*Hb.*, *Ng.*]

Tearing stitches on the right side of the chin.

Burning heat in the face, ceasing in the open air (3d d.). [*Hb.*, *Ng.*]

70. Swelling of the cheek, with swelling of a gland under the right angle of the lower jaw, with throbbing, stinging pain.

Eruption in the face.

After itching and scratching, pimples in front on the forehead (6th d.). [*Hb.*, *Ng.*]

Painless vesicles on the left side of the face (11th d.). [*Hb.*, *Ng.*]

Herpes in the face, dry and tettery. [*Rl.*]

75. The lips are contracted and seem to be fatty.

Both the lips burn like fire; also at times, burning with stinging of the upper lip (2d and 22d d.). [*Hb.*, *Ng.*]

Excoriated spot on the right side of the lower lip, with burning pain, as if sore (2d d.). [*Hb.*, *Ng.*]

Chapped lips.

Dry lips, shrunk together, they chapped, and she had to moisten them continually with the tongue.

80. Itching pimples about the upper lip (2d d.). [*Ng.*, *Hb.*]

Blisters on the upper lip, which inflame and fester (aft. 22 d.). [*Hb.*, *Ng.*]

Swelling of the gums, on the left lower row, with stitches up into the temple on that side (aft. 11 d.). [*Hb.*, *Ng.*]

Tearing in the teeth. [*Rl.*]

Tearing toothache, mostly in the evening, sometimes ceasing in bed. [*Hb.*, *Ng.*]

85. Tearing in a decayed root of a tooth, ceasing on pressure with the finger (15th d.). [*Hb.*, *Ng.*]

Stinging pain in the upper front teeth (5th d.). [*Hb.*, *Ng.*]

On the tip of the tongue vesicles, paining, as if burned.

On the tip of the tongue, vesicles, which burn like fire (3d d.). [*Hb.*, *Ng.*]

Sore throat, a stinging in the throat while swallowing and at other times (aft. 20 d.). [*Hb.*, *Ng.*]

90. Stinging in the fauces when yawning, frequently (1st d.). [*Hb.*, *Ng.*]

Swelling of the throat, without and within, with pressive pain in swallowing, and drawing, lancinating pain in the glands of the lower jaw, which are highly swollen.

In the tonsils of the throat, which are not swollen, **a throbbing**, as of a pulsating artery, with restlessness and anxiety (aft. 12 d.). [*Rl.*]

Strong throbbing in the glands of the throat, without inflammation, and swelling of the same, with **want of air in the throat** and transient heat (aft. 24 d.). [*Rl.*]

Swelling of the cervical glands (aft. 12 d.). [*Rl.*]

95. Scrapy sore throat.

Roughness in the throat, which goes off after eating. [*Hb.*, *Ng.*]

Sensation of rawness in the fauces with stinging pain (aft. 13 d.). [*Hb.*, *Ng.*]

Sensation of dryness in the throat (15th d.). [*Hb.*, *Ng.*]

Mucus in the throat, mostly early in the morning; this he can neither hawk up nor swallow down (the first 8 to 11 d.). [*Hb.*, *Ng.*]

100. In the morning, much hawking of mucus.

Taste in the mouth pappy, early on getting up (3d d.). [*Hb.*, *Ng.*]

Disagreeable taste and collection of water in the mouth (1st d.). [*Hb.*, *Ng.*]

Bitter in the mouth, the whole day (aft. 7, 8 d.). [*Hb.*, *Ng.*]

In the morning, bitter taste in the mouth, with bitter eructation, passing away after partaking of food (1st d.). [*Hb.*, *Ng.*]

105. Sourish taste in the mouth.

Early on awaking, sour taste in the mouth (14th d.). [*Hb.*, *Ng.*]

Eructation of air (soon aft. taking medicine). [*Hb.*, *Ng.*]

Pressive eructation, with taste of food partaken (aft. 22 d.). [*Hb.*, *Ng.*]

Bitter eructation, at times with the taste of food eaten, or with hiccup (5th, 11th d.). [*Hb.*, *Ng.*]

110. Belching up the ingesta [*Hb.*, *Ng.*]

In the afternoon, belching up bitter, sour water, the taste of which remained in her mouth until she again ate something (17th d.). [*Hb.*, *Ng.*]

Hiccup, very frequent, at times with stitches in the left side of the chest. [*Hb.*, *Ng.*]

Nausea (1st d.). [*Rl.*]

Nausea with inclination to vomit when taking a walk, or immediately after dinner, when it passes off through eructations and in the air. [*Hb.*, *Ng.*]

115. Nausea with pressure in the stomach, and yet inclination to eat.

Appetite almost quite lost (aft. 24 d.). [*Rl.*]

No hunger and no appetite; yet he takes his usual meals, especially his dinner, and his food has its natural taste (aft. 4 d.). [*Hb.*, *Ng.*]

In the evening, lack of appetite; she does not want to eat and yawns often (16th d.). [*Hb.*, *Ng.*]

Much thirst, especially in the evening (the first 8 d., 15th, 19th d.). [*Hb.*, *Ng.*]

120. Thirst several days and nights, when she drank very much water (aft. 24 d.). [*Hb.*, *Ng.*]

Absence of thirst, contrary to his habit (1st d.). [*Hb.*, *Ng.*]

After every meal, noon and evening, he has nausea, and the water from the stomach runs out of his mouth (water-brash), with shuddering all over (aft. 26 d.).

After meals, throbbing in the chest and fauces, with heat of the face and uneasiness.

Diarrhœa after everything partaken of, with pains in the belly, back, the small of the back and the limbs.

125. Feeling as of emptiness in the stomach, or of hunger (soon). [*Hb.*, *Ng.*]

Feeling in the stomach of fasting, yet it feels full; aggravated after breakfast (16th d.). [*Hb.*, *Ng.*]

Feeling of fullness in the stomach, with tightness, without shortness of breath, the whole afternoon, and not alleviated either by rest, or motion, or eructations. [*Hb.*, *Ng.*]

Drawing in the stomach, frequently. [*Hb.*, *Ng.*]

Sensation in the stomach, as if everything were turning over, with tendency to water-brash and great qualmishness, as if about to vomit, relieved by eructation, while walking in the open air. [*Hb.*, *Ng*]

130. Burrowing and writhing in the stomach in the morning, ceasing after breakfast (2d d.). [*Ng.*, *Hb.*]

Gnawing, or burrowing, **in the stomach**, as if there were worms in it. [*Hb.*, *Ng*]

Burning from the stomach, toward the fauces, like heartburn. [*Hb.*, *Ng.*]

Burning and pressure in the stomach, changing afterwards into stitches. [*Hb.*, *Ng.*]

Burning and stitches in the scrobiculus cordis, drawing thence into the right axilla and the upper arm. [*Hb.*, *Ng.*]

135. In both the hypochondria, intermittent pinching, both in rest and in motion (2d d.). [*Hb.*, *Ng.*]

In the region of the right ribs, stitching and burning, in the afternoon, while walking (9th d.). [*Ng.*, *Hb.*]

In the region of the left lower ribs, from time to time, stitches while spinning. [*Hb.*, *Ng.*]

Stitches in the spleen while sitting,

Colic. [*Rl.*]

140. Pressure in the abdomen.

Pressure, as if exerted by the hand, on the left side of the belly (19th d.). [*Hb.*, *Ng.*]

Heaviness in the hypogastrium, as from a load, with anxiety, as if the hypogastrium were about to burst open; passing away in sleep.

Distension of the abdomen, relieved by passing flatus, in the evening, before the menses (15th d.). [*Hb., Ng.*]

Tension and inflation of the abdomen, up to the stomach, passing away after two liquid stools; in the evening (1st d.). [*Hb., Ng.*]

145. Stitches in the left side of the hypogastrium, above the hip, while sitting and while bending forward in standing.

Cutting and lancinating pains about the navel (15th d.). [*Hb., Ng.*]

In the evening, at 7 o'clock, cutting in the whole abdomen, extending to the groin and into the small of the back, ceasing after an ordinary stool (19th d.). [*Hb., Ng.*]

Pinching in the belly, around the navel, with subsequent diarrhœa; or while standing, aggravated by stooping. [*Hb., Ng.*]

Severe pinching of the belly, quickly followed by a diarrhœic stool (at once).

150. Pinching, and pinching-grasping pain in the hypogastrium, with dyspnœa.

At every breath, pinching in the belly, passing off with the expiration (15th d.). [*Hb., Ng.*]

Early, after rising, pinching, passing around in the abdomen and the groin, as before the menses (18th d.). [*Hb., Ng.*]

Drawing, in the side of the abdomen.

Burrowing, digging, in a small spot near the navel (4th d.). [*Hb., Ng.*]

155. Burning pain in the epigastrium, in a small spot, also in the right flank, while sitting. [*Hb., Ng.*]

In the right groin, an indescribable pain, which extends often up into the hip and the small of the back (15th d.). [*Hb., Ng.*]

Sensation of distension in the groin, with painfulness in the left groin while sitting, and tension and digging in the right groin. [*Hb., Ng.*]

Pressive tension, and, as it were, pressing out in the left side of the hypogastrium, beside the abdominal ring.

Tearing, tensive pain in the region of the groin, while walking.

160. Cutting and lancinating pain in the inguinal regions, up to the small of the back, with urging to urinate, in the evening, every half hour. [*Hb., Ng.*]

Stitches in the right groin and out behind the hip, in sitting (4th d.). [*Hb., Ng.*]

Pain as of a sprain in the left inguinal region, compelling him to walk crooked (3d d.). [*Hb., Ng.*]

Pain as from ulceration in the right inguinal region, only perceptible in walking [*Hb., Ng.*]

Externally on the right side of the abdomen, a great furuncle.

165. Winding, grumbling and rumbling in the belly, sometimes with pinching, at times with the passage of much flatus. [*Hb., Ng.*]

Early, on awaking, in bed, grumbling and fermentation in the sides of the belly, up into the chest.

Frequent passage of loud sounding or fetid flatus. [*Hb.*, *Ng.*]

The stool is intermitted often for several days (on the 2d, 3d, 4th, 13th, 16th, 17th, 22d, 23d d.) with various provers. [*Hb.*, *Ng.*]

No stool for two days, with constant colic and sensation as if diarrhœa were coming on (22d, 23d d.). [*Hb.*, *Ng.*]

170. Frequent, normal stool, at times followed by burning. [*Hb.*, *Ng.*]

Solid stool, during the whole time of proving. [*Hb.*, *Ng.*]

Hard (lumpy, scanty) stool, passing with much urging, followed every time by a soft stool later on. [*Hb.*, *Ng.*]

Stool, the first part of which is hard, the later soft (9th, 14th d.). [*Hb.*, *Ng.*]

Several soft stools during the day, at times with severe urging and pain in the hypogastrium, after every new dose, and often at other times. [*Hb.*, *Ng.*]

175. Soft, yellow stool with hurried urging thereto and followed by tenesmus and burning in the anus (5th d.). [*Hb.*, *Ng.*]

Diarrhœa, with subsequent pains in the abdomen (as if sore and bruised) (5th, 8th d.). [*Hb.*, *Ng.*]

Half liquid (mucous) stools, with pains around the navel (1st, 2d d.). [*Hb.*, *Ng.*]

Green (mucous) diarrhœa in the morning (3d, 4th d.). [*Hb.*, *Ng.*]

Before the customary stool, pain around the navel (ever after 12 d.). [*Hb.*, *Ng.*]

180. With the customary stool, stitches in the anus. [*Hb.*, *Ng.*]

During and after a soft stool, much burning in the anus. [*Hb.*, *Ng.*]

In the anus, itching pain as of soreness, and beside it several pustules.

In the perinæum, tearing pain while walking.

In the evening, lancinating, tearing pain in the perinæum.

185. In the bladder, down into the urethra, a lancinating, pinching pain, while lying down.

Constant urging to urinate, beginning at 4 A. M.

Urging to urinate, but only a few drops were emitted, until with the subsequent stool the urine flowed again normally. [*Hb.*, *Ng.*]

He can emit the urine only quite slowly.

Scanty passage of urine and less frequent than usually (the first days). [*Hb.*, *Ng.*]

190. Increased micturition, even while drinking but little (2d and 9th d.). [*Hb.*, *Ng.*]

In the morning, more frequent urging to urinate and more frequent micturition.

At night he had to get up frequently to urinate, and emits an unusual quantity of urine (1st, 17th d.). [*Hb.*, *Ng.*]

The urine (discharged) is hot, and increased in quantity (the first days). [*Hb.*, *Ng.*]

Reddish, clear urine, without clouds or sediment, during the menses. [*Hb.*, *Ng.*]

195. Deep-yellow urine, with a loose cloud on the bottom (6th d.). [*Hb.*, *Ng.*]

Clayey sediment in the urine after one hour (5th d.). [*Hb.*, *Ng.*]

In the left spermatic cord, stitches and throbbing (5th d.). [*Hb.*, *Ng.*]

Frequent erections (aft. 7 d.). [*Hb.*, *Ng.*]

In the genitals, early on awaking, sensation as after nocturnal coition.

200. **The catamenia** (two days) **too early, with pains in the abdomen and the small of the back,** continuing also at night, when the blood also flows more strongly (aft. 17 d.). [*Hb.*, *Ng.*]

During the menses, much blood passes with the stool.

Leucorrhœa, with distention of the abdomen, without accumulation of flatus.

Leucorrhœa, like the white of eggs, after previous pinching around the navel. [*Hb.*, *Ng.*]

Painless discharge of brown mucus from the vagina, after every micturition (6th and 7th d.). [*Hb.*, *Ng.*]

* * * * * * * *

205. Frequent sneezing, during the day (13th and 14th d.). [*Hb.*, *Ng.*]

Sensation in the upper part of the nose, as if a cold were coming on. [*Hb.*, *Ng.*]

Continual itching in the nose, with urging to blow the nose, and a sensation as if a rough large body were sticking in the upper part of the nose, with stoppage of the same (2d d.). [*Hb.*, *Ng.*]

Coryza, with eruption in the nostrils (sore nose).

Coryza, with stoppage of the nose and loss of the sense of smell (13th and 14th d.). [*Hb.*, *Ng.*]

210. Stoppage of the nose, with pain in the right nasal cavity, at night, passing off next morning. [*Hb.*, *Ng.*]

Dry coryza, while clear water runs from the nose.

Coryza, with feeling of stoppage in the nose, while much mucus passes off, but with effort (aft. 24 d.). [*Hb.*, *Ng.*]

Coryza, only in one nostril, from which much thick, yellow matter is discharged; with tearing in the cheek-bones and the teeth of the left side.

Clear, acrid water runs from the nose, corroding the lips (1st d.). [*Hb.*, *Ng.*]

215. Hoarseness, with burning in the region of the larynx, the whole afternoon (aft. 3 d.). [*Hb.*, *Ng.*]

The chest is oppressed, as with dry catarrh.

Frequent expectoration, with ejection of little clots of mucus, with a sensation of rawness and soreness above, behind the uvula. [*Hb.*, *Ng.*]

Violent cough in the evening in bed, causing water to belch up in her mouth (3d and 4th d.). [*Hb.*, *Ng.*].

Cough, while taking a deep breath, especially while lying on the right side.

220. **Dry cough** (from tickling in the throat), in the evening and night, and also in daytime. [*Hb.*, *Ng.*]

Dry cough in the morning, with stitches in the fore part of the chest and in the region of the left lower ribs, becoming loose in the afternoon. [*Hb.*, *Ng.*]

A (dry) cough, which he had before taking the medicine, passes (aft. 15 d.) suddenly away, without expectoration. [*Hb.*, *Ng.*]

At night, lying on the back, a fit of loose coughing, with stitches in the region of the left lower ribs, so that he could not finish coughing for pain; on turning on the side it was still worse; the following day again a fit of coughing, but without stitches (aft. 21 d.). [*Hb.*, *Ng.*]

Cough, with some expectoration in the morning (1st d.). [*Hb.*, *Ng.*]

225. Expectoration of blood, following itching in the throat, for six days.

Short breath (aft. 18 d.). [*Rl.*]

Asthma, when violently moving the arms and in stooping.

She feels so heavy on the chest, while walking in the open air, that she could not get enough breath, and had frequently to stand still (2d d.). [*Hb.*, *Ng.*]

Tightness and pressure on the chest, with tendency to eructation, which came on in the open air and relieved the pressure; early on rising (aft. 19 d.). [*Hb.*, *Ng.*]

230. Pressure on the left breast, while exercising in the open air, also into the left side of the chest, when going from the warm room into the open air (3d and 19th d.). [*Hb.*, *Ng.*]

Pressure and stitches on the chest, as if a morsel swallowed down had lodged there. [*Hb.*, *Ng.*]

Stitches in the chest, here and there, at times when taking a breath or sitting bent over; at times also rythmically. [*Hb.*, *Ng.*]

Lancinating, formicating sensation of soreness in the left side of the chest, while sitting.

Beating like pulsation, on a small spot in the left thoracic cavity, only while standing, in the morning (4th d.). [*Hb.*, *Ng.*]

235. Painful tension under the right breast, with frequent intermissions, in all positions (after dinner) (15th and 16th d.). [*Hb.*, *Ng.*]

Tension or screwing together, in the lower part of the chest, without reference to respiration, while standing (1st d.). [*Hb.*, *Ng.*]

Pain as from a bruise under the right breast, of itself and also when touched, frequently intermittent, and often checking the breath (12th to 16th d.). [*Hb.*, *Ng.*]

Burning on a small spot of the chest (while walking in the open air) (soon and aft. 13 d.). [*Hb.*, *Ng.*]

Tearing in the region of the heart, passing thence into the fore-arm (15th d.). [*Hb.*, *Ng.*]

240. In the left clavicle, tearing in a small spot, with pain as from a bruise on pressing upon it (2d d.). [*Hb.*, *Ng.*]

Several spots on the left chest, sensation as of flea-bites, which immediately pass away on scratching, in the evening (11th d.). [*Hb.*, *Ng.*]

Red spots on the left side of the chest, which itched with a burning sensation, and grow pale from the pressure of the finger (10th d.). [*Hb.*, *Ng.*]

Pain in the small of the back, with obstruction of flatus.

After yawning, a sensation in the small of the back, as if something elastic, like air, was pressing to get out there (6th d.). [*Hb.*, *Ng.*]

245. Pain in the small of the back in walking, so that she cannot walk straight. [*Hb.*, *Ng.*]

On rising from stooping, pain in the small of the back.

Painful stiffness in the small of the back, even while sitting, but most on rising up after stooping.

Nocturnal pains in the small of the back, which always wake her from sleep (aft. 16 d.). [*Hb.*, *Ng.*]

Pain in the small of the back, as if bruised or crushed, in rest and in motion, **also at night in bed,** so that she can neither lie on the back nor on the side. [*Hb.*, *Ng.*]

250. Bruised pain of the coccyx, while sitting still, especially in slumber.

In the back, pain as if crushed, so that she could not lie on it at night (aft. 3 d.). [*Hb.*, *Ng.*]

Pain as if bruised and sprained between the shoulder-blades, or as if the muscles of the back were stretched apart.

Tension in the back, and as if compressed in a vise, in sitting; passing off through motion (15th d.). [*Hb.*, *Ng.*]

Drawing pressure from without inwards in the middle lumbar vertebræ, compelling her to stretch the hypogastrium forward.

255. Stitches in the left shoulder-blade, especially on lowering the shoulder and on turning the body to the left.

Stitches in the left shoulder-blade (while at rest) (4th and 9th d.). [*Hb.*, *Ng.*]

Pinching in the flesh of the right shoulder-blade (15th d.). [*Hb.*, *Ng.*]

Icy cold in the back and between the shoulders, in the spot where the former pain had been; only internally, and not to be warmed either by feathers or wool; after half a day the cold turned into itching (aft. 12 d.). [*Rl.*]

Itching in the neck, in the evening, while undressing, passing off on lying down (18th d.). [*Hb.*, *Ng.*]

260. Small, inflamed, very sensitive knot on the right shoulder-blade, not passing over into suppuration (3d d.). [*Hb.*, *Ng.*]

Furuncle on the left shoulder, with tensive pain (aft. 3 d.). [*Hb.*, *Ng.*]

Drawing in the neck, as if in the tendons (3d d.). [*Hb.*, *Ng.*]

Tension and stiffness in the neck, so that she could not move, in the evening; passing off after lying down (18th d.). [*Hb.*, *Ng.*]

Stiff neck, with pain, on turning around, extending from the neck to between the shoulders; for six days (aft. 6 d.). [*Rl.*]

265. **Tearing**, alternately in the right side and the left, then again **in both sides of the neck**, alternating with tearing in the cheeks (1st, 4th and 17th d.). [*Hb.*, *Ng.*]

Tearing stitches in the neck and in the left clavicle, on moving the head.

Tearing in the left clavicle, in a small spot, with pain as from a bruise on pressing upon it (2d d.). [*Hb.*, *Ng.*]

In the axilla a swollen gland, like a hard, red abscess, which, however, always disperses again, like a large pimple (18th d.). [*Rl.*]

Blisters as large as peas, on the right shoulder, tensive and burning, and forming a scab after three days (aft. 2 d.). [*Hb.*, *Ng.*]

270. In the shoulder-joints, first in the right, then in the left, rheumatic pain on motion.

Drawing in the right shoulder-joint, as after a cold, while resting. [*Hb.*, *Ng.*]

Beating on the right shoulder, and in the left axilla, in the morning and frequently during the day (12th and 19th d.). [*Hb.*, *Ng.*]

Burning and pressing in the right shoulder (2d d.). [*Hb.*, *Ng.*]

The right arm feels to her very heavy and as if rigid, especially in the upper arm, as if paralyzed, in the evening while spinning and in the morning (16th, 17th and 18th d.). [*Hb.*, *Ng.*]

275. Tearing in the left arm (and foot) (1st d.). [*Rl.*]

Tearing in the left arm as if in the tendons, extending down into the fingers, passing off on violent motion (9th d.). [*Hb.*, *Ng.*]

In the left upper arm, compressive pain, on leaning it on something, passing away in motion (22d d.). [*Hb.*, *Ng.*]

Tearing in the upper arm, as if in the marrow of the bone, extending down into the wrist (13th d.). [*Hb.*, *Ng.*]

Tearing in the upper arm, with sensitiveness of the arm to pressure (19th d.). [*Hb.*, *Ng.*]

280. In the lower arm, from the right elbow to the little finger, drawing, which is increased to tearing and passes away by motion (2d d.). [*Hb.*, *Ng.*]

Pressure in the left fore-arm, while lying in bed, passing off by motion, but is renewed on resting the arm on the table while writing (11th and 12th d.). [*Hb.*, *Ng.*]

Itching burning in the left fore-arm under the bend of the elbow (13th d.). [*Hb.*, *Ng.*]

Itching on the inside of the fore-arm, in the morning, and eruptive pimples in the bend of the elbow.

After scratching the inner itching side of the left fore-arm, little pimples appear, which soon disappear again (14 and 15th d.). [*Hb.*, *Ng.*]

285. Eruption of pimples on the right fore-arm, which impels by its violent itching, to continual scratching. [*Hb.*, *Ng.*]

Heaviness and feeling of going to sleep, in the right fore-arm (3d d.). [*Hb.*, *Ng.*]

In the wrist of the left arm, tearing and twitching in the tendons of the inner side, as if it would tear them out, with swelling on the dorsum of the left hand (1st d. and aft. 25 d.). [*Hb.*, *Ng.*]

On the wrist-joint little vesicles, which first itch violently, and after scratching, burn (aft. 20 d.). [*Hb.*, *Ng.*]

Large blisters and knots which are seated (on a hard foundation) in the skin, first itch violently, and after scratching, burn, inflame and form a (reddish-brown) scab, which remains inflamed a long time (with swelling of the spot), around the right wrist (aft. 12 and 19 d.). [*Hb.*, *Ng.*]

290. A violent stitch through the hand, while walking in the open air (22d d.). [*Hb.*, *Ng.*]

Stitching and beating in the left hand, worse on motion. [*Hb.*, *Ng.*]

Beating in the right palm, passing off through motion (12th d.). [*Hb.*, *Ng.*]

Paralytic feeling in the right hand, and on the right middle finger; in sitting and knitting (15th d.). [*Hb.*, *Ng.*]

Pain, as from a sprain on the dorsum of both hands, on seizing something, not in any other motion; the pain is relieved on extending the hand, and passes away with a cracking sound on pressing the joint of the thumb. [*Hb.*, *Ng.*]

295. Itching pimples on the dorsum of both hands, in the evening and night, with peeling off of the skin on this spot, the following morning (aft. 20 d.). [*Hb.*, *Ng.*]

Peeling off of the skin between the thumb and index of both hands (aft. 14 d.). [*Hb.*, *Ng.*]

In the fingers (thumbs) and their joints (twitching), tearing, increased at times by pressure or rubbing, mostly in the evening. [*Hb.*, *Ng.*]

Violent tearing in the index, when she extended it, after holding something in her hand, with stiffness after clenching it, so that she could not extend it again (during the menses) (17th d.). [*Hb.*, *Ng.*]

Tearing in the middle joint of the thumb.

300. Pain, as of cramp, in the right middle finger, as if in the tendons, on bending the fingers (11th d.) [*Hb.*, *Ng.*]

Stitches in the finger-tips and in their joints, spreading at times, with throbbing into the whole hand, and passing away by motion of the same. [*Hb.*, *Ng.*]

Stitches and painful beating **under the nail** of the left thumb (5th, 8th d.). [*Hb.*, *Ng.*]

Frequent **tingling in the tips of the fingers** (and thumbs), as from going to sleep. [*Hb.*, *Ng.*]

Violent, long-continued itching in the tip of the index, not to be relieved by scratching, in the morning (12th d.). [*Hb.*, *Ng.*]

305. In the hip, on the left side, pain, as if the tendons were too short, so that she has to limp in walking; in sitting, there is then a gnawing pain in the bones. [*Hb.*, *Ng.*]

Tearing, from the left hip down into the leg, in sitting; in the beginning relieved by rising and returning on sitting down, but later on it is not even relieved by motion (16th d.). [*Hb.*, *Ng.*]

In the legs, lassitude and weakness the whole day (the first days). [*Hb.*, *Ng.*]

Trembling of the left leg, with sensitiveness to the touch (10th d.). [*Hb.*, *Ng.*]

In the thigh, in front, tearing pain in sitting.

310. Painful tearings on the external side of the right thigh, in the evening, in sitting (15th d.). [*Hb.*, *Ng.*]

In the knee-joints, extremely painful stitches, in the evening, in sitting (3d d.). [*Hb.*, *Ng.*]

Stitching and tearing in the left knee, only in walking (11th d.). [*Hb.*, *Ng.*]

With a child, where after removing a swelling of the knee **stiffness of the knee-joints** (and curvature backward) had remained, the **mobility** was very soon restored. [*Rl.*]

The tendons in both houghs pain while walking (at times with twitching), as if too short, not while resting. [*Hb.*, *Ng.*]

315. Early, on arising from bed, the legs were contracted in the hough, as if they were dried up or too short, so that she could not get down the stairs; it passed off after longer and stronger motion (15th d.). [*Hb.*, *Ng.*]

In the legs, a drawing tension, in sitting and lying down, compelling a stooping walk, when it passes off.

Tension and drawing in the tendons of the legs, so that he can not walk well, with weariness in the legs. [*Hb.*, *Ng.*]

Spasmodic contraction about the lower part of the left leg (5th d.). [*Hb.*, *Ng.*]

Insensibility of the left leg (it is as if dead), in sitting (12th d.). [*Hb.*, *Ng.*]

320. Stinging on the inner side of the left leg, as also in the calf, in sitting (13th, 14th d.). [*Hb.*, *Ng.*]

After a four hours' walk, while resting, a stinging pain in the left calf (3d d.). [*Hb.*, *Ng.*]

The bones of the heel feel sore when treading and walking, as if stiff and bruised.

Violent tearing (and stitching), **with pain, as of a suppuration**, in the heels, at times passing of by rubbing; also at night, in bed, not alleviated by any position (4th, 17th, 19th d.). [*Hb.*, *Ng.*]

Spasmodic contraction, with pain in the right heel, in the evening in bed, also with tearing on the inside of the ankles. while sitting (14th, 15th d.). [*Hb.*, *Ng.*]

325. In the right foot, as also on the external ankle of the left foot, beating and pain, as in suppuration, in walking (9th, 11th d.). [*Hb.*, *Ng.*]

Tearing on the external border of the foot, in standing, and passing away on motion (7th d.). [*Hb.*, *Ng.*]

Feeling in the feet as if asleep, also at night (19th, 20th d.). [*Hb.*, *Ng.*]

Cold feet in the evening in bed, she can not get them warm for a long time (14th d.). [*Hb.*, *Ng.*]

In a paralyzed (already much improved) foot, pains appear. [*Rl.*]

330. Itching in the sole of the right foot, in the evening (2d d.). [*Hb.*, *Ng.*]

In the toes, especially the big toes (twitching) **tearing,** while sitting and standing. [*Hb.*, *Ng.*]

Stitches in the left small toe, in standing and walking; as also in the big toe, where it slowly decreases and increases. [*Hb.*, *Ng.*]

Pinching itching in front on the right big toe (7th d.). (*Hb.*, *Ng.*]

On the skin of the whole body, now here now there, itching (and smarting), so that she cannot scratch enough, in the evening, most before lying down, and sometimes passing away after lying down. [*Hb.*, *Ng.*]

335. In the evening, before going to bed, violent itching over the whole body, especially on the chest and the fore-arms, with little pimples on scratching (2d, 10th, 14th and 15th d.). [*Hb.*, *Ng.*]

At night and in the morning, violent itching about the hips, on the thighs, legs, and about the houghs, with miliary pimples.

Fine miliary eruption over the whole body, for two weeks (aft 16 d.).

Vesicular pimples in front on the chest and on the left leg, which first itch, then burn. [*Hb.*. *Ng.*]

All bones of the body are painful, as if bruised, while sitting still, in slumber.

340. In the whole body, especially in the back, feeling of pain as from a bruise, with tearing in both the shoulders and in the neck, early, after rising, and worse on motion (aft. 25 d.). [*Hb.*, *Ng.*]

Early on awaking, the body feels drawn together, so that she can hardly walk, but it passed away through continued walking (19th d.). [*Hb.*, *Ng.*]

Tearing, as if in the bones, on the left upper arm, and then in the right thigh, down from the hip, in sitting (10th d.). [*Hb.*, *Ng.*]

Tearing (and painful twitching) now here now there in the limbs, most of all in the (temples), arms, houghs, thighs, calves, fingers and toes, in the evening in sitting, and better after lying down; between the index and the middle finger the pain at times raged and beat as if an ulcer were about to form. [*Hb.*, *Ng.*]

In the evening, twitching tearing in the tips of the fingers and toes, then in the right upper arm, now here, now there, with anxiety; passing off on lying down (16th d.). [*Hb.*, *Ng.*]

345. Twitches (stitches) and burning **formication in the tips of the fingers and toes,** as from going to sleep, in the evening, afternoon and also at night. [*Hb.*, *Ng.*]

Stitches in the tips of the fingers and toes while walking in the open air, (22d d.). [*Hb.*, *Ng.*]

Pressive burning and stitches, now here, now there, in various places (3d d.). [*Hb.*, *Ng.*]

Stitches in the left side of the abdomen, then in the right side of the chest, then in the right shoulder-blade, and lastly in the small of the back, with chilliness and drowsiness during the day.

The limbs on the right side seem more affected than those of the left. [*Hb.*, *Ng.*]

350. She seems to feel better in the open air. [*Hb.*, *Ng.*]

His blood seems always in tumultuous activity.

Rushes of blood in the whole body, attended with anxiety, and during the whole time of proving, she feels more warm than cold. [*Hb.*, *Ng.*]

Toward evening, for one hour, a severe beating headache in the forehead, aggravated by touching the forehead; attended with weakness, so that he could hardly walk, and when he went to bed, a shaking chill.

Sudden lassitude and weakness after dinner, while moving about in the open air (19th d.). [*Hb.*, *Ng.*]

355. Very much fatigued. [*Rl.*]

Very tired in the morning. [*Rl.*]

Constant yawning without drowsiness, in the morning (7th d.). [*Hb.*, *Ng.*]

In the evening, early, great drowsiness, with closing of the eyes; passing off when the lights are lit. [*Hb.*, *Ng.*]

She cannot go to sleep before 3 A. M. (on which she sleeps in the morning and wakes up in a perspiration). [*Hb.*, *Ng.*]

360. She cannot go to sleep before midnight, on account of her cold feet.

Before midnight, she is kept awake a long time by heat in her head. [*Hb.*, *Ng.*]

In going to sleep, starting up with fright (5th d.). [*Hb.*, *Ng.*]

Uneasy sleep, after midnight, with frequent awaking and turning from one side to the other, with dreams.

She wakes up about 12 or 3 o'clock at night, and then can not go to sleep again (1st, 17th d.). [*Hb.*, *Ng.*]

365. Very restless nights. [*Rl.*]

Sleep full of dreams (aft. 3 d.). [*Hb.*, *Ng.*]

Frequently anxious, frightful dreams, at which she wakes up anxious and frightened. [*Hb.*, *Ng.*]

Dreams about falling in the water. [*Hb.*, *Ng.*]

Dreams she is sick, that she has a rash. [*Hb.*, *Ng.*]

370. **Lascivious dreams** about coition.

Voluptuous dreams (aft. 4, 5, 12 d.). [*Hb.*, *Ng.*]

At 2 o'clock at night, violent cutting throughout the abdomen, from which she wakes up (aft. 24 d.). [*Hb.*, *Ng.*]

Oft-repeated sneezing, without coryza, wakes her up at night, with formication in the throat. exciting cough and the secretion of saliva (aft. 6 d.). [*Rl.*]

Heaviness on the chest, at night, in bed, with half-unconscious awaking, in a sort of dream, as if somebody had hanged him, and pressed hard upon his chest (aft. 5 d.). [*Hb.*, *Ng.*]

375. **Excessive pains in the small of the back awake her at night** from sleep, with a paralytic pain in both hips and thighs, which parts even pain on the following morning, when touched (aft. 18 d.). [*Hb.*, *Ng.*]

At night, awaking from pains as from a sprain and a bruise in the right side of the back, extending to the middle ribs, and into the axillæ, on turning the body, stretching the arms, sneezing, yawning and breathing.

In the hip, after midnight, stitches in any position, relieved by pressure; with frequent passage of flatus, and a sensation as if the pain was caused by flatus (19th d.). [*Hb.*, *Ng.*]

At night, awaking from tearing in the right upper arm and in the legs, from the heels up into the bones (aft. 24 d.). [*Hb.*, *Ng.*]

Violent itching, at night, between the shoulders and on the left forearm, so that he felt like scratching the skin open (aft. 2 d.). [*Hb.*, *Ng.*]

380. Chilliness at night, she dare not uncover herself. [*Hb.*, *Ng.*]

Chill (and coldness), **mostly in the evening,** at times with thirst before or during the same, and a few times subsequently in the night, perspiration. [*Hb.*, *Ng.*]

In the evening, or after midnight, a chill, then (alternately) heat, then perspiration, all without thirst (3d, 13th d.). [*Hb.*, *Ng.*]

Frequent attacks of fever, chills followed by heat, with a thick, red face, and thirst during chill and heat; the intervals free of fever were of half an hour.

More heat (warmth) than cold, during the last part of the provings (aft. 17 d.). [*Hb.*, *Ng.*]

385. In the warm room and after rapid motion, heat all over, and redness of the face, but especially, externally, in front, over the whole chest; a stinging sensation of heat.

Heat, in the forenoon; thirst, early on rising. [*Hb.*, *Ng.*]

Dry heat in the head, frequently, on entering a room, with subsequent slight thirst, in the evening (19th d.). [*Hb.*, *Ng.*]

Heat in the whole body, as if perspiration was about to break out (aft. 14 d.). [*Hb.*, *Ng.*]

Frequent transient heat, with subsequent perspiration (13th d.). [*Hb.*, *Ng.*]

390. Great heat, at night, in bed; then in the morning, perspiration (18th d.). [*Hb.*, *Ng.*]

Heat in the palms, soles of the feet, and in the face; in the evening, immediately on lying down (with thirst); afterward perspiration (2d, 3d, 4th d.). [*Hb.*, *Ng.*]

Early, on arising, a feeling of heat, and some perspiration in the hands and smelling foot-sweat.

Heat in the whole body, with redness of the face and perspiration, on moving about in the open air (aft. 24 d.). [*Hb.*, *Ng.*]

Heat and perspiration, in the afternoon; then some thirst. [*Hb.*, *Ng.*]

395. Perspiration, about midnight (aft. 4 d.). [*Hb.*, *Ng.*]

Several nights, perspiration over the whole body.

Strong perspiration, early in bed (2d d.). [*Hb.*, *Ng.*]

ANACARDIUM.

(MALACCA-NUT.)

The lofty tree (*Avicennia tomentosa, semecarpus Anacardium*) which yields this fruit, grew in the time of the Arabs, on Mt. Ætna, in Sicily; now it is found in dry forests in East India. Between the outer, shining black, heart-shaped and hard shell and the sweet kernel within, which is covered with a thin, brownish-red skin, this fruit contains in a tissue of cells a thickish, blackish juice, with which the Hindoos indelibly mark their linen, and of such acridity, that even moles can be cauterized with it. It is only rarely that we get this fruit so fresh that this juice is still somewhat fluid, of the consistence of honey; usually it is quite dry. We take of this, for homœopathic use, one grain, and like other dry vegetable substances, it is brought by three hours' trituration with thrice one hundred grains of sugar of milk to the millionth powder-attenuation, and then through solution, dilution and shaking, its medicinal power is developed and potentized.

This fruit, as well as the tree which bears it, is to be carefully distinguished from another which bears a similar name, *Anacardium occidentale;* the fruit of this tree is of kidney-shape and was unknown to the Arabs, who first called attention to the medicinal powers of the heart-shaped fruit, which they called *Balador*.

During the last one thousand years this powerful and sanative remedy had fallen into total oblivion, as well as several other remedies which the more observant ancients had made good use of.

Serapio in his book, *De Simplicibus*, C. 346 (contained in *Practica Seraponis*, Venet. fol. 1550), quotes most of the writers among the Arabians who have written about the use of the juice of Anacardium. *Aben Mesuai* says: It is good when sensation and memory have been marred; *Alchalahamen:* its property is to encounter the relaxation of the nerves (paralysis); *Bedigoras:* it removes forgetfulness and sharpens sensation; *Abugerig:* it is good for paralytics and those who fear its coming. This last writer also advises carefulness in its use; it produces—*baras* (heaviness?) and leprosy and abscesses, and perhaps it kills—it is hurtful to youths and to the choleric.

If on choosing Anacardium, according to its peculiar symptoms, also one or another of the following states is found, this would only make more sure the correctness of its choice.

Hypochondriac, troubled mood; depression; unsociableness; anxiety; fear of approach of death; lack of moral sense (flagitiousness, impiety, inhumanity, hardheartedness); a condition as if he had two wills, of which the one annuls what the other impels him to do; sensation as if his spirit were unconnected with the body; feeling of the head as after a debauch; pressive headache from the temple toward the eye; headache in the occiput, from a misstep or loud noise; *weakness and dimness of the eyes;* nets and dark spots before the eyes; painful swelling of the external ear; itching in the ears; running of the ears; humming of the ears; rushing sound in the ears; *deafness;* bleeding of the nose; *fetid smell from the mouth,* without his being aware of it; waterbrash; fetid taste of the mouth; severe thirst; lack of appetite; morning sickness; weakness of the stomach; indigestion; pressure in the scrobiculus cordis, early on awaking; pressure on the liver; hardness of the abdomen; blood with the stool; varices of the anus, also painful ones; itching of the anus; humor from the rectum; burning of the glans during and after micturition; involuntary erections during the day; lack of enjoyment of coitus; leucorrhœa, with itching and soreness; sensation of dryness in the nose; stoppage of the nose; long-continued catarrh and flow of mucus from the nose; cough, with expectoration; rattling in the bronchia, while lying on the side; shooting and heaviness in the forearm; tensive pain and *weakness in the arm;* trembling of the right hand; burning in the soles of the feet; weight in the limbs, especially in the knees; tremulous weariness; want of irritability of the skin, so that it can not be excited by resins to itching and to become moist; sensitiveness to colds and draughts; *inclination to colds;* late in falling asleep; anxious dreams; chilliness; perspiration in sitting.

Camphor and ethereal spirits of nitre are but weak antidotes; but smelling of raw coffee is efficacious against the anger and violence caused by Anacardium.

Those physicians who, besides me, contributed their observations to the pure effects of Anacardium are: *Br.*, *Dr. Becher; Fz.*, *Dr. Franz; Gr.*, *Dr. Gross; Htn.*, *Dr. Hartmann; Hrm.*, *Dr. Herrmann; Lgh.*, *Dr. Langhammer; St.*, *Dr. Stapf.*

ANACARDIUM.

Sadness.

Anguish and apprehension as of imminent misfortune. [*Br.*]

Anxiety and apprehension in the evening, after cheerfulness during the day. [*Lgh.*]

A pathogenesis of Anacardium appeared in the third Vol. of the *Archiv* (1823), containing 484 symptoms obtained from the powdered bean and tincture by the seven provers mentioned above and by Hahnemann himself. His present symptom-list is made up of these and of 138 fresh symptoms obtained (in all probability) in his later manner.—*Hughes.*

Internal anguish, which did not allow him to rest, he troubled himself about every trifle, as if it would cause great injury, with solicitude about the future.

5. In walking and in standing, uneasiness, as if some one were coming behind him; everything around him seemed to him suspicious.

Timorous in all his actions; he views everything more anxiously and timidly, always thinks of being surrounded by enemies, then he becomes hot, his blood seems to boil in his chest (aft. 7, 8 d.).

Anxious apprehension and deep thoughts, on meditating over his present and his future fate. (*Lgh.*)

The future seems to him very dangerous, as if nothing were imminent but misfortune and danger; distrust in his own power, and despondency.

He is at odds with the whole world, and has so little confidence in himself that he despairs of being able to accomplish what is demanded of him.

10. In the forenoon, extremely hypochondriac, discouraged and despondent, with awkward, helpless manner; all movements are extremely clumsy and indolent (aft. 3 d.). [*Fz.*]

Anxious solicitude and moroseness. [*Gr.*]

Extremely morose and ill-humored. [*St.*]

The whole day in a peevish mood; all that surrounds him makes a disagreeable impression on him. [*Lgh.*]

Gloomy, annoyed mood, with an impulse to go into the open air. [*Br.*]

15. Very peevish and out of humor, with great sensitiveness to all offences.

He takes everything ill and becomes violent.

Passionate and contrary. [*Gr.*]

Extremely passionate at a slight offence, breaking out into violence.

Indisposed to everything.

20. Indisposition to work; he is afraid to undertake anything, he has no pleasure in anything. [*St.*]

In the afternoon he is in a better humor than in the forenoon; he is more cheerful and disposed to work, as soon as the drowsiness after dinner is passed (aft. 38 d.). [*Fz.*]

Very indifferent and unfeeling; neither agreeable nor disagreeable matters excite his sympathy; for eight days.

An excitement which is unnaturally cheerful.

He laughs, when he ought to be serious.

25. He is compelled to laugh, while engaged in very serious matters, by a titillation below the scrobiculus cordis; in laughable matters he can keep serious.

His thoughts leave him. [*St.*]

Great weakness of the memory; he could not find the words he wanted.

Great weakness of the memory; he cannot retain anything; everything immediately slips from him.

Difficult recollection; nothing remains in his memory; he has a lack of ideas, and loses his subject quickly and without perceiving it. [*Fz.*]

30. His memory is quite deficient early in the morning, especially as to single names. [*Fz.*]

In the afternoon, there is a diminution of imagination and of memory; he cannot recollect anything (aft. 5, 6 h.). [*Fz.*]

In the afternoon, his memory is better than in the forenoon, although it is slow in yielding what it ought to yield at onc; still the understanding of what he reads is very easy to him, even if he cannot quite retain it (aft. 3, 4 d.). [*Fz.*]

Increase, greater keenness of the memory; even the least circumstances of times long past come back to him, without cause; he would also be now able to easily learn by heart, if other pressing thoughts did not distract him, though he can grasp these with ease (aft. 1½ h.). [*Fz.*]

Anacardium enfeebles the understanding. [MATTHIOLUS in *Commentar. in Dioscorid.* M. M. L. V., *Cap.* V, p. 985.[1]]

35. Obtuseness of the senses, with anxiety; he hardly notices what passes around him.

His mind is very much oppressed, as if a cold in the head were coming on.

He can only think when a subject is suggested to him; he does not of himself think of anything; he cannot independently determine on anything.

Everything intellectual is hard for him, as in a dearth of ideas. [*St.*]

Obtuseness of the senses, with numb feeling of the head, and decrepitude. [*St.*]

40. In the morning, after a sound sleep, he cannot grasp the least thing; his head feels waste and empty. [*Fz.*]

Increased phantasy; something new continually occurs to him, which he must follow out.

In the evening, from 9 to 10 o'clock, his phantasy is at first unusually excited, and there are many projected ideas; he can not bridle his attention; but gradually his mental organ becomes quite blunted, so that he does not think any more of anything at all (aft. 16 h.). [*Fz.*]

The mind is much more lively than before; he enters eagerly into acute inquiries; but every exertion of this kind causes him tearing, pressive headache in the forehead, the temples, and in the occiput. [*Fz.*]

Any exertion of the mind causes him at once a sensation of prostration in the brain.

45. Delusion of fancy; he thought his name was called by the voice of his (far distant) mother and sister; at the same time an apprehension and anguish foreboding misfortune. [*Br.*]

Melancholy dejection and imagination, as if there was standing in the adjacent room a bier, on which a friend or he himself was lying.

[1] General statement of effects. (Book VI, Chap. V, p. 660 of edit. Venice, 1554.)—*Hughes.*

He mixes up the present with the future.

Numb feeling first of the left, then also of the right side of the head. [*Gr.*]

Painful, obtuse, benumbed feeling of the head, when he lies in an inconvenient position in bed. [*Br.*]

50. Dull, painful, muddled feeling of the forehead, down to the root of the nose. [*Gr.*]

Early, after rising, his head is so muddled and heavy that he can hardly carry it; he had to lie down again.

The head feels very heavy, the whole day.

Dizzy in the head, as after drinking liquor.

It whirls about in his head. [*Gr.*]

55. Vertigo on stooping, like turning around in a circle (aft. 13 h.). [*Lgh.*]

Vertigo; everything becomes black before the eyes. [*Gr.*]

After a walk, in the afternoon, violent vertigo.

While walking, vertigo, with a sensation as if all objects were too far distant.

Vertigo, as if all objects, or he himself, were staggering; he had to hold on to something (1st d.).

60. Vertigo, so that he almost fell down.

Stupefying, dizzying, pressive pain in the whole head, especially in the forehead; he was about to fall to the left side while sitting (aft. 2 to 2½ h.). [*Lgh.*]

Pressure in the head, from time to time.

Pressure in the occiput, on the right side (aft. 3 h.). [*Hrm.*]

Early, every time on awaking, pressure in the forehead, worse from walking, as if the brain were being shaken.

65. In the middle of the forehead a dull pressure, which is aggravated with slow, deeply penetrating progress, and gradually occupies the whole of the sinciput in the evening. [*Gr.*]

Severe pressure on the right side of the forehead, from within outward. [*Htn.*]

Violent **pressure in the region of the right temple.** [*Htn.*, *Hrm.*]

Dull pressure outward out of the right eminence of the forehead.

Dull **pressure, as from a peg,** on the left side of the crown. [*Gr.*]

70. Inward pressure on the left temple. [*Gr.*]

Obtuse pressure inward, here and there, in small spots of the head. [*Gr.*]

Inward pressure and squeezing in both temples, **with** constant **constriction** of the upper part of the head, passing away toward evening. [*Gr.*]

Squeezing together and dull pressure below the left frontal eminence. [*Gr.*]

Squeezing together of both temples at the same time. [*Gr.*]

75. **Constrictive headache** in the forehead, with very peevish humor, aggravated from hour to hour, with violent burrowing pain, relieved momentarily by strong pressure upon the forehead;

at last the pain occupies the whole head with a painful sensation, as if a bandage were drawn tightly from the neck toward both ears; he has to lie down, and the pains continue from 5 P. M. till next morning. [*Gr.*]

Violent pain, as from a vise, in the right side of the forehead, especially on the external border of the orbit. [*Gr.*]

Pressive, pinching headache in the sinciput, with single tearings toward the forehead (aft. 24 h.). [*Br.*]

Tearing pressure in the left temple. [*Hrm., Gr.*]

Tearing headache during arduous work (aft 4 d.). [*Fz.*]

80. Tearing pain in the brain, just over the right temple. [*Hrm.*]

Tearing, which begins quite low down on the right side of the occiput and goes up into the forehead (aft. 35 h.). [*Hrm.*]

Repeated tearing in the right side of the head, face and neck, and immediately afterward buzzing before the left ear. [*Gr.*]

Repeated tearing in the whole head, with a general shaking chill, ill-humor and restlessness, which does not allow her to remain in any one place; always returning about the third day. [*Gr.*]

Tearing headache in the occiput, in single, well-defined tearings, extending into one of the temples (aft. 1½ h.). [*Fz.*]

85. Jerking tearings and tearing pains in the occiput and the temples, especially on bending the head backward (aft. 2 h.). [*Fz.*]

Sudden, sharp, piercing and smarting tearings in the temple, extending into the brain (aft. 3 h.). [*Fz.*]

Sharp, pressive tearings in the left temple. [*Fz.*]

Tearing stitches in the forehead, over the right eye. [*Hrm.*]

Stitching jerking tearing in the left temple. [*Fz.*]

90. Sharp stitches through the left side of the head, deep into the brain. [*Gr.*]

Dull, tremulous stitches on the left side of the upper part of the head, as if it were merely incipient, but could not get to it. [*Gr.*]

Pressure in the right side of the head, interrupted by severe stitches (aft. ¾ h.). [*Htn.*]

Headache, with stitches in the left temple.

Several times on inspiring, a long-drawn stitch from the temple to the forehead (aft. 5½ h.). [*Htn.*]

95. Drawing pain on the left side of the head.

Drawing pain in the forehead, in the left side of the crown and in the occiput. [*Hrm.*]

Jerking in the left side of the head, down close before the ear, often repeated. [*Gr.*]

Single, violent jerks, extending from behind over the upper part of the head, on the left side and over the forehead so severe that he could cry out aloud, (aft. ½ h.). [*Gr.*]

Burrowing, violent headache, in the evening.

100. Painful burrowing in the right half of the sinciput, especially on the border of the orbit, moderated by strong external pressure (and during **eating**), with an unbearable pain, as if a heavy body

were squeezed in there; in the evening in bed, while lying with the painful part on the arm there is a relief, and it passes off entirely on going to sleep. [*Gr.*]

Throbbing headache.

Heat in the head.

The pains in the head are aggravated by motion. [*Fz.*]

External pressure in the forehead, over the arch of the left eyebrow (aft. 2 h.). [*Lgh.*]

105. Severe pressure in the corner, between the frontal and the nasal bone (aft. 3 h.). [*Hrm.*]

On the hairy scalp, violent itching.

Itching on the forehead.

Many tubercles, as large as lentils, on the hairy scalp, with soreness when touched and scratched. [*Lgh.*]

Painless pimples, with red areolæ, at the top of the left temple (aft. 9 h.). [*Lgh.*]

110. Pains in the eyes, without redness.

In the eyes, a sensation as if there was something between the eyeball and the upper lid, which causes friction. [*Hrm.*]

Something seems to cause friction between the eyeball and the lower lid. [*Gr.*]

Pressure on the eyeballs from before backward, or from above downward. [*Hrm.*]

Pressure below the left external canthus (aft. 2 h.]. [*Hrm.*]

115. Pressure, as of a stye, in the right inner canthus, and in the tarsal cartilages adjacent. [*Hrm.*]

Severe pressure on the eyes, especially on the left eye and in its external canthus, when looking long at an object (aft. ½ h.). [*Hrm.*]

Dull **pressure as from a peg** on the upper border of the right orbit, penetrating to the brain, with stupefaction of the whole side of the head. [*Gr.*]

Pain as if a peg were driven in under the upper border of the orbit, touching the eyeball. [*Gr.*]

Rheumatic, tearing pain in the left eye (more in the lids), extending into the temple. [*Fz.*]

120. In the morning when walking, tearing in the eyeballs and orbits (aft. 24 h.). [*Fz.*]

Twitching in the eyelids, so that it seemed to him that it must be visible. [*Gr.*]

Great sensitiveness of the eyes to the light.

The light in the evening seems to have a halo around it.

The flame of the light seems to him to be flickering, and the light seems to burn now more obscurely, then again more brightly; but on strongly straining his vision, he saw that it burned quietly.

125. Frequent flickering before the eyes.

Contraction of the pupils (aft. 14 h.). [*Lgh.*]

The pupil of the right eye became smaller for a short time (aft. 48 h.). [*Br.*]

Great dilatation of the pupils (aft. 13, 14, 19, h.) (alternate action). [*Lgh.*]

Short-sightedness; he cannot recognize anything distinctly in the distance, while he sees clearly what is held close to his face. [*Fz.*]

130. Very much diminished short-sightedness (aft. 48 h.) (curative action). [*Lgh.*]

Dimness of the eyes, as if they were full of water, which compels her to wink frequently, in the evening (aft. 16 h.). [*Htn.*]

Earache in the right meatus auditorius. [*Gr.*]

Spasmodic cramp-like pain in the external auditory meatus. [*Htn.*]

Spasmodic cramp-like contractive sensation of the left auricle (aft. ½ h.). [*Htn.*]

135. Spasmodic cramp-like contraction in the left meatus auditorius, with pressure against the tympanum. [*Fz.*]

Pressive pain upon the external ear.

Slow, dull thrusts from both sides of the ears and in their passages, as if two dull pegs, pressing inward, were about to meet in the middle. [*Gr.*]

Twitches in the left auditory meatus in short paroxysms and very painful, as if a nerve were stretched or like electric shocks. [*Gr.*]

Twitches in the external ear.

140. Drawing pain behind the left ear.

Painful drawing in the left interior auditory meatus (aft. ¾ h.). [*Hrm.*]

Tearing in the left ear, down the cheek.

Severe tearing on the upper border of the cartilage of the right ear. [*Gr.*]

Tearing stitching, dull pains in the tip of the tragus of the left ear. [*Gr.*]

145. Extremely severe, lancinating tearing in the left external ear (aft. 24 h.). [*Gr.*]

Violent stitches in the left ear.

Pain as from suppuration in the ear, especially on swallowing.

On bringing the teeth together in biting, pain in the ear as from an ulcer.

In the cartilage of the ear and the internal ear, pressive tearing and beating, as if something were about to fester; on boring in with the finger, it is aggravated, and there arises a sensation as if something obstructed the auditory meatus (aft. 10 h.). [*Fz.*]

150. Itching in the ears and running out of a brownish matter.

Sensation behind the ears as if the parts were getting sore; he has to rub them. [*Gr.*]

Roaring before the ears.

Buzzing in the ears.

Ringing in the right ear. [*Gr.*]

155. Feeling of stoppage in the left ear as from cotton; nor could he hear as well with it as with the other (aft. ½ h.). [*Hrm.*]

Sometimes he heard so ill with it that he did not notice when anyone noisily opened the door; but often so acutely that he perceived people walking in the ante-room through double doors (aft. 54 h.). [*Br.*]

In the nose, a transient pain, as is wont to come from too great cold, so that his eyes watered.

Contractive pain in the anterior part of the nose, as from great cold, with lachrymation.

Bruised sensation in the left side of the nose, seemingly in the bone. [*Gr.*]

160. Pustules with red areolæ in the corner of the right nostril. [*Lgh.*]

Red pustule on the septum in the right nostril, with soreness to the touch. [*Hrm.*]

Bleeding from the nose after blowing it strongly.

Delusion in smelling, as if he smelled lighted sponge, early on arising.

Constant smell before the nose as of the dung of pigeons or chickens, especially when he smells of his clothes or his body (aft. 2 h.). [*Fz.*]

165. **The sense of smell seems to have almost totally vanished,** though the nose is not stopped (aft. 5 h.). [*Hrm.*]

In the face, in the middle of the cheeks, a dull pressure, as if the spot were seized with pincers. [*Gr.*]

Numb pressure on the left cheek-bone. [*Gr.*]

Drawing pain on the right cheek-bone. [*Hrm.*]

Worn out, hollow-eyed appearance, with blue borders around the eyes, for several days (soon after taking the medicine). [*St.*]

170. **Paleness of the face,** without coldness (at once). [*Br.*]

Great paleness of the face, soon after taking the medicine. [*St.*]

Pale, sick, wretched complexion, without otherwise feeling ill.

Dry heat in the face and in the whole head, with benumbed feeling of the head and pale countenance; he is hot to the touch, but does not feel so. [*St.*]

White, scaly tetter on the right cheek, near the upper lip (aft. 4 h.). [*Lgh.*]

175. Itching on the forehead.

Hard, red pustules on the forehead and in the corner of the left nostril, with sore pain for several weeks. [*St.*]

About the mouth, rough, scaly, tettery skin with tingling itching. [*Gr.*]

On the lips and the corners of the mouth, dryness.

Burning dryness of the outer borders of the lips, almost as from pepper. [*St.*]

180. On the chin, externally, burning, and on its left side from below a dull pressure. [*Gr.*]

Burning between the lower lip and chin, as after scraping with a dull razor. [*Gr.*]

Suppuration and painfulness of a spot under the chin, where two years ago there was a furuncle. [*Gr.*]

In the lower jaw, frequent drawing pain, especially in the evening.

Tearing in the right ramus of the lower jaw, frequently repeated. [*Gr.*]

185. Single tearings in the articulation of the jaw (aft 42 h.) [*Fz.*]

Gum-boil.

Bleeding of the gums on slight rubbing.

Toothache in one of lower dentes cuspidati, as if he had been picking it, aggravated by touching with the tongue and in the open air (2d d.). [*Br.*]

Toothache when he takes something warm into the mouth, some jerks, but on the whole more pressive than drawing.

190. Drawing pain in the gums and the roots of the left lower molars. [*Hrm.*]

Spasmodic drawing in the right lower row of teeth, extending up into the ear (soon after taking the medicine). [*Gr.*]

Tensive drawing pain in a hollow molar, reaching up into the ear, for several days, 10 P. M. [*St.*]

Tearing in all the teeth, returning in paroxysms. [*Gr.*]

In the mouth, painful vesicles.

195. The tongue is white and rough, like a grater (aft. 3 h.). [*Lgh.*]

Heaviness of the tongue, and feeling as if swollen, so that he cannot continue talking.

In talking, some words are difficult for him to utter, just as if his tongue was too heavy.

His speech is more strong and assured in the afternoon than in the forenoon.

His throat seems raw and sore.

200. **Scraping** sensation in **the throat.** [*Gr.*, *St.*]

Pressure in the pit of the neck. [*Gr.*]

Dryness in the throat, disappearing through eating, in the forenoon. [*Fz.*]

Mucus firm and viscid in the fauces, and before the posterior nares (aft. 1 h.). [*Fz.*]

Bitter dryness in the mouth and throat.

205. Bitter taste in the mouth after smoking tobacco.

Smoking tobacco causes only smarting; he does not enjoy it.

Everything tastes like herring pickle.

Insipid, rotten taste of food, this taste is also in the mouth itself.

Flat taste of beer.

210. Loathing for food, which he else relished, so that he felt like vomiting.

He partakes of dinner, simply because it is meal-time, without being hungry, but he relishes it; though the bread tastes somewhat bitter. [*Fz.*]

Constant thirst; yet swallowing, when he drinks, takes his breath, and he has therefore to pause continually.

At times, violent hunger, at times, no appetite at all for his meals.

Good appetite, and, after meals, pressure and nausea in the stomach, even without exercise.

215. During dinner almost all his ailments vanish; two hours later they begin again. [*Gr.*]

After dinner, heat in the face, with collection of sweetish saliva in his mouth, and violent thirst. [*Fz.*]

After meals, heat in the face and a worn-out feeling. [*St.*]

Every time after meals, shuddering in the scrobiculus cordis, with every step.

After meals, pressure and tension in the scrobiculus cordis, every time.

220. During meals, intermittent, dull pressure over and beside the scrobiculus cordis. [*Gr.*]

After meals, pressure about the stomach.

After meals, pressure in the stomach, with sensation of extreme lassitude and prostration, with great thirst (aft. 3½ d.). [*Fz.*]

After a light breakfast, pressure in the region of the stomach, toward the abdomen, as if he had eaten too much.

Immediately after dinner, distension of the abdomen, as if he had eaten too much. [*Gr.*]

225. After meals, winding about of flatus in the stomach, as if from a laxative.

After a meal, urging to stool, more in the upper bowels.

After a meal, hypochondriac depression; there is a pressure in the abdomen, and he feels extremely weak in body and in spirit (aft. 6 h.). [*Fz.*, *St.*]

After dinner, while standing, quite weak in the knees, at the same time drowsy and indisposed to any exertion. [*Fz.*]

After a meal, drowsy and indisposed to work.

230. After dinner, irresistible inclination to sleep. [*Htn.*]

After a meal, tussiculation, which affects the throat as if it were raw (aft. 3½ d.). [*Fz.*]

After a meal, rawness in the throat, with a deep tone of voice. [*Fz.*]

After a meal, eructation, which burns in the throat.

Eructation, after drinks and liquid food.

235. Empty eructation, in the morning. [*Gr.*]

Eructation, with cramp-like pain in the stomach.

Hiccough. [*Fz.*]

Rising of moisture into the mouth, which chokes him, frequently repeated. [*Gr.*]

A quantity of fluid rises into his mouth and fauces, causing a feeling of nausea on the chest. [*Fz.*]

240. Heartburn, after soup, as if from sour air in the fauces, with a sensation of contraction.

Burning, rising from the stomach, up into the throat.

Nausea, in the morning, with sensation in the stomach of fasting.

In the evening, severe nausea.

Toward evening, severe nausea, constant collection of water in the mouth, and finally vomiting, with subsequent strong acidity in the mouth.

245. Nausea, with retching in the fauces, soon returning on drinking cold water, with vomiting of the same, attended with a pain, as if the fauces were pressed apart by a large ball.

Great qualmishness in the scrobiculus cordis, outside of meal-time, with distress, as from a sprain, but without any actual nausea, with a good taste in the mouth and good appetite.

At first, sensation in the scrobiculus cordis as of fasting, then pressure in the stomach the whole day, and (as it were obstructed) passage of flatus from above and below, with lack of appetite.

Pressure in the stomach, from reflection and exertion of the mind.

Slowly intermittent, painful, obtuse pressure in the scrobiculus cordis. [*Gr.*]

250. Pressive, drawing pain below the scrobiculus cordis, in walking (aft. 10½ h.). [*Fz.*]

While walking in the open air, a soft pressure, with drawing in the scrobiculus cordis, disappearing after a meal (aft. 12 h.). [*Fz.*]

Constrictive, violent stomachache, relieved by stooping, but much aggravated by lifting the arm and turning the body.

Stitches in the region of the scrobiculus cordis, on the left side, aggravated by respiration and walking, and beginning again on resuming the walk. [*Gr.*]

Sharp stitches in the region of thescrobiculus cordis, and as if from there through to the small of the back. [*Gr.*]

255. **On taking a breath, sharp stitches in the scrobiculus cordis.**

Both at inspiration and expiration compressive, painful stitches, as from a needle, in the scrobiculus cordis, not passing away in any position nor when touched (aft. 4 h.). [*Lgh.*]

Cutting, in the region of the scrobiculus cordis. [*Gr.*]

Gurgling and fermentation, in the scrobiculus cordis. [*Gr.*]

In the hypochondria, alternately on the right side, and on the left, stitches on inspiration. [*Gr.*]

260. Stitches in the left hypochondria.

Dull stitches in the region of the spleen, partly as if in the chest, partly as if in the abdominal cavity. [*Hrm.*]

In the region of the liver, pressure, an hour after eating.

About the navel, pain, **as if a dull peg were pressed** into the bowels. [*Gr.*]

Dull pressure, just below the navel, aggravated by pressure and by inspiration, soon after a meal. [*Gr.*]

265. Pressure in the region of the navel, as if something hard had formed there, with a sensation during respiration and speaking, and especially during coughing, as if the belly were about to burst open; it aches at the touch, like pressure and tension.

Hard pressure, on a little spot above and below the navel, and in the left side of the abdomen. [*Hrm.*]

Thrusts, as from a dull instrument, on the right side, near the navel (aft. 6 h.). [*Gr.*]

Stitches, very painful and dull, on the left side, near the navel. [*Gr.*]

Intermittent, dull stitches on the navel. [*Gr.*]

270. Dull stitches, in the abdominal cavity, near the navel. [*Hrm.*]

Dull, deeply pressing stitches, at the left spinous processes of the iliac bones. [*Gr.*]

Keen, sharp stitches, so that he starts, on the right side, above the navel. [*Gr.*]

Single, keen stitches in the abdomen.

It suddenly darts down, undulating into the abdomen, like lightning. [*Gr.*]

275. A rapid cut, on the right side, in the abdomen.

Cutting pinching in the abdomen, as from flatus, or from cold, with urging to stool (aft. 4 and 22 h.). [*Lgh.*]

Attacks of colic, more cutting than pinching, when flatus is checked in the abdomen.

Pinching and squeezing in the abdomen (aft. 12 h.). [*Fz.*]

Squeezing pain in the hypogastrium, seemingly in the bowels (aft. 7 h.). [*Hrm.*]

280. Pinching contraction in a small place, on the left side, above the navel, on inspiration (aft. ½ h.). [*Htn.*]

Pain, as if something was rolling together in the abdomen, with subsequent pressure (aft. 32 h.). [*Lgh.*]

The bowels pain, as if spasmodically shortened, when bending back, in the forenoon.

Externally on the right side of the abdomen, under the short ribs, rythmical, burning stitches as from needles. [*Gr.*]

In the muscles of the left side of the abdomen, immediately under the short ribs, transient, short stitches. [*Gr.*]

285. In the mons veneris, tearing.

Above the abdominal ring, intermittent, dull pressure outward. [*Gr.*]

Constant growling in the abdomen, especially in the region of the navel.

Constant growling and griping in the abdomen. [*Gr.*, *Hrm.*]

Urging to stool, frequently during the day, without being able to discharge anything, for many days.

290. Urging to stool, daily three times; he felt urging, and when he then sat down, the urging was gone; the rectum did not fulfil its functions; and he had to use great force in evacuating the fæces, though they were soft.

Urging to stool, without being able to do anything; he feels as if everything was stopped up in the rectum. [*Fz.*]

Constant urging to stool, and since the evacuation does not immediately take place, a painful twisting and turning in the bowels, transversely through the abdomen. [*Htn.*]

Daily two or three stools of the customary sort, but always discharged with difficulty.

He had to go to stool often, but only a little was discharged at a time; first soft, then hard fæces.

295. The stool was of quite a pale color (aft. 48 h.).

Diarrhœa of watery stool, often and yet with much straining.

During the stool, griping in the abdomen (aft. ½ h.). [*Hrm.*]

During stools, and more especially afterwards, a dull pressure increased by inspiration, in the muscles of the abdomen, just below the navel. [*Gr.*]

After stool, yawning and eructation.

300. In the anus frequent itching.

The varices about the anus become smaller, and do not pain any more, except that they are sore when starting to walk (curative effect).

In the urethra, itching.

Constant urging to micturition.

Frequent urging to micturition, and little discharge of urine (the first 4 h.). [*Lgh.*]

305. He has to get up at night to urinate, and he can urinate again at the usual time. [*Gr.*]

In the morning, while fasting, frequent discharge of urine, clear as water. [*Gr.*]

Frequent discharge of urine, clear as water, in small quantities. [*St.*]

The urine is turbid immediately on its discharge; it deposits a muddy sediment, and when shaken becomes of a clayey color. [*Hrm.*]

Along the penis, a pain, like a cut.

310. On the scrotum, constant voluptuous itching, exciting the sexual impulse (aft. 2 h.).

Sexual impulse, in the morning, on awaking, with erection of the penis. [*Htn.*]

Violent sexual impulse.

Unexcitableness of the sexual impulse (the first 10 d.).

Emission of prostatic juice at a hard stool.

315. In a normal stool, passage of prostatic juice.

Passage of prostatic juice, after urinating.

Seminal emission, at night, without lascivious dreams (aft. 27 h.). [*Lgh.*]

After coition, itching in the anus.

* * * * *

Sneezing. [*Gr*]

320. Stoppage posteriorly in the nose, as through much mucus. [*Fz.*]

Dry coryza.

Violent coryza, lasting four weeks.

Severe coryza, in the evening (aft. 48 h.). [*Fz.*]

Severe coryza, with catarrhal fever; she could not get warm, with heat in the head and icy coldness of the hands and feet, in the warm room; then dry heat, the tendons of the legs feel too short, cramp in the calves, and uneasiness about the heart (8th d.).

325. After frequent sneezing, a most violent, fluent coryza, with lachrymation.

Roughness in the throat.

Hoarseness after eating, with deep sound of the voice. [*Fz.*]

Tussiculation after a meal, affecting the throat as if it was raw (aft. 3 d.). [*Fz.*]

Severe croup after a meal, with vomiting of what has been eaten.

330. Cough, almost solely at night, and more severe than during the day:

For several nights, cough more severe than in daytime.

Nightly cough, with scraping in the throat.

Matutinal cough.

Suddenly at 4 A. M., and several times during the day, exhausting fits of coughing, for hours (aft. 14 d.).

335. In the evening in bed an exhausting cough, which drives the blood to the head.

Cough, with pain in the occiput.

Cough, with stitches in the forehead or side of head.

In coughing and in deep inspiration, pressive pain on the crown of the head.

Cough, with yawning after the fit.

340. Cough, with (generally ineffectual) incitation to sneezing.

Cough, beginning with formication in the bronchia and with choking.

Periodical fits of coughing, but only during daytime, taking away the breath; every three or four hours.

Shaking fits of cough, as from whooping-cough, excited every time he speaks.

Shaking cough, which does not allow him to sleep (at night).

345. Short cough, mostly in the afternoon, with ejection of a viscid, grayish yellow mass.

Short cough with ejection of pus.

He coughs up blood (4th d.).

Breath short; a choking sensation in the region of the sternum.

Asthma, especially after a meal and also in sitting.

350. Dyspnœa, asthma (aft. 10 h.).

Tightness of the chest, with weeping, by which it is relieved.

Tightness of the chest, with internal anguish and heat.

Oppression in the region of the sternum, without pain; he feels as if he could not remain in the room, but must go into the open air and be very active.

Uneasiness in the chest, as if in the heart, especially in the forenoon (4th d.).

355. Tightness on the chest in expiration, with pressure in front on the sternum (aft. 1½ h.). [*Fz.*]

Pressure on the chest like tightness, toward the axillæ, with difficult breathing (aft. 24 h.). [*Hrm.*]

Especially in sitting, pressure on the chest, with fullness, from which he feels that vomiting would relieve him (aft. 10 h.). [*Hrm.*]

Pressure above the right nipple, from without inwards. [*Hrm.*]

Quick pressure on the sternum, as if from a blow, when going to sleep in daytime.

360. Suddenly a rapid pressure on the right side of the chest, near the shoulder, which is felt at the same time in the back on the opposite side, without respect to breathing.

Dull pressure above, on the right border of the sternum. [*Gr.*]

Dull **pressure as from a large peg** in the right side of the chest. [*Gr.*]

Undulating drawing in the left side of the chest. [*Gr.*]

Sensation of soreness and rawness in the chest. aggravated by inspiration (at once). [*Gr.*]

365. Sensation of a sore spot in the chest, under the sternum.

Tearing with some pressure on the left side of the chest, reaching up toward the heart, as if it would crush the whole side, especially when sitting bent forward (aft. 10 h.). [*Fz.*]

Separate, severe stitches in the chest.

Severe stitches above, in the left breast, which keep her for some time from rising from her seat; then a sense of a pressing down load in that spot.

Dull stitches on the left side of the chest, a hand's breadth below the axilla. [*Gr.*]

370. Sharp, throbbing stitches in the chest, above the heart (aft. 80 h.). [*Gr.*]

In the region of the heart, a stitch at night, on inspiration.

Stitches about the heart, darting through and through, two at a time, following in quick succession. [*Fz.*]

In the muscles of the chest, a drawing pain.

Jerking sensation in the muscles of the chest, on moving the arm.

375. Externally, on the left false ribs, a constrictive stitch as from a needle (aft. 4 h.). [*Lgh.*]

Corrosively itching stitches as from needles in the last false rib. [*Hrm.*]

Itching on the chest.

Blunt stitches in the small of the back. [*Gr.*]

Pain from stiffness in the back on rising up from sitting, passing off by sitting bent.

380. On the right side near the spine, in the scapula, a pain as if from continued sitting bent double. [*Gr.*]

Spasmodic pressure under and beside the scapulæ, from without inwards (aft. ½ h.). [*Hrm.*]

Severe stitching pressure, close below the left scapula, unconnected with breathing (aft. 1½h.). [*Htn.*]

Keen stitches on the outer side of the left scapula. [*Gr.*]

Tearing stitches beside the right scapula, from within outward. [*Hrm.*]

385. **Dull stitches in the left scapula, returning slowly and causing a tearing pain to spread on all sides.** [*Gr.*]

Painful tearing between the scapulæ. [*Htn.*]

Formication in the scapulæ, as if from going to sleep or from ants. [*Gr.*]

Pain as from a bruise, frequently, in the right scapula and upper arm, so that she can scarcely raise her arm. [*Gr.*]

External fine and blunt thrusts, in brief paroxysms, on the right side of the external surface of the left scapula. [*Gr.*]

390. Cracking in the scapula, on lifting the arm.

In the vertebræ of the neck, a cracking, on stooping.

Stiffness of the nape of the neck.

Stiffness in the muscles of the neck, with tensive pain, especially on quickly moving the head after a period of rest; less during continued motion (aft. 52 h.). [*Br.*]

Two days in succession in the morning on awaking, painful stiffness of the neck on the right side, on which he had lain, at the least movement, and especially on turning the head to the painful side (aft. 4. 5 d.). [*Htn.*]

395. On awaking, stiffness and pressive tension in the nape of the neck, in the occiput, and between the scapulæ, both in rest and in motion.

On the left side of the nape of the neck, close to the occiput, a pinching, painful stiffness while at rest and not impeding the motion of the head nor aggravated thereby (aft. 2 h.). [*Htn.*]

Dull, intermittent **pressure, as from a heavy load,** on the right side of the nape of the neck and on the top of the left shoulder, as if it were in the bones. [*Gr.*]

Rheumatic drawing down over the neck. [*Fz.*]

In the neck, on both sides of the larynx, a hard pressure, which at times renders deglutition difficult (aft. 2 h.). [*Hrm.*]

400. Sudden, dull pressure, as from a load, on the left side of the neck. [*Gr.*]

Slowly intermitting pressure in the angle between the neck and the top of the shoulder, on the left side. [*Gr.*]

Stitches as from needles, externally, now here, now there, on the neck. [*Gr.*]

Intermittent throbbing stitches, as of needles, near the throat, and on the left side of the chest (aft. 3½ h.). [*Lgh.*]

Frequent itching on the neck. [*Fz.*]

405. In both the axillæ, a tickling itching, compelling to scratch (aft. ¼ h.). [*Gr.*]

Tickling stitches, as from needles, below the shoulders, ceasing on rubbing. [*Gr.*]

In the arms, on stretching and extending them, painful, cutting tension, from the joints down along the flexor muscles, and, when bending them back, in the joints, especially in the shoulder-joints, a cracking, with a pain as if the arms were dislocated. [*Gr.*]

Numbness of the left arm. [*Gr.*]

Sudden pressure in the right arm, as if in the muscles and the bones, with weariness therein. [*Hrm.*]

410. Tearing and drawing in the left arm.

In the right upper arm, from the shoulder to the elbow, a rheumatic drawing pain, with feeling of stiffness in the arm. [*Fz.*]

(Spasmodically) pressive pain in the muscles of the upper arm, while walking in the open air, and in the evening, on sitting. [*Lgh.*]

Dull pressure, like a threatening, on the left upper arm, almost as if in the marrow of the humerus, very keen and intermittent. [*Gr.*]

Painful jerking in the left upper arm, above the bend of the elbow. [*Gr.*]

415. Sensation as of **blows** from a heavy body, **very painful on the middle of the left upper arm** (at once). [*Gr.*]

Pimples with a red areola and pus in the tip, on the inferior portion of the upper arm, with painful itching, compelling to scratch, on moving the arms (aft. 12 h.). [*Lgh.*]

In the bend of the left elbow, pressure, which drags down the arm as if heavy, and impedes its action, on walking in the open air (aft. 13 h.). [*Fz.*]

In the forearm, now here, now there, *painful pressing* from without *inwards* (at once). [*Gr.*]

Pressive pain in the muscles of the right forearm in writing (aft. 13 h.). [*Lgh.*]

420. Pressive scratching on the bone of the forearm, at rest. [*Fz.*]

Spasmodic pressure on the left forearm, more violent when touched, and when moved it is aggravated into a tearing pressure. [*Hrm.*]

Pressive drawing on the whole upper surface of the left forearm (at once). [*Gr.*]

Cramp-like drawing in the right forearm, from the wrist toward the elbow. [*Gr.*]

Cramp-like jerking in the whole body of the forearm, beginning a hand's breadth above the left wrist (at once). [*Gr.*]

425. Cramp-like violent pain in the left forearm and on the dorsum of the hand, unaffected by motion, at night in bed. [*Gr.*]

In the wrist, jerking in the flexor tendons.

In the palm, a simple pain on moving it. [*Gr.*]

Cramp-like pain in the joints of the right hand, where the metacarpal bones join the phalanges (aft. ½ h.). [*Hrm.*]

Cramp-like pains in the joints of the left hand, where the index is joined to the metacarpal bones. [*Gr.*]

430. Cramp-like pains in the hand, in the region of the metacarpal bone of the little finger. [*Hrm.*]

Cramp-like, jerking, dull pain in the anterior extremities of the metacarpal bones, unaffected by motion. [*Gr.*]

Intermittent, bluntly lancinating, cramp-like pain on the external side of the left hand, where the little finger joins its metacarpal bone. [*Gr.*]

Spasmodic contraction in the left hand, so that she cannot straighten the fingers. [*Gr.*]

Pain as from a sprain in the metacarpal bone of the little finger of the right hand.

435. Painful grumbling between the metacarpal bone of the left index and middle fingers, just behind the knuckles. [*Gr.*]

Severe cutting in the metacarpal bones of the right index. [*Htn.*]

A pressive cramp-like pain in the muscles, across the dorsum of the left hand (aft. ½ h.). [*Lgh.*]

Pressive tearing in the dorsum of the hand (aft. 9 h.). [*Fz.*]

Pricks as of needles in the dorsum of the left hand. [*Gr.*]

440. A severe, long-continued, painfully tearing stitch in the ball of the right hand. [*Htn.*]

Keen, burning stitches on the external border of the left hand, where the little finger is joined to the metacarpal bone (aft. 36 h.). [*Gr.*]

Severe **feeling of parchedness of the hands.**

Dry, hot hands.

Itching stitches in the external knuckle of the right hand, which only passes off on scratching, continued until it is red. [*Gr.*]

445. After **nocturnal itching in the palm and between the fingers, relieved by severe rubbing,** but not removed, there appears a pimple on the side of the left index, which opens on the next day, and then passes off. [*Gr.*]

Warts all over the hands, even in the palms.

In the fingers of the left hand, **cramp-like twitching** following the rythm of the pulse, in the posterior joints. [*Gr.*]

Intermittent cramp-like pain in the posterior joints of the right thumb and index. [*Hrm.*]

Contractive lancinating pain in the muscles of the left thumb, passing off through motion and touch (aft. 2 h.). [*Lgh.*]

450. Tearing in the little finger, oft repeated. [*Gr.*]

Repeated tearing in the right thumb, going up into the elbow, as on the formation of a whitlow.

Numbness of the fingers.

Sensation of dryness in the fingers and hands.

Tickling itching on the little finger, in the evening on lying down, only relieved by strong pressing and rubbing, since it does not seem to be situated in the flesh of the muscles, but deeper within. [*Gr.*]

455. Pustules on the index, with a red areola, and stinging, voluptuous itching, spreading in the whole palm; after pressing and squeezing, to which the itching compels, there appears red and white lymph, and later a scurf, under which a clot of pus forms; in the evening, a drawing soreness in it, and the sore lasts eight days. [*Gr.*]

In the hip-joint of the right side, on moving while sitting, a loud cracking. [*Gr.*]

Pain as of a sprain or a bruise over the right hip, on rising from a seat, constant; also in moving the body while sitting; rising is then intolerable, and he has to walk stooping forward.

In the legs, here and there, after a walk, drawing, pressure and feeling of heaviness, which latter is diminished by stretching out the foot. [*Hrm.*]

Restlessness in the legs, while sitting; this restlessness runs up and down, making painful impressions in spots; passes away on walking and returns in sitting (at once). [*Gr.*]

460. **In the thighs**, painful (sharp) **dull pressure, at times in rhythmic paroxysms.** [*Gr.*]

Dull **pressure, as from a large peg,** in the gluteal muscles of the left thigh. [*Gr.*]

Cramp-like pressure in the left thigh, before and behind. [*Hrm.*]

Violent pressure in the middle of the external side of the right thigh, at every pulsation, and every time with a severe stitch (aft. 10½ h.). [*Htn.*]

Twitching pressure on the inside of the right thigh. [*Gr.*]

465. Slight twitching and drawing in the thighs, especially around and in the knees, as after a long journey on foot, with painful uneasiness, like a tremulous quivering, in sitting (aft. ¾ h.). [*Gr.*]

Drawing pain down on the external side of the right thigh. [*Gr.*]

Tearing contraction (cramp) on the outside of the left thigh in a small spot, with subsequent pain as of internal festering (aft. 11 h.). [*Fz.*]

Dull pain in the left thigh, close above the knee. [*Gr.*]

Boring stitch in the muscles of the right thigh, in front below (aft. 10 h.). [*Lgh.*]

470. Burning itching on the thighs, in the evening.

Burning pricking, as of needles, compelling to scratch, here and there, in the muscles of the thighs. [*Gr.*]

Itching stitches in the left thigh, passing off on rubbing. [*Gr.*]

In the knees, as well as in the muscles above and below the same, the most severe painfulness, after long stooping [*Gr.*]

In the knee, on the inner side, pressure in walking. [*Fz.*]

475. Pressure and drawing on the inner side of the knee, when walking. [*Fz.*]

Dull, pressive drawing on the inner surface of the right knee, when sitting. [*Gr.*]

Drawing pain in the right knee, as if under the patella, not affected by different positions (aft 1½ h.). [*Htn.*]

Painful drawing in the left knee, on bending the same (in sitting down); passing off on stretching it. [*Gr.*]

Drawing pain above the knee in sitting; in walking, it appears merely as weakness (aft. ½ h.). [*Gr.*]

480. Blunt stitches in the right knee. [*Gr.*]

Dull stitches or thrusts, close below the right knee, on setting down the foot. [*Gr.*]

Burning pain, as of a sore, as if scraped open, on the outer side of the left knee. [*Gr.*]

Dull pain, as from a sore, above the knee, when lifting the feet high, with a painful sensation of weakness about the knees, and cramp-like pinching between the hough and the calf. [*Gr.*]

Painless feeling of weakness above the knees in walking, with painful aching on sitting down, as after severely fatiguing the legs (aft. ½ h.). [*Gr.*]

485. **Painful uneasiness about the knees, with feeling of stiffness as if these parts were wrapped up** or bandaged, **when sitting.** [*Gr.*]

Paralyzed feeling in the knees, with stiffness and great weariness, so that he can hardly walk.

Itching eruption about the knees, down to the calves.

In the legs, in sitting, uneasiness as if everything there were alive and twisting about, and moving down into the feet, which felt heavy and as if about to go to sleep. [*Gr.*]

Heaviness in the legs.

490. Drawing down into the legs, very often, when sitting. [*Gr.*]
Dull, numb drawing in the legs. [*Gr.*]
Painful drawing in the tibia (aft. ¾ h.). [*Hrm.*]
Rheumatic drawing pressure in the leg, across the tibia, only in walking, while stretching the leg. [*Fz.*]
Pressive, lancinating pain sometimes with boring in the tibia and in the muscles of the leg. [*Lgh.*]
495. Pressive pain on the left tibia, when sitting, with uneasiness of the whole limb, diminished on drawing up the leg. [*Fz.*]
Tearing pressure on the anterior surface of the tibia, just above the ankle joint. [*Gr.*]
Cramp-like pressure in both calves, more outwardly toward the tibia (aft. 3 d.). [*Hrm.*]
Cramps of the calves, in walking.
Painful straining in the left calf. [*Gr.*]
500. **Tensive pain in the calf,** in walking, as if the muscles were too short, also when lying down at night, with sleeplessness.
Cramp-like, intermittent drawing in the legs, from the heels up into the calves. [*Hrm.*]
Twitching most keen, and with brief intermission, like electric shocks in the left tibia, close above the ankle. [*Gr.*]
Undulating twitches here and there **in the legs** (in sitting). [*Gr.*]
Frequent pulsations and twitches in the muscles of the legs. [*Fz.*]
505. Dull stitches, very painful, quite near the surface on the shin-bone, above the joint of the right foot. [*Gr.*]
Sore burning pain in the leg, above the heel. [*Gr.*]
Burning pain on a little spot in the middle of the leg, in front and more toward the outside. [*Gr.*]
Burning as from red-hot sparks on the legs.
In the ankle joint of the left leg, **pain on setting down the foot, as if it was sprained.**
510. Drawing pain in the ankle joint, when he sits down (aft. 32 h.). [*Fz.*]
Drawing down over the external malleoli in standing, with painfulness of the soles of the feet, so that standing is difficult to to him. [*Gr.*]
Cramp-like contortion of the sole of the right foot, out of its proper form. [*Gr.*]
Dull intermittent pressure on the inner border of the sole of the foot. [*Gr.*]
Cramp-like pressure on the left heel (aft. 30 h.). [*Hrm.*]
515. Tearing, burrowing pain in the heel, in the morning in bed.
Painful internal jerking on the dorsum of the foot. [*Gr.*]
Pricks as with needles, on the dorsum of the left foot. [*Gr.*]
Burning on the soles of the feet in sitting. [*Gr.*]
Coldness of the feet in the morning.
520. In walking, the feet, before warm, become keenly cold and the cold feet still colder.
Scratching itching, as if he was being rubbed with a woolen cloth on the dorsum of his foot (aft. 6 h.). [*Fz.*]

From the toes to the dorsum of the feet cramp-like drawing and tearing pains. [*Fz.*]

Tearing, while standing, transversely through the roots of the toes, passing off on moving them (aft. 5 h.). [*Fz.*]

Repeated tearing in the big toe. [*Gr.*]

525. Keen, intermittent jerking in the right big toe. [*Gr.*]

The skin of the body is unimpressionable as to tickling irritations.

General voluptuous itching over the whole body, which continually spreads further through scratching.

Here and there, in various places, an incitement to scratching, without itching, which immediately ceases again. [*Gr.*]

Corrosively stinging itching here and there in the body, especially on the back and the thighs, with impulse to scratch, after which it ceases only for a short time. [*Hrm.*]

530. Burning sensation here and there on the skin, impelling to scratch and thereby vanishing. [*Gr.*]

In the evening, in bed, heat in the skin of the whole body. with burning itching and irritation of the skin, such as comes through much scratching; after scratching it burns still more severely.

Burning itching in the spots affected, aggravated by scratching.

Burning and shooting in a herpes, which before was itching.

Pain, as from a furuncle, in the parts affected; he dares not touch them.

535. Stitches externally on various parts of the body, *e. g.*, on the muscles of the chest, the forehead, the wrist, etc.

Drawing and pressive pains in almost all parts of the body

(Every part of the body which is left motionless, goes to sleep.)

The symptoms always intermit for one or two days, and then again continue for a few days, so that we cannot deny a certain periodicity in their course. [*Gr.*]

He feels well while sitting, but standing causes uneasiness in the lower limbs, as if they ought to be drawn up, with anxiety. [*Fz.*]

540. While sitting still he feels in his arms, as they loosely rest on anything, yea, in the whole body, the beating of the pulse (after some bodily exertion). [*Gr.*]

General aching in the interior of the whole body.

All the tendons of the body ache, so that he cannot walk, but collapses.

In the morning, in bed, while lying still, bruised pain in all the joints, with stiffness of the nape of the neck and the small of the back and headache in the forehead and the temples; all these symptoms diminish on rising.

Intermittent, repeated tearing simultaneously through the arms and legs. [*Gr.*]

545. Heaviness in the left arm and leg, in walking.

After playing on the piano he feels heavy and full in the body.

She becomes thin, without feeling ill.

Tired and worn out; walking is a task for him in the beginning, and his feet feel heavy; by continuing his walk the sense of weariness is less and he feels better. [*St.*]

Weariness in the body; he always wants to lie down or sit down.

550. Extreme weariness, so that he can hardly move his hands; he trembles at every motion.

Very tired in going up stairs.

On a short foot-tour, he becomes so worn out that he can hardly get along, and is not able to recover himself (in sitting) for a long time afterwards. [*Gr.*]

After a short foot-tour, which came very hard to him, he is so worn out, tired and fatigued that he has to sit down at once, and would rather lie down, and he feels much relieved by laying his head down and closing his eyes. [*Gr.*]

He goes through all motions with greater emphasis and stronger energy; the muscles contract more vigorously, but the motions are as if executed with fibres too much strained, or as if there was a lack of moisture in the joints (aft. 1 h.). [*Fz.*]

555. **Paralysis of various parts of the body**. [MATTHIOLUS *in Commentar. in Dioscorid. M. M. L. U.*, Cap. V., p. 985—DACOSTA as above.[1]]

Panting, languishing condition, like paralysis, as if he was going to collapse, after a short walk, in the afternoon; in the evening, when walking briskly, and perspiring, he feels no weariness (6th d.) [*Gr.*]

While standing, there is no support from his legs; in sitting, there is painful weakness in the feet. [*Gr.*]

Weariness of the limbs as from much walking, and drowsiness as from great weakness (aft. 9 h.). [*Lgh.*]

In the evening he is tired and sleepy earlier than usual, and in the morning he wished to continue to sleep and not to leave his bed; also after dinner he is impelled to sleep. [*Gr.*]

560. In the afternoon, while sitting and reading, drowsiness and fatigue, as if he had overexerted himself by mental or bodily work (aft. 3 h.). [*Lgh.*]

After the siesta, continued indolence; he can hardly move his limbs and is vexed if he has to speak. [*Htn.*]

Sleep at night uneasy with frequent tossing about; his head now felt as if it lay too high, now too low, causing a dull, benumbed feeling of the head. [*Br.*]

For restlessness he can sleep but little every other night.

At night sleepless till two in the morning; he has to keep turning over and over (2d night).

565. Light sleep with frequent awaking.

He wakes at night for half an hour at a time, but sleeps well and refreshingly in the intervals.

Sound sleep till 9 o'clock in the forenoon (1st night).

---

1 "Paralysis of some members of the body." DACOSTA cited here without reference is not mentioned elsewhere.—*Hughes.*

At night very sound, deep sleep, and can hardly be roused in the morning.

Slumbering, day and night, with great heat and thirst; the skin hot to the touch, and muttering and moaning in his sleep.

570. He lies in a stupefied slumber without dreams, and after awaking feels quite stupid, often hot to the touch, with red cheeks and cold forehead, though he complains of heat in the head; at the same time severe thirst and dryness in the throat, paining as if sore.

He lies day and night without sleeping, but dreamy, anxious and full of business to be attended to.

He dreams that he must preach without having committed the sermon to memory; therefore there is anxious meditation, without being able to manage the matter. [*Gr.*]

Very vivid dreams full of consciousness and mental exertion; therefore on awaking there ensues a headache from being worn-out.

Vivid dreams at night; during the day it seems to him as if these things had happened to him while waking; during the first days it seemed to him as if these things had happened long ago; on the following days, as if they had happened shortly before.

575. **Vivid dreams** about old occurrences.

The dreams at night are mixed up with objects of his projected ideas. [*Fz.*]

Dreams about fire, while his sleep is otherwise sound. [*Gr.*]

Anxious dreams about conflagration. [*Br.*]

Dreams that he smelt burning tinder and sulphur, and on awaking the illusion continues, as he still thinks he smells them.

580. He dreams that his face is full of white ugly smallpox marks (aft. 21 h.). (*Lgh.*)

She dreams about loathsome diseases of other people.

Dreams of corpses, of a grave near, or of a precipitous abyss.

Anxious dreams full of danger.

He cries out anxiously in his sleep.

585. In the evening in bed while awake he starts up as if frightened (aft. 15, 16 h.). [*Lgh.*]

In the morning on awaking anxiety drives him from his bed.

At night in bed a lengthening of the teeth with pressive pain.

Severe drawing in the abdomen and the limbs, with subsequent burning, then the bones feel sore on being touched, so that she could not go to sleep.

Diarrhœa at night and subsequently constipation.

590. He cannot lie long on one side at night because his arms then pain as if bruised. [*Gr.*]

Cramp of the calves at night.

Twitchings of mouth and fingers in sleep.

After the siesta a chill of several minutes (1st d.).

Often a transient sensation as of coldness. [*Gr.*]

595. **Constant chilliness even in the warm room.** [*Gr.*]

He is averse to the open air, it is too raw for him.

Chilliness with lack of appetite. [*Gr.*]

In the morning for a few hours cold in the limbs, so that he shakes. [*Gr.*]

A shaking chill over the whole body, he only feels warm in the sun. [*Gr.*]

600. Ice-cold shudders run over him repeatedly. [*Gr.*]

Feeling of chilliness on hands and feet. [*Fz.*]

A chilly shudder over his whole body, as if he had taken cold in the wet. [*Lgh.*]

Fever-shudder over his whole body, with heat in the face, without thirst, in all positions (aft. 1½ h.). [*Lgh.*]

Fever-shudder over his whole back, as from having cold water poured over him. [*Lgh.*]

605. In the afternoon great feverish restlessness, as in catarrh, and weariness, with trembling of the limbs. [*Fz.*]

Feeling of heat, and heat in the face and the palms, without thirst. [*Fz.*]

In the afternoon quickly passing heat in the face and the brain, with redness of cheeks (aft. 8 h.) [*Fz.*]

Every afternoon at 4 o'clock heat in the face, with qualmishness and heaviness in the whole body; she has to lie down; better from eating.

He complains of great heat, without being hot to the touch (aft. 10 d.).

610. Very hot in the whole body, and yet he complains of chilliness.

Hot palms, while the backs of his hands are cold.

In the evening after supper, heat spreading rapidly over the face, without thirst and chilliness (aft. 12 h.), after half an hour thirst manifests itself. [*Lgh.*]

External heat with great thirst and dry, burnt lips.

Especially during the night great heat with violent thirst, without perspiration, so that he can not stand it.

615. On the upper part of the body great heat, with thirst and perspiration, with very hot breath; yet he complains of chilliness and shakes; his feet, which before perspired, are cold.

In the evening for two hours internal heat, with a cool perspiration all over, especially on the head, with short breath, thirst and weariness in the abdomen, and the knees as if about to collapse.

With open windows he perspires all over the body, with thirst for milk. [*Htn.*]

In the evening with open windows, warm perspiration over the abdomen, the back and the forehead, with moderate warmth over the rest of the body (aft. 12 h,). [*Htn.*]

Clammy sweat in the palms, most violent in the left hand. [*Htn.*]

620. Frequent awaking from sleep, with general perspiration (aft. 19 h.). [*Lgh.*]

Night sweats.

He perspires at night on the chest and the abdomen.

ANTIMONIUM CRUDUM.

(GRAY ORE OF ANTIMONY, TERSULPHATE OF ANTIMONY, STIBIUM SULPHURATUM NIGRUM.)

The native ore of tersulphuret of antimony is found in blocks of parallel black needles with an almost metallic lustre, and composed of twenty-eight parts of sulphur combined with 100 parts of metallic antimony. Having been first chemically tested so as to insure its freedom from the admixture of other metals, it is prepared in the manner directed at the close of the first part for dry medicinal substances and raised to the 30th potency for homœopathic use. From the pure effects on the healthy human body as laid down here, the frequent usefulness of a minimum dose of it in appropriate cases of chronic diseases may readily be perceived. It is very much to be desired that also the pure metallic antimony may be proved most carefully as to its pure effects, as we may expect of it much help, as yet unknown, and of a kind differing from that of the sulphuret of antimony; even as arsenic is different in its effects from the yellow sulphuret of arsenic, and the metallic mercury from cinnabar, each one having its own usefulness as a medicine.

The pharmaceutic remedies containing the sulphuret of antimony as kermes minerale, and sulphur auratum antimonii primæ, secundæ, tertiæ præcipitationis contain very different quantities of the sulphuret of antimony according to their varying mode of preparation.

Where the crude ore of antimony is found homœopathic in its pure effects, it will be found the more serviceable if the following symptoms are at the same time present:

Intolerance, in a child, of being touched and looked at; rush of blood to the head; troublesome itching of the head with falling out of the hair (*Htb.*); *redness and inflammation of the eyelids;* sore nostrils; heat and itching of the cheeks; *pains in the hollow teeth;* long continued loss of appetite; *eructation with the taste of the ingesta; loathing*, *qualmishness and nausea* from spoiled stomach; colic with loss of appetite, hard stool and red urine, in a child; pinching in the belly with a sensation as if diarrhœa was coming on; alternating diarrhœa and constipation in older persons (*Htb.*); difficult, hard stool; constant discharge of yellowish-white mucus from the anus

As this drug appears here for the first time, the character of Hahnemann's—and probably of Langhammer's—contributions to its pathogenesis may be inferred. But more than four-fifths of it is due to the other two physicians mentioned, who published their observations in Hartlaub and Trink's *Arzneimittellehre* (Vol. i.) in 1829, stating that they were made on healthy persons taking fractional doses of the crude substance triturated with milk-sugar.—*Hughes.*

(*Htb.*); frequent urination with much emission of mucus and burning in the urethra with pain in the small of the back (*Htb.*); cutting in the urethra during micturition; stoppage of the nose; painful inflammation of the tendons in the elbow-joint with severe redness and flexion of the arm; going to sleep of the legs while sitting still; violent pains in the lower limbs (*Htb.*); corns on the sole of the foot (*Htb.*); large, horny places on the sole of the foot, near the toes (*Htb.*); horny excrescence anteriorly under the nail of the big toe; malformations of the skin (*Htb.*); sensitiveness to cold; somnolence (*Htb.*).

Hepar sulphuris and mercury, according to Dr. Hartlaub, are the antidotes of crude antimony.

The abbreviations of the names of my fellow-provers are: *C.*, *Dr. Caspari; Htb.*, *Dr. Hartlaub; Lgh.*, *Dr. Langhammer.*

ANTIMONIUM CRUDUM.

Ill-humored and sad in the evening.

Melancholy, irritated mood the whole forenoon; the sound of bells, as well as the appearance of all his surroundings, moves him even to tears; his breathing is labored and short.

Dejection by day. [*Lgh.*]

He does not speak (2d d.). [*C.*]

5. Anxieties. [GMELIN, *allgem. Gesch. d. mineral. Gifte.*[1]]

Uneasy (2d d.). [*C.*]

Anxious meditation, during the day, about himself, his present and future fate. [*Lgh.*]

Decided impulse to shoot himself, at night, but no inclination to any other kind of suicide; he was compelled to rise from bed because he could not get rid of the thought. [*Htb.*]

Very much inclined to get frightened at a slight noise. [*C.*]

10. Ill-humor the whole day. [*Lgh.*]

Disheartened, he feels hot in the forepart of his head.

Peevish, unwilling to speak to anyone. [*Lgh.*]

Annoyed, cross without any cause (2d d.). [*C.*]

Weakness of the head. [*C.*]

15. Insanity. [HILDANUS.[2]]

Insanity; idiocy; she did not leave her bed, would not speak unless asked, demanded neither food nor drink, but she would gladly eat if anything was offered to her and she was hungry, and would refuse it if she was not hungry; at the same time she would keep pulling her neck-cloth, or fold a cloth and unfold it, or she would shred threads from the bed and gather them together; she was so deficient in sensation that she had bed-sores on several places, owing to evacuations discharged which had passed under

[1] General statement (from authors) of effects.—*Hughes.*
[2] *Observations. Cent. V., D.* 12. The case is that of sympt. 16—*Hughes.*

her; she did not feel these bed-sores, and never uttered a complaint. [CAMERARIUS, *sylloge memorabilium.*[1]]

Delirium and death, after an emetic of *Croc. metall.* [LINDESTOLPE, *de venenis.*[2]]

Continuous state of enthusiastic love and ecstatic longing for an ideal woman, which quite filled his phantasy; more while walking in the pure, open air than in the room; disappeared after several days with a seeming diminution of the sexual impulse. [*C.*]

Confused feeling in the head, as after continuous work in a cold room (4th d.). [*C.*]

20. Drunkenness. [*C.*]

Vertigo. [*C.*]

Headache, followed by some epistaxis (aft. 7½ h.). [*Lgh.*]

Light, dull headache in the sinciput and crown, increased by going up stairs. [*C.*]

Violent headache. [GARDANE, *Gazette de Santé*, 1793.[3]]

25. Violent headache, after bathing in a river, with weakness in the limbs, and aversion to food. [*C.*]

Dull, stupefying pain in the whole head, with qualmishness in the fauces, during the (customary) smoking of tobacco. [*Lgh.*]

Stupefying, dull pains in the head, more externally in the forehead, so that an anxious sweat broke out, while walking in the open air (aft. 6 h.). [*Lgh.*]

Headache as if the forehead would burst open; at the same time she was as if intoxicated, sat alone and would not speak. [CAMERARIUS, ibid.[4]]

Pain in the arch of the right eyebrow, within the skull, as if it would press everything asunder. [*C.*]

30. Pressure from without inwards, with intermittent drawing, in the left side of the forehead. [*C.*]

Momentary drawing pain over the left temporal bone, passed off by pressure, but returned immediately much more violently. [*C.*]

Tearing pain in the whole head, forward and backward, from morning to evening. [*C.*]

Violent tearing in the whole head, with heat therein, toward noon (6th d.). [*C.*]

The tearing in the head is diminished in walking and in the open air. [*C.*]

35. Constant pain in the forehead and the two temples, unchanged by touching, boring from within outward (aft. 5 h.). [*Lgh.*]

Rush of blood to the head diminished (curative action). [*C.*]

On the left parietal bone a small spot, which, on external pressure, causes pain on the bone, as if the periosteum was swollen. [*C*]

Externally on the left temple, slow throbbing, with fine

---

[1] Effects of over-dosing in adults. The last clause snould read: "So obtuse was her sensibility that when, from the acrimony of the evacuations and her position on the back, a large and foul ulcer formed over the sacrum and coccyx; she complained of no pain from it."—*Hughes.*

[2] General statement. This symptom is not found.—*Hughes.*

[3] Not accessible.—*Hughes.*

[4] Not found.—*Hughes.*

stitching several times in succession, in front toward the eyebrows, most severe when it is not particularly attended to. [*C.*]

Single, sharp stitches on the hairy scalp for one minute. [*C.*]

40. Red, hard pimple on the left temple, painful to the pressure as if sore, close to the beginning of the cartilage of the ear. [*C.*]

Little, flat nodules, as large as lentils, here and there on the hairy scalp, painful on pressure, and with formication all around. [*C.*]

Red spot, a little harder and raised, on each side of the forehead, itching like nettles, passing away and returning. [*C.*]

Close above the eyebrows, a white nodule, not itching, but painful to the touch.

Itching in the external canthus of the eye, compelling to scratch (aft. 2 h.). [*Lgh.*]

45. Quivering in the left eyelid. [*C.*]

Fine stitches, often in close succession, and without pain, in the anterior part of the eyeball, in the forenoon (9th d.). [*C.*]

Sharp, pressive stitches below the arch of the left eyebrow. [*Lgh.*]

Reddened eyelids, with fine stitches in the eyeball. [*C.*]

Redness of the left eye, with photophobia in the morning, on rising, and secretion of mucus in the inner canthus. [*C.*]

50. Red, inflamed eyes, with itching and nightly closing by suppuration.

Inflammation of the eyes. [GARDANE, *Gazette de Santé*, 1773.]

Little, humid spot on the outer canthus, which pains severely when perspiration comes in contact with it. [*C*]

Much mucus in the right canthus, in the morning, with dry eyegum in both eyelids. [*C.*]

Eyegum in the canthi, in the forenoon (aft. 3½ h.). [*Lgh.*]

55. Enlargement of the eyes. [PLINIUS; DIOSCORIDES.[1]]

Incurable blindness. [LINDESTOLPE, *de venenis.*[2]]

In the ears, stitches. [*C.*]

Drawing pain in the eustachian tube almost reaching into the mouth, after dinner (16 d.). [*C.*]

Digging and crawling in the ears, especially while lying still (5th d.). [*C.*]

60. Crawling in the right meatus auditorius (2d d.). [*C.*]

Itching stitches on the border of the right concha above the helix of the ear, ceasing on being touched (aft. 1½ h.). [*C.*]

Redness, burning and swelling of the left ear, as from the sting of a fly. [*C.*]

Swelling and redness of the whole internal concha with periodic itching. [*C.*]

Swashing in the ear, as of some drops of water, on moving the jaws.

65. Ringing before the ears (2d d.). [*C.*]

Constant buzzing of the ears, especially when there is quiet (2d d.). [*C.*]

---

[1] Dioscorides only mentions the beneficial effects of the local application of *Ant. cr.* to ulcers of the eyes; and the drug was only used topically in Pliny's times.—*Hughes.*

[2] Not found.—*Hughes.*

Buzzing in the ears, most in the afternoon. [*Htb.*]

Painful buzzing in the ears. [CAMERARIUS, ibid.[1]]

An inveterate buzzing of the ear disappeared (curative effect). [*C.*]

70. Severe din in the ears, as if someone was knocking at the door of the house.

A sort of deafness of the right ear, as if a leaf were placed before the tympanum, not to be removed by digging in it with the finger (aft. 14 h.). [*Lgh.*]

In the evening something obstructed the right ear.

Loss of hearing. [CAMERARIUS, ibid.[2]]

The nose pained in respiring, as from breathing cold air, or from inspiring acrid vapor. [*C.*]

75. Sensation of soreness in the nostrils on drawing in the air, especially in the right nostril, which is somewhat stopped. [*C.*]

Soreness of the right nostril in the front angle with painfulness, as from a cold. [*C.*]

Chapping and painfulness of the left nostril. [*C.*]

Chapping of both nostrils with formation of crusts. [*C.*]

Sore nostril with drawing pain.

80. Blowing out blood from the nose.

Bleeding at the nose, several days in succession.

Bleeding from the nose every evening.

Slight twitches in the facial muscles of the left side (aft. 9 h.). [*C.*]

Red pimple with pus in the tip, on both sides of the nose, with sensitiveness on pressure (12th d.). [*C.*]

85. Vesicular pimples in the face and on the nose, like varioloid pustules, with shooting pain on pressure. [*C.*]

Flat pimples, itching on touching, not red, with yellow scurf on both cheeks. [*C.*]

Nettle-rash in the face, especially on the cheeks.

Several pimples in the face, paining like stings of flies. [*C.*]

A bump on the right cheek as from the sting of a fly. [*C.*]

90. Red, burning, suppurating eruptions on the face. [WEPFER, *de cicuta et antimonio.*[3]]

An eruption with yellow crust, painful to the touch and easily knocked off, on the left side of the cheek toward the chin. [*C.*]

On the chin and under it, when touching it a sensation as if many little sore spots were touched, and on the skin here and there small honey-yellow granules. [*C.*]

Burning shooting as from a spark of fire on the chin and the upper lip [7th and 9th d.). [*C.*]

Formication on the upper lip as from the crawling of an insect (19th and 24th d.). [*C.*]

95. In the corners of the mouth, muscular twitches.

The lips are dry.

Furuncles in the corners of the mouth, with sore pains, returning after five, eight, twelve weeks. [*C.*]

---

[1] Preceding sympt. 73, where see note.—*Hughes.*

[2] After violent vomiting. Left ear soon recovered, but right remained permanently deaf; reporter ascribes it to rupture of membrana tympani.—*Hughes.*

[3] Cases of poisoning of men and animals.—*Hughes.*

Red pustules on the upper lip and on the right corner of the mouth, with dull pain on pressure and of itself (20th d.). [*C.*]

Many red little points, with a white little tip in the middle below the left corner of the mouth. [*C.*]

100. Toothache in a hollow tooth, worse at night than in daytime, a stinging, twitching and digging as if it were in the nerve, drawing up and down in the head; he dare not touch it with the tongue, else it aches, as if the nerve was scratched.

The toothache is renewed immediately after eating even soft foods, aggravated by being touched with cold water, and improved in the open air.

During the nocturnal toothache, great warmth as if proceeding from the chest.

Twitching toothache, in the evening in bed and after eating.

Stitches in the tooth, when drawing in air.

105. **Severe bleeding of the teeth.**

The gums are detached from the teeth, and bleed easily.

Dryness of the mouth, at night (6th d.). [*C.*]

Much salty saliva in the mouth. [WEPFER, *ibid.*]

Collection of water in the mouth. [*C.*]

110. Gathering of water on the tongue. [*C.*]

Odor from the mouth as in mercurial salivation.

Violent salivation from the nose and mouth. [*Ephemer. n. c. dec.* I. a. 3, *obs.* 270.[1]]

Salivation, without odor, from the mouth, and without looseness of teeth. [JAMES, in Simeon's *Beobachtung*, 1790.[2]]

On the tongue, anteriorly on the left margin, in close succession, some fine, sharp stitches, after dinner (aft. 33 h.). [*C.*]

115. Feeling of soreness and redness, on a small spot of the right margin of the tongue, for several days, frequently ceasing and suddenly returning (6th d.). [*C.*]

Blisters on the tongue.

Tongue coated white, in the forenoon (aft. 2 h.). [*Lgh.*]

On the palate, the whole night, a fine pinching, especially painful on deglutition and only passing away in the morning after the expectoration of mucus, which had collected through the night on the palate; only a sense of rawness remained. [*C.*]

Scraping sensation on the velum palati, as if much mucus was lying upon it, which can only be ejected after much hawking and often not at all, for several days (7th d.) [*C.*]

120. Scraping in the palate, with much expectoration of mucus by hawking (aft. 5 weeks). [*C.*]

In the throat much viscid mucus collects during the whole day. [*C.*]

Sore throat, as from a swelling or a lump on the left side of the throat.

Impeded swallowing. [GARDANE, ibid.]

Violent thirst, with dryness of the lips.

---

[1] Should be *Misc. Nat. Cur.* instead of *Ephem.* Same case as S. 421.--*Hughes.*

[2] Not accessible. (The symptom is not mentioned by James in his treatise on the Fever

125. Intense thirst. [WEPFER, ibid.]

In the evening, thirst, and inclination to drink.

Drinks much only at night.

Much thirst, at night (aft 6 d.). [*C.*]

Appetite extremely little.

130. Lack of appetite. [STAHL, *Mater. Med.*, Dresden, 1744.[1]]

Strong feeling of hunger in the region of the stomach, in the morning on awaking, without appetite, not removed by eating; at the same time a disagreeable feeling of emptiness in the scrobiculus cordis, and lack of heat in the body; for two days (aft. 4 w.). [*C.*]

During a moderate dinner a sensation as if the abdomen was very full, and a quantity of flatus arises and moves about the abdomen. [*C.*]

After a meal, indolence and an inclination to lie down. [*C.*]

The fullness and tension after a meal often alternates with lightness, cheerfulness and activity of spirit and body after a meal. [*C.*]

135. After dinner, lassitude, tremulous weariness and heaviness in all the limbs, as if coming from the abdomen, with trembling of the hands in writing, and subsequent passage of much fetid flatus, with distention of abdomen. [*C.*]

During supper, dyspnœa.

Eructation, with a raw taste. [*Lgh.*]

Loud eructation (aft. ¼ and 1½ h.). [*C.*]

Bitter eructation, like bile (aft. 5 h.).

140. Regurgitation of fluid, with a taste of the ingesta, in the afternoon (2d and 3d d.). [*C.*]

Hiccup (aft. 1 h.). [*Lgh.*]

Hiccup, frequently, while smoking tobacco (aft. 10½ h.) [*Lgh.*]

Nausea, with vertigo. [*C.*]

Nausea after drinking a glass of wine. [*C.*]

145. Inclination to vomit. [GARDANE, ibid.]

Violent loathing. [MORGENSTERN, *de usu Antim. cr.*, 1756.[2]]

Fearful vomiting, not to be stopped by anything. [LINDESTOLPE, ibid.]

Violent vomiting, with anxiety. [FRIEDR. HOFFMANN, *med. rat. et system.*[3]]

Vomiting of mucus and bile. [MATTHIOLUS; GÖTZE, in Act. Vratislaviensibus.[4]]

150. Dreadful vomiting, with convulsions. [WEPFER, ibid.]

Violent vomiting and diarrhœa. [MORGENSTERN, ibid.]

Violent vomiting and diarrhœa, attended with the greatest anguish. [BONETUS, *Polyalthea.*[5]]

In the stomach, painful sensation on external pressure upon it. [*C.*]

---

[1] Not accessible.—*Hughes.*

[2] General statement (from authors).—*Hughes.*

[3] Add Part I., § 2, Chapt. 3, of folio ed. Geneva, 1761. Statement of ill effects of antimonial emetics.—*Hughes.*

[4] Effects of Ant. cr. in a patient with syphilitic ulceration.—*Hughes.*

[5] Statement of occasional effects of Ant cr.—*Hughes.*

Pressure in the stomach, which resembles more a dull cutting, especially on drawing in the abdomen. [*C.*]

155. Pressure in the stomach, in the morning, with thirst (20th d.). [*C.*]

Pain in the stomach as from excessive fullness, but without fullness and with appetite. [*C.*]

Pain in the stomach, as after eating too much, with distended abdomen without hardness (aft. 3 d.). [*C.*]

Sensation of tightness in the stomach with empty eructations. [*C.*]

Spasmodic pains in the stomach. [FR. HOFFMANN, ibid.]

160. Cramp of the stomach. [STAHL, ibid.]

Cramp of the stomach all their life, with several persons. [WEPFER, ibid.]

Burning, cramp-like pains in the scrobiculus cordis, in paroxysms of half an hour, driving him to despair and to the determination to drown himself.

Burning in the scrobiculus cordis, like heartburn, with good appetite. [*C.*]

Pinching pain on the right side above and beside the scrobiculus cordis. [*C.*]

165. In the hypochondria, a slight tension. [WEPFER, ibid.]

In the bowels a transient, fatiguing sensation, as after violent diarrhœa. [*C.*]

Violent distention of the abdomen, especially after a meal. [*C.*]

Distended, big abdomen. [*Htb.*]

Very much distended abdomen, and pain arising thence as from an internal pressure. [*C.*]

170. The most intolerable pains in all parts of the abdomen. [GMELIN, ibid.]

Pinching pain to the left of the umbilicus. [*C.*]

Transient colic in the region of the stomach. [*C.*]

Pinching, as if rhythmically with the pulse in a small spot the left side of the abdomen, quite low down, in the afternoon d.). [*C.*]

Pinching in the abdomen, especially on the right side toward the back, beginning suddenly in the evening and aggravated by motion (aft. 3 w.). [*C.*]

175. Cutting in the abdomen, very violent (22d d.). [*C.*]

Cutting in the abdomen with qualmishness there, and collection of water on the tongue. [*C.*]

Sudden compressive colic with regurgitation of water in the mouth. [*C.*]

Cutting in the abdomen the whole day, with sensation of oppressive anxiety from the stomach, distaste for work, dry humor and pain in the stomach, during eructations. [*C.*]

Several fits of colic in the region of the stomach. [*C.*]

180. Sensation of emptiness in the bowels, ceasing after eating. [*C.*]

All the abdominal troubles commence again after two and one-half weeks. [*C.*]

In the inguinal region, pains as from a swelling, when pressing upon it; the place feels hard, like swollen glands. [*C.*]

Hard gland in the left groin, painful on pressure; it seems to lie above Poupart's ligament, and to run parallel with it. [*C.*]

Hernia. [CAMERARIUS, ibid.[1]]

185. Gurgling in the abdomen, as when air bubbles rise in water. [*C.*]

Loud grumbling in the hypogastrium (aft. 1½ h.). [*Lgh.*]

Loud grumbling in the abdomen as from emptiness, in the forenoon (aft. 3 h.). [*Lgh.*]

Flatus very frequently forms immediately after a meal, and moves about audibly, especially on the right side of the abdomen, with discharge of a portion (aft. 6 h.). [*C.*]

A quantity of rumbling and explosive flatus immediately after the meal, of which some is discharged with ill odor, the remainder rolls about in great quantities, especially on the right side of the abdomen, before it is discharged (9th d.). [*C.*)

190. With a sensation of distention, as if a copious stool were coming, a quite insignificant quantity of flatus was discharged (aft. 5½ h.). [*C.*]

Constipation for three days.

Severe, sudden urging to stool after dinner, and quick discharge of an ordinary stool, with straining (4th d.). [*C.*]

Hard stool in the morning (aft. 1 h.). [*Lgh.*]

Very difficult hard stool.

195. Difficult evacuation of a hard stool, with previous straining in the rectum for about two minutes (aft. 12 h.). [*Lgh.*]

Difficult discharge of a hard stool, without previous straining (aft. 11 h.). [*Lgh.*]

Firm stool in the evening, with violent straining in the rectum and cutting in the abdomen. [*C.*]

Stool first normal, then several small, soft stools, followed by just as small, but hard, stools with violent straining in the rectum and anus until all is over. [*C.*]

Pappy, frequent stools (aft. 1½ h.). [*Lgh.*]

200. Very thin stools. [*C.*]

The stool, which previously had been pretty firm, now becomes very thin. [*C.*]

After taking vinegar, very thin stool, with pain in the rectum at the evacuation. [*C.*]

Ineffectual urging to diarrhœa.

Diarrhœa, at night and in the morning, but each time only one discharge.

205. Mucus flows from the anus, on discharge of flatus.

Continuous passage of blood and solid fæces through the rectum. [LINDESTOLPE, ibid.[2]]

Discharge of black blood through the rectum. [MATTHIOLUS, ibid.]

During stool, pain in the rectum like soreness, or as if an ulcer had been torn open.

---

[1] "Hernia ventriculi," after violent vomiting.—*Hughes.*
[2] Not found.—*Hughes.*

Protrusion of the rectum during stool, for some time. [*C.*]

210. Drawing pain in the anus. [*C.*]

Itching in the anus. [*C.*]

Sharp itching in the rectum (7th d.). [*C.*]

Burning itching and chaps in the anus, at night (aft. 3 d.).

The varices in the anus protrude more than usual (aft. 11 d.). [*C.*]

215. Formication and burning in the varix of the anus, in the evening, in bed, until going to sleep (aft. 11 d. and 5 w.). [*C.*]

On the perinæum a furuncle, which pained and burned far around. [*C.*]

Urging to urinate, frequent and violent, with much emission of urine every time (aft. 1, 2, 2½ h.). [*Lgh.*]

Frequent micturition, with discharge of little, watery urine (4th d.). [*C.*]

Much urging to micturition, but little is discharged (aft. 5 d.). [*C.*]

220. Long continued, frequent micturition, with little discharge and quick urging (18th d.). [*C.*]

It urges to urination. [SAUNDERS, *observat. de antimon.*, *etc.*, London, 1773.[1]]

Frequent urination. [*Lgh.*]

Very copious micturition, even three times a night (10th d.). [*C.*]

Copious, frequent micturition. [WEPFER, ibid.[2]]

225. Involuntary copious micturition, with a convulsive cough (by *Sulph. aur.*). [*C.*]

Golden yellow, thin urine, with a scarcely perceptible cloud. [WEPFER, ibid.]

Brownish-red urine. [*C.*]

Dark-colored, frequent urine (aft. 7 h.). [*Lgh.*]

Little red bodies in the urine, after standing twenty-four hours. [WEPFER, ibid.]

230. In the spermatic cords, constant drawing, while a furuncle is on the perinæum; the pain was most violent in standing, and was diminished by stooping. [*C.*]

On the penis, fine itching (aft. 14 h.). [*C.*]

Violent itching of the extremity of the glans. [*C.*]

Smarting itching as from salt, on the left side of the scrotum, frequently, for 14 days (aft. 14 d.), [*C.*]

Violently excited sexual impulse, with restlessness of the whole body, so that he can not remain sitting any time (aft. 6 h.). [*C.*]

235. Later on, the sexual instinct seems to be diminished for several days. [*C.*]

Erections (aft. 6 h.). [*C.*]

Inclination to pollutions, even on leaning the back against anything.

Pollutions at night, without voluptuous dreams. [*Lgh.*]

---

[1] "But rarely," the author says.—*Hughes.*

[2] In a dog.—*Hughes.*

Pollution, with many dreams at night (11th d.). [*C.*]

240. In the womb, pressure as if something would come out.

Discharge of acrid water from the vagina, which causes smarting down the thighs.

* * * * * * * *

Stoppage of the nose, in the evening, as from catarrh, for several days. [*C.*]

Dryness of the nose on walking in the open air, so that he can hardly speak.

245. Coryza. **Stuffed coryza.** [*C.*]

Coryza with sore, encrusted nostrils. [*C.*]

Fluent coryza. [*C.*]

Fluent coryza, in the morning, for several hours, without sneezing. [*Lgh.*]

Much thick, yellowish mucus has to be drawn from the posterior nares into the fauces and ejected, all the day (9th d.). [*C.*]

250. Hoarseness.

Extreme weakness of the voice; he can only speak quite low. [WEPFER, ibid.]

Speaking and singing are unsteady and weak. [WEPFER, ibid.]

Loss of voice, as often as he became heated; it returns through rest. [WEPFER, ibid.]

In the throat, in the morning, he is very hoarse and dry (6th d.). [*C.*]

255. In his throat a foreign body seems to be suspended, which he seeks in vain to swallow or to eject. [WEPFER, ibid.]

Violent spasm in the bronchia and in the fauces, as if a plug, which at times seems to become thicker then again thinner, was filling the throat, with a sensation of soreness.

Clearing the throat and hawking while walking in the open air.

Cough in the morning after rising, in paroxysms, as if coming from the abdomen; the first fit of cough is always the most violent, the following ones become continually weaker, so that the last is only like tussiculation.

Frequent dry cough. [WEPFER, ibid.]

260. Dry, shaking cough, with involuntary copious discharge of urine (in a woman who had taken *Sulph. aur.* for a cough with copious expectoration). [*C.*]

Severe dry cough, scratching in the bronchia, in a sudden short paroxysm. [*C.*]

Cough with ejection of viscid, thin mucus; deep from the chest, in the morning. [WEPFER, ibid.]

With every cough, burning in the chest, as from a fire, with glowing hot breath from the mouth. [WEPFER, ibid.]

Deep, sighing respiration, as from fullness of the chest, for several days, in the afternoon and after a meal. [*C.*]

265. Dyspnœa after supper.

Difficulty of breathing. [GARDANE, ibid.]

Asthma. [STAHL, ibid.]
Very troublesome asthma. [WEPFER, ibid.]
Suffocating asthma with four youths. [JOUBERT, *lib. de Peste*, Cap. 19.[1]]

270. Suffocating rheum. [WEPFER, ibid.[2]]

Pressure on the chest, in the morning on awaking. [*C.*]

Pressive pain in the right breast, in the evening, while lying down. [*C.*].

Severe, pressive pain, now in the chest, now in the back, now in both at the same time. [WEPFER, ibid.]

Pressure on the chest. [*C.*]

275. Partly pressive, partly lancinating pain under the left clavicle, as if in the bronchia, while respiring. [*C.*]

Dull stitches in the chest, on taking a deep breath, first on the right side under the first two ribs, then under the upper part of the sternum. [*C.*]

Stitches in the left side of the chest, while respiring, with some cough and headache. [*C.*]

Sharp stitches in the left breast while expiring when standing (aft. 5 h.). [*Lgh.*]

Pinching stitches in the middle of the chest (3d d.). [*C.*]

280. Burning in the chest, with dry cough and tightness, as if about to choke. [WEPFER, ibid.[3]]

Violent palpitation of the heart. [GODOFR. SCHULZ *in tract. de natura tinct. bezoard.*, *Cap.* 5.[4]]

In the pectoralis major muscle, in the morning on rising and for a few hours afterward, while stretching and lifting the arm, and in pressing upon it, a pain as if crushed, or as after too great exertion (8th d.). [*C.*]

Itching on the chest, as if a vesicatory was healing. [*C.*]

Severe, continual itching on the chest the whole day. [*C.*]

285. Itching on the chest and the back. [*Htb.*]

Violent itching on the chest wakes him at night, and he feels pimples in various places. [*C.*]

When he rubs the skin on his chest on account of the itching, it feels sore; the skin is sensitive as after a vesicatory. [*C.*]

The chest feels as if sprinkled over with fine red points, with a violent itching, not removed by scratching. [*C.*]

In the small of the back, on rising from sitting, violent pains which vanish on walking.

290. Sudden pains in the small of the back, in the morning and the whole day, not at night. [*C.*]

Pain as from swelling in the cartilage or the periosteum of the upper part of the ilium. [*C.*]

In the back, tearing, the whole day, from morning till evening. [*C.*]

Spasmodic stitches in the right scapula when sitting. [*Lgh.*]

Violent itching upon the back, for fourteen days. [*C.*]

295. Little red pimples, quite on top of the right shoulder, without any sensation, passing away for a short time on pressure (7th d.). [*C.*]

Rash behind the ears extending to the nape of the neck and the scapulæ.

Red prickly heat with yellow tips over the whole right shoulder; later on they look like goose skin and scale off. [*C.*]

Brown liver colored spots on both shoulders. [*C.*]

In the nape of the neck and between the scapulæ, a straining while stooping.

300. Cramp-like drawing pains in the muscles of the neck, down into the scapulæ in the evening, after lying down, and in the morning; aroused and aggravated by stooping, exerting the arm and turning the head to the left (12th d.). [*C.*]

A hard pea-shaped body on the left side of the neck, under the skin; it can only be felt by stretching the skin in bending the head. [*C.*]

On the neck, a drawing, pressing inward, on the left side, below (19th d.). [*C.*]

Cramp-like drawing from above downward in one of the muscles of the posterior cervical region on the right side, in the evening when sitting (8th d.). [*C.*]

Single stitches in the skin of the neck, now here, now there. (2d and 3d d.). [*C.*]

305. Itching on the neck. [*C.*]

Sensitiveness of the skin of the neck; when he rubs hard on account of the itching, there is a feeling of soreness. [*C.*]

Small pimples on the neck and under the chin, painful to the touch (13th d.). [*C.*]

Hard, long continuing pustules under the throat, like little smallpox pustules, which fill up with pus not only in the tips, but all over. [*C.*]

Many red points with a little white tip in the center, with stinging pains on stroking over the hairs of the beard, on the anterior side of the throat. [*C.*]

310. Under both arms, a stitch, on walking in the open air.

Sharp itching of the inside of the left arm. [*C.*]

Itching of the arms with appearance of reddish blisters, like stings of flies, on rubbing. [*C.*]

Many light-brown little spots, like little hepatic spots on the arms. [*C.*]

On the middle of the upper arms, pimples like rash, without itching (14th d.). [*C.*]

315. Paralytic pain in the muscles of the upper arm, in bending the arms, as if they were too much contracted, or weakened by this exertion. [*C.*]

Twitching drawing in the muscles of the upper arms, which passed away not by motion but by warmth, and returned in a draught.

Sudden drawing jerking, transversely through the right upper arm (aft. 10, 20, 120 min.). [*C.*]

Light muscular twitching in the right upper arm, **in the deltoid muscle** (5th d.). [*C.*]

On the bend of the elbow, corrosively itching pimples.

320. Cracking in the elbow joint, on turning it hither and thither. [*C.*]

In the forearm drawing, in rest and in motion. [*C.*]

Drawing down the right forearm (aft. 1½ h.). [*C.*]

Paralytic drawing in the right forearm (aft. 2 h.). [*Htb.*]

Inward pressing drawing on the inside of the lower **forearm** (**19th** d.). [*C.*]

325. On the wrist of the left arm there appears at night **a large** pimple. [*C.*]

Itching heat vesicles on the left hand. [*C.*]

A blister on the styloid process of the ulna of the right **arm**. [*C.*]

A blister on the external border of the left hand. [*C.*]

Corrosively itching, eruptive pimples in the ball of the **hand, on** the muscle of the thumb.

330. Cracking in the joint of the metacarpal bone of the thumb, **on** motion (9th d.). [*C.*]

Drawing pain in the fingers and their joints. [*C.*]

Gouty pains in the joints of the third finger of the **right hand**. [*C.*]

Fine itching in the tip of the left thumb (aft. 14 h.). [*C.*]

The nails of the fingers did not grow as quickly as usual, and the skin under them was painfully sensitive [*C.*]

335. Red, pimple-like itch, stingingly painful to the touch, **with** brown scurf on the posterior joint of the right thumb (**24th d.**). [*C.*]

Pain in the right hip-joint. [*C.*]

Drawing pain in the left hip-joint, when walking, especi**ally** when bending the leg backwards; also in the evening. [*C.*]

Drawing pain in the left hip. [*Htb.*]

Painful drawing from the hip-joint toward the sacrum. [*C.*]

340. In the nates, drawing through the hip-joint, around into the **thigh** (7th d.). [*C.*]

Light twitching of the muscles in the left nates, in the evening, when sitting (5th d.). [*C.*]

Gurgling, for a few minutes, in the lower part of the right nates, when standing (aft. 4 w.). [*C.*]

Large, hard pustule on the left nates, with itching and tensive pain. [*C.*]

A little protuberance on the right nates of a child. [*C.*]

345. On the leg, white, hard tubercles, as large as lentils, arising **from** itching, and surrounded by a small, red areola. [*C.*]

Bluish spots on the thighs. [LINDESTOLPE, ibid.[1]]

On the thigh of the right leg, **quite high up**, repeated **tension, like a small spasm** (**7th d.**). [*C.*]

---

[1] **Not found.—*Hughes.***

Drawing pain in the posterior muscles of the left thigh. [*C.*]

Drawing pain in the anterior and inner side of the thigh. [*C.*]

350. Cramp-like sensation on the external border of the left thigh, as if the muscle contracted quite slowly, and then again extended itself, in the afternoon (aft. 10 h.). [*C.*]

Sharply stinging itching on the inside and the interior surface of the left thigh (aft. 4½ h.). [*C.*]

Finely stinging itching on the right thigh not passing off by scratching; afterward a small flat, yellowish pimple on the same place. [*C.*]

The stinging itching on the thighs returns every evening. [*C.*]

In the knee a pain, so that he cannot stretch the foot, but has to limp.

355. Stiffness of the knee, for eight days.

Painful stiffness of the knee; she could not stretch it for pain, and had to limp.

Pain immediately below the knee, as if tied too tight, the whole evening (aft. 13 d.). [*C.*]

A stitch in the left knee, so that he was startled and had to jerk up his leg (10th d.). [*C.*]

Sudden, violent stitch on the outside of the knee. [*C.*]

360. Drawing pain in the right knee. [*C.*]

Itching in the right knee, on the inner side, and after rubbing it, a large blister, which pains only for a short time. [*C.*]

Red pimples, like blisters, on the knee, like varioloid pustules, with a stinging pain on pressure. [*C.*]

A lump on the right knee, as from the sting of a fly. [*C.*]

In the leg, a drawing pain, reaching into the knee.

365. Drawing pain on the lower part of the left tibia. [*C.*]

Drawing pain on the inside of the left calf. [*C.*]

Painless drawing, in the evening when sitting, in the right leg, from the knee, and also from the ischium down the thigh and the tibia, even into the foot, so that he has to lift it up and bring it into another position; several times in succession (10th d.). [*C.*]

Pinching, painless and intermitting, quite low down in the right calf. [*C.*]

Sharp stitch in the shaft of the shin-bone, from within outward, in sitting (aft. 5 h.). [*Lgh.*]

370. Stitches which run low down on the tibia. [*Lgh.*]

Clucking in the posterior side of the right leg, and immediately afterward stitches in the ankle-joint (3d d.). [*C.*]

Formication down the left calf, without itching (aft. 14 h.). [*C.*]

Fine itching on the left tibia (aft. 4½ h.). [*C.*]

A spot which pains to the touch as if bruised, on the outside of the left calf, for several days (aft. 24 h.). [*C.*]

375. Bluish spots on the shin-bone. [LINDESTOLPE, ibid.[1]]

The foot is so heavy that she cannot lift it.

Going to sleep and numbness of the right foot when walking. [*C.*]

---

[1] Not found.—*Hughes.*

Pain, as if sprained, in the right external malleolus, in turning the foot outward, with frequent cracking of the joint in bending and stretching it (5th d.). [*C.*]

Drawing pain in the left heel (aft. 3 h.). [*C.*]

380. Cramp-like drawing on the outer side of the left heel (aft. 1½ h.). [*C.*]

Intolerable burning, lancinating and tearing pains in a gangrenous foot, with insensibility of the same to touch and to pricks of a needle into it. [WEPFER, ibid.[1]]

Sharp and fine prickly stitches in the sole of the foot (10th d.). [*C.*]

Painful stitches in the skin of the sole of the right foot, passing off by rubbing; in the evening in bed, after a walk of three hours (8th d.). [*C.*]

Severe itching under the right external malleolus, not immediately passing off by scratching, and leaving behind a small red spot. [*C.*]

385. Chilblains on the feet, with pain and redness in summer.

Great sensitiveness of the soles of the feet to walking, especially on stone pavements, for a long time (aft. 7 d.). [*C.*]

Large horny places on the skin of the sole of the foot, near the beginning of the toes, paining like corns, and always returning after being cut out. [*C.*]

Gangrene of the foot, which is quite black. [WEPFER, ibid.[2]]

The big toe cracks with every motion requiring an effort. [*C.*]

390. Tearing, drawing through the right big toe. [*C.*]

Rhythmical cutting under the left big toe (6th d.). [*C.*]

Burning pain on the ball of the right big toe (6th d.). [*C.*]

Fine itching on the left big toe (aft. 4½ h.). [*C.*]

A corn on the left little toe, it pains without cause, as if squeezed (7th d.). [*C.*]

395. Muscular twitching in many parts of the body.

Single, long continued, tickling, itching stitches here and there, especially on the upper arm, from within outwardly; also under the right natis, not urging to scratch.

Itching on the whole body, especially on the chest and the back. [*C.*]

Itching on many parts of the body, especially on the neck and the limbs. [*C.*]

Eruptive pimples coming on at night. [*C.*]

400. Eruptive pimples which itch on getting warm in bed at night, and thus take away the night's sleep.

Red pimples like blisters, like varioloid pustules, with stinging pain on pressure, on various parts of the skin. [*C.*]

Pustules with yellow or brown scurf here and there. [*C.*]

Eruption of red points with white tips in the middle, in various places. [*C.*]

Eruptions like rash. [*C.*]

405. Nettle rash; white bumps with red areolæ, with violent burn-

---

[1] See sympt. 388.—*Hughes.*

[2] This set in soon after violent vomiting had subsided (? embolism).—*Hughes.*

ing and fine stitches, in the face and on the limbs, except the fingers, which were swollen, with severe thirst and nausea.

Bumps and blisters as from the stings of insects, in many parts of the body, **especially in the face and in the joints** of the limbs; they arise with itching and often disappear even after a few hours. [*C.*]

Brown spots and dots, like hepatic spots, here and there, especially on the arms. [*C.*]

Discolored nails. [LINDESTOLPE, ibid.[1]]

He feels ill in the heat of the sun and the warm air, even with light motion and work. [WEPFER, ibid.]

410. Wine drinking especially aggravates his condition. [WEPFER, ibid.]

At rest and in cool air he feels better. [WEPFER, ibid.]

His symptoms all return again after the third week, but from then on they appeared more on the left side of the body. [*C.*]

Convulsive motions, especially of the head. [WEPFER, ibid.[2]]

Twitchings and trembling of the limbs. [FR. HOFFMANN, ibid.]

415. Immense swelling of the whole body. [LINDESTOLPE, ibid.[3]]

Dropsical swelling of the body. [LOTICHINO, *observationes.*[4]]

Incurable dropsy. [WEPFER, ibid.]

Excessive hemorrhages. [FR. HOFFMANN, ibid.[5]]

Emaciation and loss of strength. [WEPFER, ibid.]

420. Getting fat. [KUNKEL VON LÖWENSTERN, *laborator. chemic.*[6]]

Apoplexy, with such a violent flow of saliva that he discharged nearly a quart of water through his nose and mouth. [*Ephemer. N. c. dec.* I. a. 3.[7]]

Death, after some hours, from antimony given for cramps of the stomach. [FR. HOFFMANN, ibid.]

Death from suffocating rheum, after fifteen days, from some grains of crude antimony. [WEPFER, ibid.[8]]

Weariness, especially in the feet, with great peevishness, at 7 P. M.

425. Great weariness in the morning, and indisposition to rise. [*C.*]

Yawning, frequently three and four times in succession. [WEPFER, ibid.]

Great drowsiness during the day, and in the morning on awaking; he can not force himself out of his bed. [*C.*]

In the afternoon, sudden transient drowsiness, when sitting. [*Lgh.*]

Sleepy and peevish at 6 P. M., and at 8 o'clock he can not keep from going to sleep; at night sound sleep until morning, when he is so tired that he can scarcely open his eyes. [*C.*]

430. At 7 P. M. she is seized with almost irresistible sleep; she

---

[1] Not found.—*Hughes.*
[2] In a puppy.—*Hughes.*
[3] Not found.—*Hughes.*
[4] Case of over-dosing in an adult (lib. IV., Cap. 3, D. 5). Jaundice had preceded the emetic of Ant. cr., which was followed by this ascites. It terminated in death.—*Hughes.*
[5] Not found.—*Hughes.*
[6] Effects of continued use (p. 414).—*Hughes.*
[7] Read "*Misc. Nat. Cur.*" instead of "*Ephemer.*"—*Hughes.*
[8] See note to Sympt. 270.—*Hughes.*

sleeps all the night till morning, and then feels well, for six days in succession. [*C.*]

Somnolence in the forenoon. [*Lgh.*]

Slumber with fantastic delusions.

Slumber with fantastic delusion, as if some one was knocking at the door, and that she was called by some one.

Late in going to sleep; he could not get any sleep before 12 o'clock.

435. Wide awake in the evening in bed, so that he could not go to sleep for an hour; at the same time frequent cold shiverings, especially over the whole of the left side, on which he is not lying; or, when he gets warm, lasciviousness with erections which make him more wide awake than before; eight days in succession, and again after five weeks. [*C.*]

Little sleep (1st night). [*C.*]

At night uneasy sleep, caused by itching stitches now and then, which pass away on rubbing.

Frequent awaking from intolerable itching on the chest, where he felt pimples. [*C.*]

Frequent awaking from itching here and there, with perceptible vesicles. [*C.*]

440. Awaking about 2 o'clock at night with slight general warmth and burning itching and excoriation on the anus (3d d.). [*C.*]

Awaking from his siesta after dinner, by and with dull gnashing of the teeth (2d d.). [*C.*]

Awaking from strangury, at night.

At night, discharge of little urine in an intermittent stream, with painful erections.

He lies on his back at night. [*Lgh.*]

445. At night frequent awaking, as from fright. [*Lgh.*]

Anxious in bed, from 3-5 o'clock.

Frequent awaking at night, and when he fell asleep he dreamed of solemnities.

Anxious dreams, as if he would be wounded; he jumps up from sleep and struggles with hands and feet.

Horrible dreams of mutilations of men.

450. Dreams of his own family at home, with whom he quarreled, disturb his night's rest. [*Lgh.*]

Vexatious dreams, full of quarrels with relatives, rouse him at night from sleep. [*Lgh.*]

Lascivious dreams for several nights in succession, also with pollutions (aft. 11 d.). [*C.*]

Voluptuous images in his dreams at night, with pollution. [*Lgh.*]

Dream about seeing an old schoolmate, at which he rejoiced (aft. 23 h.). [*Lgh.*]

455. Much chill, no heat.

Unpleasant feeling of internal chilliness, so that he could never get really warm; returning after five weeks. [*C.*]

Chilly, even in the warm room. [*C.*]

Feet always cold as ice. [*C.*]

His feet do not get warm before 1 o'clock at night. [*C.*]

460. Shivering over the whole back, without thirst (aft. 2 h.). [*Lgh.*]

Shivering over the whole body, in the morning, with heat in the forehead, without thirst (aft. ½ h.). [*Lgh.*]

Severe shaking chill toward noon, with violent thirst for beer for an hour; then, after sleeping, heat and constant thirst.

By the least motion especially in the sunshine, he is overheated, and complains of excessive heat in the throat. [WEPFER, ibid.]

Goat's milk gives him an agreeable refreshment. [WEPFER, ibid.]

465. At night, in bed, he gets very hot with profuse perspiration. [WEPFER, ibid.]

General perspiration, without smell, causing the finger-tips to soften and wrinkle (12th d.). [*C.*]

Perspiration during sleep. [*Lgh.*]

In the morning, on awaking, a light perspiration over the whole body (aft. 21 h.). [*Lgh.*]

Every other morning, general warm perspiration in bed. [*C.*]

470. Perspiration, returning at the same hour for three days. [NICOLAI, *progr. ad Dissert.*, REINDEL, *de oleo* V, *et* s. s.[1]]

Pulse, now a few quick beats, then three or four slow beats (at once).

ARSENICUM ALBUM.

WHITE ARSENIC.

(The semi-oxide of metallic arsenic in diluted and potentized solution.)

As I write down the word Arsenic, momentous memories seize upon my soul.

When the All-merciful One created iron, He granted to mankind, indeed, to fashion from it either the murderous dagger or the mild ploughshare, and either to kill or to nourish their brethren therewith. How much happier, however, would they be, did they employ His gifts only to benefit one another! This should be the aim of their life; this was His will.

So also it is not to Him, the All-loving One, we must impute the wickedness practiced by men, who have dared to misemploy the wonderfully powerful medicinal substances in diseases for which they were not suitable, and besides this in doses so enormous, guided only by frivolous ideas or some paltry authorities, without having subjected them to any careful trial, and without a well-grounded selection.

[1] References not accessible.—*Hughes.*

If now a careful prover of the effects of medicines arise, they inveigh against him as an enemy to their comfort, and do not refrain from the most dishonest calumnies.

The ordinary medical art has hitherto employed *in large and frequently repeated doses* the most powerful medicines, such as arsenic, nitrate of silver, corrosive sublimate, aconite, belladonna, iodine, digitalis, opium, hyoscyamus, etc. Homœopathy cannot employ stronger substances, for there are none stronger. Now, when ordinary physicians employ them, they evidently vie with one another who shall prescribe the largest possible doses of these drugs, and even make a great boast of their mounting to such enormous doses. This practice they laud and approve in their fellow practitioners. But if the Homœopathic medical art employ the *same drugs*, not at random, like the ordinary method, but after careful investigation, only in suitable cases and in the smallest possible doses, it is denounced as a practice of poisoning. How partisan, how unjust, how calumnious is such a charge made by men who make pretensions to honesty and uprightness!

If Homœopathy now make a fuller explanation, if she condemn (as from conviction she must) the enormous doses of these drugs given in ordinary practice, and if she, relying on careful trials, insists that very much less of them should be given for a dose, that where ordinary physicians give a tenth, a half, a whole grain, and even several grains, often only a quadrillionth, a sextillionth, a decillionth of a grain is required and sufficient, then the adherents of the ordinary school, who denounce the Homœopathic healing art as a system of poisoning, laugh aloud, abuse it as childishness, and declare themselves convinced (convinced without trial?) that *such a small quantity* can do nothing at all, and can have no effect whatever, is, indeed, *just the same as nothing*. They are not ashamed thus to blow hot and cold from the same mouth, and to pronounce the very same thing to be inert and ludicrously small, which they had just accused of being a system of poisoning, whilst they justify and praise their own enormous and murderous doses of the same remedies. Is not this the grossest and most wretched inconsistency that can be imagined, invented for the very purpose of being shamelessly unjust toward a doctrine which, they cannot deny, possesses truth, consistence and agreement with experience, and which practices the most delicate cautiousness and the most unwearied circumspection in the selection and administration of its remedies?

Not very long ago a highly celebrated physician* spoke of pounds of opium being eaten every month in his hospital, where even the

*MARCUS, of Bamberg.

nurses were allowed to give it to the patients according to their fancy. Opium, mind! a drug that has sent several thousands of men to their graves in ordinary practice! Yet this man continued to be held in honor, for he belonged to the dominant clique to which everything is lawful even if it be of the most destructive and absurd character. And when, a few years since, in one of the most enlightened cities* of Europe almost every practitioner, from the physician of lofty title down to the barber's apprentice, prescribed arsenic as a fashionable remedy in almost every disease, and that in such frequent and large doses in close succession, that the detriment to the health of the people must have been quite palpable, yet this was held to be an honorable practice, though not one of them was acquainted with the peculiar effects of the semi-oxide of this metal (and consequently knew not what cases of disease it was suited for). And yet all prescribed it in repeated doses, *a single one of which, sufficiently attenuated and potentized, would have sufficed to cure all the diseases in the whole habitable world for which this drug is the suitable remedy.* Which of these two oppsite modes of employing medicines best deserves the flattering appellation of a "system of poisoning"—the ordinary method just alluded to, which attacks with tenths of grains the poor patients (who often require some quite different remedy), or Homœopathy, which does not even give a little drop of tincture of rhubarb without having first ascertained whether rhubarb is the most suitable, the only appropriate remedy for the case. Homœopathy which, by unwearied, multiplied experiments, discovered that it is only in rare cases that more than a decillionth of a grain of arsenic should be given, and that only in cases where careful proving shows this medicine to be the only one perfectly suitable? To which of these two modes of practice does then the honorary title of "thoughtless, rash system of poisoning" properly apply?

* * * * * * * *

There is yet another sect of practitioners who may be called hypocritical purists. If they are practical physicians, they, indeed, prescribe all sorts of substances that are injurious when misused, but before the world they wish to pose as patterns of innocence and caution. From their professional chairs and in their writings they give us the most alarming definition of poison; to listen to their declarations it would appear unadvisable to treat any imaginable disease with anything stronger than quick-grass, dandelion, oxymel and raspberry juice. According to their definition, poisons are abso-

*On how high a stage of lack of art must the medical art of our whole continent be, when in a city *like Berlin* they are as yet in such a state, which city nevertheless has hardly an equal in all other departments of human knowledge!

lutely (*i. e.*, under all circumstances, in all doses, in all cases) prejudicial to human life, and in this category they include (in order to prejudice against Homœopathy), as suits their humor, a lot of substances which in all ages have been extensively employed by physicians for the cure of diseases. But the employment of these substances would be a criminal offence had not *every one* of them occasionally proved of use. If, however, each of them had only proved itself curative on only one occasion—and it cannot be denied that this sometimes happened—then this blasphemous definition is at the same time a palpable absurdity. Absolutely and under all circumstances injurious and destructive, and yet at the same time salutary, is a contradiction in itself, is utter nonsense. If they would wriggle out of this contradiction, they allege, as a subterfuge, that these substances have more frequently proved injurious than useful. But did the more frequent injury caused by these substances come from these substances themselves, or from their improper employment, *i. e.*, from those who made an unskillful use of them in diseases for which they were not suitable? These medicines do not administer themselves in diseases, they must be administered by men; and if they were beneficial at any time, it was because they were at one time appropriately administered by somebody; it was because they might always be beneficial, if men never made any other than a suitable use of them. Hence it follows that whenever these substances were hurtful and destructive they were so merely on account of having been inappropriately employed. Therefore all the injury is attributable to the unskillfulness of their employers.

These narrow-minded individuals further said: "Even when we attempt to tame arsenic by means of a corrective, *e.g.*, by mixing it with an alkali, it still often enough does harm."

Nay, I reply, the arsenic must not be blamed for this; for, as I before observed, drugs do not administer themselves, somebody administers them and does harm with them. And what can the alkali do as a corrective? Is it merely intended to weaken the arsenic, or to change its character and convert it into something else? In the latter case the neutral arsenical salt produced is no longer arsenic proper, but something different. If, however, it be merely made weaker, then surely a simple diminution of the dose of the pure solution of arsenic would be a much more rational and effectual mode of making it weaker and milder, than leaving the dose in its hurtful magnitude and by the addition of another medicinal substance endeavoring to effect some, nobody knows what, alteration in its nature, as takes place when a pretended corrective is used. If you think one-tenth of a grain of arsenic too strong, what is to prevent you from diluting the solution and giving less, a great deal less, of it?

"A tenth of a grain," I hear some one say, ' is the smallest quantity the etiquette of the profession allows us to prescribe. Who could write a prescription to be made up at the apothecary's for a smaller quantity without making himself ridiculous?"

So, indeed! a tenth of a grain sometimes acts so violently as to endanger life, and the etiquette of your guild does not allow you to give less, very much less. Is it not an insult to common sense to talk in this way? Is the etiquette of the profession a code of rules to bind a set of slaves without rationality, or is it the rule among men having a free will and intelligence? If it is the latter, who hinders them from giving a *smaller quantity* where a greater might be injurious? Obstinacy? the dogmatism of a school? or what other dungeon of the intellect?

"Arsenic," "they protest, would still be hurtful, though given in a smaller quantity, even if we should be willing to descend to the ridiculous dose of a hundredth or of a thousandth of a grain, a minuteness of dose unheard of in the posologics of our materia medica. Even a thousandth of a grain of arsenic must still be hurtful and destructive, for it remains an uncontrollable poison, as we suppose, affirm, conjecture and assert."

Even if this convenient asserting and conjecturing should here for once have blundered upon the truth, still it is evident that the virulence of the arsenic cannot increase but must decrease with every further reduction of the dose, so that we must at length arrive at such a dilution of the solution and such a diminution of the dose as no longer in any way possesses the dangerous character of your regulation dose of one-tenth of a grain.

"Such a dose would, indeed, be a novelty! What kind of a dose would it be?" Novelty is indeed a capital crime in the eyes of the orthodox school, settled down upon her old lees, a school which subjects its reason to the tyranny of hoary routine.

But what pitiful rule should hinder the physician, who ought by rights to be a learned, thinking, independent man, a ruler of nature in his own domain—what in the world should hinder him from moderating a dangerous dose by diminishing its size?

What should hinder him, if experience should show him that the thousandth part of a grain is yet too strong a dose, from giving the hundred-thousandth part, or the millionth part of a grain? And should he find this last too violent in many cases, *since in medicine all depends on observation and experience* (as medicine itself is nothing but a science of experience), what should hinder him from reducing the millionth to a billionth? And if also this prove too strong a dose in many cases, who could prevent him from diminishing it to the quadrillionth of a grain, or a smaller dose still? Methinks I hear vulgar stolidity croak out from the quagmire of its thousand-year-old prejudices: Ha! ha! ha! A quadrillionth! Why that's nothing at all!

Why *not?* Can the subdivision of a substance, be it carried ever so far, bring forth anything else than parts of the whole? Must not these portions, reduced in size to the very verge of infinity, still continue to be *something*—something substantial, a part of the whole, be it ever so minute? What man of sound reason could contradict this?

And if this (quadrillionth, quintillionth, octillionth, decillionth) continue still to be really an integral portion of the divided substance, as no rational man can deny, why should even so minute a portion, seeing that it is really *something*, be unable to do *anything*, considering that the whole was so tremendously powerful? But *what* and *how much* this small part can do, can be determined by no speculative reason or unreason, but *experience alone must determine* this, and *in the domain of facts there is no appeal from experience.* It belongs to experience alone to determine if this small portion has become too weak to avail anything against diseases, too weak to remove the disease for which this medicine is in general suitable, and to restore the patient to health. This is a matter to be settled not by the dictatorial dictum from the study, but by experience *alone*, which in this case is the only competent arbiter. But experience has already decided this question and continues to do so daily before the eyes of every unprejudiced person.

But when I have done with the wiseacre, who ridicules the small doses of Homœopathy as a nonentity, as effecting nothing, and who never consults experience, I hear on the other side the hypocritical stickler for caution, with as little investigation and with the same recklessness, still inveigh against the danger of even the small doses used in homœopathic practice.

A few words then shall be added here for him.

If arsenic in the dose of a tenth of a grain be, in many cases, a dangerous dose, must it not become milder in the dose of a thousandth of a grain? And, if so, must it not become still milder with every further diminution of dose?

Now if arsenic (like every other very powerful medicinal substance) can, by merely diminishing its dose, be rendered so mild as to be no longer dangerous to life, then all we have to do is merely to find by experiment how far the size of the dose must be diminished so that it shall be small enough to do no harm, and yet large enough to fully effect its office as a remedy of the diseases for which it is suitable.

Experience, and experience alone, not the pedantry of the study, not the narrow-minded, ignorant dogmatism of the schools, which does not prove anything practically, can decide what dose, of such an extremely powerful substance as arsenic, is so small that it can be taken without danger, and yet remains so powerful as to be able to effect all that this medicine (so invaluable when sufficiently moderated in its action and selected for a suitable case of disease) was from its nature ordained to do by the beneficent Creator. It must, by dilution of its solution and diminution of the dose, be rendered so mild that the strongest man can be freed by such a dose from a disease for which it is the appropriate remedy, while this same dose will be incapable of altering perceptibly the health of a healthy infant.* This is the grand problem that can only be solved by thousandfold experiments and trials, but not settled by the sophistical dogmatism of the schools with its guessing, its assertions and its conjectures.

No rational physician can acknowledge any such limitation to his treatment as would be dictated to him by the rusty routine of the schools, which is never guided by pure experiment combined with reflection. His sphere of action is the restoration to health of the sick, and the countless forces of nature are given to him unreservedly by the Sustainer of Life as implements of healing; nothing being excluded. To him whose calling it is to vanquish the disease that brings its victim to the verge of corporeal annihilation and effect a kind of recreation of life (a nobler work than most other, even those most vaunted of mankind), to him the whole broad expanse of nature with all her creative powers and substances must be available in order to enable him to perform this curative act, if we may so call it. But he must be at liberty to employ these agents in the exact quantity, be it ever so small or ever so large, that experience and trials show him to be most adapted to the end he has in view; in any form

---

* A medicine homœopathically chosen, *i. e.*, a medicine capable of producing a morbid condition very similar to the disease to be cured, touches only the diseased side of the organism, therefore just the most excited, extremely sensitive part of it. Therefore its dose must be so small as only to affect the diseased part just a little more than the disease itself did. For this the smallest dose suffices, one so small as to be incapable of altering the health of a healthy person, who has not such points of contact sufficiently sensitive for this medicine, or of making him ill, which only large doses of medicine can do. See *Organon of Medicine*, § 277–279, and *Spirit of the Homœopathic Medical Doctrine* at the beginning of the *Materia Medica Pura*.

whatever that reflection and experience have proved to be most valuable. All this he must be able to do without any limitation whatsoever, as is the right of a free man, of a deliverer of his fellow creatures, and a restorer of life, equipped with all the knowledge pertaining to his art and endowed with a god-like spirit and the tenderest conscience.

From this God-serving and noblest of earthly occupations let all hold aloof who are deficient in mind, in the judicial spirit, in any of the branches of knowledge required for its exercise, or in tender regard for the weal of mankind and a sense of their duty to humanity; in one word, who are deficient in true virtue! Away with that unhallowed crew who merely assume the outward semblance of health-restorers, but whose heads are full of vain deceit, whose hearts are stuffed with wicked frivolity, whose tongues make a mock of truth and whose hands prepare disaster.

The following observations are the result of doses of various strength on persons of various sensitiveness:

An intelligent homœopathic physician will not give this medicine, even in its minimum dose, before he is convinced that its peculiar symptoms have the greatest possible similarity with those of the disease to be healed. But if this is the case it will surely cure.

But if in any case, from human fallibility, he should not have made his selection appropriately, smelling once or several times of Ipecacuanha, or Hepar sulphuris calcareum, or Nux vomica, according to the circumstances, will remove the ill effects.

Such a use of arsenic has shown its curative powers in numberless acute and chronic (psoric) diseases, and has then also at the same time healed the following symptoms if present:

Fits of constriction of the chest, at night, driving the patient out of bed; fear of death; peevishness; heaviness in the forehead (Hg.); headache after dinner; scurf on the hairy scalp (Hg.); *inflammation of the eyes and lids;* drawing and stitches in the face here and there; ulcers like warts on the cheek (Hg.); tumor-like swelling in the nose (Hg.); eruptions on the lips; bleeding of the gums; fetid odor from the mouth; vomiting of brownish matter, with violent colic; *vomiting after every meal;* pressure in the stomach; *burning pain in the stomach and the scrobiculus cordis;* induration of the liver; *burning in the intestines;* abdominal dropsy; ulcer above the umbilicus; swelling of the inguinal glands; burning evacuations, with violent colic; green, diarrhœic stools; constipation; paralysis of the bladder; dysuria; strangury; swelling of the genitals; menses too copious, ailments of various kinds during menstruation; acrid, corrosive discharge from the vagina; stoppage of the nose; coughing of blood;

suffocative fits, in the evening after lying down; tightness of the chest, on ascending an eminence; angina pectoris; stitches in the sternum; pressure in the sternum; drawing and tearing, at night, from the elbow to the shoulder; whitlows on the tips of the fingers, with burning pains (Hg.); tearing and stitches in the hip, the thigh and the groin; tearing in the tibia; pain as of a bruise in the knee-joint; itching herpes in the hough; old sores on the legs, with burning and stitches; weariness of the feet; ulcers in the soles of the feet (Hg.); *ulcers, with corrosive blisters on the soles of the feet and toes* (Hg.); pains as from soreness on the balls of the toes, as if rubbed open from walking; varicose and swelled veins; *burning of the skin* (Hg.); *burning pain in the ulcers;* drowsiness in the evening; at night, slow in going to sleep again, after waking up; *quotidian and intermittent fever;* shivering in the evening, with twisting of the limbs and anxious restlessness.

The abbreviations of the names of my fellow-provers are: *Bhr.*, *Baehr; Fr. H.*, *Friedrich Hahnemann; Htb. u. Tr.*, *Hartlaub u. Trinks; Hg.*, *Hering; Hbg.*, *Hornburg; Lgh.*, *Langhammer; Mr.*, *Meyer; Stf.*, *Stapf.*

ARSENICUM.

Sadness and gloominess.

Melancholy, sad mood, after a meal, with headache (aft. 80 h.).

Sad, sorrowful ideas, in the evening in bed, as if some misfortune might have happened to one's relatives.

Religious melancholy and reserve. [EBERS, in *Hufeland's Jour.*, 1813, Oct., p. 8.[1]]

5. He wept and howled, and spoke but little and briefly. [*Stf.*]

Piercing wailings, interrupted by fainting fits coming on. [FRIEDERICH, in *Hufeland's Jour.*, V., p. 172.[2]]

Piteous wailings, that a most violent constriction of the chest was taking away his breath, attended with an extremely disagreeable sensation in the abdomen; this compelled him to double up,

The inclusion of Arsenic among the antipsorics seems to have been an afterthought, as it comes in the original German edition, at the end of the alphabetical list of medicines, instead of appearing in its proper place—to which in this translation it has been restored. Its pathogenesis had already appeared in the *Materia Medica Pura*, where it contains 1,079 symptoms, of which 697 are from Hahnemann himself and seven fellow-observers, and 382 from authors. Of the two additional contributors mentioned here, "Hartlaub u. Trinks," stand for some cases of poisoning, the symptoms of which they had extracted, in the first and third volumes of their *Arzneimittellehre;* and "Hering," for a number of aggravatious and medicinal symptoms occurring in leprous patients taking the drug (*Archiv.*, XI., 2, 19). These account for 112 out of the 202 additional symptoms recorded here; the remainder are Hahnemann's, obtained in his later manner, and Wahle's (eighteen in all)—a prover unnoticed in the preface, but whose name frequently occurs among the second series of the Master's followers.—*Hughes.*

[1] Eber's observations are to be found in part 3, p. 46, and part 4, p. 3, of this volume. Effects of arsenite of potash in ague patients. This symptom not found.—*Hughes.*

[2] Poisoning of a woman. For p. 172, read part I., p. 149.—*Hughes.*

rolling here and there, then again to rise up and walk about. [MORGAGNI, *de sed. et caus. morb.*, LIX.[1]]

Fits of anguish for a long time. [TIM. A. GUELDENKLEE, *Opp.*, p. 280.[2]]

Anxiety and restlessness in the whole body (aft. 1 h.). [RICHARD, in *Schenk, lib.*, VII., *obs.* 211.[3]]

10. Anxious and trembling, he is afraid of himself, that he might not be able to restrain himself from killing someone with a knife. [MARCUS, *Ephem. d. Heilkunst, Heft.*, III.[4]]

Anxiety and heat, not allowing her to go to sleep before midnight, for many days.

Anxiety in the evening, after lying down and after midnight, at 3 o'clock, after awaking.

Severe anxiety, at night about 3 o'clock, she sometimes felt hot, then again like vomiting.

Anxiety, anguish. [MYRRHEN, *Misc. Nat. Cur.—Neue med. chir.*, *Wahrnehm*, Vol. I., 1778.—QUELMALZ, *Commerc. lit.* 1737.[5]]

15. Excessive anguish. [KAISER, in *Hb. u. Tr. Arzneimittellehre.*[6]]

The most intolerable anguish. [FORESTUS *lib.*, 17, *obs.*, 13.[7]]

Great anguish with constriction of the chest and difficult respiration. [KAISER, l. c.]

Internal anguish. [KAISER, l. c.]

Mortal anguish. [HENNING in *Hufeland's Journ.* X., 2.[8]]

20. Continual anguish, like remorse of conscience, as if he had acted in violation of his duty, without knowing in what particular.

Anguish of heart, interrupted by fainting fits coming on. [FRIEDRICH, l. c.]

Anguish and anxiety, so that he repeatedly fell into a swoon. BERNH. VERZASCH. (*Obs. med. obs.* 66.[9]]

Anguish, trembling and quivering, with cold perspiration in the face. [ALBERTI, *jurisprud. med. Tom.* II., p. 257.[10]]

Great anguish, trembling and quivering with severe tearing in the abdomen. [ALBERTI, l. c.]

25. With inexpressible anguish, he seemed on account of his increasing pains to lie at the point of death. [MORGAGNI, l. c.]

With great anguish, he rolls and tosses about in the bed. [GUELDENKLEE, ibid. BUETTNER, *Unterr. ueb. d. Toedl. d. Wund.*[11]]

He can find no rest in any place, continually changes his position, wishes to get from one bed into another and to lie, now here, now there.

---

1 Poisoning of adults. For "LIX." read Book IV., Ep. 59, §§ 3, 5, 6, 7, 8.

2 From the vapor.—*Hughes.*

3 Poisoning of adult. For obs. 211 read "*De Arsenico*," C. 4.—*Hughes.*

4 Symptoms observed in a fever patient after taking arsenite of potash. *Hughes.*

5 (To *Myrrhen* note.) From drawing solution of A. into nostrils for coryza; add *Dec.* 3, *ann.* 9, 10, C. 220. (To *Neue Med.*, etc.) Not accessible. (To *Quelmalz.*) Poisoning of girl by black oxide.—*Hughes.*

6 Poisoning of a whole family by Ars.—*Hughes.*

7 Poisoning of a woman by orpiment. This symptom is not found.—*Hughes.*

8 From application of Ars. to a diseased breast. With vomiting. Add p. 143.—*Hughes.*

9 Not accessible.—*Hughes.*

10 Poisoning of adults.—*Hughes.*

11 (For BUETTNER.) Poisonings. Add p. 179.—*Hughes.*

Restlessness, he desires to get from one bed into another. [MYRRHEN, l. c.]

Restlessness and tossing about in bed with sadness and unquenchable thirst (aft. 24 h.). [BUETTNER, l. c.]

30. Restlessness with pains in the head, in the belly and in the knees. [RICHARD, l. c.]

Full of restlessness, the child is cross and wimpers.

Restlessness, and hypochondriac anxiety as from constant sitting in a room, as if from the upper part of the chest, without palpitation (at once.)

Anguish and fear; he sees an acquaintance who is not present lie dead on the sofa, and is much afraid of him. [*Whl.*]

He sees nothing but worms and bugs crawling about on his bed, from which he desires to run away, and of which he throws out whole hands full. [*Whl.*]

35. He sees nothing but rogues in his room, and therefore always creeps under the bed. [*Whl.*]

His whole house, also under his bed, is full of rogues, which causes a cold sweat to break out, which runs down cold over his body. [*Whl.*]

In the night he runs all about the house, looking for thieves. [*Whl.*]

The greatest fear and anguish; night and day he sees ghosts.

He jumps out of bed for fear, and hides away in a wardrobe, from which he can only be gotten out with difficulty. [*Whl.*]

40. Lack of determination; he desires something, and when the endeavor is made to fulfill his desire, the merest trifle will change his determination, and then he is not willing to have it so.

Great seriousness.

When he is alone he falls into thoughts about disease and other things, from which he can not easily tear himself away.

He despairs of his life. [RICHARD, l. c.[1]]

Desponding and weeping, he thinks that nothing can help him, and he would have to die anyhow; at the same time he is cold and chilly with subsequent general weariness.

45. Super-sensitiveness and over-tenderness of mind; dejected, sad and lugubrious, she is troubled and solicitous about the merest trifles.

Very sensitive to noise.

Inclined to be frightened.

Weak in body and soul, he cannot talk, without exhibiting peevishness.

Little talking, but complains of anguish. [ALBERTI, l. c.]

50. Uncomfortable, he has no pleasure in anything.

Impatient and anxious.

Dissatisfied all day and extremely vexed at himself; he thought he had not worked enough and reproached himself most bitterly. [*Lgh.*]

Ill-humor alternating with gentle kindliness; in her ill-humor she will not look at anybody, nor listen to anything; at times also she weeps.

---

[1] Not found.—*Hughes.*

Ill-humor in the morning in bed; he pushes the pillows about in dissatisfaction, throws off the coverlet, uncovers himself, looks at no one, listens to nothing.

55. Vexed about trifles.

He is vexed at every trifle, and cannot stop talking about the faults of others.

Very peevish and dissatisfied with everything, she finds fault with everything; everything seems to her too strong and loud, all talk, every noise, all light.

Very peevish and sensitive; the least thing insults him and angers him. [*Lgh.*]

Very peevish and passionate, capricious, she takes every word ill and is cross when she has to answer.

60. Inclined to sarcastic mocking.

She became violently enraged when she was forced to eat something, while she had no appetite at all.

Her desires exceed her wants; she eats and drinks more than agrees with her; she walks farther than is necessary and is good for her.

Great indifference and lack of sympathy.

Indifference to life. [KAISER, l. c.]

65. Life seems indifferent to him, he sets no value on it.

Calm equanimity; careless about their approaching death, they neither hope nor wish to recover. (After-effects, with two suicides, who had taken arsenic.)

Calmness of soul (in a despondent, melancholy woman). [LABORDE, *journ. de Méd.*, LXX., p. 89.[1]]

Of a calm, firm mind; he retained his equanimity in all events that happened. [*Lgh.*]

Cheerful disposition; he likes to converse with others. [*Lgh.*]

70. More inclined to cheerfulness, and disposed to occupy himself. [*Lgh.*]

During the first minutes great tranquility of soul and serenity; but after half an hour excessive restlessness and anxiety; he imagined that the effects of the poison would be dreadful and desires to remain alive (in a despondent suicide). [*Stf.*]

Diminution of memory.

Very faulty memory, for a long time. [MYRRHEN, l. c.]

Forgetfulness, his memory fails him.

75. Stupid and weak in the head, about noon.

Stupid and dizzy in the head, so that he could not think. [*Mr.*]

Stupid and confused feeling in the head, as from severe coryza and vexation; the head feels like a lantern.

Stupid feeling in the head, as if he had not slept enough; from 11 A. M. to 6 P. M.

Dullness in the head, without pain.

80 Weakness of the reason. [EBERS, l. c.[2]]

Chronic weakness of mind. [EBERS, l. c[3].]

---

[1] **A woman took Ars. with a suicidal purpose. The calmness was rather mental, owing to her determination, than physical.—*Hughes*.**

[2] **Result of suppression of ague by Ars.—*Hughes*.**

[3] **Doubtful how much is ague, and how much Ars.—*Hughes*.**

Delirium. [KAISER, l. c.]

Fantastic delirium, returning from time to time. [GUILBERT, *Med. chir. Wahrnehm*, Vol. II., *Altenb.*[1]]

Crowding in of various ideas, which he is too weak to keep off so as to occupy himself with a single one.

85. The organs of sense are morbidly active. [KAISER, l. c.]

Absence of reason and of the internal and external senses; he did not see, for many days he did not speak, he heard and understood nothing; when anyone cried very loudly into his ears, he would look at those present like a drunken person awakened from a deep sleep. [MYRRHEN, l. c.]

She lay in her bed perfectly senseless, muttered unintelligible sounds, with her eyes staring, cold perspiration on her forehead; trembling in her whole body; small, hard and quick pulse. [EBERS, l. c.]

Consciousness disappears or becomes indistinct. [KAISER, l. c.]

Loss of sensation and consciousness, so that he knew not what happened to him. [PYL, *Samml.* VIII., p. 98 sq.[2]]

90. Loss of consciousness and speech. [*Misc. N. C.*, Dec. III., *an.* 9, 10, p. 390.[3]]

Ideas straying, while the open eyes are without consciousness of phantasies, either before or afterwards.

Insanity; first headache, excessive anguish, noise before the ears, as of many large bells, and when he opened his eyes, he always saw a man who sometime before had hanged himself in the garret of the house, and who incessantly motioned to him entreatingly that he should cut him down; he ran there with a knife, but as he could not cut him down, he grew desperate and wished to hang himself; being hindered in this, he became so restless that he could hardly be kept in bed; he lost his speech, though with full understanding, and when he wished to express himself by writing, he could only make unintelligible marks, whereat he trembled, wept, and with the forehead covered with the sweat of anguish, knelt down and raised his hands entreatingly. [EBERS, l. c.]

Frenzy; he has to be handcuffed and seeks to escape. [AMATUS LUSITANUS, *Curationes*, Cent II., Cur. 65.[4]]

Numb feeling of the head. [PEARSON, in *Samml. br. Abhandl. f. prakt. Aerzte*, XIII., 4.[5]]

95. The head is strongly muddled, in the evening (3d d.).

Weakness in the head, from much pain, with weakness and qualmishness in the scrobiculus cordis, so severe that she was really ill.

Dizzy in the head when walking in the open air, aggravated on re-entering the room (aft. ½ h.).

Numb feeling in the head. [BUCHHOLZ, *Beitr. z. ger. Arzneik*, IV., 164.[6]]

---

[1] Poisoning of adult.—*Hughes.*
[2] Poisoning of adult.—*Hughes.*
[3] Same case as Myrrhen's (Sympt. 14).—*Hughes.*
[4] Poisoning of a youth. This symptom not found.—*Hughes.*
[5] Effects of arsenite of potash in an epileptic.—*Hughes.*
[6] Poisoning of adults with black oxide. After antidote.—*Hughes.*

Silly in the head, after sleeping.

100. Confused feeling in the head. [*Hbg.*]

Stupefaction in the head as from precipitate haste in performing an excessive amount of work, with internal restlessness (aft. 2 d.).

Stupefaction, with loss of sensation and vertigo. [EBERS, l. c.[1]]

Sensation of reeling in the head. [ALBERTI, l. c.]

Reeling, stupid and dizzy in the head, while taking a walk, most of all in the forehead, as if intoxicated, so as to stagger now to this side, now to that, and every moment was afraid of falling (aft. 9½ h.). [*Lgh.*]

105. Vertigo. [KAISER, l. c.; THOMSON, *Edinb. Vers.*, IV.; SENNERT, *Prat. med. lib.*, 6, p. 6.[2]]

Vertigo when sitting.

Vertigo only when walking, as if he would fall to the right side. [*Lgh.*]

Vertigo every evening; she has to hold on to something when she shuts her eyes.

Vertigo, with obscuration of vision. [MYRRHEN, l. c.]

110. Vertigo, with loss of thoughts when rising. [*Stf.*]

Violent vertigo, with nausea, when lying down; he has to sit up to diminish it. [*Stf.*]

Vertigo, with headache. [KAISER, l. c.]

Pains in the head. [GRIMM, *Misc. N. C.*, Dec. III., ann. 7, 8.[3]]

Pains in the head and vertigo for several days. [G. W. WEDEL, *Diss. de Arsen. Jen.*, 1719, p. 10.[4]]

115. Headache of excessive severity. [JOH. JACOBI and RAU, *Acta N. C.*; KNAPE, *Annal. der Staats-Arzneikunde*, I., 1.[5]]

Headache in the occiput.

Semilateral headache. [KNAPE, l. c.]

Headache, for several days, immediately relieved by applying cold water, but on removing it is much worse than before.

Headache above the left eye, very severe in the evening and at night. [*Hg.*]

120. Periodic headache. [TH. RAU, l. c.]

Stupefying, pressive headache, especially in the forehead, in every position. [*Lgh.*]

Stupefying, pressive headache, especially on the right side of the forehead, just above the right eyebrow, paining as if sore on wrinkling his forehead. [*Lgh.*]

Stupefying, pressive headache, chiefly on the forehead, with fine stitches on the left temporal region, near the outer canthus, when walking and standing, passing off when sitting (aft. 2½ h.). [*Lgh.*]

---

[1] Not found.—*Hughes.*

[2] (For THOMSON) Poisoning of a woman. (For SENNERT) From inhaling realgar.—*Hughes.*

[3] From black oxide, in an adult. Add *ann.*, 7, 8.—*Hughes.*

[4] Not accessible.—*Hughes.*

[5] (For JACOBI) From suppression of ague by Ars. in a young man. (For RAU) From application of Ars. to scalp. (For KNAPE) From powdering hair with Ars.—*Hughes.*

Pain, as from a bruise, on one side of the head, in the morning immediately on rising from bed (aft. 12 h.).

125. Sensation as if beaten on the front of the head.

Pain in the forehead and above the nose, as from a bruise or sore, going off for short time by rubbing.

Heavy and confused sensation in the head, so that he cannot easily rise; he has to lie down.

Great heaviness in the head, especially when standing and sitting. [BUCHHOLZ, l. c.[1]]

Great heaviness in the head, with roaring in the ears; it goes off in the open air, **but at once returns when coming again into the room** (aft. 16 h.).

130. Excessive heaviness of the head, as if the brain was pressed down by a load, with roaring in the ears, in the morning after rising from bed (aft. 24 h.).

Heaviness of the head with pressive pain, in the morning (aft. 72 h.).

Pressive pain in the right temporal region, in all positions (aft. 3 h.). [*Lgh.*]

Pressive, drawing pain in the right side of the forehead (aft. 2¾ h.). [*Lgh.*]

Pressive, stitch-like pain in the left temple, not passing off by touching (aft. 2½ h.). [*Lgh.*]

135. Tension in the head; headache, as if stretched.

Pinching headache above the eyes, soon passing away.

Drawing headache under the coronal suture, for several hours every afternoon.

Tearing pains in the occiput. [*Bhr.*]

Tearing in the head and at the same time in the right eye.

140. Headache, composed of tearing and heaviness, with drowsy weariness during the day. [aft. 4 d.).

Tearing stitches in the left temple.

Stitch-like pain in the left temple, which ceased on touching part. [*Lgh.*]

Throbbing headache in the forehead, just above the root of the nose.

Violently throbbing headache in the forehead, on motion. [*Stf.*]

145. Violently throbbing headache in the whole head, especially in the forehead, with nausea on raising himself in bed. [*Stf.*]

Sharp, hard throbbing, like chopping, in the whole head, as if it would drive her skull apart, at night (about 2 A. M.), with an outbreak of perspiration.

Hammering, like blows of a hammer in the temples, very painful, at noon and at midnight for half hour, after which for a couple of hours she feels paralyzed in the body.

Dull throbbing headache in one half of the head, extending to above the eyes.

On motion, a sensation as if the brain was moving and beat against the skull.

---

[1] As sympt. 98.—*Hughes.*

150. On motion of the head, the brain feels as if shaking about, with pressure on it, in walking. [*Whl.*]

Clicking sensation in the head, over the ear, when walking.

The skin of the head pains when touched as if festering.

Painfulness of the hair on being touched.

Falling out of the hair of the head. [BAYLIES *in Samml. br. Abhandl. fuer pr. Aerzte*, VII., 2, p. 110.[1]]

155. Pains as from a bruise on the external head, aggravated when touched.

Contractive pain in the head.

Formication on the integument of the occiput, as if the roots of the hairs moved.

Burning pain on the hairy scalp. [KNAPE, l. c.[2]]

Swelling of the head. [HEIMREICH in *Act. N. C.* II., *obs.* 10.[3]]

160. Swelling of the whole head. [QUELMALZ, l. c.]

Swelling of the head and face. [SIEBOLD in *Hufel. Journ.* IV., part I., p. 3.[4]]

Extraordinary swelling of the head and face. [KNAPE, l. c.]

Swelling of the skin of the head, the face, the eyes, the neck and the chest, with natural color. [KNAPE, l. c.]

Itching gnawing on the head. [KNAPE, l. c.]

165. Gnawing itching on the whole head, inciting to scratch. [*Lgh.*]

Burning itching on the hairy scalp. [KNAPE, l. c.]

Painful itching like ulceration, inciting to scratching on the whole hairy scalp, which pains all over, but chiefly on the occiput, as if from suffused blood (aft. 7 h.). [*Lgh.*]

A pimple covered with scurf on the left side of the hairy scalp, inciting to scratching, and painful when rubbing as if festering underneath (aft. 2 h.). [*Lgh.*]

Eruptive pimples on the whole hairy scalp, which pain, on rubbing and touching, as if festering below, or as if suffused with blood (aft. 11 h.). [*Lgh.*]

170. Innumerable pimples, very red, upon the hairy scalp. [VICAT, l. c.[5]]

Eruption of pustules with burning pain, on the hairy scalp and in the face. [HEIMREICH, l. c.]

Pimples on the left temple, inciting to scratching, and discharging bloody water, and, after rubbing, pain as if sore. [*Lgh.*]

Two large pimples on the forehead between the eyebrows, inciting to scratching, discharging bloody water, and filled next day with pus. [*Lgh.*]

Corrosive ulcers on the hairy scalp. [KNAPE, l. c.]

175. Ulcerous scab, a finger's breadth in thickness, on the hairy scalp, falling off a few weeks later. [HEINREICH, l. c.]

Ulcerous scab, on the hairy scalp, to the middle of the forehead. [KNAPE, l. c.]

---

[1] **General statement from authors.—*Hughes.***
[2] **Effect of Ars. sprinkled on hair.—*Hughes.***
[3] **Should be "of the veins." It occurred after violent vomiting.—*Hughes.***
[4] **Effect of dressing pustular scalp with mixture of Ars. and cinnabar.—*Hughes.***
[5] **From powdering hair with Ars.—*Hughes.***

The right eye pained deep internally, with violent stitches in turning it, so that she could hardly turn her eye.

Pressive pain above the left eyelid and in the upper half of the eyeball, aggravated on looking upward.

Pressive pain under the right eye, continuing for hours, at night, so that she could not stay in bed for distress.

180. Pressure in the left eye, as if sand had got into it (aft. 2 h.). [*Lgh.*]

Drawing pain in the eyes, and quivering in the lids.

Twitching in the left eye.

Tearing in the eye, at intervals. [SCHLEGEL, in *Hb. u Tr.*[1]]

Throbbing, like pulsation, in the eyes, and at every throb a stitch, after midnight.

185. Itching about the eyes and the temple, as if picked with innumerable red-hot needles.

Smarting, corrosive itching in both eyes, compelling to scratch (aft. 3 h.). [*Lgh.*]

Burning on the edge of the upper eyelids.

Burning in the eyes.

Burning in the eyes, the nose, the mouth. [*N. med. chir. Wahrnehm.*, l. c.]

190. Red, inflamed eyes. [*N. med chir. Wahrn.*, l. c.]

Inflammation of the conjunctiva. [KAISER, l. c.]

Inflammation of the eyes. [HEUN, *allgem. med. Annalen*, 1805, Febr.[2]]

Violent inflammation of the eyes. [GUILBERT, l. c.[3]]

Swelling of the eyes. [QUELMALZ, l. c.[4]]

195. Swelling of the eyelids. [*N. med. chir. W.*, l. c.]

Œdematous swelling of the eyelids, without pains. [*Whl.*]

Swelling, first of the upper, then of the lower left eyelid, then of the forehead, the head and the neck, without pain or secretion of mucus; the swelling of the head and of the neck reached an enormous size. [*Whl.*]

Swollen eyes and lips. [KNAPE, l. c.]

Painless swelling under the left eye, which partly closes the eye, and is very soft (aft. 5 d.). [*Fr.*, *H.*]

200. Yellowness of the eyes, as in jaundice.

Yellow white of the eyes, as in a person having jaundice. [*Whl.*]

Tired look of the eyes. [KAISER, l. c.]

Dryness of the eyelids, as if they rubbed on the eyes, in reading by candle-light.

The edges of the eyelids pain on motion, as if they were dry, and rubbed upon the eyeballs, as well in the open air, as in the room.

205. Watering of the eyes. [GUILBERT, l. c.]

Constant, severe lachrymation of the right eye, for eight days (aft. 2 d.). [*Fr.*, *H.*]

---

[1] From the vapor, mingled with that of tobacco.—*Hughes.*

[2] From application of Ars. to cancerous ulcer of the cheek.—*Hughes.*

[3] Frequently recurring.—*Hughes.*

[4] As in symp. 160.—*Hughes.*

Acrid tears, making the cheeks sore. [GUILBERT, l. c.[1]]

Watering and itching **of the eyes**, some pus in them in the morning. [*Fr.*, *H.*]

Eyelids glued together in the morning.

210. The outer canthi are glued together by eyegum, in the morning. [*Whl.*]

Constant quivering of the upper eyelids, with tears in the eyes.

The (œdematously swollen) eyelids close firmly and spasmodically and look as if they were bloated. [*Whl.*]

Contortion of the eyes. [J. MAT. MULLER, in *Ephem. N. C.*, Cent. I., C. 51.[2]]

Contortion of the eyes and of the muscles of the neck. [*Eph. N.*, Cent. X., app., p. 463.[3]]

215. Protruding eyes. [GUILBERT, l. c.]

Protruded eyes. [KAISER, l. c.]

Rigid eyes, directed upward. [KAISER, l. c.]

Frightfully staring eyes. [MYRRHEN, l. c.[4]]

Wildly staring look. [GUILBERT, l. c.]

220. Wildly staring look. [*Whl.*]

Wildly staring look, without dilatation of the pupils. [KAISER, l. c.]

Wild look. [MAJAULT, *in Samml. br. Abhandl. f. pra. Aerzte.* VII., 1, 59 and 2, 69.[5]]

His eyelids close themselves; he is weary. [*Hbg.*]

Contracted pupils (aft. 1½, 5 h.). [*Lgh.*]

225. Weakness of vision, for a long time. [MYRRHEN, l. c.[6]]

Obscure vision, as through a white gauze.

He does not recognize the persons standing around him. [RICHARD, l. c.]

Obscuration of sight. [BAYLIES, l. c.]

Obscuration of sight; everything looks black before his eyes (at once). [RICHARD, l. c.]

230. Darkness and flickering before his eyes. [KAISER, l. c.]

Almost total blindness, in a weak-sighted woman, with loss of the hearing and with long continued dullness of the senses. [EBERS, l. c.[7]]

Everything becomes yellow before the eyes, during qualmishness. [ALBERTI, l. c.]

White dots or points before the eyes.

Sparks before the eyes. [EBERS, l. c.[8]]

235. Sensitiveness to light, photophobia. [EBERS, l. c.[9]]

Snow blinds the eyes, so that they water.

Otalgia. [*Bhr.*]

Cramp-like pain in the external ears.

---

[1] The eyelids also were made sore.--*Hughes.*
[2] General statement. The symptom not found.--*Hughes.*
[3] Poisoning of adult.--*Hughes.*
[4] Or "eyes distorted in a horrid manner."--*Hughes.*
[5] Poisoning with Ars., realgar and orpiment.--*Hughes.*
[6] With Sympt. 73.--*Hughes.*
[7] As Sympt. 81.--*Hughes.*
[8] With headache and vertigo.—*Hughes.*
[9] With headache and vertigo.—*Hughes.*

Tearing in the interior of the ear.

240. Drawing tearing in the left lobule.

Drawing tearing behind the ear, down the nape of the neck and into the shoulder.

Stitching tearing outwardly through the left meatus auditorius, chiefly in the evening (1st d.).

Stitches in the ear, in the morning.

Agreeable titillation in both ears, deep within, for ten days. [*Fr. H.*]

245. Voluptuous tickling in the right meatus auditorius, compelling to rubbing. [*Lgh.*]

Burning in the external ear, in the evening (aft. 5 h.).

Sensation of obstruction in the left meatus auditorius, as if from without.

Hardness of hearing, as if the ears were stopped. (aft. 16 h.).

When swallowing, something seems to obstruct the ear from within, as with deafness.

250. He does not understand what is said to him. [RICHARD, l. c.]

Deafness. [*Hg.*]

Ringing in the right ear, when sitting (aft. 1½ h.). [*Lgh.*]

Like ringing in the ears and in the whole head.

Roaring in the ears with every paroxysm of pain.

255. Roaring in the ears. [THOMSON, l. c. BAYLIES, l. c.[1]]

Violent rushing sound before the ears as from a near water-weir.

In the root of the nose, pain in the bones.

Stitches in the bones of the nose.

Violent flow of blood from the nose, owing to vexation (aft. 3 d.).

260. Violent bleeding from the nose, after severe vomiting. [HEIMREICH, *Arsen. als Fiebermittel.*]

A fetid ichor flows from the nose, which is ulcerated high up, and dropping into the mouth it causes a bitter taste. [*Hg.*]

Alternately a smell of pitch and of sulphur in the nose.

The face is sunken. [*Htb. u. Tr.*[2]]

Pale face. [MAJAULT, l. c.]

265. Paleness of the face with distorted features. [KAISER, l. c.]

Paleness of the face with sunken eyes. [J. G. GREISELIUS in *Misc. Nat.* cur. Dec. I., Ann. 2, p. 149.[3]]

Pale, yellow, cachectic appearance. [SCHLEGEL, l. c.[4]]

Deadly paleness. [HENNING, l. c.[5]]

Deadly hue of the face. [ALBERTI, l. c.[6]]

270. Yellow face with sunken eyes.

Bluish, discolored face. [MUELLER, l. c. *Eph. N. C.*, l. c.[7]]

Earthy and leaden complexion, with green and blue spots and stripes. [KNAPE, l. c.]

Distorted features, as if from discontent.

---

[1] Not found in THOMSON.--*Hughes.*
[2] From smoke of wax tapers impregnated with Ars.--*Hughes.*
[3] Symptoms observed in miners.--*Hughes.*
[4] See Sympt. 185.--*Hughes.*
[5] With violent vomiting.--*Hughes.*
[6] During vomiting.--*Hughes.*
[7] In Eph. Nat. Cur. the phrase is " face livid and lurid."--*Hughes.*

Altered and disfigured countenance. [KAISER, l. c.]

275. Death-like appearance. [ALBEREI, l. c.]

Twitches in the facial muscles. [GUILBERT, l. c.]

Pressure in the left upper jaw.

Itching in the face, causing it to be scratched till it is sore.

Bloated red face, with swollen lips. [*Stf.*]

280. Bloated, red face. [KAISER, l. c.]

Swelling of the whole face (from an external application. [*Htb. u. Tr.*]

Swelling of the face. [J. C. TENNER, in *Simon's Samml. d. n. Beob. f. d. J.*, 1788.[1]]

Swelling of the face, of an elastic nature, especially in the eyelids, and chiefly in the morning, in three persons. [TH. FOWLER, *Med. rep. of the effect of arsen.*, Sect. VIII.[2]]

Swelling of the face with swoons and vertigo. [SENNERT, *prax lib.* 6, p. 237.[3]]

285 Hard swelling like a nut on the two protuberances of the forehead; the swelling increases in the evening. [*Sr.*]

Eruption on the forehead. [KNAPE, l. c.]

Little knobs, bumps on the forehead. [*N. med. chir. Wahrn.*, l. c.]

Ulcers all over the face. [*N. med. chir. Wahrn.*, l. c.]

The lips are bluish. [BAYLIES, l. c.]

290. Bluish lips. [KAISER, l. c.]

Black-spotted lips. [GUILBERT, l. c.]

Blackish appearance about the mouth [ALBERTI, l. c.]

Pinching quivering or twitching on the one side of the upper lip, especially on going to sleep.

Itching, as if pricked with countless burning needles, in the upper lip, up to the nose, and the following day swelling of the upper lip above the red.

295. Swelling of the lips. [*Stf.*]

Bleeding of the lower lip after a meal (aft. 1½ h.). [*Lgh.*]

A brown strip of shriveled epidermis, almost as if burnt, extends through the middle of the red of the lower lip.

Red, tettery skin around the mouth.

Eruption broken out on the lips at the edge of the red, painless (aft. 14 d.).

300. Eruption about the mouth, with burning pain.

Painful knots on the upper lips.

Eruption of ulcers around the lips. [ISENFLAMM STEINNING, *Diss. de rem. susp. et ven.*, Erlangen, 1767, p. xxvii.[4]]

Eruption on the lower lip, like noma, with thick crust and a base like leaf-lard. [*Sr.*]

An ulcer eroding on the lip, with tearing pain and smarting as from salt, in the evening on lying down, in the day while moving; worst on being touched and in the open air; it prevents sleep and causes waking up at night (aft. 14 d.).

---

[1] Not accessible.—*Hughes.*
[2] Effects of arsenite of potash in ague patients.—*Hughes.*
[3] Not accessible.—*Hughes.*
[4] General statement—*Hughes.*

305. **Swelling of the sub-maxillary glands, with pain as from pressure and contusion.**

Swelling of the sub-maxillary glands, with painfulness on external pressure. [*Hg.*]

Hard swelling of the left sub-maxillary gland; the swelling is especially severe in the evening. [*Sr.*]

Toothache, more pressive than drawing.

Jerking, continuous toothache, extending into the temple, relieved or removed by sitting up in bed.

310. Tearing in the teeth and simultaneously in the head, at which she becomes so enraged as to beat her head with her fists; just before the setting in of the menses.

Pain in several teeth (in the gums), **as if they were loose and would fall out; but the pain is not increased in chewing** (aft. 1 h.).

Painful looseness of the teeth; and pain as if sore, *per se*, and more yet in chewing; so also the gums pain on being touched, and the cheek on that side swells up.

One tooth becomes loose and prominent, in the morning; its gums ache on being touched, still more in that case, the external part of the cheek, behind which lies the loose tooth; the tooth is not painful on biting the teeth together.

Convulsive gnashing of the teeth. [VAN EGGERN. *Diss. de vacill. dent. Duisb.*, 1787.[1]]

315. Gnashing of the teeth. [KAISER, l. c.]

Falling out of all the teeth. [VAN EGGERN. l. c.]

In the gums, stitches, in the morning.

Nocturnal tearing pains in the gum of the canine tooth, which is unbearable as long as he lies on the affected side, **but is removed by the warmth of the bed**; the following morning the nose is swollen and painful on being touched (aft. 3 d.).

The tongue is bluish. [BAYLIES, l. c.]

320. White tongue. [ALBERTI, l. c.]

Insensibility of the tongue, it is as if it were burnt dead, without sense of taste.

Stitching pain, as from a fish-bone in the root of the tongue, when swallowing and when turning the head.

Boring pain in right border of the tongue, while half asleep.

Pain on the tongue as if there were on it vesicles full of burning pain.

325. Erosion of the tongue at the side of the tip with smarting pain (aft. 14 d.).

On the roof of the palate, long continued feeling of roughness. [*Bhr.*]

Scrapy, scratchy sensation, behind on the velum pendulum palati, when not swallowing.

Scraping and sensation of rancidity in the throat, as from rancid fat, after the first morsel she swallowed in the morning.

In the throat a sensation as if there was a hair in it.

330. Sensation in the throat as from a lump of mucus, with a taste of blood.

---

[1] Not accessible.—*Hughes.*

Tearing pain in the œsophagus and all up the throat, also when not swallowing.

Burning in the throat. [RICHARD, l. c. BUCHHOLZ, l. c.]

Burning in the fauces. [KNAPE, l. c. KOPP, *Jahrb. der Staats-Arzneik.* II., p. 182.[1]]

Inflammation of the interior of the throat. [RAU, l. c.]

335. Gangrenous sore throat. [FELDMANN, in *Comm. lit. Nor.* 1743, p. 50[2]]

In the fauces and stomach a sensation of rolling together, as if a thread was rolled into a ball. [RICHARD, l. c.]

Sensation of constriction in the throat. [PREUSSIUS, *Ephem. N. C. Cent.* III., *obs.* 15.[3]]

Constriction of the fauces (of the œsophagus). [*N. m. ch. Wahrn.*, l. c.]

His throat feels as if pressed quite shut, as if nothing would go down his œsophagus. [ALBERTI, l. c.]

340. Deglutition very painful. [*N. m. ch. Wahrn.*, l. c.]

Difficult swallowing. [RAU, l. c.]

Sensation of paralysis of the fauces and œsophagus; the chewed roll could not be swallowed down, it went down with difficulty with a pinching pressure, **as if the œsophagus had not sufficient strength for it;** he heard it rattle down.

Feeling of dryness on the tongue. [BUCHHOLZ, l. c.]

Sensation of great dryness in the mouth, with violent thirst; but he only drinks a little at a time. [*Stf.*]

345. Sensation of dryness in the throat; she had to drink constantly, as she felt that otherwise she should perish of thirst.

Severe dryness in the mouth and violent thirst.

Severe dryness in the mouth. [THILENIUS in *Richter's chir. bibl.* V., p. 540.[4]]

Dryness of the tongue. [GUILBERT, l. c.; MAJAULT, l. c.]

Much saliva, he had to spit out frequently. [*Hbg.*]

350. The saliva ejected tastes bitter.

Bloody saliva. [*N. m. ch. Wahrn.*, l. c.]

Slimy in the mouth and throat (aft. 2 h.).

Ejection of grey mucus by hawking.

Salty expectoration (by hawking?). [RICHARD, l. c.]

355. Bitter expectoration. [RICHARD, l. c.]

Green, bitter expectoration (by hawking) in the morning.

Bitterness in the mouth, with yellow diarrhœa, [MORGAGNI, l. c.]

Bitter taste in the mouth, after a meal.

Bitter disgusting taste in the mouth, after eating and drinking.

360. Bitterness in the throat, after eating, while the food tastes normally on alternate days (**like a tertian fever**).

Bitter taste in the mouth, without having eaten anything.

Bitter taste in the mouth, in the morning. [*Hg.*]

---

1 (For KOPP.) Poisoning of adult.—*Hughes.*
2 From a plaster of Ars. applied for a quartan.—*Hughes.*
3 Poisoning of a boy.—*Hughes.*
4 Effects in a patient with scirrhous breast.—*Hughes.*

Wooden, dry taste in the mouth.
Rotten fetid taste in the mouth.
365. Putrid taste in the morning, as of putrid meat.
Sour taste in the mouth, all the food tastes sour.
All the food tastes salty.
The food tastes as if it had too little salt.
The beer tastes flat.
370. The unhopped beer tastes bitter.
Adipsia, lack of thirst.

Thirst. [PREUSSIUS l. c.; RAU, l. c.; PET DE APPONO, *de ven.*[1]]

Great thirst. [ALBERTI, l. c., Tom. II.]

Severe thirst, constant. [BUETTNER, l. c.]

375. Violent thirst. [MAJAULT, l. c.]

Choking thirst. [FORESTUS, l. c.]

Burning thirst. [MAJAULT, l. c.[2]]

Unquenchable thirst. [BUCHHOLZ, l. c.; GUILBERT, l. c.; CRUEGER.]

Unquenchable thirst, with dryness of the tongue, the fauces and the gullet. [GUELDENKLEE, l. c.]

380. Uncommon thirst, so that he has to drink much cold water every ten minutes, from morning till evening, but not at night. [*Fr.*, *H.*]

Extremely violent thirst, and drinking affords no refreshment and refection. [KAISER, l. c.]

He drinks much and often. [*Stf.*]

With great thirst, he drinks often, but always little at a time. [RICHARD, l. c.[3]]

Violent thirst, but he only drinks little at a time. [*Whl.*]

385. Violent thirst, not without appetite for eating. [KNAPE, l. c.]

Lack of appetite, with violent thirst. [STŒRK, *med. Jahrg.* I., p. 207.[4]]

Lack of appetite. [JACOBI, l. c.]

Loss of appetite. [KAISER, l. c.]

Total lack of appetite. [BUCHHOLZ, in *Hufel. Journ.*, l. c.]

390. No appetite, but when he eats he relishes food.

Lack of hunger and appetite for ten days. [*Fr.*, *H.*]

Aversion to all food, she cannot eat anything.

Loathing of food. [GRIMM, l. c.; GŒRITZ, in *Bresl. Samml.*, 1728.[5]]

Loathing of all food. [ALBERTI, l. c.]

395. Irresistible loathing of all food, so that he cannot think of eating without nausea. [EBERS, l. c.]

It is impossible for him to get his food down. [RICHARD, l. c.]

The smell of boiled meat is unbearable to him. [RICHARD, l. c.]

Repugnance to butter.

Desire for brandy. [*Hg.*]

---

[1] Effects of realgar.—*Hughes.*
[2] Not found.—*Hughes.*
[3] Not found.—*Hughes.*
[4] Effects of arsenite of potash in ague patients.—*Hughes.*
[5] Not to be found at reference.—*Hughes.*

400. Desire for sour things. [*Stf.*]
Desire for vinegar and water.
Great desire for acids and acidulous fruit.
Great desire for coffee.
Great appetite for milk, to which before she was averse.

405. While eating, a compressive sensation on the chest.
Soon after breakfast and after dinner, pressure on the stomach, with empty eructations for three hours, causing a lassitude of body which produced qualmishness.
Before eating, nausea, and after eating or drinking, distension or pressure and cutting in the abdomen.
Eructation, after taking food.
Much eructation, especially after drinking.

410. **Ineffectual efforts to eructate.**
Eructation, caused by flatus coming upward.
Constant eructation. [GŒRITZ, l. c.]
Frequent empty eructation (aft. ½ h.). [*Lgh.*]
Frequent empty eructation.

415. Constant, severe, empty eructation, with numb feeling of the head (aft. 36 h.).
Sour eructation after dinner.
Bitter eructation after eating, with belching up of greenish, bitter mucus.
An acrid liquid rises into the mouth.
Frequent hiccup after eating, every time followed by eructation. [*Lgh.*]

420. Frequent hiccup and eructation. [MORGAGNI, l. c.]
Convulsive hiccup. [ALBERTI, l. c.]
Hiccup, at night, when rising, with scratching, nauseous taste in the mouth.
Long-continued hiccup, in the hour when the fever should have come.
Qualmishness at 11 A. M. and at 3 P. M.

425. **Nausea.** [PFANN, *Samml. merkw. Fälle, Nürnb.*, 1750, pp. 129, 130; *N. Wahrn*, l. c.; KAISER, l. c.[1]]
Nausea in the fauces and stomach.
Nausea, with anguish. [ALBERTI, l. c.]
Long-continued nausea, with faintness, trembling, heat all over, followed by a shiver (aft some h.).
Qualmishness and nausea, **compelling the person to lie down**, in the forenoon, at the same time tearing about the ankle and the dorsum of the foot.

430. Frequent nausea, with a sweetish taste in the mouth, not immediately after eating.
Nausea, more in the throat, with gathering of water in the mouth.
Nausea, with abortive waterbrash, shortly before and after dinner.
Nausea, when sitting; much water collected in the mouth, as

[1] Poisoning by cobalt, "fly-powder," a mixture of metallic arsenic with arsenious acid.—*Hughes*.

in waterbrash; while walking, the nausea passed off, followed by a discharge of a copious, pappy stool (aft. 7 h.). [*Lgh.*]

Waterbrash, at 4 P. M.

435. Sickness at stomach. [MAJAULT, l. c.[1]]

Inclination to vomit. [KAISER, l. c.]

Nausea, in the open air.

Empty retching. [RAU, l. c.]

Nausea and violent vomiting. [*Htb. u. Tr.*[2]]

440. Nausea, qualmishness on raising oneself up in bed, and frequently, sudden vomiting. [*Stf.*]

Vomiting. [MAJAULT, l. c.; GRIMM, and many others.]

Vomiting immediately after every meal, without nausea. [*Fr. H.*]

The child vomits after eating and drinking, and then will neither eat nor drink, but sleeps well.

Vomiting of all the ingesta, for several weeks. [*Salzb. m. chir. Zeit.*]

445. Excessive vomiting produced with the greatest effort, of drinks, yellowish-green mucus and water, with very bitter taste in the mouth, which remained a long time afterward. [*Stf.*]

Vomiting of a thick, glassy mucus. [RICHARD, l. c.]

Vomiting of mucus and green bile. [ALBERTI, l. c.[3]]

Vomiting of a thin, bluish, smutty-yellow matter, followed by great prostration and exhaustion. [KAISER, l. c.]

Vomiting of brownish, dark matter, sometimes thick, sometimes thin, with violent efforts and increased stomachache, without subsequent relief. [KAISER, l. c.]

450. Vomiting of a brownish matter, often mixed with blood, with a violent bodily effort. [KAISER, l. c.]

Vomiting of bloody mucus. [*N. Wahrn.*, l. c.]

Vomiting of blood. [KELLNER, in *Bresl. Samml.*, 1727.[4]]

Discharged blood upward and downward. [GERBITZ, in *Ephem. Nat. Cur.*, *Dec.* III., *ann* 5, 6, *obs.* 137.[5]]

When vomiting ceases, frequent, very watery diarrhœic stools set in. [*Htb. u. Tr.*[6]]

455. Excessive vomiting and purging. [PREUSSIUS, l. c.]

Violent, continual voming, with diarrhœa. [MORGAGNI, l. c.]

Vomiting, with diarrhœa, as soon as the swoon goes off. [FORESTUS, l. c.]

During the vomiting, which continues night and day, frightful cries. [HEIMREICH, l. c.[7]]

During the vomiting, complains of severe internal heat and thirst. [ALBERTI, l. c.]

460. During the violent vomiting, severe internal burning, thirst and heat. [ALBERTI, l. c.]

Frequent vomiting, with **dread of death**. [ALBERTI, l. c.]

---

[1] Not found.—*Hughes.*

[2] As sympt. 267.—*Hughes.*

[3] Literally, "Vomiting of greenish matter at night, of whitish stuff next morning."—*Hughes.*

[4] Poisoning of a girl of twenty.—*Hughes.*

[5] From orpiment.—*Hughes.*

[6] Reference should be KAISER, l. c.—*Hughes.*

[7] Cited from CARDAN.—*Hughes.*

Pains in the stomach. [QUELMALZ, l. c.; RICHARD, and several others.]

Great painfulness of the stomach. [*N. Wahrn.*, l. c.]

Pains in the stomach, causing nausea. [RICHARD, l. c.]

465. Excessive pains in the region of the scrobiculus cordis. [S. PH. WOLFF, *Act. Nat. c.*, V., *obs.* 29.[1]]

Heaviness in the stomach, as if it were being violently distended in its whole extent and were being torn. [KOPP, *Jahrb. d. Staatsarzneik.* II., p. 182.]

Trouble in the stomach, as if it were tormented with flatus; much aggravated after vomiting and diarrhœa. [MORGAGNI, l. c.[2]]

Bloatedness and distension of the stomach and the hypochondriac region, before a stool ensues. [RICHARD, l. c.]

Bloatedness of the region of the stomach. [KAISER, l. c.]

470. The stomach begins to raise itself, and is warmer than the rest of the body. [KAISER, l. c.]

Sensation of fullness in the stomach, with distaste for eating, and stomachache after it; in the evening.

Heaviness in the stomach, as from a stone, after eating. [*Hbg.*]

Pressive feeling of heaviness in the stomach. [MORGAGNI, l. c.]

Pressure in the region of the stomach and the scrobiculus cordis; pressure on the heart. [KELLNER, l. c.; GOERTZ and many others.[3]]

475. It felt as if it would break her heart.

It felt as if it would break his heart. [*Stf.*]

Pressure on the mouth of the stomach and in the œsophagus, after eating, as if the food remained on top; then empty eructation.

Pressure about the stomach, so that he cannot stand it, whenever he has eaten anything, not at once, but some time after eating.

Pressure in the anterior wall of the stomach, on speaking (aft. ½ h.).

480. Hard pressure above the scrobiculus cordis (at once).

Cramp-like pain of the stomach, two hours after midnight.

Periodic cramp like pains in the stomach and the bowels. [KAISER, l. c.]

Cramps of the stomach, of excessive violence, with thirst. [BUCHHOLZ, l. c.]

Cramps of the stomach, with violent bellyache, diarrhœa and faintings. [LOEW, in SYDENHAM, Op. II., p. 324.[4]]

485. Cutting pain in the stomach. [THILENIUS, l. c.]

Drawing pain, in the evening while sitting, from the scrobiculus cordis to the left ribs all around, as if something were violently torn off there.

Dull tearing, transversely across the region of the stomach, when walking, in the afternoon.

---

1 Poisoning of two women. For "pains" read "anxieties," *i. e.*, anxiety.—*Hughes.*

2 Add "returning later with great violence."—*Hughes.*

3 Goertz should be GOERITZ.—*Hughes.*

4 Not found at reference.—*Hughes.*

Tearing, pressive, spasmodic pain in the stomach. [KAISER, l. c.]

Violent, tearing, boring pain and cramp in the stomach and bowels. [KAISER, l. c.]

490. Gnawing and prickling (sharp and fine throbbing) pain in the scrobiculus cordis, with sensation of tension.

Eroding, gnawing *pain in the stomach*. [RICHARD, l. c.]

Heat with pain and pressure in the scrobiculus cordis. [KAISER, l. c.]

Burning in the scrobiculus cordis. [BUCHHOLZ, l. c.; KAISER, l. c.]

Burning all around the scrobiculus cordis.

495. Burning pain in the stomach. [EBERS, l. c.[1]]

Burning in the stomach like fire. [RICHARD, l. c.]

Constant burning and severe constriction in the stomach and in the chest. [BORGES in *Kopp's Jahrb.*, l. c.[2]]

Burning in the stomach, with pressure as from a load. [MORGAGNI, l. c.]

Burning in the scrobiculus cordis, with pressive pain. [GOERITZ, l. c.]

500 Constriction in the scrobiculus cordis [*Hbg.*]

Great distress about the region of the scrobiculus cordis. [MORGAGNI, l. c.; JACOBI and others.]

Wails and lamentations about an indescribable distress in the region of the scrobiculus cordis, without distension or colic. [MORGAGNI, l. c.[3]]

Distress in the scrobiculus cordis, rising up from it, at night.

In the liver, a squeezing pressure, on taking a walk.

505. The spleen, indurated before, now swells. [*Hg.*]

Stitches in the side of the abdomen, under the short ribs, and he cannot lie on his side.

In the region of the kidneys, stitches, when respiring and when sneezing.

Pains in the abdomen of the most violent kind. [DAN CRUEGER, *Misc. N. C. Dec.* II., Ann. 4, O. 12.[4]]

Excessive bellyache and pains in the stomach. [WOLFF, l. c.]

510. Exceedingly disagreeable sensation in the whole of the abdomen. [MORGAGNI, l. c.]

Pains in the hypogastrium, with heat in the face.

Violent pain in the region of the right epigastrium. [MORGAGNI, l. c.]

Pain in the right epigastrium and the neighboring inguinal regions, which extends thence at times through the hypogastrium, at times into the right side of the flanks and the scrotum, like a renal colic; but with unchanged urine. [MORGAGNI, l. c.]

Roving pains in the abdomen, with diarrhœa and pains in the anus. [MORGAGNI, l. c.]

515. The pain in the abdomen establishes itself in the left side of the belly.

---

[1] Not found.—*Hughes.*
[2] Poisoning of an adult.—*Hughes.*
[3] *Unsaeglich*, indescribable, is in the Latin "inexplicabilis."—*Hughes.*
[4] Poisoning of adult.—*Hughes.*

Pain, as if the upper part of the body was altogether cut off from the abdomen, with great anguish and lamentation over it. [ALBERTI, l. c., Tom. IV.[1]]

Violent pains in the abdomen, with so great anguish that he had no rest anywhere, rolled about on the ground, and gave up all hope of living. [PYL, l. c.]

Fullness in the region of the epigastrium, with griping in the belly.

Distension and pains in the abdomen. [MUELLER, l. c.]

520. Severe, painless distension of the abdomen after eating; he had to lean his back against something to ease himself.

Bloatedness every morning, with passage of flatus a few hours afterwards.

Swollen abdomen. [GUILBERT, l. c.[2]]

The abdomen enormously swollen. [*Ephem. N. C.*, l. c.]

As if there were cramps and griping in the abdomen, in the evening, after lying down, with breaking out of perspiration; then passage of flatus and very thin stool.

525. Spasmodic jerk, frequently, from the scrobiculus cordis to the rectum, which makes him start.

Squeezing, cutting pains in the bowels, in the evening after lying down, and in the morning after rising; at times the pains shoot through the abdominal ring (as if they would force out a hernia) as far as the spermatic cord and the perinæum; when this colic ceases a loud rumbling and grumbling ensues.

Colics, returning from time to time. [MAJAULT, l. c.[3]]

Pinching pain, aggravated even to cutting, deep in the hypogastrium, every morning, before and during the diarrhœic stools, and continuing also after them.

Cutting pain in the abdomen. [BUCHHOLZ, l. c.; KELLNER, l. c.]

530. Cutting pain in the side of the abdomen, below the last ribs, very much aggravated by touching them.

Cutting (tearing) and gnawing pains in the bowels and the stomach. [QUELMALZ, l. c.[4]]

Cutting and tearing in the abdomen, with icy coldness of the hands and feet and cold perspiration of the face. [ALBERTI, l. c.]

Tearing in the abdomen. [PFANN, l. c.; ALBERTI, l. c.]

Tearing stitches in the left side of the abdomen, under the short ribs, in the evening soon after lying down.

535. Drawing pains in the abdomen, in the umbilical region (aft. 2 h.).

Drawing and pressing in the abdomen, as from obstructed flatus, and yet none passed off. [*Whl.*]

Twisting together of the intestines, and cutting in the belly, after previous rumbling there; then three diarrhœic stools.

Contortion of the intestines, and squeezing and rumbling in the abdomen, before and during the liquid stool. [*Mr.*]

---

[1] Add "p. 260."—*Hughes.*
[2] "Abdomen was also painful."—*Hughes.*
[3] Not found.—*Hughes.*
[4] Instead of tearing more literally in the original "lancinating."—*Hughes.*

Burrowing, with pressure, in the right side of the abdomen. [*Hbg.*]

540. Twisting colic. [RICHARD, l. c.[1]]

Twisting and griping in the abdomen. [KAISER, l. c.]

Dysenteric colic in the umbilical region. [GRIMM, l. c.[2]]

Uneasiness in the abdomen, but only during rest.

Anxious feeling in the abdomen, with fever and thirst. [MORGAGNI, l. c.]

545. **Constant chilliness, internally, in the epigastric region;** he cannot keep himself warm enough; externally the place feels warm.

Burning pain in the abdomen, at noon and in the afternoon, passing off with the discharge of a stool.

Burning in the abdomen, with stitches and cutting. [BUCHHOLZ, *Beitr.*, l. c.]

Burning in the abdomen, with heat and thirst. [ALBERTI, l. c.]

Burning in the flanks. [*Hbg.*]

550. In the groin and the inguinal region of the right side, pain in stooping, as from a sprain.

Burrowing, burning pain in the inguinal tumor, excited even by the lightest touch.

Single, severe, slow stitches in both flanks.

Weakness of the abdominal muscles.

Rumbling in the abdomen, as if from much flatus.

555. Growling in the stomach, in the morning on awaking.

Rumbling in the abdomen. [THILENIUS, l. c.]

Rumbling in the abdomen, without stool.

The flatus tends to pass upward and causes eructations.

Passage of much flatus, with previous loud growling in the abdomen. [*Lgh.*]

560. Putrid smelling flatus (aft. 11 h.). [*Lgh.*]

(Clotted, insufficient stool).

Constipation. [GOERITZ, l. c.; RAU, l. c.[3]]

Constipated abdomen.

Constipation, with pain in the abdomen. [*Htb. u. Tr.*[4]]

565. Retention of stool, despite of violent urging. [ALBERTI, l. c.]

Fruitless urging to stool.

Tenesmus, with burning. [MORGAGNI, l. c.]

Tenesmus, as in dysentery; a constant burning, with pain and straining in the rectum and anus.

Unperceived discharge of stool, as if it were flatus.

570. Stools pass without his knowledge. [BUETTNER, l. c.[5]]

Involuntary passage of fæces. [KAISER, l. c.]

Copious stools. [KAISER, l. c.]

Pappy fæces pass, now more, now less (aft. 6, 13 h.). [*Lgh.*]

Diarrhœa. [MAJAULT, l. c.; KELLNER, l. c.]

575. Diarrhœa, which frequently becomes very severe. [KAISER, l. c.]

---

[1] Not found.—*Hughes.*

[2] The Latin is "tormina circum umbilicum."—*Hughes.*

[3] In Rau's case, "for four days."—*Hughes.*

[4] Observations on a patient. *Hughes.*

[5] Not found.—*Hughes.*

Diarrhœa, with violent burning in the anus. [THILENIUS, l. c.]

Diarrhœa, alternating with constipation. [*Stf.*]

Yellow, watery, scanty diarrhœic stools, with subsequent tenesmus, as if more stool would pass, and painful colic about the navel. [*Stf.*]

Yellow, diarrhœic stool, with tenesmus and burning pains in the rectum and anus.

580. Small stools, with tenesmus, first with dark-green fæces then of dark-green mucus, with previous colic.

Evacuation of lumps of mucus, with tenesmus, with cutting pains in the anus, as of blind piles.

Mucous, thin stools, as if hacked.

Mucous and green evacuations. [PHILENIUS, l. c.]

Viscid, bilious matter is often discharged with the stool, for two days. [PHILENIUS, l. c.[1]]

585. Greenish, dark-brown, diarrhœic stool, with a smell as of fetid ulcers. [*Hg.*]

A black fluid, burning in the anus like fire, is discharged after much restlessness and pain in the abdomen. [RICHARD, l. c.]

Black, acrid, putrid stools. [BAYLIES, l. c.]

A spherical lump, which seemed to consist of undigested tallow with layers of tendinous matter, went off with the stool. [MORGAGNI, l. c.[2]]

Watery blood is discharged with the fæces and envelops them.

590. Bloody discharge with the stool, almost every moment, with vomiting and excessive colicky pains. [GRIMM, l. c.]

Dysentery. [CRUEGER, l. c.]

Before the diarrhœic stool, cutting and contortion in the bowels.

Before the diarrhœic stool, sensation as if he would burst. [ALBERTI, l. c.]

During the stool, painful contraction close above the anus, toward the small of the back.

595. After the stool, cessation of the colic. [RICHARD, l. c.]

After the stool, burning in the rectum, with great weakness and trembling in all the limbs.

After the stool, distension of the abdomen.

After the stool, palpitation and tremulous weakness; he has to lie down.

The rectum is spasmodically protruded and pressed out, with great pains.

600. After a flow of blood from the anus, the rectum continues to protrude.

Itching of the anus.

Scraping or erosive pain in the anus, with itching.

Pain of the anus as of soreness, on being touched.

Burning in the anus.

605. Burning in the anus. [MORGAGNI, l. c.]

---

[1] **Not found.—*Hughes.***

[2] **Instead of "tallow," we may translate "fat."—*Hughes.***

Burning in the anus, for one hour, going off after the discharge of a hard, clotted stool.

The hemorrhoidal veins are painfully swollen, with tenesmus. [MORGAGNI, l. c.]

Blind piles, with pains like slow pricks with a hot needle.

Varices on the anus, with pricking pain, when walking and sitting, not during the stool.

610. **Hemorrhoidal lumps at the anus, which,** especially at night, **pain and burn like fire** and permit no sleep; during the day the pain becomes aggravated and changes into violent stitches; worse when walking than when sitting or lying down.

On the perinæum eroding itching, compelling him to scratch (aft. ½ h.). [*Lgh.*]

Suppression of urine. [GUILBERT, l. c.; *N. Wahrn.*, l. c.]

Retention of urine, as from paralysis of the bladder.

Retention of urine despite of internal urging to urinate. [ALBERTI, l. c.]

615. **Frequent urging to urinate,** with copious flow of urine (aft. 2 to 17 h.). [*Lgh.*]

Urging to urinate every minute, with burning in the bladder.

He has to rise at night three or four times to urinate, and each time he passes a good deal, for several days in succession.

Involuntary micturition at night, when sleeping, wetting the bed. [*Hg.*]

Involuntary micturition. [KAISER, l. c.]

620. Involuntary micturition; she could not get to the utensil before the urine ran from her, though it was but a little.

Diminished micturition. [FOWLER, l. c.[1]]

But little water passes, and it scalds during the flow.

Increase of urine. [FOWLER, l. c.[1]]

Very copious and burning hot urine. [*Hg.*]

625. Almost colorless urine.

Exceedingly turbid urine (aft. 5 d.).

Greenish, dark-brown urine, turbid already when passed, like cow-dung stirred into water, without settling. [*Hg.*]

Bloody urine. [O. TACHENIUS, *Hipp. chym. cap.*, 24.[2]]

When beginning to urinate, burning in the anterior part of the urethra; in the morning. (aft. 24 h.).

630. **During micturition, burning in the urethra** [MORGAGNI, l. c.; *N. Wahrn*, l. c.]

During micturition, contractive pain in the left iliac region.

After micturition, sensation of great weakness in the epigastrium, so that she trembled.

In the urethra, a stinging pain.

Frequent pain, like tearing, deep in the urethra.

635. In the genitals, itching.

Burning anteriorly on the prepuce, with erection.

Stinging itching, anteriorly on the prepuce.

Severe itching on the glans, without erection.

---

[1] "Sometimes," FOWLER says; but of § 623, he says, "often."—*Hughes.*

[2] From inhaling sublimated Ars.—*Hughes.*

Eroding itching posteriorly on the penis, compelling him to scratch. [*Lgh.*]

640. **Inflammation and swelling of the genitals, even to mortification**, with excessive pains. [DEGNER, *Act. Nat.* C. VI., app., pp. 8, 9.[1]]

Sudden mortification of the male genitals. [STAHL, *Opusc chym. phys. med.*, p. 454.[2]]

Exceedingly painful swelling of the genitals. [*N. Wahrn*, l. c.]

The glans is bluish-red, swollen and cracked in chaps. [PFANN, l. c.]

Swelling of the testicles. [ALBERTI, l. c.[3]]

645. Erection in the morning without pollution. [*Lgh.*]

Pollution at night, with voluptuous dreams. [*Lgh.*]

Pollution, at night, without voluptuous dreams, followed by long continued erection. [*Lgh.*]

Emission of prostatic juice during a diarrhœic stool.

Sexual furor in a woman; she desires coitus twice a day, and when it is not accorded, a discharge takes place of itself.

650. **Menses too early.**

The menses set in twice too early, returning in twenty days.

Menstruation too profuse.

During the menses, pinching, lancinating cutting from the scrobiculus cordis down to the hypogastrium, also in the back and in the sides of the abdomen; she had to bend herself double, standing and cowering down, with loud eructation and with loud groaning, wailing and weeping.

During the menses, sharp stitches from the rectum into the anus and the pudenda.

655. Instead of the menses, which were suppressed, she had pains in the region of the anus and the shoulders. [*Sr.*]

After the menses, a flow of bloody mucus.

A discharge of leucorrhœa while standing, with discharge of flatus (aft. 24 h.).

Discharge from the vagina about a cupful in twenty-four hours of yellowish, thickish matter, with smarting erosion and excoriation of all the parts it touches; for ten days.

Stitches from the hypogastrium down into the vagina.

* * * * * * * *

660. Frequent sneezing, without coryza (aft. 11 h.). [*Lgh.*]

Severe, continuous sneezing.

Dryness of the nasal cavity.

Coryza, with sneezing, quickly transient; every morning on awaking.

Fluent coryza, with frequent sneezing (aft. 11 h.). [*Lgh.*]

665. Severe, fluent coryza.

Fluent coryza, combined with dry coryza.

Excessive coryza, with hoarseness and sleeplessness.

The watery nasal-mucus discharged smarts and burns in the nostrils, as if they became sore from it.

---

[1] Effects of applying solution of Ars. for itch, in two men.—*Hughes.*
[2] The "Brand" mortification, is *sphacelatio*. Poisoning of two adults.—*Hughes.*
[3] It was the scrotum, not the testicles, that was swollen.—*Hughes.*

Flow of an acrid liquid from the nose. [MYRRHEN, l. c.]

670. Dryness of the larynx.

The voice is tremulous. [GUILBERT, l. c.]

The voice unequal, now strong, now weak. [KAISER, l. c.]

Rough voice and hoarseness.

Roughness and hoarseness of the throat, in the morning.

675. Very viscid mucus on the chest, difficult to cough up.

Constant tickling in the whole of the windpipe, inciting to cough, even when not respiring.

Cough, with a sensation of constriction in the upper part of the windpipe, as from vapors of sulphur.

Frequently a quite dry, short, scratching cough, with a choking sensation in the larynx, as from vapors of sulphur.

Tussiculation, without expectoration, excited in the windpipe. [*Lgh.*]

680. Cough without expectoration, after previous twitching in the hip, which seems to call it forth.

Cough, especially after drinking.

When he drinks, without being thirsty, it causes cough.

Cough, causing him to lose his breath, on moving the body.

Cough, when she comes into the cold, open air.

685. On walking in the open air he feels choked, so that he has to cough.

Morning-cough, of a very severe kind.

In the morning a short cough, after the (usual) drinking of tea.

In the evening, cough with asthma, without expectoration.

In the evening, cough after lying down.

690. In the evening, in bed, for several minutes, constant cough, with nausea and rising in the throat, as if to vomit.

In the evening, just after lying down, cough, so that she has to sit up again; then a contractive pain in the region of the stomach and the scrobiculus cordis, which sustained the cough, until it made her weary.

Nocturnal cough, causing him to sit up, as soon as it starts.

The cough wakes him at night; severe fits, so that he felt like choking, and his throat swelled up.

After midnight, deep, dry, short, incessant cough.

695. Dry tussiculation. [STŒRK, l. c.]

Dry, fatiguing cough. [STŒRK, l. c.]

Dry, very violent cough (aft. 2 h.).

Dry, retching cough, with short, difficult breathing, and a pain in the scrobiculus cordis, even to the middle of the chest, as if from a festering sore.

A croaking cough, the mucus loosened with difficulty, causing a pain on the chest, as from chaps.

700. Tussiculation, with pain on the chest and salty expectoration, after previous tightness of the chest. [EBERS, l. c.[1]]

Bloody streaks in the mucus that is coughed up.

Expectoration of mucus, with bloody streaks, then nausea.

[1] As sympt. 81.—*Hughes.*

With severe coughing, much water comes out of the mouth, as from waterbrash.

In coughing, a pain, as from a bruise or a contusion in the abdomen.

705. In coughing, a lancinating pain in the scrobiculus cordis.

In clearing the throat, a drawing, lancinating pain under the left hypochondrium up into the chest.

In coughing, increased stitches under the ribs and increased headache, as from heat therein.

In coughing, heat in the head.

In coughing, stitches, first in the side of the chest and then (after two days) also in the side of the abdomen.

710. In coughing, a lancinating pain up into the sternum.

Immediately after coughing, the breath is always short, as if it drew the whole chest together.

The breath very short. [*Htb. u. Tr.*[1]]

Painful respiration. [*N. Wahrn*, l. c.]

Difficult respiration. [TACHENIUS, l. c.[2]]

715. Difficult breathing with great anguish. [KAISER, l. c.]

Anxious, groaning breathing. [GUILBERT, l. c.[3]]

Frequent, distressing, pressive dyspnœa in all positions.

Severe oppression of breathing. [PYL, l. c.[4]]

Asthma of long duration. [GUELDENKLEE, l. c.]

720. Asthma returning frequently. [MORGAGNI, l. c.]

Asthma, when he gets vexed.

Asthma as from anguish, when he has tired himself out.

Tightness of the chest. [RAU, l. c.[5]]

Tightness of the chest, dyspnœa. [THILENIUS, l. c.]

725. Tightness in the region of the sternum makes breathing difficult, for eight days.

Tightness of the chest, when walking fast, when coughing or going up stairs.

Breathing is checked by pain in the scrobiculus cordis.

Breathing is checked by an intolerable anguish and a very distressing sensation in the abdomen, causing piteous wailings. [MORGAGNI, l. c.]

His breath leaves him at once in the evening, if he gets into bed ever so carefully and lies down, and there is as fine whistling in the constricted windpipe as if a fine string (in an instrument) sounded.

730. Constriction of the chest. (PREUSSIUS, l. c.]

Constriction of the chest, so that he could hardly speak a word, and almost fainted (3d d.). [*Htb. u. Tr.*[6]]

Constant contraction of the chest and tussiculation. (*Htb. u. Tr.*[6]]

As from compression of the chest, his breath is rendered difficult during the abdominal pains.

---

[1] As sympt. 267.—*Hughes.*
[2] See sympt. 625.—*Hughes.*
[3] Literally, "breathing difficult, and often interrupted by sighs.—*Hughes.*
[4] For a long time.—*Hughes.*
[5] Latin is: "anxietates pectoris."—*Hughes.*
[6] Both these are SCHLEGEL'S, see § 183.—*Hughes.*

Grievous anguish as if everything was being constricted, with anguish in the scrobiculus cordic.

735. Constriction of the chest with great anguish and restlessness, in the evening.

Tightness of the chest, threatening suffocation, for one hour. [GREISELIUS, l. c.[1]]

Asthma (angina pectoris); her breath constantly grows weaker and shorter, so that she can only, by leaning her chest forward, breathe and speak very low. [*Whl.*]

She thinks every moment that she will suffocate, attended with so great a weakness that she is unable to breathe deeply. [*Whl.*]

Sudden tightness of the chest, threatening suffocation, with dyspnœa, when walking, with weakness and extreme exhaustion. [MAJAULT, l. c.[2]]

740. **Catarrh threatening sudden suffocation, at night.** [MYRRHEN, l. c.]

He is about to suffocate, his tongue sticks out. [WEDEL, l. c.]

Suffocating rheum. [*Misc. n. e., Dec.* III., *an.* 9, 10.[3]]

Pains in the chest. [PEARSON, l. c.]

Severe pains in the chest. [*N. Wahrn.*, l. c.]

745. Interior pains in the upper part of the chest (aft. 5 h.).

Tensive pain in the chest, chiefly while sitting.

Pressure on the chest. [BUCHHOLZ, *Beitr.*, l. c.]

Stitches in the side, under the short ribs, and he can not lie on this side.

Stitches in the upper right part of the chest, especially in breathing, as it were a pressure ending in a stitch (aft 1½ h.).

750. Stitches in the left breast, when taking a deep breath, compelling him to cough.

Stitches in the left breast, only when expiring, which is thus rendered difficult. [*Lgh.*]

Dull stitches in the chest on stooping.

Stitching tearing pain in the uppermost right rib.

Formication in the chest.

755. Sensation of soreness and rawness in the chest.

A sensation of coldness internally in the chest, in the evening, also after supper.

Great heat in the chest, extending into the midriff. [*Hbg.*]

Burning in the chest. [STOERK, l. c.]

Burning in the region of the sternum, long continued. [STOERK, l. c.]

760. Burning in the right side of the chest, extending into the flanks, where there is a pressure. [*Hbg.*]

The beat of the heart is excited. [KAISER, l. c.]

Palpitation of the heart. [MAJAULT, l. c.]

Excessive, very burdensome palpitation. [*Stf.*]

Violently raging palpitation. [KAISER, l. c.]

765. When he lies on his back, his heart beats much more quickly and strongly. [*Stf.*]

---

[1] In self, from inhaling vapors.—*Hughes.*

[2] [Latter part of symptom should be: "With much lassitude and oppression in breathing in walking."]—*Hughes.*

[3] Same case as MYRRHEN'S (see S. 14), and same symptom as S. 740.—*Hughes.*

Irregular heart-beat, but so strong that he thinks he can hear it, at 3 o'clock at night, with anguish. [*Mr.*]

Violent palpitation, at night. [*Bhr.*]

Yellow spots externally on the chest. [WEDEL, l. c.]

Lack of strength in the small of the back.

770. Painful stiffness in the small of the back, all the day.

Pain in the small of the back as from a bruise.

Pain in the back, with restlessness and anxiety. [BUETTNER, l. c.]

Stiffness in the spine, extending up from the coccyx.

Pain in the back as from a bruise, and over the scapulæ as if beaten (aft. 4 d.).

775. Drawing pain in the back, in the forenoon (aft. 6 d.).

Drawing, up and down the back.

Drawing pain between the scapulæ, **compelling him to lie down.**

Drawing pain in the back, from the small of the back into the shoulders, with stitches in the sides, while flatus moves about in the abdomen, pressing upward; then eructation and relief.

Strongly clucking motion in the muscles of the left side of the back, only when lying on the right side (aft. 3 h.). [*Lgh.*]

780. In the nape of the neck, stiffness, as if bruised or from over-lifting, with a like pain above the hips; at night and in the morning.

In the neck, tensive stiffness. [*Bhr.*]

Distortion of the cervical muscles. [MUTTER, l. c.[1]]

Swelling of the external neck, without pain. [*Stf.*]

The artery of the left side of the neck swelled out extraordinarily, on stooping. [*Bhr.*]

785. Itching on the neck, below the jaw.

Colorless, smarting eruption all around the neck, on the shoulders and in the sides. [*Fr. H.*]

Soreness in the axillæ. [KLINGE, in *Hufel. Journ.*, VI., p. 904.[2]]

Tearing, stitching pain in the right axilla.

Swelling of the glands in the axilla. [*Hg.*]

790. In the arms, drawing pains. [*Hg.*]

Pain in the arm, on the side on which he is lying, at night.

Tearing in the arms, especially in the elbow and wrist, at night, in bed.

The right arm goes to sleep, when he sleeps on the right side.

A painful lump on the right arm. [*N. Wahrn.*, l. c.]

795. On the fore-arm, near the wrist, eroding itching, impelling to scratch. [*Lgh.*]

The hands are stiff and void of feeling. [PYL, l. c.[3]]

Drawing pain in both wrists, every evening.

Drawing pain in the metacarpal bones, in the morning.

---

[1] Not found.—*Hughes.*
[2] Observations on miners in Ars.—*Hughes.*
[3] For a long time.—*Hughes.*

Tearing stitches in the bones of the hand and of the little finger.

800. Cramp in the hand on moving it.

Cold hands. [*Stf.*]

Painful swelling of the hands. [*N. Wahrn.*, l. c.]

Severe formication in the hands, at night.

Fine tickling in the left palm, compelling to scratch. [*Lgh.*]

805. Little lumps, tubercles on the hands. [*N. Wahrn.*, l. c.]

Large suppurating boil on the hand, between the thumb and index, very broad, pale red, and extremely painful, especially in the evening. [*Hg.*]

The finger-joints are painful on moving them.

Cramp in the fingers of the right hand, when he stretches them straight out.

Cramp in the fingers, especially at night, in bed.

810. Painful cramp in the posterior joints of all the fingers.

Painful cramp in the tips of the fingers, from morning till noon (aft. 5 d.).

Rigidity of the fingers as if they were stiff.

Drawing pain in the middle fingers.

Drawing twitching, and tearing from the finger-tips up into the shoulders.

815. Tickling itching on the right middle finger, compelling him to scratch. [*Lgh.*]

Hard swelling of the fingers, with pains in their bones. [*Hg.*]

Discolored nails. [BAYLIES, l. c.]

Gout in the hips. [BORELLUS, *hist. et obs.*, *Cent.* III., *obs.* 36.[1]]

Violent, drawing tearing pain in the hips and in the left foot, in the morning, after a sleepless night (3d d.). [*Htb. u. Tr.*[2]]

820. In the lower limbs, especially in the joints, violent pains. [MAJAULT, l. c.]

Unbearable pains in the lower limbs. [*Htb. u. Tr.*]

Drawing tearing in the lower limbs, from the front side of the thigh to the knee and ankle-joint, when walking.

Tearing in the lower limbs, especially in the joints of the knees and the feet, only in motion.

Tearing in the lower limbs. [PYL, l. c.]

825. Tearing in the lower limbs, from above downward; he could not tread, nor sit, nor lie, either in bed or on a bench, but had either to keep the foot swinging to and fro, day and night, or limp around with it, not being able to rest; worse at night.

Tearing stitches as if in the periosteum, down the whole lower limb, even to the tip of the big toe.

Restlessness in the lower limbs, so that he can not lie still at night; he had to lay his feet now here, now there, or walk about for relief.

Restlessness in the lower limbs, before going to sleep, passing off when lying down.

---

[1] From carrying Ars. in the pocket.—*Hughes.*

[2] As sympt. 183.—*Hughes.*

Formication in the lower limbs, as if from going to sleep.

830. Cramp, spasm in the lower limbs. [PYL, l. c.]

With a spasmodic pain, certain bundles of muscles in the thighs and in the calves contracted, and the toes were drawn backward, making him very tired, in the evening, in bed.

Spasmodic pain in certain spots in the muscles of the thighs and legs, in jerks, with twitching; on touching it, it feels like something alive.

Convulsions of the lower limbs and knees. [ALBERTI, l. c.]

Weariness in the lower limbs.

835. Sensation as if the lower limbs were about to give way, on going up stairs. [*Htb. u. Tr.*[1]]

Paralysis of the lower limbs. [EBERS, l. c.[2]]

Coldness of the lower limbs, especially of the knees and feet, with cold perspiration on them; they could not get warm.

Swelling of the lower limbs, with unbearable pains. [*Htb. u. Tr.*]

On the thighs, eroding itching, impelling to scratch (aft. 13 h.). [*Lgh*]

840. Eroding itching on the right thigh, near the groin, with incitation to scratching (aft. 4½ h.).

Soreness between the thighs, with itching. [KLINGE, l. c.]

About the knees, sensation as if the lower limbs were tightly bandaged there.

Tension in the houghs, as if the tendons were too short, when sitting and standing, but not in walking.

Pain, as from bruising, on the side of the knee, only when touched, and in sitting, not when walking; a sensation as if the flesh there was detached.

845. Pain in the left knee, as if from a bruise or a sprain, especially on rising from a seat.

Stitching pain in the knees (aft. 2 h.). [RICHARD, l. c.]

Weakness in the knees, so that he could only with difficulty seat himself.

Great want of firmness in the right knee, it gives way under him.

Paralysis of knees. [J. B. MONTANUS, in *Schenk's lib.* 7 *obs.* 200.[3]]

850. In the right leg, drawing tearing, from the hough down into the heel, as if from a sprain.

Drawing pain in the legs, when they rest perpendicularly in sitting.

Drawing, tearing and twitching in the leg, from the ankle up into the knee.

Twitching in the legs, in the afternoon, when sitting.

Sharp, tearing drawing in the tibia.

855. Single, sharp tearings in the tibia, making him cry out.

Tearing pain in the right calf, when sitting (aft. 11 h.). [*Lgh.*]

---

1 As in symp. 183.—*Hughes.*
2 Not found.—*Hughes.*
3 Poisoning of a woman.—*Hughes.*

Tearing stitches low down on the inner side of the leg, in a small spot.

Boring pain in the right tibia.

Pressive pain in the calves.

860. Spasmodic pain in the leg, in the morning, changing into a tingling and humming therein.

Cramp in the calf, when walking (aft. 2 h.).

Cramp in the calves, chiefly at night, in bed.

Hardness in the calf, and sensation as if pressed flat, with unbearable pain, almost like cramp, from which she screamed for one and one-half hours; the whole leg was cold, insensible and stiff, so that she could not move it at all; there remained tension in the calf, and a sort of paralysis in the leg (aft. 50 h.).

Paralysis of the legs, so that he can scarcely walk. [FORESTUS, l. c.]

865. Heaviness of the legs, so that he can scarcely lift them.

Heaviness, weariness and drawing in the legs, with knuckling, lack of firmness and weakness of the knees, chiefly in the morning.

Emaciation of the legs. [MAJAULT, l. c.]

Swelling of the legs up above the calves; preceded by tearing in the calves, passing off on applying warm cloths.

Twitching pains, from above downwards, in the legs. [*Hg.*]

870. Ulcer on the left leg, below the knee. [*Hg.*]

Ulcer on the leg, covered with a gray scurf, burns painfully and has an inflamed border.

Pains in the feet. [GUELDENKLEE, l. c.]

Painfulness of the ankles on being touched. [*Htb. u. Tr.*[1]]

Pains of the heels, in the morning on awaking, as if they had lain on a hard surface.

875. The pains of the feet are aggravated by motion. [*Bhr.*]

Pain in the ankle-joint, above on the instep, as if ricked or sprained, when treading.

Pain in the foot, as from a sprain, when she does not set it down right or makes a misstep. [*Bhr.*]

Drawing in the foot, so that he cannot keep it still; at the same time he cannot step quickly, but only very gently and carefully.

Tearing in the ankles.

880. Tearing in the heels. [*Bhr.*]

Tearing around the ankles and on the dorsum of the feet, when lying down, with nausea.

Tearing and stitches in both the ankle-joints; when treading and walking, shooting pains, as if the feet were sprained, so that she is likely to fall; the ankles pain as if sore, when touched.

Lancinating pains on the outer border of the foot.

Stitches in the sole of the foot (aft. 1½ h.).

885. Stitches on the bottom of the left heel, when treading, extending up into the thigh.

Numb pains in the right foot; she can only lift it up, when sitting, by raising it up with her hand. [*Bhr.*]

---

[1] As sympt. 183.—*Hughes.*

Numbness, stiffness and insensibility of the feet, with swelling and great pain, from time to time. [PYL, l. c.]

Paralysis of the feet, after vomiting. [CARDANUS, in vol. VII of *Opera omnia Leyden, 1663.*[1]]

Cold feet, continually, when he is sitting still; he can hardly warm them in bed.

890. Coldness of the feet, with contracted pulse. [MORGAGNI, l. c., §8.]

Sensation of cold in the soles of the feet.

Swelling of the feet. [JACOBI, l. c.]

Swelling of the ankles, without redness, with tearing pains, relieved by external warmth.

Shining hot swelling of the feet, up above the ankles, with round red spots, which cause a burning pain (aft. 3 d.).

895. Hard reddish blue, greenish-yellow and very painful swelling on both feet (aft. 28 d.). [*Htb. u. Tr.*[2]]

Itching on the swelling of the feet.

The skin of the soles of the feet becomes insensible, thick as cork, and the soles chap. [*Hg.*]

Blisters break out in the night over the whole of the soles of the feet, as from applying cantharides; they crack open, discharging light-yellow fetid water. [*Hg.*]

Ulcers on the heels, with bloody pus. [GUILBERT, l. c.[3]]

900. All the toes become stiff, so that she could not tread. [*Hg.*]

Tickling, running itching on the right big toe, as when a wound is healing, compelling him to scratch (aft. 1½ h.). [*Lgh.*]

All her limbs ache.

All his limbs ache, whether walking, sitting or lying down.

Excessive pains in the limbs. [PFAUN, l. c.]

905. Pains in the whole body, chiefly in the evening. [*Sr.*]

Indescribably painful, excessively disagreeable sensation of illness in all the limbs.

Pain in the whole trunk, mostly in the back and in the sacrum, especially after riding on horseback (in a good rider.)

Gouty pains in the limbs, without inflammation.

Numb pain on the whole side of the body. [*Bhr.*]

910. Drawing pains in the joints of the knees, of the feet and of the hands.

Drawing pains, in the evening, in bed, in the middle finger and in the foot.

Severe tearing in the arms and lower limbs, while he cannot at all lie on the painful side; most endurable while moving the suffering part to and fro.

Tearing pains in the long bones.

Tearing pains in the bones. [*Bhr.*]

915. Sudden, tearing twitching or lancination, changing into burning, in the thumb or in the big toe, in the morning, in bed.

A thumping and tearing pain drawing up from the abdomen toward the head, where it was still more severe; then into the left

---

[1] General statement from authors.—*Hughes.*

[2] As sympt. 183.—*Hughes.*

[3] "Blutigem Eiter" (bloody pus), is "ichorose stoff" in the original; *i. e.*, ichorous matter.—*Hughes.*

side, where it was a lancinating, jerking pain, with two or three stitches.

Throbbing, drawing and stitching pain, at night, in the back, the sacrum and in the legs.

Beating in all the limbs and also in the head.

Burning pains, chiefly in the inner organs, in the skin and in ulcers.

920. Burning pains. [QUELMALZ, l. c., and others.]

Burning, eroding pains. [PREUSSIUS, l. c.; GABEZIUS, l. c.[1]]

In the suffering part, pain, as if the bone there was rubbed sore and swollen; perceptible when seated.

Ulcerous pain in the suffering parts, as if it was suppurating and would break open; sensible while sitting.

The pain in the suffering part wakes him up during the night, from time to time, especially before midnight.

925. **The pains are felt during the night, even in the midst of the sleep.**

The pains seem to the patient unbearable and make him frantic.

The pains and ailments frequently return, like intermittent fever, at certain hours.

Renewal of the same arsenical ailments, after the type of the quartan fever, at the same hour. [MORGAGNI, l. c.[2]]

With the paroxysms of pain other secondary ailments frequently arise.

930. To many ailments, a shiver is added.

With the pains, a shaking chill, and after them thirst.

With the outset of the pains, heat of the face and the body.

With the outset of the pains, roaring in the ears.

In ailments which are even slight, an excessive prostration and sinking of strength.

935. Many ailments only come on in the evening, after lying down; some a few hours after midnight, not a few in the morning after getting up.

After dinner, especially while sitting, many pains see renewed or aggravated.

The talking of others to him is intolerable, because it enormously aggravates his pains.

The ailments chiefly appear when sitting and lying down, and are diminished by standing and by motion.

Only by walking about can he make the nightly pains endurable; when sitting, and most of all in lying still, they are not to be endured.

940. **The pains may almost always be relieved by external warmth.**

By compressing the suffering parts, the pains are diminished and relieved.

During a sitting occupation, such uneasy restlessness in the body that she must rise and walk about.

---

[1] No reference for Gabezius, and he cannot be traced.—*Hughes.*

[2] This recurrence took place once only.—*Hughes.*

In the evening from 6 to 8 o'clock, violent pressing and squeezing in the head, excessive lack of appetite, transient perspiration and great anguish.

Great weariness and anxiety; she cannot recollect; it is difficult for her to give attention to everything; at the same time she feels like reeling.

945. Exhaustion when in ill-humor; with returning cheerfulness, she feels stronger.

Exhaustion. [BUCHHOLZ, *Beitr.* l. c.]

Fainting fits. [BUCHHOLZ, l. c. FORESTUS and many others.]

Violent swooning. [*Guilbert*, l. c. MORGAGNI, l. c.]

Profound swoons. [TENNERT. *prax. med. lit.* 6., p. 6, l. 9.]

950. Frequent swoons with weak pulse (aft. 3 h.). [FERELIUS, l. c.[1]]

Faint, in the morning, and anxious and weak.

Faintness comes on. [FRIEDRICH, l. c.]

Great weakness, especially in the legs. [PYL, l. c.]

Excessive weakness. [GOERITZ, l. c.]

955. **Sinking of the strength.** [STOERK, l. c., RAU and many others.]

Extraordinary weakness, especially in the legs, which can hardly be moved along. [KAISER, l. c.]

The strength sinks more and more. KAISER, l. c.]

Weakness, as if from lack of nourishment; there was lack of strength.

The strength of the hands and feet seems to have, as it were, gone, and they are extremely tremulous in the morning.

960. Extraordinary weakness in the knees, if he walks ever so little.

Paralytic weakness of the limbs, daily at a certain time, as in intermittent fever.

From weakness, walking becomes very difficult; he feels as if he should tumble down. [*Hbg.*]

Weakness, so that he can hardly cross the room without sinking down.

Great weakness, he cannot cross the room without sinking down. [*Stf.*]

965. Weakness, so that he could hardly cross the room. [EBERS, l. c.]

So weak, that he could not walk alone at all, before vomiting. [ALBERTI, l. c.]

He falls down on attempting to walk, while retaining consciousness. [PYL, l. c.]

Extraordinary weakness and bruised feeling in the limbs, compelling him to lie down. [GOERITZ, l. c.]

Weakness of the body for several days, with weak pulse, so that he has to lie down. [WEDEL, l. c.]

970. He must lie down and keep his bed. [*Fr. H.*]

Lying down. [ALBERTI, l. c.]

He lies down constantly during the day.

---

[1] With vomiting.—*Hughes*

He could not leave his bed, because of tremulous debility. [EBERS, l. c.[1]]

He could hardly get up from bed for several days. [*Stf.*]

975. He wants to get up, but on rising he cannot keep on his feet.

When she rises from bed, she at once sinks down from weakness and dizziness, with aggravated headache.

Merely from sinking of strength—death ensues, without vomiting and convulsions, and without pains. [MORGAGNI, l. c. and several others.]

With extreme asthenia, with violent vertigo, constant vomiting and hematuria; a rapid extinction of life (without cramps, without fever and without pain). [HALL, *Allg. Lit. Zeit.*, 1815, No. 181.[2]]

Emaciation. [STOERK, l. c.; JACOBI, l. c.[3]]

980. Total emaciation. [GREISELIUS l. c.]

She becomes very much emaciated, with earthy sallow complexion; blue rings around the eyes; great weakness in all the limbs; disinclination for all work, and constant inclination to rest (aft. 8 d).

Emaciation of the whole body, with profuse sweats.

Consumption. [MAJAULT, l. c.[4]]

Consumptive fever. [STOERK, l. c.[5]]

985. Gradually wasted away (and died within a year). [AMAT. LUSIT, l. c.]

Consumption, ending in death. [SALZB, *Med. Chir. Zeit.*[6]]

Jaundice. [MAJAULT, l. c.]

Dropsy of the skin. [EBERS, l. c.[7]]

Complete general anasarca. [EBERS, l. c., p. 56.]

990. Severe swelling of the face and of the whole body. [FERNEL, l. c.]

Swelling of the whole right side of the body, down to the hips, with swelling of the left leg. [THILENIUS, l. c.]

Swellings on various parts of the body, of an elastic kind. [FOWLER, l. c.]

Swelling of the face and of the feet, dry mouth and lips, distended abdomen, diarrhœa, colic, vomiting. [EBERS, l. c.[8]]

Cholera. [WOLFF, l. c.[9]]

995. **Cramps.** [HENNING l c.; KELLNER, l. c.]

Tetanus [KAISER, l. c.]

Attacks of tetanus. [*Salz M. C. F.*, l. c.]

With and without spasms—death. [KAISER, l. c.]

Convulsions. [CRUEGER, l. c.; WEDEL and others.]

1000. Convulsions before death (after-effect?). [ALBERTI, l. c.; BONETUS, l. c.]

---

[1] As symptom 81.—*Hughes.*

[2] From inhaling arseniuretted hydrogen in a man. (Death did not occur till the seventh day.)—*Hughes.*

[3] As symptom 81.—*Hughes.*

[4] With symptom 987.—*Hughes.*

[5] As symptom 81.—*Hughes.*

[6] From application of ars. to a fungus on the head.—*Hughes.*

[7] As symptom 81.—*Hughes.*

[8] As symptom 81.—*Hughes.*

[9] That is constant vomiting and diarrhœa, with sharp nose, cold limbs, cramps and death.—*Hughes.*

Convulsions of an extremely violent kind. [VAN EGGERN, l. c.]

Convulsions and piteous contortions of the limbs. [MORGAGNI, l. c.]

Convulsions, which are caused from time to time by violent pains in the soles of the feet. [PFANN, l. c.]

Convulsive paroxysm; at first she struck outwards with the arms, then she lost all consciousness, lay like a dead person, pale, yet warm, turned her thumbs inward, turned her clenched hands, slowly drew up her arms and then slowly laid them down; after 10 minutes she drew the mouth hither and thither, as if she waggled her jaw; at the same time no respiration could be perceived; after a quarter of an hour the fit ended with a jerk throughout the whole body, like a single thrust forward with arms and feet, and at once her full consciousness returned, only great prostration remained.

1005. Epileptic convulsions. [CRUEGER, l. c.; BUETTNER, l. c.]

Trembling of the limbs. [BONETUS, l. c.; GREISELIUS and many others.]

Trembling. [KAISER, l. c.]

Trembling of the limbs, even after a moderate walk. [*Htb. u. Tr.*[1]]

Trembling and quivering with perspiration in the face. [ALBERTI, l. c.]

1010. Trembling over the whole body. [GUILBERT, l. c.]

He trembles in every part of the body. [*Hbg.*]

Trembling in all the limbs. [JUSTAMOND on Canc. Disorders, London, 1750.[2]]

Trembling of the limbs after the vomiting. [CARDAMUS, l. c.]

Trembling of the arms and the lower limbs.

1015. **Stiffness and immovableness of all the joints.** [PET. DE APPONO, *de venen*, c. 17.]

She becomes quite rigid, can not stir or move herself, but merely stand still.

Stiffness of all the joints; he cannot stretch himself, because everything in the body is tense; the knees are so stiff and cold that he bandages them in cloths, as they else would pain him and disturb his sleep. [*Hg.*]

Stiffness and immovableness of the limbs with severe tearing pains. [*Htb. u. Tr.*[3]]

Stiffness, especially of the knees and feet, alternating with tearing pains. [*Htb. u. Tr*[3].]

1020. As if paralyzed in all the limbs; he cannot tread firmly. [*Hbg.*]

Paralysis, he could not walk any more. [CREUGER, l. c.]

Paralysis, contraction. (*Pet. de Appono*, in SCHENCK, *lib.* 17, *obs.* 214).

---

[1] As sympt. 183.—*Hughes.*

[2] From ars. given to a woman with cancer on tongue. For "on canc. disorders" read "Surgical Essays, p. 333."—*Hughes.*

[3] As sympt. 183.—*Hughes.*

Contraction of the limbs. [HAMMER in *comm. lit. Nor.* 1773. Hebd, 24.[1]]

Paralysis of the lower limbs. [BERNHARDI. *Annal., d. Heilk.* 1811, Jan., p. 60.[2]]

1025. Paralysis of the lower limbs, with loss of sensation. [HUBER, *N. act. n. c.* III. *obs.* 100.[3]]

Paralysis of the feet. [HEINREICH l. c.[4]]

The skin on the whole body peels off in large scales. [*Hg.*]

Painfulness of the skin of the whole body.

Stitches in the skin as if from needles [*N. Wahrn.* l. c.]

1030. Slow stitches here and there on the skin as if from a red hot needle.

Fine stitches all over the body.

Much itching on the right thigh and on the arms.

Itching crawling sensation as from fleas, on the thighs up to the abdomen, also on the loins and nate, compelling to scratch.

Burning itching on the body.

1035. Burning itching, with painfulness of the spot on scratching.

Intolerable burning on the skin. [HEINREICH, l. c.]

Burning on the skin (of the finger), excessively violent, as if the spot had been burned with boiling fat (after dipping the hands in a cold solution of arsenic.)

Spots here and there on the skin. [BAYLIES, l. c.]

Blue spots on the abdomen, on the genitals, and in the white of the eye. [KAISER, l. c.]

1040. Inflamed spots like measles over the body, chiefly on the head, the face and neck. [THOMSON, l. c.]

Eruption on the skin: [MAJAULT, l. c.[5]]

Eruption like red petechiae, from the size of a flea-bite up to that of a lentil, sharply defined, in the evening, painful, quite dry, only humid and burning after scratching. [*Sr.*]

Miliary eruption all over the body, falling off in scales. [GUILBERT, l. c.]

Red, scorbutic, miliary rash. [Hartmann, *dissert. æth.* ant. et ars. Halle, 1759.[6]]

1045. Pimples like millet, with white points over the whole body, even over the hands and feet. [DESGRANGES, in *Phys. med. Jour.* 1800, Apr., p. 299.[7]]

Little pointed pimples break out, with itching which passes off on scratching.

Whitish, pointed pimples, with watery humor in the tip, break out with a burning itching, as from the stings of flies, on the hands, between the fingers and on the abdomen; by scratching, the humor flows out and the itching ceases.

Small pimples on various parts of the body, also on the forehead and under the chin, causing burning pain and some itching.

---

[1] Poisoning of a girl of 20.—*Hughes.*
[2] Not accessible.—*Hughes.*
[3] Statement that author knows a woman so affected by ars.—*Hughes.*
[4] Cited from CARDAN; same sympton as 888.—*Hughes.*
[5] Not found.—*Hughes.*
[7] Not accessible.—*Hughes.*
[7] From rubbing ars. into head.—*Hughes.*

Eruption of pimples with severe burning, so that she can hardly contain herself for distress.

1050. Eruption of itch, especially in the houghs. [*Hg.*]

Fine sandy tickling itch on the whole body. [*Hg.*]

Little lumps which heal with great difficulty. [AMAT. LUSITAN, l. c.[1]]

Dense eruption of white tubercles, larger and smaller than a lentil, of the color of the rest of the skin, with a smarting pain, usually worse at night. [*Fr. H.*]

Cutaneous eruptions similar to nettle-rash. [FOWLER, l. c.[2]]

1055. Black pocks, which cause burning pain. [PFANN, l. c.]

Very painful black pocks. [VERZASCH, l. c.]

Ulcer which is painful, especially in the morning, with dark-brown, thin, bloody pus under a thin scurf, and with single stitches while sitting, alleviated by standing and still more by walking.

Cancerous ulcer, which compels the amputation of a limb. [HEINZE in EBERS, l. c.[3]]

The ulcer comes to have very elevated borders.

1060. Painful sensitiveness of old ulcers which hitherto were painless.

Tearing pain in the ulcers.

Burning pain in the ulcers.

Burning pain in an ulcer. [HARGENS in *Hufel Journ.* IX, I.]

Burning in an ulcer as from a red hot coal.

1065. Burning in an ulcer, which comes from itching. [HEUN, l. c.]

Burning around the border of an ulcer, with subsequent itching in the ulcer.

Burning like fire around an ulcer, which is very fetid and suppurates a little; attended with exhaustion and drowsiness in the day-time.

Inflammation of an ulcer in its border; it bleeds on being bandaged and a superfical dry scab forms. [HARGENS, l. c.]

The ulcer discharges much black, coagulated blood.

1070. Proud flesh forms in the ulcers (on the finger) and quickly putrefies, becomes blue and green with a sticky ichor, which spreads an intolerable stench. [*Hg.*]

Great indolence and indisposition to the lightest movement. [*Hg.*]

Weariness and pain of the joints, in the forenoon, more when sitting than when walking.

Great weariness after eating.

Great weariness after dinner, and excessive yawning.

1075. Yawning and stretching as if he had not slept enough. [*Lgh.*]

Very frequent yawning.

Yawning, almost uninterrupted.

Yawning and exhaustion after eating, so that he had to lie down and sleep.

Frequent fits of sleep, in day-time, while sitting.

---

[1] Not found.—*Hughes.*
[2] Slight.—*Hughes.*
[3] In a refiner of ars.—*Hughes.*

1080. Strong inclination to sleep; he falls asleep again just after conversing; for four days (aft. 6 d.). [*Fr. H.*]

Great, almost irresistible inclination to sleep, alternating with great restlessness. [KAISER, l. c.]

Drowsiness, interrupted by uneasy dreams and severe anxieties.

Feels as if he had not slept enough, in the morning. [*Hg.*]

She has not slept enough in the morning and there is weariness in her eyes so that she cannot get out of bed in the morning.

1085. Toward morning, involuntary mental activity, hindering him from sleeping, much as he requires sleep.

Sleeplessness. [BUCHHOLZ, l. c.; KNAPE and several others.]

Sleeplessness, with fainting fits from time to time. [GUELDENKLEE, l. c.]

Sleeplessness, with restlessness and moaning.

Sleepless tossing at night, with crawling in the abdomen.

1090. At night, lancinating pain in the left meatus auditorius, as from within outward.

At night, soon after going to sleep, toothache, from which he awakes.

At night, while lying in bed, severe stinging tearing in the corn.

After midnight, from three o'clock on, he tosses about and only sleeps in fits.

At night, she cannot get warm in bed.

1095. After midnight, sensation of anxious heat, with tendency to uncover himself.

The whole night, much heat and restlessness, with pulsation in the head, so that she cannot go to sleep.

During the night, much thirst, on account of great dryness in the throat, which ceases in the morning.

Before going to sleep at night, she feels in the larynx as if choking, as if from fumes of sulphur, causing tussiculation.

On going to sleep, violent twitching in the limbs.

1100. **Twitches of various kinds on going to sleep**, in the evening.

On going to sleep in the evening, startling twitches, like shaking thrusts in the parts affected, which are excited by a slight ailment in a distant part, by a tearing, an itching, etc.

Immediately on lying down, sudden contractive twitching in the knee, with awaking as from an electric shock, caused by dreaming that he is about to knock his foot against a stone.

In sleep, a spasmodic starting of the whole body (aft. 36 h.). [THOMSON, l. c.[1]]

Much violent starting and awaking frightened from his sleep. [THOMSON, l. c.[2]]

1105. During sleep, in the evening, loud moaning.

---

[1] Should be "in bed" and not "in sleep," and "after 12" and not "36" hours.—*Hughes.*
[2] After opium had been taken as an antidote.—*Hughes.*

In sleep, moaning, with tossing in bed, especially about the third hour after midnight.

He talks and scolds in his sleep.

In sleep, he gnashes with his teeth.

In his slumber, in the morning, he hears every sound and every noise, and yet he continues to dream with it all.

1110. In his sleep, a general sensation of illness, two nights in succession.

In sleep, he lies on his back, the left hand supporting his head.

In sleep, he moves his fingers and his hands.

The sleep is uneasy and she wakes up very early. [*Bhr.*]

During frequent awakings at night, **burning in all the arteries.**

1115. On awaking in the morning, much ill-humor; she did not know what to do for vexation; she pushed away the pillows and the coverlet and would not look at anyone or listen to anyone.

On awaking early in bed, a dull headache, passing away on rising.

On awaking early in bed, a sensation of qualmishness, of nausea all the way up in the chest, then vomiting of white mucus, but with bitterish taste in the mouth.

Early in bed, at sunrise, general heat, perspiration of the face and dryness of the anterior part of the mouth, without thirst.

He wakes up at night in a dream, during a pollution, without being able to remember his dream. [*Whl.*]

1120. Dreams at night, full of threats or fears or repentance.

Anxious dreams; he wakes up and dreams about the same thing on going to sleep again.

Anxious, dangerous dreams, from each of which he awakes, sometimes with a loud cry, whereupon he then always dreams of something else.

Anxious, sorrowful and fearful dreams disturb his sleep.

Anxious, fearful dreams at night.

1125. Anxious dream, at once on going to sleep; he wishes to scream, but can hardly get out a word and awakes suddenly from his own cry, which he still hears.

Many grievous dreams at night. [*Htb. u. Tr.*[1].]

Continuous dreams of thunder-showers, conflagrations, black water and darkness.

Vivid, vexing dreams. [*Lgh.*]

Delirium, at night. [SIEBOLD. l. c.]

1130. Dreams, full of wearying reflection.

Coldness of the limbs. [RICHARD, l. c.; FERNELIUS, l. c.]

Coldness in the hands and feet, and even in the abdomen, in the evening.

General coldness, with profuse perspiration of the skin. [KAISER, l. c..]

Coldness of the body and dryness of the skin alternate with cold sweat. [KAISER, l. c.]

---

[1] **Reference ought to be** [BORRI, l. c.]—*Hughes.*

1135. Shivering. [BUCHHOLZ, *Beitr.*, l. c.]
Febrile rigor. [*M. N. Zeit.*, 1798, Sept.[2]]
Febrile rigor, chill.
Shivering without thirst. (At once).
Loathing shivering after drinking. [ALBERTI, l. c.]
1140. **After drinking, shivering** and chill. (At once).
After dinner, shivering.
After dinner the shivering ceases. (A more rare alternate action).
Every afternoon at five o'clock, the shiver returns.
In the evening, shivering, just before lying down.
1145. Every evening a febrile rigor.
A shiver before going to bed.
When going into the open air shiverings come on.
Shiverings all over the body, with hot forehead, warm face and cold hands [*Lgh.*].
Shiverings all over the body, with warm forehead, hot cheeks, and cold hands. [*Lgh.*]
1150. **During the rigor there frequently arise other ailments or pains.**
During the rigor, tearing in the legs.
Chilliness in the external skin, over the face and the feet.
Chilliness, even up to the most severe chill. [KAISER, l. c.]
Violent shaking chill. [FERNELIUS, l. c.]
1155. Chill, without being able to get warm, with peevishness and a flying heat running over the body while speaking or moving; then she became red in the face, and yet was chilly.
Chill with cold feet, he began to perspire.
Every afternoon at 3 o'clock, chill with hunger; after the meal, the chill was aggravated.
In the afternoon, internal chill, with external heat and red cheeks.
Toward evening, chilliness with coldness.
1160. In the evening, chilliness in the legs, from the calves down to the feet.
In the evening after lying down a severe chill in bed.
In the evening, he cannot get warm in bed; he thinks he caught cold in bed.
During the chill, no thirst.
In the afternoon—chill, colic and diarrhœic stool; and after this, continued colic.
1165. She is either too cold all over the body, and yet is nowhere cold to the touch, or she is too warm, and yet is nowhere hot to the touch, except perhaps in the palm.
Heat, internal and external, through the whole body, as from drinking wine, with thirst for beer. [*Mr.*]
Internal heat. [GŒRITZ, l. c.]
Internal heat, with thirst, after diarrhœa. [MORGAGNI, l. c.]
Severe heat. [KAISER, l. c.]
1170. Dry heat of the skin. [KAISER, l. c.]

[2] Not accessible.—*Hughes*.

Anxious heat. [PET. DE APPONO, l. c.[1]]

General anxious heat. [*Hbg.*]

In the evening about seven o'clock, heat in the face, for an hour.

Nocturnal heat, without thirst and without perspiration.

1175. After the heat, nausea.

Perspiration. [MAJAULT, l. c.[2]]

Perspiration with excessive thirst, so that he continually desires to drink. [*Hbg.*]

Perspiration, which exhausts him in bed, even to fainting.

Cold, clammy sweat. [HENNING, l. c.[3]]

1180. Perspiration, during which the skin and especially the eyes are colored yellow. [EBERS, l. c.[4]]

In the forenoon, perspiration with heaviness of the head, roaring of the ears and trembling.

Night-sweats. [*Hg.*]

Night-sweats, three nights in succession.

At night, profuse sweat on the lower limbs, especially about the knees.

1185. Itching and slight perspiration on the back, all the night.

In the beginning of the sleep, in the evening on lying down, perspiration, which ceases in the subsequent sleep.

In the beginning of sleep, perspiration, only on the hands and thighs, which passes away in the subsequent sleep (aft. 6 h.).

Morning-sweat, all over the body from the time of awaking till rising.

In the morning, on awaking, sweat only in the face.

1190. In the morning, perspiration on the legs (the 1st night).

Fever of a very violent kind. [KNAPE, l. c., DEGNER, l. c.]

Fever. [HENN, l. c.[5]]

Fever, terminating in death. [AMAT. LUSIT, l. c.[6]]

Fever with violent thirst. [MORGAGNI, l. c.]

1195. Paroxysms of fever, returning several days at the same hour.

Toward evening, he has an unpleasant sensation in his body, like fever, and when he lies down, his head becomes hot, and especially the ears, but the knees are cold (aft. 36 h.).

Fever, chill in the evening and morning, without thirst, with much micturition, little stool, and stretching in all the limbs. [*Hg.*]

Fever, external chilliness of the limbs, with intermal heat, with anxious restlessness, and weak, changeable pulse. [ALBERTI, l. c.]

Fever, a brief chill, at night, then severe heat with delirium, without thirst. [*Hg.*]

1200. Febrile rigor, in the morning, alternating with heat.

Febrile rigor and shivering, with heat of the external ear, at the same time anguish and gnawing in the scrobiculus cordis, combined with nausea.

---

1 Latin, "exæstuatio."—*Hughes.*
2 Stated as effect of antidote, (aniseed.)—*Hughes.*
3 With violent vomiting. (See S. 19 and 268).—*Hughes.*
4 As sympt. 81.—*Hughes.*
5 **Not found.—*Hughes.***
6 **Not found.—*Hughes.***

Fever, in the afternoon, shivering of the external head, with stretching and drawing in the limbs, then chill with goose-skin, from 8–9 P. M.; heat in the body, especially in the face, without perspiration, with cold hands and feet.

Fever, when he comes from the open air into the room; first a chill, then long-continued hiccup, then general perspiration, then again hiccup.

Fever toward evening; chilliness with drowsiness and a disagreeable sensation of illness all through the body, as after a fit of fever quite or nearly gone; then after midnight, a profuse sweat on the thighs; it returned after two days, at the same time.

1205. Fever, much chilliness during the day, after it thirst, in the evening much heat in the face.

Febrile rigor first, then dry heat of the skin. [KAISER, l. c.]

Fever, alternately chills and heat. [ALBERTI, l. c.]

Fever in the forenoon; violent rigor without thirst, with spasms in the chest, pains throughout the body, and a sort of lack of the power of recollecting; then heat with thirst; then sweat with roaring in the ears.

Fever, every other day; the first afternoon about 6 o'clock a chill, with weariness and a feeling of bruisedness in the thighs; the third afternoon at 5 o'clock, at first inclination to lie down, then a shaking chill all over without thirst, then heat without thirst, with pressive headache in the forehead.

1210. Fever in the evening at 10 o'clock; heat with redness in the whole body; then sweat. [*Stf.*]

Fever at night at 2 o'clock; increased warmth of the whole body, perspiration in the face and on the feet, and a tension with colic-like pains in the hypochondria and the epigastrium, causing anxiety.

Burning fever, so that cold water gives no relief; after the heat, sweat, especially in the nape of the neck; appearing sometimes every fourteen days, a few days at a time. [*Hg.*]

When the fever is at an end, the perspiration always follows at its termination.

In the paroxysm of fever, increased tension in the hypochondria, so that he can hardly lie on the side at all.

1215. Inordinate rush of blood. [GRIMM, l. c.[1]]

Feeling as if the blood ran through the arteries too rapidly and too hot, with small, quick pulse. [*Stf.*]

Pulse exceedingly feverish. [KNAPE, l. c.]

Pulse excited and frequent, not full. [KAISER, l. c.]

Quick, small, hardish pulse. [KAISER, l. c.]

1220. **Quick, small pulse.** [N. WAHRN, l. c.; MAJAULT, l. c.]

Quick, weak pulse. [MAJAULT, l. c.[2]]

Quick, weak, intermittent pulse. [GUILBERT, l. c.[3]]

Tense pulse. [KNAPE, l. c.]

Little and weak pulse. [KAISER, l. c.]

1225. Little, frequent, weak pulse. [MORGAGNI, l. c.]

---

[1] Latin "exæstuatio" as in S. 1171.—*Hughes.*

[2] Not found.—*Hughes.*

[3] Pulse was "irregular," not "intermittent."—*Hughes.*

Exceedingly slow pulse, down to thirty-eight beats. [PEARSON, l. c.[4]]

Intermittent, small pulse. [KAISER, l. c.]

Intermittent, unequal, small pulse, which finally vanishes entirely. [KAISER, l. c.]

Absence of pulse, attended with frequent, very excited heart-beat. [KAISER, l. c.]

1230. After death, the lips and the nails on the hands and feet are blue, as well as the glans and the scrotum; the whole body, especially the limbs, are rigid and contracted, and the large intestine very much constricted. [PYL, l. c.]

The body after sixteen days was still fresh and undecomposed. [PYL, l. c.]

AURUM, GOLD.

(THE WELL-KNOWN METAL.)

Just as superstition, inexact observations and credulous conjectures have been the source of innumerable untrue statements as to the virtue of medicines in the materia medica, so also lack of proving and groundless theoretic reasons of physicians have with just a little reason denied to exceedingly powerful, and therefore highly curative substances, all medicinal powers, and have thus deprived us of these remedies.

Here I will only mention gold, and, indeed, not the gold changed through the ordinary chemical processes, neither that dissolved by acids, nor that which is separated again by precipitation (the fulminating gold), both of which were also stated to be, if not useless, still utterly injurious substances; probably because they could not be given in a so-called *justa dosis*, *i. e.*, in an excessive quantity, without incurring danger.

No! I speak of the pure gold, unchanged by any chemical process.

This the modern physicians have declared to be entirely without effect, and have finally omitted it altogether from all their teachings of materia medica, and have thus deprived us of all its great curative powers.

It was stated, that "it cannot be dissolved in the gastric juice, and that it is, therefore, altogether without power or use." This was their theoretical supposition, and such *theoretical dicta* have

[4] Pulse had not been previously counted.—*Hughes.*

always, in medicine, had the force of *conviction.* As they do not question experience—the only possible revealer in the healing art, which rests altogether on experience—*because it was more convenient merely to assert*, they usually put bold affirmation, theoretic, empty supposition and arbitrary decrees in the place of well-founded truth.

The excuse, that older physicians also supposed gold to be without any use or efficacy, will not here avail them. So, *e. g.*, FABRICIUS (in *Obs. med.*) says: "How could the slight heat of our stomach have any effect on leaf-gold, when it loses nothing even in the most violent fire?" Or NIC. MONARDES (*de ferro*, pp. 32, 33): "The patients may believe me and save the expense of putting gold into their medicine; they will in no wise gain from it any medicinal virtue in their diseases." Or again, ALSTON (*Nat. Med.*, I., p. 69): "Since gold in its metallic state is not dissolved and can not be changed by our vital force, it can not, therefore, have any medicinal power, except such action as it may exert on the bowels by means of its weight, hardness and mechanical form. Or, finally, J. F. GMELIN (*Appar. med. min.*, I., p. 445): "Since gold is indestructible, cannot be dissolved into vapor, and cannot therefore combine with the juices of the animal body, it cannot therefore have any curative power."*

Nor can it serve them as an excuse if they can adduce many other old physicians as deniers of the medicinal powers of gold, and can name men like ANT. MUSA BRASSAVOLUS, FEL. PLATERUS, HIER. CARDANUS, JO. BRAVUS PETRAFIT, FRANC. PIC. MIRANDOLA, MERINUS MERCENIUS, DURETUS, CAMERARIUS, CORDOSUS, CONRINGIUS, LEMARY, ANGELUS SALA, and even JOH. SCHROEDER, so credulous in other matters.

They are all wrong, and with them all the modern physicians.

Gold has great medicinal virtues which cannot be supplied by anything else. At first I allowed myself to be kept back by these deniers from hoping to find any medicinal virtues in pure gold; but as I could not be satisfied in believing that any metal was, in itself, without medicinal virtues, I first made use of gold in solution. From this experiment were derived the few symptoms of the solution of gold. I then would give, where the symptoms would lead me to its homœopathic use with patients, one quintillionth or a sextillionth

---

* It was very silly to desire to decide theoretically the question whether gold *could* have any curative virtues; all that was necessary was but to gather conviction by trials and experience, whether gold has or has not medicinal powers. If it has medicinal virtues then all the theoretical hypotheses of denial are ludicrous.

of a grain of gold solution as a dose, and found even here a similar curative virtue as I afterwards discovered in pure gold.

But I am in general, on the score of pure simplicity, unwilling, where I can avoid it, to use the metals combined with acids, as they must surely suffer a change of their virtues through these acids. This may be seen at once on comparing the medicinal powers of the corrosive sublimate with those of the blackish protoxid of mercury. It was, therefore, to me a welcome fact to find a series of Arabic physicians who unanimously extolled the virtues of gold used in a *fine powder*, and this in states of disease which sorely need help, and in which the solution of gold had already in part done wonderful service; a circumstance which was bound to give me confidence in the asseverations of the Arabs.

The first trace of this use of gold we find as early as the eighth century, where GEBER (*de Alchimia traditio*, *Argent. ap.* ZETZNER, 1698, *Lib.* II., P. III., Cap. 32) praises gold as a "*materia laetificans et in juventute corpus conservans*" (a substance that gladdens and preserves the body in youth).

At the end of the tenth century SERAPION the younger (*De simplicibus comment.* Venet. fol. ap. Junt. 1550, Cap. 415, p. 192) says: "Powdered gold serves in melancholy and in weakness of the heart."

Then, in the beginning of the eleventh century, AVICENNA (*Canon*, *Lib.* II., Cap. 79) says: "Powdered gold is added to medicines against melancholy; it cures the fetid odor of the mouth, and taken internally, it is even a curative in the falling out of the hair; it strengthens the eyes, helps in cardialgia and palpitation of the heart, and is extremely useful in asthma."*)

The preparation of such a gold powder is first described in the beginning of the twelfth century by ABULKASEM (ALBUCASIS) (in *libro servitoris de præp. med.*, p. 242): "The gold must be rubbed on rough linen in a basin full of water, and the fine powder that settles at the bottom of the water must be used." JOHANN VON ST. AMAND (in the thirteenth century) teaches the preparation in the same manner, in the apendix to MESUE, *Opera*, *Venet.*, 1561, p. 245, 4 E.

ZACUTUS, the Portuguese, imitated this and he describes (*Hist. medic.*, lib. I., obs. 33) the case of a nobleman, who had been for a long time tormented by melancholy phantasies, and whom he cured

*This latter word is in Arabic an ambiguous expression, meaning, according as the word is accentuated, either: "talking with oneself" or "asthma." The curative virtue of gold, as shown by experience, shows that the latter is here the true meaning of the word.

within a month *solely* by the finely comminuted powder of gold, pre pared on a grindstone.

We do not now need the further praises of the gold powder and of gold, as found in Jo. PLATEARIUS (*quaest. therap.*), RODERICUS A CASTRO (*de Meteor. microcosm, Cap.* 3), ABRAHAM A PORTA LEONIS (*dialog. de Auro*), ZACCHARIAS A PUTEO, JOH. DAN. MYLIUS *Anatomia Auri*), HORN (*Ephem. Nat. Cur. Dec.* II., *ann.* 3, *obs.* 159), FR. BACO (*Histor. vitæ et mortis*), FR. JOSEPH BURRHI (*Epist.* 4 *ad. Thom. Barthol. de oculis*), JO. JACOB WALDSCHMIEDT (*Diss. de auro ejusque in medic. viribus, Gryphisv*, 1703), LEMNIUS, PET. FORESTUS, OL. BORRICHIUS, ROLFINCK, ANDR. LAGNER, ETTMUELLER, TACKIUS, HELCHER (*Diss. de Auro*, Jen., 1730), POTERIUS, J. D. HORSTIUS, HOLLERIUS, HŒFER and ZWELFER (*Pharm. August*). I believed that I might well prefer the testimony of the Arabians concerning the curative virtues of the fine powder of gold to the theoretic doubts of the moderns supported by no experiment; I therefore rubbed the finest leaf-gold (of 23 carat 6 grains fineness) with 100 parts of sugar of milk for a full hour, in order to apply it to internal medicinal use.

I do not wish to decide whether in this fine powder the gold was merely still further comminuted, or was also somewhat oxidized by this vigorous trituration. It is sufficient that in proving this preparation 100 grains of this powder (containing one grain of gold) sufficed with some healthy adults, with others, however, 200 grains (containing two grains of gold) dissolved in water, to excite very strong changes in the state of their health, and to cause the symptoms enumerated below.

From these it will be seen that the asseverations of the Arabs cannot have been without foundation, as even small doses of this metal, used in the form mentioned, caused very similar symptoms of disease in healthy persons to those which these orientals (who are not without merit in discovering medicines) had healed (unconsciously in accordance with the Homœopathic principles).

Of melancholies, resembling that caused by gold, I have since cured quickly and permanently several persons who were seriously entertaining suicidal intentions, and, indeed, by small doses, which for the whole cure did not contain more than $\frac{3}{100}$ or $\frac{9}{100}$ of a grain of gold. So I have also cured several other difficult maladies, which in their symptoms showed similarities to those of gold. I have no doubt that much more attenuated preparations of the gold powder will be quite sufficient to attain this same purpose.

* * * * * * * *

Some time after closing this preliminary account I had the opportunity of convincing myself that a hundredfold attenuation of the above-mentioned preparation (the gold triturated with 100 parts of sugar of milk), thus the .0001 part of a grain of gold as a dose proved itself no less effective in causing a cure, especially in caries of the bones of the palate and nose, produced by the abuse of salts of mercury. The symptoms of gold for this homœopathic cure may easily be found in this list.

By further triturations and dilutions, the virtue of gold is still more developed and spiritualized, so that I now need for such curative effects but a very small part of a grain of the decillionth attenuation.

Would the ordinary proceedings of our physicians, which consist in fabricating medicinal virtues from airy hypotheses, and who decry this product in their Materia Medica, have ever succeeded in discovering the wonderful virtues of a metal, which their learned art of conjecture had already condemned as totally powerless? Or by what other favorite method of our manufacturers of Materia Medica could we ever have found out the curative side of gold, if its symptoms creating a similar morbid state had not loudly and with full certainty taught it to the homœopathic physician?

Poor, fabulous Materia Medica of the ordinary kind! How far do you stay behind those revelations which medicines unequivocally reveal of their effects on the healthy human body in causing those morbid symptoms which the homœopathic physician is sure to be able to apply with unfailing success in the cure of natural diseases!

The period of activity of gold in moderate doses is at least twenty-one days.

An antidote to its excessive effects has been found in the smelling of a potentized preparation of crude coffee, and more especially of camphor.

Gold has especially proved itself useful in chronic diseases when the following ailments predominate, or at least were simultaneously present.

Hypochondria; melancholy; surfeit of life; impulse to suicide; *rush of blood to the head* [*Lh.*]; caries of the bones of the palate and the nose; obscuration of the vision through black dots floating before the eye; *toothache from rush of blood to the head with heat in it;* inguinal hernia; induration of the testes of long-standing; prolapsus and induration of the uterus; *rush of blood to the chest;* falling down unconscious, with blueness of the face [*Lh.*]; fit of suffocation with severe

* This same curative effect from the internal use of gold against injuries from mercury was witnessed by ANT. CHALMETEUS in *Enchiridon chirurg.*, p. 402.

constrictive tightness of the chest [*Lh.*]; injuries from abuse of mercury; pains in the bones, at night; nodosities from gout.

The abbreviations of the names of my fellow provers are: *Fz.*, *Dr. Franz; Gr.*, *Dr. Gross; Fr. H.*, *Dr. Friedrich Hahnemann; Hpl.*, *Dr. Hempel; Hrm.*, *Dr. Hermann; Lgh.*, *Dr. Langhammer; Lh.*, *Dr. G. Lehmann; Mch.*, *Dr. Michler; Rl.*, *Dr. Rummel; Wl.*, *Dr. Wislicenus.*

AURUM FOLIATUM.

Dejected and sad.

He is dejected and seeks solitude.

He believes that he has lost the love of others, and this mortifies him even to tears. [*Fz.*]

Discontent with all conditions; he thinks that he everywhere finds an impediment, caused now by an opposing fate, then again by himself, which latter mortifies him and renders him dejected. [*Hpl.*]

5. Melancholy; he imagines that he is not fitted for the world, he therefore longs for death, of which he thinks with the most intense delight. [*Fz.*]

Great anxiety springing from the region of the heart, and which drives him from one place to another, so that he cannot long remain in a place. [*Fz.*]

Great anxiety and weakness, so that he is thought to be near death. [J. H. SCHULZE, *praelect. in pharm.*, *Aug.*, p. 46.[1]]

Frequent attacks of anguish of heart and tremulous anxiety. [*Ephem. Nat. Cur. Ceut.*, 10, *obs.* 35.[2]]

Extraordinary anxiety with palpitation of the heart, weariness in all the limbs and drowsiness.

10. **Great anguish, mounting even to suicide** with spasmodic contraction in the abdomen.

Restlessness and hurried impulse to bodily and mental activity; he can not work fast enough; he could not act so as to satisfy himself. [*Hpl.*]

He is driven to constant activity, and is sorry for his inaction, although he cannot do anything. [*Fz.*]

Restless and undecided, without perceptible ebullition of the blood; he always thinks he is neglecting something for which he will be reproached; he seems to carry with him this internal restlessness, and it took from him all perseverance and energy. [*Hpl.*]

Aurum first appeared in the *Materia Medica Pura*, and all but two of the provers named above co-operated with Hahnemann in obtaining the pathogenesis there given—he contributing 157 symptoms, they 198. The first trituration was used, and of this as many as 100 or 200 grains were taken by the provers. In the following symptom-list there are eighty-two fresh symptoms, of which seventy-five are Hahnemann's, and the remainder Lehmann's and Rummel's, possibly provings with the 30th dilution.—*Hughes.*

[1] No accessible.—*Hughes.*

[2] Not observation about Aurum occurs at this reference.—*Hughes.*

Anxiousness; even a noise before the door makes him anxious; he is afraid some one might come in; as if afraid of men.

15. Shyness.

Pusillanimity.

The least thing discourages him.

Dispirited ill-humor; he thinks he cannot succeed in anything. [*Wl.*]

Dispirited and despondent; he thinks that everything goes awkwardly with him, and nothing will succeed with him. [*Hpl.*]

20. Discouraged and at odds with himself.

Crying and wailing; she thinks that she is irretrievably lost. (Surfeit of life.)

Constant sullen seriousness and reserve. [*Lgh.*]

Peevishness and dislike to talking. [*Hrm.*]

25. Contrary mood.

Some persons excite his extreme antipathy.

Choleric and quarrelsome.

Excessively disposed to take offense; even the least thing seeming offensive to him, affected him deeply and caused resentment. [*Hpl.*]

He gets excited in his thoughts about some absent persons.

30. Peevish and **irascible; the least contradiction excites him to the greatest anger.** [*Gr.*]

If he is left undisturbed, he sits by himself in a corner, quiet, reserved, as if melancholy; the least contradiction excites him to the most violent anger, which he manifests at first with quarreling and much talking, but afterwards with a few abrupt words (aft. 3 d.). [*Hrm.*]

He trembles, when he cannot give way to his anger.

He tries his best to quarrel with somebody and to revile him.

Passionateness and violence.

35. Now weeping, now laughing, in the evening, as if she had not full control of herself.

Silent peevishness and cheerfulness alternate frequently (aft 1 and 3 h.). [*Hrm.*]

Good humor the whole day, with talkativeness and self-satisfaction (alternative action). [*Lgh.*]

Serene, contented mood; he always wishes to converse with others. [*Hrm.*]

Considerable merriment and agreeable, comfortable feeling (aft. 2 h.). [*Gr.*]

40. Tremulous quivering of the nerves, as with a joyous hope. [*Fz.*]

The thinking faculty is more acute and the memory more faithful (curative effect).

She feels impelled to think deeply over one subject and another; but it renders her weak, tremulous, cold and damp over the body.

Lost in thought, he says something absurd in talking with a person.

Mental labor affects him very much; he feels very much exhausted.

45. Mental work causes him nausea, which occupies his whole being.

Confusion of the head. [*Hrm.*]

Confusion of the head, in the morning on rising, with heaviness in the occiput. [*Wl.*]

A sort of hypochondriac intoxication; the head, especially toward the nape of the neck, feels as if full of compressed air.

(In talking, he involuntarily smiles.)

50. Vertigo, in stooping, as if everything turned around with him; it went off on raising himself. [*Lgh.*]

Vertigo when standing, compelling him to sit down. [*Hrm.*]

Vertigo when taking a walk, as if he were intoxicated and as if he would fall to the left side; it obliged him to lie down, and returned even then for some time at the slightest motion (aft. 43 h.). [*Lgh.*]

Headache, as from a cold coming on.

Stupefying pressive headache, as from a violent wind. [*Lgh.*]

55. Headache, from the morning onward, as if the brain were bruised, which is aggravated by reflection and reading, but especially by speaking and writing, to extreme violence and to a complete confusion of ideas; it diminishes every time on ceasing to reflect, speak and write, until it entirely vanishes at 7 P. M. (aft. 6 h.).

Headache, partly like a pain from a bruise, partly like a painful pressure in some part of the brain, and then again it is felt like tearing, increasing from early in the morning, and disappearing at 3 P. M. (aft. 24 h.).

Pressive pain in the temples.

Pressure in the left side of the forehead (aft. 1½ h.). [*Hrm.*]

Pressive tearing in the head, here and there, especially in the forehead, with a sensation of vertigo. [*Hrm.*]

60. Pressive tearing in the right side of the head, from the occiput to the forehead (aft. 3 h.). [*Hrm.*]

Tearing pressure in the right occiput. [*Hrm.*]

Tearing pressure in the left side of the crown, aggravated by motion. [*Hrm.*]

Tearing headache auteriorly in the forehead and the temples, deep within the brain, alleviated in the open air. [*Gr.*]

Tearing in the left side of the crown (aft. 1½ h.). [*Hrm.*]

65. Tearing in the right side of the crown (aft. 3 h.). [*Hrm.*]

Tearing in the left temple. [*Fz.*]

Tearing in the left side of the forehead, aggravated by motion. [*Hrm.*]

Fine tearing in the forehead. [*Hrm.*]

Fine tearing from the right side of the occiput through the brain, even into the forehead; worse on motion (aft. 1 h.). [*Hrm.*]

70. Cutting, tearing pain in the right side of the crown (aft. 17 d.). (*Hrm.*]

Burrowing, boring and dull sound in one side of the head, early on awaking, aggravated by coughing and by bending the head back.

Semi-lateral, sharply beating, hacking headache.

Prickling sensation in the sinciput.

Rush of blood to the head.

75. Violent rush of blood to the brain (aft. ¾ h.).

Violent rush of blood to the head, on stooping, passing off on raising the head (aft. 8 d.). [*Hrm.*]

Raging and roaring in the head, as if he was sitting by a rushing water (aft. 14 d.).

The bones of the head ache on lying down, as if broken, so that it took away all his vital spirit.

Small osseous tumor, on the left side at the top of the forehead.

80. **A small osseous tumor on the right side of the crown, with boring pains, aggravated by touching.**

Externally on the forehead, pressive pain (aft 10 h.). [*Hrm.*]

Pressive pain, externally on the left temple (aft. 32 h.). [*Hrm.*]

Pressure on the left temple, aggravated by touching (aft. ¼ h.). [*Hrm.*]

A stitch in the middle of the forehead, where the hair begins.

85. Pricking externally on the forehead, as from needles (aft. 24 h.). [*Hrm.*]

Stitches on the frontal bone, like a slow drawing (aft. 6 h.). [*Fz.*]

He shakes his head sideways, up and down.

In the eyes, while looking, a sensation as when strongly heated, as if the blood pressed on the optic nerve.

Sensation of weakness and pressure in the eyes.

90. Pressure on the left eye from without inward (aft. 8 d.). [*Hrm.*]

Pressive pain on the right eyeball, from above downward. [*Hrm.*]

Pressive pain on the right eyeball from without inward, aggravated by touching (aft. 6 h.). [*Hrm.*]

Pressure in the eyes, as if a foreign body had got into it.

Enormous, spasmodic pressure in the posterior part of the left orbit. [*Gr.*]

95. Sensation as if the left eyeball was being pressed out, in its interior, superior angle. [*Fz.*]

Tension in the eyes, which impedes vision (aft. 1 h.). [*Hrm.*]

Inordinate tension in the eyes, with diminution of the visual powers, aggravated when fixing the eyes upon any object, relieved when he closes them (aft. 9 d.). [*Hrm.*]

Fine tearing within the right orbit, near the external canthus (aft. 5 h.). [*Hrm.*]

Dull stitch in the left orbit, below, from within outward.

100. Several single stitches in the inner canthus, and in the lid of the left eye (aft 36 h.). [*Hrm.*]

Smarting pain in the left upper eyelid.

A sort of burning in the eye.

Itching and burning in the right canthus.

Painless, smooth nodule on the border of the right lower eyelid.

105. Swelling of the lower eyelids. [*Fr. H.*]

Bluish appearance of the inner canthi.

Distended and protruding eyes.

Contraction of the pupils (aft. 2, 4 h.). [*Lgh.*]

Dilatation of the pupils (aft. 3½ h.). [*Lgh.*]

110. Indistinct vision, as if a black gauze was drawn before the eyes (aft. 6 d.). [*Hrm.*]

His vision leaves him for a moment.

Half-vision, as if the upper half of the eye was covered with a black body, so that he could see only the objects situated lower down with the lower half of the eye, while the superior ones remained invisible. [*Hrm.*]

He cannot distinguish anything clearly, because **he sees everything double, so that one object presents itself to him commingled with another,** with violent tension of the eyes. [*Hrm.*]

Sparks of fire before the eyes.

115. In the ears, tension.

Pressive tearing in the left external meatus auditorius (aft. ¾ h.). [*Hrm.*]

Crepitation in the left ear.

Humming before the left ear.

Roaring in the ears, in the morning in bed.

120. The parotid gland is painful when touched, as if from pressure or contusion.

The nasal bone on the right side and the adjacent part of the upper jaw are **painful to the touch,** especially where the facial nerve comes out.

Itching in the nostrils.

Twitching on the septum of the nose, from above downwards. [*Wl.*]

Smarting pain in the lower part of the nose. [*Fr. H.*]

125. Smarting pain in the lower part of the nose, so that tears come in his eyes, as in an impulse to sneezing in the bright sunlight, or in exalted religious melancholy, or in the highest degree of pity. [*Fz.*]

Tickling formication in the alæ naris, as in coryza, at times with an impulse to scratching. [*Lgh.*]

Feeling of soreness in the nose. [*Fr. H.*]

Sensation of soreness in both nostrils, especially on seizing the nose.

Ulcerated, agglutinated, painful nostrils, so that he can get no air through the nose.

130. Ulcerated crust in the right nostril, almost painless, yellowish and almost dry. [*Fr. H.*]

Swelling of the nose in the room, after taking a walk.

Swelling and redness on and below the right nostril. [*Fr. H.*]

Dark, brown-red spots on the nose, but litttle raised above its surface, on touching them there is a pressive pain (aft. 24 h.). [*Hrm.*]

Olfaction very acute; everything with him smells too strong.

135. The vapor from the candle affects his sense of smell unpleasantly.

Frequently a sweetish odor in the nose.

Transient smell of brandy in the nose, with tightness of the chest.

Putrid smell in the nose, on blowing it.

In the face, violent tearing in the zygoma. [*Gr.*]

140. Tearing drawing in the left side of the face (aft. 2 h.). [*Wl.*]

Tension in the cheekbones and the ears.

Lancinating pain in the one cheek (1st d.).

Burning stitches in the zygoma.

Itching pricks, as from needles, in the right side of the face.

145 **Eruption of fine pimples in the face,** with tips filled with pus, for several hours.

Bloated, shining face, as from perspiration, with eyes distended and protruding.

Swelling of both cheeks, with swelling of the lips and nose, in the morning.

Swelling of one cheek, with drawing and tearing in the upper and lower jaw-bone, and a sensation of threatening pain and of hacking in the teeth, which seem too long.

In the lower lip a burning vesicle, in the red part.

150. On the chin, tearing in the right half of the same. [*Gr.*]

On the lower right jaw a tearing pressure, passing away by pressing upon it. [*Hrm.*]

Intermittent, dull stitches on the outer border of the lower jaw. [*Gr.*]

A gland on the lower jaw is painful, as if swollen.

Dull, pressive pain *per se* and while swallowing, in a gland under the angle of the lower jaw.

155. The teeth of the upper front row are very sensitive in chewing.

In chewing, suddenly a violent, dull pain in an upper molar.

Threatening pain and hacking in the teeth, with swelling of the cheek.

Twitching pain in the upper row of teeth. [*Fr. H.*]

Dull tearing in the two posterior molars of the right upper jaw, caused by touching and eating during a painful swelling of the gums. [*Hrm.*]

160. Toothache, from air penetrating into the mouth.

Single stitches in the teeth.

Sensation of dullness in the molars (aft. ½ h.).

Looseness of the teeth, even of the anterior ones, in sudden paroxysms.

Swelling of the gums on the molars of the right upper jaw, with pressive pain, as of soreness, on touching them and on eating. [*Hrm.*]

165. Painful pustules on the gums, as if a fistula in the gums was coming on.

Gum-boil, with swelling of the cheeks (aft. 10 d.).

In the region of the palate, a sort of pressure, for several hours.

Paroxysms of stretching apart of the fauces, as in vomiting, but without nausea.

A painful impediment to swallowing in the left side of the fauces.

170. Lancinating pain, as of soreness in the throat, only in deglutition.

Agreeably sweetish saliva gathers in the mouth. [*Fz.*]

Much mucus in the fauces, for several days.

Frequently, mucus in the fauces; it can be hawked out, indeed, but yet impedes the inspiration (aft. 2 h.). [*Fz.*]

Fetid odor from the mouth in the evening and night, without his becoming aware of it himself.

175. Smell from the mouth, as of old cheese.

Putrid smell from the mouth.

The taste in the mouth is insipid.

Sweet taste anteriorly on the tongue.

Agreeable milky taste in the mouth.

180. Putrid taste in the mouth, as of high game, when not eating.

Sourish taste in the mouth at times (aft. 2½ h.).

Bitter taste in the mouth, with sensation of dryness (aft. 8 h.). [*Lgh.*]

Much thirst for 6 days. [*Fr. H.*]

No appetite for anything; he can only eat rolls and milk.

185. Aversion to all meat.

Great desire for coffee.

He is impelled to eat very fast, especially at the beginning of the meal.

He relishes his food well, but it does not quite satisfy his appetite, and he could have eaten again, right away.

During eating the anxiety of his mind passes away. [*Fz.*]

190. Sickness at the stomach and in the throat. [*Hrm.*]

Feeling of qualmishness an uneasiness from the stomach and the abdomen.

Retching, as if about to vomit, with pressure in the abdomen. [*Fr. H.*]

Eructation, with the taste of what he has drunk (beer).

Pain in the stomach, as from hunger.

195. Pressure in the region of the stomach at noon.

Swelling of the scrobiculus cordis, and of the whole epigastrium, with lancinating pain on pressing upon it or when firmly constricting it.

In the hypochondriac region, constant pressure, as from flatus, especially after partaking of some food or drink, often aggravated by motion and walking; passes off without discharge of flatus.

Stitches in the left hypochondrium, like stitches in the spleen.

In the abdomen, heaviness, with ice-cold hands and feet.

200. Pressure in the abdomen.

Tensive pressure in the hypogastrium, just below the navel, in the lumbar region, with sensation of fullness (aft. 53 h.). [*Hrm.*]

Tensive pressure in the hypogastrium and the lumbar region, with urging to stool (aft. 6 d.). [*Hrm.*]

Pinching pain in the hypogastrium, now here, now there (aft. 12 h.). [*Hrm.*]

Colic of dull pinching and cutting in the belly, then diarrhœic stool, and after the stool distension of the abdomen.

205. Painful feeling of contraction in the abdomen.

Single tearing in the right side of the abdomen, extending up under the ribs, as if everything there was being crushed, compelling him to bend double, when sitting (aft. 36 h.). [*Fz.*]

Pain as from a bruise in the right hypogastric region, when sitting, passing off when he rises or draws up his leg (aft. 24 h.). [*Fz.*]

Colic in the abdomen. [*Ephem. nat. cur.*, *Dec.* II., *ann.* 6, *app.*, p. 6.[1]]

Twitching squeezing in the left side of the nates, frightening and startling him (aft. 6 h.). [*Wl.*]

210. Pain in the groin, as from a swollen inguinal gland.

Want of mobility, and stiffness in the bend of the groin and in the tendons of the lumbar muscles, when walking and spreading out the legs, as after a long foot-tour (aft. 3½ h.).

Drawing from the groin down into the thighs.

Drawing pain in the mons veneris.

Burning pain in the abdominal ring, which else has been healthy.

215. Cutting thrusts in both groins, compelling him to draw in the abdomen and to draw up the legs. [*Wl.*]

Weakness in the groin.

Urging in the right abdominal ring as if a hernia was about to protrude, when sitting, on stretching out the body; it passes off on rising. [*Fz.*]

Protrusion of an inguinal hernia, with great pain, like cramp; flatus seems to pass into the hernia.

Much tormented with flatus, it accumulates under the left rib, with lancinating pains.

220. Colic from flatus, soon after partaking of the lightest food most moderately.

Flatulence, colic after midnight; a quantity of flatus forms quickly, which, finding no egress, presses and strains painfully here and there, and causes distress; unchanged by rest or motion.

Rumbling in the abdomen.

Grumbling in the belly.

Grumbling in the hypogastrium. [*Hrm.*]

225. Rumbling and grumbling in the belly (aft. 1 h.). [*Hrm.*]

Much passage of flatus (1st d.).

Discharge of much fetid flatus (aft. 8 d.). [*Hrm.*]

Uneasiness in the abdomen, with sensation as if he wanted to go to stool, especially after a meal (aft. 36 h.). [*Hrm.*]

Constipation for three days. [*Gr.*]

230. Very large-formed stool, and difficult discharge of faeces.

---

[1] A casual mention of there being an "*aurea colica.*"—*Hughes.*

Every day very hard, clotted stool (the 1st days).

Every morning soft stool with some griping.

Unusually profuse stool, in the evening (aft. 10 h.).

Frequent, but ordinary stool (aft. 16 h.). [*Hrm.*]

235. Diarrhœa. [*Fr. H.*]

Nocturnal diarrhœa with much burning in the rectum.

(Whitish-yellow stool.)

The border of the anus painfully swollen.

In the anus and the rectum sharp stitches. [*Hrm.*]

240. Constant urging to urinate, whereby little urine, but of normal nature is passed. [*Gr.*]

More urine passes than his amount of drinking warrants.

Turbid urine, like buttermilk, with deep sediment of mucus.

In the urethra, dull, lancinating tearing. [*Hrm.*]

Sexual impulse much increased, while it had been long dormant.

245. Much inclination for coitus, early on rising, with violent erections.

He could not sleep all the night for the excitation of his sexual impulse, until he had quieted it by coitus (1st night).

Two nights full of excitement of lascivious phantasy, with relaxed, small penis (2d, 3d nights).

Erections, many nights in succession.

Nocturnal erections, without emission of semen (1st n.). [*Wl.*]

250. **Nightly erections and pollutions.** [*Gr.*]

Pollutions, at night (the 1st night). [*Wl.*]

Nightly pollutions, with voluptuous dreams (aft. 7 d.). [*Hrm.*]

Pollutions, three nights in succession, without subsequent debility.

The prostatic juice is emitted from the relaxed penis.

255. In the penis, painful twitching, from before toward the posterior parts.

On the glans, pricking as from needles about its extremity, and after every stitch there follows a similar one above the navel toward the scrobiculus cordis (aft. 3 h.). [*Wl.*]

Shooting tearing on the glans, when there is an urging to urinate (aft. 3 h.). [*Wl.*]

On the scrotum, itching.

In the right testes, pressive, tensive pain, as from a contusion (aft. 3½ h.). [*Lgh.*]

260. **Swelling of the right testicle,** with pressive pain only when touched and rubbed, beginning for several evenings at 6 P. M. and ceasing about 11 P. M. (aft. 5 d.). [*Hrm.*]

Labor-like pains in the abdomen, as if the menses were about to set in.

* * * * * * * *

Sensation of stoppage of the nose as in dry coryza, and yet sufficient air passes through (aft. 2½ h.). [*Lgh.*]

The nostril seems to him to be stopped, though he can get air through it. [*Fr. H.*]

Coryza. [*Fr. H.*]

265. Severe, fluent coryza.

Dry catarrh, firmly seated on the chest, early on awaking; only with much exertion he can by coughing detach some very tough mucus, and this also only after rising from bed (aft. 16 h.).

Mucus firmly adhering to the top of the windpipe, detached by retching with difficulty.

Frequently, mucus deep down in the windpipe, below the larynx, which he cannot cough up despite his greatest efforts. [*Gr.*]

Mucus deep down in the lungs, which is thrown up copiously and easily; with subsequent free respiration and expansion of the chest (while before he was very asthmatic)

270. Cough. [*Fr. H.*]

Cough on account of lack of breath, at night. [*Hrm.*]

In cough, compression of the chest and of the abdomen.

In coughing, stitches under the left ribs.

Frequent deep respiration.

275. In deep breathing and yawning, painful stitches under the ribs, which impede the yawning and respiration; ceasing on going to sleep.

In respiration, stitches in the left side of the chest.

In breathing, sharp stitches seemingly in the side of the bladder.

In expiration, grumbling in the upper part of the chest, extending down into the abdomen and the groin; then rapid palpitation, with weariness and anxiety; then slumber.

Shivering in the right breast on yawning.

280. Dyspnœa.

Severe tightness of the chest.

Severe asthma, on taking a walk.

Asthma, when laughing, or when walking briskly, as if the chest were too narrow to inspire, and too flat and low in front (aft. 44 h.). [*Gr.*]

Enormous tightness of the chest, with difficulty of breathing, at night. [*Hrm.*]

285. **Tightness of the chest,** also when at rest, and not lightened by any position; **he always takes a deep breath, and cannot get enough air.** [*Gr.*]

Tightness of the chest, with dull stitches in it on taking breath. [*Hrm.*]

Tightness of the thoracic cavity, with anxiety (aft. 3 d.). [*Hrm.*]

Pressure on the right side of the chest, with violent anguish. [*Fz.*]

Pressure on the sternum, with eager, anxious bearing, as if some great joy were about to come to him. [*Fz.*]

290. Pressure as of something hard on the sternum, with drawing tearing pains toward the shoulders. [*Fz.*]

Pressure on the left side near the scrobiculus cordis, below the cartilages of the uppermost false ribs, more violent during expiration (aft 7 d.). [*Hrm.*]

Obtuse, constricting shooting, below the cartilages of the first three ribs of the right side of the chest, which sometimes continues like a peg sticking there, sometimes slowly ceases, and is felt less when walking; externally this spot is red (aft. 16 h.). [*Gr.*]

Some very violent stitches in the chest over the heart (aft. 72 h.). [*Gr.*]

Sharp stitches on the sternum (aft. 2 h.). [*Wl.*]

295. Dull stitches on both sides of the chest, with heat and tightness in the chest, aggravated on inspiring. [*Wl.*]

Obtuse, lancinating and cutting pain, on the right side by the sternum, under the last true ribs. [*Hrm.*]

Obtuse, cutting pain in the left side, near the sternum, more severe during inspiration (aft. 9 d.). [*Hrm.*]

The heart seems to shake in walking, as if it was loose. [*Fz.*]

At times a single, very severe beat of the heart.

300. **Palpitation of the heart** (aft. ½ h.).

Violent palpitation (aft. 4 d.). [*Hrm.*]

On the internal side of the ischium, pinching pain. [*Wl.*]

In the small of the back, pain as from weariness (aft. 3 h.).

Cutting over the small of the back, when sitting, as if it was pressed with something sharp. [*Fz.*]

305. In the spine, in the morning, a pain so severe that he could not move a limb.

Pressure on the left side, near the lumbar vertebræ, and upon the upper border of the os innominatum. [*Hrm.*]

Merely on inspiring, a sharp, piercing pain in the right loin.

Fine, tearing lancination on the right side, beside the lumbar vertebræ, passing away every time he presses on it. [*Hrm.*]

Painful pricks, as from needles, close under the right scapula, beside the spine (aft. ½ h.). [*Gr.*]

310. Tearing pain on the inner side of the scapula and below it, on bending the body backward and to the left (aft. 10 h.). [*Hrm.*]

In the nape of the neck, tension as if a muscle were too short, even when at rest, but more severe when stooping (aft. 10 h.). [*Wl.*]

On the neck, a tearing pressure on the right side, on the lower part, near the clavicle (aft. 14 d.). [*Hrm.*]

Jerking, tearing lancination in the left external cervical muscles (aft. 7 d.).

Eruption of fine pimples, with tips full of pus, on the neck and the chest, for several hours.

315. Under the axilla, tearing tension. [*Wl.*]

On the top of the shoulder fine stitches. [*Wl.*]

Pain on the top of the shoulders, as from soreness, even without touch and motion. [*Fz.*]

Extending down the left arm, a pain, incumbent on the bone, passing off on motion. [*Fz.*]

Pressure on the left upper arm, in the periosteum (aft. 48 h.). [*Hrm.*]

320. Pressure on the lower surface and in the middle of the right upper arm. [*Hrm.*]

Tearing pressure on the anterior surface of both upper arms (aft. 15 d.). [*Hrm.*]

Fine tearing in the left upper arm, most severe on baring it (aft. 3 h.). [*Wl.*]

In the elbow-joint of the right arm, spasmodic tearing. [*Gr.*]

The fore-arms are heavy when at rest, but not when in motion (aft. 12 h.). [*Wl.*]

325. Pressure on the anterior surface of the right fore-arm. [*Hrm.*]

Pressure on the external side of the right fore-arm (aft. 12 d.). [*Hrm.*]

Intermittent, tearing pressure on the inside of the left fore-arm. [*Hrm.*]

In the bones of the wrist, tearing (aft 8 h.). [*Hrm.*]

Tearing in the metacarpal bones. [*Hrm.*]

330. Cramp like tearing in the bones of the wrists of both hands, deep within, drawing from the lower row to the upper, chiefly at night, but also in daytime. [*Gr.*]

Cramp-like pain in the metacarpal bones of the left hand, especially of the thumb, without impeding motion. [*Gr.*]

Pricking, very rapid and almost stinging, between the thumb and index.

Itching on the hand, between the thumb and index.

In the finger-joints, drawing. [*Hpl.*]

335. Tearing in the posterior joints of the right fingers (aft. 4 d.). [*Hrm.*]

Tearing on the posterior joint of the left little finger. [*Hrm.*]

Fine tearing in the fingers of the right hand. [*Hrm.*]

Fine tearing in the anterior joint of the right thumb. [*Hrm.*]

Dull tearing in the joints of the fingers of both hands, spreading often into the phalanges (aft. 5 d.). [*Hrm.*]

340. In the hip-joint an extraordinary, paralytic pain, only when rising from a seat and in walking; not when sitting.

Cramp-like pain in the region of the hip, on the inner brim of the pelvis, aggravated by rubbing (aft. 36 h.). [*Wl.*]

A fine stitch darts in a tortuous manner through the gluteal muscles downward, several times in succession (aft. 16 h.). [*Wl.*]

The thigh feels as if paralyzed and cannot be raised, on account of a stiffening pain above in the tendons of the psoas-muscle.

Weakness of the thigh when walking.

345. Pain in the shaft of the right thigh, as if it were broken, when he throws the right thigh over the left. [*Fz.*]

When he is sitting and throws the left leg over the right, the muscles of the posterior side of the right thigh seems to be in a twitching motion. [*Gr.*]

Pressive, tensive pain in the muscles of the left thigh, when taking a walk, not relieved by touching or by standing or walking, but by sitting. [*Lgh.*]

Cramp-like drawing in the tendons of the psoas-muscle, which bends the thigh, extending down into the thigh, when sitting; passing away in rising. [*Fz.*]

Tearing in the thigh, as from growing, merely when moving, not in sitting (aft. 24 h.).

350. A spot which pains as if excoriated, comes at night when lying down, on the outer side of the left thigh. [*Gr.*]

In the right knee, a simple pain, while walking.

Painful stiffness and paralyzed feeling in the knees, both in rest and in motion.

Pain in the knees, as if they were tightly bandaged, in sitting and walking.

The right knee becomes weak from walking, so that when he treads, and also after walking, in every position, a drawing pain is felt in it (aft. 24 h.). [*Gr.*]

355. Unsteadiness of the knees.

On the left tibia, a pressure on stretching the leg. [*Fz.*]

Dull, gnawing pain on both sides of the leg above the ankles, with single sharp stitch in the tendo Achillis during rest, passing off in motion (aft. 14 h.). [*Wl.*]

Little elevations on the leg and under the knee, from slight rubbing; these degenerate into thick, hard knots under the skin (5th, 8th d.). [*Rl.*]

Knots under the skin, like an insect-bite, on the leg, above the heel and behind the knees, with severe itching, so that it is almost intolerable while walking (11th d.). [*Rl.*]

360. Smaller and larger elevations on the legs and calves, which look like nettle-rash, burn severely and feel like hard knots, of dirty yellow color, at the same time transient, disappearing in a few hours, and appearing less in the room than in the open air. [*Rl.*]

Hard, red swelling of the leg from the ankle to the calf, from a little rubbing of the boot, passing off again after a short rest. [*Rl.*]

On the foot, on the hollow of the sole, pressure, as from something hard.

Tensive pressure beside the inner side of the right ankle (aft. 5 d.). [*Hrm.*]

Drawing pain on the feet. [*Rl.*]

365. Severe drawing in both heels, in the evening on going to sleep. [*Rl.*]

Paralytic drawing in the metacarpal bone of the big toe, as far as the extremity of the toe. [*Hrm.*]

Tearing pain on the back part of the sole of the right foot (aft. 30 h.). [*Hrm.*]

Violent stitches on the dorsum of the foot, behind the toes.

The heels pain as if festering within, or as if suffused with blood.

370. Itching on the ankle-joints and on the soles of the feet. [*Rl.*]

Itching on the ankle-joints, especially when walking (7th d.). [*Rl.*]

In a former chilblain, a burrowing pain (aft. 1 h.).

In the big toe, in the posterior joint, pain, as if bruised and sprained, when walking.

Drawing in the joints of the toes. [*Hpl.*]

375. Paralytic drawing in the toes of the right foot. [*Hrm.*]

Fine tearing in the toes of the right foot. [*Hrm.*]

All the joints feel as if beaten, in the morning and in the whole forenoon.

Early, at daybreak, in bed, simple pain, or pain as from a bruise in all the joints, especially in the small of the back and in the knees; this increases the longer he lies still, but soon passes after he rises.

Pain as from a bruise in the head, **and in all the joints in the morning in bed,** most severe in perfect rest, passing away immediately on rising.

380. Going to sleep, numbness and insensibility of the arms and legs, early on awaking, more while lying still than when in motion.

In the arms and lower limbs, transient drawing pains from time to time. [*Rl.*]

Painful drawing in the veins and lassitude, in the afternoon.

Remarkable ebullition of blood, as if it boiled in all the arteries (aft. 24 h.).

All the blood seems to pass at once from the head down into the lower limbs, which feel paralyzed, she sinks down and has to seat herself at once.

385. Internal emptiness and weakness in the whole body.

Excessive sensitiveness in the whole body and susceptibility for every pain, which he seems to feel from merely thinking about it, with a sensation as if all things were intolerable. [*Hpl.*]

All his sensations are subtle and acute. [*Hpl.*]

When he thinks of a motion, he unconsciously makes slight motions.

Comfortable feeling in the whole body (curative effect).

390. Even in the most unpleasant weather, he feels well in the open air and it agrees with him. [*Fz.*]

Formication in the body, now here, now there. [*Hpl.*]

Transient but intense itching on the abdomen, the hips, the knees, the arms and the wrists. [*Rl.*]

Itching, burning radiations, darting hither and thither, almost like stitches.

Eruptions of pustules in the face, on the neck and on the chest.

395. Very tired in the morning; her legs pained, so that she would have liked to have lain down at once.

Very weak, early on awaking.

Great weariness in the afternoon, suddenly, when sitting and reading; he went to sleep with it, and when he awoke, the weariness had vanished (aft. 9 h.). [*Lgh.*]

Drowsiness during the day.

Slumberous sleep, with weakness of the head when sitting, during the day.

400. Irrepressible sleep after dinner, and during this slumber he had to think much (aft. 4 h.). [*Fz.*]

All night long, wide awake and without sleep, though without pains, and in the morning he still was not sleepy or exhausted.

Early from 4 o'clock onward, he cannot sleep soundly any more, he throws himself uneasily from side to side, because he cannot remain long in any one position, and the hand on which he lies soon gets tired. [*Gr.*]

He could not lie at night either on the left or on the right side.

He feels the pains during the sleep of the uneasy night.

405. At night, painful accumulation of flatus, chiefly in the left hypochondriac region.

He moans loudly in his sleep [*Gr.*]

Frequent awaking at night, as if from fright. [*Lgh.*]

He awakes in violent dreams.

Frightful dreams about thieves, with loud screaming during the sleep.

410. **Frightful dreams.**

Frightful dreams, at night. [*Gr.*]

A dream at night, causing horror.

Dreams that he was about to fall from a great height.

Dreams about dead men.

415. Dreams full of quarrels.

Dreams with erections, all the night.

Agreeable and very rational dreams, but he cannot well remember them.

Vivid dreams, not easily remembered, at night. [*Lgh.*]

In the evening, immediately on going to sleep, while still half awake, she dreams much, as if some one was talking with her.

420. She dreamt the whole night that she was in the dark.

After 3 A. M. the child became wide awake and spoke in bold tones deliriously, with rapid utterance and red face: "Mother, thou art my gold daughter!" "What kind of a dog is that?" "What head is that on the wall?" "What is that running about in the room?" and thus her ravings all consisted of questions.

Very sensitive to cold in the whole body.

Coldness in the whole body, in the morning, especially on the arms and hands down from the shoulders, with blueness of the nails, but without fever.

Coldness of the body, especially of the hands and feet.

425. Coldness of the hands and feet, in the evening, in bed.

Coldness of the soles of the feet and of the patellæ, as soon as he gets into bed in the evening. [*Hpl.*]

Coldness of the whole body and afterward increased warmth, without fever.

Coldness of the body, almost the whole day, with blue nails, insipid taste and nausea, then increased warmth, but without any sensation of fever.

Chill between the scapulæ.

430. Shaking chill in the back.

Shivering through the whole body, with goose-skin on the thighs and with concussion of the brain under the frontal bone. [*Fz.*]

Chill in the evening in bed, with coldness of the legs up to the knees; he can not get warm all night, sleeps little, always only a half hour at a time, with anxious dreams that cannot be recalled (aft. 16 d.).

In the evening in bed, before going to sleep, a febrile rigor through the whole body as if he had taken cold in a draught, he could hardly get warm (aft. 16, 19 h.). [*Lgh.*]

In the evening febrile rigor over the whole body, with dry coryza, without heat and without thirst after it. [*Lgh.*]

435. In the evening after lying down, shivering and chilliness; before lying down, headache.

In the evening, a febrile rigor all over, with coldness of the hands, and warmth of the face and the forehead, without thirst. [*Lgh.*]

Chills and heat alternately. [*Fr. H.*]

Heat in the face, with cold hands and feet.

Slight perspiration at night like vapor and moistness only between the thighs like sweat (aft. 10 h.).

440. Morning—sweat all over

AURUM MURIATICUM.

(SOLUTION OF CHLORIDE OF GOLD.[1])

Drawing headache in the forehead (aft. 2 h.).

A tickling itching on the forehead (aft. 1 h.).

In the left eye, a tearing pain.

Ringing in the ears (aft. 6 h.).

5. After the ringing, dullness of hearing, as if the ears internally were wide and hollow, and so could not perceive anything distinctly.

In the nose a crawling, as if something was running about in it.

A burning and itching pain externally in the upper part of the nose.

Redness and itching inflammation on the nose which afterwards desquamates.

Red swelling of the left side of the nose; the cavity of the nose is ulcerated deep in, with a dry, yellowish scab and a sensation of stoppage, although sufficient air passes through.

10. Red swelling on and under the right nostril; with a painless ulcer-scab within and with a sensation of stoppage, though air passes through. [*Mch.*[2]]

Discharge of a greenish-yellow matter from the nose, without bad smell, for 7 days (aft. 10 d.).

In the teeth a twitching pain, partly on the side and partly in the upper incisors.

Twitching toothache also in the anterior upper row of teeth. [*Mch.*]

Distension of the abdomen.

*   *   *   *   *   *   *   *

15. The breathing is short and as if stopped in the larynx, for several days.

---

[1]This medicine stands here as in *Materia Medica Pura.—Hughes.*

[2]Michler.—*Hughes.*

Several stitches close above the heart.

In the wrist a swelling without pain *per se.*, tension only in bending back the hand; on grasping with it, he has stitches in it.

Tearing pain in the middle finger after dinner.

FULMINATING GOLD.[1]

Bellyache, especially in children, with apprehension (*Pharmac. Wirtemb.* II., p. 28.[2])

Sinking of the strength, syncope, cold sweat on the limbs, violent vomiting, convulsions. [FR. HOFFMANN, *Med. rat. Syst.* II., p. 287.[3]]

Violent diarrhœas. [LUDOVICI, *pharmac. med. sec. appl.* pp. 182, 188.[4]]

BARYTA CARBONICA.

(Crystalline muriate of baryta is finely powdered, boiled for a few minutes with 6 parts of alcohol, to remove any muriate of strontia that may be present; the remaining powder is dissolved in six parts of boiling distilled water and precipitated with weak ammonium, say a solution of sal ammoniac in water. The precipitated baryta is washed several times with distilled water and then dried.)

One grain of this bartya is first brought to the millionth powder attenuation, and then being dissolved, it is diluted and potentized to the decillionth degree (X) as taught in the *direction* for the preparation of dry antipsoric remedies in part I.

A few of the smallest pellets, moistened with this medicine and put into a powder of sugar of milk, form a dose which will prove efficient of good for over 40–48 days, if the medicine was selected homœopathically suitable to the case of disease.

This antipsoric medicine may be used very advantageously in many cases, and is especially serviceable where the following ailments are among the chronic ills to be cured:

Weeping mood; anxiety about domestic affairs; shyness as to strange persons and as to social meetings; headache close above the eyes; the head easily catches cold; eruption on the head; *baldness of*

[1] This medicine stands here as in the *Materia Medica Pura.—Hughes.*
[2] Not accessible.—*Hughes.*
[3] Statement as to pernicious effects. These symptoms ended in death.—*Hughes.*
[4] Not accessible.—*Hughes.*

the head; eruption on the ears, and behind them; tubercles behind the ears; eruption on the lobule of the ear; roaring and ringing before the ear; pressure in the eyes: inflammation of the eyeballs and eyelids with photophobia; the eyelids closed by suppuration; flying webs and black spots before the eyes; dimness of vision, he cannot read; the eyes are dazed by the light; scurf under the nose; eruption on the face; single jerks in the teeth; burning stitches in the hollow tooth, when anything warm touches it; *dryness of the mouth;* constant thirst; eructation after a meal; sour eructation; *water-brash;* long continued nausea; *pressure on the stomach*, both when fasting and after a meal; pain of the stomach, on touching the scrobiculus cordis; difficult knotty stool; hard and insufficient stool; urging to urinate and frequent micturition; *weakness of the sexual powers;* leucorrhœa just before the menses; coryza; troublesome dryness of the nose; *nocturnal cough;* mucus on the chest with nocturnal cough; excessive secretion of mucus in the chest; palpitation of the heart perceptible *per se; pain in the small of the back;* stiffness of the small of the back; *stiffness of the nape of the neck;* stitches in the nape of the neck; pain in the deltoid muscle, on lifting the arm; the arm goes to sleep, while lying on it; going to sleep of the fingers; drawing and tearing in the legs; ulcers on the feet; *fetid sweat of the feet*; painful lymphatic swelling on the ball of the big toe; twitching and jerking of the body in daytime; heaviness in the whole body; asthenia; general weakness of the nerves and the body; tendency to take cold; WARTS; raving when asleep; at night, twitching of the muscles of the whole body; *night-sweat.*

The names of my fellow-provers are marked as follows: *Ad.*, *Dr. Adams; Gr.*, *Dr. Gross; Htb.*, *Dr. Hartlaub, Sen.; Hn.*, *Dr. Hartmann; Ng.*, *anonymous; Rt.*, *Dr. Rueckert; St.*, *Dr. Stapf; Rl.*, *Dr. Rummel.*[1]

The symptoms marked with a dash before them (—) were caused by acetate of baryta.

Smelling of a solution of camphor proved an alleviation of the excessive effects of baryta, and smelling of a highly potentized solution of zinc removes the troublesome symptoms of baryta.

---

[1] The few symptoms marked *Sr.* are reported by *Dr Schreter*, of Hungary, cf. Preface to *Borax.—Transl.*

Baryta carbonica first appeared in the edition of 1828, where it contains 286 symptoms. The present list is made up of these; of the results of proving the acetate reported by Adams, Gross, Hartmann, Rueckert and Stapf in Vol. III. of the *Archiv.* (1824); and of a pathogenesis of the carbonate furnished by Hartlaub and Nenning to the third Vol. of Hartlaub and Trink's *Arzneimittellehre.* The manner of these last two provings is unknown. A few symptoms are added by Rummel, who doubless proved the 30th dilution.—*Hughes.*

BARYTA CARBONICA.

Dejected, he did not want to speak.

Dejection and unsociableness. [NEUMANN, *krankh. d. vorstellungs vermœgens*, p. 345[1]]

—Misanthropy. [*Gr.*]

—She suspected, that when walking in the street, men found fault with her, and judged her amiss, which made her anxious, so that she dared not look up, she looked at nobody, and perspired all over. [*Gr.*]

5. —Sad mood. [*Gr.*]

Sad and anxious; all manner of gloomy ideas as to his future fate rise in his mind, and he believes himself totally forsaken; in the evening (aft. 35 d.). [*Ng.*]

—An evil fearful foreboding comes suddenly upon his soul, as if, *e.g.*, a beloved friend might suddenly have fallen fatally ill. [*Gr.*]

—Grief at every trifle. [*Gr.*]

—Great solicitude and anxious apprehension. [*Gr.*]

10. —She is very anxious and solicitous about things quite trifling, which else are indifferent to her. [*Gr.*]

—Anxious and fearful; a little noise on the street seems to him at once like fire alarm, and he is frightened by it, so that it darts through all his limbs. [*Gr.*]

—The greatest irresolution; he proposes to himself a brief journey, and as soon as he is to make his preparation, he is sorry for it, and prefers to stay at home. [*Gr.*]

—Long wavering between opposing resolutions (aft. several days. [*Gr.*]

—During the day she determines to attend to some particular matter; but scarcely has the time come, when she is sorry for it, and she knows not for irresolution what to do or to leave undone. [*Gr.*]

15. —All self-confidence has vanished. [*Gr.*]

Great timidity and cowardice.

Extremely discouraged and pusillanimous; she thinks she will die, and weeps (7th–10th d.). [*Ng.*]

Pusillanimity and anxiety. [NEUMANN, l. c.]

Great ennui and ill-humor. [*Ng.*]

20. —Cross and peevish. [*Gr.*]

Indisposed to play, of children. [NEUMANN, l. c.]

—Peevish, cross, indisposed to work. [*Ad.*]

Cross and quarrelsome. [*Ng.*]

—Extremely contrary, irritable humor, passionate about trifles (very soon). [*St.*]

25. —Sudden, excessive, but quickly transient burst of anger and wrath, even to rage, even from slight causes, easily provoked even to violence (aft. several d.). [*Gr.*]

Mirthfulness, passing over into wantonness.

Lack of memory (aft. 16 h.).

---

[1] Observations on scrofulous children treated by baryta.—*Hughes.*

Great forgetfulness, he does not know what he has said just before (aft. 27 d.). [*Ng.*]

—**Forgetfulness, he forgets the word he is about to utter.** [*Gr.*]

30. —In the midst of her talk she often cannot think of quite a common word. [*Gr.*]

Inattention of a child in studying. [NEUMANN, l. c.]

Dullness in the head.

—Stupid in the head. [*Ad.*]

Gloomy in the head, early on awaking and the whole forenoon (aft. 27 d.). [*Ng.*]

35. Numb feeling of the head, when sitting; passing off in the open air (20th d.). [*Ng.*]

—Numb feeling of the head, spreading toward the temple and the forehead. [*Ad.*]

—Numb feeling, dullness and heaviness of the head. [*Gr.*]

Numb feeling and heaviness of the head, in the evening, with drowsiness; the head always tends to fall forward; at the same time peevish and tired (aft. 46 d.). [*Ng.*]

—Stupid in the head, with tensive numbness in the forehead and the eyes, chiefly in the inner canthi. [*Gr.*]

40. Reeling sensation in the head, so that he had to sit down and hold on to something, with nausea.

Vertigo. [*Rt.*]

Vertigo, early after rising, everything turns around with her, with fainting nausea in the stomach (8th–11th d.). [*Ng.*]

Vertigo, with nausea, from stooping.

Vertigo, with headache, from stooping (aft. 25 d.).

45. Vertigo on raising up the head from stooping. [*Ng.*]

Vertigo, so that he knew not where he was, from walking over a little bridge. [*Ng.*]

—Vertigo on moving the body. [*Ad.*]

Vertigo, so that everything seemed to turn around, suddenly on raising the arms. (12th d.). [*Ng.*]

Headache, in the evening, so that every noise, especially the voices of men, caused pain to her brain (5th d.).

50. —Pressive pain in the left temple (aft. several d.). [*Gr.*]

—Pressive pain through the right half of the brain, from the neck to the protuberances of the forehead (aft. 1½ h.). [*Htn.*]

Pressure in the brain under the crown, toward the occiput, on awaking from sleep, with stiffness of the nape.

—Dull, pressive pain in the occipital bone, from the cervical vertebræ, behind the right ear, obliquely into the parietal bone; at 4 P. M., returning at the same hour the following day. [*Htn.*]

—Stupefying, dull pressure in the forehead, close above the the root of the nose. [*Gr.*]

55. —Pressive pain in the forehead, close above the right eye. [*Htb.*]

Pressive pain in the forehead, from within outward (12th d.). [*Ng.*]

—Pressive, pushing thrust in the left temple, outward (aft. 2½ h.). [*Htn.*]

—Pressive, aching pain, outward, in the whole forehead, especially in the orbits of the eyes, very much aggravated on holding the head upright, ceasing on stooping (aft. 10 h.). [*Htn.*]

—Violent pressure in the whole head, as if it were about to burst; especially violent in both the frontal protuberances and above the orbits of the eyes (aft. 4½ h.). [*Htn.*]

60. Pressure, with heaviness on the right side of the sinciput. [*Ng.*]

—Feeling of heaviness in the whole occiput, especially close to the nape, with tension therein, without change from motion (aft. 4 h.). [*Htn.*]

Feeling of tension about the skin of the whole forehead, as if too tight; after dinner. [*Ng.*]

Tension, with burning on a little spot on the left parietal bone (aft. 1 h.). [*Ng.*]

Painful compression of the head from both sides, as from screwing in a vice, then tearing in a little spot of the left parietal bone and later in the occiput of the left. [*Ng.*]

65. Sharp drawing over the left eye, extending from the nose toward the temple, in the evening. [*Htb.*]

—Sudden intensely painful drawing, from the occiput over the right ear down to the lower jaw. [*Gr.*]

Tearing in the crown. [*Htb.*]

Fine tearing on a small spot of the right parietal bone, deep in the bone. [*Ng.*]

Tearing in the left side of the occiput, relieved by bending back the head. [*Ng.*]

70. Tearing, with twitching in slight intermissions, deep in the brain, behind the right ear, instantly renewed by touching it. [*Ng.*]

Rheumatic pain in the occiput, with glandular swellings in the nape of the neck. [*Ng.*]

—Twitching deep within the temple, the orbit and the ear of the left side. [*Gr.*]

Twitches in the head, beginning at once from the heat of a stove. [*Ng.*]

Violent dull stitches in the left frontal protuberance, on stooping in washing. [*Ng.*]

75. Sharp stitches in the whole head, decreasing and increasing (3d d.).

Stitches in the side of the head, also after dinner and in the evening, when it is worse on the left side. [*Ng.*]

Dull stitches over the right temple in the morning, in yawning. [*Ng.*]

Dull stitches in the left side of the head, from the occiput into the frontal protuberance, or alternating, now here, now there. [*Ng.*]

Violent stitches in the brain, with heat and formication in the head (aft. 15 d.). [*Ng.*]

80. —Small severe stitches in the right frontal protuberance, outward (aft. 9 h.). [*Htn.*]

Pressive stitches on the crown, spreading through the whole head as often as she stands in the sun. [*Ng.*]

—A stitch producing dilatation, beginning in the left side of the head, passing through all the left side of the occiput, and terminating in the vertebræ of the neck (aft. 9 h.). [*Htn.*]

—Drawing stitches, aggravated intermittingly in the left mastoid process in a small spot, which also violently pains afterward, especially on touching it, or on turning the head. [*Gr.*]

A burning stitch in the right temple. [*Ng.*]

85. Beating, with stitches in the left side of the head (7th d.). [*Ng.*]

Throbbing in the occiput, extending into the frontal protuberance; in the evening (5th d.). [*Ng.*]

Violent throbbing in the sinciput, deep in the brain, on stooping (aft. 30 d.). [*Ng.*]

—Burrowing headache in the forehead and the temples. [*Gr.*]

—Burrowing headache in the upper and anterior parts of the head, almost daily, early on arising, continuing during the forenoon, and quiescent in the afternoon; in shaking the head, the brain seems loose and detached. [*Gr.*]

90. Sensation of looseness of the brain, which on moving the head seems to fall to and fro (aft. 45 d.). [*Ng.*]

In stooping, a sensation as if everything was about to fall foreward into the forehead (aft. 16 d.). [*Ng.*]

On knocking the foot against anything, concussion in the brain.

Much rush of blood to the head; it feels as if the blood stopped and could not circulate (aft. 27 d.).

Humming in the head as if from boiling water (aft. 27 d.). [*Ng.*]

95. Heat in the head, early on rising, and stabs as from knives (17th d.). [*Ng.*]

Early on waking, first heaviness, then after rising, heat in the head, with coldness in the hands and feet.

Feeling of coldness in the right side of the head, as of ice, and yet at the same time a sensation of burning. [*Ng.*]

—Without feeling cold, a shivering thrill over the hairy scalp, as if the hairs stood on end. [*Gr.*]

—The skin of the head aches at every touch. [*Rt.*]

100. Pain as if the hair was being pulled upward, on a small spot of the right parietal bone. [*Ng.*]

The hair of the head comes out in combing (aft. 4 d.). [*Rl.*]

—On the hairy scalp, here and there, slow fine stitches, compelling him to scratch. [*Gr.*]

Itching and gnawing on the hairy scalp and on the temples (aft. 3 d.).

Itching, crawling here and there on the head, passing off by scratching. [*Ng.*]

105. Formication as from ants, in the whole scalp in the evening. [*Ng.*]

Small pimples on the sides of the hairy scalp. [*Ng.*]

Small furuncle on the forehead. [*Ng.*]

Eruption on the forehead (like herpes?) with more of a burning than an itching sensation. [*Ng.*]

An old lump on the hairy scalp, hitherto painless, begins to enlarge and to pain on being touched, as if festering underneath.

110. Eruption on the right eyebrow, which on being touched causes a stinging pain.

The eyeballs are painful. [*Htb.*]

Violent pains in the left eye and from there over the temple into the ear (aft. 20 h.).

—Pain and weariness of the eyes, with pressure in them. [*Gr.*]

—Pressure deep in the eyes, aggravated when she looks at one particular point or upward and to the side, but relieved by winking or looking downward (aft. several d.). [*Gr.*]

115. —Constant pressure on the eyeballs. [*Gr.*]

—Dull pressure in the left eye, after twitching headache in the left temple and orbit, with a sensation as if water was about to gather in the eye, and a sort of weakness, compelling her to close it frequently; at last the same takes place in the right eye.

Pressure in the external canthus, as if a grain of sand was in it. [*Ng.*]

Pressure in both eyes, with itching, as from dust. [*Ng.*]

Tearing in the eyes. [*Htb.*]

120. Twitching tearing in the right upper eyelid. [*Ng.*]

Twitching stitches in the external canthus. [*Ng.*]

A stitch through the left upper eyelid.]*Ng.*]

Itching on the edge of the upper eyelid. [*Ng.*]

Itching in the eyes.

125. Itching, burning, pressing and feeling of soreness and dryness in the eye.

Dry heat and pressure in the eyes. [*Htb.*]

Burning of the eyes on straining the sight. [*Ng.*]

Burning of the eyes in the inner canthi and severe lachrymation of the same. [*Ng.*]

Sensation as if a burning spark darted from the upper border of the right orbit down to the root of the nose. [*Ng.*]

130. Internal inflammatory redness of the eyelids.

Redness in the white of the eye and a white pimple thereon, near the cornea. [*Htb.*]

Reddish, white of the eye and lachrymation.

Swelling of the eyelids in the morning.

The eyes are swollen in the morning.

135. Pus externally on the eyelids, especially in the morning.

Agglutination of the eyes in the external canthi at night. [*Ng.*]

The eyes are closed by suppuration.

Difficulty in opening the eyelids in the morning.

Closing of the eyes in the evening twilight.

140. —Rapid change from dilation to contraction of the pupils, during which they seem not to be quite round, but with some obtuse angles (aft. 5 min.) [*Gr.*]

—Everything appears to her for several minutes as in a mist, when she closes her eyes on account of pressive pain in the eyeballs and presses a little with the hand upon the eyeballs. [*Gr.*]

Like gauze before the eyes, in the morning and after dinner.

Frequent obscuration of the eyes.

Black spots before the eyes (aft. 24 h.).

145. The candle-light has a halo with rainbow colors.

Sparks before the eyes in the dark.

Sparks of fire before the eyes and tearing in them. [*Htb.*]

In the ears, a drawing, a sort of otalgia.

Tearing in the left ear, outward. [*Ng.*]

150. **Tearing** with boring and drawing **in the bone before the right ear.** [*Ng.*]

Tearing behind the right ear. [*Ng.*]

Stitches deep in the left ear. [*Ng.*]

Severe continual stitches in the ear for two days (aft. 28 d.).

—Violent stitches, so that she has to scream, several times a day under the right ear beside the ramus of the lower jaw (aft. 24 h.). [*Gr.*]

155. Boring in the right ear, so violent that she would like to scream. [*Ng.*]

Throbbing like pulsation in the (left) ear, on which he lay at night. [*Ng.*]

Throbbing and severe pressure after midnight, deep in the right ear on which he lay, and on turning over on the left side, it goes to the left ear. [*Ng.*]

Beating before the left ear, when he lies on it.

Itching in the ears (aft. 24 d.).

160. Severe itching in the left ear. [*Ng.*]

Crawling and quivering in the left ear. [Ng.]

Crawling pain in the bone before the right ear. [*Ng.*]

Eruption on the ears.

The right parotid gland is swollen and painful to the touch.

165. Cracking in the ear when walking briskly, when swallowing, sneezing, etc.

A snapping sound in the ear, as if it was broken, when swallowing.

A snapping sound in both ears, on swallowing.

He could not lie on his left ear, else there would be in it a clucking sound passing through to the right ear, preventing him from sleeping (aft. 11 d.).

Sound of explosion in the ears at night.

170. Stunning noise in the ears (aft. 2 d.).

Ringing in the ears. [*Htb.*]

Loud, continued ringing of the ears.

Roaring and buzzing before the ears (aft. 28 d.)

Severe roaring in the ears, in the evening, like the ringing of bells and the rushing of a storm.

175. An echo in the ears from severely blowing the nose.

Resounding in the ear, even on taking breath, as on a sounding board (aft. 2 d.)

Sensation as of deafness. [*Rl.*]

Hardness of hearing (the first days).

Her nose feels swollen and agglutinated within. [*Ng.*]

180. Crawling sensation on both sides of the nose.

Burning on a small spot on the back of the nose, as from a drop of hot fat. [*Ng.*]

Bleeding at the nose, several times a day (aft. 24 h.).

Frequent bleeding at the nose.

Frequent and profuse bleeding of the nose (aft. 24 h.).

185. Bleeding at the nose early in bed, of light-red blood. [*Ng.*]

On blowing the nose, every time a stream of blood follows. [*Ng.*]

The nose bleeds readily, on blowing and clearing it.

The sense of smell is very sensitive. [*Htb.*]

In the face, sharp stitches. [*Ng.*]

190. —Painful stitches in the face. [*Rl.*]

Quivering in the left side of the face. [*Ng.*]

Running or crawling on the left cheek (1st d.). [*Ng.*]

Feeling of tension in the whole skin of the face. [*Ng.*]

—Tension in the face, drawing down the eyelids, with inclination to throw out sputa. [*Gr.*]

195. —Tensive sensation in the whole face, with loathing and diarrhœic stool (aft. 1½ h.). [*Htb.*]

—Sensation as if the skin of the whole face was covered with cobwebs. [*St.*]

—Very disagreeable sensation, over the skin of the whole face and over the hairy scalp, and especially in the temporal region, as if something closely fitting was drawn over it, with a sensation of cold in the face (very soon). [*St.*]

Sensation of swelling in the face. [*Ng.*]

—Sensation as if the whole face was swollen thick, but this was only slightly the case, although the folds of the face, which at other times were deep, had totally disappeared, and the face seemed smooth for several hours (aft. ½ h.). [*St.*]

200. Swelling of the left cheek and of the region behind the ear, with pain in the temple (aft. 30 d.).

—Sensation of heat in the face, without redness of the same. [*Htb.*]

Heat and redness of one cheek, while the other frequently was cold.

Redness of the face, in the evening (12th d.). [*Ng.*]

Severe redness in the face, with deep-red lips and strong ebullition of the blood (at once).

205. Rough dry place on the right cheek. [*Ng.*]

Small pimples in the face, like furuncles, but without sensation. [*Ng.*]

The lips are dry, early after rising. [*Ng.*]

Feeling of dryness in the lips and in the gums, not relieved by drinking. [*Htb.*]

Burning on a small spot on the red of the lower lip (17th d.). [*Ng.*]

210. Sensation of swelling in the upper lip. [*Ng.*]

—Sensation in the upper lip, as if it was about to swell up, but on its inner side and on the palate a sensation as if it was burnt or turgid. [*St.*]

Swelling of the upper lip with burning pain. [*Ng.*]

Cracked upper lip. [*Htb.*]

A burning chap on the lower lip. [*Ng.*]

215. A cluster of small itching pimples with a red base, below the left corner of the mouth. [*Ng.*]

A blister on the lower lip. [*Ng.*]

—A broad red spot on the upper lip, under the skin, very painful to the touch. [*Ad.*]

—Pustule in the right corner of the mouth, painful to the touch. [*Ad.*]

Under the chin, pressure, aggravated by touching and by moving the lower jaw. [*Ng.*]

220. He cannot close the lower jaw without great pain in the articulation of the jaw.

A tearing pain in the lower jaw. [*Ng.*]

A stitch in the middle of the lower jaw. [*Ng.*]

Painful gnawing in the left lower jaw. [*Ng.*]

The glands on the lower jaw are painful.

225. Swelling of the glands of the lower jaw (aft. 39 d.).

Toothache in the evening in bed, not during the day (aft. 8 d.).

Tensive and laucinating pain in the whole of the right row of teeth.

Threatening pain in a molar. [*Ng.*]

Tearing in the molars. [*Ng.*]

230. Painful gnawing in the roots and the gums of the molars. [*Ng.*]

Boring in the teeth, as if they were being burst in pieces, when anything cold or warm is brought in the mouth.

Drawing, jerking, throbbing toothache, as if something was lodged under the teeth, drawing into the ear and the right temple.

Throbbing pain, with great sensitiveness in a lower molar, early after rising. [*Ng.*]

Burning pain, now in an upper, then in a lower tooth of the left side, with gathering of much saliva in the mouth; he can not lie on this side, because the side of the head then seems to him as it were squeezed in, and there is throbbing in the left ear.

235. Formicating burning in the left lower row of teeth (aft. 36 d.). [*Ng.*]

Painful formication in the crown of the teeth, in the evening (6th d.). [*Ng.*]

Sore pain in the tooth, she dared not touch the tooth.

A sound tooth begins to be loose, and pains during eating and for some time afterwards.

(A tooth becomes hollow rapidly.)

240. **Severe bleeding of the teeth, frequently.**

The gums bleed and seem to recede from the teeth. [*Rl.*]

—Swelling and painfulness of the gums of an upper molar on the right side; it only looks reddish and has a narrow, dark-red border near the tooth; on drinking anything cold, the tooth pains acutely, as well as the neighboring ones. [*Gr.*]

The buccal cavity feels numb in the morning (3d and 4th d.). [*Ng.*]

The whole mouth is filled with inflamed vesicles, especially the palate and the inside of the cheeks.

245. On the tongue, early on awaking, roughness; when he touches the palate with it, it feels like a grater (31st d.). [*Ng.*]

Hardness of a spot on the middle of the tongue, with burning on being touched, for several days (aft. 18 d.). [*Ng.*]

A chap, with burning pain, on the tip of the tongue (4th d.). [*Ng.*]

A crack, as if torn, on the left border of the tongue, which pains as if sore.

Pain on the side of the tongue, as from vesicles.

250. Pointed vesicles, on the middle of the tongue.

Burning vesicles on the tip of the tongue, of long duration (aft. 6 d.). [*Ng.*]

A vesicle under the tongue. [*Ng.*]

Thickly coated tongue.

Dryness of the tongue, in the morning, with a sensation as if the throat was swollen, on deglutition.

255. In the palate, pricks, as from neeedles (9th d.). [*Ng.*]

Dryness in the mouth, early on rising. [*Ng.*]

Glutinous sensation in the mouth.

Much thick mucus in the mouth. [*Ng.*]

Constant spitting of saliva, for eight days (aft. 38 d.). [*Ng.*]

260. —Constant spitting of saliva, without nausea. [*Gr.*]

The mouth is always full of water, rising up from the stomach (14th d.). [*Ng.*]

In the throat, scratchy and rough, worse after swallowing (2d d.). [*Ng.*]

Roughness and excoriation in the throat, after previous night-sweat, more painful in empty deglutition than while swallowing soft food (aft. 48 h.).

Sore throat, with excoriation on deglutition, but chiefly on empty deglutition; the neck is also painful externally on both sides, on being touched.

265. Lancinating sore throat on empty swallowing and in swallowing food.

Shooting in the throat (aft. 14 d.). [*Ng.*]

Shooting in the throat, worse when swallowing, with dryness, in the evening (6th d.). [*Ng.*]

Dryness and severe painful, shooting and pressure, as from a swelling, posteriorly in the left side of the throat, only on deglutition (4th d.). [*Ng.*]

Pressive sore throat in swallowing.

270. Choking or contraction in the throat, with interception of breath, so that he has to unbutton his clothes during dinner (26th d.). [*Ng.*]

Fits of choking in the throat, after dinner, while sitting and writing, with a sensation as if the thyroid gland was pressed inward, and the breath thus impeded (aft. 28 d.).

Contraction in the throat, with a sensation in swallowing as if a plug was in the region of the larynx, worse in the afternoon. [*Ng.*]

Sensation in the fauces, as if a delicate leaflet was lying before the posterior nares, early on awaking (2d d.). [*Ng.*]

In sneezing, a sensation in the fauces as if in the upper part of the throat a piece of flesh had become detached, with burning in the spot (4th d.). [*Ng.*]

275. Sensation as of much mucus in the throat, and, therefore, much tendency to drink, so as to become rid of this sensation.

Sensation in the fauces after previous scraping there, as if there was a plug in the throat, or as if a morsel of food had lodged there.

Sensation of swelling in the throat, in the morning, on deglutition, with dryness of the tongue.

Swelling of the left tonsil.

After chill and heat and bruised feeling in all the limbs, inflammation of the throat with thick swelling of the palate and the tonsils, which pass into suppuration, on account of which he cannot open his jaws, nor speak, nor swallow; with dark-brown urine and sleeplessness (aft. 18 d.).

280. Sense of taste quite lost, for several days. [*Ng.*]

Perverted taste in the mouth, every morning, with thickly coated tongue.

Perverted, bitter taste and smell in the mouth.

Bitter and slimy sensation in the mouth, with coated tongue (6th d.). [*Ng.*]

—Very bitter taste in the mouth, while food has its proper taste. [*Gr.*]

285. Sour taste in the mouth, in the evening.

Sour taste in the mouth before eating, not afterwards.

Sour taste in the mouth, early after rising (48th d.). [*Ng.*]

Sweet taste posteriorly on the root of the tongue (aft. 19 d.).

Salty taste in the mouth and throat, in the afternoon.

290. —Scratchy taste in the throat, during the (customary) smoking of tobacco (aft. ¾ h.). [*Htn.*]

Unbearable, fetid smell from the mouth, which he himself did not perceive (5th d.). [*Ng.*]

Thirst, with dryness in the mouth. [*Ng.*]

Lack of appetite. [*Htb.*]

Appetite scanty, for several days. [*Ng.*]

295. Lack of appetite for three weeks (aft. 26 d.).

—Little appetite, but food tastes good; no hunger. [*Gr.*]

—Satiety the whole day; whatever she eats, she eats without hunger. [*Gr.*]

—Slight appetite, and if he eats anything, it will not go down; the food has its proper taste, but is repugnant to him; and eating it makes him uncomfortable. [*Gr.*]

Indifference to sweet things.

300. Aversion to fruit, especially to plums.

—Aversion to eating, and yet a sensation of hunger. [*Rt.*]

Sensation of hunger in the stomach, but no appetite (aft. 10 d.). [*Ng.*]

Hunger, at once in the morning on rising (2d d.). [*Ng.*]

Insatiableness.

305. (Lickerishness.)

—Good appetite, every day, and hunger soon returns, if he only satisfies himself moderately; but if he satisfies himself fully, there is great discomfort and indolence. [*Gr.*]

During dinner, several of his ailments seem to decrease. [*Ng.*]

When eating and drinking, heat overpowers him.

—After eating he feels prostrated, weary and uncomfortable, with constant tenesmus and anxious feeling in the lumbar region, as when resting.[1] [*Gr.*]

310. After dinner he feels very warm and uncomfortable, and feels a pressure in the right side over the stomach.

After dinner, great indolence and indisposition to work. [*Htb.*]

After dinner, there seems to be a gauze before his eyes.

After dinner, much urging to urinate.

After dinner, incomplete eructation, with subsequent spasmodic, contractive pain in the stomach (17th d.). [*Ng.*]

315. —Rising of air, with a sensation in the region of the stomach, as if the air had difficulty there in pressing through, causing a pain as of soreness, until eructation without taste follows afterward. [*Gr.*]

Frequent eructation.

Constant eructation.

Eructation from the afternoon till late at night, so that he could not go to sleep (aft. 40 d.).

Empty eructation wakes him early from sleep (aft. 42 d.).

320. Much empty eructation, in the afternoon (aft. 25 d.).

—Empty, tasteless eructation (aft. ¼ h.). [*Htn.*]

—Empty eructation, with disagreeable taste, and gathering of water in the mouth, without nausea. [*Gr.*]

Violent eructation, with pressure in the stomach, as if a stone came up with it and then fell back again. [*Ng.*]

Frequent eructation of air, with a sensation, as if a lump, the size of a filbert, was coming up with it, in the morning (aft. 19 d.). [*Ng.*]

325. Frequent, bitterish eructation. [*Ng.*]

Sourish eructation, daily, a few hours after dinner.

Rancid eructation. [*Ng.*]

—Heartburn after a single eructation. [*Ad.*]

Belching up of sweetish or bitter water after dinner. [*Ng.*]

330. Violent hiccup, in the forenoon and after dinner. [*Ng.*]

Hiccup.

Nausea, in the morning, fasting, with palpitation and anxiety.

Nausea, as from a spoiled stomach, in the morning. [*Ng.*]

—Feeling of nausea about the stomach, qualmishness. [*Ad.*]

335. —Inclination to vomit, discomfort, with a sort of qualmishness. [*Gr.*]

---

[1] Doubtless misprint, "Ruhe" for "Ruhr;" as in dysentery," cf. Sympt. 414. *Translator*

—Inclination to vomit, in the stomach, when walking, aggravated by touching the region of the stomach, without gathering of saliva. [*Ad.*)

Vomiting of mucus, frequent.

Pains in the stomach. [*Rt.*]

Sensitiveness of the scrobiculus cordis, every time on setting her foot hard on the ground, she has a sense of pain there. [*Gr.*]

340. Fullness in the stomach after eating, as if he had eaten too much. [*Htb.*]

Feeling of over-repletion in the stomach. [*Ng*]

—Heaviness in the stomach, with nausea, in the morning, fasting; passing off after breakfast (aft. several d.). [*Gr.*]

—Heaviness in the scrobiculus cordis, as from a load, which makes respiration difficult, aggravated by carrying a slight load. [*Gr.*]

—Even if she eats ever so little, she feels full at once and feels a painful weight in the stomach, as from a stone, with painful gnawing; the pain is only transiently relieved by stretching or by bending backwards; by sitting bent it is much aggravated. [*Gr.*]

345. Pressure in the stomach, as from a stone, relieved by eructation. [*Ng.*]

Severe pressure in the stomach with nausea, after eating bread, not after cooked food, even when she eats little, with gathering of saliva in the mouth.

Pressure and choking on the right side of the stomach extending up into the chest, as if a hard body was laboriously pushing itself upward, from the morning till the afternoon. [*Ng.*]

—Pressure in the scrobiculus cordis, with dyspnœa and a sensation as if in taking a deep breath, the breath was arrested there, at the same time hoarseness, only transiently relieved by clearing the throat, and aggravation of the pressive pain from slightly partaking of food. [*Gr.*]

Contractive pain in the stomach, in the afternoon. [*Ng.*]

350. Pain in the stomach as from ulceration, on external pressure applied to it.

—**Pain as of soreness in the scrobiculus cordis** on externally pressing upon it and in respiration (1st d.). [*Gr.*]

—**Painful writhing sensation in the stomach when, in eating, the morsel gets down there, as if it had to squeeze its way through and impinged on sore places.** [*Gr.*]

—Even when fasting, she feels pains as of soreness in the stomach for several days. [*Gr.*]

—The pressive sensation of soreness and gnawing in the stomach is most severe when standing and walking, as also in sitting bent forward; in lying on the back, in stooping forward or pressing with the hands on the stomach, she feels a painful pressure, but not the gnawing. [*Gr.*]

355. Fine stitches through the stomach, extending to the spine. [*Ng.*]

—Painful dull stitches, close under the scrobiculus cordis,

near the ensiform cartilage, which continue then as a simple pain. [*Gr.*]

—Sudden drawing pain in the scrobiculus cordis, from time to time. [*Gr.*]

Drawing tearing in the scrobiculus cordis, with the sensation as if a heavy burdening body rested there, on straightening up after stooping (aft. 17 d.). [*Ng.*]

Feeling of weakness in the stomach, passing away after dinner. [*Ng.*]

360. Burning in the region of the stomach, in the afternoon. [*Ng.*]

Feeling of coldness and sensation of emptiness in the stomach. [*Ng.*]

Violent dull stitches in the left hypochondrium. [*Ng.*]

Pain below the right ribs, with coldness of the hands and feet, and heat and redness of the cheeks (aft. 2 d.).

Pressive pain in the region of the liver, worse on motion and still worse when touched.

365. —Pressive pain in a small spot of the right hypochondrium, only on inspiring, especially on taking a deep breath; the place is also painful on pressure (2d d.). [*Htb.*]

Tensive pain from the back forward, under the ribs of the right side, on rising from a seat, and on stooping low (to raise something).

Short stitches under the right hypochondrium, unaffected by respiration (aft. ½ h.). [*Htb.*]

Bellyache, so violent that it draws in the navel and he had to bend double, in the evening. [*Ng.*]

He could not sleep at night for pains in the abdomen, as soon as he moved at all, the pains returned again (aft. 27 d.). [*Ng.*]

370. The pains in the abdomen are relieved partly by eructations partly by warm applications. [*Ng.*]

—Disagreeable sensation in the epigastrium, as before vomiting. [*Rt.*]

Fullness of the abdomen (aft. 19 d.). [*Ng.*]

Distension of the abdomen.

Painful Distension of the abdomen.

375. Sensation in the abdomen, as if something in it was swollen.

Large, inflated abdomen.

Inflation of the abdomen with sensitiveness of the abdominal integuments, when touched. [*Ng.*]

Pressure in the abdomen above the ossa pubis, in the morning, in bed, while lying on the back. [*Ng.*]

Pressure in the right side of the abdomen, in the morning, after awaking in bed; it passes off after rising.

380. Contraction of a spot on the left epigastrium, a handbreadth in width (2d d.). [*Ng.*]

—Sudden contractive pain in the hypogastrium, over the groin, aggravated by intermissions and then gradually passing off (aft. 5 min.). [*Gr.*]

—Sudden violent squeezing pain in the region of the transverse colon, as if flatus was pressing through by force. [*Ad.*]

Griping in the abdomen, with nausea.

Griping about the navel, at the least motion which is made in the night while lying down, and while sitting down in daytime; passage of flatus alleviates and walking removes the pain (aft. 27 d.). [*Ng.*]

385. Griping about the navel, more while sitting than in motion. [*Ng.*]

—Griping bellyache through the whole abdomen, spreading from above downward. [*Ad.*]

—Griping in the left epigastric region, in a small spot close below the left hypochondrium, aggravated by pressure with the finger (aft. ¼ h.). [*Htn.*]

Cutting bellyache, at night.

Painful cutting in the abdomen, especially about the navel, in the evening (15th d.). [*Ng.*]

390. Cutting pain in the hypogastrium, at night, with urging on the rectum, with a dilating pain in the intestines and fullness above the ossa pubis, as if everything was stopped up and the abdomen would burst, when lying straight; followed first by a hard, knotty stool, then by a liquid stool with much urging, with a remission of the pains in the belly and subsequent burning in the anus (2d d.). [*Ng.*]

—Violent colic, as if diarrhœa was coming, moving here and there in abdomen, and only transiently relieved by loud rumbling in the abdomen. [*Ad.*]

—Sensation in the abdomen, as if she was to have diarrhœa, with a febrile rigor. [*Gr.*]

—**Anxious feeling, with discomfort and restlessness in lumbar region, like tenesmus**; only transiently removed by passage of flatus or eructation of air; at last followed by a soft stool with brief intermissions. [*Gr.*]

Several drawing cuts, upward in the left epigastrium.

395. Drawing pain deep in the hypogastrium, along down the right groin, as by a string (2d d.). [*Ng.*]

A stitch on the right side of the abdomen, and at the same time in the small of the back (2d d.). [*Ng.*]

Sudden stitches under the umbilicus (4th d.). [*Ng.*]

Stitches in the right side of the abdomen, during hiccup, while turning the body, yawning, and taking a deep breath; not while walking.

—Sudden, sharp stitches on the right side of the abdomen, so that she feels like screaming. [*Gr.*]

400. —Suddenly, a violent stitch from the right groin into the abdomen, causing her to start. [*Gr.*]

Externally, around the abdomen, a pain as if soreness, coming from the sacrum. [*Ng.*]

Pressing pain anteriorly in the abdomen, as if outside of the bowels, in the muscles, especially in the evening; aggravated so as to be unbearable during motion and walking, quickly relieved by sitting and lying down, but at once returning on walking (aft. 24 h.).

In the abdominal ring, straining outward during motion and during stool.

Itching on the spot where the hernia protrudes.

405. (Inflammation of the place of protrusion) (aft. 3d d.).

Many troubles in the abdomen, owing to flatulence; the varices protrude, and are painful in sitting.

—Grumbling and rumbling in the abdomen. [*Ad.*]

—Loud grumbling and clucking in the abdomen. [*Gr.*]

—Clucking in the abdomen, when moving the same, as from much liquid, though she has not drunk anything, in the afternoon. [*Gr.*]

410. Emission of fetid flatus. [*Ng.*]

Very frequent tenesmus.

Hurried urging to stool; she cannot keep back the stool, because it surprises her too quickly.

—Frequent urging to stool, but she does not have more evacuations than usual, and the stool then is natural. [*Gr.*]

—**Frequent urging to stool, with painful aching in the lumbar region**, and shivers passing over the head and the legs, **as in dysentery; then a soft stool with brief intermissions**, with constant pains in the loins *with renewed tenesmus.* [*Gr.*]

415. —Urging to stool, with violent pain in the abdomen, as if the intestines were being dilated; then soft stool, followed by **renewed tenesmus** (aft. 1 h.). [*Htb.*]

Soft stool, after very hurried urging (after a hard stool had already preceded), with subsequent burning and dilatation of the rectum (1st and 2d d.). [*Ng.*]

—Soft, granular stool, without any attendant trouble. [*Gr.*]

—Soft and, at last, diarrhœic stool. [*Ad.*]

Diarrhœic stool (1st and 30th d.). [*Ng.*]

420. Diarrhœic stool mixed with blood, in a child.

Light-colored stool.

Viscous stool.

Hard stool, with burning in the anus. [*Ng.*]

Very hard stool, discharged with difficulty, with pain in the rectum and bloody mucus. [*Htb.*]

425. The stool is sometimes omitted for a day. [*Ng.*]

Discharge of ascarides.

Discharge of a round worm in the stool. [*Ng.*]

During a (normal) stool, burning in the anus. [*Ng.*]

After a (sufficient) stool, much empty eructation (aft. several h.).

430. After the stool, humid varices.

In the anus, varices as large as filberts, with excoriating and lancinating pains.

Discharge of blood from the anus frequently, with distension of the abdomen.

Crawling in the anus.

Smarting in the anus.

435. Burning in the anus. [*Rl.*]

Pain as of soreness and burning around the anus, toward evening. [*Rl.*]

Painful soreness around the anus as if from excoriation (aft 5 d.) [*Rl.*]

Stitches in the rectum, the whole day, and hard stool.

Hurried urging to urinate, she cannot check micturition, it overtakes her too hurriedly.

440. Frequent micturition, every second day (aft. 29 h.). [*Ng.*]

Increase of urine, she has to rise to urinate twice every night; the discharge copious every time (aft. 19 d.). [*Ng.*]

—Increased secretion of urine. [*Ad.*]

—Frequent and copious micturition, in the morning, fasting, without having drank anything. [*Gr.*]

—He has to pass urine frequently, though little at a time; the urine is clear as water. [*Stf.*]

445. Rare and scanty micturition with burning in the urethra (8th and 17th d.). [*Ng.*]

Urine, with yellow sediment.

In micturition, burning in the urethra (15th d.). [*Ng.*]

During micturition, pinching in the abdomen. [*Ng.*]

After micturition, renewed urging, when she emitted each time a few drops of urine; passing off while sitting.

450. Burning in the left testicle (aft. 13 d.).

Violent itching on the right side of the scrotum, so that he cannot scratch enough. [*Ng.*]

—Profuse sweat of the scrotum. [*Ad.*]

—Red, excoriated, humid, burning hot spot between the scrotum and the thigh. [*Ad.*]

—A testicular excrescence, swollen previously, again swells up very severely. [*Ad.*]

455. Numbness of the sexual organs for several minutes (aft. 28 d.).

The sexual instinct is quiescent (the first days).

—Diminished sexual impulse. [*Ad.*]

Very much increased sexual instinct (in after-effect). [*Rl.*]

He goes to sleep over the coitus, without seminal effusion (aft. 21 d.).

460. Tardy erection (aft. 9, 14 d.).

Erection, in the morning before rising, else a rare occurence (aft. 17 d.). [*Ng.*]

Erections every night (aft. 30 d.). (After-effect?)

In the evening sudden erection, more violent than for a year, with a shiver and such violence, that coitus became necessary (aft. 10 h.).

Pollution in an aged man, and then a feeling of dryness all over the body (aft 10 d.).

465. Several pollutions in quick succession (in a married man) with subsequent lassitude (aft. 35 d.).

Profuse nightly pollution, after a coitus shortly before (aft. 4 d.).

With the woman, constantly increased sexual desire (curative effect).

With the woman, more inclination to coitus and far more excitation and perseverance during it (curative effect).

Menses extremely weak.

470. The menses flow very scantily and only for one day, while else they continued 2 or 3 days. [*Ng.*]

—The menses somewhat more copious and continued than usual, and take place without any of the former pains (curative effect). [*Gr.*]

The catamenia appear 2 days sooner. [*Ng.*]

The catamenia set in too early and flow very copiously.

During the catamenia, a pressure like a heaviness over the ossa pubis, in every position. [*Ng.*]

475. During the menses, cutting and pinching in the abdomen. [*Ng.*]

During the menses, pain as from a bruise about the sacrum. [*Ng.*]

Emission of some bloody mucus from the vagina, with anxious palpitation, uneasiness in the abdomen, pains in the sacrum and weakness even to syncope.

Painful tearing in jerks, in the pudendum, so that she felt like screaming, in the evening (4th d.). [*Ng.*]

* * * * * * * *

Sneezing, so violent that the brain is shaken by it, and a sensation of vertigo remains behind (1st d.). [*Ng.*]

480. Frequent sneezing, in quick succession in the evening. [*Htb.*]

Stoppage of the nose.

Troublesome dryness of the nose. [*Rl.*]

A constant coryza, with sensation of stoppage in the nose (aft. 15 d.). [*Ng.*]

Frequent but brief attacks of coryza, scarcely longer than a half hour.

485. Fluent coryza, coming quickly and passing off soon. [*Htb.*]

Fluent coryza, with hollow deep voice and dry cough, in the morning and in daytime, but not at night.

Frequent discharge of mucus from the nose. [*Ng.*]

Frequent urging to blow the nose, with secretion of thick mucus in the nose, followed every time by a sensation of dryness (aft. 8 d.). [*Ng.*]

Discharge of thick, yellow mucus from the nose. [*Htb.*]

490. In the windpipe, stitches (2d d.). [*Ng.*]

—Pressure just below the larynx, unconnected with swallowing (aft. 3 h.). [*Htn.*]

In the throat, sensation, as if he inspired nothing but smoke (aft. 27 d.). [*Ng.*]

Hoarseness for fourteen days.

Hoarseness, or rather aphony, for several weeks.

495. —Voice husky, from viscid phlegm, which nearly always occupies his fauces and larynx, for many days; he only ejects a little by hawking, and clears his tones thereby only for a short time. [*Gr.*]

Roughness of the throat, and thence some paroxysms of coughing (aft. 1 h.). [*Ng.*]

Tickling in the throat, inciting to constant tussiculation. [*Ng.*]

Cough, excited by continual speaking (aft. 35 d.). [*Ng.*]

Cough after midnight. [*Ng.*]

500. Dry cough, soon after arising, with a sensation after it, as if a hard body fell down into the chest (aft. 20 d.). [*Ng.*]

Dry cough for three days, excited by a tickling in the windpipe and in the region of the heart; the only intermission is after midnight, and somewhat after dinner. [*Ng.*]

Dry, short cough, in the evening.

Violent, dry cough, in the evening, with following weakness in the head. [*Ng.*]

Choking cough.

505. Cough, with expectoration of phlegm. [*Htb.*]

Cough, from unceasing irritation, with mucous expectoration. [*Ng.*]

A loose cough, with salty, starch-like expectoration, which had lasted for four weeks, passed away (curative action). [*Ng.*]

While coughing, feeling of soreness on the chest. [*Ng.*]

Arrest of breathing during coughing and without it (9th d.). [*Ng.*]

510. Fullness in the chest, with short breath, especially in ascending a height, and with stitches in the chest, especially on inspiring. [*Ng.*]

Fullness in the chest, and painfulness as if bruised on the left side. [*Ng.*]

Pain in the chest. [*Htb.*]

The pains in the chest are relieved partly by eructation and partly by application of warm cloths. [*Ng.*]

Pressure and tickling in the chest, with dry cough, pass away (curative effect). [*Ng.*]

515. —Pressive heaviness, transversely across the chest, increased by inspiring, and then causing a lancinating pain under the upper end of the sternum (aft. ½ h.). [*Htn.*]

Stitches in the left part of the chest.

Slight stitches in the left side of the chest, at every inspiration (aft. 19 d.). [*Ng.*]

A violent stitch in the left side of the chest, on raising a heavy load with both hands (aft. 20 d.). [*Ng.*]

Sudden stitching and burning, deep in the left side of the chest, so that she was startled, in the evening (4th d.). [*Ng.*]

520. Transient stitches in the right breast, causing her to scream, in the evening (2d d.). [*Ng.*]

—Transient stitches in the right side of the chest, between the sixth and seventh ribs. [*Htn.*]

Dull stitches under the sternum, deep in the chest, with subsequent pain, as from a bruise on that spot (1st d.). [*Ng.*]

Stitches from the chest, coming out through the shoulders. [*Hth.*]

Pains as from soreness in the chest, and externally in the same. [*Ng.*]

525. Transient burning in the left side of the chest. [*Ng.*]

Throbbing, with lancinating pain in the left side of the chest, extending from the scrobiculus cordis upward. [*Ng.*]

Violent beats of the heart, at times (in the first 14 d.).

Sensation of a violent beating of the heart, anteriorly in the chest. [*Ng.*]

Palpitation of the heart on lying on the left side.

530. Palpitation, which is renewed on thinking about it; for then she feels anxious; chiefly about noon.

Externally, in the breasts, tearing and lancination (aft. 19 d.). [*Ng.*]

Burning, externally, on the whole chest, with redness of the skin. [*Ng.*]

—Itching on the chest. [*Htb.*]

Pain in the small of the back (aft. 12 d.).

535. Heaviness in the sacrum and the loins, as from a cold.

Painful drawing in the sacrum, as if a heavy body was moving downward there (6th d.). [*Ng.*]

Tensive pain in the sacrum, worst in the evening, so that he could not rise from his seat nor bend backward.

Stitches in the sacrum, worse when sitting than in motion (aft. 11 d.).

A violent stitch in the region of the sacrum. [*Ng.*]

540. —A threatening throbbing in the lower part of the sacrum.

Pain in the back as if he had been lying on too hard a bed.

Great pain in the side of the back, on lying down.

Weakness and lack of mobility in the spine, it feels as if it would collapse on prolonged sitting. [*Htb.*]

Pain, as from a bruise between the shoulders (5th and 10th d.). [*Ng.*]

545. Pain, as from a sprain in the left scapula.

—Sudden, transient cramp-like pain in the left scapula. (aft. ½ h.). [*Htb.*]

Dull stitches through the left scapula coming out through the chest in front (3d d.). [*Ng.*]

—Transient stitch in the left shoulder-blade and on the outer side of the right thigh. [*Htb.*]

Burning stitch on the outer border of the right scapula (2d d.). [*Ng.*]

550. Burning in the upper part of the right scapula. [*Ng.*]

Burning on the loins, drawing transversely through the body.

Burning in a small spot on the left side of the lumbar vertebræ, and at the same time in the lower part of the left scapula, worse when rising from a seat, better when walking; also at night, so that he can only lie on one side (17th, 19th d.). [*Ng.*]

Throbbing in the back, a strong pulsation, chiefly while at rest, and especially after emotions (the first 3 d.).

Throbbing, alternating with tearing, now on the left shoulder, then between the scapulæ, also at night (aft. 19 d.). [*Ng.*]

555. Severe itching on the back, day and night.

Much itching, with eruption on the back.

Itching on the left scapula, with small pimples after scratching. [*Ng.*]

In the nape, stiffness, on awaking from the nap after dinner (aft. 24 h.).

Boring pain in the bones of the neck, neither aggravated nor diminished either by motion or touch (aft. 3 d.).

560. —Pressive, tensive pain on the left side of the nape, when at rest and in motion. [*Htn.*]

Swelling in the nape, which gradually extends all over the head, with redness and ulcerative pain of the skin and severe swelling of all the glands in this region, for several days (aft. 7 d.). [*Ng.*]

Several swollen glands in the nape, near the occiput.

Itching pimples in the nape, close to the hair of the head (aft. 3 d.).

In the axillæ, under the arms, frequent pain in the glands

565. In the shoulder-joint, an audible cracking at every motion of the left arm (aft. 18 d.). [*Ng.*]

—Painful digging in the left shoulder-joint. [*Gr.*]

The arms are heavy and tremulous.

Going to sleep of the arms, on resting them on the table. [*Rl.*]

Going to sleep of the left arm; she could only rehabilitate it after much rubbing.

570. —Painful drawing in all the long bones of the right arm. [*Gr.*]

Tension here and there in the arms, always only in a small spot (2d d.). [*Ng.*]

Swelling of the right arm, with pain in the axillary glands.

—Acute pain in the humerus, in a small spot. [*Htb.*]

Pain in the humerus, as if an ulcer was about to form there.

575. —Pain in the middle of the left humerus, as if it had been beaten in two. [*Gr.*]

Pain as if from a blow, above the left elbow. [*Ng.*]

On the elbow, pain as from a contusion.

Twitching tearing in the bend of the right elbow. [*Ng.*]

Quivering, almost like shaking, in the bend of the left elbow, extending to the middle of the upper arm and of the fore-arm. [*Ng.*]

580. In the left fore-arm, painful tearing, from its middle to the wrist. [*Ng.*]

—Short painful drawing in the left fore-arm, as if in the bone, both when at rest and in motion (aft. 1½ h.). [*Htb.*]

—Pain as from a bruise, intermittently aggravated, in the back of the fore-arm, seemingly in the long bone (aft. many d.). [*Gr.*]

Paralytic pain in the fore-arm and in the hand, passing away through motion and returning in rest. [*Ng.*]

In the wrist-joint and in other parts of the right arm, tension or drawing. [*Ng.*]

585. Drawing in the left wrist, up to the middle of the upper arm. [*Ng.*]

—Twitching in the coronoid process of the ulna, in slow, undulating intermissions, in the morning, while lying in bed. [*Gr.*]

—Rhythmical, twitching pain in the styloid process of the radius. [*Gr.*]

Squeezing pain in the hand. [*Rl.*]

—Cramp-like pain in the right wrist, from within outward (aft. 3½ h.). [*Htn.*]

590. Tearing, sudden pain in the wrist. [*Ng.*]

—Tearing in the wrist, extending into the finger-tips. [*Gr.*]

Dull stitches in the left wrist, relieved by motion. [*Ng.*]

Pain as from a sprain, on the back of the hand. [*Ng.*]

The hands tremble, when writing. [*Ng.*]

595. The skin of the hands is dry, like parchment (aft. 5 d.).

Rough, dry skin on the back of both hands. [*Ng.*]

Peeling off of the skin on the back of both hands (aft. 20 d.). [*Ng.*]

Distended veins on the hands, and redness of the same (12th d.). [*Ng.*]

Perspiration of the palms of the hands and of the fingers, in the afternoon (18th d.). [*Ng.*]

600. At first formication of the hands, then going to sleep of the same [*Ng.*]

—Intolerable formication and gnawing in the hollow of the hand, so that she has to rub it continually. [*Gr.*]

—Burning formication on the back of the hands and of the fingers, during the day, only transiently removed by scratching. [*Gr.*]

Itching pimples on the wrist. [*Ng.*]

On the index, drawing as if paralyzed, with a feeling on bending them as if it was turgid, especially at the tip. [*Htb.*]

605. Drawing pain in the posterior joint of the thumb. [*Ng.*]

Tearing in the posterior joint of the thumb and also in the fourth finger, as violent as if the finger had been torn out. [*Ng.*]

Tearing under the nail of the thumb. [*Ng.*]

Stitches in the posterior joint of the thumb, and suddenly in the tip of the thumb, so violent as to startle him. [*Ng.*]

—Violent, small, slight stitches in the posterior joint of the index of the left hand, both when at rest and in motion (aft. 9½ h.). [*Htn.*]

610. Beating in the middle joint of the middle finger, as from a hammer. [*Ng.*]

Cracking of the joint of the thumb and of the little finger, on moving them. [*Ng.*]

Paronychia on the fourth finger of the left hand (aft. 2 d.).

Chapping and peeling off of the skin on the finger tips. [*Ng.*]

—Pustules on the left middle finger, with painfulness to the touch, as from a sore. [*Gr.*]

615. In the hip-joint of the right side, pain on taking a walk.

Cramp-like pain in the right hip joint, as if stiff or compressed in a vice, the pain spreading down the front side of the thigh. [*Ng.*]

Sudden stitches in the hip-joint, as if dislocated, with pain, as if about to give way, in walking.

On the nates, burning.

Drawing pain in the right natis, as if the flesh were being pulled off. [*Ng.*]

620. Violent stitches in the natis. [*Ng.*]

Stinging itching in the nates. [*Ng.*]

A small furunculus on the nates. [*Ng.*]

—Intermittent tearing downward in the right natis. [*Gr.*]

In the legs, much cramp.

625. Tension in the lower limbs up to the hips, as if all the tendons were too short, worst in standing, relieved by lying down (37th d.). [*Ng.*]

Tension and tearing in the lower limbs, relieved by walking (aft. 16 d.). [*Ng.*]

Tearing and tension in the bones of the lower limbs down to the heel; somewhat relieved when walking (aft. 15 d.). [*Ng.*]

—Tearing down along the lower limbs, most long-continued and painful in the knees, but then also in the other joints, the nates, the hips and the ankles. [*Gr.*]

—**Drawing pain down the whole of the left lower limb.**

630. Weariness in the legs, in the morning, as if he was about to collapse (10th d.). [*Ng.*]

—Weariness in the legs, and jerking in the foot, when sitting, with acute pain in the posterior surface of the thigh, aggravated by treading, and darting down into the foot. [*Gr.*]

Sense of pressure from without inward, in the bend of the right thigh. [*Ng.*]

Burning in the bend of the thigh as if in the bone, when sitting. [*Ng.*]

Drawing down the anterior side of the thigh, as if in the bone, relieved when walking (27th d.). [*Ng.*]

635. Tearing in the right thigh, in the morning after arising, relieved by the warmth of the bed (19th d.). [*Ng.*]

—Tearing down the external and anterior side of the thigh, down to the knee, under the skin, when walking (aft. 7 h.). [*Htb.*]

Violent stitches in the right thigh, so that he could hardly walk (aft. 4 d.).

Sudden dull stitches on the inner surface of the thigh, startling him (aft. 4 d.). [*Ng.*]

A blow on the thigh above the right knee when standing, so that she thinks she is about to fall forward. (*Ng.*]

640. Violent pain as from a bruise in the middle of the right thigh, which gradually extends to the whole leg, and continues from the afternoon till midnight. [*Ng.*]

Quivering in the thigh above the right knee. [*Ng.*]

Severe itching on the thighs, also at night (aft. 11 d.).

In the right knee, at times a swift, momentary pain like gashes with a knife, paralyzing the leg.

—Painful aching on the inner side of the left knee, on lifting and advancing the leg in walking (aft. several h.). [*Gr.*]

645. —Pressive pain in the left knee, more toward the inner side, while sitting; by stretching out the foot, this pain changes into a dull pressive sensation. [*Htn.*]

Tearing on the inner side of the knee down to the middle of the tibia, going off while walking, returning when seated. [*Ng.*]

—Tearing from the knee downward, under the skin, when walking (aft. 7 h.). [*Htb.*]

Lancinating pain in the knee-joint.

—Sharp stitches on the inner side of the left knee suddenly, so that she is startled. [*Gr.*]

650. Violent stitches dart through the left knee on going up stairs and leave behind them a painful paralysis in the same. [*Htn.*]

Cutting burning in the right patella.

In the leg, especially in the right tibia, a paralytic pain; relieved by resting the leg in an elevated position, *e. g.*, on the sofa. [*Rl.*]

Tension in the tibiæ, on descending a mountain (aft. 16 d.). [*Ng.*]

Tension in the tendons of the calf, as if they were too short (15th d.). [*Ng.*]

655. Cramp in the calves, on stretching the legs.

Drawing pain, as if in the bones of the leg; in the evening, when sitting; he must rise and walk about.

—Painful drawing on a small spot of the left tibia (aft. 3/4 h.) [*Htb.*]

Quivering in the right calf. [*Ng.*]

Formication in the left calf, as if from its going to sleep, when sitting. [*Ng.*]

660. —Sensation as if a draft of cold air blew on the tibiæ, down to the ankles. [*Gr.*]

Restlessness in the feet.

Restlessness in the feet, while sitting; he has to keep moving his leg, to relieve the tension in the thigh and the burning in the groin. [*Ng.*]

Trembling of the feet in standing, so that he must hold to something, to keep him from falling (10th d.). [*Ng.*]

Pain, in the ankle-joint, as if sprained.

665. Pain, as if sprained, in the ankle-joint and on the dorsum of the foot, even while at rest, with severe lancination when in motion.

Cramp-like pain in the soles of the feet. [*Htb.*]

Drawing pain in the foot, only while walking.

—Drawing pain in the sole of the left foot. [*Htb.*]

Tearing in the feet, up into the knees, worse when moving. [*Ng.*]

670. Stitches, deep in the ball of the right foot. [*Ng.*]

Stitches in the heel.

Burning in the soles of the feet, the whole night, and yet he can bear no cooling of them. [*Ng.*]

Pain as of ulceration on the ball of the foot, on treading, especially in the morning on rising. [*Ng.*]

The hard skin on the sole of the foot pains acutely in walking, like a corn.

675. Corns, with pinching pain.

Burning stitches in the corns.

She gets corns on the toes.

In the toes a drawing pain (aft. 5d.).

Violent tearing in the right big toe, towards its extremity. [*Ng.*]

680. A tearing and a stitch in the left big toe, on the nail, with continuing sensitiveness of this spot; with great peevishness (1st d.). [*Ng.*]

Cramp in the toes, on stretching the foot.

In the joints, a very disagreeable lack of tone.

Stitches, at times, in the joints.

General great exhaustion. [*Htb.*]

685. Excessive acuteness of all the senses. [*Htb.*]

The whole body feels bruised in the morning on awaking (aft. 11 d.).

As if bruised all over the body, and very much exhausted (aft. 24 h.)

—The whole body feels bruised, with weariness and heaviness of the lower limbs. [*Gr.*]

—Dull pressure, as if from bruising, slowly increasing and decreasing, here and there, in small spots. [*Gr.*]

690. Drawing, alternately in the right shoulder, the leg, the arms, the occiput and in the eyes, with heaviness of the occiput, great indolence and dizziness, causing drowsiness. [*Htb.*]

—Drawing in the whole body, now here, now there, especially in the joints. [*Gr.*]

Tearing in the whole body, now here, now there (aft. 7 d.). [*Ng.*]

Squeezing, pressive pain in several parts of the body. [*Rl.*]

Sense of tightness and tension in the whole body, with anxiety, in the forenoon. [*Ng.*]

695. Going to sleep of the arm, the foot, etc., when lying on them, [*Rl.*]

She cannot lie on the left side, on account of ebullition of blood and strong pulsation of the heart, with a sensation of a wound in the heart, and great anxiety.

—The ailments (tearing, drawing, dull, threatening pain) in the head and in the limbs are most felt on the left side. [*Gr.*]

Many troubles come on when sitting, are relieved when standing, and pass off by motion. [*Ng.*]

Many troubles vanish in the open air. [*Ng.*]

700. On the skin of the whole body, pricking, as from needles.

—Painful, fine stitches here and there on the skin. [*Htb.*]

—**Crawling and burning pricks, as of needles, here and there,** often sudden, in a small spot, **not relieved by scratching and rubbing,** to which they incite. [*Gr.*]

—Unbearable crawling all over the body, especially on the back, the hips, the legs, the ankles, and on the dorsum of the feet, and on the back of the fingers, wakes him at night, and compels a continual scratching, which relieves only transiently; for three nights in succession. [*Gr.*]

Burning on several places of the skin, now here, now there (aft. 17 d.). [*Ng.*]

705. Burning itching here and there. [*Ng.*]

Itching in the evening, in bed, now in the face, now on the back, now on the hands.

Severe itching all over the body, keeping her from sleeping for several hours at night (aft. 29 d.).

Itching here and there, sometimes disappearing from scratching, sometimes not. [*Ng.*]

Itching here and there, and from scratching there ensues a violent pain. [*Rl.*]

710. Pimples in many places, *e. g.*, on the arms, the hips, the nose, the upper lip, forehead, etc. [*Htb.*]

A small wound often makes trouble, *e. g.*, a finger which had a splinter in it, which has been extracted, does not heal up; it suppurates and throbs, so that she cannot sleep for it at night.

Great sensitiveness to cold (aft. 12 d.).

Liability to take cold, and from it, especially inflammation of the throat.

Colds cause sore throat; a sharp lancinating pain on swallowing (aft. 7 d.).

715. Taking a walk is troublesome to him; but the farther he went, the easier it became.

From taking a walk, headache.

After the (customary) walk, colic, and then an exhausting night-sweat (aft. 5 d.).

On taking a walk, the right foot gets cold, and he has tension in the calf.

A little walk tires him very much; he has to sleep immediately after it.

720. Great weariness and lassitude of the body, so that he almost sinks down, in the evening at eight o'clock. [*Htb.*]

When lying down, the weakness, which shows itself as heaviness, is least insupportable. [*Ng.*]

—Great weariness; he would like to continually lie or sit down. [*Gr.*]

—Lack of steadiness and strength; his knees give way in standing, the spine is painful, especially in the lumbar region, as if he had been taking a long ride on horseback; he feels uncomfortable in the whole body, and would like to sit continually, or rather still to lie down; not to stand, rather to walk. [*Gr.*]

Quivering through the whole body, in the morning on rising.

725. Much yawning, every morning.

Frequent, violent yawning. [*Ng.*]

—Frequent yawning, while her eyes water. [*Gr.*]

—Yawning, stretching, and drowsiness. [*Ad.*]

Great drowsiness after dinner, every day. [*Ng.*]

730. Great drowsiness in the evening, so that his eyes close. [*Htb.*]

—Irresistible drowsiness. [*Rt.*]

—Drowsy weariness, in the forenoon [*Gr.*]

—She cannot help falling asleep in the afternoon, and nods continually. [*Gr.*]

Late in falling asleep in the evening, and then uneasy sleep, with dreams. [*Ng.*]

735. In the evening, the thought, that she had during the day made up her mind to sleep very soundly during the night, kept her from going to sleep.

Sleeplessness at night, from a sensation of great heat. [*Ng.*]

Frequent awaking, at night, at all hours. [*Ng.*]

Frequent awaking at night, the child called for its parents.

—Although very tired and sleepy when he went to bed, his first sleep was very uneasy and frequently interrupted; he frequently woke up, without any cause. [*Ad.*]

740. —She wakes up at night more frequently than usual; she feels very hot, she uncovers herself, and her feet ache, as if she had been standing for days; this passes off after rising and walking. [*Gr.*]

All night, frequent drawing in the ear.

In the morning's nap, saliva runs from the mouth.

Violent colic awakes him at midnight.

Pain in the lower limbs at night, as if he had been exhausted by excessive walking or dancing.

745. Fainting sensation, at night; she had to vomit violently, and felt qualmish even the following day (2d night).

Anxious, in the evening in bed; she had to open her night-dress.

In a weeping mood, at night.

Extravagant fancies and stupefaction, at night, as in a fever.

In the morning, on awaking, he is as it were stupefied.

750. Not refreshed by his afternoon nap; heavy, as if bruised, the head is painfully muddled; constant yawning (aft. 4 h.).

—In the morning, on awaking, he feels in no way strengthened by his sleep; his limbs were weary as if bruised; improved after rising. [*Ad.*]

Dreams, nearly every night.

Confused dreams, for several nights, so that in the morning, on rising, she has first to collect her thoughts. [*Htb.*]

—Confused dreams, with uneasy sleep, frequent awakings, and great weariness. so that he soon falls asleep again. [*Gr.*]

755. —She dreams about things chaotically confused. [*Gr.*]

—Vivid, adventurous dreams. [*Ad.*]

Anxious dreams, nearly every night, and restless sleep.

Anxious dreams, at night, and heaviness of the head, in the morning.

—Dreams about dead people (which, however, did not cause him any fear), and murmuring in his sleep (1st n.). [*Htb.*]

760. Dreadful dreams about fire and the like (aft. 8 d.).

Dreadful dream, from which she awoke in a sweat. [*Ng.*]

Frightful dream. [*Ng.*]

Starting up, as from terror, in the evening, on going to sleep, so that it caused the whole body to start up. [*Ng.*]

Chill, on entering the room from the open air. [*Ng.*]

765. Chilliness with thirst, in the afternoon (7th d.). [*Ng.*]

Chilly hands, and then they itch. [*Ng.*]

At 8 P. M., chill in the whole body, with shaking, commencing with the feet, and horripilation (20th d.). [*Ng.*]

Sudden febrile rigor, with goose-skin, external cold and horripilation, in the forenoon. [*Ng.*]

Shivering in the arms, passing off by the warm stove, but is aggravated by the least draught, in the afternoon. [*Ng.*]

770. —Chilliness, especially in the arms, with goose-skin and yawning in repeated fits. [*Gr.*]

—Shaking chill in the head, with dull tension in the zygomata as if goose-skin must come in the face, and as if the hair stood on end. [*Gr.*]

—Chilliness, in the forenoon; cold rises with painful pressure into the pit of the stomach, so that it seems to her to draw her hair together, and then it slowly goes down the arms and legs, even to the feet. [*Gr.*]

—Chill and cold down through the whole body, repeatedly, with cold hands (aft. 7 h.). (*Gr.*]

Constant cold, as if she had cold water poured over her, worse in the afternoon (7th–10th d.). [*Ng.*]

775. Burning sensation of coldness in the forehead, in the forenoon (7th d.). [*Ng.*]

In the forenoon, chilliness; toward evening he feels too warm in the whole body, and the blood pulsates in the head.

Icy-cold in the feet, from the afternoon to the evening, and after lying down, heat in the whole body (7th d.). [*Ng.*]

Now chill, now heat, the whole night. [*Ng.*]

Alternately chills and heat, toward evening.

780. —After repeated light chills, starting from the scrobiculus cordis, the whole body with the exception of the feet, which remain cold, becomes agreeably warm; ten minutes later the chill returns. [*Gr.*]

—Short shaking chill, with quick flushes of heat, chiefly in the back; the chill seems to start in the face, where there is tension (aft. 1 h.). [*St.*]

Alternate heat by day (aft. 9 d.).

Transient heat often rises in her head (4th d.). [*Ng.*]

Dry heat of the face, in the afternoon (12th d.). [*Ng.*]

785. **Heat, at night, and anxiety,** that he cannot contain himself, till morniug, when he rises (5th d. and aft. 14 d.). [*Ng.*]

Dry heat the whole night, with sleeplessness, and when she puts her hand out of the bed, she feels cold, chilly and thirsty (aft. 12 d.). [*Ng.*]

—Transient flush of heat over the whole body, with subsequent exhaustion, so that she would like to let her hands sink down; at the same time her face and hands are hot, the other parts almost cool [*Gr.*]

—Sensation of heat on the back. [*Htb.*]

Severe heat and sweat in the head, then thirst, in the evening (11th d.). [*Ng.*]

790. Almost every evening, at 6 o'clock, thirst (aft. 16 d.). [*Ng.*]

Excessive lassitude in all the limbs, in the afternoon; then, toward evening, perspiration, and at night vomiting; all repeated according to the tertian type. [*Htb.*]

Severe sweat on the left side, especially on the head. [*Htb.*]

Several nights, after midnight, sweat (aft. 7 d.). [*Ng.*]

Exhaustive night-sweat (aft. 13 d.).

BORAX, BIBORATE OF SODA.[1]

This crystalline salt is useful for soldering and as flux in technical works. This salt in its crude form was originally for several centuries, brought by the Venetians from the East Indies, especially from lakes in Thibet; therefore it is still called *borax veneta;* it afterwards was refined by the Dutch, by a process which they kept secret, and was then brought into commerce. In later times, however, it has been manufactured by the French, by an addition of soda to a kind of boracic acid brought from some hot springs and lakes of Tuscany in the neighborhood of Sasso.

Borax consists of 22 parts boracic acid, 32 parts soda and 46 of water in the hundred; it is consequently not fully neutralized by its acid (*acidum boracicum, sal sedativum Hombergii*), which appears in shiny scales, of a taste slightly acid, and which is yet to be proved as to its pure, and surely important, symptoms.

In household practice, borax has been for a long time empirically used in solution against the aphthæ of children and for facilitating the labor-pains of parturient women.

Antidotes of borax are: *Coffea cruda* against its sleeplessness and headache; *Chamomilla* against the pains of the swelling of the cheeks. *Wine* aggravates the symptoms, especially those of the chest, and *vinegar* reproduces the ailments that have been already removed, especially the stitches in the chest.

The symptoms marked (*Sr.*) were observed by Dr. Schrèter, of Hungary, in various persons.

BORAX VENETA.

Great anxiety with great drowsiness; the anxiety increased till 11 P. M. when the person became dizzy and went to sleep.

Anxiety, with weakness, trembling in the feet and palpitation (while being mesmerized) (3d d.). [*Sr.*]

---

[1]Borax appears for the first time in this edition, and Hahnemann's symptoms contributed to its pathogenesis were doubtless observed on patients. Some at least of "the several persons" on whom *Schreter* observed his symptoms would seem to have been of this kind, though 107 of the latter, first appearing in Hartlaub and Trink's *Annalen*, may have come from provings on the healthy with the usual 30th dilution.—*Hughes.*

Anxiety with rumbling in the abdomen (aft. 10 h.). [*Sr.*]

Very timid, in driving down a mountain; quite at variance with his customary bearing; he felt as if it would take his breath away (the first 5 weeks). [*Sr.*]

5. The child is timid while being dandled; when it is rocked up and down in the arms it makes a very frightened face during the downward motion (the first 3 w.). [*Sr.*]

Apprehension and fear of infection.

Timid, both he and she are startled by a shot at a distance. [*Sr.*]

Timid, an anxious scream causes terror to fall on all his limbs (aft. 4 w.). [*Sr.*]

The suckling is startled at expectoration and sneezing. [*Sr.*]

10. Irritability in an important business (8th d.). [*Sr.*]

Very serious (1st d.). [*Sr.*]

Peevish and cross (2d d.). [*Sr.*]

The child is cross, weeps and cries, contrary to its habit (the first days). [*Sr.*]

Very cross at 4 P. M. and peevish, even when he was in a good humor before, and he then reproaches people for slight matters, for several days (aft. 8 d.). [*Sr.*]

15. Passionate, cross, takes offence easily (the first days). [*Sr.*]

Passionate, he scolds and swears about trifles (the first days). [*Sr.*]

He is not vexed, and is indifferent about matters which else vexed him seriously (curative effect) (aft. 15 d.). [*Sr.*]

The child weeps periodically very violently, after some minutes it stops, and is then very friendly and laughs. [*Sr.*]

Very merry, cheerful, tender, with pleasure and enjoyment in all work, in the forenoon (6th d.). [*Sr.*]

20. Disinclination to work, he only does what he has to do, as if compulsorily (the first 8 weeks). [*Sr.*]

He fritters away the afternoon, without getting to any real work, goes from one work to another, from one room to another, without remaining at *one* thing. [*Sr.*]

Pleasure and joy in his work (curative effect) (aft. 5 weeks). [*Sr.*]

He several times lost the train of his thoughts (4th d.). [*Sr.*]

He had to think a long time before he recollected all that he had done during the day, and for quite awhile it is not clear to him, whether it was yesterday or to-day that he was in a certain place (aft. 6 d.). [*Sr.*]

25. Fits of vertigo with loss of presence of mind (3d d.). [*Sr.*]

Vertigo, in the morning, in bed (aft. 5 d.). [*Sr.*]

Vertigo, in the evening, while walking, as if some one pushed him from the right side to the left (5th d.). [*Sr.*]

Dizzy, with fullness in the forehead, in the morning, so that he at once loses his humor (4th d.). [*Sr.*]

Vertigo and fullness in the head, on ascending a mountain or the stairs (5th d.). [*Sr.*]

30. Fullness in the head and pressure about the eyes, as if they were held fast, and could not be moved. [*Sr.*]

Fullness in the head and pressure in the sacrum, while sitting; at the same time drowsiness in the eyes (aft. 17 d.). [*Sr.*]

Fullness in the head, in the morning, with want of clear ideas and of presence of thoughts, so that he could do no mental work, nor had he any desire for it; after a walk it was better, but he felt afterwards a great weakness in the feet and joints (2d d.). [*Sr.*]

Heaviness of the head (the first days). [*Sr.*]

Light, serene mood (6th d.). [*Sr.*]

35. Headache in the crown and in the forehead, in the evening (2d d.). [*Sr.*]

Headache, with numb feeling of the whole head, and stitches in the left ear, in the evening (1st d.). [*Sr.*]

Headache in the forehead, with stitches in the left ear, and in a hollow molar on the left side, below, in the evening (14th d.). [*Sr.*]

Aching in the whole head, with qualmishness, nausea, and trembling of the whole body at 10 a. m., with two female provers at the same time (2d d.). [*Sr.*]

Pressive headache over the eyes, quickly passing when taking a walk (4th d.). [*Sr.*]

40. Pressure above the eyes, from time to time (aft 10 d.). [*Sr.*]

Dull pressive headache, in the morning, especially in the forehead (the first days). [*Sr.*]

Dull pressure in the forehead (aft. 6 d.). [*Sr.*]

Pressive drawing headache in the forehead, above the eyes and toward the root of the nose, at times drawing even into the nape of the neck; in stooping, it presses severely against the frontal bone, and in writing and reading, the pain becomes much more violent, with pressure in the region of the spleen (6th d.). [*Sr.*]

Drawing pain in the forehead, toward the eyes (4th d.) [*Sr.*]

45. Twitching pain in the forehead, with nausea and tearing in both eyeballs, in the afternoon (1st d.). [*Sr.*]

Tearing in the crown, in the forenoon, with severe roaring in the ears (aft. 8 d.) [*Sr.*]

Tearing in the left half of the head, starting from a hollow tooth (4th d.). [*Sr.*]

Stitches from the right temple into the left half of the forehead. [*Sr.*]

Transient stitches, in the left side of the head, in the crown, followed later on by transient stitches in the sexual organs, and in the night by lewd, disgusting dreams, in a married woman (1st d.). [*Sr.*]

50. Lancinating headache over the eyes and in the temples, with alternate heat and cold, so that sometimes she has quite hot hands, then quite blue hands, with stitches in the swollen cervical glands, which then became softer and smaller (14th d.). [*Sr.*]

Stitches deep in the right side of the head, with running of pus from the right ear and such violent stitches, that he involuntarily drew back his head; with this, a tickling in the left ear as before the discharge, followed by very acute hearing (aft. 32 d.). [*Sr.*]

Pressive stitches in the right temple (aft. 11 d.). [*Sr.*]

Rhythmical, pressive, obtuse stitches into the right temple (aft. 40 d.). [*Sr.*]

Boring in a small spot beside the crown (aft. 20 d.). [*Sr.*]

55. Beating in both temples (aft. 4 d.). [*Sr.*]

Beating in the forehead. [*Sr.*]

Beating headache in both temples, especially in the right (aft. 16 d.). [*Sr.*]

Beating headache in the occiput, as if something were going to fester there, with shivering all over the body; during the whole night and the following day (aft. 2 d.). [*Sr.*]

Pulsating ebullition of the blood in the occiput (aft. 16 d.). [*Sr.*]

60. **Hot head of a suckling,** with hot mouth, and hot palms (4th to 7th d.). [*Sr.*]

As in a plica polonica, the hair of a child gets entangled at the tips and becomes agglutinated, so that it cannot be separated, and if these bunches are cut off, the hair gets entangled anew, for ten weeks. [*Sr.*]

Sensitiveness of the outside of the head to cold and to the weather.

In the eyes, sensation as if something was pressing in; disappearing on rubbing (7th d.). [*Sr.*]

Sensation in the right eyelid, while sitting, as if something was pressing from within outward, beneath the skin, coming from the temple; then at once, pressure about the eyes (4th d.). [*Sr.*]

65. Pressive pain in the upper eyelid, on opening the eye. [*Sr.*]

Pressure in the right eye, very painful, as if it were being pressed into the orbit, in the morning (aft. 5 weeks). [*Sr.*]

Cutting in the left eye, lengthwise, suddenly coming and going (aft. 37 d.). [*Sr.*]

Tearing in both eyeballs, with twitching in the forehead, and nausea, in the afternoon. [*Sr.*]

Stitches in the left eye, in the evening (3d d.). [*Sr.*]

70. Stitches in the eyeball, with contraction of the upper eyelid (aft. 8 d.). [*Sr.*]

Itching in the inner canthus, so that she must rub it frequently (the first days). [*Sr.*]

Itching in the eyes, with the sensation, at times, as if there was sand in them (aft. 4 d.). [*Sr.*]

Soreness in the outer canthi (aft. 5 w.). [*Sr.*]

Burning in the eyes and momentary contraction of the same, as soon as he puts on his spectacles (aft. 6 d.). [*Sr.*]

75. Pressive burning in the right eye, in the afternoon (aft. 3 d.). [*Sr.*]

The suckling, in crying, becomes quite red around the eyes (aft. 4 d.). [*Sr.*]

The eyelashes turn inward into the eyes and inflame them, especially in the outer canthus, where the edges of the lids **are quite sore** (aft. 6 w.). [*Sr.*]

Inflammation of the right eye in the outer canthus, with derangement of the eyelashes, and agglutination of the eyes by night (aft. 35 d.). [*Sr.*]

Inflammation of the left eye in the inner canthus, with nightly agglutination (the first days). [*Sr.*]

80. Inflammation of the edges of the eyelids, with a suckling; he rubs his eyes, and they are agglutinated in the morning (the first days). [*Sr.*]

At night, the eyes are glued together with quite hard, dry eyegum, which irritates the eyes like sand (aft. 5 w.). [*Sr.*].

In the morning, the eyes are agglutinated, and they water (aft. 5 d.). [*Sr.*]

Lachrymation (aft. 8 d.). [*Sr.*]

In the evening she can hardly close the eyes, and in the morning she can only open them with difficulty (aft. 5 w.). [*Sr.*]

85. Flickering before the eyes, in the morning, in writing, so that he does not see anything clearly; there are, as it were, pellucid waves now moving from the right to the left side, then from above downward; several mornings in succession (aft. 24 d.). [*Sr.*]

Obscuration before the left eye, in the evening; she must strain her eyes, and yet does not see anything (9th d.). [*Sr.*]

Sensitiveness of the eyes to candle-light, in the evening (aft. 3 d.). [*Sr.*]

Otalgia, a painful pressure behind the right ear (aft. 6 d.). [*Sr.*]

Stitches in the ears (aft. 6 w.). [*Sr.*]

90. Stitches in the ears, when washing them with cold water in the morning (aft. 3 d.). [*Sr.*]

Stitches in the left ear, on waking up unusually early (4th d.). [*Sr.*]

Stitches in the left ear, with two provers (aft. 14 d.). [*Sr.*]

Itching in the left ear, and after removing the ear-wax, pain as of soreness; in the evening when taking a walk; at the same time a sort of stitch in the left side of the neck (19th d.). [*Sr.*]

Pain as of soreness in the ear, on boring in it with the finger (aft. 32 d.). [*Sr.*]

95. Inflammatory, hot swelling of both ears, with running out of pus from the same (27th d.). [*Sr.*]

Discharge of pus from the ears, with lancinating headache (aft. 32 d.). [*Sr.*]

Discharge of pus from both ears, after previous itching in the occiput (19th d.). [*Sr.*]

A previous discharge from the ears ceases (curative action). [*Sr.*]

Smacking sound in the left ear, as if a thick salve were in it, which stopped the ear, which then opened again, in the evening (10th d.). [*Sr.*]

100. He feels suddenly as if the ears were covered or muffled.

Deafness in the left ear, in a child of five years (9th d.). [*Sr.*]

Ringing and whistling in the right ear, afterward changing into a roaring. (aft. 20 d.). [*Sr.*]

Ringing and buzzing in the right ear (8th d.). [*Sr.*]

Roaring in the ears, and very much harder hearing (18th and 19th d.). [*Sr.*]

105. Rushing in the left ear, as from a storm (3d and 4th d.). [*Sr.*]

Dull drumming in the left ear, as above a subterranean vault (aft. 14 d.). [*Sr.*]

Itching and crawling, in the nose, he has to put his finger into it (aft. 12 d.). [*Sr.*]

The suckling rubs his nose hard with his hands, and then his eyes (aft. 15 d.). [*Sr.*]

Ulcer in the left nares anteriorly, in the upper part toward the tip, with pain as of soreness, and swelling of the tip (10th d.). [*Sr.*]

110. Red and shining swelling of the nose, with a sensation of beating and throbbing.

Many dry scabs in the nose, which on being removed with the finger, are continually reproduced (aft. 16 d.). [*Sr.*]

In blowing the nose, some blood is always discharged, after previous itching of the nose (aft. 18th d.). [*Sr.*]

Bleeding of the nose (aft. 25 d.). [*Sr.*]

Bleeding of the nose, in the morning, and in the evening, throbbing headache (aft. 6 d.). [*Sr.*]

115. Complexion of the suckling wretched, pale, earthy (the first days). [*Sr.*]

Dull tearing in the left cheek, starting from a hollow tooth, with pressure in the forehead and in the two eyeballs (aft. 4 d.). [*Sr.*]

Sensation on the right side of the face, by the mouth, as if cobwebs were laid on it. [*Sr.*]

Twitching of the muscles near the right commissure of the mouth, several times. [*Sr.*]

Burning heat and redness of the left cheek (aft. 4 d.). [*Sr.*]

120. Erysipelas in the face (aft. 34 d.). [*Sr.*]

Swelling, heat and redness of the cheek, with tearing pains in the zygoma and great pains in the swelling, when laughing (aft. 31, 33 d.). [*Sr.*]

Swelling of the face, with eruptive pimples on the nose and lips (the first days). [*Sr.*]

Eruptive pimples in the face (aft. 4 d.). [*Sr.*]

Red eruptive pimples on the cheeks and around the chin, in a suckling (aft. 5 w.). [*Sr.*]

125. The mouth of the suckling is quite hot. [*Sr.*]

In the corners of the mouth, pain, as if they would ulcerate (aft. 20 d.). [*Sr.*]

On the lips, crawling as from bugs (aft. 2 d.). [*Sr.*]

Burning on the upper lip, under the left nares, in the morning in bed (7th d.). [*Sr.*]

Burning pain on the lower lip, quickly passing off, in the evening (3d d.). [*Sr.*]

130. Red, inflamed swelling, as large as a pea, on the lower lip, which on being touched, pains with a sore burning (aft. 41 d.). [*Sr.*]

Large patches of herpes around the mouth, and the upper lip, after burning heat, became covered with porrigo.

Toothache in an upper hollow tooth, with swelling of the cheek, which on being touched, was painful with tension (aft. 7 d.). [*Sr.*]

Toothache in hollow teeth, with dull griping, in wet, rainy weather, with five provers. [*Sr.*]

Contractive griping in a hollow tooth (aft. 4 d.). [*Sr.*]

135. Tearing and griping in an upper hollow tooth, which seems to be longer, so that she cannot bite on it, nor bring her teeth together; at the same time the gums are inflamed and swollen, as if a gum-boil was coming; in the evening the pain spread also into the lower teeth, and only passed off on falling asleep (aft. 4 d.). [*Sr.*]

Tearing from the hollow teeth, extending into half the head, when she touches them with the tongue, or takes cold water into the mouth. [*Sr.*]

Pressure in the hollow teeth, in bad weather (aft. 40 d.).

Dull, pressive boring in a hollow tooth, in the evening, in cool air (the first days). [*Sr.*]

Pressive and grinding toothache, coming after every supper and breakfast, and relieved by smoking tobacco; for several days (aft. 40 d.). [*Sr.*]

140. Drawing pain in the teeth.

Lancinating toothache in a lower hollow molar, on the left side, with stitches in the left ear and headache in the forehead, in the evening (aft. 14 d.). [*Sr.*]

Fine, intermittent stinging in all the teeth, but chiefly in a hollow, lower molar, on the left side (2d d.). [*Sr.*]

Crawling and tickling in the upper and lower incisors, and then gathering of saliva in the mouth (aft. 7 d.). [*Sr.*]

A little piece of her hollow tooth broke off of itself (aft. 6 d.). [*Sr.*]

145. The teeth feel as if too long (the first days). [*Sr.*]

The gums of the upper teeth bleed, without other pains (aft. 6 d.). [*Sr.*]

Swelling of the gums, for three days, with pressure in the hollow teeth, in bad weather (aft. 40 d.). [*Sr.*]

Inflamed, intense swelling on the outer side of the gums, which pains severely, a gum-boil, with dull pains in a hollow tooth, with swelling of the cheek, and of all the left side of the face, up to below the eyes, where it is raised into a watery blister (smelling of chamomilla removes the pains) (aft. 36 d.). [*Sr.*]

Mucous in the mouth (the first days). [*Sr.*]

150. **Aphthæ in the mouth** (aft. 4 w.). [*Sr.*]

Aphthæ on the inside of the cheek, bleeding during eating (aft. 30 d.). [*Sr.*]

Aphthæ on the tongue (aft. 33 d.). [*Sr.*]

On the tongue red vesicles, as if the skin were pulled off; they pain at every movement of the tongue, and when anything salty or sharp comes on it (aft. 5 w.) [*Sr.*]

Dryness of the tongue, in the afternoon (3d d.). [*Sr.*]

55. Cramp on the tongue, like stiffness and going to sleep, so that it impeded the breathing. [*Sr.*]

The palate of the suckling is contracted almost into wrinkles and he often screams when sucking (aft. 4 w.). [*Sr.*]

The mucous membrane of the palate is shrunk anteriorly, as if burnt, and pains, especially in chewing, for several days (aft. 6 d.). [*Sr.*]

In the throat, dryness (5th d.). [*Sr.*]

Roughness in the throat, as if there was a grater in it. [*Sr.*]

160. Burning in the throat, compelling him to swallow saliva, when it pains (9th d.). [*Sr.*]

Much mucus gathers in the throat, so that he has to hawk it up. [*Sr.*]

Tough mucus in the throat, which is detached with difficulty (aft. 18 d.). [*Sr.*]

Tough, whitish mucus in the fauces, which is only loosened after much exertion, for many days (aft. 5 d.). [*Sr.*]

Much tough mucus in the throat, which he expectorates with so much exertion, that he vomits (aft. 6 d.). [*Sr.*]

165. Hawking up mucus, in the morning; the mucus is detached easily in lumps. [*Sr.*]

Green, loose mucus is hawked up by him from the throat (aft. 12 d.). [*Sr.*]

He hawks up a lump of phlegm, covered with a streak of blood (aft. 9 d.). [*Sr.*]

The taste in the mouth is insipid and disagreeable (aft. 5 d.) [*Sr.*]

Bitter taste in the mouth; if she eats anything, or swallows saliva, all tastes bitter (2d d.). [*Sr.*]

170. She has no sense of taste, when she eats anything, for several weeks (aft. 8 d.). [*Sr.*]

Thirst, in the morning; he must drink much (aft. 14 d.). [*Sr.*]

Appetite for eating, much less than usual (aft. 5 d.). [*Sr.*]

Little hunger and appetite (the first 5 w.). [*Sr.*]

Diminution of hunger and appetite; often, however, hunger without real appetite (aft. 5 d.). [*Sr.*]

175. He has little appetite, especially for supper (aft. 8 d.). [*Sr.*]

She has little appetite in the evening, for several weeks (aft. 8 d.). [*Sr.*]

No appetite for dinner (12th d.). [*Sr.*]

He eats very little. [*Sr.*]

He did not relish his soup at dinner, and it caused him perspiration (8th d.). [*Sr.*]

180. Loathing for food, at noon, with coldness, drawing headache and colic, disappearing after three diarrhœic stools (aft. 20 d.). [*Sr.*]

No more relish for smoking tobacco (2d d.). [*Sr.*]

After smoking, a sensation as if diarrhœa were coming (6th d.). [*Sr.*]

Increased appetite for breakfast (aft. 4 d.). [*Sr.*]

Much appetite in the evening.

185. Desire for acid drinks (14th and 15th d.). [*Sr.*]

During a meal, restlessness of the whole body, with nausea,

so that he had to compel himself to eat; stretching backward brought relief (aft. 20 d.). [*Sr.*]

During the meal, nausea (19th d.). [*Sr.*]

After every meal, distension from flatus (aft. 5 d.). [*Sr.*]

After eating, which he relished, severe distension; he feels uncomfortable, ill and peevish; in the evening, on taking a walk, somewhat relieved (aft. 41 d.). [*Sr*]

190. After supper, distended abdomen (5th d.). [*Sr.*]

After eating stewed apples with mutton, fullness of the stomach, with peevishness and ill humor, and fullness in the head, as if the blood were violently pressing in (19th d.). [*Sr.*]

After eating pears, especially in the morning or forenoon, pressure in the scrobiculus cordis, with discomfort. [*Sr.*]

Immediately after a meal, pain in the abdomen, as if diarrhœa were coming; this passes after the siesta (2d d.). [*Sr.*]

After dinner, rumbling in the abdomen and diarrhœa (3d d.). [*Sr.*]

195. Immediately after dinner, diarrhœa, with weakness in the joints and legs, relieved after walking (1st d.). [*Sr.*]

Soon after breakfast, cutting in the right hypochondrium, transversely through the abdomen downwards, then diarrhœa, and, indeed, a sudden evacuation at once (3d d.). [*Sr.*]

After breakfast, diarrhœa four times in succession (4th d.). [*Sr.*]

Hiccup after eating (aft. 8 d.). [*Sr.*]

Severe hiccup, so that the throat is made rough from it.

200. The suckling has hiccups very frequently. [*Sr.*]

Nausea and little appetite (4th d.). [*Sr.*]

Nausea and qualmishness, as if about to faint, in the morning (6th d.). [*Sr.*]

Frequently feels qualmish and faintish, in the afternoon (aft. 12 d.). [*Sr.*]

Nausea in the stomach, with pain in the sternum, from three P. M. till evening, several days in succession (aft. 5 d.). [*Sr.*]

205. Nausea, with occasional urging to vomit (5th d.). [*Sr.*]

Nausea, in the morning, with inclination to vomit; passing off after dinner (6th d.). [*Sr.*]

Nausea even to vomiting, while driving (1st d.). [*Sr.*]

Nausea immediately after awaking, with great impulse to vomiting, but this will not come, until he drinks some water, when, with much exertion, he vomits up a great mass of phlegm, and at times something bitter (after 17th d.). [*Sr.*]

Nausea, with subsequent vomiting of mucus, with heat and quick, feverish pulse (aft. 23 d.). [*Sr.*]

210. Vomiting of sour phlegm, after breakfasting (on cacao) (2d d.). [*Sr.*]

In the stomach, pain as from bad digestion, with external pressure on the scrobiculus cordis (2d d.). [*Sr.*]

Pain in the region of the stomach, after lifting something heavy; the pain extended to the sacrum, where it became lancinating, so that she can only with great pain turn over at night; in the morning she felt better (two days before the menses) (13th d.). [*Sr.*]

Pressure in the stomach, after every meal (the first days). [*Sr.*]

Pressure in the scrobiculus cordis, passing off in walking. [*Sr.*]

215. Pressive lancination in the scrobiculus cordis, with tightness of the chest, compelling him to take a deep breath, which he can not do, however, on account of a sharply compressing, griping pain in the right side of the chest. [*Sr.*]

Contractive pain in the stomach-region, every day, from 4 A. M. to 12 at noon, a rolling together, which passes into the spine and there causes stitches, for several days. [*Sr.*]

Contraction in the scrobiculus cordis (6th d.). [*Sr.*]

In the hypochondrium of the left side, as it were a strong pressure with the hand, on riding in a wagon without springs. [*Sr.*]

In the left hypochondrium, after the siesta, a pressure from the last rib to the hip-bone, aggravated by external pressure, till evening (2d d.). [*Sr.*]

220. Pressive pain in the left hypochondrium, as if a stone was lying there, during dancing; it passed off on continued dancing (aft. 15 d.). [*Sr.*]

Painful pressure in the splenic region (1st d.). [*Sr.*]

Pressure, and at times burning, with a sensation in the left hypochondrium, when breathing deeply, as if something was drawn up into the chest from the region of the spleen, which, on expiration, again sank down (aft. 6 d.). [*Sr.*]

Cutting in the left hypochondrium, in walking fast, as if there was a hard, sharp, movable piece, with a sensation in the abdomen, as if nothing but hard pieces were there, which were jumbled together (6th d.). [*Sr.*]

In the region of the kidneys, pressure and stitches, increased by turning (aft. 3 d.). [*Sr.*]

225. Stitches in the right lumbar region, increased by stooping, in the morning, on walking out; relieved on sitting down (1st d.). [*Sr.*]

Colic, several times during the day, as if diarrhœa was setting in. [*Sr.*]

Weakness in the abdomen (4th d.). [*Sr.*]

Griping bellyache, with shivering and goose-skin (aft. 6 d.). [*Sr.*]

Pinching in the abdomen at various times. [*Sr.*]

230. Pinching, contracting colic, above the navel, so that she had to bend double, which stopped it, every day, in the morning, for five minutes (aft. 8 d.). [*Sr.*]

Pinching in the abdomen, with diarrhœa (aft. 20 d.). [*Sr.*]

Formation and frequent emission of flatus. [*Sr.*]

Much flatus. [*Sr.*]

Loud rumbling in the abdomen, at night, relieved by emission of flatus, upward and downward. [*Sr.*]

235. Frequent urging to stool, with rumbling in the abdomen and diarrhœic evacuation (the first days). [*Sr.*]

Frequent urging to stool, with pinching in the abdomen, and easy, pap-like evacuation. [*Sr.*]

Urging to stool, in the morning, with stools at first hard, then diarrhœic, with burning in the anus (1st d.). [*Sr.*]

Frequent, very easy stools, every day (first days). [*Sr.*]

He went to stool once every hour, and this was soft, mucous, and without any trouble (3d d.). [*Sr.*]

240. Soft stools (the first 3 days). [*Sr.*]

Very soft stool, in the morning, in the evening customary evacuation (aft. 7 d.). [*Sr.*]

Somewhat soft, light-yellow, mucous stool, every day three times, with languor and weakness (the first days). [*Sr.*]

Diarrhœa, two, three times, without pain (1 h. after taking medicine). [*Sr.*]

Diarrhœa, six times from the morning till 2 P. M., painless (5th d.). [*Sr.*]

245. Diarrhœa, without pain, twice a day, with subsequent discharge of mucus and blood (16th d.). [*Sr.*]

Diarrhœa, with rumbling in the abdomen (the first days). [*Sr.*]

Diarrhœa towards noon, with rumbling and grumbling in the abdomen (4th d.). [*Sr.*]

Diarrhœic stool, in the afternoon, with much flatus, after a hard stool (5th d.). [*Sr.*]

The child has loose stools, three times a day, the last like yellow water. [*Sr.*]

250. The first effect of borax is to cause soft stools, then a few days no stool, later hard stools, once a day. [*Sr.*]

Hard stool, with straining (aft. 16 d.). [*Sr.*]

Costiveness and evacuation like sheep's dung, for ten days (aft. several d.). [*Sr.*]

Green stool in a suckling, with previous screaming (aft. 6 d.). [*Sr.*]

Discharges of ascarides.

255. Before the stool, which ensued easily in the afternoon, he was peevish, cross, lazy, discontented; after it cheerful, contented with himself and with the world, and looking brightly into the future (aft. 20 d.). [*Sr.*]

With the stool, pale mucus was discharged, four times in the morning, once also involuntarily (14th d.). [*Sr.*]

With the stool, tough, viscid, yellowish mucus (18th, 19th d.). [*Sr.*]

Brown mucus in the anus, after the stools (9th d.). [*Sr.*]

Reddish, liquid mucus, with the stool, as if the stool was colored with blood (aft. 21 d.). [*Sr.*]

260. Discharge of blood and mucus from the anus (aft. 9 d.). [*Sr.*]

In the anus a varix, like a goose-quill, soft to the touch and painless (aft. 23 d.). [*Sr.*]

Itching in the anus, in the evening (7th d.). [*Sr.*]

Itching in the anus, as from the mucus of piles (aft. 16 d.). [*Sr.*]

Contraction in the rectum, with itching (aft. 40 d.). [*Sr.*]

265. Boring, lancinating pain in the anus and in the sacrum (aft. 15 d). [*Sr.*]

Stitches in the rectum, in the evening (2d d.) [*Sr.*]

Urging to urinate, without being able to discharge a drop, with cutting in the genital organs and distension in both hips, for two hours, in the evening (1st d.). [*Sr.*]

Violent urging to urinate, at night, se ral times (25 d.). [*Sr.*].

Very hurried, violent urging to urinate, so that he could hardly contain the urine (the first days). [*Sr.*]

270. Frequent micturition (the first days) [*Sr.*]

The suckling urinates almost every ten or twelve minutes, and often he weeps and screams before the urine comes; for some time (aft. 6 d.). [*Sr.*]

Hot urine in a suckling (aft. 4 d.) [*Sr.*]

Sharp smell of the urine (the first days). [*Sr.*]

Sharp, striking smell of urine (the first 2 w.) [*Sr.*]

275. After micturition, burning tension in the urethra. [*Sr.*]

After micturition, pains as from excoriation in the urethra (15th, 20th and 30th d.). [*Sr.*]

After micturition, the extremity of the urethra is painful. [*Sr.*]

Along the urethra, pain as from excoriation, especially on touching it (aft. 26 d.). [*Sr.*]

Dark-blue spot at the orifice of the urethra, as if the skin was off, with stinging pains during micturition (aft. 24 d.). [*Sr.*]

280. The orifice of the urethra feels as if glued shut with gum. [*Sr.*]

Quite indifferent to coitus (the first 10 d.). [*Sr.*]

Quite indifferent to coitus (the first 5 w.). [*Sr.*]

While innocently holding his hands on a sick woman, he had lascivious fancies, without desire for coitus (3d d.). [*Sr.*]

Frequent excitement in the sexual organs, without desire for coitus (the first days).

285. Lascivious mood (aft. 5 w.). [*Sr.*]

Tensive erection in the morning on awaking (4th d.). [*Sr.*]

Pollution, with a dream as if he was engaged in coitus, while the semen is emitted rapidly, causing him to awake. [*Sr.*]

During the emission of semen in a pollution, cutting pains in the urethra, and the semen is so thin that he thinks he is urinating. [*Sr.*]

After a pollution, urging to urinate, and in urinating, cutting in the urethra. [*Sr.*]

290. During coitus, the semen is emitted very quickly, and there continues an excitation in the sexual organs (aft. 5 w.).

He has to wait quite a while during coitus, before the semen is emitted (aft. 5 w.).

On the penis, on a spot where there was formerly a chancre,

lancinating pain as from soreness, espeically when touched (aft. 24 d.). [*Sr.*]

The menses appeared a day sooner, without any trouble (aft. 4 d.). [*Sr.*]

Menses four days early, without trouble; only the evening before, and the morning before their appearance, heaviness at the chest, with arrest of breath and more severe roaring in the ear (aft. 26 d.). [*Sr.*]

295. Menses three days too soon, painless (aft. 7 w.). [*Sr.*]

The menses, which had been suspended for six weeks, came at once on taking borax, lasted one day and disappeared; but at their appearance they were so copious as to be more like a hemorrhage [*Sr.*]

Menses four days too early and very copious, with griping in the abdomen, nausea and pain in the stomach, extending to the sacrum, lasting till midnight, when a copious sweat set in, after which she fell asleep (8th d.). [*Sr.*]

Menses for two days, very scanty, but on the third very copious, with pale-red blood, till the sixth day, with lassitude, so that she could hardly stand. [*Sr.*]

Suppression of the menses, for fifty-four days, without trouble, then they set in without trouble, only at first somewhat pale, but in the afternoon more red and copious, ceased the third day in the night and came back on the fourth day. (The courses ought to have set in three weeks after taking the medicine.) [*Sr.*]

300. The menses did not appear in the second month after taking the medicine, but when she had taken another dose of borax in the sixth week, they set in on the day following, with pinching in the body. [*Sr.*]

During the menses, throbbing in the head, and roaring in the ears. [*Sr*].

During the menses, spasmodic urging and lancinating pain in the groin.

After the menses, on the second day, pressure, as from a stone in the region of the right ribs, even to the scapula, whence the pain extended spasmodically into the stomach and sacrum, with subsequent vomiting. [*Sr.*]

Leucorrhœa, white like mucus, without other troubles, fourteen days after the menses (aft. 5 w.). [*Sr.*]

305. Leucorrhœa, like the white of eggs, with a sensation, as if warm water was running out, for several days (aft. 12 d.). [*Sr.*]

Leucorrhœa, thick like paste and of white color, for five days (aft. 4 d.). [*Sr.*]

A woman who had been sterile for fourteen years, and who, on account of a chronic, excoriating leucorrhœa, had, after several remedies, finally received borax, conceived, and the leucorrhœa improved. [*Sr.*]

Easy conception, during the use of borax, observed in five women. [*Sr.*]

In the uterine region, stitches (2d d.). [*Sr.*]

310. In the clitoris, a dilatation and stitches, at night (6th d.). [*Sr.*]

* * * * * * * *

Sneezing, with great painfulness; he has to try to suppress it, as there were with it violent stitches in the right side of the chest, for three weeks (aft. 6 d.). [*Sr.*]

Sneezing and fluent coryza (the first days). [*Sr.*]

Fluent coryza, with severe crawling in the nose (aft. 16 d.).

Discharge of much greenish, thick mucus from the nose. [*Sr.*]

315. In the larynx, tearing, for two hours, in the evening (3d d.). [*Sr.*]

Rough throat, in the morning.

Roughness in the pit of the throat, with drawing stitches there, when coughing and sneezing, with alleviation on hawking up phlegm (11th d.). [*Sr.*]

Tearing from the throat down into the chest, inciting to cough (aft. 5 w.). [*Sr.*]

Tickling in the throat, inciting to dry cough (aft. 4 w.). [*Sr*].

320. Scratching in the throat and thence dry cough (aft. 9 d.). [*Sr.*]

Dry tussiculation in a child. [*Sr.*]

Dry cachectic cough, as in old people, chiefly in the morning, on rising, and in the evening, on lying down, with stitches in the right side of the chest and the right flank; washing the chest with cold water brought the most relief; but on drinking wine, the pains increased; for twelve days (aft. 3 w.). [*Sr.*]

Cough, with scraping in the throat and pressure in the chest (1st d.). [*Sr.*]

Tussiculation and violent cough, with slight expectoration, of mouldy taste and smell, with every fit of coughing (3d d.). [*Sr.*]

325. Nocturnal cough.

Cough, with expectoration of mucus, chiefly in the morning, with pain in the region of the liver, continuing also after coughing till noon (4th d.): [*Sr.*]

Bloody streaks in the phlegm, on coughing up white phlegm, which was detached with difficulty (aft. 18 d.). [*Sr.*]

In coughing, he has to press with his hand on the right side of the chest and the right flanks, whereby the pains become less intolerable (the first 3 w.). [*Sr.*]

At every fit of coughing, stitches in the right breast, about the nipple; in the evening (3d d.). [*Sr.*]

330. **At every cough, and every deep breath, stitches in the chest** (aft. 7 d.). [*Sr.*]

The breathing is rendered more difficult (aft. 18 d.). [*Sr.*]

The breathing is more difficult; it compels him to take deep breaths, but this he cannot do, on account of stitches in the chest (the first days). [*Sr.*]

Every three to five minutes he must take a quicker, deeper breath, followed every time by a stitch in the right side of the chest, with a subdued sigh of pain and slow expiration (aft. 7 d.). [*Sr.*]

Tightness of the chest, with constrictive oppression of the

breath on going up stairs; he has then to take a deep breath, when he every time receives a painful drawing stitch in the right side of the chest (6th d.). [*Sr.*]

335. Shortness of breath, after going up stairs, so that he cannot say a word, and every time he speaks a stitch darts into the right side of the chest, so also in running and in every heating exertion of the body (aft. 8 d.). [*Sr.*]

Arrest of breath while lying in bed; he has to jump up and gasp for breath, when he, every time, receives a stitch in the right side of the chest (aft. 7 d.). [*Sr.*]

With every breath, stabs in the left side of the chest, as from a knife (2d d.). [*Sr.*]

At every effort to breathe, her chest is contracted (14th, 15th, 17th d.). [*Sr.*]

On taking a deep breath, a sensation as if something were drawn along with burning pressure from the left hypochondrium into the chest, and in expiration, it sank down again. [*Sr.*]

340. On the chest, a heaviness, so that at times she has no breath (aft. 6 w.). [*Sr.*]

Anguish on the chest, in the evening in bed (1st d.). [*Sr.*]

Pressure in the chest. [*Sr.*]

Pressive squeezing, while sitting bent forward, moves from the scrobiculus cordis into the chest; it takes his breath, with stitches in the lungs (aft. 7 d.). [*Sr.*]

Lancinating pressure in the sternum, after dinner, much aggravated by deep breathing (aft. 40 d.). [*Sr.*]

345. **Stitches in the chest, in yawning, coughing and deep breathing** (aft. 7 d.). [*Sr.*]

Stitches in the chest, as from obstructed flatus (the first days). [*Sr.*]

Pricks as with fine needles, from the back into the chest, in the evening (aft. 8 d.). [*Sr.*]

Stitches in the region of the left ribs, with aching in the interior of the chest. [*Sr.*]

Stitches between the ribs of the right side, so that he could not lie on this side for pain, with painful drawing and obstruction to breathing, so that he has to gasp for breath; if he lies on the painful side, the pains at once wake him from sleep (the first 4 w.). [*Sr.*]

350. Pain draws at once into the right side of his chest, with lancination, when he raises the arm upward (aft. 7 d.). [*Sr.*]

The drawing lancinating pain in the right side of the chest goes down into the right flank, where he then feels a violent pain in hiccupping, sneezing, coughing and yawning (aft. 3 w.). [*Sr.*]

Drawing pain in a small spot in the intercostal muscles, which on bending to the left side, changes into a pain, as from a violent blow. [*Sr.*]

Drawing pains in the right intercostal muscles, in bending forward or to the right (aft. 6 d.). [*Sr.*]

When he holds the painful side with his hand, during the pain in the chest, it becomes less intolerable. [*Sr.*]

355. On lying still, outstretched on his back, his chest feels somewhat easier. [*Sr.*]

The pains in the chest are most relieved by slowly walking about the room, and he feels easiest there. [*Sr.*]

Weakness in the chest, with dryness in the throat (9th d.). [*Sr.*]

Sensation as if the heart was on the right side, and was being squeezed off (7th d.). [*Sr.*]

Pain in the major pectoralis muscle, as if from a hard couch, with painfulness to the touch, at night (3d d.). [*Sr.*]

360. In the left mamma a griping, and at times lancination, and when the child has done drinking, she has to press the breast with her hand, because it aches from being empty. [*Sr.*]

Contractive pain in the left breast, while the child is drinking in the right one (the first days). [*Sr.*]

The milk in the breast increases (aft. 4 d.). [*Sr.*]

Much milk runs from the breast, so that the bed gets wet (aft. 32 d.).

The milk that runs from the breasts becomes caseous and curdles (the first days). [*Sr.*]

365. On the coccyx, violent itching and crawling, so that he cannot bear it without scratching; afterwards discharge of mucus from the anus (aft. 32 d.). [*Sr.*]

Pain in the sacrum, when sitting and stooping, as if from pressure (3d d.). [*Sr.*]

Pains in the sacrum, while walking (1st d.) [*Sr.*]

Pains in the sacrum, with much discharge of mucus with the stool (19th d.). [*Sr.*]

Dull pain in the sacrum when stooping (aft. 6 d.). [*Sr.*]

370. Dull pressure in the sacrum (7th d.). [*Sr.*]

Burning in the sacrum, when sitting (5th d.). [*Sr.*]

In the back, pressive pain, on both shoulders [*Sr.*]

In the nape, rheumatic, drawing pain, passing thence into the left shoulder and then into the scapula, in the evening, while walking out (aft. 41 d.). [*Sr.*]

In the axilla of the left side, a boil.

375. On the shoulder and between the scapulæ, a drawing tearing pain, so that she cannot stoop down, for eight days (aft. 5 w.). [*Sr.*]

Pricks as with needles, in the right shoulder, at once. [*Sr.*]

On the upper arm, a burning pain, a hand's breadth around the whole limb (2d d.). [*Sr.*]

In the palms, a stitching, with a sensation in the whole hand up to above the wrist, as if the arm was asleep; in the evening (2d d.). [*Sr.*]

Tearing and breaking in the fore part of the right hand, seemingly rheumatic (aft. 15 d.). [*Sr.*)

380. Sensation on the skin of the hands, as if covered with cobwebs. [*Sr.*]

Two hard indurations like warts, on the palms, after beating hard with a cane on something (aft. 30 d.). [*Sr.*]

Itching here and there on the back of the hand, inciting to scratch, as from flea-bites. [*Sr.*]

In the tip of the thumb, a throbbing pain, day and night; frequently rousing from sleep at night (2d and 3d d.). [*Sr.*]

Long-continued suppuration of a spot under the thumb-nail, where she had pricked herself with a needle, and painfulness on touching it. [*Sr.*]

385. Violent itching on the backs of the finger-joints, so that he must scratch violently. [*Sr.*]

Burning, heat and redness of the fingers, from slight cold, as if they had been frozen (aft. 24 d.). [*Sr.*]

Pustules with red areolæ on the middle finger of the right hand, with swelling and stiffness of the finger, which also continued to suppurate and to pain for a long time after the pustule had opened (aft. 30 d.). [*Sr.*]

On one natis a boil (a corrosive blister?) (aft. 15 d.). [*Sr.*]

Eruption of herpes on the natis of the child (aft. 4 w.). [*Sr.*]

390. On the right thigh near the pudenda, a burning, aggravated by coughing and by laying the hand upon it (3d d.). [*Sr.*]

Burning pain on the left thigh, a hand's breadth around that limb (aft. 8 d.). [*Sr.*]

Transient tearing in the right femur, from the middle downwards, and then up again, from morning till noon, and again in the evening (7th d.). [*Sr.*]

In the left leg numbness, with sensation of heat.

Erysipelatous inflammation and swelling on the left leg and foot, after a good deal of dancing, with tearing, tension and burning, and increased burning pain on touching it; the redness momentarily disappears on pressing with the finger (17th d.). [*Sr.*]

395. In the foot where the erysipelas had been, there is tension on the dorsum of the foot, so that standing became burdensome; she is not impeded in walking (aft. 22 d.). [*Sr.*]

Pain in the left ankle and the left toes on treading, as if something pressed her (aft. 20 d.). [*Sr.*]

Stitches in the sole of the foot, with two persons in the same way (2d d.). [*Sr.*]

Sensation of heaviness in the feet, on going up stairs, in the evening (1st d.). [*Sr.*]

Itching in the ankles (2d, 9th, 10th d.). [*Sr.*]

400. Pain in the heel, as if sore from walking. [*Sr.*]

Suppuration on a spot in the heel, rubbed open by a shoe. [*Sr.*]

On the big toes, especially on the balls, an acutely pressive pain, especially on treading (aft. 41 d.). [*Sr.*]

Burning heat and redness of the toes, when there is but slight cold, as after freezing them (aft. 24 d.). [*Sr.*]

Inflammation and itching on the ball of the little toe, as from being frozen (aft. 15 d.). [*Sr.*]

405. Inflamed pimple on the back of the little toe, paining like a corn (aft. 15 d.). [*Sr.*]

In the corns, frequent stinging, especially in rainy weather (the first days). [*Sr.*]

Boring stinging in the corns, relieved by pressure (the first 5 w.). [*Sr.*]

The skin does not heal; small wounds fester and suppurate. [*Sr.*]

Tendency of old wounds and ulcers to suppurate. [*Sr.*]

410. Whitish pimples of the size of hemp-seed, with red areolæ on the chest and the throat, extending to the nape of the neck (aft. 6 w.). [*Sr.*]

In the erysipelatous inflammation of the leg, first coldness, febrile rigor and thirst, with vomiting of food and bile, then heaviness in the head, and throbbing in the temples, with sleep uneasy at night, only like slumber, and later (on the sixth day), bleeding of the nose. [*Sr.*]

Every evening, lack of appetite, nausea, drawing in the head from the crown into the temple, and drawing in the abdomen toward the groin, for several days (aft. 5 w.). [*Sr.*]

Restlessness in the body, which does not allow him to sit or lie long in one place (1st d.). [*Sr.*]

The suckling becomes pale, of earthy complexion; the flesh, before solid, becomes relaxed and flabby; he cries much, rejects the breast, and often anxiously screams out in his sleep (the first two weeks.) [*Sr.*]

415. Lack of strengh in the joints (5th d.). [*Sr.*]

She feels altogether weak and without strength (aft. 5 w.).

Weakness, especially in the abdomen and the thighs (4th d.). [*Sr.*]

Broken down, weary and indolent, with heaviness in the feet (the first days). [*Sr.*]

Formication and trembling of the feet, with nausea and tendency to faint; it ceases in the open air (14th d.). [*Sr.*]

420. After an exciting conversation, restlessness of body, nausea, stupefaction and vertigo (3d d.). [*Sr.*]

During reflection, while at work, trembling all over the body, especially in the hands, with nausea and weakness in the knees (8th d.). [*Sr.*]

Weary, lazy, cross, thirsty after the noonday nap, with heat on walking in the open air, and perspiration on the head and face, with benumbed feeling of the head, pressure in the forehead and the eyes, which pain to the touch, as if sore; attended with a tendency to take deep breaths; during which there are stitches in the intercostal muscles, with hard, quick pulse. [*Sr.*]

Drowsiness at noon, and deep sleep of two hours (8th d.). [*Sr.*]

The child at the breast sleeps more than usual, but awakes frequently (the first days). [*Sr.*]

425. In the evening, very sleepy and tired.

In the evening, gets sleepy early, and early falls into a long sleep; for four weeks (aft. 8 d.). [*Sr.*]

In the morning, he feels as if he had not slept enough.

In the evening twilight, drowsy, but when he went to bed, his sleep altogether went away, although he had had severe exercise during the day, and slept but little the night before (aft. 7 d.). [*Sr.*]

Very wide awake, in the evening.

430. Late in falling asleep, and early in waking up in the morning (aft. 6 d.). [*Sr.*]

Uneasy sleep, she could not go to sleep, and tossed about in the bed (aft. 21 d.). [*Sr.*]

Uneasy sleep, with thirst and coldness (1st d.). [*Sr.*]

Restless nights, he could not sleep well on account of rushes of blood to the head, restlessness in the body, rumbling in the abdomen and diarrhœa (the first days). [*Sr.*]

At night, he had to rise several times to urinate (aft. 34 d.). [*Sr.*]

435. He can only sleep on his left side, for as soon as he turns on his right side, drawing lancinating pains in the intercostal muscles of the right side wake him up (aft. 7 d.). [*Sr.*]

He wakes up before midnight and can not go to sleep again before two A. M. [*Sr.*]

He woke up at one o'clock at night, and could not go to sleep again for abundance of ideas, until four A. M. (9th d.). [*Sr.*]

Unusually early awaking, in the morning about three o'clock, then she could not go to sleep again for two hours, on account of the heat in the whole body, especially in the head, and perspiration of the thighs (11th and 12th d.). [*Sr.*]

He wakes early at four o'clock and is wide awake, so that he goes cheerily to his work (aft. 5 w.). [*Sr.*]

440. The child often screams out in his sleep, and throws his hands about, clutching at things. [*Sr.*]

The five-year-old child tosses about, screams all night till four A. M.; frequently starts from sleep and is then, in the morning, in a whining mood (4th d.). [*Sr.*]

The suckling often screams out in his sleep, and anxiously clings to his mother, as if he had had frightful dreams (the first 2 w.). [*Sr.*]

Vexatious dreams. [*Sr.*]

Dreams about sore throat and other diseases.

445. Lascivious dreams (aft. 30 d.). [*Sr.*]

She dreams of coitus, but without voluptuous sensation (aft. 4 d.). [*Sr.*]

Shivering all over the body, during the night and the following day, with throbbing headache in the occiput, as from an ulcer (2d d.). [*Sr.*]

Chilliness in the whole body, especially in the back, without thirst, with disagreeable taste, roughness of the throat, stitches in the chest while breathing, exhaustion, worn.out feeling, stretching and extension of the limbs, with contracted, quick pulse; attended with heat, heaviness and stupefaction of the head, and burning of the eyes, with sensitiveness to the light (23d d.). [*Sr.*]

Febrile rigor, at night, from 2–4 o'clock, with trembling, vomiting of food, tearing in the thighs and pain in the femur, as if it were broken; then, after sleep, heat and thirst, followed at

9½ A. M. by bitter vomiting, and then sweat, with diminution of the thirst (2d d.). [*Sr.*]

450. Chill with headache and subsequent heat, without thirst; on walking in the open air, the headache ceases, and she then felt quite well (14th d.). [*Sr.*]

Chill, every second day, in the afternoon, with thirst and sleep; then on awaking, heat, with pressive pain in the inguinal region, without subsequent sweat (aft. 38d.).

Chill, in the afternoon from 2 to 6 o'clock (after thirst in the forenoon); then heat, with pressive pain in the left hypochondrium till he goes to sleep (aft. 5 w.). [*Sr.*]

Chill, immediately after dinner, with more thirst than appetite for dinner, and with a retractive tension round about the hypochondria, and with heat quickly mounting to the head when taking a deep respiration; then at 6 P. M. heat, with which he had to lie down till 10 P. M., then sweat and after the sweat, thirst; for four days (aft. 15 d.). [*Sr.*]

Now chills, now heat, often with sweat in the face, while a chill runs down his back, with stretching and extension of the limbs, with exhaustion and drowsiness, so that he has to lie down in the afternoon, but without being able to sleep; on taking a walk he drags his feet along, and is peevish and taciturn. [*Sr.*]

455. Transient heat, often in the morning, with nausea and inclination to vomiting (2d d.). [*Sr.*]

Heat in the head, in the evening, while writing, with thirst and a sensation as if sweat was coming (aft. 7 d.). [*Sr.*]

Heat, when she puts her hands under cover, but as soon as she puts her hands out she feels cold (aft. 5 d.). [*Sr.*]

Heat in the evening in bed, and sweat; as soon as he gets up he feels cold (aft. 17 d.). [*Sr.*]

Sweat during his morning sleep; on dressing he feels cold, gets a dry cough, with rawness on the chest, as after a cold (aft. 15 d.). [*Sr.*]

460. Slight perspiration at night.

CALCAREA CARBONICA, LIME.

Break in pieces a clean, somewhat thick oyster shell, take one grain of the softer, snow-white calcareous substance found between the outer and the inner harder shell. This is prepared in all the degrees of potencies up to X in the manner directed as to the preparation of dry medicinal substances for homœopathic use, given at the conclusion of Part I. This is preserved from sunlight and great warmth, to be used for its various purposes.

For the sake of comparison I have also observed the symptoms of acetate of lime, and have given them marked with a dash in front (—).

Lime when thus potentized belongs among the most effective antipsoric remedies, especially in cases where the following symptoms are prominent:

Dejection; inclination to weep; lack of cheerfulness, with heaviness of the lower limbs; anxiety when sweating; restless anxiety; *anxiety;* shivering and horror *when evening approaches;* anguish, excitable by thoughts; anxiety after hearing of cruelties; nervous excitation; *timidity;* fits of despondency about shaken health; sensitive peevishness; self-will; indifference; difficulty in thinking; long-continued numb feeling of the head, as if a board was before the head; dizziness and trembling before breakfast; vertigo when going up stairs; vertigo when mounting high, *e. g.*, on the roof; heaviness and pressure in the forehead, so that he has to close the eyes; headache from reading and writing; headache from overlifting; boring in the forehead, as if the head would burst; *beating* headache in the occiput; throbbing in the middle of the brain; hammering headache after walking in the open air, compelling him to lie down; headache and humming in the head, with heat of the cheeks; icy cold in the right side of the head; *evening-sweat in the head; falling out of the hair; pressure in the eyes;* burning and excoriation of the eyelids; burning and cutting in the eyes during reading by candle-light; cutting in the eyelids; stitches in the eyes; itching of the eyes; *closing of the eyes by suppuration;* suppuration of a fistula lachrymalis; *lachrymation* in the open air or in the morning; quivering in the upper and lower eyelids; agglutination of the eyelids every morning; obscuration of the sight when reading; obscuration of the eyes, after eating; dim vision, feathers before the eyes; dim-sightedness as from gauze; mist before the eyes, when straining the eyes and reading; long-sightedness, he cannot read without convex spectacles; dazzling of the eyes by a bright light; stitches in the ears; running of pus from the ears; cracking in the ears, when swallowing; *throbbing in the ears;* ringing in the ears; humming before the ears; roaring in the ears; rushing in the ears, with hardness of hearing; thundering in the ears; obstruction in hearing; *hardness of hearing;* sore nose; obstruction of the nose with yellow, fetid pus; *bleeding at the nose;* bad smell and fetor from the nose; smell of dung before the nose; faceache; *itching and eruption of the face;* freckles on the cheeks; itching and itching pimples in the whiskers; eruptions on the mouth, pain in the glands of the lower jaw; toothache, whenever drinking something cold; drawing toothache, with stitches, day and night, renewed by cold and by warmth; toothache, like digging and soreness; difficult teething of children; painful sensitiveness of the gums; stitches in the gums; gum-boils; bleeding of the gums; *dryness of the tongue*, at night, or in the morning on awaking; aphthæ under the tongue; accumulation of mucus in the mouth; hawking up mucus; constriction in the throat; bitter taste in the mouth in the morning; lack of appetite; *lack of appetite, with constant thirst;* aversion to his customary smoking of tobacco; aversion to warm food; long-continued aversion to meat; hunger immediately or soon after eating; voracious hunger in the morning; she cannot eat enough, she cannot get it down; after meals, heat; eructation after eating; bitter eructation; water-brash; weakness of digestion in the stomach; *pressure in the stomach, fasting and after eating;* nocturnal pressure in the scrobiculus cordis; stinging pressure in the stomach after eating; cramps in the stomach; pinching and cutting in the scrobiculus cordis; during pressure in the stomach, a pressing out under the last rib; inability to bear tight clothing over the scrobiculus cordis; swelling of the scrobiculus cordis, with pressive pain; the scrobiculus cordis painful to the touch; tension in both hypochondria; pressive, lancinating colic, without diarrhœa; colic in the epigastrium; in the afternoon, cutting and griping in the abdomen, with vomiting of food eaten at dinner; coldness in the abdomen; *inflation and hardness of the abdomen; obstruction of flatus;* pressure of flatus to the abdominal ring, as if hernia was about to come; constipation; costiveness; stool scanty and hard; stool twice a day; frequent, continual soft stool; involuntary discharge of foaming stool; during stool protrusion of the varices of the rectum, with burning pain; after the stool, lassitude and feeling, as if bruised all over; itching of the anus; *ascarides in the rectum;* burning in the urethra; too frequent urination; hæmaturia; flow of blood from the urethra; wanton, lewd ideas; lack of sexual instinct; deficient sexual powers; lack of pollutions; too brief erections during coitus; stinging and burning in the male genitals during the emission of semen in coitus; pressive pain in the vagina; pressure upon the prolapsed womb; stitches in the os uteri; itching on the pudenda and anus; distended veins on the labia pudendi; after-pains or milk fever after parturition; *bloody flux from the uterus;* (suppressed menses;) *menses too early and excessive;* during the menses, cutting in the abdomen and griping in the sacrum; *leucorrhœa before the menses; leucorrhœa*, like milk, in jets; *burning, itching leucorrhœa;* during the flow of leucorrhœa, itching on the pudenda.

Frequent sneezing; *troublesome dryness of the nose;* constant coryza; *delayed flow of the coryza; dry coryza;* dry coryza in the morning; stoppage of the nose; ulceration of the larynx; hoarseness;

mucus on the chest; evening-cough in bed; *night-cough* during sleep; cough in the morning; *dry cough;* yellow fetid expectoration; during cough, pressure on the stomach; arrest of breathing in stooping; pressure on the chest; *stitches in the side of the chest on moving;* stitches in the left side, on bending to that side; burning in the chest; prickling stitches in the muscles of the chest; *palpitation of the heart,* also at night; pain in the sacrum; pain as of a sprain in the back; *stiffness and rigidity in the nape of the neck;* swelling of the cervical glands; goitre; pressive pain in the right upper arm; nocturnal drawing and tearing in the arms; *sudden exhaustion of the arms, like paralysis;* dying off [numbness] in the hands on grasping; swelling of the hands; *sweat of the hands;* arthritic nodosities on the wrists and the joints of the fingers; formication as from going to sleep of the fingers; numbness of the fingers and sensation as if they were dead, also in the warmth; awkwardness of the fingers; frequent paralysis of the finger; heaviness of the legs; stiffness of the legs; cramps in the legs; going to sleep of the legs in sitting; ulcers of the legs; stitches in the thigh on treading; distended veins in the thighs; stitches in the knees, when standing and sitting; stitches and tearing in the knee; drawing pain in the knee, when sitting and walking; swelling of the knee; red spots on the legs; burning of the soles of the feet; swelling of the soles; coldness of the feet, in the evening; *foot-sweat;* dying off [numbness] of the feet, in the evening; sensitiveness of the big toes, corns; pains in the corns; going to sleep of the limbs; cramps in the arms and legs; pain as of bruising in the upper arms, also in the middle of the thighs, on going up stairs; tearing in the limbs, in the arms and legs; tendency to strain oneself, making the nape of the neck rigid and stiff, with headache; tendency to strains, with sore throat thence; great fatness and corpulence with youths; exhaustion from speaking; *lack of strength, lassitude;* lassitude in the morning; great exhaustion after every little walk; attacks of epilepsy at night during full moon, with cries; great fatigue from moderate walking in the open air; copious perspiration on moderate exertion of the body; great sensitiveness to cold; *tendency to take cold;* visible twitching in the skin, from the feet up to the head, causing dizziness; dry feeling in the skin; roughness of the skin, as it covered with miliary eruption; bran-like covering of the skin; furuncle; *warts;* drowsiness in daytime; *drowsiness early in the evening;* frequent waking up at night; insomnia; at night, tossing in bed; thirst at night; at night, pressure in the scrobiculus cordis and rising from there to the larynx and the head; nocturnal pain in the back and in the arms; nocturnal asthma; nocturnal palpitation of the heart; heat and anguish at night; horrible fantastic visions before going to sleep, in the evening in bed; anxious dreams; fantastic exaltation and delirium at night; chill in the morning after rising; frequent rushes of heat; rushes of heat with palpitation and anguish of heart; tertian, evening fever, at first, heat in the face then chill.

Calcarea when potentized has a long-continued action. When nitric acid, given previously, though selected apparently properly, yet acts in some respects unfavorably, then Calcarea may generally be profitably employed; so also any unfavorable effects of Calcarea, even when selected apparently homœopathically, may be neutralized by following it with nitric acid, and the effects will be changed into favorable ones Especially is nausea, produced by Calcarea, removed by smelling of the spirits of nitre; this is almost a specific and much more effective than smelling of camphor. There are, however, troublesome effects which call for the smelling of nux vomica. Calcarea is frequently useful after the use of sulphur, also when the pupils of the eyes are apt to dilate.

If the catamenia usually come several days before the period and are excessive, Calcarea is frequently the indispensable curative, and the more so, the more abundant the flow. But if the menses always appear at the right period or later, even if the menses are profuse, Calcarea is yet but rarely useful. Calcarea can rarely be advantageously repeated with older persons, even after other intervening medicines, and very rarely, yea, hardly ever, can its doses be repeated at once, without injury. But with children, when it is indicated by the symptoms, it may be repeated several times, and the younger they are, the more frequently.

The symptoms marked with a dash (—) before them were the effects of acetate of lime.

The names of my fellow-provers are designated by the following marks: *Fr.*, *Dr. Franz; Gr.*, *Dr. Gross; Htn.*, *Dr. Hartman; Lgh.*, *Dr. Langhammer; Rl.*, *Dr. Rummel; Stf.*, *Councillor of Medicine Stapf; Wl.*, *Dr. Wislicenus; Sr.*, *Dr. Schréter.*

CALCAREA CARBONICA.

Dejected and melancholy in the highest degree, with a sort of anxiety.

Melancholy, not really mournful feeling, about the heart, without cause, with a sort of voluptuous tremor all over the body.

Of the fellow-observers mentioned above, *Franz, Hartmann, Langhammer and Wislicenus* assisted *Hahnemann* in proving a solution of oyster-shells in vinegar, which he called CALCAREA ACETICA. Their results were published in the *Materia Medica Pura* and are incorporated here with *Hahnemann's* later observations on patients made with Calcarea carbonica, and with undescribed contributions from *Gross, Rummel, Schreter* and *Stapf.—Hughes*

—Mournful, almost to tears, with solicitous occupation with the present and the future. [*Lgh.*]

Troubled, oppressed humor, with irresistible inclination to weeping.

5. Inclination to weep, in the evening (aft. 5 d.).

Much crying, in a suckling, whose mother had taken *Calcarea*. [*Sr.*]

Weeping, on being admonished.

Weeping about trifles, with sensitive, irritated humor.

Grief and complaints over insults long past.

10. Anxious about every trifle, and inclined to weep.

Anxiety in the afternoon, after qualmishness and headache in the morning.

—Anxious about the present and the future, with deep reflection, at the same time indifferent to things outside, but not without inclination to work. [*Lgh.*]

—Anxious at heart, as if he had done wrong, or had to apprehend reproaches, with constant inclination to work. [*Lgh.*]

Great anguish and palpitation.

15. A sort of sweat of anguish, with some nausea.

With the anguish, frequent jerks in the scrobiculus cordis.

Anxious restlessness and feverish activity; she ever wishes to do many things, and gets to nothing; after this zeal she feels relaxed.

Restlessness in the mind, with gloom and anxiety.

Restlessness and ebullition of blood.

20. Extremely restless, in the evening, after nausea, in the afternoon, during which she had been very thoughtless.

Solitude is a burden to him, with coldness of the face, of the hands and feet.

Timid and restless, as if evil was impending over her (aft. 4 d.).

Fearful, anxious forebodings, as if evil would befall him or some one else, and as if he could in no way evade it (aft. 23 d.).

—Anxious, sad mood, as if he had to expect sad news. [*Lgh.*]

25. His heart is agitated with fear and anxiety for the future, with fear of consumption.

She is afraid of losing her reason.

She is afraid people may notice the confusion in her head.

Hypochondriac, she conceives herself fatally diseased, and yet cannot complain of anything (the first days).

Despairing mood, with fear of sickness and misery, with forebodings of sad events.

30. She despairs of her life, and believes she has to die; her heart is sad with weeping, and frequent attacks of sudden, general heat, as if she had hot water poured over her.

Irritation and anxiety, in frequent paroxysms.

Irritable, exhausted and dejected, in the morning, after little work.

Very much affected by noise.

Every noise near him startles him, especially in the morning.

35. Impatient, desperate.

Unnaturally indifferent, unsympathetic, taciturn (aft. 8 d.).

—Indisposed to talk, without being ill-humored (aft. 6½ h.). [*Htn.*]

Peevishness and constant obstinate self-will, for three days (aft. 28 d.).

—Very peevish and indisposed to speak, as soon as he comes from the open air, where he feels well, into the room; with increased headache. [*Fr.*]

40. —As soon as he is idle and sits still, he becomes peevish and drowsy, and everything goes against him. [*Fr.*]

—Peevish, morose, very cross and most indifferent to the most important things; he also did everything repugnantly and as if by compulsion. [*Lgh.*]

Intolerable ill-humor and perverse disposition.

Contrary mood.

Contrary, dejected humor.

45. Everything is repugnant to her, with much crossness.

Troubled and cross, she looked at the worst side of thing, and sought out all the evil.

Cross without cause, for two successive evenings.

Cross mood, without cause, especially in the morning.

Cross and restless.

50. Very cross (aft. some h.).

Often cross, and then she throws out saliva.

So cross about trifles, that she was dizzy the whole evening, went to bed early, but could not sleep (aft. 20 d.).

Very cross and irritable (after taking a cold).

Vexed about trifles and very irritable, in the morning, before the stool; he twists everything, so as to become angry.

55. Thoughts of former vexations irritate him to anger.

Aversion, dislike and repugnance to most men.

Indisposed to all work.

Aversion and repugnance to work, with great irritableness and heaviness of the feet.

—Lack of determination and yet consciousness of power (aft. 7 d.).

60. —During the day, peevish and cross; in the evening, humorous and talkative. [*Lgh.*]

—The first part of the day anxious, the latter part cheerful and self-contented. [*Lgh.*]

He is cheerful, and would like to be among men, to talk with them (aft. 10 h.). [*Htn.*]

His ideas flit away; his memory is short.

Very forgetful (aft. 48 h.).

65. Great weakness of the imaginative faculty; with a very slight exertion in speaking, he felt as if his brain was paralyzed, chiefly in the occiput; he could not think, nor recollect what was spoken of, with muddled feeling in the head.

She confounds words and is apt to use wrong expressions.

Cannot remember, is dizzy as after turning in a circle.

—Silly in the head, as from long whirling around, from 1 A. M. to 4 P. M. (aft. 25 d.).

Unconsciousness and delusion about her abode, as if her room were a hall in a garden.

70. In the evening, two fits of loss of consciousness in walking; she would have fallen down, if she had not been held up (5th d.).

Loss of consciousness, with anxious pressure in the stomach, from which she suddenly starts up as if through a violent fright.

In stooping and moving the head, she seemed not to know where she was.

Confused, tremulous feeling in the head (1st d.). [*Rl.*]

As if confused in the head.

75. Sense of silliness in the head, every morning on rising from bed.

Great confusion of the head, after the noon nap.

Dull, persistent **numb feeling in the head.**

Painful numb feeling of the head, so that she cannot understand what is read, nor what is spoken.

Constant numbness of the head, as if too full.

80. Insensibility and dullness of the senses in the whole head, as if from a violent cold.

Dizziness in the head, in the morning on rising, with qualmishness and roaring before the ear, and a sensation as if he would fall down unconscious (aft. 22 d.).

A dizziness in the forenoon, so that everything seems to him as if in a half dream.

Stupefaction, with unconsciousness of external objects, with undulating humming in the top of the head.

Stupefaction of the head, like vertigo, all the afternoon (aft. 24 d.).

85. Dizzy staggering, in the evening, when walking out, so that he reels to and fro.

Feeling of vertigo, as if he was lifted high up and thrust forward.

Vertigo, as if about to fall down, with exhaustion. [*Gr.*]

—Vertigo, as if the body did not stand firm (aft. 6 h.). [*Wl.*]

—Slight passing vertigo (aft. ¼ h.). [*Htn.*]

90. —Fit of stupefying vertigo; the body bent forward to the left side, both when at rest and in motion (aft. ¾ h.). [*Lgh.*]

Vertigo from vexation.

Vertigo on quickly turning the head, and also when at rest.

Quickly passing vertigo, mostly when sitting, less when standing and still less when walking.

Violent vertigo in stooping, then nausea and headache.

95. Vertigo, as if about to fall over, after stooping, while walking and standing; she has to hold to something.

Vertigo after walking, while standing and looking around, as if everything turned with her.

Vertigo on walking out, as if about to stagger, **especially in quickly turning the head.**

—**Vertigo, on taking a walk in the open air** (also aft. 26 h.).

—Vertigo, on taking a walk in the open air, as if about to fall to the right (aft. 2 h.). [*Lgh.*]

100. Vertigo and painful whirling in the head as if in a circle, in the morning on rising; especially very dizzy when walking and standing, with chill and pin-pricking in the left side of the head.

Headache, also at times with vertigo, every morning on awaking.

Headache in the forehead, over the nose.[1]

Headache in the occiput, when she ties anything firmly around the head.

Frequent semi-lateral headache, always with much empty eructation.

105. Headache, with nausea (aft. 12 d.).

Headache only in the side on which he is lying (a burning?).

—Sensation every time he stoops, as if headache was beginning in the right side of the head. [*Htn.*]

Dull pain in the forehead, with waste confusion in the head, in the morning on awaking, with dry, slimy tongue (5th d.). [*Rl.*]

First dull, then pressive headache in the temples, in the morning on awaking, with much empty eructation. [*Rl.*]

110. Violent dull headache, first in the sinciput, then also in the occiput, for several days (aft. 8 d.).

Stupefying pressure in the upper part of the head, as after whirling around quickly (aft. 24 d.).

Stupefying pressive aching in the forehead, as in vertigo, both when **at rest and in motion** (aft. 1½ h.).

—**Stupefying pressive pain in the forehead,** with lack of the power of recollection and fogginess of the whole head, **during reading;** he had to stop in reading and knew not where he was. [*Lgh.*]

—Stupefying, pressive pain in the whole body, in the morning, after rising from bed, as if he had not slept enough, or had been spreeing at night (aft. 24 h.). [*Lgh.*]

115. —The stupefying pressive aching in the (right) side of the forehead is aggravated chiefly by stooping (aft. 50 h.). [*Lgh.*]

Constant feeling of fullness in the head.

Painful feeling of fullness in the forehead, with throbbing in the temples.

Heaviness in the forehead, aggravated by reading and writing.

Heaviness and heat of the head, almost only in the forehead.

120. Heaviness of the head, in the morning on awaking, for several mornings (aft. 20 h.).

Great heaviness of the head, in the morning on awaking, with heat therein; both symptoms much aggravated by motion of the head and raising up the head (aft. 27 h.).

—Great heaviness of the head, with violent jerks in both temples, and painfulness of the whole head in stooping, passing off on raising the head (aft. 9½ h.). [*Htn.*]

Heaviness and pressure in the occiput (aft. 13 h.).

—Headache from heaviness, after some stooping, when stand-

[1] In the original: "In the nose above the forehead."—*Transl.*

ing, with pressure in the whole forehead, outward, especially over the left eye (aft. 5½ h.). [*Htn.*]

125. Pressure in the head, now above, now in the temple (aft. 12 d.).

—Pressive, squeezing pain in the whole head, especially in the two temples (aft. 9 h.). [*Htn.*]

Pressure in the temple every day, for eight days.

—Pressure in the left temporal bone, as if it was being crushed in; the pressure is both internal and external simultaneously (aft. 7½ h.). [*Htn.*]

—Pressure in the right temple, close to the eyes, as if something pressed on it severely (aft. 5½ h.). [*Htn.*]

130. Severe pressive pain in the crown wakes him every morning at 5 o'clock, and then passes off in an hour.

—Pressure in the vertex of the head, extending into the eyes.

Pressure in the forehead.

Pressive headache, chiefly in the forehead, increased in the open air.

Pressive pain in the forehead, as if it was quite thick there.

135. —Pressive headache in the forehead, especially over the left eyebrow, on walking in the open air. [*Lgh.*]

—Pressive headache in the right protuberance of the forehead, extending to the right eye and compelling this to close involuntarily (aft. 1½ h.). [*Htn.*]

—Pressive pain, suddenly darting through the occiput, disappearing only gradually. [*Htn.*]

Pressure in the sinciput (4th d.).

Pressing outward in the forehead, very severe and like vertigo; relieved by pressure with the cold hand, and disappearing when walking in the open air (aft. 9 d.).

140. —Pain pressing outward in the left temporal region and the whole left side of the head, as also in the right side of the occiput. [*Htn.*]

—Jerking pressure outward in the left side of the occiput, extending to the nape of the neck (aft. 14 h.). [*Htn.*]

—Sensation in the occiput as if it was pressed asunder. [*Htn.*]

Violent, almost lancinating pain, pressing outward in the region of the crown, on stooping (aft. 14 d.).

Painful straining outward in the whole head, with sensation as if the brain was pressed together (aft. 15 d.).

145. Compressive, pinching headache on the left side.

Tensive, sharp pain in the forehead.

Tension over the upper part of the head.

The head aches, as if tense.

Tension and pressure in the right side of the head, as from a blunt instrument, which is being pushed through it, with jerks from above downward.

150. Cramp-like pain, drawing from the forehead toward the vertex (after a cold) (aft. 6d.).

Cramp-like drawing under the crown, in the upper part of the head, with stitches in the temples and heat in the ears (aft. 48 h.).

—Cramp-like pain in the right temple (aft. 6 h.). [*Wl.*]

—Cramp-like pain in the left temple (aft. 8, 14 h.). [*Lgh.*]
Pinching pain in the forehead. [*Rl.*]

155. Pinching, drawing pain in the left temple, toward the parietal bone, with heat in the face. [*Rl.*]

Drawing pain in all the right side of the head, in the zygoma and the jaw (4th d.).

—Drawing pain in the right side of the forehead, above the eye and in the occiput, on straining the mind (aft. 2 d.). [*Fr.*]

Drawing pain in the upper part of the head.

Almost constant drawing pain under the crown of the head.

160. Drawing pain under the crown and in the temples, seeming to come up from the back.

Headache, drawing up from the nape of the neck.

Drawing pain in the occiput, always toward the side to which he moves his head; passing away on sneezing (aft. 12 d.).

—Drawing and pressive headache in the region of the left eyebrow, or in the temporal bone [*Fr.*]

—**Pressive, drawing headache in the right temporal muscle**, also in the evening; at times with pressure on the upper row of the teeth; by pressure on the temple, the pain is changed into a pressive headache in the forehead. [*Fr.*]

165. —Drawing, pressive headache in the left side of the occiput, with sensation of stiffness in the nape. [*Fr.*]

—Drawing, pressive, at times also tearing headache, now in the forehead, now in the occiput, now in the temples, passing of on pressure, and on exerting the thoughts, it vanishes (aft. 3 d.). [*Fr.*]

Tearing pain, the whole day, in the temples, in the bones of the orbit, and in the cheek, which swells up thick.

Digging and pressure in the head, spreading to the eyes, the nose, the teeth, and the cheeks, with great sensitiveness to noise, with slight attack of fainting.

Gnawing sensation in the occiput.

170. Cutting pain in the occiput and in the forehead, as if something sharp were being pushed in, aggravated by walking and by pressure of the hand upon the part (aft. 5 d.).

Stitches in the head.

Transient stitches in the head, here and there.

Stitches in the head, in the evening, with stitches in the legs.

Stitching pains in the brain, with sensation of emptiness in the head, for three days (aft. 28 d.).

175. Single stitches through the head, with great chilliness.

Lancinating headache, outward from the eyes (the first days).

Lancinating headache on the right side, extending into the eye.

Stinging headache in the one-half of the forehead, improved while lying down.

Stitches in the whole head, for half an hour, when she raises herself up after lying flat on her back, and so also after stooping.

180. **Lancinating headache on the left side,** over the temple (aft. 2 d.).

Frequent stitches in the temples (aft. 7 d.).

Stitches through the left temple into the head, and out through the right temple (aft. 5 h.)

Stitches on the right side of the upper part of the head, extending into the right eye (aft. 29 d.).

—Fine stitches on the vertex, externally (aft. 7 h.). [*Wl.*]

185. Stitches in the right side of the occiput (aft. 11 d.).

—Intermittent needle-pricks in the left side of the forehead, both when at rest and in motion. [*Lgh.*]

—Violent jerking stitches through the whole of the right side of the brain, often renewed, and leaving behind them a tensive, dilating sensation. [*Htn.*]

—Dull, pressive stitches, into both of the temples (aft. 24 h.). [*Wl.*]

—Dull, pressive stitches in walking, occupying chiefly the left side of the forehead, and passing off again on continuing the walk. [*Lgh.*]

190. —Digging stitches in the left temple, near the eyebrow, on moving the lower jaw (aft. 5 h.). [*Lgh.*]

—Boring, stitching pain in the left side of the forehead, when sitting, passing off at once when going, or standing, and on being touched (aft. 12 h.). [*Lgh.*]

—Boring pain in the middle part of the forehead, extending into the brain (aft. 3 h.). [*Wl.*]

—Rhythmically intermittent stabs of a knife, boring outward in the left temporal region, going off by touching the part and by sitting down. [*Lgh.*]

—Pulsating stitches in the left parietal bone (at once). [*Wl.*]

195. Single jerks or thrusts through the brain.

Cramp-like, jerking pain in the right temple.

Momentary jerks in the head.

Throbbing headache in the middle of the brain, every morning and continuing all day.

Beating pain in the forehead.

200. Lancinating beating in the head, when walking briskly.

—Violent beating in the upper part of the head in the region of the vertex, as from an artery, with cutting thrusts outward. [*Wl.*]

Rushes of blood to the head, with heat of the face, for seven hours after a meal.

Heat in the head and strong ebullition of blood.

Heat in the left side of the head.

205. Heat about the head, in the evening.

Icy cold in and **on the head** (aft. 4 h.).

Crepitation, audible to him for several minutes, in the occiput, toward noon, and then a warm sensation up the neck.

Concussion in the brain, on violent motion, with dull tearing pain (12th d.).

Painful concussion in the brain, especially in the right side of the occiput, at a slight shaking of the head, and at every step.

210. —Concussion in the brain, when making a step, like an echo in the head.

In the left parietal bone, a sudden pain, as if the bone were cut to pieces, with a shudder over the whole body. [*Rl.*]

Externally on the right side of the head, a numb place.

Several places of the head pain on touching (aft. 14 d.).

—The whole skin of the head painfully sensitive on moving the frontal muscles to and fro (aft. 1½ h.). [*Wl.*]

215. —Sensation of soreness on the occiput, when touched, as if the spot was festered below. [*Lgh.*]

Pain on the head, as if the skin was detached, down to the nape of the neck.

Tearing in the head and eyes, with redness of the whole face, every afternoon from 3 or 4 to 9 or 10 o'clock.

Great tendency of the head to catch cold and from it a headache, as if a board lay on the head, with straining pain in it and chilliness of the body (aft. 6 d.).

Itching on the hairy scalp

220. Itching on the occiput.

Itching behind the ear, with dizziness of the head after scratching.

Itching of the hairy scalp on taking a walk in the open air.

—Tickling itching of the hairy scalp compelling to scratch, with painfulness to the touch of the roots of the hair. [*Lgh.*]

—Crawling and itching on the hairy scalp, not removed by rubbing (aft. 10 h.). [*Wl.*]

225. Burning itching on the hairy scalp (aft. 13 d.).

Burning itching as from nettles, with severe crawling on the hairy scalp, and on the lower part of the face, in the evening before going to sleep.

The scalp on the vertex becomes scaly.

Eruption on the hairy scalp, with swelling of the cervical glands.

Severe eruption on the head. [*Rl.*]

230. **Eruptive pimples on the forehead.**

Painless tumor on the right side of the head (aft. 15 d.).

Tumor below the left temple (aft. 15 d.).

Tumor on the right temple, in the morning, passing away in evening (aft. 15 d.).

Thin, moist porrigo on the hairy scalp. (aft. 12 d.).

235. A furuncle on the forehead, where the hair begins (the first days).

The hair of the head comes out, when she combs it.

—A pustule over the left eyebrow. [*Lgh.*]

The eyes pain, ss that she must close them, with a sensation as if she ought to press them inward (aft. 8 d.).

Painful sensation as if a small, foreign body had gotten in the eye (aft. 17 d.).

240. Pain in the eyes, as if they were being pressed inward.

Pressure in the eyes, in the evening.

Severe pressure, day and night, as if there was a grain of sand lodged under the upper eyelid (aft. 19 d.).

Pressure in the eye, in the evening, after lying down, and in the night, as if a grain of sand had lodged in the eye.

Pressure and burning in the eyes, and lachrymation.

245. Tension in the muscles of the eyes on turning them or on straining them in reading.

Twitching and beating in the eyes, by jerks (aft. 20 d.).

Stitches in the eye and in the head (during the menses) (aft. 8 d.).

Severe stitch in the eye which has a fistula lachrymalis.

Stinging and smarting in the eye.

250. **Stitches in the inner canthus,** then alternately stitches and throbbing in the eyes, and after the pain goes off, several times a blowing of the nose.

—Stitches in the external and internal canthus. [*Fr.*]

—Itching stitches in the inner canthi, going off by scratching (at once). [*Wl.*]

—Violently tearing stitches in the right eye, as if inflamed. [*Fr.*]

—Boring stitch in the upper border of the orbit (aft. 5 h.). [*Wl.*]

255. Itching on the edges of the eyelids.

Itching in the eyes, in the evening, but pressure in the morning.

Severe itching of the eyes.

—Itching in the canthi.

Itching in the right inner canthus.

260. —Itching of the eyes in both canthi.

—Tickling itching in the right outer canthus, compelling to rub (aft. 25 h.). [*Lgh.*]

Excoriating pain in the lower eyelid

Smarting in the eyes (aft. 7 d.).

Sensation of coldness in the eyes (at once).

265. Sensation of heat in the eyes, with heaviness in the upper lids.

Burning in the eyes, when he closes the lids.

—Burning in the left upper eyelid, toward the inner canthus (aft. 6 h.). [*Htn.*]

Burning of the inner canthi, with stitches in them.

Burning and itching in the eyes (aft. 8 d.).

270. Itching burning in the eyes, on the head and in the throat (aft. 7 d.).

Redness of the edges of the eyelids.

Redness of the white of the eye.

Reddish white of the eye, with pressure in the eyes (aft. 20 d.).

Inflammation and swelling of the left canthus, and lower lid, with lancinating and throbbing pains and itching round about (aft. 10 d.).

275. —Violent inflammation of the eyes, the white of the eye is quite red, and in the eyes, especially the outer canthi, much eyegum all the day; the outer canthi are, as it were, sore and suppurated for fourteen days (2d d.).

Swelling and redness of the eyelids, with nocturnal suppuration; in the day they are full of eyegum, with sensation of heat and pain of excoriation, and lachrymation (aft. 11 d.).

Swelling of the lower eyelids, in the morning, after rising.

Lachrymation, when writing.

Lachrymation, and the eyes are affected (aft. 7 d.).

280. Lachrymation in the morning.

Smarting water runs from the left, reddened eye.

Sensation as of fat in the eyes.

Mucus-like matter (eyegum) is constantly in the eyes, she has to wipe them often.

Dry pus in the edges of the eyelids and in the canthi.

285. —Eyegum in the canthi, for two days (aft. 10 h.). [*Lgh.*]

—Stickiness of the eyelids, on moving them, with pressure in the canthi, and especially the outer ones (aft. 55 h.). [*Lgh.*]

Eyes closed by suppuration.

The eyelids of the eyes which look watery, are glued together with eyegum in the morning, and the eyes pain when he looks at the light (aft. 24 h.).

—Eyes closed by suppuration, early on awaking from sleep (aft. 24 h.). [*Lgh.*]

290. Some blood exudes from the eye, which is much reddened in its white part, but painless.

Quivering in the upper eyelids, with sensation as if the eye moved involuntarily (aft. 18 d.).

Stiffness in the left eyeball, in the morning, after rising; it cannot be moved without a disagreeable sensation.

She has to wink with her eyes while reading; they constantly tend to close (were red and exuded water).

Dilatation of the pupils.

295. —First dilated, then contracted pupils. [*Lgh.*]

An obscurity or darkness at times glides over her eyes.

Dimness of the eyes (after a cold in the head) (aft. 6 d.).

Dimness of the vision, while she wants to shut her eyes, without sleepiness (6th d.).

Sensation as of feathers before the eyes.

300. Sensation as of a gauze before the sight, in both the inner canthi, going off through lachrymation.

Something comes before her eyes like a shadow, with pupils very much dilated, so that objects on one side seem to her, as it were, obscure and invisible; so, *e. g.*, she saw only one eye in a man.

Sudden blindness, just after dinner; he could not even see the table, at which he sat; with sweat of anguish and nausea, and at the same time a brightness before her eyes; the symptom passed off after half an hour's sleep.

In the dark, he seems to see, as it were, electric sparks before the eyes.

Far-sightedness; she has to use convex spectacles in reading.

305. **Far-sightedness**; while she before could see well, both near and far, she cannot distinguish anything fine when near; she cannot thread a sewing-needle (the first 9 d.).

—Far-sightedness in a man who is short-sighted; he could recognize all things at a considerable distance, the whole day. [*Lgh.*]

Small objects she distinguished better than large ones.

A black point followed the letters in reading.

At times, he sees a black spot, before the left eye, which goes off in a few minutes.

310. In great bodily efforts, she often sees black spots before the eyes (aft. 11 d.).

He sees a halo around the candle and around the moon.

The letters dance before the eyes.

Flickering before the eyes and dullness of vision.

Flickering and like fiery sparks before the eyes, in the morning on awaking.

315. Light blinds her.

Looking into candle-light, affects the eye and the head.

Otalgia, as if something was pushing through.

Pressure in the ears.

Cramp-like pain in the ears (7th d.). [*Rl.*]

320. —Cramp-like sensation on the posterior part on the concha (aft. 9 h.). [*Htn.*]

Jerks in the right ear, with hissing rushing, every minute, and so violent that it sometimes jerks up the body with it.

—Twitching in the cartilage of the ear (aft. 48 h.). [*Wl.*]

Drawing, dull pain in the ears.

Stitches in the left ear and the temple, going off when at rest with closed eyes.

325. Stitches and pain in the right ear.

—Stitches in the ears.

Tearing stitches in the right ear (aft. 3 d.).

Throbbing in the ears (the first days).

Crawling in the right ear (aft. 7 d.).

330. Itching in the concha of the ear.

Burning itching in both ears.

Frequent chilliness externally in the ears.

Heat in the interior of the ears, like hot blood (aft. 29 d.)

Heat, as it were, streams out of the left ear (aft. 5 d.).

335. Burning pain about the ear.

Swelling in the left ear, with itching.

Severe swelling of the right ear.

Swelling of the inner ear and of the right side of the face, with frequent secretion of earwax.

The bone behind the left ear feels swollen and itches; but on touching the place it pains, as if festered.

340. Eruption behind the right ear; it becomes moist.

Tumor before the left ear, which is painful to the touch, like a furuncle.

—A tumor under the tip of the ear, which causes tensive pain in the jaw on chewing.

A little water drips from the ear which hears well, while the other, well provided with earwax, is very hard of hearing.

When blowing the nose, there is an obstruction felt before the ear.

345. On violently blowing the nose, the ear feels obstructed, so that she cannot hear with it (this vanishes on swallowing).

—Sensation in the right ear, as if something had pushed itself before the membrana tympani, without diminution of the hearing (aft. 15 h.). [*Lgh.*]

Impaired hearing (the first 3 days).

Hardness of hearing for a long time. [*Sr.*]

Sensitiveness of the brain, to loud sounds.

350. —Sensitive to noise, in the evening on going to sleep.

Tinkling before the ears.

Singing in the ears, followed by crepitation.

Now singing, then cracking in the left ear.

Singing and roaring in the ear.

355. Ringing in the left ear and in the head.

Buzzing in the left ear.

Loud roaring in the ear, with hard hearing, in the morning (aft. 2 d.).

Sound of spitting (of cats) before the left ear.

—Light whirring in both ears, with confused feeling in the whole head (aft 1½ h.). [*Wl.*]

360. **Squashing sound in the ears, on swallowing** (the first days).

Flapping sound in the ear, as if skin was detached in it.

A sort of grunting in the ear, on swallowing.

Cracking sound in the ear, when chewing.

In the nose, a twitching of the external muscles (aft. 14 d.).

365. —Gnawing pain in the root of the nose (aft. 1 h.). [*Wl.*]

Itching of the nose, without and within (aft. 2 d.).

Pain as of soreness on the margin of the nostrils, and especially on the septum.

The nostril, almost sore, pains like stinging, on being touched.

Soreness of the right nostril.

370. Red spot on the tip of the nose.

Inflammation, redness and swelling on the anterior part of the nose.

Swelling of the nose, especially of its root, frequently going off and returning (aft. 6 d.).

Swelling of the right ala nasi, with painfulness on moving.

Eruption on the nose.

375. Painful pimple in the left nostril, with itching, lancinating pain.

Pimple in the right nostril, only painful on moving the muscles of the face and nose; the wing of the nose is red and itches externally and internally.

—Pimples in both nostrils, with scurf.

Sore, ulcerated nostrils; preceded at times by frequent sneezing.

The skin of the nose feels as if covered with oil (aft. 25 d.).

380. When blowing the nose, blackish blood.

Severe bleeding of the nose (aft. 10 d.).

Some bleeding of the nose, at night (aft. 18 d.).

Bleeding of the nose, in the morning (aft. 7 d.).

Violent bleeding of the nose, as in a severe venesection, almost to fainting. [*Sr.*]

385. The sense of smell is dulled.

Very sensitive sense of smell (aft. 22 d.).

Very bad smell in the nose (aft. 25 d.).

Fetor before the nose, as from rotten eggs or gun-powder (aft. 1 h.). [*Lgh.*]

The complexion is pale, with blue rings around the eyes (the first days).

390. Pale, thin face with sunken eyes, with dark borders (aft. 14 d.).

Yellowness of the face.

—Yellowish complexion.

Frequent deep redness and heat of the face.

Constant bloated redness and heat of the face.

395. Erysipelas on the (swollen) cheek.

Pain in the face, and then swelling of the cheek, causing the pain to pass off (aft. 10 d.).

—Dull pain in the muscles of the left cheek (aft. 2 h.). [*Lgh.*]

—Pressive pain in the right side of the jaw while chewing (aft. 3 h.). [*Htn.*]

With cramp-like compressive pain, her right cheek is spasmodically drawn sideways (aft. 30 d.).

400. Twitching in the muscles of the face.

—Fine twitching, extending from the upper border of the orbit down to the nose.

Tearing in the bones of the face and head.

Tearing in the left cheek bones.

Violent tearing in the right side of the upper jaw (aft. 9 h.). [*Htn.*]

405. Stitches in the right cheek, very violent, the whole day (aft. 5 d.).

—Pulsating throbbing on both cheek bones (aft. 2 h.). [*Wl.*]

Prickling in the face and neck.

—Fine formication in the face, below the eye, and on the side of the nose. [*Wl.*]

Severe itching on the whole face; she had to scratch constantly (the first 7 d.).

410. Burning in the whole face.

Sensation of swelling in the face, especially below the eye, and around the nose, without visible swelling.

—Sensation of tension in the right cheek, as if swollen (aft. 2 d.). [*Tr.*]

Swelling under the left eye, painless.

Painless swelling of the cheeks, early, on rising (2d d.)

415. Swelling of the face, without heat, with pricking as of needles, here and there.

White spots on the face, with itching.

Eruption of small, painless pimples in the whole face (aft. 5 d.).

Miliary eruption in the face, near the eyes and on the nose.

Many pimples in the whole face, with severe itching.

420. Itching pimples on the forehead, with itching in the whole face.

Itching pimples on both cheeks, on the zygoma, for several weeks.

—Pimples in the middle of the cheek, which became moist on scratching, and left a greenish scurf (aft. 48 h.). [*Lgh.*]

—A boil on the cheek, with stinging pain.

The lips and the mouth are spasmodically contracted, so that she could not open the mouth.

425. At first a slight drawing in the lower lip, then it was as if dead, white and numb, with a sensation as if it was getting thick and hanging down, for five minutes. [*Stf.*]

Stinging itching about the upper and lower lips.

—Itching crawling on the upper lip, which on rubbing at once re-appears on another spot near by (aft. 1 h.). [*Wl.*]

—Roughness and dryness of the lips, especially the upper lip, as if it would chap (aft. 49 h.). [*Lgh.*]

Chapped lips, with fissures and excoriation in the tongue (aft. 48 h.).

430. Chapped upper lip.

Swelling of the upper lip, in the morning.

Eruption on the vermilion of the lower lip (aft. 32 d.).

Pimples on the upper lip.

Eruption of pimples around the mouth and in the commissures of the lips.

435. Pimple under the right commissure of the lips.

Scurfy pimple on the margin of the vermilion of the lower lip.

—Large, humid scurf under the right commissure of the lips.

Ulcerated commissure of the lips, for fourteen days.

The right commissure of the lips is closed by ulceration, and and pains as if sore.

440. On the chin, itching.

Tickling itching on the border of the right side of the lower jaw, with incitation to scratch. [*Lgh.*]

Eruptional pimple in the middle of the chin.

Fine eruption about the chin and the neck, with itching.

On the left side of the lower jaw, thick swelling, with drawing pains (aft. 12 d.).

445. Glandular swelling on the lower jaw.

Hard swelling of a submaxillary gland, as large as a hen's egg, with painful tension when chewing, and stinging pain when touched (aft. 41 d.).

—Swelling of the submaxillary gland, with a pressive sensation in it. [*Fr.*]

Toothache, only while eating.

Toothache, excited by hot and cold things, but chiefly by a draught, day and night, with flow of much saliva from the mouth, and stitches darting out at the ears and the eyes, so that she cannot sleep at night (aft. 8 d.).

450. Toothache in all the teeth (as of fine needle-pricks) aggravated by cold air penetrating the mouth; it wakes him at night from sleep.

The teeth cannot bear the air, nor cold.

Toothache, only when cold air or drinks come into the mouth.

The tooth is painfully sensitive to every touch.

The toothache is increased by external noise.

455. Drawing in the teeth.

Drawing pain in a front tooth, for some minutes, and returning at intervals (aft. 17 d.).

Drawing cutting in all the teeth (aft. 11 d.).

Tearing in the teeth, as if the roots were being torn out (aft. 20 h.).

Tearing in the teeth upward into the head, into the temple, chiefly at night.

460 Single tearing pains in hollow teeth, in paroxysms of half an hour, worst when partaking of something warm; also at night; it tears in the whole cheek.

Gnawing toothache, worst in the evening.

—Gnawing toothache in the right upper molars, as if they were becoming hollow, in all positions (aft. 6 h.). [*Lgh.*]

Smarting pain in the teeth.

Much tickling toothache in the hollow tooth.

465. Boring toothache, with stitches toward the nasal bone, day and night, and with swelling of the gums and cheek.

Boring and stinging toothache up into the eye and the ear, enormously aggravated by driving in a carriage (22d d.).

At first stitches in the posterior molar, two hours after dinner, then boring, relieved by eating.

Severe stitches in a tooth, up into the right eye and the right temple; only in daytime; with it, a tendency to touch the tooth with the tongue, which, however, causes every time a severe stinging jerk in the tooth, so that she started, and it shook her (the first 5 d.).

—Stitches in the teeth.

470. Twitching toothache (24th d.).

Twitching in the left teeth and the left side of the head.

A push against the teeth, as with a fist.

Tendency to chatter with the teeth, as in a chill.

Beating toothache in a canine tooth, only while eating.

475. —Throbbing toothache, with sensitiveness of the tooth to the touch, and a gum-boil, which pained on being touched (aft. 7 d.).

Looseness of an old stump under the swollen gums, with stinging pain as of soreness when touched.

Soreness of the teeth; only when she bit on them, they pained violently.

The teeth feel as if elongated.

Bad smell from the teeth.

480. The gums itch. [*Rl.*]

—Fine stitching in the gums of the whole upper jaw (aft. 2 h.). [*Lgh.*]

—Boring in the upper gums on the right side, with subsequent swelling of the same, with pressive drawing in the right temporal muscle. [*Fr.*]

Severe throbbing in the gums.

Beating in the swollen gums.

485. Soreness of the gums, with painfulness of the roots of the teeth.

Swelling of the gums in a hollow tooth.

Painful swelling of the gums, without toothache; also with swelling of the cheek, which is painful when touched (aft. 3 d.).

Swelling of the gums (and the jaw); chiefly on a broken tooth a lump swells up, from which the pains extend to the ear.

Pustules in the gums, over one molar, like a dental fistula (after a cold?) (aft. 24 d.).

490. Ulcer on the gums (aft. 14 d.).

Bleeding of the gums, also at night (aft. 2, 3 d.).

In the mouth, swelling of the right cheek into a thick lump, with drawing tearing pains in it every evening.

Blisters in the mouth, which break open and form ulcers (aft. 12 d.) (after vexation?).

Blisters in the mouth, and ulcers arising thence on the inside of the cheek (after a cold?)

495. Little vesicles on the inner side of the cheek, where the teeth strike.

Whitish-yellow little ulcers, on the right tonsil in the mouth.

The tongue pains on the side and in its lower surface, especially when chewing, swallowing and spitting out (7th d.). [*Rl.*]

Pain under the tongue, on the left side, behind the os hyoides, in swallowing. [*Rl.*]

Burning pain on the tip of the tongue, as from soreness; she could not take anything warm into her mouth, on account of the pain (aft. 6 h.).

500. Violent pain on the tongue and in the whole mouth.

—Sensation of roughness and soreness of the tongue, which is coated white. [*Lgh.*]

Thick tongue, quite white, with sensation as if it was totally without skin, and sore.

Swelling of one side of the tongue, impeding deglutition.

Vesicles on the tongue, which trouble him in eating.

505. —Vesicles on the tongue, with burning pain and heat in the mouth.

White coated tongue (the first days).

Impeded mobility of the tongue.

Talking is difficult for her.

He moved his mouth as if he would talk or scream, but could not utter a word.

510. In the palate, stinging.

—Roughness and scraping, posteriorly in the palate, inciting to cough, but not removed thereby (aft. 12 d.). [*Wl.*]

Sore throat, with glandular swelling under the jaw.

Pain in the throat, as if the uvula impeded swallowing, even in empty deglutition; but in speaking, less pain, and none at all while lying in bed.

Sore throat, as if swollen within, extending up to the ears (aft. 14 d.).

515. Sore throat, as from a lump in the throat, in swallowing.

Sensation as of a foreign body in the pharynx, always compelling him to swallow (aft. 15 d.).

Obstruction in the throat to swallowing, as of a body pressing there.

Spasmodic constriction of the œsophagus.

Sensation in the œsophagus in the afternoon, as if the food had lodged in it, and had not got into the stomach, with a sort of qualmishness.

520. Pressure in the œsophagus, after deglutition.

Stitching and pressure in the throat, on swallowing.

Violent stitches in the throat, even into the ear, on deglutition, and more yet in speaking.

Stitches in the throat on deglutition, she cannot get bread down.

—Violent stitch on the right side at the top of the œsophagus, when not swallowing (aft. 3/4 h.). [*Htn.*]

525. Roughness and burning in the throat, with a sensation as if the whole œsophagus, down to the orifice of the stomach, was rough and sore.

Sensation as if the throat and the uvula were sore and quite excoriated.

Rawness and soreness of the whole œsophagus; he can hardly swallow anything (aft. 29 d.).

Swelling of the tonsils, with elongation of the uvula, and a sensation of tightness of the œsophagus in swallowing, and a feeling of soreness with stitches (aft. 5 d.).

Swelling and inflammation of the palate; the uvula is dark-red and full of vesicles.

530. Swelling and dark redness of uvula.

Great dryness of the mouth and tongue, with a rough, stinging sensation [*Rl.*].

—Dryness in the mouth, as from lime. [*Fr.*]

Dryness of the tongue, early on awaking (aft. 13 d.).

—Sensation of dryness on the tongue (aft. 5 d.).

535. Dry and bitter in the throat, the whole day, chiefly in the morning.

Sensation of dryness in the palate, causing him to hawk up mucus.

Much gathering of saliva in the mouth, but not so as to spit it out.

Saliva collects several times in the mouth, in the forenoon, with qualmishness (4th d.).

—Much collection of saliva in the mouth, he could not swallow enough (aft. 1 1/2 h.). [*Lgh.*]

540. Much mucus in the mouth, with sensation of dryness. [*Rl.*]

—Sensation of much mucus in the fauces, when swallowing, with dryness in the mouth (aft. 1 1/2 h.). [*Lgh.*]

Phlegm in the mouth, in the morning, not easily removed by rinsing the mouth (aft. 24 h.).

Mucus in the throat, with taste of iron.

Expectoration of mucus, at night, with scratching in the throat.

545. Hawking up mucus, in the morning.
The taste is blunted.
Everything tastes to her as if unsalted.
—The food has too little taste for him, especially the meat. [*Fr.*]
Insipid, watery taste in the mouth, while the taste of food is abnormally acute.
550. **Bad taste in the mouth**, in the morning, as from a spoiled stomach.
Taste as of manure in the mouth, and fauces.
Unclean, bitterish taste in the mouth.
In the morning, two hours after rising, bitter taste in the mouth.
Bitterish taste, back in the mouth (5th d.).
555. Sweet taste in the mouth, as from sugar, day and night (aft. 12 d.).
Metallic taste, taste of lead in the mouth, in the morning (aft. 6 d.).
Taste of iron in the mouth.
Taste of ink in the mouth, in the morning on awaking.
Sour taste in the mouth.
560. Sour taste in the mouth, with much viscid saliva.
Sour taste of the saliva, which she continually spits out (aft. 2 d.).
Sour taste of all food, without any sour taste in the mouth (after a cold?).
Salty taste in the mouth, and much thirst (aft. several h.).
Great thirst.
565. Intense thirst, in the afternoon (aft. 3 h.).
Much thirst, and brown urine.
Much thirst after beer.
—In the morning, thirst.
—Unusual thirst and dryness in the throat.
570. —Intense thirst, with desire for cold drinks, especially for water; he has to drink much for eight hours (aft. 8 to 55 h..) [*Lgh.*]
—The appetite is less; she feels acridity in the stomach.
Entire lack of appetite (aft. 24 h.).
Constant fullness.
She has no desire for eating anything cooked.
575. Inordinate appetite, with great weariness, in the evening.
Much voracious hunger, with weak stomach.
Rabid hunger, in the morning.
Great desire for salty things.
Much appetite for wine, which she did not else care for.
580. Lickerishness.
The customary tobacco is not relished, and on being smoked, causes headache and nausea.
Milk does not agree with him, causes qualmishness and nausea.
—Milk tastes sour, and is repugnant to him. [*Htn.*]
He relishes milk. [*Htn.*]

585. The milk which he partook of, regurgitates, tasting sour (aft. 3 d.).

After milk, water from the stomach runs out of his mouth (water-brash).

—After drinking milk in the morning, qualmishness rises from the stomach, as if the stomach was spoiled.

After every meal, she has for several hours afterwards an almost intolerable burning of the throat, with or without eructation.

After scarcely eating half enough for dinner, he feels qualmish; the ingesta regurgitate into the mouth, with nauseous taste, and constant eructation follows, for three hours (aft. 20 d.).

590. Regurgitation of food.

As soon as he had just eaten enough, nausea came on, but passed away, when he then quite stopped eating (aft. 9 to 12 d.).

After all food, eructation, with the taste of the ingesta.

After a meal, much eructation.

After dinner, at once distended, hard abdomen.

595. After little eating and drinking, distension of the stomach and abdomen.

After partaking of thin liquid nourishment, in the evening, he is as if stuffed full, with much cramp-like pressure.

After supper, colic.

During dinner, pinching in the belly, starting from the navel (aft. 18 d.).

During the meals, loud rumbling, just above the navel.

600. After supper, cramp-like pressure of the stomach, and when it ceases, a sensation in the intestines, as if diarrhœa was coming, but it does not appear (aft. 7 to 8 d.).

After dinner, stitches in the region of the scrobiculus cordis (aft. 9 d.).

After dinner, pressure in the crown and in the forehead.

—After a meal, the drawing pressive headache around the temple is always aggravated, and comes even while eating, with a great sensitiveness of the teeth; when chewing, he feels as if these were loose and were being bent over. [*Fr.*]

Two hours after dinner, rush of blood to the head, with heat of the face.

605. After dinner, strong heart-beats.

After a meal, he feals the heart-beats, without laying the hand on his chest.

After dinner, exhaustion and sensation of weakness (aft. 9 d.).

After dinner, drowsiness; he takes a nap.

After eating, an irresistible sleep; then a shaking chill and a cough from tickling.

610. **After supper, strong inclination to sleep.**

After dinner, cold feet.

After supper, perspiration all over the face.

Much eructation, even in the morning, on awaking while fasting.

—Frequent empty eructations. [*Lgh.*]

615. Frequent eructation, with the taste of the ingesta.

Even after six hours, risings with the taste of the food, eaten at dinner.

Regurgitation of the ingesta.

Bitter eructation.

Eructation, with taste of bile, in the afternoon.

620. Sour eructation in the morning.

—**Sourish**, disgusting **eructation.** [*Lgh.*]

—Constant sourish eructation. [*Htn.*]

Gastric acid rises even into his throat, a sort of heartburn, all day.

Belching up of acid stuff, late in the evening.

625. Belching up of brownish, acid liquid, with burning, coming up from the scrobiculus cordis (heartburn) (aft. 8, 9 d.).

Rancid eructation, scratchy heartburn.

Heartburn (aft. 1 h.).

Burning, rising up the throat after every **meal**, especially after hard, dry viands.

Eructation, with hiccup.

630. Hiccup the whole day, till evening (aft. 29 d.).

—Frequent hiccup [*Lgh.*]

—Violent hiccup, for a quarter of an hour (aft. 5 h.). [*Wl.*]

Qualmishness in the stomach, with collection of saliva in the mouth (aft. 3 h.). [*Lgh.*]

Nausea, in the morning (aft. 2 h. and aft. 5 d.).

635. Nausea every morning, with diminished appetite.

Nausea, in the morning, fasting, with loathing, horror and shuddering.

Nausea in the scrobiculus cordis, in the morning, fasting, with things becoming black before the eyes, so that he had to sit down.

Feeling of nausea, in the forenoon.

Violent nausea in the scrobiculus cordis, in the afternoon, as from great emptiness in the stomach.

640. Nausea, in the evening, and heat, with very uneasy sleep.

—Nausea, with cough and a sort of heartburn, wakes him up about midnight.

Nausea, with anxiety (aft. 8 d.).

Nausea, like fainting, frequently.

Nausea, with emission of sourish water from the mouth.

645. At 11 A. M. qualmishness and nausea.

Tendency to choking in the throat, without nausea, with collection of water in the mouth, like water-brash.

Water-brash and colic (aft. 44 h.).

—Nausea, with eructation and gathering of water in the outh, with a sort of vertigo in the head (at once). [*Htn.*]

Nausea, with vomiting of the ingesta, with exhaustion, fainting and unconsciousness. [*Sr.*]

650. Vomiting in the morning, with nausea, the whole day, with digging pain in the abdomen.

Vomiting of sour water, at night.

Black vomiting (aft. 9 d.).

The region of the stomach is painful to the touch.

Quick pain in the stomach, as if it would distend it.

655. Fullness of the stomach in the afternoon.
Distension of the region of the stomach, toward **the left side.**
Pressure in the stomach, the whole day (aft. 7 d.).
Pressure in the stomach, even fasting.
Pressure, transversely across the stomach.
660. Pressure in the stomach, as of a body lying there, **heavy and fast.**
Pressure in the stomach, as if there were a lump in it, **after a** moderate supper, for an hour.
Pressure in the stomach, with collection of saliva **in the** mouth.
Pressure in the stomach, in the evening before lying **down**, like choking.
Severe pressure in the stomach, like cramps, for two **hours**; she could not stay in bed for it, but had to rise.
665. Cramps in the stomach, with nausea, eructation and yawning (aft. ¾ h.).
Severe cramp in the stomach in the afternoon, till sweat broke out all over.
Cramp in the stomach and abdomen, cutting and compressive.
Contractive pain in the stomach for several days, **at times** with pressure after a meal.
Griping in the scrobiculus cordis.
670. Gnawing and, as it were, jerks in the stomach.
Lancinating pain in the scrobiculus cordis, on **pressure**, especially severe after a stool.
Stitches, transversely through the region of the stomach.
Pain, as of soreness in the stomach.
Burning in the stomach.
675. —Anxious pain in the scrobiculus cordis (aft. 6 h.). [*Wl.*]
—Anxiety, as if coming from the stomach, when sitting, with a hot burning in the abdomen; soon disappearing in walking or standing (aft. 26 h.). [*Lgh.*]
In the hypochondria, tension.
As if constricted, below the hypochondria, with trembling and beating in the region of the stomach.
—Tensive squeezing pain in the whole hypochondrial region and in the scrobiculus cordis (aft. 10 h.). [*Htn.*]
680. —Dull, pinching choking, close under the scrobiculus cordis (at once). [*Htn.*]
—Griping, pinching sensation in the whole hypochondriac region, extending to below the sternum, here it becomes lancinating, causing eructation (aft. ¾ h.). [*Htn.*]
—Violent pinching in the hypochondriac region and the chest, terminating now and then in a little stitch (aft. ½ h.). [*Htn.*]
—Griping in the hypochondriac region, below the scrobiculus cordis, with chill of the whole body.
Close fitting clothing about the hypochondria is intolerable.
685. In the region of the liver, tensive pain.
Tension and pressure in the region of the liver, **as if it was** very thick there, ready to burst.
Thickness and elevation of the right side of the abdomen (in

the hepatic region?); she always feels there a pressure and a heaviness; she dare not lie on that side; with obstruction of flatus.

Pressive pain in the liver, especially at night, when its hardness is also most sensible.

Pressure in the region of the liver at every step in walking.

690. Drawing pain in the posterior hepatic region, toward the back, like darting tearing.

Drawing pain in the right hypochondrium toward the symphysis pubis.

Twitching pain in the hepatic region (7th d.).

Stitches in the hepatic region, during or after stooping.

Transient stitches in the right hypochondriac region, in the forenoon, for an hour.

695. Stitches in the right hypochondriac region, drawing thence into the back, in the evening (aft. 30 d.).

—Long stitches in the right side below the ribs (aft 13 h.). [*Htn.*]

Shaking stitch from the hepatic region into the chest (aft. 10 h.). [*Fr.*]

Excoriative, lancinating stitch in the hepatic region, by the last false rib.

Pain as of rawness, in the liver.

700. In the left hypochondrium, frequently during the day, paroxysms of ¼ of an hour of pressive throbbing (beating), both when at rest and in motion.

Sharp pinching together in the region of the left lower ribs.

In the abdomen, in its middle, an enormous aching from qualmishness, without inclination to vomit, for a quarter of an hour (aft. 27 d.).

Pain in the abdomen, above the hips, when walking and breathing (aft. 6 d.).

Aching in the hypogastrium, even when only walking a few steps, with sensation of heat in the whole body (aft. 5 d.).

705. **Pressure in the abdomen**, from the scrobiculus cordis downward.

Pressive bellyache below the navel early after rising, like a pressing into the abdomen, with constipation (aft. 12 d.).

Severe pressure in the hypogastrium, and hard stool (the first days).

Pressure in the hypogastrium, during violent bodily exertion.

Pressive colic in the hypogastrium, with nausea (for 8 days).

710. Pressure in the abdomen, with stitches in the scrobiculus cordis downward.

—Pressure in the hypogastrium, which muddles the head.

Fullness in the abdomen, especially after a meal.

Distension of the abdomen, only after dinner, not after supper, though she eats much.

Inordinate distended abdomen.

715. Severe distension of the abdomen, with colic, frequently during the day.

Fullness of the belly, in the evening, so that he can hardly move, with violent colic.

Distended, hard abdomen.

Distended, full abdomen, with contraction of the rectum, holding back the flatus.

Tension in the abdomen, with inflation, the whole afternoon, without sensation of flatulence; it passed off on discharge of flatus (aft. 20 d.).

720. Tension in the abdomen (the first days).

Tension in the abdomen, while sitting after violent exercise.

Tension and cutting in the hypogastrium (aft. 15 d.).

Squeezing and straining, close below the navel, after supper, aggravated by walking, and later passing into inflation of the abdomen.

Contractive pains in the abdomen, toward the sacrum (aft. 40 d.).

725. Contractive colic in the epigastrium, so that she had to walk crooked, excited chiefly by deep breathing (aft. several d.).

Contractive sensation in the abdomen and in the scrobiculus cordis, with appetite now too strong, now too weak.

Contraction of the abdomen toward the chest, at once in the morning, for one hour (aft. 18 h.).

Gnawing, griping in the abdomen and stomach, starting from the chest.

Frequent severe cramp in the intestinal canal, but especially in the evening and night, with coldness of the thighs (aft. 8, 29 d.).

730. Cramp-like contortion and convolution about the navel (aft. 4 d.).

Snatching together in the hypogastrium toward the womb, for several days, with discharge of bloody mucus in the stool (aft. 17 d.).

Writhing in the intestines.

Writhing, cutting pain in the abdomen.

Colic, frequently during the day, for several minutes, like pinching, followed by nausea.

735. Pinching in the belly (the first days).

Pinching in the hypogastrium (aft. 8 d.).

Pinching deep in the hypogastrium, in the region of the bladder, with pain at every step, as if the internal parts were drawn down by a weight. [*Sr.*]

—Pinching in a small spot below the navel, which on being rubbed, passes over into a clucking (aft. ½ h.). [*Htn.*]

—Pinching deep in the hypogastrium, as if in the region of the bladder, frequently repeated, and always with the emission of some flatus. [*Htn.*]

740. Cutting in the left side of the abdomen, going off after a soft stool.

Violent cutting in the abdomen, in the morning on awaking.

After the passing away of a severe cold lasting two days, **frequent attacks of colic**, with great exhaustion and wretched complexion, for many days, which is then suddenly quite removed by dipping into cold water (aft. 19 d.).

—Cutting in the abdomen, every morning, also in the evening

and night; after the meal it ceased, but later there was grunting in the belly.

—Cutting pain in the right lumbar region, pressing outward; going off only transiently by touching. [*Fr.*]

745. Stitches, transversely through the abdomen, below the navel, on inspiring.

Stitches in the abdomen (aft. 17 d.).

Stitches in the belly, extending through to the back, with arrest of breathing.

Transient stitches in the abdomen, especially on inspiring.

Stitches in the hypogastrium.

750. Stitches in the left side of the abdomen toward the sacrum, more frequent in the evening and on turning the body, or when stooping.

Drawing, in the abdomen, and restlessness in it, in the morning on awaking.

Jerking tearing, down in the side of the abdomen (aft. 36 d.)

Pain as of soreness in the hypogastrium, with painful tension on holding the body straight, or on bending it backward (aft. 16 d.).

Burning in the abdomen, frequent.

755. Burning pain below the navel, for some hours, in the afternoon.

Pain, at times burning, at times lancinating below the navel, into the flank, which is inflated, more in the left side.

In the groin, aching, as from a concussion (aft. 24 h.).

—Pressive tension, in the region of the left groin (aft. 8 h.). [*Htn.*]

Heaviness and drawing pain in the groin.

760. Twitching pain in the right groin, when sitting (aft. 18 d.).

Cutting pain in the groin, around the os pubis (aft. 21 d).

Straining in the groin, in the hernia, in the rectum and the back, with stitches in the chest.

Stitches in the groin, in the place of the hernia, as if the inguinal hernia was about to protrude.

Pain as of excoriation in the right inguinal region.

765. —Pain as from soreness, on both sides of the groin, as if a glandular swelling was forming, especially sensible when walking; on touching it, an elevation of the glands was sensible (aft. 10 h.). [*Lgh.*]

In the inguinal glands, straining, also when sitting (aft. 40 d.).

—Tearing in the inguinal glands, when sitting and walking (aft. 9 h.). [*Fr.*]

Sensation of swelling in the inguinal glands. [*Rl.*]

Slight glandular swellings in both groins.

770. Painful glandular swelling in the groin, the size of a horse-bean (aft. 20 d.).

—Swelling of the glands in the left groin (aft. 22 d.).

In the muscles of the abdomen, twitching, during the stool.

—Tearing in the muscles of the abdomen, increased by respiration. [*Wl.*]

—Pinching, almost cramp-like pain in the abdominal integuments of the right groin; in a small spot, only while speaking; also painful on being pressed with the finger (aft. 8 h.). [*Htn.*]

775. Tension in the muscles of the epigastrium, on leaning back, with painfulness on stroking the epigastrium with the hand, as if the skin was sore (aft. 10 d.).

Pricking as from needles, in the abdominal muscles, below the ribs, from within outward, especially on inspiring.

Much rumbling in the abdomen.

—Loud rumbling and grumbling in the abdomen, as if from emptiness. [*Lgh.*]

Grumbling in the abdomen on inspiration and on expiration.

780. Continual grumbling in the left epigastrium (aft. 4 d.).

Grumbling in the abdomen and then eructation.

Constant cooing in the belly.

Clucking in the left side of the abdomen, with restlessness in the abdomen, painless.

—Audible churning in the right side of the abdomen, as if diarrhœa was coming. [*Lgh.*]

785. —Frequent audible rumbling and crawling straining upwards in the right side of the abdomen, as from flatus, which also passed off. [*Fr.*]

Much fermenting in the abdomen.

Very frequently obstructed flatus, with rumbling in the abdomen (aft. 19 d.).

Obstructed flatus, with pain in the sacrum (aft. 19 d.).

Obstructed flatus, with much vertigo (aft. 6 d.).

790. The flatus passing off, is very fetid.

Constipation during the first days; she has no stool without an enema.

Constipation, aggravated from day to day.

Constipation. [*Rl.*]

—Constipation, lasting for two days (aft. 7 d.).

795. —The second day, he has no stool. [*Fr.*]

No stool, with constant tenesmus, and with this, gloominess in the head.

Fruitless urging to stool (8th d.). [*Rl.*]

Diminished stool (aft. 24 d.).

Costiveness (aft. 7, 18, 24 d.).

800. **Hard, undigested stool**, and not every day.

Hard, black stool (aft. 4 d.).

Hard stool, with mucus, burning during the discharge.

Stool of unusually large formation.

Frequent discharge of stools, at first hard, then pappy, then thin.

805. —Frequent stools, first firm, then pappy, then thin, painless; the following two days, costiveness. [*Lgh.*]

Painful tenesmus, day and night.

Continual urging to stool, which she can satisfy only by great efforts, while only little passes (aft. 24 h.).

Urging, as if diarrhœa was coming, and yet normal stool.

First thin, then lumpy stool, without colic. [*Htn.*]

810. Diarrhœic stool (1st, 3d, 5th d.).

Diarrhœa, the first eight days.

—A diarrhœa, which does not weaken, two, three, four times a day, for many days (aft. 2 d.).

Undigested stool, more thin (aft. 6 d.).

Undigested, hard, intermittent stool.

815. Stool, fetid, like rotten eggs.

A liquid, smelling like herring-pickle, drips from the anus.

Quite white stool.

White stools, with streaks of blood, with much ill-humor, and much pain in the liver, excited by breathing and touch.

Stool scanty, mixed with blood (aft. 26 d.).

820. Much loss of blood from the anus, with the evening stool.

Discharge of blood from the rectum. [*Rl.*]

The varices of the anus are swollen, pain when sitting, and also discharge blood.

The varices of the anus swell suddenly.

The varices of the rectum swell and protrude daily during the first days, but not on the following days.

825. Protrusion of a large varix of the rectum.

The swollen varices of the rectum protrude and make even the stools which are not hard, painful.

The varices of the rectum protrude and pain severely while walking, less during stool.

The rectum, with its varices, protrudes during the stool like a scroll.

Ascarides of the rectum. [*Rl.*]

830. Infestation from ascarides in the rectum.

An ascaris crawls out from the rectum, with itching and formication. [*Rl.*]

Ascarides, during stool.

Before the stool, nausea.

During stool, burning in the anus.

835. Pain in the rectum, as if torn open, even when the stool is not hard.

—At the passage of the stool, straining at the termination of the rectum, with grumbling and rumbling in the belly. [*Wl.*]

After tenesmus, there is still a continued pressure on the rectum and dyspnœa.

After the stool, anxious oppression of the chest.

After the forenoon-stool, severe stitches in the scrobiculus cordis, on pressure.

840. After the stool, sensation of tiredness.

After the stool, drawing cutting, in and about the anus.

After a healthy stool, drawing and cutting in the lower part of the rectum, with sensation of heat there.

After a profuse stool, burning in the rectum, in the morning.

After the stool, a burning itching in the anus.

845. In the lower part of the rectum, sensation of heaviness.

Grumbling in the rectum.

Pressure in the rectum, in the evening, while sitting (aft. 22 d.).

Violent pressure in the rectum (after several h.). —Pressure in the anus.

850. Pressure in the rectum, as if diarrhœa was coming.

Straining in the anus and painful urging in the rectum.

Straining, almost cutting, bearing-down pain in the rectum, soon after dinner.

Cramp in the rectum, the whole forenoon, a pinching together and stinging, with violent, anxious oppression, so that she could not sit still, but had to walk about (aft. 10 d.).

Twitching in the rectum.

855. Tensive, twitching pain in the rectum, unconnected with stools, in the evening.

Stitches toward the rectum (aft. 13 d.).

Lancinating pain, as from soreness, on the outside of the anus.

Transient pain, as from excoriation on the anus (aft. 16 d.).

Burning in the rectum.

860. **Burning in the anus, even during the noon nap.**

Burning and feeling of dryness on the anus.

Crawling in the anus.

Crawling in the rectum, as from ascarides.

—Severe itching on the anus.

865. Inflamed, burning painful, eruption like grapes, on the anus (aft. 19 d.).

Soreness on the anus and between the thighs.

—Soreness between the nates, when walking.

In the urinary passages, pain after the feet have slightly got wet.

Pain in the bladder, and cutting micturition during the night (aft. 11 d.).

870. **Stinging** in the female urethra.

Cutting stinging in the urethra, with tenesmus.

Urging to urinate, especially while walking.

The boy is urged to urinate, though the urine does not flow at once; then again he cannot restrain it, but allows some drops to pass.

Frequent urging to urinate, soon again after micturition, with little discharge.

875. —Frequent urging to urinate, with little, sometimes very little, emission of urine (aft. 26 h.). [*Lgh.*]

Urging to urinate, and he feels as if he could not restrain the urine.

Wetting the bed (aft. 3 d.).

Frequent nocturnal micturition.

Nocturnal micturition, with burning in the orifice of the urethra.

880. Micturition, frequent, through the whole night. [*Sr.*]

Frequent micturition (in a suckling whose mother had taken *Calcarea*). [*Sr.*]

Very frequent micturition (aft. 8 h.).

Frequent and copious micturition, in the forenoon and afternoon. [*Rl.*]

The whole day, she emits an unusual quantity of watery urine.

885. —Frequent urging to urinate, with passage of much urine. [*Lgh.*]

Sensation as if he could not finish urinating, and as if always some urine remained behind in the bladder.

In micturition, always something remains behind, and when he thinks he is done, it continues dripping. [*Rl.*]

Dripping of urine after micturition.

Very dark-colored urine, without sediment.

890. —The urine looks turbid, after standing, like clay-water. [*Wl.*]

Much passage of mucus with the urine, like leucorrhœa, but the mucus does not appear otherwise.

Frequent deposition of a white powder, like flour, in the urine (aft. 11 d.).

Fetid, dark-brown urine, with white sediment.

Very fetid urine (aft. 2 d.).

895. Fetid, smarting smell of the urine, which yet is very clear and pale (25th d.).

Sharp smell of the urine.

Much sourish-smelling urine at night.

During micturition, cutting in the urethra (the first days).

During micturition, burning in the urethra.

900. During micturition, burning and pain as from soreness in the urethra.

Before and after micturition, burning in the urethra.

After micturition, burning in the urethra and constant urging to urinate.

After micturition, pain as from soreness in the pudendum.

In the male organ, disagreeable twitching, in the morning and evening in bed.

905. In the glans, violent stitches (3d d.). [*Rl.*]

Cutting pain in the tip of the glans (4th d.).

Severe burning in the tip of the glans (aft. 10 d.).

Itching anteriorly in the glans, especially after micturition (aft. 28 d.)

—Tickling itching on the tip of the glans, compelling him to rub it (aft. 10 h.). [*Lgh.*]

910. —Tickling itching on the prepuce, compelling him to rub the part (aft. 9 h.). [*Lgh.*]

The prepuce is red and inflamed, with burning pain at micturition and when touched (4th d.).

In the right testicle, a pressive pain.

Pain as from pressure or contusion in the left testicle (aft. 12 d.).

Pain as from contusion in the testes.

915. —The left testicle is drawn up spasmodically to the abdomen, with painful pressure and pain in the left groin; it is also painful to the touch.

Cutting, excoriative pain in the testes, starting from the groin.

Stitches in the testes (formerly indurated), in periods of two minutes.

The scrotum hangs down relaxed.

Severe itching on the scrotum.

920. A sore spot on the scrotum.

In the spermatic cord, pain, as if it were contracted

Sexual instinct very much increased.

Very active sexual instinct (aft. 21 d.).

Strong excitement to coitus, especially when walking, in the forenoon (aft. 17 d.).

925. Violent sexual instinct, due only to wanton fancies, while the organ lacks stiffness, so that erection was only effected through application; scarcely had it entered, when the semen was emitted; this was followed by excessive prostration and great excitation of the nerves; he was discontented, irascible, and the knees seemed ready to give way for weakness (4th d.).

Erections in the morning after rising, with much inclination for coitus.

Pollutions much more frequent in the first days, then continually less so.

Pollutions are frequent in the first eleven days, in a man of forty-three years, who had not had any for eighteen years.

Pollution the first night, and then improved health.

930. —Frequent pollutions.

—Emission of semen, the first night. [*Fr.*]

—Two seminal emissions the following night, with voluptuous dreams. [*Htn.*]

—Two seminal emissions in one night, without any voluptuous dreams. [*Lgh.*]

Prostatic fluid flows out after micturition.

935. After the stool and the micturition, prostatic juice flows out.

During coitus, the emission of semen is very tardy (aft. 7 d.).

During coitus, the semen is not squirted out in the voluptuous moment, but only runs out, as it were, afterward.

During coitus, a normal emission of semen, but without any thrilling voluptuous sensation (aft. 5 d.).

During coitus, so violent a titillation on the tip of the glans, that he had to draw back the organ.

940. After coitus, stinging in the anus.

After coitus, on the following day, the head is greatly affected.

After coitus, for several days very much exhausted and affected.

After coitus, weakness and trembling of the legs, especially above and below the knees.

In the female pudenda, itching and stinging.

945. Itching of the internal and external labia.

—Itching on the pudenda.

Burning in the pudenda, two days before the menses (aft. 39 d.).

Burning pain, as of a sore in the genitals.

Burning smarting, with soreness in the female pudenda.

950. Inflammation, redness and swelling of the pudenda of a little

girl, with pus-like discharge, without pain during micturition.

Stitching burning nodule on the border of the labia (aft. 8 d.).

Moistness, like copious sweat in the fold between the pudenda and the thigh, with smarting.

Voluptuous sensation in the female genitals (in the afternoon, without cause), and effusion of fluid, followed by great exhaustion (aft. 7 d.).

Flow of blood, outside of the period of the menses (9 days before) for two days (aft. 12 d.).

955. —Flow of blood from the uterus of an old woman, who had not menstruated for years; in the last quarter of the moon (aft. 7 d.).

Flow of bloody water from the vagina, in an old woman, with pain in the sacrum, as if the menses were about to appear again.

The menses, which had long been suppressed, appear with the new moon (in a woman of 32) (aft. 6 d.).

The menses which had long ceased (in a woman of 52) reappeared with the new moon (aft. 6 d.).

The menses come the first time (aft. 14 d.) two days sooner, but the next time they only appear on the 32d day. (aft. 46 d.).

960. The menses are three days too soon (aft. 17 d.).

Menses four days sooner, lasting eight days.

The menses, always before regular, on taking *Calcarea*, appeared seven days too soon.

Two times in succession, the menses flowed profusely, and with a sort of labor-pains, they caused the expulsion of a small fœtus, as an abortion, with violent tenesmus and cutting and pressing in the abdomen.

The menses, which were usually too copious, were moderated (curative effect).

965. Before the menses, in the night, a very voluptuous dream.

The day before the menses, headache.

The day before the menses, she was strongly affected; a trifle served to terrify her.

The evening before the menses (after supper), a strong chill and then colic, continuing all night.

During the menses, vertigo, in stooping and raising the head up again.

970. **During the menses, rush of blood to the head and heat there.**

During the menses, pressive pain on the vertex of the head.

During the menses the eyes were closed by suppuration and they watered; her head was heavy and she could not well grasp her thoughts.

During the menses, sore throat; a pain as from soreness while swallowing, soreness in the fauces, on the uvula and behind it.

During the menses violent burning in the throat, with hoarseness.

975. During the menses, an attack of toothache.

During the menses, boring in a hollow tooth, which on stooping turns to throbbing (16th d.).

During the menses, nausea and tenesmus.

During the menses, drawing, pressive pains, with stitches in the abdomen, and in other parts of the body, now here, now there, with restlessness, even to fainting (aft. 10 d.).

During the menses, when the flow of blood ceased for a few hours, contractive, pinching colic.

980. During the menses, the urine passes involuntarily at every movement.

Immediately after the menses, toothache, drawing and stitches, day and night, worst when she bends the head to the right, the left, or backwards; it hinders her from sleeping and wakes her up (aft. 50 d.).

Leucorrhœa, like mucus (aft. 5, 16 d.).

Leucorrhœa, like milk (the first 3 d.).

Milky leucorrhœa, which flows most during micturition.

985. —The leucorrhœa, already present, is increased.

*   *   *   *   *   *   *   *

Frequent sneezing. without a cold.

Repeated sneezing, daily.

Much sneezing in the morning.

—Without a cold, frequent sneezing. [*Lgh.*]

990. Dryness of the nose (aft. 22 d.).

Dry nose, at night; moist during the day.

Stopped nose (aft. 18 d.).

Total stoppage of the nose, in the morning, on rising.

Stoppage of the nose and a cold.

995. *Dry coryza* (1st d. and aft 12 d.).

Dry coryza, with much sneezing (the first 7 days).

Attacks of dry coryza, with sneezing, for several weeks.

—Dry coryza, with frequent sneezing (aft. 72 h.). [*Lgh.*]

Severe, dry coryza, with headache (aft. 32 d.).

1000. A cold; heaviness in all the limbs.

Violent cold, for eight days (aft. 36 d.).

Violent coryza, with pains in the hypogastrium. [*Sr.*]

Severe fluent coryza (almost at once and aft. 4 d.).

The fluent coryza flows more strongly.

1005. An excessive fluent coryza, with previous sneezing, often abortive. [*Rl.*]

—Fluent coryza, with much sneezing (aft. 27 h.).

Fluent coryza, lasting three days, with ulceration of the left nostril (aft. 9 d.).

—Coryza, with painful sensitiveness of the nose and internal heat in the head (aft. 72 h.). [*Wl.*]

Severe coryza, with heat in the head and cough (aft. 13 d.).

1010. **Violent cold, with headache** and tightness of the chest (aft. 10, 16 d.).

—Fluent coryza, with headache (at once relieved by camphor) (aft. 5 d.).

Severe coryza, going off after two days, and turning into violent colic, lasting several days (aft. 17 d.).

Fluent coryza, with great lassitude.

A severe coryza, and at the same time a flow of blood from the anus.

1015. Copious flow of mucus from the nose, while it is obstructed (aft. 14 d.).

The throat is rough, especially in the morning.

Roughness of the larynx, with pain on deglutition.

Painless hoarseness, so that she cannot talk, especially in the morning (aft. 11 d.).

—Hoarse, rough throat, for three days (aft. 24 h.).

1020. —Tickling in the windpipe, inciting to tussiculation. [*Lgh.*]

Whooping, hoarse cough, which, as far as can be heard, strikes against no phlegm.

Mucus in the larynx, detached by clearing the throat.

Mucus on the chest, without cough (aft. several h.).

Sibilus in the windpipe, in the evening, after lying down.

1025. —Loud rattling in the windpipe on expiring, as from mucus on the chest (aft. 37 h.). [*Lgh.*]

Cough, with cold.

Tickling cough, as from feathery dust in the throat.

Cough, excited by a sensation as if there was a plug in the throat, moving up and down.

Excitation to cough, on inspiring.

1030. Cough, excited by eating.

Cough, always excited by playing on the piano.

In the evening, especially in bed, dry tussiculation (aft. 2 d.).

Nocturnal cough (aft. 6 d.).

Constant nocturnal cough, with hoarseness (aft. 39 d.).

1035. At night, on awaking, severe cough for two minutes.

At night, in bed, after the first awaking (about 10 P. M.) a continuous, violent, scraping cough (7th d.).

At night, after midnight, **dry cough**, so that heart and arteries throbbed.

Nocturnal cough, without awaking.

Cough, mostly in sleep; with it, at first, dry, then fluent coryza.

1040. Constant short hacking cough, in single paroxysms.

Convulsive cough, in the evening.

Dry cough, especially at night.

Cough, with expectoration in the day, but no expectoration at night.

Cough with expectoration, all the day.

1045. Cough, with much viscid expectoration, without taste and smell, in the morning and evening, in bed.

Much cough, with expectoration of mucus, in the evening, after lying down, and at night; during the day but little, and then dry cough.

Mucous cough, from time to time.

Mucous expectoration, in the morning, with tussiculation.

Cough, with much expectoration of thick mucus, at night.

1050. Expectoration of mucus, sweet of taste, through coughing.

Cough, in the morning, with yellow expectoration (aft. 5 d.).

—The cough becomes loose, and whole pieces are ejected, like pure pus. [*Gr.*]

Expectoration of blood by coughing and hawking, with sensation of rawness and soreness in the chest.

Expectoration of blood by a hacking cough (short tussiculation), with vertigo and unsteadiness in the thighs, in quick motions.

1055. After he had choked in the morning, during breakfast, he had to cough violently, when he threw out blood several times, with subsequent stitches in the palate.

In coughing, a darting, several times through his head, like a tearing pain.

In coughing, there are stitches in the head.

With every fit of coughing, there is a painful concussion of the head, as if it would burst.

During a violent coughing fit, in the evening, there is a rising, and he throws up a sweet substance.

1060. Very violent cough, at first dry, then with frequent salty sputa, with pain as if something was being torn off in the throat.

In coughing, pain in the chest, as if it was raw, in the evening and night.

Arrest of breathing, while walking in the wind; and also in the room, tightness of the chest, which increases as soon as she walks a few steps.

Want of breath in lying down, then sibilant breathing.

Frequent necessity of deep breathing.

1065. He has to breathe deeply, and then there are stitches, now in the right side, now in the left of the chest and lower ribs.

Violent urging to take a deep breath, with expansion and contraction of the abdomen and pain in the belly and chest (aft. 3 d.).

Desire to hold the breath.

Difficult, loud breathing through the nose, when walking.

Difficult breathing (aft. 7 d.).

1070. —Difficult breathing, facilitated by bending the shoulders backwards.

Shortness of breath, worse in sitting, than in motion.

Shortening of the breath at the least ascent. [*Rl.*]

Short, almost hiccuping breath, in sleep, after previous weeping.

Tightness of the chest; she lacks breath.

1075. **Tightness of the chest, as if it were too full, and filled with blood.**

Tight feeling of fullness in the chest, early on rising, as if the lungs could not sufficiently expand for breathing; going off after some expectoration.

—Tight, anxious sensation the whole day, as if there was not enough room in the chest for breathing, with stoppage of the nose (aft. 13 d.).

Dyspnœa in the chest, with stitches in it.

Tightness of the chest, soon after rising in the morning; he could not go two steps without having to sit down (aft. 24 d.).

1080. Asthma, in the forenoon, when taking a walk in the open air (aft. 48 h.).

—Severe **anxious asthma and difficult breathing, like tension in the lower part of the chest; it took his breath away while moving and sitting, for an hour; almost to suffocation** (aft. 30 h.). [*Lgh.*]

Tightness and tension on the chest.

Hot breath with heat in the mouth, yet without thirst.

The whole chest is painfully sensitive to the touch and during respiration. [*Wl.*]

1085. Pressure in the chest, especially below the right nipple.

Pressure on the chest in front, also when not respiring.

Pressure in the right side of the chest, as it were by thrusts, after exercise for an hour.

Pain as if pressed upon, in **the sternum.**

Cramp in the left intercostal **muscles;** he has quickly to bend to the side, to be relieved.

1090. Cutting in the chest, when taking breath (aft. several h.).

—Pains cutting from within outward in the last ribs, increased by inspiring. [*Wl.*]

Stitches in the chest, toward the neck, for several hours.

Stitches in the left side of the chest, especially in the evening (aft. 11 d.).

Stitches through the chest from the left to the right side, with feeling of contraction of the chest; he breathed hard, and as he breathed, the stitches became more violent (aft. 4 d.).

1095. **Stitches in the left part of the chest**, almost every time she takes breath, and mostly passing off by rubbing (aft. several h.).

Stitches in the left side of the chest, on inspiring and during bodily motion.

Stitches deep in the right side of the chest, in the evening, especially while taking breath.

Stitches and drawing in the left side of the chest, up into the left submaxillary gland.

Twitching stitches in the chest, mostly on the left side.

1100. —Itching stitches on the chest, most severe while expiring, going off on rubbing (aft. 48 h.). [*Wl.*]

—Sharp stitches in the right side of the chest, from within outward, without regard to respiration (aft. 7 h.). [*Wl.*]

—Sharp stitches in the left side, under the axilla, outward from the chest, most severe while inspiring (aft. 2 h.). [*Wl.*]

—Broad stitch in the thoracic muscles upward, with every heart-beat. [*Wl.*]

—Dull thrusts from the posterior walls of the thoracic cavity up to between the scapulæ, in the rhythm of the heart-beat, with great oppressive anguish (aft. 8 h.). [*Wl.*]

1105. Gnawing pain on the left side of the chest, as if external, upon the ribs and the sternum, but little aggravated by inspiration (aft. 1 h.). [*Wl.*]

Pain as of soreness in the chest, especially during inspiration.

Pain as from rawness in the chest, after much **speaking** and **walking, also in coughing.**

Weakness in the chest, **after some loud speaking.**

Anxious oppression in the chest (the first days).

1110. —Anxious oppression in the chest, as if it was too narrow, with short breath, especially in sitting, and pressure on the chest, especially during an inspiration; the heart beats anxiously and tremulously. [*Wl.*]

In the heart, anxiety (aft. 2 d.).

Palpitation of the heart.

Severe palpitation.

Excessive palpitation, with unequal pulsation.

1115. Severe palpitatation, with an anxious fear that he has an organic disease of the heart.

Severe palpitation, with excessive anguish and restlessness, tightness of the chest and pain in the back; with every breath she utters a loud sound, as if there was a lack of air, with coldness of the body and cold sweat. [*Gr.*]

Painful pressure in the region of the heart.

Spasmodic contraction in the region of the heart, taking the breath away, with subsequent violent thrusts (aft. 16 d.).

Stitches in the heart, which arrest the breath and leave a pressive pain in the heart.

1120. —Lancinating, drawing pain in the region of the heart (aft. 9½ h.). [*Fr.*]

External itching on the chest (aft. 10 d.).

Pimples below the chest, with excoriation on rubbing them.

The female breasts are painful, as if festered, especially when touched.

Pain as of soreness in the right nipple, at the lightest touch.

1125. Swelling and inflammation of the left nipple, with fine stitches in it (aft. 4th d.).

Swelling and external heat of the right breast.

Swelling in the glands of the right breast, with pain on touching it.

The milk in the breasts of a nursing woman dries up (aft. 48 h.).

Pain in the sacrum (aft. 6, 8 d.).

1130. Intolerable pains in the sacrum.

Severe pains in the sacrum, so that she can neither sit nor lie down.

Pain in the sacrum, so that he could hardly rise again after sitting down.

Pain in the sacrum, at once in the morning after rising.

Pain in the sacrum, as from a strain in lifting.

1135. Pain in the sacrum, from heavy lifting.

Constant straining in the sacrum toward the rectum.

Drawing in the sacrum (aft. 4 h.).

Drawing pain in the sacrum, while sitting

Spasmodic twitching pain from the sacrum towards the anus.

1140. —Twitching stitches in the sacrum, and at the same time on the leg above the ankle (aft. 2 h.). [*Wl.*]

—In a spot above the sacrum, stitches on being touched

Eruptive pimples on the sacrum and the nates.

In the region of the kidneys and the loins, aching on taking a drive.

Pressive pain in the renal region.

1145. The spine pains on bending backward.

Pain as from being bruised, in the back and chest.

Pain as from a sprain, in both sides of the back.

As from a strain in lifting, the spine pains in the renal region on stretching. [*Rl.*]

Painful stiffness in the spine, with laziness and heaviness of the legs, in the morning on awaking and after rising (aft. 17 d.).

1150. Pressive pain in the middle of the back and below the scapulæ (aft. 27 d.).

Pressive pain in the spine, between the scapulæ, with short breath, aggravated in respiring, with pain in the spinal vertebræ on being touched.

Pressure between the scapulæ on motion, **obstructing the respiration.**

Pressure under the right scapula upward.

Stitches in the back.

1155. Single, violent stitches in the upper part of the back in respiring.

—Violent pricks, as from needles, in the middle of the spine, almost causing him to cry out, on taking a walk in the open air, somewhat relieved by standing. [*Lgh.*]

—Severe stitches from the thoracic cavity through the spine, out between the scapulæ. [*Wl.*]

Stitches in the left scapula in the cardiac region (2d d.)

Itching stitches in the right scapula.

1160. —Sharp stitches within the shoulder-blade. [*Wl.*]

Pinching contraction between the scapulæ (aft. 30 d.).

Drawing pain between the scapulæ.

Twitching in both scapulæ and in the chest.

Tearing between the scapulæ (aft. 3 h.).

1165. Cutting pain between the scapulæ, when resting (aft. 6 d.).

Painless jerks in the right side of the back, in respiring, with a chill and a cold shiver (aft. 7 d.).

Coldness and feeling of numbness on the side of the back, on which he lay during his siesta.

Itching, and itching pimples on the back.

Pustules on the back.

1170. The neck feels stiff.

Stiffness of the nape of the neck and of the neck.

Sensation of stiffness in the side of the nape. [*Rl.*]

On bending, the nape of the neck is as it were rigid.

Tension in the neck, so that she cannot turn her head.

1175. Stitches in the nape of the neck and the scapulæ, with gloominess of the head.

Itching, stitching, burning in the nape and between the scapulæ, with heartburn (aft. 5 d.).

Swelling and painfulness of the lowest cervical vertebræ, in the nape.

Painless glandular swelling of the size of a hazelnut in the neck, where the hair begins (aft. 5 d.).

On the neck, on turning or twisting the head, pain as if a hernia or a tumor would protrude.

1180. Sudden pain in the neck, as from a sprain, on turning and twisting the head.

Swelling of a left gland on the neck, as large as a pigeon egg, with stitching sore throat on deglutition.

Swelling of the neck on the left side, with painfulness on touching, and on turning the head, with sore throat.

The cervical glands are painful.

Hard swelling of the cervical glands (aft. 13 d.).

1185. The shoulder-joint is painful, in the evening and night.

—Pain in the top of both the shoulders.

Pain in both shoulders and in the elbow-joint, as after great fatigue.

Pressure on the shoulder (aft. 24 h.).

Pressive pain in the right shoulder-joint, only when resting, not in lifting and moving the arms.

1190. Tearing in the left shoulder-joint and elbow-joint (aft. 14 d.).

Stitches in the left shoulder-joint, the whole day (aft. 4 d.).

—Severe stitches in both axillæ (aft. 4 d.). [*Wl.*]

The arms are painful, as if bruised, on moving them, and on grasping with them.

Cramp in the whole of the one arm or the other, for a quarter of an hour (aft. 5 d.).

1195. Twitching pain in the right arm, in the evening (13th d.).

Drawing, tearing in the right arm, from the shoulder to the hand (aft. 3 h.).

Tearing in the right arm, from above downward.

Burning, paralytic pain in the whole right arm, from the finger-joints to the shoulder (aft. 6 d.).

Restlessness and anxious distress in the joints of the arms and wrists.

1200. Going to sleep of the arm on which he is lying, with pains.

Weakness and a sort of paralysis of the left arm; he finds it difficult to move it or to lift it; of itself it always tends to fall down again.

Burning, itching on the left arm, from morning till evening.

The upper arm is painful, just below the shoulder-joint, so that he cannot lift it high, nor bring it to his back.

Pain in the middle of the upper arm, as if the flesh was drawn tight to the bones.

1205. —Spasmodic pain (with tearing) in the muscles of the upper arm (on taking a walk in the open air). [*Lgh.*]

Drawing pain in the left upper arm, while sitting (and sewing).

—Fine twitching in the left upper arm. [*Wl.*]

Tearing pain in the middle of the upper arm, in a small spot.

—Tearing, twitching in the upper arm (aft. 7 h.). [*Wl.*]

1210. —A tearing stitch in the muscles of the left upper arm, when sitting. [*Lgh.*]

In the fore-arm, a painful pressure in the muscles, while walking, passing off at once on touching it, or on standing and sitting (aft ¼ h.). [*Lgh.*]

—Tearing pressure in the muscles of the left fore-arm, both in rest and in motion (aft. 3 h.). [*Lgh.*]

Drawing pain in the left fore-arm.

Drawing pain in the fore-arm, from the bend of the elbow to the wrist, chiefly in rest.

1215. **Spasmodic tearing pain** on the outer side **of the fore-arm,** from the elbow to the wrist, as soon as he seizes anything with the hand.

—Cramp-like tearing in the muscles of the left fore-arm (aft. 40 h.). [*Lgh.*]

—**Cramp-like pains in the fore-arm,** before the elbow-joint (aft. 1 h.). [*Wl.*]

—Cramp-like pains in the outer side of the fore-arm, near the wrist (aft. 1, 13, 29th). [*Lgh.*]

—Fine tearing and boring stitches in the muscles of the left fore-arm. [*Lgh.*]

1220. Swelling of the fore-arm and the back of the hand, with tension on moving it.

The hands pain in the morning and are quite relaxed.

Severe pain in the knuckles of the hand, as if excoriated with caustic.

Like a sprain in the right wrist-joint.

Pain as from a sprain in the right wrist-joint, or as if something was wrenched or strained.

1225. Pain in the right wrist-joint, as if strained, with stitching and tearing therein, on motion. [*Rl.*]

—Pain as of a sprain, close above the wrist-joint, more severe when at rest than in motion. [*Lgh.*]

Cramp in the hands, at night, until rising in the morning.

Cramp in the left hand.

Twitching thrusts in the wrist-joint.

1230. Drawing pain in the wrist-joint and the metacarpus.

Drawing pain in the hand.

Jerking drawing in the wrists and from there up the arms, even in the morning in bed.

Tearing pain in the palm of the hand.

Stinging in the palm, in the morning in bed, for two minutes.

1235. —Sharp stitches in the outer protuberance of the wrist. [*Wl.*]

Trembling in the hands for several hours, in the afternoon (2d d.).

Sweat in the palms, even in slightly moving the body.

The veins in the hands are distended, with burning sensation on the back of the hands.

—Crawling and stitches on the wrist. [*Wl.*]

1240. —Itching, stinging tickling in the right palm, inciting to scratching. [*Lgh.*]

—Itching tickling on the border of the left hand, inciting to scratching. [*Lgh.*]

A furuncle on the back of the left hand, with lancinating pain when touched.

The fingers, when stretched out, seem as if strained and clinched, as if they were glued together.

Cramp-like contraction of the fingers.

1245. Cramp in the fingers, without their being clinched.

Cramp-like pain in the posterior joint of the index. [*Lgh.*]

Cramp-like pain between the third and fourth fingers of the right hand. [*Htn.*]

Twitching pain in the fingers.

Involuntary twitching of the left thumb.

1250. Tearing in the finger-joints (aft. 28 d.).

Transient tearing pains in the finger-tips.

Numbness[1] of the fingers.

Numbness[1] of the three middle fingers; they become white, cold and insensible; preceded by a slight drawing therein (aft. 3 h.). [*Stf.*]

Pain of the finger-joints as if they were swollen, on awaking from the (evening) sleep, without visible swelling.

1255. Burning itching on the fingers of the left hand (aft. 13 d.).

—Tickling itching on the index, inciting to scratching. [*Lgh.*]

Large, painful furuncle on the posterior joint of the ring finger (twice on two different doses. [*Sr.*]

Around the nail of the middle finger, suppuration.

Incipient paronychia on the right index (aft. 6 d.).

1260. Several agnails.

—On the border of the iliac bone, pinching. [*Wl.*]

In the nates, pain as if festered, when touched; less in sitting than in walking (aft. 48 h.).

Drawing, cramp-like pains on the right side of the nates, toward the anus.

Painful muscular twitching in both the nates, in sitting and standing.

1265. Burning itching on one of the nates.

In the hip-joint, tension, with drawing pain in the hip-bone, during the evening's walk.

—Drawing pain as of a sprain in the hip-joint, when walking. [*Fr.*]

—Pinching twitching on the posterior side of the hip-joint, worse in rest than in motion. [*Wl.*]

Stitches over the right side of the hip.

1270. Stitches in the hip-joint, on stooping.

Stitches in the hip-joint up from the patella, when treading in starting on a walk.

—Cutting in the acetabulum of the hip-joint, when sitting (aft. 3 h.). [*Wl.*]

—Tearing in the hip-joint and around the anterior crest of the ilium, extending into the groin, in motion. [*Fr.*]

---

[1] Literally, "dying off."—*Transl.*

Pain as of inside festering in both hip-joints, on walking in the room.

1275. Sensation of numbness on the right hip and the thigh, with a sensation as if these parts were brittle, and as if too short and small.

In the lower limbs and around the pelvis, muscular twitchings.

Drawing pain in the muscles of the lower limbs, on the back of the thigh and in the calves, in the evening (aft. 36 h.).

—Drawing in the lower limbs, extending into the tips of the toes.

Tearing in both lower limbs, from the hip down into the ankle (aft. 14 d.).

1280. A lancinating jerk into the right lower limb, so that it suddenly darted up (aft. 30 d.).

Restlessness in the lower extremities, with much eructation.

Heaviness of the lower extremities (aft. 8 d.).

Painful weariness of the lower extremities, especially of the thighs, as after a fatiguing walk (aft. 17, 19 d.).

Fatigue and bruised feeling in the lower limbs, especially in the joints (aft. 20 d.).

1285. Pain as from a bruise in the shaft bones of the lower limbs.

—Pain as from a bruise in the lower extremities, especially in the legs, when lying down. [*Fr.*]

Going to sleep of the lower extremities in the evening, when sitting.

Sensation of numbness in the left lower limb (aft. 7 d.).

On the right thigh, in a small spot, painful twitching.

1290. Cutting pain in the upper part of the left thigh, as from straining a muscle, especially on motion.

—Tearing pain on the inner side of the thigh on moving it. [*Fr.*]

Stitches in the thigh, in the knee and in the heel, only at night.

—Pressive stitches on the inner side of the left thigh, when sitting (aft. 3 h.). [*Htn.*]

—Cramp-like stitching in the muscles of the right thigh, in standing and walking, going off in sitting. [*Lgh.*]

1295. —Sharp stitch on the outer side of the thigh, above the left knee (aft. 3 h.). [*Wl.*]

—Tearing stitches on the inner side of the thigh, above the knee, in sitting (aft. 12 h.). [*Fr.*]

Weariness and, as it were, rigidity in the anterior muscles of the thigh, in the morning, on starting to walk.

Pain as from a bruise in the muscles of the right thigh, when retiring after walking.

—Pain as from a bruise in the muscles of the thighs, when walking.

1300. **Itching on the thighs** (aft. 12 d.).

Violent itching on the lower part of the thigh, at night.

Stinging itching in a small spot of the left thigh (aft. 20 d.).

Fine stinging itching on the thighs.

Burning itching on the left thigh, from morning till evening.

1305. Eruptive pimples on the thighs (aft. 11 d.).

In the knee, a sensation as if she could not sufficiently stretch the limb (aft. 16 d.).

Pain in the patella, when rising from sitting (4th d.). [*Rl.*)

—Pain of the knees, in turning, twisting and in touching them.

—Pain in the left knee-joint, even when at rest.

1310. Pain as from a sprain in the right knee (aft. 14 d.).

—Pain as from a sprain in the left patella, when sitting, going off on walking and standing (aft 12 h.). [*Lgh.*]

Tension below the knee on cowering (crouching) down.

Pressive pain in the knees.

Dull pressive pain in the patella.

1315. Drawing pain about the knee, just above the hough.

—Drawing, cramp-like pain on the patella (aft. 2 d.). [*Fr.*]

Tearing and tension on the inner side of the knee, on rising from sitting.

Transient tearing pain in the knees.

Lancinating and throbbing pain in the left knee, in the morning, more when sitting than when walking; he had to limp.

1320. —Sharp stitches in the right knee-joint (aft. 4 h.). [*Wl.*]

Stitches in the left knee for one-half hour (5th d.).

Pain as from a bruise in the knee (10th d.).

—Pain as of a bruise, close below the patella, on taking a walk in the open air (aft. 13 h.). [*Lgh.*]

Sensation of numbness in the knees, in the afternoon siesta, going off on awaking.

1325. Perspiration of the knees.

Swelling of the knees.

—Below the patella, an inflamed swelling.

The leg pains in the calf in walking and in treading, on touching and on bending the foot.

Pain as from a strain in the anterior muscles of the tibia, when walking (aft. 21 d.).

1330. Tension in the calf.

Straining in the leg, from the foot to the knee, as if the leg was asleep (during a pressive cramp in the stomach).

Cramp in the right leg, for an hour, while the foot was bent inward and doubled up (aft. 4 d.).

Cramp in the muscles of the tibia, at night.

—Cramp-like pains, close beside the shaft of the tibia, when sitting. [*Lgh.*]

1335. **Violent cramp in the calf, at night.**

Cramp in the calves and houghs, on stretching the leg (in putting on the boot), it is relieved on bending the leg, but returns on stretching it.

Cramp in the calf and the foot, when moving it briskly, with lancinating pain.

Dull pressive pain in the muscles beside the tibia, in walking.

—Pressive pain on the left tibia, near the ankle, on taking a walk in the open air (aft. 52 h.). [*Lgh.*]

1340. —Intermittent pressive pain in the calf. [*Fr.*]
Drawing and crushing pain in the tibia.
Tearing drawing in the calf.
—Tearing twitching anteriorly in the leg, below the knee, when at rest. [*Wl.*]
Twitching upward of the leg.
1345. Cutting above the tibia.
Stinging and weakness in the calf.
—Pain as of a bruise of the legs, as if overfatigued; he has to keep changing his seat. [*Wl.*]
A stinging crawling on the legs.
Much itching on the legs and feet.
1350. **—Itching below both the calves.**
Burning itching on the right tibia. [*Rl.*]
Erysipelatous inflammation and swelling of the leg, with chill of the body.
Large, dark-red itching tetter on the legs, with some swelling on it.
Red streaks on the tibia, consisting of miliary granules, with severe itching, and burning after rubbing (aft. 7 d.).
1355. Several ulcers on the legs (aft. 7 d.).
In the ankle-joint, pain as if it was broken, in walking, especially in the afternoon.
Pain in the right ankle, when treading, as if the foot was about to be sprained.
Pain as of a sprain in the left foot (aft. 13 d.).
Pain, as if the foot was too tightly bandaged, above the left ankle.
1360. Tension in both the ankles on the inner side.
Cramp in the sole of the left foot.
—Cramp in the soles, after some walking, relieved by walking a little longer, and vanishing when sitting.
—Cramp in the soles and toes, at night, and in the daytime when pulling on the boots (aft. 11 d.).
—Cramp-like pain in the sole of the left foot (aft. 5 h.). [*Htn.*]
1365. Severe tearing in the soles of the feet.
Severe cutting on the outer side of the sole of the right foot, in the evening and the whole night (aft. 10 h.).
Painful sensitiveness of the soles of the feet, even in the room, as if softened by hot water, with great painfulness when walking.
Pain as from internal festering in the soles of the feet.
Burning in the soles of the feet.
1370. Burning of the feet, in the evening.
Sudden, quite hot sensation on the dorsum of the left foot and on the leg, as if a very hot breath was being blown on it.
Sweating of the feet.
Sweating of the feet, toward evening.
Inflammatory swelling on the dorsum of the left foot, with burning pain and severe itching around it.
1375. Swelling of the feet, for eleven days.
—Swelling of the outer side of the ankle on the left foot.

Itching around the ankles and below the calves (aft. 13 d.).

Itching in the ankle of the diseased foot.

Violent burning itching on the ankle of the right foot, from morning till evening (aft. 15 d.).

1380. Blisters come on the left heel, in walking, which turn into a sort of large blood-boil, with stinging and itching pain (aft. 8 h.).

The toes ache, as from the pressure of boots. [*Rl.*]

Violent pain on the tip of the right big toe (aft. 21 d.).

Cramp in the toes.

Visible twitching in the left big toe, in the evening, in bed.

1385. Tearing in the toes.

Tearing in the big toe. [*Rl.*]

Transient tearing pains in the toes.

Stitches in the big toe.

—Violent stitch in the left little toe, as if it was outside of it (aft. 14 h.). [*Htn.*]

1390. —Sharp stitch in the posterior joint of the big toe, when resting (aft. 24 h.). [*Wl.*]

—Intermittent, cramp-like needle-pricks in the toes of the right foot, in sitting and standing, but disappearing in walking (aft. ½ h.). [*Lgh.*]

Violent burning in the tip of the big toe (aft. 21 d.).

Under the nails of the big toe, a burning pressure.

In the corns, a burning pain as from a sore.

1395. All over the body, a sensation of painful tension.

Quivering of the muscles.

Painless twitching of single limbs, in daytime.

Single, involuntary movements and jerks in the right thigh, in the left shoulder and the left arm.

Drawing pressure in the joints. [*Rl.*]

1400. Painless drawing in the limbs, in the afternoon.

Tearing in the limbs.

Tearing in the arms and legs, but always only in a small spot.

Burning in the palms and the soles of the feet.

Stitches in the upper arms, under the arms, in the back and in the lower limbs.

1405. The hands and feet go to sleep.

The parts on which he was sitting, during his afternoon siesta, went to sleep.

Paralytic pain as from a bruise of the bony shafts and of the joints of the lower limbs, as also of the sacrum, while moving; also while sitting and standing, the sacrum pains as if bruised, and the muscles of the legs are painful to the touch.

He is apt to get strained; heavy lifting gives him at once pain in the sacrum.

The pains are very violent, but pass by quickly.

1410. His chronic ailment is worse and better every other day.

After working and washing in water, the ailments are aggravated and renewed.

Orgasms of blood.

Twice in succession, warm rushes of blood from the scrobiculus cordis, extending to the head.

Very much heated, in the morning, after rising.

1415. Rush of blood to the head and chest, after painful stiffness in the spine.

Rush of blood to the head, with discharge of blood at the anus, for several days in succession.

He feels the need of walking much.

Restlessness, so that she had to move the hands and feet.

Great restlessness, in the evening, especially in the legs; he cannot let them lie still.

1420. Restless motion in the whole body, owing to incomplete eructation.

Trembling in the morning.

Anxious trembling, with lassitude.

Continual trembling of the body, which became worse, when he came into the open air.

Great clumsiness of the body.

1425. Sensation of illness in the whole body; she has to spit much, and shuns the open air (aft. 22 d.).

Great desire to be mesmerized.

Uneasiness in the evening, as before an attack of chills and fever.

Much affected; the hands and feet often cold, paleness of the face and frequent palpitation; all of which was removed by bodily exercise.

Attack of the nature of a general breaking down, with numb feeling in the head, vertigo, pain of the sacrum, and chill over the whole body, for six hours (aft. 22 d.).

1430. So much frightened at a little prick on her finger from a needle, that she feels sick; her tongue, lips, and hands, quite white and cold, with coldness of the forehead and of the face, with obscuration of the vision, restlessness, rush of heat and trembling; she had to lie down (mesmerizing helped her quickly) (aft. 18 d.).

While it became black before his eyes, he was suddenly overcome in the evening (from 7 to 9 o'clock) for four times by a sweet sleep, with nausea, continuing even after lying down, but without vomiting.

Fainting fit, in the evening, while things become black before her eyes, while sitting down.

Fainting fit, with coldness and indistinct vision (aft. 3 d.).

Fainting fit, with large drops of sweat on the face.

1435. Worn-out feeling and lassitude in the limbs, especially in the knees.

Very weak.

Weakness in the thighs and groins, in walking.

He soon becomes very tired, during bodily exertion.

After walking, he is wearied even to fever, and is seized by chilliness and thirst after it.

1440. In taking a walk, great asthenia, especially in the lower extremities, with languid sweat.

She could not go up stairs, and was quite exhausted from it (aft. 14 d.).

She becomes weak from talking; she has to cease.

Weakness in daytime, so that she hardly knew how to endure the oppressed, anxious state; only the breathing of the fresh open air improved and strenghtened her (aft. 12 d.).

She lay for ten days entirely worn out and languid, so that she could neither move nor occupy herself; with the most violent spasms of laughter.

1445. Fit of epilepsy; while occupied in manual labor, he suddenly fell over to the ground to one side unconscious, and found himself, on returning to consciousness, lying down with outstretched arms; then followed heat and some perspiration (aft. 9 d.).

Great sensitiveness to cold air; the feet are, as it were, dead in the evening.

At a slight sensation of cold air, goose-skin on the thighs and legs, even so that it was painful.

The damp open air does not agree with her; her skin is immediately affected by it.

Great tendency to catch cold.

1450. Symptoms of a cold; stiffness of the nape of the neck and of the cervical muscles, stinging in the neck and head, above the eyes, and cough (soon).

Every time she walks out in the open air, she becomes sad and has to weep.

On taking a walk in the open air, pressive headache in the crown, lasting till going to sleep.

On taking a walk, visible inflation of the abdomen.

During a walk, palpitation and pain in the chest (aft. 19 d.).

1455. While walking out, a sensation of drawing through the whole body, extending to the head, compelling her to sit down (aft. 30 d.).

After taking a walk in the open air, a boring pain, externally in the left side of the forehead.

After a walk, feels unwell, hoarse, with tightness of chest.

The whole skin of the body is very painful to the touch, chiefly in the feet.

Itching all over the body (aft. 23 d.).

1460. Violent itching of the parts perspiring, especially between the scapulæ.

Violent itching, in the evening in bed, on the back, in the scrobiculus cordis, in the neck, the chin, the left eye, the hairy scalp, the mons veneris and the scrotum.

Itching in the mouth, in the nose, and around the anus.

Itching on a dry, hot skin, as if it was covered with salt and ashes.

Burning in the skin, with itching over half the back, on the nates, and the posterior side of the thighs (aft. 10 d.).

1465. Stinging in the skin, as from needles.

Urticaria, which always goes off in cool air.

Itching eruption of vesicles over the whole body, especially over the hips.

Eruption of red, raised spots, of the size of a lentil and larger, mostly on the cheeks and elbows, with great heat, much thirst and little appetite; on the third day they disappeared, leaving behind dark spots, as if suffused with blood (with a suckling whose mother had taken *Calcarea*). [*Sr.*]

Scurfy spots on the legs, with burning in daytime (aft. 24 d.).

1470. The herpes quickly reappear.

The former herpes under the two axillæ in the bend of the left elbow and in the hough reappear after twenty days.

—In the place of a herpes, disappeared years before, there appears again an itching (aft. 5 d.).

An old sore on the leg now pains, throbbing, with tearing around it, and begins to smell like rotten eggs (aft. 7 d.).

The skin is unhealthy, readily ulcerating, even slight lesions pass into suppuration and will not heal again.

1475. **Many** very small **warts appear here and there.**

Excrescences like warts (behind the ears) inflamed, and became ulcers.

A wart in the bend of the elbow became inflamed, pains like a furuncle, then dried up and disappeared.

Unusual lassitude, relieved by walking.

Great general lassitude, in the evening, for half an hour.

1480. Weariness with yawning (aft. 4 d.).

Frequent yawning.

Long continued, almost interminable yawning, and then a shaking throbbing in the head, abdomen and chest, with severe heat in the face.

Constant yawning, with drowsiness (aft. 4d.).

—Constant yawning, as if he had not finished sleeping (aft. 56 h.). [*Lgh.*]

1485. **Inclination to stretch in the morning.**

Drowsiness, in the morning.

Still sleepy and tired in the morning when he should rise, he can hardly rouse himself.

Not easily roused, in the morning on awaking.

—Great sleepiness in the morning, with peevishness, and pressive headache about the whole of the forehead (aft, 2 d.). [*Fr.*]

1490. **Drowsiness during the day and weariness**; he went to sleep several times in the forenoon (aft. 9 d.).

At noon, a very long sleep.

The whole day, very tired and sleepy (aft. 11 d.).

During the day ,sleepy and fatigued, with chill and headache.

—Very drowsy, weary in daytime; but he cannot get to sleep.

1495. In the evening, sleepy very early (aft. 3 h.).

In the evening, drowsy weariness in all the limbs with chill; he cannot keep off sleep, but yet he did not sleep soundly, but kept waking up, for sixteen hours; in the morning much sweat, and dryness in the throat, without thirst (aft. 4 d.).

—In the evening great sleepiness and peevishness. [*Fr.*]

Often very late in getting to sleep, in the evening.

He cannot get to sleep before 2 or 3 A. M.

1500. She cannot get to sleep at night, and when asleep, she yet wakes up soon again.

She cannot get to sleep, if she goes to bed late; she is as i were taken from her rest.

He cannot get to sleep in the evening for a long time; he feels too hot, though he is only lightly covered, in a cold room (aft. 11 d.).

—He could hardly get to sleep all night, tossed about, and perspired all over his body (aft. 10 h.). [*Lgh.*]

He tossed about in bed all night.

1505. On account of his vivacity of mind, he cannot get to sleep before midnight.

Difficulty in getting to sleep, for involuntary abundance of thoughts.

He cannot get to sleep in the evening for a long time, nor rid himself of his thoughts, which are in part wanton, in part vexatious; they even follow him still in the morning on awaking.

Restless wakefulness, in the evening in bed, full of horrible fantastic visions (6th night).

—Before going to sleep in the evening, anxious thoughts, which passed and came again; he also supposed the objects around to be different from what they were, feared the dark and endeavored to look into the light; all of this ceased on the passage of flatus.

1510. On going to sleep, fantastic delusion, as if she heard a rumbling and rattling above her bed, which caused her to shudder.

As soon as she closes her eyes at night, fantastic visions appear before her imagination.

On closing her eyes, horrible faces appear to her.

On lying down in the evening, as soon as she has laid down her head, dull toothache for an hour, then sleep.

Before going to sleep, in the evening in bed, palpitation and oppressive anxiety.

1515. On going to sleep in the evening, a starting up of the whole of the upper part of the body, with jerks, extending even to the head; then humming and hissing in the ear.

At night, very anxious and fantastic, she is frightened in her dream and is anxious about it with trembling, even after she wakes up (aft. 20 d.).

At night, anguish, as if she was or was becoming insane; then for some minutes a febrile rigor, and then a sensation in the body as if she was annihilated, beaten to pieces.

Horrible things appear to her at night, which she cannot ward off.

At night, soon after going to sleep, he raises himself in bed, unconsciously, but, with open eyes, occupying himself with his hands.

1520. At night, much orgasm of blood, and many dreams.

At night, orgasm in the blood, with uneasy sleep, chiefly during the menses.

At night, with uneasy sleep, palpitation of the heart.

At night, internal heat, especially in the feet and hands, **and in the morning dry tongue,** without thirst, with external **heat** of the head (6th, 7th d.).

At night, violent vertigo, with flitting before her eyes, continuing till noon.

1525. In the night, stupefaction of the head, at which he wakes up; these become continually more severe, almost to fainting, then trembling of the limbs and continual lassitude, so that he cannot go to sleep again.

Every night, on awaking, itching of the head.

At night, a tearing pain in the gums, and on biting the teeth together, sensation as of looseness of the teeth.

At night, boring drawing pain in most of the molars.

Nocturnal toothache, more like pressure or a rush of blood to the teeth, beginning immediately on lying down (the first three nights).

1530. At night, when lying down, severe eructation; she had to rise up to be relieved.

At night, on awaking, eructation.

At night, cramp of the stomach, from which he awakes.

At night, much colic, without diarrhœa (aft. 12 d.).

For many nights, much accumulation of flatus in the abdomen (aft. 5 d.).

1535. At night, at the beginning of sleep, the shoulder-joint becomes stiff; he has to lay his arms over his head.

At night, a twitching or lancinating pain in the arm and wrist, hindering him from sleeping.

At night, lassitude in the knees.

At night, burning in the soles of the feet.

At night, drawing pain in the feet, from which he awakes.

1540. In sleep, she laid her arms above her head.

Snoring groans, the whole night, in a slumber without remembrance and from which he cannot be awaked, with constant tossing; before going to sleep, copious sweat in the face.

In sleep, he often chews, and then swallows.

At the noon siesta, palpitation while sitting up, at which he awakes.

Talking, in a sleep full of dreams (aft. 10 d.).

1545. Talking in sleep, in a giddy confusion, with uneasiness from dreams and heat.

Crying out at night, in an uneasy sleep.

Uneasy sleep, with sweat.

Uneasy sleep toward morning (aft. 15 d.).

Uneasiness of body does not allow her to lie long in one place.

1550. Uneasy half-sleep, at night, with dry heat, confusion in the head, as in fever, and constant awaking.

—Uneasy sleep, with talking in sleep and frequent awaking. [*Htn.*]

Frequent awaking from sleep.

—While tossing about, he often awakes from sleep; he thinks, he got turned around in his bed. [*Lgh.*]

—Frequent awaking from sleep, as from disturbance. [*Lgh.*]

1555. —Frequent awaking from sleep, as if he had done sleeping. [*Lgh.*]

Short sleep, she cannot sleep after 12 o'clock, but tosses about restlessly.

Sleeps only from 11 P. M. to 2 or 3 A. M.; then she cannot sleep any more, but remains wide awake.

Anxious awaking after midnight, with heavy breathing (aft. 12 d.).

Anxious awaking during the night, frequently from anxious dreams (aft. 36 h.).

1560. Screaming and starting up, from anxious dreams.

Starting up frightened, in the evening, soon after going to sleep, till she becomes wide awake.

The child raises itself up in its bed after midnight, crying: Father! it commences to cry and wishes to jump up; the more it is talked to, the worse is its screaming and opposition; it rolls on the floor and does not wish to be touched.

On waking up, in the morning, confused in the head.

On awaking in the morning, numb feeling in the head, with quivering throughout the body and rush of blood to the head.

1565. On awaking in the morning, after an uneasy sleep, orgasm in the blood, several mornings (during the first days).

On awaking in the morning from an uneasy sleep, he feels the blood coursing in all the blood-vessels, which are also distended, with sensation of bruisedness all over the body.

On awaking in the morning, he is unrefreshed.

On awaking from a deep sleep in the morning, very much exhausted, so that the slumberous state continued even after rising from bed.

Sleep at night, full of dreams.

1570. Vivid dreams, every night.

—Vivid, confused dreams, which he does not remember. [*Lgh.*]

—Vivid dreams, full of contentions and quarrels. [*Lgh.*]

—Many vivid dreams of former occurrences, with long, deep sleep in the morning. [*Wl.*]

Confused, anxious dreams.

1575. Half-wakeful dreams, in the evening, soon after going to sleep, with great anxiety.

Anxious and frightful dreams, of which he cannot rid himself after awaking.

Anxious dreams, that he was bitten by a dog, on which he wakes up, then he goes to sleep again and wakes up again over an equally anxious dream, and thus several times every night.

Several anxious dreams in one night, seven nights in succession.

Anxious dream of fire and murder, toward morning.

1580. **Frightful dreams the whole night**, and at last a voluptuous dream, with a (very rare) pollution (aft. 10 d.).

Frightful dream, as of falling down or being cast down.

—Horrible, fearful dreams. [*Lgh.*]

Dreams of dead persons and of cadaverous smells.

—Dreams of sick men and corpses, with violent weeping, while sleeping (a woman who else never dreams). [*Stf.*]

1585. Quick pulse, without sensation of fever.

Great internal chilliness; she has to wrap up her cold hands, but her feet are warm.

Great constant chilliness, with much thirst.

She is cold, when she leaves her bed.

Very chilly, in the evening.

1590. Internal chill, with restlessness and trembling anguish.

—Frequent chilliness, with yellow complexion.

Chill in the evening, for several hours (aft. 10 h. and 13 d.).

For two evenings, chill of a quarter of an hour, without subsequent heat or sweat.

Chill, in the evening, in bed.

1595. Chill, in the evening, in bed, so that he, although covered with feather-beds, could yet not get warm, as if from a lack of vital heat (aft. 30 d.).

Febrile rigor, at night.

Febrile rigor, first over the face, with horripilation, then passing over the whole body, with sensation of chill. [*Rl.*]

—Febrile rigor over the whole back (aft. 24 h.). [*Lgh.*]

—Febrile rigor over the whole body, as if he had taken a cold, with frequent yawning. [*Lgh.*]

1600. —Febrile rigor over the whole body, with warmth or heat of the forehead and face, with cold hands (aft. 3 and 48 h.). [*Lgh.*]

Feeling of heat in the interior of the body.

Often a flying heat.

A flying heat, some two or three times a day, all over, but especially in the face and the hands; it overcomes her in sitting, as if from anguish, with perspiration of the face and hands for ten to fifteen minutes at a time.

Heat for several evenings, from six to seven o'clock.

1605. —In the evening, on lying down, external heat, with internal chill.

At night, dry heat (aft. 12 h.).

Toward morning, dry heat (aft. 6 d.).

Heat in the chest and the head, with cold on the rest of the body, the whole day (aft. 24 d.).

—Glowing heat and redness of the face, with hot forehead, cold hands and severe thirst, for several hours. [*Lgh.*]

1610. Almost constant heat, which first makes weak and anxious, till sweat breaks out.

Sweat often breaks out during the day.

Almost constant sweat.

Much sweat, as well in daytime, while walking, as also at night, in bed.

—Exhaustive sweat, day and night, for three days.

1615. Copious sweat, during the day, in cold air.

Sweat during the day, at the least movement.

In the evening, in bed, he feels warm at once, and sweats the whole night.

Night-sweat, chiefly before midnight, with cold legs.

Night-sweat in the back.

1620. Night-sweat only on the lower limbs, clammy to the touch (aft. several d.).

Violent morning-sweat, many mornings in succession.

Morning-sweat (the next morning after taking the medicine).

Morning-sweat, three mornings in succession.

—**Morning-sweat, every morning** (aft. 7 d.).

1625. Fever: now chill, then heat; she has to lie down.

Fever, in the forenoon; **chills and heat alternate.**

Fever heat and burning thirst, alternating with chills.

Evening fever: externally chills, with internal heat and violent thirst; he was cold also in bed, and he sweated at the same time, and yet he could not get warm; at last a copious sweat (aft. 10 h.).

In the forenoon, at first headache, which continually increased, with sudden sinking of the strength, so that he could hardly get home, with great heat in the forehead and the hands, with much thirst for acidulous water; then, after lying down, ice-cold hands, with quick pulse (aft. 21 d).

1630. Every forenoon at 11 o'clock, feverish heat, without previous thirst or chill, for an hour; she felt hot and was hot to the touch, with face somewhat red; then anxiety and slight perspiration, especially in the hands and feet and in the face; four days in succession (before the appearance of the menses).

Fever from the morning till noon or afternoon; first tearing in the joints and heaviness of the head, then lassitude, scarcely allowing her to raise herself up in bed, with heaviness of the limbs, stretching and extending the limbs, heat and sensation as if she was going to perspire always, with trembling and unrest in all her limbs.

CARBO ANIMALIS, ANIMAL CHARCOAL.

[To prepare the animal charcoal, lay a thick piece of ox-leather between the red-hot coals and allow it to burn, until the last little flame disappears and then quickly place the glowing piece between two flat stones, so that it may be suddenly extinguished, as else it would continue to glimmer in the open air, destroying the coal for the most part.]

However much similarity there may be found in the effects of animal charcoal and of vegetable charcoal on the state of human health, there are, nevertheless, so many variations in the effects of animal charcoal from those found in vegetable charcoal, and so many particular symptoms, that I have thought it useful to add here what I have been able to observe.

The animal charcoal is prepared like the other antipsoric remedies up to the decillionth, potentized attenuation, and one or two small pellets, moistened with it, are given as a dose in the various degrees of potency. Camphor has proved itself an antidote and a means of relieving its too violent action with persons who were too sensitive.

In treating diseases to which this medicine is appropriate the following symptoms have been relieved or cured:

Timidity; morning-vertigo; pressure in the whole of the brain; pressure on the head after a meal; eruptions on the head; roaring in the ears; discharge from the ears; erysipelas in the face; stinging in the cheek-bones, the lower jaw and the teeth; drawing pain in the gums; bleeding of the gums; *suppurating blisters* on the gums; dryness of the palate and of the tongue; *bitter taste in the mouth;* incomplete eructations, with pain; sour eructation; hiccup after a meal; faintish qualmishness; nocturnal nausea; weakness of digestion in the stomach, where almost everything partaken of causes trouble; pressure in the stomach, as from a load; clutching and *griping* in the stomach; pressure and cutting in the hepatic region; rumbling in the abdomen; obstruction of the flatus; frequent stools every day; stinging in the anus; fetor of the urine; *leucorrhœa*; burning, smarting leucorrhœa; stoppage of the nose; dry coryza; painful induration of a gland in the chest; burning in the back; induration of a cervical gland, with lancinating pain; herpes under the axilla; gouty stiffness of the finger-joints; pain in the hip, causing halting; drawing and stitches in the legs; sensitiveness to the open air; tendency to strains; chilblains; sweat when walking in the open air; fatiguing sweats, especially on the thighs; morning sweat.

The symptoms marked *Ad.* were observed by *Dr. Adams*, in Russia; those marked *Whl.* by the Practitioner *Wahle;* those with *Htb. und Tr.* by *Drs. Hartlaub* and *Trinks*, in their *Reine Arzneimittellehre.*

CARBO ANIMALIS.

Extremely melancholy mood, with a sensation of being deserted.

He feels, in the morning, as if he was deserted, and full of homesickness.

Homesickness.

Great disposition to sadness.

5. Pusillanimous and sad; everything seems to her so lonely and sad, that she would like to weep (3d d.). [*Htb. u. Tr.*]

Inclination to solitude, sad and introverted, she always only

---

A pathogenesis of this substance, probably (as with its vegetable congener), made with the 3d trituration, first saw the light in Vol. VI of the second edition of the *Materia Medica Pura* (1827). It contained 191 symptoms contributed by *Hahnemann* himself and a *Dr. Adams.* It reappeared in Vol. III of the *Chronic Diseases.* The symptoms of *Hartlaub* and *Trinks* (254 in number), in the third volume of their *Arzneimittellehre*, have no name attached, but are probably *Henning's.* From these printed sources, from his own later observations on patients and from 23 symptoms (probably of the same kind), supplied by *Wahle*, Hahnemann has compiled the present list.—*Hughes.*

wishes to be alone, and she shuns every conversation (the first 4 d., and after 8 d.). [*Htb. u. Tr.*]

Morose thoughts and ill-humor, not to be driven away, concerning things present and past, even to weeping.

Disposition to weep.

He can not weep enough.

10. Melancholy and anxious, in the morning, on awaking.

Very anxious and dejected, especially in the evening and night; she cannot for internal anguish sleep quietly; she feels best in the morning.

For anguish, he has to rock backward and forward in his chair.

Restlessness and hurry.

Shy and timid.

15. Timid and fearful, all day.

He feels horror in the evening, even to shivering and weeping.

Thoughts of death.

Hopelessness.

Despairing mood, day and night.

20. Peevish, she talks only with repugnance (1st d.). [*Htb. u. Tr.*]

Peevish, at once in the morning on awaking (the first days).

Greatly disposed to vexation.

Taking things ill. [*Ad.*]

Angry and malicious. [*Whl.*]

25. Self-willed; no one can do anything to please him. [*Whl.*]

Unsympathizing, in the beginning; later, increased excitability for passionate impressions.

At times inclined to weep, at times absurdly merry.

Extremely merry. [*Ad.*]

Involuntary loud whistling.

30. Weakness of memory; he forgets the word in his mouth. [*Htb. u. Tr.*.]

He cannot write a letter, nor express his thoughts.

The objects on the street seem to him changed, *e. g.*, farther apart and brighter than usual, as in an empty, abandoned city.

Gloominess in the head, in the morning, and everything she looks at vexes her. [*Htb. u. Tr.*]

Dizzy in the head, and as if she had not done sleeping, in the morning. [*Htb. u. Tr.*]

35. In the morning, he is quite confused in his head, knows not whether he has been asleep or awake.

Stupefied, in the morning, and as if in a confused dream.

Great stupefaction, while sitting at the table, and flightiness of the head, with anxious fear that he might fall down unconscious at any moment.

Sudden stupefaction, several times he heard and saw nothing, and had no thoughts.

Sudden stupefaction, in moving the head and in walking.

40. Dizzy, as from beating the head to and fro.

Vertigo while sitting, as if she would fall backward over her chair, with silliness. [*Htb. u. Tr.*]

Vertigo, in walking, with mist before the eyes; she felt impelled to walk fast and toward the right. [*Htb. u. Tr.*]

Vertigo, while things turn black before the eyes.

With sensation of vertigo in the head, as if some sickness was coming on him, a mist comes over his eyes suddenly like a watery gauze, repeated twice.

45. Vertigo, with nausea, on raising up the head after stooping.

Vertigo about 7 P. M.; when she raised up her head, everything turned around with her. She had always to sit bent forward, and in rising, she staggered to and fro; she felt, as it were, gloomy in the head, and as if objects moved about; when lying in bed, she did not feel anything all night, only in the morning again, on rising.

In the head, a sensation as of something weighing down in the forehead, or like a board before it; a sensation as when stepping from great cold at once before a hot stove in a room, in the morning.

Headache on awaking, as after intoxication from wine.

Heaviness of the head. [*Ad.*]

50. **Heaviness of the head, in the morning**, with dimness of vision and watery eyes. [*Htb. u. Tr.*]

Heaviness in the head at night, with weariness of the feet, which she could hardly lift (aft. 2 d.). [*Htb. u. Tr.*]

Heaviness in the forehead, on stooping, with a sensation as if the brain would fall forward; on raising her head, vertigo, so that she soon fell down. [*Htb. u. Tr.*]

Painful feeling of heaviness in the whole occiput. [*Htb. u. Tr.*]

Heaviness of the head, especially **of the occiput** and of the left temple, with a numb feeling.

55. Pain in the upper part of the head, where the spot is also sensitive externally; on stooping, the pain passes into the forehead. [*Htb. u. Tr.*]

Headache, which presses down the eyebrows.

Stupefying headache in the forehead, while spinning, going off after dinner. [*Htb. u. Tr.*]

Pressure and feeling of numbness in the whole head, after dinner till evening. [*Htb. u. Tr.*]

Pressure and feeling of heaviness in the occiput, whence the pain draws forward into the crown; better in the open air (during the menses). [*Htb. u. Tr.*]

60. Pressure in the left side of the occiput, both when at rest and in motion, frequently intermitting. [*Htb. u. Tr.*]

Pressive headache in the occiput. [*Ad.*]

Pressive pain in a small spot of the occiput.

Pressive headache in the nape of the neck, while writing.

Dull pressure in both parietal bones near the vertex, in a small spot, daily, unintermittent for several hours, mostly in the forenoon, especially excited by the exhalation from unclean clothes and much relieved in the open air.

65. Pressive headache in both temples.

Tension in the head, almost daily.

Pinching pain in the lower part of the temple. [*Ad.*]

Pain in the vertex, as if the skull there was burst or torn apart, so that she had to hold her head with her hand, for fear of its falling apart; also at night, and especially in wet weather. [*Htb. u. Tr.*]

Jerking, tearing, darting to and fro in the left side of the occiput, in the evening. [*Htb. u. Tr.*]

70. **Tearing on the right side of the head.**

Frequent tearing on the right side of the head, in the day-time.

Severe tearing in the external parts of the head.

Tearing and beating in the whole head, in the orbits, the ear, the left side of the face, the cheek bones and in the lower jaw; starting immediately after dinner, relieved by pressing on it with the hand, and quickly ceasing when the cheek swelled up (aft. 28 h.).

Painful tearing and stitches on the right side of the occiput, both when at rest and in motion, in the evening. [*Htb. u. Tr.*]

75. Pain as from a bruise over and in the root of the nose, *per se* and when touched. [*Htb. u. Tr.*]

Boring pain in the temporal bone, extending into the zygoma. [*Ad.*]

Boring drawing pains on the head and tearing pains there; when the head becomes cool, it is worse, especially toward the ear (aft. 7 d.).

Shooting pains in the head, especially in the temples.

Sharp stitches in the vertex, in the evening (2d d.). [*Htb. u. Tr.*]

80. Stitches in the temple, with contractive pain or straining. [*Htb. u. Tr.*]

Pecking headache on the left side of the forehead, in the morning on rising, better in the open air. [*Htb. u. Tr.*]

Stitches and **beating in the occiput.** [*Htb. u. Tr.*]

Intolerable throbbing and lancinating pain in the vertex, as if the head would burst, when walking.

Rush of blood to the head, with numb feeling of the same.

85. Sensation of heat and heaviness in the forehead, which yet externally is cold to the touch, in the afternoon. [*Htb. u. Tr.*]

Heat in the head, with anxiety, in the evening in bed; she had to get up and then felt better. [*Htb. u. Tr.*]

Sensation of painful looseness of the brain, on motion. [*Htb. u. Tr.*]

Splashing in the left half of the brain, when walking fast.

The external head is painful on the left side, as if festered underneath.

90. Pain in the head and neck at night; as if both had gone to sleep and were sprained.

Everything he had on his head, weighed him down, and even his neckcloth oppressed him (aft. 18 d.).

Involuntary anxious upward drawing and tension of the skin on the forehead and vertex.

Drawing in the forehead, above the eyebrows.

Sensation in the forehead, as if something were lying above the eyes, so that she could not look up.

95. Violent itching on the hairy scalp, so that she would like to scratch till it bled, but this does not make it go away. [*Htb. u. Tr.*]

Hard tumor on the forehead.

Falling out of the hair (aft. 18 d.).

The eyes pain pressively, in the evening at candle-light.

Pressure in the inner canthus (aft. 72 h.).

100. From above downward, pressive, lancinating pain over the left eye, in the eyelid and in the upper half of the eyeball. [*Ad.*]

Stitches in the eyes.

Stitches, burning and lachrymation of the eyes, after itching and rubbing of the same. [*Htb. u. Tr.*]

Stinging and smarting in the left inner canthus, in the morning after rising, improved by rubbing. [*Htb. u. Tr.*]

Itching in the upper eyelid, going off by scratching. [*Htb. u. Tr.*]

105. Smarting itching in the eyes, with burning after rubbing. [*Htb. u. Tr.*]

Itching and pressing in the eyes, in the day-time.

Excoriative burning in the outer canthus.

Weakness in the eyes.

In the evening, great weakness in the eyes; she could not occupy herself with anything for which vision is necessary.

110 Quivering in the upper eyelid.

Quivering in the right eye, with a sensation as if a body, moving within it blinds her, with a drawing down of the upper eyelid; it goes off after rubbing, but returns once more, leaving behind it a sensitiveness of the upper border of the orbit, when touched. [*Htb. u. Tr.*]

Disagreeable sensation in the left eye, as if something had flown in, that hindered his sight; he has always to wipe it; at the same time the pupil is extremely dilated, with great far-sightedness, that he could not clearly recognize anything held near.

The left eye is glued together, all the forenoon. [*Htb. u. Tr.*]

Lachrymation of the eye, in the morning on rising. [*Htb. u. Tr.*]

115. Dimness before the eyes, as if she saw through a mist. [*Htb. u. Tr.*]

The eyes seem to lie quite loosely in the sockets and he has not the strength to see clearly, despite all his efforts; this makes him uneasy.

Continually misty vision all day.

Nets seem to float before the eyes.

Many small black and yellow points are seen by candle-light, in regular rows before his eyes.

120. Light hurts his eyes, in the evening.

Cramp in the ears, extending down to the fauces, on the left side, impeding deglutition. [*Ad.*]

Cramp-like pain in the interior of the left ear. [*Ad.*]

Drawing in the ear.

Drawing in the outer ear and in the left cheek-bone.

125. Tearing in the lobule of the right ear and boring in the ear. [*Htb. u. Tr.*]

Transient tearing pain in the left ear. [*Htb. u. Tr*]

Stitches in the ears. [*Htb. u. Tr.*]

Burning, like fire, in the lobule of the right ear. [*Htb. u. Tr.*]

A sort of periosteal swelling behind the right ear, which stings, from 7 P. M. onward every evening.

130. The gland by the right ear is swollen (2d d.).

Swelling of the parotid glands. [*Rust's Magaz. f. d. Heilk.*, Vol. XXII, *H.* 1, p. 198.[1]]

The hearing is weak and dull.

Weak, confused hearing; the sounds are confounded; he knew not from which side they came, and it seemed to him, as if they came from another world.

Tingling in the ears, the whole night.

135. Tingling in the right ear, on taking a walk in the open air. [*Htb. u. Tr.*]

Whistling in the ears, when blowing the nose.

In the side of the nose, fine tearing. [*Htb. u. Tr.*]

Itching of the tip of the nose, not to be stopped by scratching. [*Htb. u. Tr.*]

The tip of the nose is red, and painful when touched.

140. Red, chapped, burning and tensively painful tip of the nose (during the menses). [*Htb. u. Tr.*]

Redness and swelling of the nose, it feels sore on the inside.

Swelling of the nose and mouth.

Swelling of the nose, with pimples within and without, which form scabs of long duration.

Dryness and peeling off of the skin on the tip of the nose. [*Htb. u. Tr.*]

145. Vesicles on the right nostril. [*Htb. u. Tr.*]

Furuncle, with tension in the nostril. [*Htb. u. Tr.*]

Blood flows frequently from the nose, when blowing it.

Bleeding of the nose, in the morning while sitting, and in the afternoon.

Bleeding of the nose in the morning, several mornings, with preceding vertigo.

150. Bleeding of the nose, whole cupfuls of bright-red blood. [*Whl.*]

Bleeding of the nose, after pressure and dullness of the head [*Whl.*]

The skin of the face pains, especially on the cheeks, around the mouth and chin (after shaving). [*Ad.*]

Tearing, oft repeated, now in the upper, now in the lower jaw, on the right side of the face. [*Htb. u. Tr.*]

---

[1] Statement as to the effect of crude substance on healthy persons.—*Hughes.*

Transient tearing pains in the left zygoma, toward the temple. [*Htb. u. Tr.*]

155. Heat in the face and head, in the afternoon.

Often a transient heat in the cheeks, with redness.

Frequently, a rising heat with redness and burning of the cheeks, in the evening. [*Htb. u. Tr.*]

Eruption of small pustules on the left cheek and forehead. [*Htb. u. Tr.*]

Eruption on the cheeks, like red spots.

160. Yellowness of the face.

Copper-colored eruption in the face. [RUST'S *Magaz.* l. c.]

Pimples in the face in abundance, without sensation.

The mouth is swollen.

Ulceration of the one corner of the mouth, with burning pain.

165. Swelling of both lips, with burning of the same. [*Htb. u. Tr.*]

Dryness of the lips, as from too great heat, in the morning. [*Htb. u. Tr.*]

The lips are cracked.

Bleeding of the lips.

Blisters on the lips.

170. On the chin, a little red nodule with yellow point. [*Htb. u. Tr.*]

The nerves of the teeth are sensitive, when the crown of the teeth is touched.

Drawing in the teeth, with flying heat in the face.

Constant drawing in the left molars, especially in the afternoon.

Drawing in a left lower molar, at night, as often as she awakes. [*Htb. u. Tr.*]

175. A drawing forward and backward in the teeth, also in the front teeth.

Suddenly, while eating bread, drawing and lancinating pains in the nerves of the molars.

Tearing toothache, chiefly in hollow teeth, also at night, disturbing the sleep. [*Htb. u. Tr.*]

Painful griping in the teeth of the left side, increased in the open air. [*Htb. u. Tr.*]

Muttering pain in the teeth, worse when touching them, and in the evening. [*Htb. u Tr.*]

180. Pecking toothache, on drinking something cold, and then waggling of the teeth.

The hollow tooth is sensitive, and as if it was prominent ; it pains on biting, and more yet in the evening in bed, with much saliva in the mouth.

The upper and the lower teeth are too long and waggle.

The teeth of the right upper row are as if too long and loose, without any pain, for several days. [*Htb. u. Tr.*]

Great looseness of the teeth, so that she cannot chew the softest food without pain.

185. Looseness of the teeth and tearing therein, most violent in the evening, in bed.

Looseness of the lower teeth, with pains in their gums.

The gums are pale, and pain as if ulcerated. [*Htb. u. Tr.*]

The gums are red and swollen and very painful.

Blisters in the mouth, causing burning.

190. She frequently bites the inside of her cheek in her mouth, wounding it. [*Htb. u. Tr.*]

Burning on the tip of the tongue, as if it was sore. [*Htb. u. Tr.*]

Burning on the tip of the tongue, and roughness in the mouth. [*Htb. u. Tr.*]

Little blisters on the edges of the tongue. [*Htb. u. Tr.*]

Vesicles on the tongue, which pain as if burned.

195. Mouth and tongue feel as if immovable, with troublesome, slow and very low speech (aft. several h.).

Sore throat, with pains as from an ulcer, on deglutition.

Pain in the throat, when swallowing, as if there was a blister there. [*Htb. u. Tr.*]

Scraping in the throat, with ptyalism.

Scraping stinging in the throat.

200. Sensation of rawness in the whole fauces and the œsophagus, extending to the scrobiculus cordis, not aggravated by swallowing.

Pain as from soreness and burning, like heartburn, in the throat, extending down into the stomach, worse toward evening, at night and in the morning; better after rising and after eating and drinking. [*Htb. u. Tr.*]

Roughness in the throat, nearly every morning, going off after breakfast. [*Htb. u. Tr.*]

Burning sensation in the throat.

Pressure in the throat, only while swallowing.

205. Pressure in the fauces, extending into the stomach.

Pressure in the throat, and dryness of the tongue.

A rising in the œsophagus into the throat, where there was a choking and pressing sensation with sensation of roughness. [*Htb. u. Tr.*]

Dryness in the throat and mouth, without thirst, almost the whole day (2d and 3d d.). [*Htb. u. Tr.*]

Mucus in the mouth, in the morning; going off after rising. [*Htb. u. Tr.*]

210. Sensation of mucus in the throat, early on awaking, compels her to prolonged hawking; it goes off at noon. [*Htb. u. Tr.*]

Much phlegm in throat and frequent sneezing and hawking (aft. 24 h.).

Foaming saliva.

Bad smell from the mouth.

Ill-smelling breath, without his perceiving it himself.

215. Taste of manure in the mouth, in the morning.

Bitter taste every morning.

Bitterness in the mouth at times, also in the morning.

Bitter taste in the mouth, in the morning, going off after rising. [*Htb. u. Tr.*]

Bitterish putrid taste in the mouth.

220. Bitter, sour taste in the mouth.

Sour taste in the mouth.

Slimy sour taste in the mouth, in the morning after awaking. [*Htb. u. Tr.*]

Offensive taste in the mouth, in the morning. [*Htb. u. Tr.*]

Thirst, at once in the morning, quite unusual (6th d.). [*Htb. u. Tr.*]

225. Great thirst, especially for cold water, with dryness and heat in the throat.

Little desire for eating, but the appetite comes while eating.

The appetite quickly passes off when eating.

No appetite, everything tastes to her alike. [*Whl.*]

There is hunger, but no relish for the food.

230. Repugnance to cold drinks.

Repugnance to fat.

Fat meat altogether spoils his appetite.

Appetite for raw sour-krout, while otherwise without appetite.

Desire for sour and refreshing things.

235. Increased appetite (1st, 2d, and 9th d.). [*Htb. u. Tr.*]

Intense hunger in the morning.

Ravenous hunger.

After an abundant dinner, in two hours there is again a good appetite and in the evening again hunger, and later on, thirst.

From smoking tobacco, nausea and repugnance to it.

240. **After eating meat, long qualmishness,** with nausea and much empty eructation.

At the beginning of a meal, an internal chill.

During eating, sudden weariness of the chest and the organs of mastication.

At dinner, much heat and sweat in the face.

During eating, perspiration.

245. He gets tired from eating.

After eating, anxiety on the chest.

After little eating, with good appetite, soon fullness of the stomach.

After eating, pressure in the stomach

After a moderate dinner, violent distension of the abdomen. [*Htb. u. Tr.*]

250. Immediately after eating, boring in the right side of the abdomen.

After eating, asthma.

Soon after eating, anguish and restlessness in the back, without pain.

After breakfast, palpitation, and also after other meals.

All the ailments of the forenoon go off through eating dinner (2d d.). [*Htb. u. Tr.*]

255. Frequent eructation. [*Ad.*]

Much eructation from the stomach.

Frequent, empty eructation, changing to belching up.

Empty eructation after every meal. [*Htb. u. Tr.*]

Eructation, with the taste of the food eaten long before.

260 Putrid, fishy eructation.

Almost continual putrid eructation. [*Htb. u. Tr.*]

Hiccuping eructation at dinner. [*Htb. u. Tr.*]

Sourish taste in the fauces, but not in the mouth.

Rising heartburn from the stomach.

265. Scratching heartburn.

Qualmishness (in the abdomen) toward evening, with rising heat (aft. 10 d.).

Nausea, after much walking, when he gets to sit down.

Sick and nauseous at the stomach, in the morning on arising, with heat, anxiety and rising of sourish water in the mouth, with general lassitude. [*Htb. u. Tr.*]

Tendency to waterbrash, with nausea in the stomach, at night. [*Htb. u. Tr.*]

270. Attack of waterbrash, with flow of salty water from the stomach through the mouth, with retching and a spasmodic sensation in the jaws, then violent, empty eructation with cold feet, and then hiccup for half an hour.

Pressure in the stomach, also before breakfast.

Severe pressure in the stomach, in the evening, after lying down in bed; she had, in order to relieve herself, to press with her hand on the region of the stomach (aft. 16 h.).

Pressure in the stomach, with heaviness and fullness, with tendency to waterbrash. [*Htb. u. Tr.*]

Sudden transient pressive pain in the scrobiculus cordis, when taking a deep breath.

275. Contracting cramp in the stomach.

Sensation as from a bruise in the scrobiculus cordis, as after a violent cough (aft. 6 d.).

Frequent stitches in the stomach. [*Htb. u. Tr.*]

Sharp stitches on the right side, near the scrobiculus cordis, also during inspiration, and better while walking. [*Htb. u. Tr.*]

Tearing stitch from the scrobiculus cordis into the chest, on raising the head after stooping. [*Htb. u. Tr.*]

280. Boring pain in the stomach, almost as if from fasting, extending into the abdomen. [*Htb. u. Tr.*]

Clucking, as from bubbles, in the stomach. [*Ad.*]

Audible rumbling in the stomach, in the morning on awaking. [*Ad.*]

In the liver, pressure, even while lying down.

Severe pressive pain in the liver, almost like cutting; this region is also painful externally to the touch, as if sore.

285. Under the left ribs, pressive stitches.

Pressive pain in the left side of the abdomen.

Pain in the region of the kidneys, when walking. [*Htb. u. Tr.*]

Repeated lancinating pecking in the renal region. [*Htb. u. Tr.*]

Feeling of heaviness in the abdomen, as from a lump, also fasting, for several days.

290. **Severe inflation of the abdomen.**

The belly is always much inflated.

Inflations here and there in the belly, like hernias. [*Fr. u. Hbg.*]

Painful tension in the abdomen, with pain to the touch under the ribs, as if there was an ulcer and as if the places festered underneath.

Pain in the abdomen, as if festered inside.

295. Sensation as if constricted in the abdomen, while fasting, with sensation of great emptiness, but without hunger and appetite.

Pinching constriction, deep in the hypogastrium.

Griping and restleness in the abdomen.

Griping in the umbilical region.

Pinching in the belly, about the navel, with a sensation as if a stool was coming. [*Htb. u. Tr.*]

300. Pinching in the right side of the epigastrium, with stitches, while sitting. [*Htb. u. Tr.*]

A lancinating pinching in the epigastrium, every morning, chiefly in bed.

Lancinating pinching above the navel and in the scrobiculus cordis, every morning in bed, as if flatus had accumulated; passage of flatus, evacuations and micturition relieve it, but it also goes off of itself, and even in walking, it is but little perceptible.

Partly cutting, partly stitching in the abdomen, very painful all day, and returning frequently during the day.

Colic in the forenoon.

305. Brief cutting, deep in the hypogastrium. [*Htb. u. Tr.*]

Violent cutting in the belly, with frequent urging to stool and even tenesmus, while only flatus passes; from morn till noon. [*Htb. u. Tr.*]

Digging and writhing in the epigastrium.

Heat about the abdomen.

Burning in the abdomen, while walking.

310. Colic, as if diarrhœa was coming.

In the right hypogastrium, painful sensation, as if something was trying to squeeze through.

In the groins, straining; at times like the burning in dysury. [*Htb. u. Tr.*]

Sensation in the left flank, while sitting down, as if a large, heavy body was lying there; after pressing upon it, it is relieved by passage of flatus. [*Htb. u. Tr.*]

Cutting in the right flank, when sitting; better when walking and when respiring deeply. [*Htb. u. Tr.*]

315. **Stitches in the groins**, also at night, disturbing the sleep and awaking her. [*Htb. u. Tr.*]

The hernia protrudes and is painful in walking and moving, and when touched.

Movement of flatus, with sensation as if something were moving in the abdomen, as if contused and torn.

Much torment from flatus.

Movements in the inflated belly, with passage of fetid flatus. [*Htb. u. Tr.*]

320. Audible grumbling, as from accumulated flatus, which finds no egress. [*Htb. u. Tr.*]

Audible rumbling in the belly. [*Ad.*]

Audible rumbling and grumbling in the large intestines, passing up under the stomach and thence down again. [*Ad.*]

Rumbling and grumbling in the right hypogastrium, after drinking warm milk, now above, now below, with fruitless efforts at emitting flatus. [*Ad.*]

Grumbling in the rectum. [*Ad.*]

325. Fermentation in the intestines.

Clucking and fermentation in the belly.

Frequent emission of fetid flatus, while out walking after supper. [*Ad.*]

Frequent emission of fetid flatus, in the forenoon. [*Htb. u. Tr.*]

Moving about of flatus in the stomach, with tenesmus. [*Htb. u. Tr.*]

330. Frequent pressure on the rectum as for a stool, but only flatus is emitted and then the pressure returns again.

Frequent, but fruitless urging in the lower part of the rectum. [*Ad.*]

Too much urging to stool, though every time a little is discharged, but with difficulty.

Violent urging to stool, which passes with difficulty, is hard and mixed with bloody streaks. [*Htb. u. Tr.*]

Scanty and light colored stool (the first times.). [*Htb. u. Tr.*]

335. **Scanty and delaying stool,** for several days.

Scanty stool, after 24 hours, hard and lumpy.

Hard, lumpy stool, which she can only get rid of with much effort, as if owing to the inaction of the abdominal muscles, with obstruction of the breath, in the evening. [*Htb. u. Tr.*]

Very hard stool, after a previous shudder in the head, as if from having cold water poured over him. [*Htb. u. Tr.*]

First part of the stool too hard and passing with difficulty, with the sensation as if it was too little, and if something more was to come, but the rectum has not sufficient strength to discharge it.

340. Four stools on the 3d day, every time preceded by colic.

First, firm, then soft stool, afterward, burning in the anus. [*Htb. u. Tr.*]

At night, a stool, after midnight. [*Htb. u. Tr.*]

Soft stool with mucus, which looks like coagulated albumen.

A soft stool, after previous urging toward the ossa pubis (aft. 27 d.). [*Htb. u. Tr.*]

345. Soft green stool, with bellyache before and during the same. [*Htb. u. Tr.*]

Liquid stool, followed by tenesmus (7th d.). [*Htb. u. Tr.*]

Diarrhœa, after pinching in the belly, with burning in the anus. [*Htb. u. Tr.*]

During the stool, tearing from the pudenda up into the abdomen (aft. 22 d.).

350. During the evacuation, stinging in the anus as from needles. [*Ad.*]

During the stool, violent cutting in the varices of the anus.

During the stool, discharge of blood.

During a hard stool, a stitching pain in the groins, as from flatus. [*Htb. u. Tr.*]

During the stool, pain in the sacrum, with inflation of the belly, extending up to the chest. [*Htb. u. Tr.*]

355. With the hard stool, a piece of tape-worm is discharged. [*Htb u. Tr.*]

After the stool, severe scraping in the rectum.

After the (second) stool (on the same day), great weakness and pain in the intestines, as if they were being screwed together.

After the stool, a shudder (in the evening). [*Htb. u. Tr.*]

After the stool, urging to urinate (the urine smelled very strong), then lassitude and early sleepiness in the evening, without being able to fall asleep (on lying down); she started up again right away, with a ringing in her ears, as if she would faint; then a febrile rigor.

360. **The varices of the anus swell severely and pain in walking.**

Large varices of the anus, which burn painfully.

In the rectum, severe burning, in the evening.

Burning in the anus.

Painful contraction of the anus.

365. **Stitches in the** (sore) **anus.**

Soreness of the anus, with oozing out of moisture, the whole evening.

A furuncle on the anus (aft. 16 d.).

A viscid, odorless liquid presses out from the rectum.

From the perinæum, behind the scrotum, there exudes much sticky, odorless moisture.

370. He readily gets sore on the buttocks from riding on horseback, causing large blisters.

Pinching, digging pain in the perinæum.

Cutting drawing from the anus through the coccyx, unconnected with stools.

Tearing, transversely across the ossa pubis and then through the pudenda to the anus (aft. 14 d.).

Single jerks from the coccyx toward the bladder, compelling micturition.

375. Strong pressure on the bladder, at night.

Sudden urging to urination. [*Ad.*]

Intense urging to urinate; she had to hurry frequently in urinating, and feels after micturition a voluptuous titillation in the urinary passage.

With slight pressure, the urine is emitted almost involuntarily (aft. 16 d.).

The emission of urine is much increased.

380. She passes urine frequently, without having drunk much (1st d.). [*Htb. u. Tr.*]

Very profuse discharge of urine, in the morning, after awaking

Very much urination; he had to rise three times in the night to urinate.

Increased passage of urine, with **frequent nocturnal micturition**; she urinates much more than she has drunk. [*Htb. u. Tr.*]

Copious passage of urine, after the nocturnal heat.

385. Turbid, orange-colored urine.

The urine, turbid at once when passed, soon leaves a turbid sediment (4th d.). [*Htb. u. Tr.*]

Yellow urine, soon depositing a loose sediment (the first d.). [*Htb. u. Tr.*]

Diminished quantity of urine (aft. 4 d.). [*Htb. u. Tr.*]

The stream of urine is intermittent. [*Htb. u. Tr.*]

390. Scanty urine.

Scanty and hot urine, at night, scalding during the discharge.

The urine scalds in the urethra on urinating.

During micturition, burning pain, as of soreness in the urethra.

After urinating, burning in the urethra.

395. Itching above the pudenda.

On the scrotum, stitches on both sides.

The sexual instinct is lacking for a long time, even when an effort is made to excite it.

Total relaxation of the genitals and feeling of debility therein.

The customary morning-erection is lacking (2d d.). [*Htb. u. Tr.*]

400. Pollution, at 4 P. M. (5th d.). [*Htb. u. Tr.*]

Pollution, the first time after a very long intermission, with voluptuous dreams, without erection. [*Ad.*]

Frequent pollutions (the first days).

Three nights in succession, copious pollutions, such as had not taken place for years.

After a pollution, in the morning, on awaking, a cramp-like pain along the urethra, especially in its posterior part. [*Ad.*]

405. After a pollution, very much exhausted in mind and body, and very anxious, as if evil was impending.

Menses, 4 days too early, with headache before they set in.

Menses, scanty the first day, the second day more profuse than usual, and the blood darker (8th d.).

Menses 4 days too early, with pain in the sacrum and the groins. [*Htb. u. Tr.*]

Catamenia, more profuse than usual. [*Htb. u. Tr.*]

410. Menses, not copious, but they last longer than usual, and flow only in the morning.

Menses, shorter than at other times, and 5 days late.

Before the menses set in, anxious heat.

Before and during the period, feeling in the thighs of being greatly worn out. [*Htb. u. Tr.*]

During the menses, violent pressure in the groins, in the sacrum and the thighs, with fruitless attempts at eructation, with chilliness and yawning. [*Htb. u. Tr.*]

415. During the menses, great inflation of the abdomen.

After the menses appear, so great a lassitude that she could hardly speak, accompanied with yawning and stretching.

Leucorrhœa (aft. 14 d.).

Discharge from the vagina, which stains the linen yellow (aft. 21 d.).

Watery **leucorrhœa**, while walking and standing. [*Htb. u. Tr.*]

* * * * * * * *

420. Sensation in the nose as in the beginning of a cold, after eating; increasing in the evening. [*Ad.*]

Dry coryza; he cannot draw any air through the nose.

Dry coryza in the forenoon till the evening (1st d.). [*Htb. u. Tr.*]

Dry coryza, early on awaking, going off after rising. [*Htb. u. Tr.*]

Stoppage of the left nostril, in the forenoon (2d and 3d d.). [*Htb. u. Tr.*]

425. Fluent coryza, with loss of the sense of smell; yawning and much sneezing. [*Htb. u. Tr.*]

Fluent coryza (aft. 10 d.).

Fluent coryza of much watery mucus. [*Htb. u. Tr.*]

Excessive fluent coryza, several hours in the evening.

Frequent discharge of mucus from the nose, with dry coryza.

430. Cold, catarrh, and scraping in the throat, especially in the evening and night, chiefly in swallowing.

Symptoms of a cold, with rough throat.

In the windpipe, pain as after much coughing.

Hoarseness, worse in the evening.

Roughness and hoarseness **in the throat, early after rising** with dry cough. [*Htb. u. Tr.*]

435. After hoarseness in day-time, she becomes aphonous at night, wakes up with coldness, swelling of the scrobiculus cordis, severe cough, difficult expectoration and obstruction of the breath with anxious sweat; she could not get her breath at all.

Tickling in the windpipe, with cough, diminished after eating. [*Htb. u. Tr.*]

Excitation to cough, with constriction of the throat and spasms of the chest.

Tickling, causing cough.

Cough without expectoration, from titillation in the larynx, in the evening, for 3 days. [*Htb. u. Tr.*]

440. Rough cough, with pain in the throat, as if sore.

Cough, from dryness of the throat, in the morning; as soon as phlegm is ejected it ceases.

Short tussiculation frequently, from tickling in the larynx (1st d.). [*Htb. u. Tr.*]

In the evening, hacking cough, chiefly in bed.

Cough which intercepts the respiration.

445. Suffocating cough, in the evening, an hour after going to sleep.

Only at night, while lying on the right side, **dry cough,** for several nights. [*Htb. u. Tr.*]

Dry cough, day and night.

Severe dry cough, early on rising, and almost the whole day, shaking the hypogastrium, as if everything was coming out; she has to hold the abdomen with the hands, and sit still; there is a rattling on the chest, before she detaches something by coughing.

The cough, before dry, becomes loose (2d d.). [*Htb. u. Tr.*

450. Cough with expectoration.

Yellowish white mucus is expectorated. [*Whl.*]

Cough, with expectoration of thick pus (aft. 14 d.). [*Whl.*]

Cough, with expectoration of greenish pus, excited only in a small spot, an inch square, in the right side of the chest. [*Whl.*]

Expectoration of green pus, after dry cough. [*Whl.*]

455. Ejection of thick green pus from a *vomica,* which appears in the right side of the thoracic cavity. [*Whl.*]

From cough, pleuritic stitches. [*Whl.*]

After a dry cough the pleuritic stitches cease and she can then cough several times without feeling it again. [*Whl.*]

From coughing, pain in the hypogastrium, as if sore.

Rattling and wheezing in the chest for hours, in the evening in bed.

460. Panting while breathing, with tightness of chest.

Asthmatic oppression of the chest, after a meal.

Sudden tightness of the chest, when she wished to take a deep breath. [*Htb. u. Tr.*]

The person feels as if the breath stuck in her chest. [*Whl.*]

Tightness in the chest; the whole chest feels oppressed or too much strained.

465. Her chest feels contracted.

Constriction of the chest, as if about to suffocate, in the morning in bed; she thought she was dying; speaking gave her stitches in the heart, and on moving her arms there was a sensation as if her heart and chest were about to be torn.

Anguish in the chest in the morning.

Pain, as if the middle of the chest were squeezed together, *per se,* and on being touched, with oppression of the breathing, for a quarter of an hour. [*Htb. u. Tr.*]

Violent compression of the chest, with obstruction of respiration, while sitting in the morning. [*Htb. u. Tr.*]

470. Pressure in the middle of the chest. [*Htb. u. Tr.*]

Violent pain in the whole of the chest as if it would burst, with pain in it as of soreness. [*Htb. u. Tr.*]

Stitches below the right breast so that she cannot sit still, while sitting and writing; after rising it ceases.

Stitches in the right side of the thoracic cavity. [*Whl.*]

Stitches in the right side of the chest with every breath, as if there was an ulcer. [*Whl.*]

475. Stitches in the left side of the upper thorax and, at times, in the right. [*Whl.*]

Stabs in the sternum, as from knives, mostly when moving.

Stitches in the back part of the right side of the chest, extending into the axilla. [*Htb. u. Tr.*]

Sharp, burning stinging in the left side of the chest, also when sitting. [*Htb. u. Tr*]

Stitches, with obstruction of the respiration, at times below the left breast, then in the right shoulder-joint, then in the right flank; with some dry cough, which increases the pain, in the morning. [*Htb. u. Tr.*]

480. Digging, pinching and tension in the upper part of the chest.

Painful writhing in and below the chest.

Trembling in the chest, like moaning.

Sensation of coldness in the chest (aft. 7 d.).

Burning in the chest, more on the right side.

485. Burning in the chest, with pressive pain.

In the heart a pressure, almost like pinching.

Palpitation in the evening, without anxiety (aft. 24 d.).

Violent palpitation, and every beat was felt in the head.

Violent palpitation during singing in church.

490. Violent palpitation in the morning on awaking; she has to lie quite still, without opening her eyes and without speaking.

In the female breast, in the lower part, lancinating pain, increased by pressure, obstructing the breath. [*Htb. u. Tr.*]

Painful knots in the breasts. [*Rust's Magaz.* l. c.]

On the coccyx, pain, which on touching the place becomes a burning pain.

Straining pain, as from a bruise on the coccyx.

495. Pain as from a bruise and pressure in the crest of the left ilium, aggravated in the evening, so that she had to bend double. On external pressure the place pained as if ulcerated. [*Htb. u. Tr.*]

Pain as from an ulcer under the skin, on the lower end of the spine, mostly only when sitting and lying.

Pain in the sacrum in sitting, as if the catamenia would appear. [*Htb. u. Tr.*]

Violent pains in the sacrum.

Pressive pain in the sacrum.

500. Stiffness in the small of the back.

Drawing pain in the sacrum, and a sensation as if it was broken, in walking, standing and lying.

Sharp drawing transversely through the sacrum, very sensible at every step.

Stitches close above the sacrum, when taking a deep breath.

A stitch in the sacrum, passing down the thighs at every breath.

505. A severe stitch in the sacrum.

The back is painful on the left side, so that she cannot lie on it for three nights. [*Htb. u. Tr.*]

Pain in the lower part of the back.

Violent pain in the loins, when she rises after sitting.

parts had been strained or had suffered injury, with a like pain in the front part of the chest on moving the arm.

510. Painful tension between the scapulæ, relieved by rubbing. [*Htb. u. Tr.*]

Lancinating tension in the right scapula. [*Htb. u. Tr.*]

Intermittent stitches in the back, above the right hip.

Stitches between the scapulæ. [*Htb. u. Tr.*]

In the nape of the neck a sensation as if her skin was being pulled up in a small spot. [*Htb. u. Tr.*]

515. Tension in the nape.

Stiffness in the nape of the neck.

Stiffness in the left side of the nape.

Swelling of the cervical gland.

The axillæ exude much moisture.

520. Violent itching in the right axilla.

The shoulders feel weighted down and tired.

In walking the shoulders and chest feel loaded down and pressed.

Tearing in the shoulders (going off by motion and rubbing). [*Htb. u. Tr.*]

In the arms and hands, a drawing pain.

525. Digging down into the arm, as if it was working in the bones; less perceptible when she lay on this arm.

In the right upper arm, violent tearing on lifting the arm.

Tearing in the middle of the right arm, after midnight, on lying on this side; she could not go to sleep for pain. [*Htb. u. Tr.*]

Painful tearing in the right humerus, toward the elbow. [*Htb. u. Tr.*]

In the olecranon of the ulna drawing stitches; the skin there pains as if sore, even at the lightest touch; but when grasped strongly it does not pain at all.

530. Lancinating pain below the bend of the left elbow, and out through the palm. [*Htb. u. Tr.*]

Burning and straining on the bend of the right elbow, in the evening. [*Htb. u. Tr.*]

In the left forearm, burning and stitches, often repeated, and at times passing even into the shoulder-joint; by rubbing it is only relieved for a short time. [*Htb. u. Tr.*]

Itching on the inner side of the right forearm, where after three days there appears an itching eruption, which occupies a large surface. [*Htb. u. Tr.*]

Hard, elevated, itching spot, transversely around the forearm, near the wrist. [*Htb. u. Tr.*]

535. **The wrist-joint pains, as if sprained.**

Straining pain in the wrist-joint, on moving it.

Tearing in the hands.

Pricking as with needles in the left palm, as also in the right ball of the hand. [*Htb. u. Tr.*]

Drawing shooting pain on the outer edge of the hand, where the skin pains as if sore, when touched lightly, but does not hurt when strongly grasped.

540. Often a very painful boring in the knuckles of the hand.

The hands go to sleep, every day.

The hand goes to sleep, when at rest.

Numbness of the left hand in the morning in bed, going off after rising.

Burning heat in the left hand when he came in the evening from his room into the open air and sat down. [*Htb. u. Tr.*]

545. Troublesome heat in the palms, in the morning.

Itching on the back of the hands and the fingers, for many days.

White, itching nodules on the dorsa of the hands, which burn and are red after scratching. [*Htb. u. Tr.*]

The middle finger-joints pain on moving them.

Straining in the posterior joint of the middle finger, on moving it.

550. Tearing on the back (and in the bones) of the fingers, passing off by rubbing. [*Htb. u. Tr.*]

Stitches in the tips of the fingers.

An exceedingly violent stitch in the tip of the index, like a wasp-sting.

Stinging in the fingers. [*Htb. u. Tr.*]

The fingers go to sleep; later on, the whole hand.

555. Itching of a wart on the finger.

Chilblain on the little finger.

In the right hip, cramp, when walking.

Stitches in the left hip, when sitting.

The lower limbs cannot be stretched, owing to straining and contraction in the groins.

560. Disagreeable tension of the skin of the lower limbs, with sensation of burning or of icy cold.

Cold legs during the day.

Pinching pains, here and there, on the lower limbs.

In the thighs, jerking pain.

Drawing and tearing in the muscles of the thigh.

565. Tearing in the thighs, under the hips, from morning till evening, but worse in the forenoon and when sitting. [*Htb. u. Tr.*]

Painful tearing, while standing, as if in the marrow of the left thigh; going off when sitting (during the menses). [*Htb. u. Tr.*]

A violent tearing stitch in the middle of the right thigh, on the inner side, while standing; in the evening. [*Htb. u. Tr.*]

Fine, burning, transient stitches, here and there, in the thigh and sacrum, the whole day. [*Htb. u. Tr.*]

Boring and drawing, in the upper part of the right femur, after an uneasy night.

570. In the right hough a sensation when walking, as if the tendons were too short; goes off in sitting. [*Htb. u. Tr.*]

Painless drawing with crooking of the right hough, which pains on stretching it; goes off after continued motion. [*Htb. u. Tr.*]

Cramp in the right knee, when walking.

Pain in the right knee as if compressed in a vice, while standing; with a sensation as if it would draw the leg crooked or contract it, in the evening. [*Htb. u. Tr.*]

Tearing above the right knee; also above the left, as if in the bone, where it only goes off transiently by rubbing. [*Htb. u. Tr.*]

575. Tearing and formicating stitches in the right knee, which on rubbing goes down into the tibia, where it is only transiently improved by rubbing. [*Htb. u. Tr.*]

Painful stitches in the left hough, on taking a walk. [*Ad.*]

Pain as of soreness in the knee on bending it, day and night.

Pain as of soreness in the right knee, worse when walking.

In the leg, anteriorly, beside the tibia, cramp, when walking.

580. Cramp in the calves, in the morning, for several days.

Painful cramp in the calves, after taking a walk.

Painful tension in the calves, while walking.

Painful contraction of the tendo Achillis, frequently repeated, in the evening (3d d.). [*Htb. u. Tr.*]

Pressure in the tibia, when walking.

585. Pain as from a bruise in the tibia, while taking a walk in the open air, intermittently, with tension in the calf.

Drawing in the tibia, by jerks. [*Ad.*]

At night, a painless drawing extending up her left leg.

A tearing in the right leg, especially in the knee-joint and ankle-joint.

A tearing downward in the left tibia, as also on the outer side of the right leg, and afterward in the big toe. [*Htb. u. Tr.*]

590. Painful stitch in the right toe on rising from her knees; this darts through the whole body, and startles her. [*Htb. u. Tr.*]

The legs go to sleep as far as the calves, in daytime.

The foot turns in walking, as if from weakness of the ankles.

Lack of strength in the ankles in walking, causing the foot to turn.

Feeling of stiffness in the ankle-joint, in the morning on rising.

595. Tension on the dorsum of the foot, as if a tendon was too short; the day after, the spot is swollen and painful to the touch. [*Htb. u. Tr.*]

Drawing and tearing in the tendons of the right heel. [*Htb. u. Tr.*]

Sharp stinging in the sole of the left foot. [*Htb. u. Tr.*]

Pain, as if festering inwardly, in the heels.

A stinging crawling in the feet, as from going to sleep, in the morning.

600. Cold feet, in walking, in the forenoon.

Extremely cold feet, also in the evening continuing for a long time while in bed.

Very hot feet.

In walking, her feet burn; in sitting, they swell up.

Inflammatory swelling of the foot, breaking open on a toe.

605. Swelling and tension of the feet. [*Htb. u. Tr.*]

Profuse foot-sweat.

In the toes, often during the day, cramp; on walking over a rough road it feels as if they turned.

Pain as of a sprain in the posterior joint of the toes, in walking and on every motion.

Tearing in the right big toe. [*Htb. u. Tr.*]

610. Violent cutting burning in the toes, chiefly in the little ones.

Violent itching of the toes formerly frozen (aft. 24 d.).

Swelling of the ball of the big toe, in the morning; much heat in it, and it pains, as if formerly frozen and ulcerated.

She easily gets sore between the toes in walking.

Corns appear, which are painful to the touch.

615. Stitches in a corn, for many days.

Pressive pains in the joints and muscles.

Pressure in the stomach, in the chest and at times in the abdomen.

Pain as if from the pressure of fingers, on the arms and legs.

Tearing drawing pains in the fingers and toes.

620. Stiffness of the limbs, after sitting.

Frequent sensation as if the hands and feet were going to sleep. [*Htb. u. Tr.*]

Going to sleep, now of the right arm, now of the right foot, in the evening in bed [*Htb. u. Tr.*]

The arms go to sleep when resting the head upon them, and the legs when crossed.

Feeling of numbness of all the limbs, but especially also in the head.

625. Sensation as of **a bruise in all the limbs**, especially on moving them.

The ligaments of the elbows and knees are painful when lying down.

The joints of the body feel bruised and severed, without strength.

Sensation of severance in the joints.

Cracking of the joints.

630. The joints are apt to get sprained.

The gait is tottering, as if caused by an external force.

Attack, from 10 A. M. to 4 P. M.; she feels very uncomfortable; she feels confused in the head and unsafe on the feet, with paleness of the face, qualmishness, and blue rings around the eyes.

Heaviness and trembling of the arms and legs.

Often heaviness in all the limbs.

635. Throbbing and beating in the whole body, worse in the evening.

Orgasm of blood, without heat.

Easily heated, the whole day.

Weakness and lack of energy of the whole body, with numb feeling in the head.

He eats and drinks, yet his strength decreases from day to day. [*Whl.*]

640. Easily exhausted by walking.

Much affected by walking, she became fatigued at once, chiefly in the hypochondria.

In the afternoon, so much anxiety and heaviness in the body, that he found it very hard to walk.

While taking a walk, much perspiration.

After a walk, tired and sleepy.

645. But little sensitiveness to the sharp, wintry air (after-effect).

Itching spreads all over the body, especially in the evening in bed.

Stings, like flea-bites, all over the body; by scratching it is always driven to another place. [*Htb. u. Tr.*]

Stitches in a cicatrix from a burn.

Several small knots on the wrist, in the nape of the neck, and on the dorsum of the foot; they itch violently; on scratching they burn with itching, and pass off after three days. [*Htb. u. Tr.*]

650. Attack: vertigo, she screams, opens her mouth and bends to the right and backward, with raised hands. [*Whl.*]

She is about to tumble over, opens her mouth, and looks upward; then heat all over the body, with perspiration in the face, and tearful mood. [*Whl.*]

Indolence and indisposition to mental and bodily work, the whole day.

Relaxed, anxious and melancholy, especially in the afternoon. [*Htb. u. Tr.*]

As in a slumber, the whole day, and therefore lazy, deaf, dim-sighted, peevish and brooding morosely.

655. In the forenoon, stupid and sleepy, worse after dinner. [*Htb. u. Tr.*]

In the forenoon, general lassitude, ready to sink down.

In the morning, especially in the lower limbs, as it were, tired and worn out. [*Htb. u. Tr.*]

In the morning, after a sound sleep, still very tired, on awaking.

In the morning, laziness in all the limbs.

660. In the morning, on rising, very weary, with such sadness she could have cried.

Sleepiness, with frequent yawning, the whole forenoon. [*Htb. u. Tr.*]

Drowsiness in the evening, with photophobia (the first days).

She could not go to sleep in the evening, and had in general only a very light sleep. [*Htb. u. Tr.*]

He could not get to sleep before 5 A. M., and yet, after two hours' sleep, on awaking he felt refreshed.

665. He cannot sleep at night for heat and restlessness.

Restless and anxious she tosses about all night, without finding rest, with frequent awaking. [*Htb. u. Tr.*]

Very restless night, he cannot find a restful position in bed.

Restless night; already at 2:30 A. M. the sleep was gone, from internal unrest.

Very uneasy sleep; he was very much excited and could not get to sleep before 2 A. M.

670. Very uneasy sleep, with frequent awaking.

Before going to sleep in the evening, he sees horrible faces in his phantasies.

On going to sleep, she starts up, as if she was about to fall down.

Before going to sleep in the evening in bed, fear of suffocation while lying down, closing her eyes; this fear only passed away as she sat up and opened her eyes; this hindered her from sleeping all night; her throat at the same time was full of mucus.

At night an anguish and a rush of blood, so severe that she had to sit up.

675. At night, much pain in the joints.

At night, tearing in the outer side of the thigh, going off on rising.

At night, cramp in the thighs and legs.

At night, cramp of the calves disturbs the calm sleep.

At night, tearing in the knee, going off by rising.

680. At night, on awaking and turning his lower limb in bed, a sudden pain, as if the leg was broken in two, upon which the lower limb became heavy, like lead.

At night, on lying down, the right limb goes to sleep, down to the toes, while lying on this side, with the sensation as if this leg was the longer. [*Htb. u. Tr.*]

At night, pain in the tibia; in the morning on awaking this pain had gone off.

At night, epistaxis for a quarter of an hour.

At night, much passage of urine.

685. At night, feeling of the whole body as if worn out, as if beaten all over. [*Htb. u. Tr.*]

After midnight, on awaking, sweat in the houghs, and swollen fingers.

On going to sleep, in the evening, an internal trembling of the limbs, and involuntary twitching in the knees, legs and feet; they moved visibly and he had to draw them up.

On going to sleep, in the evening, frequent starting up. [*Htb u. Tr.*]

In sleep, running out of saliva.

690. Groaning in sleep. [*Htb. u. Tr.*]

Loud talking in sleep. [*Htb. u. Tr.*]

Weeping at night, in sleep, and on awaking, sobbing.

Very vivid dreams, at night. [*Ad.*]

Vivid dreams concerning scientific matters; he worked out themes in his thoughts, and spoke aloud. [*Ad.*]

695. **Sleep full of vivid fantastic enthusiasm.**

Many fantastic and confused dreams during the night, so that he hardly slept at all.

Vivid, frightful dreams, for seven nights in succession.

Dreams of murders. [*Htb. u. Tr.*]

Anxious dreams at night, with crying and weeping, followed by sad dreams, then voluptuous ones, with pollution.

700. **Great chilliness**, by day.

Chilly, for a long time, after dinner. [*Htb. u. Tr.*]

He can hardly get warm in the morning.

She feels chilly as soon as a little air gets into the room. [*Htb. u. Tr.*]

Always chilly, with ice-cold feet. [*Htb. u. Tr.*]

705. **Very cold feet**, from 9 A. M. to 3 P. M.

In the evening, very cold feet, when she got into bed (aft. 10 h.).

In the evening, cold hands and feet.

At night, in bed, febrile rigor, which awakes her.

Chill and cold running over him in the afternoon, and trembling as from within, without thirst, for three hours; then burning in the skin of the body and in the eyes, with some thirst.

710. Rigor, up the back; this seems to start from the chest, every afternoon (aft. 4 w.). [*Whl.*]

Every second day toward evening some chill and thirst, then very violent dry heat, so that she imagines that sparks of fire dart from the eyes; the following night, a little sweat. [*Whl.*]

In the evening, a chill without thirst, then heat; going off after lying down. [*Htb. u. Tr.*]

In the evening at 9 o'clock, chill over the whole body; then after lying down, heat, during which she falls asleep, but frequently wakes up with thirst; toward morning, sweat. [*Htb. u. Tr.*]

In the evening, in bed, a chill; then sweat, while sleeping.

715. In the evening from 5 till 8 o'clock, chill, with goose-skin; then at 11 P. M. awaking with profuse sweat, which permits uncovering, and lasts till 2 A. M. [*Htb. u. Tr.*]

At night in bed his head and trunk were hot, but the lower limbs were cold and grew warm only gradually; toward morning, a chill, in bed (1st d.).

At night, heat and thirst without chill before and without subsequent sweat. [*Htb. u. Tr.*]

She cannot bear to be uncovered during the febrile heat, as she gets chilled at once. [*Htb. u. Tr.*]

Heat, at night, with moisture of the skin.

720. Sweat, while eating and while taking a walk.

Profuse sweat while walking and while partaking of warm viands.

Sweat which colors the linen yellow.

Profuse night sweat.

At night, sweat on the head.

725. Morning sweat, on awaking (2d d.). [*Htb. u. Tr.*]

Fatiguing night sweats. [*Whl.*]

Fetid night sweats. [*Whl.*]

As soon as he shuts his eyes a very profuse sweat breaks out. [*Whl.*]

CARBO VEGETABILIS, WOOD CHARCOAL.

The charcoal of any kind of wood, thoroughly heated to redness, seems to manifest itself uniformly in its effects on the human health, when it has been prepared and potentized in the manner which Homœopathy uses. I employ the charcoal of birch wood; in some of the provings by others the charcoal of the red beech was used.

Formerly charcoal was considered by physicians as non-medicinal and powerless. Empiricism only added it in its most highly composite powders, *e. g.*, for epilepsy, the charcoal of the linden tree, without being able to adduce any proof of the efficacy of this particular substance. Only in recent times, since LOWITZ, in St. Petersburg, discovered the chemical properties of wood charcoal, especially its power of removing from putrid and mouldy substances their bad odor, and of preserving fluids from fetid smell, physicians began to use it externally (iatro-chemically). They advised rinsing the mouth of fetid odor with powdered charcoal, and covered old putrid ulcers with the same powder, and the fetor was in both instances almost instantaneously alleviated. Also when administered internally in the dose of several drachms it removed the fetor of the stools in autumnal dysentery.

But this medicinal use was, as before mentioned, only a chemical use, but not a dynamic employment penetrating into the internal sphere of life. The mouth rinsed out with it only remained odorless for a few hours; the ill smell returned every day. The old ulcer was not improved by its application, and the fetor, chemically removed from it for the moment, was always renewed; it was no cure. The charcoal powder taken in autumnal dysentery only chemically removed the fetor of the stools for a short time, but the disease remained and the nauseous smell of the stools quickly returned.

In such a coarse, pulverized state, charcoal can exercise no other than a chemical action. A considerable quantity of wood charcoal in its ordinary crude form may be swallowed without producing the slightest alteration in the health.

It is only by prolonged trituration of the charcoal (as of many other dead and apparently powerless medicinal substances) with a non-medicinal substance, such as sugar of milk, and by dissolving this preparation and potentizing (shaking) these solutions, that the dynamic medicinal power concealed within, and which in the crude state is combined, and so to say slumbering and sleeping (latent), can be awakened and brought to life; but then its material external must vanish.

The various degrees of potency are employed according to the varying intention in healing, down from the decillion-potency to the million-powder-attenuation, using one, two or three fine pellets moistened therewith as a dose.

Arsenic, camphor and raw coffee have been found antidotes of charcoal, but the spirits of nitre seem to be more efficient.

In healing the diseases to which this remedy is homœopathically appropriate, the following symptoms were chiefly relieved or removed:

Anguish, irritability; fearfulness; *fear of ghosts* at night; peevishness; headache from overheating; heaviness of the head; rush of blood to the head; headache from nausea; tendency of the head to colds; eyeache from strained vision; burning in the eyes; heat and *pressure in the eyes;* burning and pressure in the canthi; closing of the eyes by suppuration, at night; roaring in the ears; suppuration of the inner ear and discharge from it; itching of the nose; continued epistaxis; herpes in the face; chapping of the lips; bleeding of the gums; toothache from taking cold or warm things in the mouth; contractive toothache; gnawing toothache; clucking toothache; chronic looseness of the teeth; dryness, or gathering of saliva in the mouth; stomacace [or aphthæ]; scraping in the throat; hawking up of much phlegm from the throat; bitter taste in the mouth; salty taste in the mouth; long-continued loathing of meat; lack of appetite; *excessive hunger* or thirst; empty eructation; bitter eructation; eructation tasting of the fat eaten; regurgitation of the ingesta; perspiration while eating; acidity in the mouth after a meal; chaotic sensation and pressure in the stomach after a meal; nausea in the morning; constant nausea; waterbrash, at night; *stitches under the ribs;* lancinative pain in the liver; stitches in the spleen; pain as from a bruise in the hypochondria; tension of the abdomen; inflation of the abdomen; pain above the navel, when touched; colic from driving out; excessive discharge of flatus; thin, pale stool; light-colored *mucous stools;* scant stools; constipation; *itching of the anus; varices* of the anus; pain in the varices of the anus; blood from the anus at every stool; diminished secretion of urine; frequent anxious tenesmus of the bladder, by day and night; wetting the bed; urine too dark; excoriative pain in urinating; pressure in the testes; *too frequent pollutions;* unnatural abundance of voluptuous thoughts; too rapid emission of semen in coitus; soreness and itching on the pudenda; itching and burning of the genitals; swelling of the pudenda; *too early menses; menses too copious;* scanty menses; paleness of the blood in the catamenia; vomiting during the menses; flux from the vagina; leucorrhœa before the menses; *stoppage of the nose;* discharge of water from the nose; severe cold; constant hoarseness; morning-hoarseness; catarrh and sore throat with the measles; *asthma, dyspnœa;* short breath during walking; dropsy of the chest; stitches in the chest; chaps and pains as from soreness in the chest; brownish spots on the chest; drawing pain in the back; itching pimples on the back; *stiffness of the nape of the neck;* pain in the elbow on grasping it; heat in the hands; restlessness in the legs, the knees go to sleep;

herpes on the knee; cramp in the calves, at night; continued insensibility of the feet; *sweat of the feet;* redness and swelling of the toes, with lancinating pains as after freezing them; pain in the limbs as from spraining and straining; pain in the left hypogastrium from a strain in lifting; the limbs go to sleep; *worn-out feeling of the limbs, in the morning on rising from bed;* throbbing here and there in the body; tremulousness; jerking of single limbs, by day; after-effects from yesterday's wine-spree; chronic ailments from the abuse of cinchona bark; tendency to take cold; neetle-rash; herpes; ulcers (on the legs) fetid and bleeding readily; *great drowsiness by day;* sleep in the forenoon; insomnia on account of restlessness of the body; phantasies at night and starting from anxious dreams; *frequent rushes of transient heat;* coldness and chill of the body; night-sweat; morning-sweat.

Any excessive action can be quickly removed by *repeated smelling of camphor*, and still more surely by smelling of *spirits of nitre.*

The symptoms marked *Ad.* were observed by *Dr. Adams*, a physician of St. Petersburg; those marked *Gff.* by the Royal Counselor, Baron von Gersdorff, M. D., and those with *C.* by the late *Dr. Caspari*, of Leipzig.

CARBO VEGETABILIS,

Anxious, as it were oppressed in the chest, for several days.

Very much oppressed and full.

Inexpressibly weighed down with anguish, every afternoon from four to six o'clock.

In the evening for several hours increasing anguish, with heat in the face.

5. In the evening, restlessness.

Restless the whole day.

He trembled for restlessness and anxiety, and could not stay long anywhere.

For restlessness and anguish every afternoon, he trembled all over the body; he felt as if he had committed a great crime, this dissolved itself into copious weeping, even before strangers on the street.

He felt like weeping, everything seemed to him dreadful, and he felt in despair.

10. Great disposition to weep; he wishes to shoot himself.

She wishes to die, she feels so unhappy.

Pusillanimous and timid.

If she has to speak before people, her pulses throb, her pale face becomes bloated and bluish red.

Impatient.

Vegetable charcoal appeared with the animal variety in the *Materia Medica Pura* and the first edition of the *Chronic Diseases.* Its pathogenesis obtained with the 3d trituration shows 720 symptoms in the former, 930 in the latter work. The fresh symptoms both here and there were *Hahnemann's*, obtained in his later manner, as the three physicians mentioned all made their contributions to the original list.—*Hughes.*

15. Great irritability.

Excessive excitation, as if she was too much hurried, or overworked in business.

Irritation and ill humor, with lassitude of mind (aft. 10 h.). [*C.*]

Irritability and sensitiveness. [*Ad.*]

Very irritable during the day and inclined to be annoyed.

20. Very sensitive and moody (aft. 4 h.). [*Gff.*]

Peevish, impatient, desperate, so that he would like to shoot himself.

Peevish irritableness, with numb feeling in the head. [*Gff.*]

Peevishly irritable, the whole day (2d d.).

Violent irritable disposition.

25. **Passionate and peevish, in the forenoon.**

Very peevish, irritable and inclined to anger.

Involuntary angry ebullitions (aft. 36 h.).

Sensitive mood, inclined to weep.

Very irritable and easily put into bad humor, he can easily weep over sad events, and just as easily laugh over the merest trifle, so that tears stand in his eyes.

30. Sensitive, easily irritated humor, which however, when cause is given, is wont easily to turn into awkward gayety, when to the laughter is added relaxation of the muscles of the arms and the hands. [*Gff.*]

Excessively cheerful, but easily put out of humor. [*Ad.*]

Out of humor (after a meal). [*Ad.*]

Indifferent, unsympathetic. [*Ad.*]

Indifferent he listens to everything without pleasure or displeasure, and without thinking of anything.

35. The mind is indolent and indisposed to think (aft. 10 h.). [*C.*]

Music, which he loves, does not affect him all day. [*Ad.*]

Freedom of spirit, lightness and general good health (curative effect after chaotic state of the head, as from a cold, and general heaviness of the limbs and of the body) (aft. 4 h.). [*C.*]

Lack of memory, periodically occurring.

Sudden lack of memory, he could not recollect what he had just said to somebody, and what he had recounted to him. [*Ad.*]

40. Slow flow of ideas, which always revolve around one subject, with a sensation as if the head was bandaged too tightly. [*Ad.*]

Numbness in the head, which makes thinking difficult.

Severe numb feeling in the head in the morning, at once after rising; he can not think well, and has to tear himself with difficulty, as it were, from a dream; after he lay down again, it went off. [*Gff.*]

Numb feeling in the head, for several days without pain.

Numb feeling in the occiput, as after a spree. [*Ad.*]

45. Numb feeling in the head, after dinner. [*C.*]

Numb feeling in the head, in the evening, after a walk (aft. 19 h.). [*C.*]

Numbness of the occiput like an outward tension (aft. ½ h.). [*Ad.*]

Dullness in the head, after awaking from the noon-day nap. [*Ad.*]

50. Dizzy in the head, as after a spree, spreading from the occiput to the front, worse in the evening, and occupying the whole head, with aggravation by walking. [*Ad.*]

Dizzy, befogged, giddy (3d d.).

Turning around in the head, all day.

Vertigo at the least motion.

Vertigo at a quick movement of the head.

55. Vertigo so that he had to hold on to something (aft. 15 d.).

Vertigo and staggering, when walking.

Dizzy, while walking and sitting (4th d.).

Vertigo, when stooping, as if the head wagged to and fro.

Vertigo, when stooping, when turning over in bed, and when gargling.

60. Vertigo in bed, on awaking from sleep.

Dizzy in the evening, while sitting, after sleeping, with trembling and vibration in the whole body; on rising from his seat, he was as it were in a faint, which continued even while he was lying down, for a quarter of an hour.

Vertigo, only while sitting, as if the head swayed to and fro.

Headache, as with an incipient cold.

Headache which occupied the whole right side of the head and face, with chill, coldness and trembling of the body and of the jaws.

65. Headache, from quick alternation of warm and cold weather.

Dull headache, with heaviness before the forehead. [*Gff.*]

Dull headache on the occiput. [*Gff.*]

Headache which as it were rises from the stomach into the head, and robs her of consciousness for a short time.

Heaviness in the head.

70. The head feels as heavy as lead.

Pain in the head as if too full.

Tension in the brain; it feels more numb than painful.

Cramplike tension in the brain.

Pressive headache, first in the nape of the neck, then in the forehead, then lachrymation of the eyes, with closing of the lids.

75. **Pressure in the occiput**, especially after supper. [*Ad.*]

Violent pressive pain on and in the occiput, at the bottom. [*Gff.*]

Pressive pain in the occiput from time to time.

Constant pressive pain **on top of the vertex, with aching when the hair is touched.** [*Gff.*]

Pressive headache in the upper part of the right side of the occiput, with pressure in the eyes. [*Gff.*]

80. Pressive pain in single spots of the head, in light attacks passing quickly; they seemed to be in connection with flatus (aft. 48 h.). [*C.*]

Pressive headache in the forehead, especially close above the eyes, which hurt on moving, the whole afternoon. [*Gff.*]

Pressive headache in the forehead, it passes off and returns. [*C.*]

Pressure on the top of the head, every afternoon.

Pressive headache above the eyes, extending into them. [*Gff.*]

85. **Pressure in both temples**, and on top of the head.

Pressure in the left temple, from within outwards, for several hours. [*Ad.*]

Pressure above on the head, then drawing in the whole head, but more on the left side.

Pressure and drawing in the head, in paroxysms.

Compressive headache.

90. Pressure, as if something lay on the vertex, or as if the integuments of the head were constricted together, spreading then also into the forehead. [*Ad.*]

Headache as from contraction of the integuments of the head.

Headache, as from contraction of the integuments of the head, chiefly after supper. [*Ad.*]

Contractive pain in the head, especially on motion.

The hat presses on the head, like a heavy load, and when he takes it off, he still retains the sensation, as if the head was bandaged together by means of a cloth. [*Ad.*]

95. Tension in the brain, the brain feels more numb than painful.

Spasmodic tension in the brain.

Severe headache for five days, on stooping; the brain seemed about to come out, in the occiput and in front. (Pain in the right side of the head on shaking it.)

Squeezing and cutting headache, above and behind the left ear. [*Gff.*]

Pinching headache in the occiput.

100. Drawing headache here and there, especially in the forehead, extending up beyond the root of the nose. [*Gff.*]

A confusing drawing in the whole of the head, starting from the occiput (aft. ½ h.). [*C.*]

Drawing and tearing in the left occiput. [*Gff.*]

Drawing tearing in the upper anterior part of the head. [*Gff.*]

Tearing through the head, starting from a little spot on the occiput. [*Gff.*]

105. Tearing pains in frequent paroxysms, in the inside of the head, toward the right temple. [*Gff.*]

Tearing in the left half of the head, starting from the left half of the nose. [*Gff.*]

Short, sharp, tearing pains through the whole left side of the head. [*C.*]

Dull tearing headache on the crown and in the temples, in paroxysms. [*Gff.*]

Short tearing pains in the right side of the occiput. [*C.*]

110. Tearing in the left half of the head, with drawing in the left arm. [*Gff.*]

Tearing in the temples, extending to the molar teeth. [*Gff.*]

Violent tearing in the forehead, in a small spot, beside the temples. [*Gff.*]

The tearing pains in the head start at times from the limbs, and seem to terminate in the head. [*C.*]

Smarting pressive headache, like the sensation in the nose from abortive sneezing, in the morning on awaking, in the right half of the head on which he was lying and in the occiput; on raising the head, the pain was only alleviated, but on rising from bed, it vanished entirely. [*Gff.*]

115. Stitches here and there into the head, with general painfulness of the surface of the brain.

Stitches in the upper part of the head, from reading.

Violent stitches in the upper part of the head.

Stitches in the head, toward the temples, upward.

Stitches in the forehead, over the right external canthus (aft. 2 h.). [*Ad.*]

120. Lancinating headache, above the right eye.

A dull tearing stitch, from time to time, deep into the brain, on one side of the head, as from a nail driven in.

Burning stinging in a small spot on the occiput. [*Gff.*]

Boring headache below the left temple.

Boring and pressive headache in the sinciput.

125. Twitching headache.

Pecking headache, very violent, in the occiput, as if there was a festering underneath, from morning till evening (aft. 9 d.).

Beating headache, in the evening in bed, with heavy breathing.

Beating in the temples, and fullness of the brain, on awaking from a long, deep noon siesta. [*Ad.*]

Beating headache, in the afternoon.

130. Throbbing headache in the forehead, after a meal, with pressure in the occiput, heat in the head, and eructation.

Rush of blood to the head.

Rush of blood to the head, with hot forehead and confused feeling in the head.

Intense pressure of blood to the head, with chaotic feeling and hot forehead (aft. 6 h.). [*C.*]

Heat and burning in the forehead.

135. Burning in the forehead and heat in the mouth, with pains in the eyes.

A spot on the head very hot to the touch, as large as a hand, with constant headache.

Burning and violently pressive headache, in the evening in bed, especially on the vertex, and toward the front, even to the forehead. [*Gff.*]

Buzzing in the head, as from bees.

Cracking in the occiput when sitting.

140. Severe noise in the head, from reading.

Externally on the head, pains drawing here and there. [*Gff.*]

Frequently repeated, short, drawing pain on the right side of the occiput (aft. 2½ h.). [*Gff.*]

Tearing pain on the left side of the head, above the temple. [*Gff.*]

Tearing in the right side of the occiput (aft. 4 h.). [*Gff.*]

145. Tearing in an old scar from a sabre wound, on the top of the head. [*Gff.*]

Pressive pain on a small spot on the right side of the forehead, where there had been a wound (aft. 4 h.). [*Gff.*]

Tearing in the bones of the head (aft. 24 h.).

Headache over the whole crown, in the morning in bed, with painfulness of the hair to the touch; going off after rising.

Crawling on the integuments of the occiput, as if the hair was moving. [*Ad.*]

150. **The hair on the head falls out very much.**

Eruptive pimples on the temples.

Red, smooth, painless pimples, here and there on the forehead. [*Gff.*]

Painless pimples on the forehead (5th d.).

Red pimples on the forehead, near the hairy scalp, painful only when touched. [*Gff.*]

155. White little nodules in the skin of the forehead, like little glands (aft. 3 d.). [*C.*]

Tension and pressure in both temples and on the forehead; he cannot keep his eyelids open.

The muscles of the eyes are painful on looking upward. [*Gff.*]

Dull pain in the left eye. [*Gff.*]

Pressure in the eyes, with numb feeling in the head (aft. 6½ h.).

160. Pressure in the upper eyelids and in the upper half of both eyeballs, on taking exercise in the air. [*Ad.*]

Sensitive pressure on the right eyeball, from above downward (aft. ½ h.). [*Gff.*]

Pressure as from sand in the right eye, with sensation of soreness in the canthi (aft. 36 h.). [*C.*]

Pressure in the eyes as from a grain of sand, with sensation of soreness, chiefly in the canthi, and with smarting in the right eye. [*Gff.*]

A smarting pressure in the outer canthus of the right eye [*Gff.*]

165. Tearing pressure on the left eye. [*Gff.*]

Drawing in the right eyelid (aft. 13 d.).

Drawing above the right eye, through the head.

Pain in the eye, as if it would be torn out, with headache.

Violent stitches in both eyes.

170. **Itching around the eyes.**

Itching on the edges of the eyelids.

Itching on the inner canthus of the left eye. [*Gff.*]

Itching on the right eye (aft. 36 h.). [*C.*]

Itching on the right eye, with great dryness of the eyelid (aft. 14 d.).

175. **Itching in the left eye; after rubbing, a smarting, especially in the inner canthus.** [*Gff.*]

Smarting itching, chiefly in the outer canthus of the right eye. [*Gff.*]

Smarting in the left canthus. [*Gff.*]

Smarting in the eyelids, with some redness on their edge (aft. 24 h.). [*C.*]

Burning in the eyes.

180. Inflammation of the right eye.

Swelling of the left eye.

Profuse lachrymation and smarting in the right eye (aft. 24 h.). [*Gff.*]

The eyes closed from suppuration, in the morning.

Quivering of the left eyelid (aft. 9 d.).

185. Quivering of the upper eyelid.

At night, she could not open the eyes, when she could not go to sleep.

The left eyelid seemed to him agglutinated, but was not.

A weight upon the eyes, so that he must strain very much in reading and writing, to make it out.

After straining his eyes, he for a time becomes short-sighted.

190. Great short-sighteness; he can only recognize an acquaintance at a few steps' distance (aft. 3 d.).

Flickering before the eyes, at once in the morning on rising. [*Gff.*]

Black, flying specks before the eyes.

Rings before the eyes, with a lighter colored center.

Otalgia in the left ear. [*Gff.*]

195. Otalgia in the right ear, in the evening. [*Gff.*]

A straining outward in both ears (aft. 17 d.).

Fine pinching in the left ear. [*C.*]

Tearing in the inner part of the right ear. [*Gff.*

Tearing pain in the pit behind the right ear. [*Gff.*]

200. Burning tearing pain on the lobules of the left ear. [*Gff.*]

Tearing jerks or single stitches in the right internal meatus auditorius. [*Gff.*]

Stitches passing inward in the left meatus auditorius (aft. 48 h.). [*C.*]

Itching on the upper part of the external ear, which then becomes hot.

Itching in the ears, with tendency to seek to diminish it by swallowing.

205. Violent crawling itching in the internal right ear, continually recurring after boring in it with the fingers. [*Gff.*]

Itching behind the ear.

Throbbing in the ears.

Heat and redness of the left ear, every evening.

Severe swelling of the parotid gland, extending to the angle of the lower jaw.

210. A thick brown matter is discharged from the right ear.

Discharge of a thickish, flesh-colored fetid liquid from the ear.

His ears feel obstructed, as from two little sandbags lying before the meatus auditorius. [*Ad.*]

A weight lies in and before the ears; they seem to him obstructed, but without diminution of hearing (aft. ½ h.). [*Ad.*]

Loud talking affects the hearing and is disagreeable. [*Ad.*]

215. **Ringing in the ears.**

Ringing in the left ear, with a whirling vertigo.

Fine tinkling in the left ear, in the afternoon (aft. 40 h.). [*C.*]

Roaring in the ears.

Severe buzzing before both ears.

220. Chirping in the ears, as from locusts (7th d.).

Rustling in the ear as from straw, at every motion of the jaw (at breakfast).

In the root of the nose, a drawing.

Sensation of heaviness of the nose.

Trembling of the skin and the muscles, on the right side of the root of the nose.

225. Formication in the nose for two days.

Constant formication in the left side of the nose, in the evening.

Eruption in the corner of the ala nasi.

White itching pimples about the nose.

Itching about the nostrils.

230. Scabby nose-tip.

Much mucus always comes from the posterior nares.

Epistaxis, at night, with ebullition of the blood (aft. 52 h.).

Epistaxis, every forenoon, 10 to 12 drops.

Severe epistaxis in the morning in bed, and immediately afterwards pain in the chest.

235. Profuse epistaxis which can hardly be stopped (aft. 48 h.).

Severe epistaxis for two weeks, daily several times, with great paleness of the face every time before and afterwards.

The complexion becomes greyish yellow.

Extremely pale complexion.

Aching of the facial bones of the upper and lower jaw.

240. Pain in the left side of the cheek, as if it were being bored and burned, in paroxysms (aft. 6 d.).

Drawing pain in the cheek, for two days.

Drawing pain in the upper and lower jaw, on both sides, with drawing in the head and feeling of obtuseness in the same (aft. 2 h.). [*Gff.*]

Jerking pain in several parts of the face.

Jerking drawing pain in the cheek and the jaw (1st d.).

245. Tearing in the face.

Tearing facial pain in the left cheek.

Tearing pain in the left corner of the mouth and from there into the cheek. [*Gff.*]

Tearing by jerks in the left zygoma, before the ear, in the evening in bed. [*Gff.*]

Tearing by jerks in the bones of the upper jaw on the right side. [*Gff.*]

250. Fine tearing stitch on the right cheek (aft. 3 h.). [*Gff.*]
Glowing heat in the face, after sitting a short time.
Swelling of the cheeks.
Swelling of the face on the chin, for 2 hours.
Many pimples on the face and on the forehead. [*C.*]
255. Single white nodules on both the temples (aft. 4 d.). [*C.*]
A white pimple on the lower part of the cheek.
Swelling on the lips.
Swelling of the upper lip and cheek, with twitching pain.
Twitching in the upper lip.
260. Painful eruption on the upper lip; the red part is full of pimples.
Pustules, with a burning sensation below the red part of the upper lip.
Eruption in the left corner of the mouth, like itching herpes.
Ulceration of the right corner of the mouth.
Eruptions on the chin; boil below the jaw and before the ear.
265. Drawing toward the chin, starting from the right corner of the mouth.
On the lower jaw, cramp-like pain (aft. 13 d.).
Tearing jerks in the left lower jaw (aft. 4 d.). [*C.*]
Toothache, with dry lips.
Aching of the roots of the teeth, above and below.
270. Toothache in the sound incisors. [*Ad.*]
Toothache, as if from acid things, especially in the gums, as often as she eats anything salty. [*C.*]
Toothache, the teeth are as if rubbed sore, and the pain, when the teeth are touched with the tongue, is as from an ulcer; the pain is renewed on eating.
Pinching pain in the right lower molars. [*Gff.*]
Pressive toothache in the left upper molars.
275. Drawing pain in a hollow tooth.
Drawing pain in an upper incisor. [*Gff.*]
Frequently repeated drawing pains in the teeth which are sound. [*C.*]
Frequent drawing in the hollow molars (aft. 3 d.). [*C.*]
A smarting drawing pain in the upper and lower incisors, more in the gums. [*Gff.*]
280. Subdued drawing in the right molars, with violent jerks [*Gff.*]
Violent drawing jerk in a hollow molar. [*Gff.*]
Drawing and tearing toothache in all the molars. [*Gff.*]
Gnawing and drawing pain in a hollow tooth, with swelling of the gums.
Pain as from soreness, with drawing in the first molar of the left upper row. [*Gff.*]
285. A tickling stinging and drawing in the first upper molar on the left side [*Gff.*]
Stinging pain, every moment, in teeth quite sound, passing quickly and giving place to a short lancinating pain in the abdomen (3d d.).
Bleeding of the teeth, when cleaning them.

Bleeding of the teeth and gums, on sucking with the tongue. [*Gff.*]

For several days, frequent bleeding of the teeth and gums. [*Gff.*]

290. The gums are painfully sensitive in chewing.

Drawing pain in the gums.

Heat in the gums.

Pain in the gums, as from soreness, by day.

Swelling of the gums, on a hollow tooth.

295. **A pustule on the gums.**

Recession of the gums from the lower incisors.

The gums are detached from the incisors, and the roots are laid bare (cured by mercury) (aft. 6 d.). [*C.*]

Detachment of the gums from the upper and lower incisors; (with a young girl, cured by mercury). [*C.*]

The gums are detached from the teeth and sensitive.

300. Very violent bleeding of the gums.

Bleeding of the gums, after sucking (aft. 2 d.). [*C.*]

On sucking the gums with the tongue, there is a taste of blood in the mouth, and the saliva is bloody (aft. 51 and 85 h.). [*C.*]

On sucking the gums, pure blood gathers in the mouth, in the forenoon, returning several days at the same time (aft. 5 d.). [C.]

The tongue is coated white.

305. Tongue coated with yellowish brown mucus.

Cramp-like pain on the left side of the root of the tongue.

Fine tearing pain on the right side of the tongue.

Sensitiveness of the tongue, and sensation as of rawness.

Stinging on the tongue.

310. Soreness on the (right) side of the tongue, with lancinating pain.

Difficulty in moving the tongue, and in speaking. [*Ad.*]

Heaviness of the tongue and lack of mobility, so that talking becomes very difficult to her.

Heat and dryness of the tip of the tongue. [*C.*]

Heat in the mouth, with roughness and dryness of the tip of the tongue (aft. 1, 2 d.). [*C.*]

315. Sensation in the mouth and on the tongue as after copious drinking of wine in the evening (aft. 10 h.). [*C.*]

Heat in the mouth, especially on the upper lip.

Dryness in the mouth, without thirst.

Dryness of the mouth, in the morning.

Great dryness of the mouth, in the morning on awaking.

320. Increased collection of saliva in the mouth (aft. 1/4 h.). [*C.*]

Bitter mucus in the mouth, in the morning.

Back on the palate, a pressive pain. [*Gff.*]

Pressive pain, close behind the palate in the fauces.

A tearing pressure in the back part of the fauces and on the left side of the root of the tongue. [*Gff.*]

325. Smarting in the back part of the fauces, as in the beginning of a cold, but smarting even more sharply. [*Gff.*]

Frequent smarting and burning in the fauces and in the palate. [*Gff.*]

Burning in the upper part of the fauces. [*Gff.*]

Burning in the fauces and behind in the pharynx, as in a cold (aft. 10 h.). [*C.*]

Bitterness in the palate, with dryness of the tongue.

330. A blister in the upper part of the palate.

Much tough mucus in the fauces, which he has to hawk out.

Much hawking of mucus.

Mucus in the fauces, of disagreeable taste and smell.

In the throat and the fauces, violent scratching and formication, only transiently relieved by clearing the throat. [*Gff.*]

335. Scraping in the throat.

Scratching in the throat.

Scraping and rawness in the throat, for several days.

Feeling of dryness in the throat, on deglutition.

A sort of fullness and pressure in the gullet, extending down into the stomach, almost like heartburn.

340. Pressure in the œsophagus; also when not swallowing, as if it were contracted and constricted. [*Gff.*]

In the œsophagus, sensation as if contracted or constricted.

Contractive sensation deep in the œsophagus.

Sensation of contraction and an inner swelling of the throat.

Sore throat, as from swelling of the palate, with painful deglutition, for 4 days.

345. Painless impediment to deglutition; the saliva swallowed goes down only gradually. [*Gff.*]

Food cannot be swallowed easily; the throat is as it were constricted by a spasm, but without pain.

In deglutition, and in coughing and in blowing the nose, the fauces and the posterior nares are painful as if sore.

Pains as from soreness in the throat, when eating.

Sensation of coldness down the throat.

350. Inflammation of the throat, with a sensation as if something had lodged in it, with stitches.

Inflammation and swelling of the uvula, with stitches in the throat.

Insipid, watery, unpleasant taste in the mouth.

Salty taste in the mouth, the whole day.

Bitterness in the mouth, with eructation.

355. Bitterish taste in the mouth, before and after eating.

Sour taste in the mouth after eating.

Appetite, little, and no sense of taste, as in a cold.

Little appetite, with heat in the mouth and roughness and dryness on the tip of the tongue (after 42 h.). [C.]

She cannot eat anything in the morning, till noon, then she relishes it; but she cannot then eat anything in the evening.

360. The lack of appetite is combined with a sensation of lack of tone and weakness of the muscles in the limbs. [*C.*]

Lack of hunger; he could have done without eating. [*Gff.*]

Scanty appetite; she is satiated at once; she feels an aching in the scrobiculus cordis, and as if too empty in the stomach, for half an hour.

Entire lack of appetite, with coated tongue, and great lassitude. [*C.*]

Lack of appetite and frequent eructation, with numb feeling in the head.

365. Toward noon, diminution of appetite, with nausea (aft 3 d.).

At noon, little appetite, and slight colic (aft. 4 d.). [*C.*]

Hunger, and still there is repugnance to dishes which are agreeable to him.

The appetite for coffee is lost.

Repugnance to fat meat.

370. Aversion to butter.

She is averse to milk, and it causes flatulence.

Desire for sweet and for salty things.

A little wine at once causes heat. [*Gff.*]

During eating, perspiration on the forehead.

375. During eating, sudden throbbing in a tooth.

At every meal, nausea.

After a meal, nausea, with pressure in the stomach and then a pulling down pain about the navel, from above downward.

After eating, a painful hiccup in the œsophagus. [*Ad.*]

After a moderate dinner, hiccup, and while sitting bent forward, fine pinching in the abdomen along the spinal vertebræ on the left. [*C.*]

380. After eating, severe palpitation of the heart.

After dinner, weariness (aft. 4th d.).

After dinner, invincible drowsiness, with burning of the eyelids on closing the eyes (7th d.).

After eating, great sleepiness.

After supper, sleepiness, with red, hot face.

385. **After dinner, the abdomen very much inflated** (9th d.).

When he eats or drinks, **he feels as if his abdomen would burst.**

After eating but little, inflation of the abdomen and rumbling in it. [*Gff.*]

After a moderate breakfast, at once full and satiated. [*C.*]

After a moderate breakfast, fullness, eructation, general heaviness; writing proceeds slowly and with difficulty. [*C.*]

390. During and after eating, pinching in the belly. [*Gff.*]

After enjoying breakfast, weakness.

After every dinner, great heaviness in the feet, for 8 days.

After a moderate breakfast, a general sweat.

After and during a meal, anxiety.

395. After eating, headache.

Eructation (aft. 1½ h.). [*C.*]

Severe, almost constant eructation.

Very frequent eructation, as well before, as after a meal, chiefly in the afternoon, for 8 days (aft. 4 d.). [*C.*]

Frequent empty eructation, the whole day, chiefly in the afternoon. [*Gff.*]

400. **Frequent empty eructation, and preceded by transient pinching in the belly.** [*Gff.*]

Empty eructation after soup, and every time he drinks.

Eructation, after eating and drinking.

Eructation is always empty, and connected, especially in the afternoon, with accumulation of flatus in the abdomen. [*C.*]

By eructation, a mouth full of mucus is belched up, always a few hours after dinner.

405. Sweet eructation.

Bitter, scraping eructation.

Sour eructation toward evening, in the open air.

Sour eructation, after drinking milk.

Sour eructation, with burning in the stomach.

410. Sensation of constant heartburn; acid always rose up into the mouth.

Frequent sensation, in the forenoon, of something hot and acrid rising up the œsophagus.

Hiccup, especially after every movement.

Great tendency to hiccup, at the slightest occasion.

Nausea and lack of appetite, also before breakfast, still more after a meal, with anxiety, dizziness, obscuration of the eyes, and a white tongue; toward evening he had to lie down, without sleepiness (aft. 6, 7 d.).

415. Momentary attack of nausea.

Nausea, in the morning, an hour after awaking, with qualmishness in the stomach.

Nausea, every forenoon, about 10 or 11 o'clock.

Nausea, before dinner, even to retching.

Nausea, after every meal.

420. Nausea, at night.

Continual nausea, without appetite and without stool.

Nausea, with inclination to vomit (4th d.).

Often, an inclination to vomit, but he did not.

Waterbrash.

425. The region of the stomach is very sensitive.

Heaviness of the stomach, and, as it were, trembling therein.

Painfulness of the stomach, in walking and standing, as if heavy and pendant.

Aching in the scrobiculus cordis, in the evening, with sensitiveness of the same to the touch, with nausea and loathing if she only thought of eating.

The stomach seems tense and full.

430. Tension and pressure, extending transversely across the stomach from the ribs.

Pressive sensation in the region of the stomach, going off by the passage of flatus, with rumbling. [*C.*]

Pressure in the stomach, after rumbling in the abdomen.

Pressure in the stomach as from an ulcer, worse if touched.

Pressive sensation below the scrobiculus cordis (aft. 24 h.). [*C.*]

435. A constant painful pressure in the scrobiculus cordis and the epigastrium, seemingly in the stomach, after 7 P. M. [*Gff.*]

An anxious pressure in the scrobiculus cordis (aft. 4 d.).
Pinching in the scrobiculus cordis, as from flatus.
Cramp in the stomach, with incessant sour eructation.
Cramps in the stomach and cardialgia, with a nursing woman.

440. **Contractive spasm of the stomach**, even at night, rising up into the chest, with inflation of the abdomen; she had to double up, and could not lie down, because this aggravated it; the pain came by fits and took away her breath.

Contractive sensation under the stomach.

Contractive pain beside the scrobiculus cordis, on the right side; in the morning and afternoon.

A constrictive pain below the scrobiculus cordis, aggravated by the pressure of the finger. [*Ad.*]

On lying on the back and in taking a walk, he perceives the acidity of his stomach.

445. Gnawing in the stomach, in the morning, before breakfast.

Scratching in the stomach, extending up the throat, like heartburn.

Burning sensation in the stomach.
Constant burning in the stomach.
Throbbing in the scrobiculus cordis.

450. In the right hypochondrium, a short but violent pain. [*Gff.*]

The hepatic region is very sensitive and painful to the touch.

Pain, as from a bruise, in the liver.

Tension in the hepatic region, as if something was too short, on awaking from the noon siesta.

Pressive pain in the liver, on taking a walk in the open air.

455. Violent tearing pain in the liver, causing an outcry.

Violent stitches in the hepatic region (aft. 48 h.).
In the left hypochondrium, a pressive pain.
Pressive lancinating pain under the left breast.
Drawing pain under the left ribs.

460. In both hypochondria, painful, lancinating tearing, radiating from a point close below the scrobiculus cordis, toward both sides. [*Gff.*]

Both the hypochondria are painful to the touch.

When he stoops down, it seems to him, as if sausages were lying to the right and left beside the stomach.

Pressure under the short ribs, after breakfast. [*Gff.*]

Every piece of clothing, fitting tightly to the hypochondria, presses and is unbearable to him.

465. **Bellyache, as after catching cold**; it is aggravated before the passage of flatus, and continues even afterward.

Heaviness in the abdomen.
The abdomen seems to him very heavy.

Sensation as if the abdomen hung down heavily; she has to stoop forward in walking.

Pain over the whole abdomen down to the os pubis, as if all the muscular fibres were tense or indurated, which makes him very anxious.

470. **Tension of the abdomen, constant.** [*Gff.*]

Tension of the abdomen from accumulated flatus, which, however, passes copiously and easily in the afternoon. [*C.*]

The abdomen feels full and oppressed, and as if it were filled with food, day and night, with eructation.

Tensive and pressive pain in the right epigastrium, extending all over the stomach.

Tensive and pressive pain all over the whole abdomen, with continual restlessness and weeping, as from despair.

475. **Pressive colic in the hypogastrium.**

Pressive pain in the umbilical region.

Dull, pressive pain in a small spot in the abdomen. [*Gff.*]

A disagreeable pain in the abdomen, so that she would like to hold it always with her hands.

Pressive colic, with tenesmus and passage of hot flatus, which relieves it. [*Gff.*]

480. Pressive colic, with rumbling, and with the passage of warm, humid, odorless flatus, which removes it. [*Gff.*]

Pressive pain in the left side of the abdomen, moving about in the abdomen with pinching.

A pinching pressure, deep in the right side of the hypogastrium, toward the hip. [*Gff.*]

A squeezing pressure, deep in the hypogastrium. [*Gff.*]

Sqeezing colic in the hypogastrium. [*Gff.*]

485. Frequent, squeezing colic, especially in the right side of the abdomen. [*Gff.*]

Pinching pain in different parts of the abdomen, frequently passing quickly. [*C.*]

Fine pinching of the abdomen, while sitting crooked. [*C.*]

Violent pinching about the umbilical region, after partaking of a little harmless food; it quickly goes off through eructation and the emission of flatus. [*Gff.*]

Pinching about the navel, extending into the stomach, four days and nights (at first in the morning on rising); she had to lie down, could not stand upright for pain, with constant chill; only in the second night diarrhœa set in, worst at night (aft. 6 d.)

490. Pinching in the stomach, with good stool.

Pinching and lancinating pains in the left hypogastrium. [*Gff.*]

Constant pressive pinching in the epigastrium. [*Gff.*]

The pinching in the abdomen arises almost only in the afternoon and evening, and seems caused by flatus, after the passage of which it passes away. [*C.*]

Contractive sensation in the abdomen.

495. Cutting in the abdomen, like colic, in the evening.

Colic.

Cutting in the abdomen, only momentary, but very frequent.

Cutting in the abdomen, darting like lightning through the abdomen.

Tearing in the hypogastrium, up toward the navel (aft. 48 h.). [*Gff.*]

500. Tearing stitch in the hypogastrium, extending up to the navel. [*Gff.*]

Lancinating pain, aggravated by breathing, in the left side of the abdomen and chest. [*Gff.*]

Crawling, running stitches deep in the hypogastrium (aft. 28 h.) [*Gff.*]

Dull, pinching stitches, as if from below outward, in the abdomen. [*Gff.*]

Burning in the abdomen.

505. Burning about the umbilical region. [*Gff.*]

Great anguish in the abdomen.

Pain in the abdomen, as from straining in lifting, even when she only does something with her hand whereby the arm is stretched up a little; also on touching it, the same pain appears.

Pain in the abdomen, as from straining or spraining, as soon as she lies on her side; chiefly in the left side of the abdomen.

Externally on the hypogastrium, pain as from soreness, also when touching it (aft. 4 h.). [*Gff.*]

510. Pain as from soreness, in a spot under the navel. [*Gff.*]

Burning pain in the skin near the navel, often renewed (aft. 4 h.). [*Gff.*]

Pain as from a bruise in the abdominal muscles.

In the right inguinal region, pressive pain. [*Gff.*]

Pinching pain in the right inguinal region. [*Gff.*]

515. **Accumulation of flatus in the left epigastrium, more toward the back, with a squeezing pain.**

The flatus is obstructed here and there in the abdomen, below the short ribs, in the region of the bladder, causes squeezing and pressure, and gradually goes off with sensation of heat in the rectum. [*C.*]

The flatus inflates the abdomen in the afternoon. [*C.*]

The flatus causes intermittently a paralytic sensation in the left thigh (aft. 5 d.). [*C.*]

Colic from flatus, with passage of odorless flatus. [*Gff.*]

520. The flatus moves about in the abdomen, and there are single stitches now here now there, especially in the left side, toward the ribs. [*Gff.*]

Much flatus, with rumbling and audible moving about in the abdomen, in the afternoon. [*C.*]

Flatus keeps moving in the abdomen (at once). [*Gff.*]

Flatus keeps moving about deep in the hypogastrium. [*Gff.*]

There is a moving about in the abdomen, and much flatus, partly loud, partly noiseless and somewhat moist, passes. [*Gff.*]

525. Clucking in the left side of the hypogastrium. [*Gff.*]

Audible rumbling works about slowly in the abdomen (aft. 3 h.). [*Gff.*]

Loud rumbling and noise in the abdomen, for eight days. [*C.*]

Audible rumbling in the umbilical region. [*Ad.*]

Audible rumbling in the abdomen with some pinching. [*Ad.*]

530. After the rumbling, discharge of much flatus. [*Ad.*]

Unceasing noises in the abdomen, without tenesmus.

Fermentation in the abdomen, then diarrhœic stool with discharge of flatus of putrid odor.

Discharge of much odorless, loud flatus, with frequent eructation (aft. 4 d.). [*C.*]

Discharge of some odorless flatus, with much working about of flatus in the abdomen (aft. ½ h.). [*C.*]

535. In the afternoon, suddenly a great quantity of flatus, passing without trouble (aft. 36 h.). [*C.*].

Excessive discharge of odorless flatus, in the morning on awaking.

Even what else was easily digested, causes much flatus and inflation of the abdomen.

Flatus of putrid odor (aft. 1½ h.). [*Gff.*]

Much very fetid flatus (aft. 1 d.). [*C.*]

540. Discharge of flatus of a putrid odor, and lastly also humid, with painful bearing down toward the sacrum and thence to the abdomen (aft. 2 h.). [*Gff.*]

The urging to stool terminates with a loud discharge of flatus. [*Gff.*]

Sensation as if a stool should come, with burning in the anus and discharge of flatus. [*Gff.*]

On one day no stool, the next day two.

Totally constipated (aft. 67 h.). [*C.*]

545. Ineffectual urging to stool (aft. 80 h.). [*Gff.*]

Ineffectual urging to stool; only flatus was discharged, with painful pressure in the rectum.

Ineffectual urging to stool, in the evening (aft. 36 h.).

Sudden urging to stool, as if from fullness in the rectum, which soon went off. [*Ad.*].

Sensation in the abdomen and sacrum, like an ineffectual call to stool. [*Gff.*]

550. Violent urging to stool, with formication in the anus, and pressure on the bladder, toward the sacrum, like a hemorrhoidal colic, recurring in fits; instead of a stool, there follow violent labor-like pains in the hypogastrium, toward the front and the back, with burning in the anus, and a sensation as if diarrhœa were coming on; after these labor-like pains, with much effort, some fæces discharged, consisting of soft pieces, followed by a cessation of the pains. [*Gff.*]

A call to stool after breakfast; the stool, though not hard, passes only with much straining. [*Gff.*]

Violent urging to stool, but only a scanty and hard stool is passed. [*Gff.*]

Much straining at the stool, in the rectum.

Stool is unusually late in the evening, at 10 o'clock, with rumbling in the abdomen (aft. 44 h.). [*C.*]

555. The first week, rare stools, only every two or three days.

Every two or three days, a hard stool.

Hard stool. [*Gff.*]

Hard, delayed stool, with much straining (aft 30 h.). [*Gff.*]

Tough, scanty stool, not sufficiently homogeneous, with inactivity of the rectum (aft. 6 d.). [*C.*]

560. Stool, a second time (aft. 14 h.). [*C.*]

Pappy stool, with burning in the rectum.

Thinner stool than usual, with urging thereto (aft 20 h.). [*C.*]

Diarrhœa (aft. 48 h.).

Acrid stool, with coated tongue.

565. Discharge of mucus, with forcing toward the anus.

Mucus precedes the stool, then hard, followed by soft fæces, then cutting pain in the abdomen; during the first week.

Much mucus is discharged with the stool.

Much mucus is discharged from the rectum, for several days.

Yellowish, threadlike mucus is woven around the fæces, which in their latter portion are quite bloody. [*Ad.*]

570. Every six or seven minutes, the child screams out very loudly, while every time instead of fæces mucus with blood is discharged.

Before the stool, colic.

Before the stool, pains passing transversely through the abdomen. [*C.*]

With every stool, discharge of blood.

Flow of blood from the anus, with the stools.

575. During the stools (of scanty, hard, lumpy fæces) burning in the anus. [*C.*]

During stool, cutting in the anus. [*C.*]

During stool, stinging in the rectum, as from needles.

With hard stool, cutting pain in the anus. [*Gff.*]

After stool, repeated pains in the abdomen, extending toward the sacrum and the bladder, almost as after rhubarb. [*Gff.*]

580. **After stool**, forcing or griping **colic**. [*Gff.*]

After a hard, scanty morning-stool, pinching stinging in the left side of the hypogastrium, and incomplete urging to stool, like a pressure on the rectum, all day (aft. 4 d.). [*Gff.*]

After the stool, a total emptiness in the abdomen, especially sensible when walking. [*C.*]

After the stool he feels swollen in the abdomen, as from induration (2d d.).

After stool, burning in the anus.

585. After stool, lassitude.

After stool, anxiety, with tremulous sensation and involuntary motions.

After stool, tremulous weakness.

On the anus, smarting. [*Gff.*]

Pressive pain in the anus. [*Gff.*]

590. Gnawing in the rectum, between the stools.

Pinching in the rectum, between the stools.

Stitches toward the anus.

Several violent stitches in the anus, in the evening. [*C.*]

A very painful stitch through the rectum and anus, starting from the coccyx, as with a hot needle (aft. 6 d.). [*C.*]

595. Formication in the rectum, and torment from ascarides.

Discharge of ascarides.

Itching in the anus, in the morning in bed, increased by scratching, and followed by burning. [*C.*]

Itching in the anus, and after rubbing, a burning there. [*Gff.*]

Burning on the right side of the anus (aft. 6 h.). [*Gff.*]

600. Burning at the anus, with disagreeable sensation of dryness there (aft. 7 d.). [*C.*]

Burning and stinging at the anus.

Rush of blood to the anus.

Swollen, painful varices of the anus.

On the varices of the anus, tickling itching.

605. Flow of pure blood from the rectum, with tearing pains for several days; (with a young wife who had never had the like (aft. 7 d.). [*C.*]

Flow of an acrid, corrosive humor from the rectum (aft. 24 h.).

A viscid, musty-smelling fluid escapes at night in considerable quantity from the anus.

Moisture of the anus, with pressure upon it, during micturition.

Excoriation at the anus.

610. Excoriation, on the perinæum, with painful itching when touched.

Excoriation with itching and moisture of the perinæum, at night.

Shooting pain in the perinæum, near the anus. [*Gff.*]

Pressive pain as from soreness below the coccyx. [*Gff.*]

A large red blotch, close to the anus, with a black pimple on it, itching a little.

615. The urine passes much more sparingly (aft. 48 h.). [*Gff.*]

Much inclination to urinate, but the urine passed slowly.

Urging to urinate, almost every hour.

Pressure on the bladder, often by day, but she could retain the urine.

He must rise several times during the night to make water, and more urine is discharged, with pressure on the bladder.

620. Copious discharge of urine, after drinking but little (aft. 6 h.). [*Gff.*]

Copious light-yellow urine (aft. 24 h.). [*C.*]

Some thick, milky urine when about stopping to urinate.

Dark-colored urine.

Dark, red urine, accompanied with roughness of the throat. [*Gff.*]

625. **Dark-red urine, as if it was mixed with blood** (aft. 2 d.).

Reddish, turbid urine.

The urine remains clear, but nevertheless deposits some fine gravel.

Red sediment in the urine.

Very strong smell of the urine.

630. During micturition, itching of the female pudenda.

During micturition, stinging in the female pudenda.

Burning in the urethra during micturition.

During micturition, extremely painful burning and pinching in the urethra.

During micturition, often a tearing in the urethra; the last drops consist of mucus and give pain in passing.

635. After micturition, in the morning, tearing and drawing in the urethra. [*Gff.*]

Constriction of the urethra, every morning.

Pinching pains in the urethra (almost at once).

On the prepuce, itching and soreness.

Severe itching, soreness and a vesicle, on the inner side of the prepuce.

640. Formication in the testes and in the scrotum.

Itching near the scrotum on the thigh; with exudation of moisture (aft. 24 h.).

Swelling of the scrotum, hard to the touch.

Severe itching on the mons veneris.

Sexual instinct quite lacking, in the morning; not even excitable through sensual ideas (aft. 24 h.). [*Gff.*]

645. More lively sexual instinct (aft. 49 d.).

Frequent erections (aft. 24 d.). [*C.*]

Frequent, persistent erections, for three days in succession.

Persistent erections at night, without voluptuous sensation or fancies. [*Gff.*]

Pollution without dreams

650. Frequent pollutions, without much sensation.

Violent pollution, painfully affecting the nerves, and then violent burning, anteriorly in the urethra, with severe cutting and burning while urinating; this pain continued a long time and was renewed at the slightest external touch. [*Gff.*]

During coitus, quick emission of the semen, and then orgasm of the blood in the head.

Emission of prostatic juice, on straining to emit the stool.

On the female pudenda and on the anus, itching.

655. Heat and redness in the pudenda.

Burning on the female pudenda.

Severe soreness on the female pudenda, anteriorly, in the evening.

Aphthæ on the pudenda.

Red, sore spots, looking like little ulcers, on the pudenda; these do not pain, but merely itch, with emission of leucorrhœa.

660. Pain, as from excoriation, on the female pudenda, with discharge of leucorrhœa, for two days; then appearance of the menses which had not made their appearance for many months previously; these flowed for three days, but quite black; then only a very little leucorrhœa, without excoriation.

Menses five days too early (aft. 21 d.).

Menses six days too soon (2d d.).

Menses appear five days late (after-effect) (55th d.).

The menses, which appear six days late, were, as it were, excoriating, and made the parts sore.

665. The blood discharged at the menses was thick and of strong odor.

Before the menses set in, severe itching of a tetter.

Just before the menses, an itching eruption on the neck and between the shoulders.

Just before the menses, drawing pain from the hypogastrium into the sacrum.

Before the appearance of the menses, colic, like cramps, from morning till evening.

670. During the menses, cutting in the hypogastrium.

While the menses are flowing more sparingly, much colic, pain in the back, and pain in all the bones, as from a bruise.

During the menses, violent headache, contracting the eyes.

During the menses, burning in the hands and in the soles of the feet.

Leucorrhœa, flowing after micturition (12th d.).

675. Flow of white mucus from the vagina (aft. 4 d.).

Very much thin leucorrhœa, in the morning on rising, and then no more the whole day.

Milk-colored, excoriating leucorrhœa (aft. 12 d.).

Thickish, yellowish-white discharge from the vagina.

Greenish discharge from the vagina (6th d.).

680. Bloody mucus from the vagina (6th d.),

During the discharge from the vagina, soreness and rawness in the pudenda.

* * * * * * * *

The breath smells bad.

Frequent sneezing, with constant and violent formication and tickling in the nose, and catarrhal roughness in it and in the upper part of the chest, at night when in bed. [*Gff.*]

Repeated violent sneezing (aft. 5 h.). [*C.*]

685. Very frequent sneezing, without a cold. [*Gff.*]

Sneezing, with lachrymation of the left eye, causing smarting in the inner canthus. [*Gff.*]

Violent sneezing and then violently smarting pain above and in the nose, with lachrymation of the eyes, as when a severe cold breaks out; also when blowing the nose, there is pain. [*Gff.*]

Incomplete, ineffectual urging to sneeze, now stronger, now weaker. [*Gff.*]

Sneezing, with stitches in the abdomen. [*Gff.*]

690. Sneezing, with burning in a large part of the right side of the abdomen. [*Gff.*]

Ineffectual incitation to sneezing, with formication in the left half of the nose, which then became moist, but after blowing it, the right nostril remained stopped up, with a formication and smarting (as if from coryza) in the left side of the palate (aft. 5 d.). [*Gff.*]

Stoppage of the left nostril, for an hour. [*Gff.*]

Stoppage of the left nostril (aft. 1½ h.). [*C.*]

Stoppage of the left nostril, after sneezing. [*Gff.*]

695. **Stuffed coryza.**

Stuffed coryza, with scraping in the throat.

Stuffed coryza, for several days.

Sensation of an incipient cold, in the root of the nose. [*Ad.*]

Pressure in the root and the bones of the nose, as in a severe cold; but he can draw air through the nose. [*Ad.*]

700. Irritation to coryza for several days, at night, and in the morning on awaking; this (with the exception of occasional sneezing) went off during the day. [*Gff.*]

Itching irritation in the nose, with increased moisture (aft. 7 h.). [*C.*]

Increased moisture in the nose, after previous stoppage (aft. 3 h.). [*C.*]

Discharge of mucus from the nose, with formication in the right nostril; then violent sneezing, lachyrmation of the right eye and coryza. [*Gff.*]

Discharge of green mucus from the nose.

705. Fluent coryza, with sneezing (almost at once). [*Gff.*]

Fluent coryza, every evening.

Violent fluent coryza.

Cold, with catarrh (aft. 7 d.).

Severe coryza, with hoarseness and rawness in the chest (2d d.).

710. Sensation of dryness in the throat and the posterior nares.

Unusual sensation of dryness in the windpipe, not relieved by hawking, for several days (aft. 3 d.). [*C.*]

Hoarseness, in the evening (aft. 12 d.).

In the morning, almost aphonous.

Catarrh, so that he can hardly speak aloud (aft. 8 d.).

715. Sudden great hoarseness in the evening, so that he could hardly utter a sound, with violent tightness of the chest, which almost took all his breath away, when taking a walk (aft. 6 d.)

Hoarseness and roughness of the larynx, so that she could not speak aloud without great effort.

Slight roughness of speech, as if he felt oppressed, or affected by speaking (aft. 3 d.). [*C.*]

Severe roughness of the larynx, with deep roughness of the voice, which fails him when he exerts his voice, but without pain in the throat. [*Gff.*]

Roughness on the chest, and frequent irritation to cough. [*Gff.*]

720. Sensation of roughness in the throat, posteriorly (aft. 3 d.). [*C.*]

Scraping in the throat (aft. 3 d.). [*C.*]

Scraping in the throat, evening and morning, exciting her to a dry cough.

Scrapy feeling in the throat, with some cough, causing lachrymation, especially in the left eye. [*Gff.*]

Severe formication in the throat, only transiently relieved by clearing it, with much collection of saliva. [*Gff.*]

725. Crawling in the upper part of the windpipe, as if something adhered there, which excites coughing (aft. 3 h.). [*Gff.*]

Crawling and itching in the larynx, with wheezing during respiration; the mucus adheres firmly to his chest, and he has to cough (dry) in the evening on lying down.

After the coryza is past, there is a heavy sensation on the chest, and boiling and rattling; he cannot stay in bed at night for lack of air, and the cough, which comes on in fits so as almost to make him vomit detaches mucus only with difficulty.

In the morning, on rising, he feels a heavy oppression on his chest, like catarrh, and he has to cough a few times violently, but pains then dart through his head.

Light fits of coughing, a few impulses at a time (after five minutes); they are repeated about the same hour on the third day. [*C.*]

730. Cough, caused by tickling in the larynx (with tough, salty[1] expectoration), in the evening when going to sleep, and in the morning, an hour after rising. [*C.*]

Irritation to cough, returning frequently, posteriorly in the throat, with a short cough. [*Gff.*]

Violent tickling cough, with whitish expectoration, in the morning after awaking.

Half voluntary rough cough, with constant sensation of roughness and formication in the throat. [*Gff.*]

Cough, caused by irritation and formication in the throat, in several deep impulses, whereupon the chest pains as if pressed in. [*Gff.*]

735. Irritation to cough, as from sulphurous fumes, with retching.

Repeated cough, from irritation in the upper part of the chest, and roughness and scraping in the throat (aft. 3 d.). [*C.*]

After every expiration, he has a fit of dry cough, with a flush of heat and sweat.

Cough, after taking the least cold, in the morning on rising from bed, or when she comes from a warm room into a cold one.

Cough every time, when he has eaten to satiety.

740. **Evening cough,** in bed, and before going to sleep.

Nocturnal cough in repeated fits, with ever recurring irritation to cough.

Short hacking cough, in the evening.

He has often to clear his throat in the evening, so that his larynx becomes raw and sore.

Frequent fits of short cough. [*Gff.*]

745. **Spasmodic cough,** daily in three or four fits.

Spasmodic cough in the evening, for five hours (from walking too briskly?) (6th d.).

Cough which fatigues, with tightness and burning of the chest.

Cough, causing vomiting and retching in the evening.

Rough cough, without any expectoration.

750. Expectoration of mucus from the larynx, by a short hacking cough.

Expectoration of whole pieces of green mucus.

Severe cough, with much expectoration of yellow pus, and lancinating pain in the left hypochondrium on breathing, followed by violent stitches in the upper part of the left side of the chest,

[1] The original has *satzigem*, "leaving a sediment;" probably a misprint for *salzigem* "salty"—*Transl.*

With a rough cough, pain in the upper part of the chest. [*Gff.*]

In coughing, pain on the chest, as if flesh were raw.

755. In coughing, severe pain in the larynx and in the region of the thyroid cartilage, as if from an ulcer.

In coughing, painful stitches through the head.

During the excitation to cough, in the evening, a chilliness and a drawing in the cheeks.

Her respiration ceased, just as she began to go to sleep, with increased vertigo.

On turning over in bed, she gets out of breath.

760. Urging to take a deep breath, with groaning.

He has to take a deep breath, with an effort of his chest, abdomen, back, nape and head, with drawing up of his feet.

Difficult breathing, more while sitting down.

Difficult breathing, in the evening, while lying down, with throbbing in the head.

Dyspnœa, from phlegm on the chest.

765. Difficult breathing, fullness of the chest and palpitation, even from slight exercise, chiefly toward evening.

Short breath and anxious oppression of the chest; he could not sit down, but had to walk about continually, for ten days.

On account of much tightness of the chest, she had to walk more slowly than usual.

Very tight and fatigued on the chest, on awaking.

Tightness of the chest and short breath, as from flatus pressing upward (aft. 41 h.). [*Gff.*]

770. Tight, oppressed sensation on the chest, as if coming from the abdomen and from flatus. [*C.*]

Sensation of tightness on the chest, which passes off at once after eructations.

Spasmodic tightness and contraction of the chest, for three or four minutes.

As if pressed together in the breast and shoulders, in the morning on rising from bed.

Constriction of the chest, in frequent fits, with obstruction of the breath.

775. Breath quite cold; also coldness in the throat, the mouth and the teeth.

In inspiring, pressure in the windpipe.

On respiring, painful throbbing in the head and in the teeth.

In the chest, pain as from obstructed flatus.

Pain, on expanding the chest.

780. Dull pain on the sternum, on a small spot, just above the scrobiculus cordis, excited as well in stooping forward, as in touching it. [*Gff.*]

Dull pain, first in the left, then in the right side of the chest, more noticeable in expiring than in inspiring. [*Gff.*]

Dull pain on the right side of the chest (aft. 6 h.). [*Gff.*]

Rheumatic pain extending from the left ribs, down to the hip. [*Gff.*]

Pressive rheumatic pain in the right side, on the short ribs, for a quarter of an hour. [*Gff.*]

785. **Pressive pain in the upper part of the right side of the chest**, extending into the right scapula. [*Gff.*]

Pressure on the left side of the chest. [*Gff.*]

Frequently, a squeezing pressure on the chest. [*Gff.*]

Pinching in small spots on the chest, caused by flatus. [*C.*]

A pressive tearing on the left side of the chest (aft. 26 h.). [*Gff.*]

790. Tearing from the chest toward the back, in the morning, in bed, extending into the arms and the left ear, with internal heat, especially in the head.

Tearing in the right side of the chest. [*Gff.*]

Drawing rheumatic pain on the right short ribs. [*Gff.*]

Painful drawing in the chest (the shoulders and the arms), more on the left side, with sensation of heat and rush of blood to the head, while she is cold to the touch.

Lancinating pain in the cardiac region (7th d).

795. Lancinating pain, increased on inspiration, in the right side of the chest and abdomen. [*Gff.*]

Deep stitch in the right side of the chest, on taking a deep breath. [*Gff.*]

Very painful stitches through the chest, obstructing the breath, when going to sleep. [*Gff.*]

Obtuse stitch in the left part of the chest, toward the short ribs. [*Gff.*]

Violent obtuse stitches, as if stabbing outward, deep down in the right side of the chest. [*Gff.*]

800. Severe stitches under the left breast; she could not sleep nor walk for them; they also continued when sitting (without chill or heat).

Contractive stitches in the lower part of the left side of the chest, obstructing the breath (3d d.).

Obtusely lancinating, oppressive pain in the cardiac region, going off with an audible rumbling in the left side, as from obstructed but now released flatus (aft. 3 h.). [*Gff.*]

Sense of weakness and fatigue of the chest.

On awaking, he feels as if his chest were wearied.

805. Itching, internally in the chest.

Rush of blood to the chest, in the morning on awaking, with coated tongue.

Ebullition in the blood, and rush of blood to the chest, with hoarseness and hawking.

She constantly felt as if the blood was rising to the chest, while her body felt cold.

Warm orgasm in the chest, with oppression, caused by accumulated flatus in the abdomen (aft. 9 d.). [*C.*]

810. Rush of blood to the chest and burning in it.

Severe burning in the chest, as from glowing coals, almost uninterruptedly.

Burning on the left side of the chest, and on the right side near the scrobiculus cordis.

More burning is felt in the cardiac region than stinging pains.

Palpitation of the heart, chiefly in sitting.

815. Frequent palpitations, several quick throbs.

Excessive palpitation, for several days.

Palpitation and intermitting pulse, in the evening on going to sleep, for several days.

Pulsation in the chest, with restlessness and anxiety; she plainly felt the heart beat, with her hand.

Externally on the left side of the chest, on touching it, a pain like tension and pressure.

820. In the region of the coccyx, a pricking itching, in the evening in bed.

In the sacrum, sensation of coldness, numbness and tension.

Tensive pain and stiffness in the sacrum.

Severe pain in the sacrum; she cannot sit, for it then feels as if there were a plug in her back; she must put a pillow under her.

Tearing pressure in the sacrum. [*Gff.*]

825. Tearing pressive pain on the left side beside the hip, extending into the back. [*Gff.*]

Tearing pain in the sacrum, at times drawing into the hips (aft. 3 d.). [*C.*]

Tearing in the hips, with intermission (aft. 3 d.). [*C.*]

Drawing pressive pain in the sacrum down into the coccyx (aft. 24 h.). [*C.*]

Above the right loin, a pain that obstructs respiration.

830. Violent burning, externally on the right hip. [*Gff.*]

The back pains on the side, as if bruised.

Weakness in the back.

Heaviness in the back, and tightness of the chest.

Jerking of the muscles in the left side of the back. [*Gff.*]

835. Painful stiffness of the back, in the morning on rising.

Pressive pain, beside the lowest part of the back.

A squeezing pressive pain, beside the lowest part of the spine.

Painful pinching, beside the spine.

Drawing pain in the back, mostly in sitting down.

840. Drawing pain in the back, in the evening.

Rheumatic drawing in the back, especially when stooping, for several days. [*C.*]

Rheumatic pain at the upper part of the left scapula after the (accustomed) washing with water (not cold). [*C.*]

Rheumatic sensation in the whole of the left scapula, when writing (aft. 6 h.). [*C.*]

Violent tearing in the left scapula, on bending back the arm. [*Gff.*]

845. Tearing in the lower part of the back, beside the sacrum. [*Gff.*]

Stitches between the scapulæ, obstructing the breathing, at night.

Warmth in the spine, up to the neck.

Burning in the left side of the upper part of the back.

Burning in the right scapula. [*Gff.*]

850. In the cervical muscles, an obtuse burning pain. [*C.*]

The neck and the head shake and tremble, in paroxysms.

Painful pressive pain in the cervical muscles (aft. 4 d.). [*C.*]

Pressive and tensive pain in the nape, seemingly in the cervical vertebræ.

Drawing pain in the nape of the neck, ascending to the head, and into it, causing nausea with running of water from the mouth.

855. **Tearing in the cervical muscles.** [*Gff.*]

Tearing pain in the cervical muscles of the left side, especially when moving (aft. 3 d.). [*C.*]

Pressive tearing in the cervical muscles of the left side, for two days (aft. 3 d.). [*C.*]

On the neck, pressive pain (aft. 6 d.).

Violent pressive pain in the cervical muscles (of the right side). [*Gff.*]

360. **Pressive tearing in the cervical muscles.** [*Gff.*]

The cervical glands swell and pain, especially the posterior ones toward the nape.

Lancinating itching on the throat and neck, and red spots there (aft. 38 h.). [*C.*]

Single, scattered, red unequal little spots on the neck, with painful itching in the evening (aft. 48 h.). [*C.*]

Eruption of pimples on the neck.

865. Under the right axilla, a pressive, drawing pain, especially noticeable on motion. [*Gff.*]

Burning pain in the right axilla. [*Gff.*]

Itching, moisture and excoriation in the axillæ.

In the shoulder, a drawing pain.

Drawing pain in the left shoulder-joint. [*Gff.*]

870. Painful drawing in both shoulder-joints, as well in motion as in rest (aft. 26 h.). [*C.*]

Rheumatic drawing in the right shoulder. [*Gff.*]

Violently tearing pain in the right shoulder-joint, especially on motion, with drawing in the shafts of the arms. [*Gff.*]

Tearing pain in the shoulder-joint (aft. 10 h.). [*C.*]

Paralytic tearing in the right shoulder-joint, often recurring.

875. Stitches in the right shoulder, by day and by night.

Burning on the top of the right shoulder. [*Gff.*]

Burning on the shoulder-joint (aft. 3 h.). [*Gff.*]

Paralytic weakness of the right shoulder and the right arm (aft. ¼ h.). [*C.*]

The arms are heavy and lazy in moving (aft. 4 h.). [*C.*]

880. Heaviness in the arms, with drawing in the back.

Pain as from a bruise in the right arm.

Cramp in the arms.

Drawing in the right arm.

The arms and hands frequently go to sleep in daytime, but chiefly at night, so that she don't know, when in bed, where to lay them.

885. His upper arm feels especially heavy. [*C.*]

Drawing pain in the upper arm, with burning. [*Gff.*]

Obtuse drawing on the inner side of the left upper arm (aft. 4 h.). [*C.*]

Drawing pains from above downward, in the right upper arm (aft. 4 h.). [*C.*]

Tearing in the left upper arm (aft. 5 h.). [*Gff.*]

890. Tearing in the left upper arm, in single paroxysms (aft. 4 d.). [*C.*]

Violent tearing in the right upper arm, especially on moving it (aft. 5 d.). [*C.*]

Burning in the upper part of the upper arms (aft. 5 h.). [*Gff.*]

Burning itching, frequently repeated, on the lower part of the inner side of the left upper arm, only transiently removed by scratching (aft. 54 h.). [*C.*]

A large furuncle on the upper arm, and many itching pimples around it (aft. 7 d.).

895. In the elbow-joints of both arms, pains as if crushed, at once early in bed.

Burning on the right elbow. [*Gff.*]

In the forearm, drawing pain, down the shaft of the radius toward the wrist (at once). [*C.*]

Tearing in the whole of the right forearm. [*C.*]

A drawing tearing in the left forearm, from the elbow to the hand (aft. 48 h.). [*Gff.*]

900. Drawing tearing in the left radius (aft. 14 h.). [*C.*]

Drawing tearing in the upper side of the left forearm, near the elbow; this spot is also painful on pressing on the shaft of the bone (aft. 3 h.). [*Gff.*]

The drawing and tearing in the forearm extends, especially while moving, into the hand and the fingers. [*C.*]

Burning itching on the forearm, near the elbow. [*Gff.*]

On the back of the hand, a pressive pain (aft. 4 d.). [*C.*]

905. Sensation in the left wrist-joint, as if the tendons were too short, in certain motions.

Spasmodic contraction of the hand.

Drawing pain in the wrist.

Drawing in the right metacarpal bone (aft. ¾ h.). [*C.*]

Tearing in the left palm, from the root of the little finger inward. [*Gff.*]

910. **Tearing in the right or the left wrist.** [*Gff.*]

Throbbing pain in the hand, in the metacarpal bone of the middle finger. [*Ad.*]

Icy cold hands (aft. 48 h.). [*Gff.*]

Sweaty balls of the hands.

The hands go to sleep.

915. Sensation on washing in the morning as if the hands would go to sleep.

Tendency of the hands to grow numb.

Pain as from being bruised on the back of the left hand. [*Gff.*]

Paralytic pain in the wrist, on motion.

A pain as from straining in the right hand and wrist, as if he had overstrained it by grasping too strongly (aft. 3 d.). [*C.*]

920. Sensation in the hands as if their muscular power was weakened, especially sensible in writing (aft. 6 h.). [*Gff.*]

Writing proceeds slowly and with difficulty (aft. 4½ h.). [*C.*]

A small swelling on the side of the bend of the wrist.

Severe itching in the palms, at night.

Fine, itching eruption on the hands.

925. After a severe stitch in the hand (in the evening) her second and third fingers were spasmodically drawn over each other, making the others further distant.

Tearing in the fingers of the left hand.

Tearing pains in several fingers, in the evening. [*C.*]

Tearing in the fingers of the right hand (aft. 6 h.). [*Gff.*]

Fine tearing in the second and third fingers of the right hand. [*Gff.*]

930. Tearing in the joints of the last two fingers. [*Gff.*]

Tearing in the right little finger, aggravated by motion. [*Gff.*]

Violent tearing in the posterior joint of the left index. [*Gff.*]

Fine tearing in the middle joint of the right index. [*Gff.*]

Tearing in the tip and under the nail of the left fourth finger (aft. 48 h.). [*Gff.*]

935. Tearing under the thumb-nail. [*Gff.*]

Fine tearing in the right thumb, as if in the bone. [*C.*]

Fine burning tearing in the tip of the right thumb. [*Gff.*]

Gouty pain in the anterior joint of the thumb.

Drawing in the right index, toward the tip.

940. Stitches in a finger, on rising from a seat.

Stitch in the posterior joint of the left middle finger (aft. ¾ h.). [*C.*]

Sudden, deep stitch in the anterior joint of the right middle finger (aft. 41 h.). [*C.*]

Stitches, as from a splinter, in the distal phalanx of the fourth finger. [*C.*]

Stitches in the ball of the thumb, starting from the wrist.

945. Fine stitches in the skin of the right index, renewed by flexing the arm (aft. 2 h.). [*C.*]

Tearing shooting in the middle joints of the fingers.

Boring pain in the proximal joints of the middle finger and the thumb. [*Ad.*]

Boring pain in the middle joint of the left index, at rest; but on motion or on flexing it, a fine pricking pain, as from a splinter, for six hours. [*Ad.*]

Throbbing on the back of the thumb, repeated. [*C.*]

950. A slow throbbing pain in the distal phalanx. [*Ad.*]

Chilling burning in the proximal phalanges of the right middle and ring fingers. [*Gff.*]

The finger-tips are covered with a cold sweat.

Swelling of the distal phalanx of the left middle finger, with drawing pains in it.

Paralysis and weakness of the right fingers, in grasping something. [*C.*]

955. Violent itching on the outer side of the left thumb.

In the right hip, tearing. [*Gff.*]

Tearing pressive pain under and beside the left hip, toward the back and the sacrum, often recurring. [*Gff.*]

Drawing pain in the hip-joint down the thigh, aggravated by walking.

The lower limbs are painful, both of them, especially the legs, while sitting and lying, so that he knows not where to place them.

960. Tearing in the thighs and legs. [*Gff.*]

Tearing in the right lower limb, from the thigh down through the leg. [*C.*]

Tearing in the lower limbs; this seems aggravated by accumulation of flatus. [*C.*]

Sensation of drawing in the lower limbs, especially in the legs. [*Gff.*]

Severe paralytic drawing pain from the abdomen down the left lower limb. [*Gff.*]

965. Sensation of restlessness in the right thigh and leg, which compels him to continually shift his position in sitting. [*C.*]

The lower limbs go to sleep (3d d.).

Numbness and insensibility of the lower limbs.

Lassitude and sensation of paralysis in both the lower limbs (aft. 40 h.). [*C.*]

Sensation of rigidity in the lower limbs after the evening nap, so that he was unsteady in his walk until he had walked awhile.

970. Relaxation in the lower limbs, so that he could not lift them up, from noon till evening.

Heaviness in the lower limbs (aft. 5 d.).

In the thighs rigidity above the knee, early on rising.

Rigidity in the thigh and drawing, like paralysis or dislocation (the first 4 days).

Cramp-like pain in the lower and outer part of the left thigh, when walking, and especially when raising the thigh and going up-stairs; the parts are also painful to the touch (aft. 35 h.). [*C.*]

975. Contractive pain in the thigh, down to the knee, so that it gives way in walking.

Muscular subsultus on the posterior part of the left thigh, in morning in bed. [*Gff.*]

Tearing pain in the middle of the thigh, often recurring. [*Gff.*]

Rheumatic drawing in the left thigh, in the evening in bed, alleviated by lying on it. [*Gff.*]

Stitches dart down the thigh in walking (12th d.).

980. Obtuse pain in the upper part of the thigh. [*Gff.*]

Burning on the thigh, at night, in bed.

Burning sensation in the upper and outer part of the thigh.

Numbness of the thighs in walking.

On slightly knocking the knee against anything, severe pain in the bone.

985. Pain in the knees on going up-stairs.

Tension in the knees and ankles (aft. 5th d.).

Tension in the houghs, as from weariness, without previous exercise.

Stiffness and weakness in the knee.

Drawing pain in the knees, while standing.

990. Pressive tearing in both knees and legs.

Shooting pains in the patella, after rising from sitting, with a sensation as if the knee was swollen.

Burning pain on the inner side of the left knee. [*C.*]

Severe burning on the right knee. [*Gff.*]

Paralytic pain on the knees, while sitting and on rising trom a seat, also at night while lying in bed, when she turns over or stretches out the knee.

995. Lassitude and sensation of unsteadiness in the knees, while walking and standing. [*G.ff*]

Paralytic sensation in the knee-joints after walking.

Itching pimples on the knee.

In the leg, a severe cramp, especially in the sole of the foot, on taking a walk.

Severe cramp in the whole (lower) leg, at night in bed, especially in the sole of the foot.

1000. Drawing sensation in the leg from the knee downward. [*Gff.*]

Rheumatic drawing in both legs, down to the metatarsal bones (aft. 45 h.). [*C.*]

Drawing and gnawing in both legs; he cannot let them lie still, and at one time he has to stretch them, at another to draw them up, for half an hour.

Drawing in the left leg, with restlessness in it. [*C.*]

Tickling restlessness in the legs, in the evening.

1005. Tearing in the right leg. [*Gff.*]

Tearing in the leg, from the calf down, to the inner ankle. [*Gff.*]

Stitches in a nodosity in the calf.

Swollen spot in the calf, painful to the touch.

Paralytic sensation in the left leg.

1010. Itching blotches on the calves.

In the soles of the feet, cramp, in the evening after lying down; it drew his toes crooked.

Pain in the metatarsal bones, as if they were being torn, when treading.

Tearing in the bone above the left ankle. [*Gff.*]

Drawing in the feet, chiefly when sitting.

1015. A stitch at times in the left ankle, as if sprained.

Burning in the soles of the feet after standing.

Burning in the soles of the feet, on sitting and walking.

Copious foot-sweat (aft. 9 d.).

Sweating feet when walking.

1020. Swelling of the sick foot.

Restlessness in the left foot; he had to move it to and fro.

In walking, the soles of the feet pained, as if too soft. [*Gff.*]

In the toes of the right foot, tearing pain, aggravated in walking. [*Gff.*]

Tearing in the middle toes of the right foot. [*Gff.*]

1025. Severe tearing under the toe-nails, from evening to night; it extended into the soles (the first 4 days.).

Pain under the nail of the right big toe. [*Gff.*]

Pain in the joint of the big toe.

A stitch darted into the right big toe.

Lancinating pain in a corn of the little toe.

1030. Rigidity in the knee-joints and hip-joints, in the morning on awaking.

Tension in the knees and in the left hand as if fatigued by too great exertion.

Drawing pain in the limbs.

Drawing pain in almost all parts of the body, especially below the chest, in the nape and in the arms.

Drawing in the back and the feet, only in sitting.

1035. Drawing pain in the sacrum, the abdomen and the left side of the back, extending up into the arms; the left side of his body was drawn together quite crooked.

Drawing in the joints of the wrist, the elbow and the shoulder, chiefly in the morning wind and going off when moving.

Rheumatic drawing in the whole body, with coldness of the hands and feet. [*Gff.*]

Drawing pain in the hands and feet.

Tearing in various parts of the body, at night in bed.

1040. Tearing in the left shoulder in the morning on awaking, then in the right hand, then in the right upper jaw, in the incisors. [*Gff.*]

Frequent tearing pains here and there, *e.g.*, in the left half of the occiput and of the face, in the left shoulder, the left thigh, etc., with severe pressure in the arms and legs. [*Gff.*]

Tearing and drawing pains in various parts of the body. [*Gff.*]

To these drawing and tearing pains in the limbs are gradually added slight burning pains. [*C.*]

When these tearing, drawing, burning pains even for a short time attacked the external chest, they always brought with them a sensation of tightness of breath. [*C.*]

1045. Most of the pains appear on talking a walk in the open air.

With the pains great anguish and heat.

With every slight pain she feels unhappy.

After the pains, great lassitude.

After two days' duration of the (rheumatic) pains an excessive sensation of lassitude in the parts seized. [*C.*]

1050. The blood is in a state of great ebullition.

Formication in the whole body.

The limbs go to sleep.

The limbs on which he lies are apt to go to sleep.

Bruised feeling of all the limbs.

1055. Sensation of great bruisedness in the joints, the limbs feel better when stretched, in the morning on awaking, in bed; the sensation gradually goes off on rising. [*Gff.*]

Great heaviness in the left arm and leg like paralysis.

After long sitting, he feels, on rising, heaviness and stiffness in the limbs which goes off after a little walking.

Lack of energy in the motions of the muscles (aft. 1 h.). [*C.*]

The bends of the joints seem unable to sustain the body (aft. 5 d.). [*C.*]

1060. Every limb in the body aches, so also the back, with much headache and great weakness.

Tremulousness of the body with feeling of decrepitude.

Indisposed to bodily exertions. [*C.*]

Lassitude, especially in the legs. [*Ad.* and *Gff.*]

General relaxation toward noon; inclination to lean the head against something and to rest; emptiness of the head, with sensation of hunger (aft. 12 h.). [*C.*]

1065. Sensation of great lassitude in the morning, with trembling of the limbs and around the stomach, as after much drinking of wine (aft. 24 h.). [*Gff.*]

Painful weakness in the body in the evening, as from the loss of much blood.

He is fatigued and languid as if he had risen from a severe illness.

Weakness as from stupefaction in the forenoon.

The lassitude is chiefly observable in walking; less in sitting, and then chiefly in the arms while writing. [*C.*]

1070. Lassitude after a short slow walk in the open air. [*Gff.*]

Sudden lassitude while walking in the open air; but this soon vanished (aft. 3 d.).

Fits of sudden fainting weakness.

Very often only momentary fits of fainting as if about to sink down, also at times with vertigo; then colic and griping in the abdomen as if diarrhœa was coming, but only an ordinary stool came (aft. 24 h.)

Attack of vertigo in the forenoon with nausea and obscuration of the eyes, ringing before the ears; trembling; a warm sweat all over the body which stood in drops on the forehead; shortly before the fit, epistaxis in a few drops.

1075. An attack: in looking out of the window, he is suddenly seized with nausea and vertigo; he falls down unconscious and lies thus for several minutes, and when he regained his senses he felt as if he had lain in a deep sleep from which he can hardly rouse himself; after waking up, inclination to vomit, which obliged him to lie down for two hours, and was renewed when he rose up; then he became very lachrymose and desperate (aft. 6 d.).

An attack: the boy becomes hoarse, turns up his eyes (as if there were stitches in them) when he wants to speak, and water collects in them; then his cheek gets red, he has pain on deglution, breathes loudly in his sleep; he coughs, vomits up the milk, becomes obstinate and cries often (aft. several hours).

In the warm room he is apt to sweat on the trunk and then he easily catches cold.

Itching all over the body, day and night.

Severe itching on the arms, the hands and between the fingers, so that he could not sleep at night, but without any eruption.

1080. Itching stitches on the side on which he is lying, in the evening in bed.

Itching as from flea-bites in various parts of the body. [*C.*]

Fine slight stinging all over the body, when she becomes warm in bed.

Itching and stinging in various parts of the body. [*C.*]

Itching and burning in various parts of the skin, on the back, the chest, the navel, the thighs, etc. [*Gff.*]

1085. **Burning on various parts of the skin**, at night in bed.

Slightly burning pains on various parts of the skin. [*C.*]

Burning on the skin, as from a mustard-plaster, here and there on the back, in the sides, on the right side of the abdomen, etc. (aft. 12 h.). [*Gff.*]

Nettle-rash, for several weeks (aft. 4 d.).

An old wound from a stab begins again to bleed, at various times.

1090. A spot rubbed sore, which was almost covered again with epidermis, began again to be denuded and to become moist.

An ulcer on the leg now feels pressed upon and tense.

A healed ulcer again breaks out, and discharges instead of pus, lymph mixed with blood; the part is hard and painful when touched.

The ulcer of the fontanelle discharges a corrosive humor.

The pus of the ulcer becomes fetid like carrion.

1095. Lassitude, in the morning in bed. [*Gff.*]

In the morning great lassitude and stretching of the limbs.

Languid and unrefreshed she rises in the morning from her sleep, but after a few hours she feels stronger.

Sensation of great lassitude in the morning in bed, especially in the joints; going off after rising. [*Gff.*]

Lazy, languid, tremulous in the limbs, in the morning, and easily thrown into perspiration (aft. 2 d.). [*C.*]

1100. In the evening, lassitude.

Laziness in the evening, drowsiness and indisposition to everything.

Yawning. [*Ad.*]

Much yawning and stretching. [*Gff.* and *C.*]

Frequent stretching and extending the limbs, whence he feels better (aft. 5 d.). [*C.*]

1105. Sleepiness with frequent yawning. [*Gff.*]

Sleepiness, which passes off by exercise, in the forenoon, while sitting and in reading. [*Ad.*]

Inclination to sleep, after dinner, without being able to get to sleep.

Great sleepiness by day; he had to sleep before and after noon; at night his sleep was full of phantasies (aft. 8 d.).

After a meal a sleep lasting for hours, uninterrupted, but made uneasy by anxious dreams. [*Ad.*]

1110. After eating, excessive drowsiness.

In the evening, very early, inclination to sleep.

In the evening, excessive drowsiness.

Late in falling asleep, not before 1 A. M.

He cannot get to sleep at night, though his eyes are full of sleep.

1115. She cannot fall asleep at night, nor can she open her eyes.

Insomnia, on account of restlessness of body.

Uneasy sleep, without refreshment; in the morning, light perspiration.

Uneasy sleep and frequent awaking (1st night).

Awakes at 4 A. M.

1120. Restless sleep, with frequent awaking, and early in bed headache, with burning here and there on the body. [*Gff.*]

In the evening after lying down he is overcome with anguish, so he can hardly remain abed (aft. 9 d.).

In the evening after lying down, anguish, as from oppression of the chest, with heat in the head, heat in the hands and sweat on her forehead; she could not remain abed, for feeling as if her heart would be crushed; the objects around seemed to her to become ever closer and smaller, and when it was dark in the room extremely frightful forms appeared before her vision.

In the evening in bed, shooting headache, extending even into the occiput (aft. 16 h.).

In the evening after lying down, his eyes ached.

1125. In the evening in bed, a drawing sensation in both his lower limbs.

In the evening in bed, restlessness in her lower limbs; she often had to stretch them.

Several evenings in bed, violent twitching in the arms and legs, which for a long time kept her from going to sleep.

On going to sleep he starts up and is startled.

In the evening, very cold feet and hands.

1130. In the evening in bed, the feet will not get warm before one o'clock.

At night in sleep, illusion of hearing; he thinks he hears somebody walking, who comes before his bed; this wakes him up with anxiety.

At night, with a shudder in his back he is startled at a noise.

At night he wakes up several times on account of pulsation of the head, as if about to have a stroke of apoplexy; immediately after awaking he was composed, and felt that it was an illusion, for the throbbing in the head had ceased; but when he attempted to observe in slumber what should happen, his legs and knees were drawn up involuntarily and his back bent; and he felt that if he had not aroused he would have fainted.

At night, after going to sleep, he wakes up in several attacks, with a sensation of a rush of blood to the head, with hair on end; anxiety, accompanied with a shiver, and a feeling as if some one stroked with the hand over his body, and as if ants were running over his skin at every movement in bed; at the same time the hearing was so sensitive and acute that the slightest sound re-echoed in the ear.

1135. At night, headache.

At night, severe pain in the occiput and boring in the sinciput, with sweat, very pale face, cold, trembling hands and nausea at the stomach.

At night, a pressure below the stomach, with restless sleep and anxious dreams.

At night he awakes every hour with erections.

She is waked up very early by urging to micturition.

1140. At night, continual sneezing.

At night, heaviness in the back and in the limbs, like weariness.

At night, drawing pains in the arm, on which he is lying.

At night, restless, with drawing pains in the limbs.

She cannot rest quiet at night, except by drawing up her legs to her body.

1145. At night in bed, the corns ache with pressive pain.

At night she often awakes with coldness in the limbs and knees.

At night she often awakes with heat and thirst.

Before midnight, profuse sweat of the body and even of the head.

In the morning on awaking, tremulous anxiety.

1150. At 3 A. M., on awaking from a restless sleep with many anxious dreams, a violent squeezing colic, like labor pains, which especially pressed upon the sacrum (and the bladder), with rumbling in the belly. [*Gff.*]

In the morning in bed, shooting pains under the left ribs and from there radiating into the belly, the scrobiculus cordis and the chest, pressing upon the larynx; aggravated by breathing and when passing off, renewed by a pressure upon the abdomen. [*Gff.*]

On awaking from quite a long sleep, itching on the anus, aggravated by scratching and turned into burning (aft. 32 h.). [*C.*]

Nights very full of dreams (aft. 16 h.). [*Gff.*]

Very many dreams (the 1st night). [*C.*]

1155. Very vivid, disquieting dreams (2d n.). [*C.*]

Vivid, but unremembered, dreams. [*Gff.*]

A very vivid lascivious dream (2d n.).

Frightful dreams.

Disquieting dreams in a restless sleep. [*Gff.*]

1160. Extremely anxious dreams. [*Gff.*]

Anxious, frightful dreams.

Tormenting dreams disturb the sleep.

Much connected talking in sleep, on which he awakes and remembers his dream.

Feverish coldness in the evening; he does not perceive the the warmth of the stove.

1165. Coldness in the left arm and in the left leg.

Anxiety like a fever, the hands are cold and she trembles with it.

Frequent chilliness; especially at night, chilliness and cold.

In the evening, chilliness.

Shaking chill of one hour, frequently.

1170. Chill and thirst.

Internal chill, with severe thirst.

In the evening, febrile rigor and weariness, and even before he goes to sleep, a flying heat (aft. 10 d.).

Chilliness and heat toward evening (aft. 12 d.).

Febrile rigor in the morning, with thirst, shaking and blue finger nails till in the afternoon; then in the evening heat and sweat, without thirst.

1175. For several days at 11 A. M., a chill; at 6 P. M., heat.

In the evening, sensation of heat, with great anguish, though she was cold to the touch all over.

In the evening, general burning heat, with great weariness and delirium at night.

Much heat the whole day, but the feet always cold.

In the evening, very much excited, with distended blood-vessels.

1180. At night in bed, heat.

At night she could not sleep for heat in her blood.

Very much inclined to sweats. [*C.*]

Frequent profuse sweat in the face (in a boy of two years). [*C.*]

In the morning, on awaking, increased sweat (3d d.). [*C.*]

1185. Warm sweat in the morning (aft. 29 h.). [*C.*]

Night sweat of putrid odor.

Sour-smelling sweat (aft. 8 d.).

Frequent pulse (aft. 2 h.). [*C.*]

Weak, languid pulse.

CAUSTICUM, CAUSTIC SUBSTANCE.

Lime, in the state of marble, owes its insolubility in water and its mildness to an acid of the lowest order which is combined with it; when heated to red heat the marble allows this acid to escape as a gas. During this process the marble, as burned lime, has received (besides the latent heat) another *substance* into its composition, which substance, unknown to chemistry, gives to it its caustic property as well as its solubility in the water, whereby we obtain lime-water. This substance, though itself not an acid, gives to it its caustic virtue, and by adding a fluid acid (which will endure fire), which then combines with the lime by its closer affinity, the watery caustic (Hydras Caustici?) is separated by distillation.

Take a piece of freshly burned lime of about two pounds, dip this piece into a vessel of distilled water for about one minute, then lay it in a dry dish, in which it will soon turn into powder with the development of much heat and its peculiar odor, called lime-vapor. Of this fine powder take two ounces and mix with it in a (warmed) porcelain triturating bowl a solution of two ounces of bisulphate of potash, which has been heated to red heat and melted, cooled again and then pulverized and dissolved in two ounces of boiling hot water. This thickish mixture is put into a small glass retort, to which the helm is attached with wet bladder; into the tube of the helm is inserted the receiver half submerged in water; the retort is warmed by the gradual approach of a charcoal fire below and all the fluid is then distilled over by applying the suitable heat. The distilled fluid will be about an ounce and a half of watery clearness, containing in concentrated form the substance mentioned above, *i.e.*, *Causticum;* it smells like the lye of caustic potash. On the back part of the tongue the caustic tastes very astringent, and in the throat burning; it freezes only in a lower degree of cold than water, and it hastens the putrefaction of animal substances immersed in it. When Muriate of Baryta is added, the causticum shows no sign of sulphuric acid, and on adding oxalate of ammonia it shows no traces of lime.

Of this distillate put one drop in vial filled about 2/3 with 99 or 100 drops of alcohol, potentize the mixture by ten successive strokes and continue in this manner through 29 similar vials with alcohol, developing each attenuation and potency with ten successive strokes, carrying it to the decillionth (causticum X) dynamic development.

One or at most two of the smallest pellets moistened with this fluid constitute the dose of this mighty antipsoric; the duration of its action often extends far beyond 50 days.

In the second volume of the "*Reine Arzneimittellehre*" there is mentioned a (less pure) preparation of causticum under the name of Caustic-tincture, but the proving of this remedy as to its peculiar effects on the changes of human health was yet very imperfect. But after I had recognized its antipsoric virtues, its proving was completed in the following list of symptoms, and thus the homœopathic selection of this great antipsoric for the appropriate cases was rendered possible, which with the lesser number of symptoms was frequently impossible without making injurious mistakes.

As an antidote to its too violent action with very excitable patients, smelling of sweet spirits of nitre will serve, presumably also the tincture of crude coffee.

Causticum may be advantageously repeated after the intermediate use of other antipsoric remedies, when it is again homœopathically indicated; but it should always be used in a different degree of potency.

In healing the diseases to which this medicine is homœopathically appropriate, the following symptoms were either relieved or removed:

Hypochondriac dejection; melancholy; sorrowful thoughts at night and weeping by day; anxiety; distrust of the future; hopelessness; tendency to get frightened; passionateness; peevishness; dizzy vertigo; dull, gloomy pressure in the brain occupying the head; shooting in the head; stitches in the temples; shooting in the upper part of the head with rigid fullness; lachrymation; inflammation of the eyes; *suppuration about the eyes;* incipient amaurosis; dark webs floating before the eyes; flickering before the eyes; growling and humming before the ears and in the head; roaring in the ears; eruption on the tip of the nose; old warts on the nose or eyebrows; painful teeth, protruding from their sockets; chronic suppuration of some one spot on the gums; fistula dentalis; mucous troubles in the fauces and behind the palate; mucous expectoration through hawking or a hacking cough; repugnance to sweet things; qualmishness like fainting fits; vomiting of sourish water; pressure on the stomach after eating bread; pressing and griping in the stomach; cramplike pains in the stomach; stitches in the scrobiculus cordis; pressure in the epigastrium; pressure in the whole of the abdomen after eating; distention of the belly in children; inflation of the abdomen; obstruction of flatus with hard stool; chronic constipation; tough stool, shining like fat; light-colored and white stool; during stool, cutting in the rectum; during stool discharge of blood; itching of the anus; protrusion of the varices of the rectum; fistula of the rectum in the nates; urging to urinate, with thirst; *involuntary micturition by day and night; involuntary emission of urine when coughing, sneezing and walking;* many pollutions; lack of erections; *aversion of females to coitus; delaying menses;* menses too scanty; soreness between the legs and the pudenda; *vaginal discharge; stoppage of both nostrils;* continual stuffed coryza; chronic hoarseness; short *cough;* inability to eject the detached mucus; short breathing; *stitches about the heart;* painful stiffness of the back, chiefly when rising from a seat; stiffness in the nape of the neck and the sacrum; drawing and tearing in the scapulæ; rigidity in the nape of the neck; swelling of the cervical glands like a goitre; drawing in the arms; eruptions on the arms; pressive pain above the elbow; sensation of fullness in the hand in grasping; shooting in the fingers, extending to the elbows; pains in the sole of the foot, the back, the ankles and toes of the feet when walking; *cold feet; swelling of the feet;* pain in the distended veins and varices; unsteadiness in the walk of a child, and tendency of same to fall; restless in the body; palpitation;

tremulous weakness; anxious dreams; chilliness; sensitiveness to cold; night-sweat.

The names of those who contributed to the following symptoms are indicated by the following abbreviations: *Br.*, *Becher; Fr.*, *Franz; Htm.*, *Hartmann; Hrn.*, *Herrmann*; *Hbg.*, *Hornburg; Lgh.*, *Laughammer; Ng.*, *anonymous; Rl.*, *Rummel; Stf.*, *Stapf.*

CAUSTICUM.

Mournful, lachrymose, sorrowful mood, as if beside himself.

Melancholy mood.

The child is apt to cry at every trifle.

Excessively compassionate; at the relations of others and of the cruelties inflicted upon them, she is beside herself for weeping and sobbing, and cannot content herself.

5. The mind is sad and somewhat anxious.

Anxiety the whole day, as if he had done something wrong, or had to fear it, or as if a misfortune had happened. [*Lgh.*]

Anxious, restless mood, as if something disagreeable was impending, which keeps him from working. [*Br.*]

Great anxiety during the day (aft. 13 d.).

Anxiety about bodily ailments.

10. Álways anxious and perspiring. [*Ng.*]

Anxious and as if stupefied in the head. [*Ng.*]

The greatest anguish for twelve hours.

Anxiously careful as to all occurrences.

Great apprehensions as to whatever happens.

15. Despondency, indisposition to everything, extreme lassitude and decrepitude. [*Rl.*]

Lack of courage.

Full of fearful ideas, in the evening.

Timidity, at night.

When she closes her eyes, she always sees frightful visages and distorted human faces before her.

20. Extreme anxious timidity; she is so much afraid of a dog near her, which did not harm her at all, that she trembled over the whole body; every noise in the street made her afraid, and

---

The pathogenesis of Causticum has quite a history belonging to it. In the *Fragmenta de Viribus* (1805) Hahnemann published thirty symptoms as obtained by him from a substance he called "Acris tinctura." In the first and second editions of the *Materia Medica Pura* appears a more extensive pathogenesis of this preparation now called "Aetzstoff Tinctur—Tinctura acris sine Kali." To this (in its latest form containing 307 symptoms) belong the observations of Becher, Franz, Hartmann, Herrmann, Hornburg, Langhammer and Stapf and over 100 of Hahnemann's. In the third edition (1833) the drug is not included, and consequently it is not to be found in Dudgeon's translation of the work. This was because in 1830 Hahnemann had transferred its pathogenesis to the *Chronic Diseases* where it has 1014 symptoms, among which are those already published, the new ones being furnished by himself and Rummel. It is now called simply Aetzstoff" or "Causticum," and is differently prepared. In Volume III of their *Arzneimittellehre* Hartlaub and Trinks give, from Nenning's hand, nine symptoms from the older and seventy-three from the newer preparation. From these materials with Hahnemann's own later observations is made up the symptom-list now translated.—*Hughes.*

when she saw boys climbing she was very uneasy lest they might get hurt.

Her fear and anxiety cause her to wish that she might not live.

He occupies himself with thoughts of death, with restlessness and great solicitude.

Extreme excitability of spirit; the least vexation darts through her body, so that her knees give way.

Discontented with himself, of gloomy countenance. [*Rl.*]

25. Long, morose silence (aft. 6 h.). [*Hbg.*]

Peevish, taciturn and introverted, while before he was very gay (at once). [*Ng.*]

Sullen and ill-humored, in the forenoon. [*Ng.*]

Peevishness. [*Hbg.*]

Very peevish and indolent.

30. Peevish, all day, at odds with himself, dissatisfied, anxious and yet not indisposed to mental work. [*Lgh.*]

Peevish the whole day; all that was around him made a disagreeable impression on him. [*Lgh.*]

Morose and dejected, without being peevish (1st d.).

Very peevish (aft. 48 h.).

Peevish, irritable **mood**. [*Rl.*]

35. Peevish, irritable, does not enjoy music.

Peevish, lachrymose.

Bad, irritable humor (aft. 4 d.).

Very sensitive, hot and passionate.

Unbounded inclination to take things ill.

40. Sensitive and inclined to anger, while the nerves are much affected; inclined to be chilly, and easily heated by exercise.

Apt to be very passionate after his noon siesta, with great ill-humor.

Incensed at trifles.

Inclined to scold and to bluster, with sullen mood. [*Hbg.*]

Inclined to quarrel and to be noisy, without being vexed. [*Fr.*]

45. Constant scolding (aft. ¼ h.).

Obstinacy.

Furiously self-opinionated and quarrelsome.

Indisposed to work (aft. 10, 20 h.).

At times merry, and soon after, a peevish mood.

50. At times excessively merry, soon after, dejected.

The first twelve hours, cheerfulness, light-hearted mood, easy flow of ideas;* but after twenty-one hours (in the morning, on awaking, and the whole forenoon) anxious, tremulous, sleepy, obtuse in the head, with pressive heaviness in the occiput and in the forehead, heaviness in the limbs, with almost constant pains in the joints and muscles in the fingers, arms, shoulders, knees and feet. [*Stf.*]

Although (*e. g.*, political) disputes were started with him, he

---

***So far it seems to have been a curative action on a previous opposite state of mind and spirit.**

remained pretty calm; he felt himself excited indeed, but avoided speaking of it, or getting into a passion (curative action, the first hours). [*Stf.*]

The whole day, good humor, contented with himself and very talkative; he always desires to converse with some one (curative action). [*Lgh.*]

Bright and talkative, in the forenoon. [*Ng.*]

55. **Weakness of memory.**

Distractedness and thoughtlessness. [*Fr.*]

Inattention and distraction.

He is inattentive and distracted.

Indisposed to give attention. [*Fr.*]

60. A momentary abstraction of thought, during which it seemed as if he thought of something, without thinking (aft. ½ h.). [*Fr.*]

A sort of absent-mindedness; while doing one thing, he always felt as if he had to do something else, more important, and yet he knew not what; he reflected about it, and yet thought nothing. [*Fr.*]

Weakness of thought, slow flow of ideas. [*Fr.*]

He often mispronounces words and interchanges syllables and letters (as, *e. g.*, "cluent foryza" instead of "fluent coryza"), for several days. [*Rl.*]

Stupor in the head, as if it were (screwed in a vise or) intoxicated, with redness of face. [*Ng.*]

65. Misty mind.

Obtuseness of the head from the morning, all the day, as if in a musty room in which clothes are washed and dried; aggravated by stooping; not going off in the open air, but on returning to the room.

Obtuseness and heat of the head (aft. 7 d.).

A momentary (painfully tensive) obtuseness of the head; almost like a slight, throbbing headache, going off after a meal. [*Stf.*]

Dizzy in the morning on awaking, with painful obtuseness of the head. [*Stf.*]

70. Dizzy in the head. [*Stf.*]

Stupid in the head and as if he had a cold.

Feels stupefied and intoxicated in the head (aft. 24 h.).

Feels intoxicated and giddy, with distraction of the thoughts.

He always feels as if he would fall, without vertigo.

75. Vertigo, as if from spirituous liquors. [*Hbg.*]

Vertigo, almost like unconsciousness, after walking, in sitting; he almost fell over.

Vertigo, whirling with heaviness of the head, in standing and sitting.

Giddy in the head, with anxiety in the whole body. [*Ng.*]

Vertigo, with weakness in the head.

80. Vertigo, forward and sideways.

Vertigo, in the morning, on rising from bed.

Vertigo, and falling over without cause. [*Rl.*]

Vertigo, while looking attentively at one point.

Vertigo, while looking upward (at a high tower), so violent that he falls over. [*Rl.*]

85. Momentary vertigo, while sitting, as if he was about to stagger (aft. 3½ h.). [*Stf.*]

Vertigo, while stooping, going off when raising the head. [*Ng.*]

Vertigo, when standing.

Vertigo, in the open air, everything runs around with her, and persons seem to her larger than at other times; it goes off in the room. [*Ng.*]

Vertigo, which diminishes in the open air. [*Stf.*]

90. Headache, with nausea.

A stupefying pain in the forehead, when sitting and reading, not removed when walking and standing. [*Lgh.*]

Pain in the upper part of the head, as if the brain were torn or crushed, especially in the morning on awaking (aft. 3 h.).

The whole brain aches, on shaking the head.

Sensation as if the brain were loose, and was shaken by taking a walk in the open air.

95. Aching of the head at night, as if there was an ulcer in it.

A morning headache, which had existed for a long time previous, disappears (curative effect). [*Ng.*]

Headache, as if something was forcing itself in between the frontal bone and the anterior part of the brain, or as if the part behind the frontal bone was hollow. [*Fr.*]

A pressure at times deep in the head, with heaviness of the head.

Pressive pain in the right **frontal protuberance.**

100. Pressive headache from all sides, with pinching in the ear and boring toothache.

Pressive pain in the right parietal bone and in both temples.

Pressive pain in the right side of the head, extending into the eyes.

Pressive pain in the right temple.

Pressive headache on the upper border of the temporal bone. [*Fr.*]

105. Slow pressure above the right orbit. [*Hbg.*]

Sharp pressure in the left side of the forehead. [*Fr.*]

A sudden pressure, as from a sharp stone falling upon it, in the vertex, in the region of the coronal suture. [*Hbg.*]

A painful drawing pressure, anteriorly in the forehead. [*Htm.*]

A drawing pressure in the right side of the occiput and of the cervical muscles, aggravated by a brisk walk; it originated in the open air. [*Fr.*]

110. Contractive pressure in the forehead in the open air, aggravated the more briskly he walks, and disappearing suddenly, when he stoops low down. [*Fr.*]

Compressive headache. [*Hbg.*]

Dizzy, as from compression of the head, the whole week.

Headache in the temples, pressing outward, night and day, with nausea, causing vomiting (aft. 9 d.).

Sensation of the head as if screwed in a vise, and heaviness, going off in the open air. [*Ng.*]

115. Sensation in the head, as if everything was coming out in front, on stooping. [*Stf.*]

Headache, with a feeling of fullness and rigidity up from the nape of the neck (aft. 24 h.).

Tensive and drawing headache between the eyes.

Tension in the right temple and the eye, which felt paralyzed.

Tension on the left side of the head.

120. Drawing pain in the occiput. [*Rl.*]

Frequently a drawing on the left side of the upper part of the head.

Drawing in the left side of the forehead.

Violent drawing pain in the temple, gradually increasing to the highest degree and then suddenly vanishing (aft. 24 h.). [*Rl.*]

Tearing in the head, neither aggravated nor relieved by motion or rest, for several days, now weaker, now stronger.

125. Tearing pain in the middle of the forehead and the cervical vertebræ, by day, in a heated room and while smoking tobacco; but especially at night, when he could not sleep for it.

Tearing in the left side of the head, especially in the forehead and temple, commencing in the evening and continually increasing, with swelling of the painful side (16th d.).

Violent tearing in the left side of the head, especially (at 4 P. M.) in the temple. [*Ng.*]

Painful tearing in the right temple. [*Ng.*]

Shooting tearing toward the left side of the crown (6th d.). [*Ng.*]

130. Shooting tearing in the head, beginning in the forehead and drawing toward the right side through the whole head. [*Htm.*]

Shooting in the head and warmth therein. [*Ng.*]

Shooting in the temples.

Stitches in the left side of the head, for several evenings.

Stitches along through the right side of the head, for half an hour.

135. Violent stitches in the occiput, for half an hour.

Obtuse stitches in the left temporal bone, which every time spreads into a circle, where the pain is alleviated or lost (aft. 9 d.)

Shooting headache, in the morning, on awaking, and almost the whole day.

Slow stitches drawing about in the left side of the sinciput, above the eye.

Straining shooting, from the lower part of the forehead into the upper part of the head (aft. 10 d.).

140. A painful, pressive cutting arises at once in the frontal bone, when he moves the arms violently, while stooping. [*Fr.*]

A painless **digging in the whole head.**

Twitching headache in the right side of the forehead and the head. [*Rl.*]

Twitching, pinching pain through the head. [*Rl.*]

Jerks and severe shocks in the head, every minute, in any position, in rest and in motion.

145. Beating and throbbing in the whole crown, as if everything was coming out, in the morning on rising. [*Ng.*]

Beating pain, a very painful throbbing in the arteries of the brain.

Throbbing in the crown, intermixed with stitches, in paroxysms.

Throbbing pain in the right side of the occiput, which goes off by rubbing toward the vertex, where it then pains as if bruised. [*Ng.*]

Severe throbbing in the forehead, for three days, more in the afternoon, with stiffness in the nape of the neck (aft. 12 d.).

150. Throbbing headache in the right temple on motion; *per se*, it is only pressive.

Painful pressive throbbing in the forehead, as with a dull point. [*Hbg.*]

Dull, painful throbbing of the arteries in the head, above the orbits. [*Fr.*]

Ebullition in the head, and sensation as if intoxicated, going off in the open air. [*Ng.*]

Rushing of blood in the head, in the evening.

155. Rush of blood to the head, with heat there.

Internal warmth and heat in the head, without external heat, especially after dinner, in the forehead. [*Ng.*]

Internal warmth in the forehead and back, as if perspiration would break out. [*Ng.*]

Burning in the right temple and right side of the forehead and in the region of the vertex. [*Ng.*]

Frequently a chilling burning before the vertex. [*Ng.*]

160. Burning headache in the forehead, as if the anterior part of the brain was inflamed, after returning from the open air into the room. [*Fr.*]

Sudden pain in the occipital bone, while sitting, as if something in the muscles there had been displaced. [*Fr.*]

Sensation in the occipital bone, as if these parts were numb, pithy, or dead (aft. ¼ h.). [*Fr.*]

Pain on a small part of the crown, as if contused or beaten, only when touched.

Pain on the upper part of the head, on pressing or touching it.

165. Painfulness of the hairy scalp, on rubbing it.

Between the eyes, often, drawing and pressure.

Tension and warmth on the forehead and nose, with slight drawing in the eyes from time to time.

The skin of the head is tense and stretched.

On the hairy scalp, before the vertex, a tearing burning. [*Ng.*]

170. Sensation as of shaking or trembling in the skin of the right temple, lasting till going to bed. [*Ng.*]

Movement of the skin of the head toward the forehead (aft. 13 d.).

Crawling sensation upon the crown.

Itching of the hairy scalp.

Itching of the forehead.

175. Shooting itching on various parts of the head, on the right and left parietal bone, on the forehead, on the right cheek, behind the left zygoma toward the ear, and on the upper part of the temporal bone. [*Fr.*]

Involuntary nodding with the head, just as if some one pressed it down (during writing). [*Fr.*]

Falling out of the hair of the head.

In the eye, a pressive pain, which is aggravated on touching it.

Pressive pain into the eyes, starting from the forehead.

180. Pressure in the orbits and behind the eyes. [*Fr.*]

A very painful pressure in the eyes, in the morning, before he can keep his eyes open; when he shuts them again, the pain is relieved.

Pressure in the eyes as if there was sand in them.

Pressure in the upper eyelid, as if a stye were forming.

Pressure in the upper eyelid, as from a swelling, as if a stye were forming. [*Fr.*]

185. Pressure in the right eye, as if from a swelling of the eyelids. which are actually red, with watery eyes. [*Fr.*]

Pressive pain above the right eye, as if the upper eyelid was about to be pressed down (aft. ¾ h.). [*Htm.*]

Pressure in the eyes, as if they were pressed from without inward and would come out.

Pressure in the left eye, as if it were being gouged out. [*Fr.*]

An internal pressure in the eye, as if it were being distended. [*Fr.*]

190. Distending pain in the right eyeball. [*Fr.*]

Drawing in the arch of the right eyebrow.

Tearing and pressure in the eyes.

Itching above the eyes.

Itching in the eyes and in the canthi, which goes off by rubbing them (with subsequent lachrymation of them). [*Ng.*]

195. Itching in the right eyeball, in the morning. [*Ng.*]

Itching of the eyes, especially of the lids. [*Fr.*]

Itching on the lower eyelid, and on its internal surface; with burning as soon as he touches the eye or moves it.

Itching like a flea-bite in the inner left canthus, with excitation to scratch. [*Fr.*]

Voluptuous itching on the right canthus, compelling to rub it for an hour (aft. 8 h.). [*Lgh.*]

200. Smarting in the eyelid. [*Rl.*]

Sensation in the eyes, as from salt. [*Stf.*]

Smarting and pressure in the eyes, which feel heavy, with redness of the eyelids.

An itching pain as from soreness in the inner canthus of the right eye, in the morning, after awaking, as if from salt that has got in the eye, compelling violent rubbing, and yet much aggravated thereby, so that water exudes, without redness of the eye. [*Stf.*]

Excoriative pain of the left eyelid (aft. 4 d.). [*Rl.*]

205. Heat in the eyes.

Burning in the eyes, without redness.

Burning and dryness in the eyes, in the afternoon; or also in the evening with pricking in them as from needles, together with photophobia. [*Ng.*]

Burning in both the inner canthi (3d, 4th d.).

Burning of the left eyelid. [*Rl.*]

210. Burning pain on the edge of the eyelids, as from burning with gunpowder. [*Hbg.*]

Inflammation of the eyes, with burning and pressive pains (aft. 4 d.).

Inflamed eyelids from time to time, with hardened eye-gum between the lashes.

Inflammation of the eyes with pressure therein by day, while they are closed by suppuration in the morning.

Eyes closed by suppuration, in the morning. [*Ng.*]

215. Sensation of dryness with pressure in the eyes. [*Stf.*]

Friction in the eyes as of sand.

First dryness and stiffness in the eyes in the morning, then lachrymation of same. [*Stf.*]

Lachrymation of the eyes, especially in the open air (2d and 3d d.). [*Ng.*]

Lachrymation of the eyes, even in the room, but chiefly in the open air.

220. Unusual lachrymation of the eyes in the room, without redness in them. [*Br.*]

The eyes, lachrymating before, become better (curative action). [*Ng.*]

Eye-gum in and about the canthi. [*Lgh.*]

Quivering of the left eyebrow (aft. 2 d.).

Visible twitching of the eyelids and of the left eyebrow.

225. Sensation as if the eyelids were swollen, chiefly in the morning. [*Hrn.*]

Sensation of heaviness in the upper[1] eyelid, as if he could not well raise it, or as if it was agglutinated to the lower lid, and could not be loosed easily.

Tendency to close the eyes; they closed involuntarily.

The opening of the eyes is rendered difficult, with a sensation as if the lids were swollen, chiefly in the morning.

Weary in the eyes.

230. Sensation as if the eyes would close for weariness.

The pupils in the beginning seem contracted, but after ten to twelve hours to be dilated. [*Stf.*]

Dilated pupils. [*Fr.*]

Things become black before the eyes, for half an hour (aft. 5 d.)

Momentary **obscuration of the eyes, while blowing the nose.**

235. Frequent obscuration of the eyes, especially when he looks where it is bright, as if he then was blinded by the light, and could see nothing at all. [*Fr.*]

---

[1] By misprint the original has *lower* eyelid.—*Transl.*

Obscuration of the eyes; it descended from the head down into the left eye, and the light appeared as if there were many points of light in a dark circle.

While reading, some letters become invisible. [*Rl.*]

Obscuration of the eyes, frequently, as if they were covered with a fine membrane.

Obscuration of the eyes in the morning, while blowing the nose, as if a membrane was drawn before the inner canthus up to one-half of the pupil.

240. **Obscuration of the eyes, as if a gauze was drawn before them,** in standing. [*Fr.*]

Darkening of the eyes at times, as from gauze.

Dimness of vision, as if a thin membrane were drawn over the eyes or as from a mist before them, aggravated by wiping and rubbing them. [*Htm.*]

Dimness of the eyes. [*Rl.*]

Dimness of vision, as from a thick fog before the eyes, also in the morning, after awaking, until he washes himself. [*Ng.*]

245. Far-sighted the first day, he can no more read without spectacles.

Small round forms arise before his vision, even before his open eyes, while lying down. [*Fr.*]

If he looks too long at anything the objects flit before his eyes, and everything gets mixed up, causing a pressive pain in the eyes.

Flitting before the eyes, like a swarm of insects.

Flickering before the eyes.

250. Flickering before the eyes, as if a gauze was before them.

Sparks of fire before the eyes, even in bright daylight.

When winking, he sees sparks of fire, even in bright daylight.

Photophobia; the eyes pain on moving them, when he looks into the bright daylight.

Photophobia the whole day, he has continually to wink with his eyes.

255. Otalgia, in the evening, in the right meatus auditorius (aft. 48 h.).

When cleaning the ear, the meatus feels as if sore and ulcerated. [*Rl.*]

Pressive pain before the ear, on the mastoid process.

Tension behind the ear. [*Hbg.*]

Sensation in the ear of a pressing outward. [*Rl.*]

260. Pain in the ear, as if everything was pressing outward, and as if the ears would burst open, like a tearing, mixed with itching.

Sensation in the left ear and in that whole side of the head in the evening, on lying down, as if the parts were too tight; he cannot go to sleep lying on this side; on touching it, it felt as if the flesh was severed from the bones, but it was relieved by a stronger pressure.

Straining pain in the ear.

Tearing in the left ear (12th d.). [*Ng.*]

Tearing in the tympanum, with tensive gloominess in the head.

265. Boring pain in the right ear. [*Ng.*]

At times boring, then pulsating throbbing, behind the left ear (4th d.).

Stabs, as from boring knives, externally behind the left ear, often with a very sudden general sweat, lasting up to eight minutes, every day several times (aft. 7 d.).

Stitches in the right ear, jerking and in quick succession. [*Stf.*]

Sharp, intermitting stitches before the right ear, on the mastoid process.

270. A tearing, shooting pain in the ear, with a rushing as from a tempest.

Shooting on the outer margin of the ear, with burning pain, chiefly in the evening in bed.

Crawling in the left ear, as from an insect, with itching. [*Ng.*]

Itching in the left ear. [*Rl.*]

Itching in the ear, starting from the throat, in the Eustachian tube.

275. A shooting itching in the anterior part of the right meatus auditorius. [*Fr.*]

Itching of the lobule of the ear, as from a small tetter. [*Rl.*]

Sensation as of a cold wind blowing on the orifice of the right ear. [*Ng.*]

A tumor behind the ear.

Swelling of the external ear, with contractive pain.

280. Swelling of the meatus auditorius, with straining earache and discharge of a bloody humor.

Running and suppuration of the internal ear, with a bad smell.

During eructation air darts into the ear. [*Rl.*]

Feeling of stoppage in the right ear.

Sensation of stoppage in the ears, in the morning.

285. Re-echoing in the ears, every morning.

Her words and steps echo in the ears.

The sounds echo in the ear, and he is hard of hearing.

Ringing in the left ear. [*Ng.*]

Ringing before the right ear, in the evening.

290. Whistling in the left ear. [*Ng.*]

Shrill singing in the ears, like crickets in the distance, then beating, then again singing (aft. 8 h.). [*Stf.*]

Roaring before the ears (aft. 5 d.).

Roaring in the right ear. [*Ng.*]

Roaring before the ears, frequently, by day.

295. Rushing, in the evening, shortly before going to sleep, first before one ear then before the other, for a minute.

Rushing before the ears, as from water rushing over a dam, with hardness of hearing.

Detonations in the right ear.

In the ala nasi, a drawing, starting from the external right canthus.

Cutting tearing through the right ala nasi. [*Ng.*]

300. Tickling in the left nostril, going off on external pressure. [*Ng.*]

Itching in the nose.

Itching in the nostrils.

Severe itching on the nose.

Itching on the tip of the nose and the ala nasi. [*Fr.*]

305. The septum of the nose is painful to the touch.

Pain as from soreness on the lower part of the nose, as in violent coryza.

Soreness in the interior of the nose.

Swelling of the nose, frequently in the morning, going off in the evening.

Pimples on the tip of the nose.

310. Pimples on the root of the nose. [*Rl.*]

Falling out of the hairs about his nostrils, of which he had many.

In blowing his nose in the morning a bloody substance is expelled for several mornings successively (aft. 24 h.).

Severe epistaxis (aft. 7, 9 d.)

Violent bleeding from the left nostril (aft. 8 h.). [*Lgh.*]

315. The sense of smell is lacking, the nose being wholly stopped up.

The face looks very sickly (aft. 7 d.).

Very **yellow complexion** (aft. 21 d.).

Discoloring of the face, yellowish about the temples, with pale-blue lips.

Short violent drawing pain in the right cheek and then in the ear (aft. 2 d.). [*Rl.*]

320. Tearing in the left cheek bone.

Tearing in the left cheek, under the ear. [*Ng.*]

Tearing and shooting in the cheek.

Shooting in the cheek, by the lower jaw.

Beating and twitching in the muscles of the cheek, but little visible (aft. 3 d.).

325. Painful burning on the upper part of the cheeks, before the ears, as if an eruption was coming there. [*Fr.*]

Burning and chilling burning on the zygomata. [*Ng.*]

Swelling of the cheeks with throbbing pain.

Itching of the face.

Itching of the head, the nose and the chin.

330. Much itching on the nose, the chin and the neck, below the ears.

Itching of both eyebrows, of the left zygoma, of the temples and the ears, going off by scratching. [*Ng.*]

Burning itching beside the nose. [*Ng.*]

Eroding itching in the face, with rush of blood to the face, with heat and redness, and then the formation of many little red pimples. [*Stf.*]

Eruption in the face.

335. Fine eruption in the face, more noticeable to the touch than to the sight. [*Rl.*]

A pimple between the eyebrows and above the nose.

Pimples on the left cheek, with severe itching.

Red pimples on the left side of the forehead, the left temple, the nose, and the middle of the chin; they are filled with pus, stinging when touched, and when healing covered with scurf.

Burning vesicles in the face, which when touched exude an erosive humor, drying up into scurf. [*Stf.*]

340. Cramp-like sensation in the lips.

Fine tearing in the lips. [*Ng.*]

Pain on the lip as if sore. [*Stf.*]

Red spot above the upper lip, which looks as if chapped, and causes a burning pain (aft. 6 d.).

Soreness in the left corner of the mouth (aft. 7 h.). [*Rl.*]

345. Itching about the mouth.

Swelling of the lower lip with a pimple which stings and tingles.

Pimple in the left corner of the mouth, with tingling stinging.

Little pimples below the left corner of the mouth, for twenty-four hours. [*Ng.*]

Pimples beside the upper lip.

350. Eruption of vescles in the right corner of the mouth, which is very painful while eating.

An ulcer, with burning pain, on the inner side of the upper lip.

Tetter on the lower lip.

On the chin, not far from the lower lip, a pustule with a red areola (aft. 27 h.). [*Lgh.*]

Tensive drawing pain on the lower part of the chin. [*Fr.*]

355. Tearing in the lower part of the chin.

Tearing in the middle of the chin, in the bone.

Burning, cutting pain in the chin, on the right side, as if there was a piece of glass in it, which was cutting its way out (aft. 3 h.). [*Fr.*]

Inflammatory swelling below the chin, as if an abscess was forming, with burning pain.

In the articulation of the lower jaw on the right side, painfulness (aft. ½ h.). [*Stf.*]

360. **Sensation of tension and pain in the jaws, so that she could open her mouth only with difficulty**, and could not eat well, because a tooth also stood too high.

He cannot without trouble get his jaws apart, nor open his mouth sufficiently; it feels as if there were a swelling or tension below the lower jaw on the neck.

Drawing first from the right then from the left branch of the lower jaw to its articulation and thence back in the direction of the respective corners of the mouth

Tearing in the right lower jaw. [*Ng.*]

Gouty pains in the lower jaw (aft. ¼ h.).

365. Prickling digging in the lower jaw. [*Hbg.*]

Burning pain in the lower jaw.

Toothache in the upper and lower molars. [*Fr.*]
Toothache, with much spitting of saliva (aft. 24 h.).
Painful sensitiveness of the teeth to the touch.

370. In the morning, the teeth and gums are very sensitive.
On opening the mouth, pain darts into the teeth.
Pain in a sound tooth as the air rushes in.
Peculiar sensation in the roots of the teeth, compelling him to gnash his teeth. [*Ng.*]
Pain in the teeth, as from ulceration, at night, and also by day, when she moves her mouth.

375. Severe pain in the teeth, as from soreness, in the morning; then throbbing in them; the pain disappeared when the gums began to bleed.
Pressive toothache.
A dull pressure as if from without, in the roots of the two anterior upper molars (aft. ½ h.). [*Fr.*]
Drawing in the teeth (aft. 26 h.).
Drawing toothache in the second right molar tooth, seemingly more on its outward surface, and extending into the temple. [*Fr.*]

380. Violent drawing toothache, with itching in the empty places between the teeth. [*Rl.*]
Drawing pain in the teeth of the left lower row. [*Ng.*]
Tearing in the roots of the teeth of the lower jaw, in the morning, renewed every four minutes. [*Br.*]
Tearing toothache extending into the head and the left eye.
Tearing toothache in both rows on the right side, extending to the zygoma, with pain as from bruising in the jaws on that side, when pressing on them and chewing. [*Ng.*]

385. Tearing pain in all the teeth, as if they would fall out. [*Ng.*]
Tearing in a rotten root of a tooth of the lower left row. [*Ng.*]
Tearing in the posterior molar of the left upper row, worse in the open air. [*Ng.*]
Shooting toothache (aft. 16 d.).
Shooting in the tooth, when biting on it (aft. 12 h.).

390. Dull stitches in the upper molars, passing upward.
Dull stitches in the lower molars, passing downward.
Boring pain in a lower molar, extending into the nose and eye.
Painful pricking digging in the lower molars, extending to the ear (aft. 1 h.). [*Hbg.*]
A severe jerk in the teeth, almost at once.

395. **Throbbing toothache**, with painful gums, so that he could not chew.
Throbbing aching in the affected molar tooth.
Burning pain in the hollow teeth, while eating and drinking.
Toothache, composed of pressing, tearing and shooting, day and night, with red (erysipelatous) swelling of the cheek, and a swollen lump on the gums, which passes into suppuration; for seven days.
Looseness of several teeth.

400. **Painful looseness of the incisors.**

Looseness of the incisors. [*Rl.*]

The gums are painfully sensitive, without toothache.

Dull, drawing pains in the gums of the lower jaws. [*Fr.*]

Swelling and painfulness of the gums, both in front and behind.

405. Swelling of the gums, on the left side, with great sensitiveness while eating, and cramp-like pains in the evening.

Swelling of the gums.

Swelling of the gums, with acridity in the pudenda while urinating (aft. 16 d.).

Severe bleeding of the gums (aft. 10 d.).

In the mouth, swelling of the inner side of the cheek; in chewing he bites into it. [*Rl.*]

410. On the tongue, on the left side, pain, as if he had bitten into it. [*Rl.*]

Pain, as of soreness upon the tongue and below it, and on the palate.

Pain, as from burning, on the tip of the tongue, and on its edge. [*Stf.*]

Burning, scrapy feeling on the tip of the tongue, as after burning it with something red-hot, with much flow of saliva, and disagreeable taste in the mouth, not going off from eating. [*Stf.*]

Burning on the tip of the tongue. [*Ng.*]

415. Dry tongue and thirst (aft. 10 h.).

Vesicles on the edge of the tongue. [*Stf.*]

Painful blisters on the tongue.

Painful blister on the tip of the tongue.

In the upper part of the palate, a spot paining as if sore.

420. Pain, as from soreness and burning, on the palate. [*Ng.*]

Anteriorly on the palate a spot, which when touched with the tongue pains as if ulcerated. [*Fr.*]

Stitches on the left side of the palate. [*Ng.*]

Crawling and burning pricking on the back part of the palate. [*Ng.*]

Roughness in the mouth, as if covered with a membrane, after a scraping sensation on the tongue. [*Stf.*]

425. Burning, scraping sensation in the mouth (on smelling the drug.) [*Stf.*]

Dryness in the mouth and on the lips, but without thirst.

Severe dryness in the mouth, without thirst, the whole forenoon.

Dryness in the mouth, with thirst, all the day. [*Ng.*]

Burning dryness in the mouth.

430. Much collection of saliva. [*Stf.*]

Gathering of watery saliva in the mouth, in the forenoon, with qualmishness (2d d.).

Gathering of water in the mouth (aft. 1 h.). [*Ng.*]

Gathering of water in the mouth, with rancid taste. [*Ng.*]

Mucus comes into her throat, which she cannot eject by hawking, but has to swallow down, one-half hour after dinner. [*Ng.*]

435. Hawking of mucus.

Frequent hawking up of mucus, which is, however, replaced at once. [*Ng.*]

Hawking and expectoration of much phlegm, with sensation of soreness and burning in the fauces, from 5 P. M. till night. [*Ng.*]

Hawking up of tough mucus, which is first detached with difficulty, later on easily. [*Ng.*]

Dryness in the back part of the throat, for three days. [*Ng.*]

440. Dryness in the throat, without thirst.

Dryness of the throat in the morning.

Dryness of the throat, with dry tussiculation. [*Ng.*]

At times dryness, then again moisture in the throat. [*Ng.*]

Dryness in the throat, sensible in swallowing, then scratching extending down the throat.

445. Scrapy sensation in the fauces, especially observable in the evening and in deglutition.

Scrapy and scratchy in the throat, with heartburn. [*Rl.*]

Rough in the throat, with a sensation like heartburn. [*Ng.*]

Rough in the throat, with a sensation of lack of air in breathing. [*Ng.*]

Scraping, scratchy soreness of the throat, with a sensation during empty deglutition, as if he had to swallow over a protuberance. [*Rl.*]

450. Rough, hoarse throat, with pain as of soreness, as well, *per se*, as in speaking and swallowing.

Sensation of soreness in the throat, behind the palate.

Sore throat, paining as from excoriation.

A burning shooting pain as of soreness in the œsophagus and in the uvula, aggravated on deglutition.

Sensation as if torn within the throat, not when swallowing, but when straining the head, as also when lifting and carrying.

455. Sensation as if swollen in the throat and rough (aft 2 d.).

The fauces feel too narrow and as if closed by swelling.

She has to swallow all the time; she feels as if the throat was not wide enough, and in swallowing she feels dryness in it.

Continual inclination to swallow.

Sore throat as from a lump in it, with lancinating pain.

460. Pressure in the throat, behind the palate and in the epiglottis.

Dull pressure in the œsophagus, as if behind the sternum, as if he had swallowed too large a morsel. [*Fr.*]

Choking pressure in the œsophagus, in the morning on awaking, as from swallowing a crust of bread not sufficiently masticated.

Violent sore throat, so that he can scarcely swallow, because it then pricks him as with needles; after dinner much relieved. [*Ng.*]

Sore throat, as if the attachment of the tongue had grown fast.

465. Contractive sensation of the throat, frequently.

Sensation of coldness in the throat, which rises quickly and spreads over the palate, with frequent collection of saliva. [*Stf.*]

Audible creaking, deep in the throat.

Taste in the mouth as from a spoiled stomach, in the afternoon, for several days. [*Ng.*]

An acrid fluid comes into the mouth.

470. Bitter taste in the mouth, but only for a short time. [*Ng.*]

Smeary, clayey taste in the mouth (aft. 4 d.).

Fatty taste in the mouth.

Putrid taste in the mouth.

Violent thirst, for many days (aft. 2 d.).

475. Several mornings, much thirst.

Severe thirst for cold drinks, from morning till afternoon. [*Ng.*]

Violent thirst for beer.

He eats too hastily.

Unusually early hunger. [*Ng.*]

480. A sort of ravenous hunger.

Enormous hunger, which gives him headache, removed by eating.

Little appetite, but he relishes food.

Continual sensation of satiety and lack of appetite, and an hour afterward hunger, and relish of the food eaten.

Little appetite, but much thirst, especially after eating.

485. Diminished taste in the food eaten.

Appetite is lacking; he has hunger, but does not relish his food, for three days.

She has an appetite, but it seems as if she did not dare to eat, but without any loathing for it.

Even if he started to eat with appetite, and began to eat, the appetite vanished at once.

He has appetite, but when eating, he at once loathes the food.

490. Even when he starts to eat there is loathing.

Repugnance to sweet things.

He can only eat smoked things; after eating fresh meat, he gets sick, as if he should vomit.

When she eats anything, while her hunger is lacking, she feels at once, as if sated and full, with the sensation that the stomach does not desire anything, and would feel better, if she had not eaten anything.

After eating, while out walking, water collects in the mouth, and there is more moisture in the nose.

495. After a meal she feels as if the food remained lodged in her throat.

After a meal the taste of the food long remains in her mouth.

After a meal, mucus collects in the throat.

After supper, heartburn.

After eating supper with appetite, nausea.

500. Even while eating, nausea.

After breakfast, pressure on the stomach (aft. 5 d.).

Soon after eating, cutting from the scrobiculus cordis toward the abdomen, with the taste in the mouth of the food eaten, and eructation tasting of the ingesta, with obtuseness of the head, diarrhœa and chilliness; he had to lie down.

Even while eating, a cutting pinching in the abdomen, which vanished at once on the discharge of flatus (aft. 6 h.). [*Lgh.*]

After eating, a severe distention of the abdomen.

505. After eating and drinking, the abdomen feels full at once, with restlessness and drawing in it.

After eating, the stomach being too full, grumbling in the abdomen.

Immediately after dinner, a call to stool, which goes off with straining and is hard.

After dinner, itching of the anus.

After drinking, the nose is moist and secretes more moisture.

510. After dinner, frequently a sharp pressure on the chest, without reference to respiration, chiefly in walking (the first 3 w.).

After a meal, shooting in the left side of the chest.

After supper, trembling and anxiety.

After meals, chilliness.

After meals, chilly. [*Rl.*]

515. After a meal, chilly, with heat in the face.

After a meal, warmth and redness in the face. [*Hbg.*]

After a meal, much heat in the face and in the eyes (aft. 8 d.).

Sensation as of a spoiled stomach, with inflation of the abdomen (aft. 15 d.).

Eructation of air (aft. ½ h.). [*Ng.*]

520. **Empty, tasteless eructation of mere air.** [*Stf.*, *Hbg.*]

Very frequent and mostly **empty, eructation** (aft. 9 d.)

Frequent audible eructation, long continuing. [*Ng.*]

Eructation, with the smell of the ingesta.

Eructation tasting of the ingesta, five hours after eating.

525. **Eructation, as if from food remaining undigested.**

Eructation, with taste of the breakfast-soup. [*Ng.*]

Eructation, with agreeable, almond-like taste. [*Ng.*]

Eructation, with smell of musk. [*Ng.*]

Violent eructation, with acrid taste (aft. 14 d.).

530. Abortive eructation; it only rises to the middle of the throat, where it stops.

She always feels as if she should eructate, but it does not come, causing various troubles.

Eructation, with choking in the œsophagus, so that it impedes the respiration; it goes off after another eructation. [*Ng.*]

Burning hot eructation, in the afternoon and evening, without any bad taste.

Heartburn. [*Ng.*]

535. A burning sensation frequently rises from the throat, as if he had eaten pepper

Hiccup (aft. ¼ h.). [*Ng.*]

Sensation of continual ebullition, as if lime was being slaked in his stomach, with rolling eructation of air. [*Ng.*]

Frequent belching up of ill-tasting water, or rising of the same into the mouth, with nausea, going off on eructation. [*Ng.*]

Belching up of water, several times, with aching in the anus. [*Ng.*]

540. Waterbrash, several times in the forenoon, with salty taste of the water rising up (aft. 17 d.).

A sort of waterbrash; in the evening, while lying down, cool water rises up from the stomach, which she has to spit out continually.

Qualmy and weak in the stomach, with alternation of chill and heat. [*Ng.*]

Sensation of fasting in the stomach. [*Ng.*]

Qualmishness about the stomach (aft. several h.).

545. Sensation of loathing in the throat.

Sick at stomach, as if qualmish, without excitation to vomit. [*Ng.*]

Qualmishness (at once).

Qualmishness, with anxiety.

Sensation of qualmishness, before a meal, with hunger.

550. Qualmishness, and a half hour later, hunger, in the afternoon.

Nausea, every morning.

Nausea and excitation to vomiting, all the afternoon till evening.

Sick at stomach, as if about to vomit, with frequent belching up of water into the mouth, compelling spitting continually. [*Ng.*]

Inclination to vomit, with sensation of emptiness in the stomach and sourish, bitterish taste in the mouth.

555. Sour vomiting, and after it still sour eructation.

Vomiting of coagulated blood, at night.

Stomachache, with belching up, going off after dinner. [*Ng.*]

Sensation of emptiness in the stomach, although she had eaten enough, in the afternoon. [*Ng.*]

Violent pains in the stomach, in the morning, soon after rising, increased by every quick motion; with heat in the right side of the head; she has to lie down, and the pain seemed to be now in the stomach, now in the chest (aft. 27 d.).

560. Pains in the stomach, quieted by lying down.

Pain, as from bruising, in the stomach, observable also when pressing it. [*Ng.*]

Pressure in the stomach, in the morning, after rising from bed, and only when sitting.

Pressure on the stomach, in the morning when fasting, and soon after, a contractive sensation in the abdomen (aft. 2 d.).

Pressure about the orifice of the stomach, increased by pressing against the edge of the table, as also by reading aloud, by much speaking, by lying on the back, and when the air touches the abdomen.

565. **Pressure in the scrobiculus cordis.** [*Fr.*]

Severe pressure in the scrobiculus cordis.

A rhythmical, chilling pressure in the scrobiculus cordis, as from an icicle. [*Hbg.*]

A continual shooting pressure in the scrobiculus cordis. [*Htm.*]

Tensive pain in the scrobiculus cordis.

570. Cramp in the stomach.

Cramp in the stomach, like pressure and contraction, in the morning, on awaking from a frightful dream, with nausea and collection of water in the mouth (aft. 21 d.).

Contractive, not very painful, sensation in the region of the stomach. [*Ng.*]

Sudden griping in the scrobiculus cordis.

Griping snatching in the scrobiculus cordis, when taking a deep breath.

575. Stitches in the stomach, for ten minutes.

Stitches in the scrobiculus cordis, which seem to contract the heart.

Formication in the region of the stomach.

Constant sensation of agreeable warmth in the stomach and abdomen. [*Ng.*]

With increasing pain in the stomach, she shudders.

580. In the left hypochondrium, acute stitches. [*Ng.*]

Violent stitches on the first false ribs. [*Ng.*]

Short, burning pain the left hypochondrium.

In the liver, a tensive, pressive pain, when lying on the back.

Stitches in the hepatic region, in the afternoon, for four hours (aft. 12 d.).

585. Stitches in the hepatic region when driving out, on a spot as large as a hen's egg, which causes lancinating pains also when touched, with great inclination to sleep and general lassitude.

Lancinating pain under the right ribs, in the evening.

Violent stitches below the last true rib, on the right side. [*Htm.*]

Painful tearing in the liver, in the evening (17th d.).

Colic, in the morning.

590. In the abdomen, pressure, extending up into the fauces, in the evening (aft. 10 d.).

Pressure in the stomach and abdomen, below and above the navel, with nocturnal diarrhœa, three times, and periodical stitches obstructing respiration and extending from the back forward into the right side of the abdomen (aft. 2 d.).

Pressure in the abdomen, many afternoons in succession, so severe that she could not attend to her domestic duties.

Pressure in the hypogastrium, as from a load.

Dull, pressive pain, deep in the hypogastrium, at last with fever, anguish and restlessness, so that he could neither sleep nor lie down at night; the hypogastrium was painful to the touch, as in gastric inflammation.

595. Pressive pain in the abdomen and short breath, in the morning, after rising.

Inflation of the left subcostal region.

Inflation on the left side of the abdomen, extending to the groin (aft. 6 h.).

Inflation and distention of the belly, so that she can only with difficulty draw breath, at the same time frequent discharge of flatus. [*Ng.*]

Great inflation of the abdomen, so that she has to loosen her clothes, with frequent discharge of loud flatus, which, however, relieve only for a short time. [*Ng.*]

600. Strong inflation of the abdomen, especially in the evening. [*Ng.*]

Inflated belly, with internal pressure, especially when taking a deep breath.

Full hard abdomen, in the evening.

Distended abdomen, in the evening (aft. 10 h.).

Painful distention of the abdomen, so that she has to loosen her clothes; at the same time pains in the abdomen, like cramps.

605. Tension in the right side of the abdomen.

Tension and pressure in the epigastrium.

Contractive tension in the stomach and abdomen.

Contractive sensation about the epigastric region.

Pain in the abdomen as if it was being drawn together with a rope, when breathing.

610. Jerking contraction in the abdomen, at noon (aft. 9 d.).

Pain as if constricted, in the two loins.

Pinching bellyache, with paleness of the face,

Pinching about the navel, in the morning in bed, going off after rising. [*Ng.*]

Pinching about the epigastrium, frequently recurring. [*Ng.*]

615. Pinching in a small spot of the right side of the abdomen, below the navel, after a meal. [*Ng.*]

Pinching and cutting in the right side of the abdomen, as from diarrhœa. [*Ng.*]

Violent pinching and cutting in the whole belly, with yawning. [*Ng.*]

Cutting in the abdomen and discharge of flatus, on inspiring. [*Fr.*]

Cutting in the epigastrium, in a space like a small band, with soft stool; going off after dinner. [*Ng.*]

620. Cutting colic, in the morning, and then three soft stools, and during the whole day, a sensation in the abdomen, as if diarrhœa were setting in. (aft. 8 d.).

Cutting pain in the groin, on motion, especially on walking. [*Fr.*]

Stitches in the abdomen, one after the other, for a long time, so that he could not keep his seat.

Stitches in the right side of the abdomen, in the evening.

A stitch in the right side of the abdomen, through the abdomen and out at the sacrum. [*Ng.*]

625. A violent stitch in the left side of the abdomen. [*Stf.*]

A transient stitch in the left side of the abdomen.

Sharp stitches in the left loin, by the last false rib.

Sharp stitches above the left hip, by the last false rib.

Sharp stitches in the right loin above the ilium; they wind upward toward the ribs, but pass quickly, like an electric spark.

630. Obtuse stitches above the ilium, below the last false rib.

Dull lancinating pain in the right side of the abdomen, when lying down. [*Rl.*]

Dull stitch in the right side of the abdomen, and then pain as of bruisedness in the left lower ribs, which is also sensitive in pressing upon it. [*Ng.*]

Pricking all over the abdomen as from needles. [*Ng.*]

Pain as from a bruise and pinching **in the right side of the chest,** then pains shooting outward through the pudenda, frequently. [*Ng.*]

635. Sensation of emptiness in the abdomen, relieved by pressing upon it.

Formication in the navel, with a sensation as if diarrhœa was coming on. [*Ng.*]

Formication and moving about in the abdomen, as after a purgative. [*Ng.*]

Throbbing in the abdomen.

Sensation of coldness in the abdomen with cracking and crepitation in it. [*Hbg.*]

640. Burning pain in the abdomen, around the region of the stomach, waking him from sleep; but transient. [*Stf.*]

Swelling of the navel, with painfulness round about when touched.

Tendency to catch cold in the abdomen; when the air touches it, there is pressure on the stomach and diarrhœa.

Quivering or muscular twitches, on the lower left side of the abdomen, when bending forward in sitting (aft. 4 h.).

Shooting burning on the right side of the abdomen, with sensation as if something was detaching itself there. [*Ng.*]

645. In the flanks, pain as from bruising, at times with shooting. [*Ng.*]

Shooting pain down the right flank, as if a hernia was forming, after breakfast. [*Ng.*]

Forcing toward the front from both inguinal regions, with abortive urging to urinate; when sitting. [*Ng.*]

Much obstruction to flatus, with hard stool (1st week).

Accumulation of flatus in abdomen after a moderate meal; this causes the varices of the rectum to protude, which are painful and moist (aft. 5 d.).

650. Working about in the abdomen with cutting, going off after a soft stool. [*Ng.*]

Rolling noise in the abdomen, with discharge of flatus. [*Ng.*]

Loud rumbling in the abdomen, when sitting, as if from emptiness (aft. 1 h.). [*Lgh.*]

Audible grumbling and croaking in the abdomen, as from frogs.

Flatus breaks out upward and downward.

655. Too frequent discharge of the flatus (aft. 4 d.).

Frequent loud discharge of flatus, the whole afternoon. [*Ng.*]

Frequent discharge of flatus without troubles in the abdomen. [*Ng.*]

Frequent discharge of flatus, after breakfast. [*Br.*]

Frequent discharge of fetid flatus, without troubles. [*Stf.*]

660. No stool (2d and 3d d.). [*Ng.*]

Constipation (aft. 24 h.).

Ineffectual urging to stool, frequently, with many pains, anxiety, and redness in the face (aft. 4, 10, 30 d.).

Frequent call to stool, without anything but flatus being discharged (aft. 3 d.). [*Rl.*]

Urging to stool, but the anus is spasmodically and painfully contracted, so that no stool at all resulted; but the pressure still continued (2d d.).

665. Tenesmus, with grumbling in the abdomen. [*Ng.*]

At call to stool, anxious apprehension that some ill might happen to him.

The stool is more readily discharged while standing.

Hard, firm stool (3d, 4th d.). [*Ng.*]

With the sensation as if merely flatus would pass, fæces were discharged.

670. He has to get up at night for stool, which is very soft. [*Ng.*]

The stool came in lumps, then the rectum was contracted, and a soft stool came, formed very thin, like a quill (aft. 16 h.).

Soft stool, with discharge of flatus. [*Ng.*]

Half-thin stool. [*Hbg.*]

Half-liquid (diarrhœic) stools. [*Ng.*]

675. Liquid stool.

Liquid stool, in the morning. [*Ng.*]

Diarrhœa, with tenesmus and burning in the anus. [*Ng.*]

Cold in the abdomen is apt to cause diarrhœa.

Evening diarrhœa. [*Ng.*]

680. Nocturnal diarrhœa.

Stool, with an ascaris. [*Ng.*]

Stool, with white mucus (aft. 6 d.).

Mucus and bright blood come together, with knotty, difficult stool, without any sign of varices.

Painless passage of blood, with soft stool.

685. Bloody stool, with burning and feeling of soreness in the rectum.

Before the stool, writhing pain in the abdomen. [*Rl.*]

During stool, stinging in the rectum.

After stool, burning in the anus, anxious pulse, and palpitation of the heart.

After stool, burning in the anus, making him weak.

690. After stool, tremulous lassitude and palpitation.

After stool, anxious oppression, heat in the face, and inclination to perspire.

After stool, in the evening, **anxious oppression on the chest**, and abdomen very much inflated.

After stool, anxiety.

After the (first hard, then soft) stool, first succeeds dyspnœa, then inflation and pinching in both hypochondria, especially in the right, at every step.

695. After stool, often qualmishness.

After the stool (the third on that day), salty and mucous water flowed from his mouth (waterbrash).

After stool, emission of prostatic juice.

In the rectum, pressure, all day.

Continual pressure in the rectum and anus, worse after every stool.

700. Frequently a sudden, piercing, pressing pain in the rectum.

Sensation of something hard lodged in the rectum, like a kernel of a fruit. [*Rl.*]

Sensation in the rectum, as of fæces lodged there, which would come away. [*Rl.*]

Cramp in the rectum, making it impossible to walk; she was at once obliged to sit still (aft. several h.).

Stitch of the anus (before a meal).

705. Itching of the anus. [*Ng.*]

Excessive itching of the anus, day and night (aft. 2 d.).

Severe itching in the rectum and the pudenda.

Itching and stinging of the rectum.

Tingling itching of the anus.

710. Formication in the rectum (aft. several h.).

Smarting pain in the anus, after stool.

Violent burning in the anus, during stool.

Pain as of a sore on the anus, and moisture there. [*Rl.*]

Varices on the anus, impeding the stool (aft. 13 d.).

715. Large painful varices. [*Rl.*]

Pains as from a sore of the varices of the anus, intolerably aggravated by walking and by reflection.

Hard varices of the anus, shooting and burning, extremely painful when touched; when walking, standing and sitting they are equally painful; relieved by stool; for fourteen days (aft. 19 d.).

Swollen varices of the anus, with itching, stinging and much oozing moisture.

Large, painful boil, near the anus, discharging much pus and blood, attended with much fatigue. [*Rl.*]

720. **Pain in the perinæum.**

Severe throbbing in the perinæum.

In the bladder, pains; he cannot pass urine, and even if a few drops are discharged, he feels violent pains in the urethra, with constipation and cramps in the rectum.

Tenesmus of the bladder, and if a few drops are discharged there is violent pain in the bladder, and (after much walking, undertaken to improve it,) also cramps in the rectum (21st d.).

Tenesmus of the bladder, after long waiting only a little is passed, and the urging is soon renewed, without any pains. [*Ng.*][1]

725. **Frequent urging to urinate.**

Urging to urinate after walking.

Frequent urging to micturition and after it a shaking chill in the open air, going off in the room. [*Ng.*]

Very often urging to urinate, with involuntary dripping of urine.

Frequent urging to urinate without discharge; then, when sitting, an involuntary discharge (1st d.).

730. He is frequently urged to urinate at night (aft. 15 d.).

He has to get up twice at night to urinate, and the urine passes copiously; there is also diarrhœa, repeated in the morning. [*Ng.*]

Wetting the bed, with violent erection, without any voluptuous sensation. [*Ng.*]

At night in sleep urine passes from her (aft. 7 d.).

Involuntary passage of urine while coughing and while blowing the nose.

735. The urine is intermittent in its discharge. [*Ng.*]

Retarded emission of the last drops of urine.

Little urine attended with much thirst. [*Ng.*]

The urination proceeds so easily, that he hardly feels the stream, and in the dark he does not know that he is urinating. [*Ng.*]

Frequent micturition.

740. Unusually abundant passage of urine (5th d.).

Frequent, very much increased urination; the urine soon deposits a yeast-like sediment. [*Ng.*]

Frequent discharge of much urine. [*Rl.*]

The urine is often discharged under great pressure and in far greater abundance than corresponds to what he drinks.

Very frequent discharge of little urine, without pain or urging. [*Stf.*]

745. Colorless urine, like water.

Pale urine, like water. [*Ng.*]

Often dark brown urine.

Reddish urine, but without any sediment. [*Ng.*]

The urine becomes turbid and cloudy in standing.

750. Much mucus in the urine, it can be drawn out in threads.

During micturition, pain in the urethra.

Scalding of the urine. [*Ng.*]

Scalding of the urine in the region of the frænulum.

Scalding of the urine after a pollution.

755. During micturition, burning in the urethra or in its root. [*Ng.*]

During and after micturition there is acridity; it erodes the pudendum like salt (aft. 11, 17 d.).

After micturition, in the evening, pain in the urethra, with dull aching on the upper part of the head.

Itching at the orifice of the urethra (8th d.). [*Ng.*]

Cutting in the urethra.

760. Burning sensation in the urethra. [*Rl.*]

Sudden burning in the urethra, at night.

In the penis, burning pain.

Large, red spots on the penis.

Increased smegma about the glans; an excessive quantity is secreted behind the glans.

765. Itching of the frænulum. [*Rl.*]

Itching on the inner surface of the prepuce, sometimes tickling, sometimes stinging.

Vesicles under the prepuce, which turn into suppurating ulcers.

Itching scurf on the inner surface of the prepuce. [*Rl.*]

In the testes, pressive pain, at noon.

770. Pressive pain, as from contusion, in the right testicle.

Tearing pains in the testes.
Stitches in the right testicle (aft. 6 d.).
The scrotum itches and perspires.
Itching of the scrotum and of the skin of the penis. [*Fr.*]
775. Itching, cutting pain on the septum of the scrotum. [*Fr.*]
Excitation of the sexual instinct (aft. several h.).
Increased sexual instinct (the 1st days). [*Ng.*]
Increased, very active sexual instinct, with indisposition to all work. [*Rl.*]
Sexual instinct but little active (aft. 32 d.).
780. There is no stiffness of the penis in coitus; he was impotent (aft. 27 d.)
Voluptuous twitches of the organ, with semi-rigidity.
Frequent, slight erections, in the morning, after coitus. [*Rl.*]
Erection, with urging to coitus, in the morning (2d d.). [*Ng.*]
Stiffness of the penis, all the forenoon (2d d.). [*Ng.*]
785. Excitation to emission of semen.
Violent pollutions and incontrollable erections, at night and the whole forenoon (aft. 50 d.). [*Ng.*]
Pollutions several nights in succession, also in the afternoon siesta (with an impotent man) (aft. 3 d.).
Frequent pollutions in an old man (aft. 7 d.).
Pollution, and then scalding of the urine.
790. After pollution he feels stupid during the day.
During the emission of semen in coitus, blood passed from the urethra (aft. 21 d.).
After coitus, spasmodic drawing pain in the rectum (anus).
In the female pudenda, burning. [*Stf.*]
Delays the menses by ten days, but then they flow more fully.
795. Delays the menses, which usually were regular, by two or three days (aft. 11 d.).
Delays the menses, which were just expected (at once).
Hastens the appearance of the menses by eleven days, while else they were two or three days late (aft. 24 d.).
At night, no blood passes during the menses.
Increased flow of blood during the menses.
800. When the menses are already completed, for several days afterward, from time to time, a little flow of blood is perceived.
The menstrual blood has a bad smell, and excites itching on the pudenda.
Before the menses, she feels melancholy; everything looked dark to her.
Before the menses, the last two days, much pain in the sacrum and anxious dreams.
Just before the menses and on the first day of the menses, a pain drawing to and fro in the abdomen.
805. **At the appearance of the menses, colic** without diarrhœa, with tearing in the back and sacrum, especially during motion.
During the menses, colic and diarrhœa.
During the menses, pain in the abdomen, as if everything

was broken in two, with pain in the sacrum as if bruised, and discharge of blood in large lumps.

During the menses, pain in the back.

During the menses, a sort of lancinating pain below the left breast.

810. During the menses, she is quite yellow in the face.

During the menses, very ill-humored and weary.

During the menses, vertigo and turning around in the head, worse on stooping forward, relieved in the afternoon. [*Stf.*]

Vaginal discharge at night (aft. 3 d.).

Very profuse vaginal discharge; it shoots out like the menses and with a similar smell (aft. 14 d.).

* * * * * * * *

815. **Frequent sneezing, in the morning.**

Frequent sneezing in the morning, after rising. [*Ng.*]

Frequent sneezing (at once).

Abortive sneezing. [*Fr.*]

Itching in the nose, as if a cold was coming. [*Fr.*]

820. Burning in the nostrils, as from an incipient cold.

Stoppage of the nose.

Stuffed coryza, with severe stoppage of the nose; inspiration through the nose and mouth is impeded.

Coryza with stoppage of the nose and sneezing (2d d.). [*Ng.*]

Short coryza, with sneezing (almost at once). [*Rl.*]

825. Discharge of fetid mucus from the nose and sneezing. [*Ng.*]

Profuse fluent coryza and eyes agglutinated in the morning (aft. 17 d.).

Profuse fluent coryza, for two weeks, with painful nocturnal cough and seven days' headache.

Coryza and hoarseness, so that she could not speak aloud (aft. 14 d.).

Severe stuffed and fluent coryza with roughness of the throat, and excoriation in the chest from violent coughing (aft. 32 d).

830. Severe coryza and cough, with pain in the chest, drawing in the limbs, frequent awaking at night and chill.

Irritation in the larynx as in incipient cold, with general feverish motions.

Acute pressive pain in the larynx when blowing the nose.

Painful drawing in the larynx, without cause.

Dryness in the larynx.

835. Sensation of dryness in the windpipe.

Burning and roughness in the throat, with hoarseness. [*Ng.*]

Rough throat, mucus on the chest, and feverish chill.

Mucus in the chest (the windpipe), after eating.

Rawness of the chest, in the morning.

840. Scraping on the chest.

Hoarseness and roughness in the throat, in the morning. [*Ng.*]

Hoarseness.

Severe hoarseness especially in the morning and evening, with scraping in the throat.

Hoarseness for many days, she could not speak a word aloud

845. The voice is obstructed for several mornings, as if there was a wedge in the larynx, which he ought to throw out.

The laryngeal muscles refuse to act; despite of all efforts, he cannot utter words aloud.

Catarrh, with nocturnal dryness of the throat and stoppage of the nose, when lying down (aft. 16 d.).

Catarrh, with coughing and scratching in the throat.

Frequent desire in the larynx, to clear away something.

850. Hawking of mucus, with pain in the pit of the throat.

Hawking of mucus, in the morning.

Irritation to cough, at once, early in bed.

Tickling cough, frequently (aft. 4 d.).

Cough, excited by unceasing tingling.

855. Cough, excited by tingling, or when he stoops to pick up something.

Cough in short fits, from mucus in the throat, which tickles there. [*Ng.*]

Cough, from tickling in the throat and roughness, without expectoration, or this only comes long afterward. [*Ng.*]

Tussiculation from continued tickling in the throat. [*Ng.*]

Cough, with scraping in the throat, without expectoration.

860. Excitation to cough at every expiration.

Cough, excited every time he talks.

Cough, after getting cold, when she becomes warm again.

Irritation to cough, on awaking in the morning in bed.

In the morning on awaking, constant, fatiguing dry cough, as after taking a cold; this did not allow him to go to sleep again. [*Lgh.*]

865. Cough, only at night, on awaking.

Every night at 2 o'clock a two hours' cough with much expectoration; by day but rare and little cough.

Also at night, severe cough.

Cough wakes her from sleep, in the evening and morning; by day, little or no cough.

Short cough with some expectoration of mucus, especially after eating.

870. Cough, with retching, attended with dyspnœa.

Hoarse cough, mostly in the morning and evening, not at night.

Dry cough, causing burning on the chest.

Frequent dry tussiculation, only rarely with expectoration of mucus. [*Ng.*]

Dry, hollow cough, five or six impulses in succession, with pain as from soreness, along a space like a band in the inside of the windpipe, where it pains at every cough and almost checks the breathing.

875. Hollow cough, especially at night and in the morning, with mucus adhering to the chest, which pains both while coughing and at other times, with a stinging sorenesss and as if festering underneath; with stuffed coryza and stoppage of the nose (aft. 24 d.).

Violent cough, at times quite dry, with pain in the right side of the abdomen.

Before the beginning of a coughing fit, short breath.

During coughing, the chest pains as if sore.

During coughing, stitches in the left side of the chest.

880. **During coughing, a loud rattling in the chest** (aft. 24 h.).

Cough, with rattling at every breath, as if there was much mucus on the right side of the chest, in the forenoon.

During coughing, pain over the left hip, as if it were going to burst open there.

Obstruction of respiration, while talking and while walking briskly; **she has to quickly catch her breath.**

Sudden obstruction of breath in the open air (while hunting), with very rapid palpitation; he could not hold himself upright, but had to kneel down, sweating all over; the breath became very short, the blood rushed to the head, the face became bluish-red, as if he should have a stroke of apoplexy; for one hour (4th d.).

885. Shortness of breath, when taking a walk in the open air.

Shortness of breath in the morning, with pressive pain in the abdomen, going off during the day (aft 6 d.).

Short breath and tightness of the chest.

Lack of breath, with weakness of the thighs (aft. 9 d.).

Difficult and deep respiration. [*Hbg.*]

890. Sensation of tightness and lack of air in the throat, with inflation of its left side: he has to loosen his cravat. [*Ng.*]

Sensation on the chest, as if the clothes were too tight.

Sensation as if the chest was too tight.

Asthma, chiefly when sitting.

Asthma, after lying down.

895. Tightness of the chest, with hoarseness and roughness of the throat. [*Ng.*]

Tightness of the chest; he has often to take a deep breath (1st d.). [*Rl.*]

Spasmodic asthma.

Painful tightness of the chest, in the afternoon, going off by dancing (aft. 16 d.).

Tightness of both sides of the chest, as if they were being pressed together. [*Fr.*]

900. Painful compression of the chest from both sides, toward the sternum, with oppressed breathing and weakness of voice.

Frequent fits of choking on inspiring, as if some one was constricting the windpipe, so that it obstructed the breath, when sitting. [*Htm.*]

Great oppression of the heart, with melancholy.

In the chest, on the lowest rib of the left side, a pressive pain.

Pressive pain in the right side of the chest in the evening.

905. Pressure in the costal muscles, transversely over the chest, on stooping forward.

Pressure over the chest and stomach.

Pressure on the chest, just above the scrobiculus cordis.

Pressure on the right side of the chest (aft. 24 h.).

Pressure on the chest, with short and labored breath. [*Ng.*]

910. Pressive pain above the xiphoid cartilage, straight upward.

Tearing pain anteriorly on the chest, almost only in the open air, or at least aggravated there.

Tension about the chest, long continuing (2d d.). [*Ng.*]

Painfulness, like a drawing internally in the upper part of the chest, after too violent running or singing, with a sense of a weight upon it (aft. 3 h.). [*Stf.*]

Rheumatic pain in the chest and the abdomen. [*Ng.*]

915. Lancinating tearing in the left side of the chest. [*Ng.*]

Stitches in the right side of the chest, on inspiring (aft. ½ h.). [*Htm.*]

Dull stitch in the right side of the chest, near the clavicle.

Stitches in the left side of the chest, below the nipple.

Violent stitch in the left side of the chest, on inspiration. [*Ng.*]

920. Shooting below the left breast, going off by rubbing. [*Ng.*]

Dull stitches in the left side of the chest, opposite the xiphoid cartilage. [*Htm.*]

Obtuse stitch in the left side of the chest, above the heart, on motion.

Sharp, slow stitches in the left part of the chest, horizontally with the scrobiculus cordis. [*Htm.*]

Stitches at night, without obstructing the breath, as if from a knife, thrust in anteriorly in the chest, and into the back behind, with great anguish and restlessness, so that he has continually to toss about, without being able to sleep.

925. **Shooting in the sternum, on taking a deep breath** and on lifting things.

A stitch in the sternum, when taking a deep breath and during bodily labor (aft. 16 d.).

A stitch, first, one continuing for eight minutes on the lower part of the sternum on inspiring and expiring, then a stitch in the sternum continuing all the forenoon with alternating violence, most observable on expiration; this stitch was connected with a constant dull stitch in the left shoulder joint, which was also most sensible at expiration.

Stitches in the chest as from a nail. [*Hbg.*]

Shooting, deep in the chest, on taking a deep breath, for an hour in the forenoon (aft. 14 d.).

930. Stitches from the depth of the chest, going out at the back.

Stitches as with needles, on the chest, while taking a walk in the open air. [*Lgh.*]

Sensation in the chest as if cut to pieces, in the morning, with burning. [*Ng.*]

Pain in the right side of the chest, as if the lungs were being torn off from the pleura, almost constant, even when lying down.

Pain as of a bruise, below the right mamma, unchanged by respiration. [*Ng.*]

835. Pain as from a sprain in the lower muscles of the left side of the chest, on moving the left arm (aft. ½ h.). [*Fr.*]

Rushing sound in the left side of the chest, in the cardiac region, for several mornings in bed, till rising; it, indeed, is diminished with every movement, but returns on lying down.

Heat internally in the chest.

Heat in the chest, at times extending up into the throat. [*Ng.*]

Burning pain in the chest, and at times shooting.

940. Under the skin of the chest, short, acute stitches.

Sharp stitches in the chest, beside the nipple, which always quickly draw toward the navel, especially on inspiring.

Stitches in the chest, under the arms, even to the scrobiculus cordis, with anxiety (and then rumbling in the abdomen, and pinching toward the chest, which vanished altogether after the discharge of flatus) (aft. 29 d.).

Obtuse stitches beside the axilla, toward the chest.

Severe itching about the breasts.

945. Palpitation with lassitude (aft. several h.).

Severe palpitation, in the morning, with irregular pulse and backache.

Severe palpitation, in the evening, with great anxiety, which caused a great shortness of breath, without any peculiar thoughts (6th d.).

Anxious palpitation, with rhythmical contraction of the abdomen.

In the region of the coccyx, a dull, drawing pain. [*Fr.*]

950. Twitching pain in the coccyx (aft. 7 d.). [*Rl.*]

Pain as from a bruise in the coccyx. [*Fr.*]

Pain in the sacrum; she painfully feels every motion of the body in her sacrum.

Pressive pain in the sacrum, when sitting.

Pressive pain in the sacrum, so that he had to remain bent down (with pressive pain in the abdomen).

955. Violent tensive pain in the sacrum.

Pinching, cramp-like pain in the sacrum and the nates. [*Rl.*]

Pressive, cramp-like pain in the sacrum and the renal region, when sitting (4th d.).

Violent tearing in the sacrum. [*Ng.*]

Sensation as from a bruise in the sacrum, when walking; going off when sitting. [*Ng.*]

960. Pain as from a bruise in the sacrum, toward evening, for several hours, with discharge of leucorrhœa (aft. 31 d.).

Violent pain in the sacrum, as from a strain caused by lifting, on motion (aft. 2 d.). [*Rl.*]

Stiffness in the lumbo-sacral articulation (aft. ¼ h.). [*Fr.*]

Single itching stitches in the sacrum. [*Fr.*]

Pain as from soreness in the sacrum, with subsequent pressure in the hypogastrium, as if everything was coming out at the rectum and the pudenda; like a flatulent colic; (from straining in lifting).

965. Frequent throbbing in the sacrum.

Pain the back, a pressure in the middle of the back.

Pressive cramp-pain in the back, in the renal region.

Violent pressive pain, combined with tearing, toward the back, on the edge of the right scapula, increased by bending back the right upper arm and the head, finally at **every movement of the** body, even when the part is shaken only a little, but most severe when the head is turned to the left side.

Stinging, piercing twitching in the back and sacrum, taking his breath.

970. Drawing, in the back and as if bruised; thence the pain extended to the sacrum and the abdomen, where much flatus accumulated with bellyache, and as the flatus was discharged leucorrhœa appeared.

Tearing in the back in a small spot. [*Ng.*]

Tearing in the vertebræ of the back, between the scapulæ, extending into the right scapula and then also into the left.

Stitches in the back (aft. 20, 27 d.).

Stitches in the back, as from needles, when sitting down.

975. A stitch in the back, then backache.

Crawling in the back. [*Ng.*]

Itching in the skin of the back (aft. 10 h.). [*Stf.*]

Itching of the back and some perspiration.

Much itching of the back and of the calves.

980. A furuncle on the back.

Between the scapulæ, pain from stiffness (aft. 5 d.). [*Rl.*]

Severe tensive pain, in the upper part of the scapulæ, during motion.

Tearing in the right scapula. [*Hrn.*]

Painful tearing between the scapulæ. [*Ng.*]

985. Drawing in the left scapula.

Pressive drawing in the scapulæ.

Violent stitches in the left scapula, as from needles

A pressive shooting pain, beside the right scapula, in deglutition and in hawking, as well as in exerting oneself in speaking.

Burning in the middle of the right scapula. [*Ng.*]

990. In the cervical muscles, a tension, when quickly raising the body, and turning the head.

Tension in the nape, as if someone was drawing her backward by the ears. [*Ng.*]

Stiffness of the neck, that he could not move his head.

Stiffness of the nape and of the neck, with pains in the occiput, the muscles felt bound, so that she could hardly move her head (12th d.).

Twitching motion in the neck, toward the head.

995. Shooting in the nape at night, when lying down.

Shudder in the nape of the neck, extending into the brain, in the evening.

Pain in the neck as from a bruise (aft. 4 d.). [*Rl.*]

Miliary eruption in the nape, between the scapulæ, and on the back, with itching.

A nodule with tension, in the nape of the neck. [*Ng.*]

1000. Very much itching and a humid tetter in the nape of the neck.

In the cervical muscles, tension and jerking, also when at rest. [*Hbg.*]

Constant tension in the right side of the neck and chest, so that it draws the body to the right side. [*Ng.*]

Pinching pain on the right side of the neck. [*Rl.*]

Pain from stiffness in the right side of the neck. [*Rl.*]

1005 Stiffness of the right side of the neck with tensive pain. [*Fr.*]

Pressure in the pit of the throat, when taking a deep breath.

Burning on a small spot of the right side of the neck, with a red spot there. [*Ng.*]

In the axilla, shooting burning. [*Ng.*]

The shoulder pains all the day, on moving the right arm. [*Ng.*]

1010. **Pressure on the shoulder.**

Stiffness in the shoulders.

Tearing in the left shoulder-joint.

Tearing in the right shoulder, with pain as from a bruise on the inner edge of the right scapula, on moving the right arm or on turning the head to the right; if she turns the head to the left, the spot is tense. [*Ng.*]

Sharp stitches in the top of the shoulders, on the right and the left side.

1015. Obtuse stitch in the left shoulder. [*Ng.*]

The left shoulder pains as if sprained, from morning till evening. [*Ng.*]

Paralytic pain in the left shoulder. [*Ng.*]

The left arm twitches repeatedly. [*Rl.*]

Convulsive movements in the (left, weak) arm, up and down, after some slight exertion, then great heaviness of the arm, then a sort of rumbling down in the muscles, even into the leg, like the running of a mouse, whereby the twitches vanished.

1020. Pressive pain in the right arm.

Drawing in the right arm, which feels heavy, as if paralyzed (aft. 14 d.).

Drawing pains in the muscles of the arms. [*Stf.*]

Dull tearing in the arms and hands.

Severe tearing in the arms and the hands, extending into the back.

1025. Arthritic drawing, here and there, in the joints of the arms and the wrists, and in the shoulders, seemingly aggravated by motion. [*Stf.*]

Single stitches in the arm, extending into the left side of the chest.

Slowly tearing stitch in the right arm, from the shoulder down into the hand (aft. 1¼ h.). [*Htm.*]

Tendency of the left arm to grow numb at night in sleep, waking him up. [*Ng.*]

The left arm grows numb, when raised up over the head, and held up for a time; it is as if the blood in it flowed back, and in the right side of the chest there is a pain, as if the muscles were shortened.

1030. Great heaviness and weakness in the arms.

Heaviness in the right arm, as if in consequence of a violent blow on the thickest part of the fore-arm.

Weakness in the right arm, with a troublesome crawling, in front of both shoulders. [*Ng.*]

Trembling of the right arm, if he holds anything with outstretched arm.

Weakness, almost like paralysis, of the right arm, with sensation of stiffness, especially when writing. [*Fr.*]

1035. **Itching of the arms.**

The muscles of the upper arm are painful, as if sprained (aft. 7 d).

Drawing pain in the left humerus.

Drawing pain in the deltoid muscle, extending toward the clavicle, now in the one arm, then in the other. [*Stf.*]

Drawing pain in the muscles, in the lower part of the left upper arm. [*Lgh.*]

1040. Tearing in the left upper arm and in the shoulder-joint.

Tearing in the left upper arm and in the right, close below the shoulder-joint (at once).

Tearing in the left humerus to elbow-joint, in which the pain is most severe.

Drawing cutting in the deltoid muscle of the right arm. [*Fr.*]

Pinching in the deltoid muscle of the upper arm, with sensation of coldness, terminating in burning. [*Hbg.*]

1045. Shooting pain in the left humerus, at the top, near its head, toward the outside.

Stitches in the deltoid muscle of the upper arm, when she carries anything.

Shooting pain in the right upper arm, on raising the arm.

Sharp stitches in the left upper arm, near the shoulder.

Acute shooting pain on the right upper arm, at times going off by rubbing. [*Ng.*]

1050. Burning on the outer surface of the left upper arm. [*Ng.*]

The elbow-joint is painful, as if he had knocked it against something. [*Stf.*]

Pain in the bend of the left elbow, on stretching the arm, as if a tendon was too short. [*Rl.*]

Quivering on the outer side of the elbow-joint, on resting the arm on something (aft. 3 h.).

Drawing pain in the elbow-joints and the lower arms.

1055. Boring in the olecranon process of the ulna, with a sensation as if it would bend the arm double. [*Ng.*]

Pain, as from a bruise, in the bend of the elbow and the pectoral muscles, much aggravated by external pressure. [*Rl.*]

In the fore-arm, tearing, in the bones.

Tearing in the fore-arms. [*Ng.*]

Tearing in the tendons of the right fore-arm. [*Ng.*]

1060. Tearing in the left fore-arm, down from the elbow.

Throbbing, tearing in the left fore-arm. [*Ng.*]

Contractive pain in the muscles, on the lower part of the left fore-arm. [*Lgh.*]

Shooting upward in the tendons of the inner side of the right fore-arm. [*Ng.*]

Painfully drawing stitches in the muscles of the lower part of the left fore-arm. [*Lgh.*]

1065. Boring and tearing, on a small spot of the right fore-arm, just under the elbow, as if in the bone. [*Ng.*]

Burning, transversely over the fore-arm, close by the wrist. [*Ng.*]

Sensation of coldness and rigidity of the right fore-arm and the fingers; he could not warm his hand even on the warm stove.

Paralysis of the fore-arms; he could hardly raise them owing to their heaviness and sensation of rigidity. [*Fr.*]

Paralytic pain in the shaft of the right ulna. [*Ng.*]

1070. Short, tremulous twitches on the right fore-arm, during writing (2d d.).

Swelling of the fore-arm, seemingly in the periosteum, only aching when pressed upon. [*Rl.*]

Small, itching pimples on the fore-arms.

Formication in the skin of the right fore-arm, going off by rubbing. [*Ng.*]

Itching (at times with burning after scratching) and itching pimples and vesicles on the fore-arms. [*Ng.*]

1075. In the hands, cramp-like sensation.

Cramp-like weakness in the hands, in the morning on awaking.

Sensation of fullness in the left palm, on grasping anything.

Swelling of the hands at night, with formication in them.

Drawing pain in the wrist.

1080. Drawing pain in the left wrist, on the outer side. [*Stf.*]

Drawing pain, extending from the right wrist-joint into the fingers.

Drawing pain, extending from the wrist through the metacarpal bone into the little finger, in the tip of which it is most severe; on stretching out the hand, the pain is even greater, and involuntarily draws the finger together, while the drawing from the wrist also seizes upon the other fingers, and gradually draws them all double, sometimes more, sometimes less.

Tearing in the right wrist. [*Ng.*]

Tearing on the dorsum, now of the one hand, now of the other.

1085. Very painful tearing on the back of the hand, extending into the middle finger with cramp-pain. [*Ng.*]

Tearing on the inner edge of the right hand, toward the little finger, as if in the bone. [*Ng.*]

Tearing in the hands and fingers (aft. 24 h).

Tearing in the hand, in the metacarpal bone of the left and the right thumb.

Stitches in the left palm, with tingling in the fingers. [*Ng.*]

1090. Tingling shooting in the right wrist and the second and third fingers.

Twitching stitches in the muscles of the left hand, right across its dorsum, on moving the arms (aft. 9 h.). [*Lgh.*]

Pain as from a sprain or a strain, in the right wrist, in grasping, (aft. 18 d.).

A shooting pain as from a sprain, in the left wrist, while working (aft. 10 d.).

A tensive pain as from spraining, right across the left hand, on moving it (aft. 26 h.). [*Lgh.*]

1095. Coldness of the hands; in the left arm this extends almost to the elbow.

The hand goes to sleep, with tingling therein (aft. 5 d.). [*Rl.*]

Trembling of the hands (aft. 21 d.). [*Hbg.*]

Great heaviness in the right hand.

Paralytic sensation in the right hand, for several weeks. [*Rl.*]

1100. Lack of strength in the hands, in a room which is too warm.

Itching in both hands.

Itching on the back of the left hand. [*Stf.*]

Much itching in the palms.

Itching in the palms, and after scratching, itching vesicles, containing water. [*Ng.*]

1105. The posterior joints of the fingers are tense, when they are flexed, in the forenoon.

Little twitches of the fingers, while writing.

Drawing twitches in the left fingers. [*Stf.*]

Like electric shocks, repeated dartings from the abdomen into the fingers, bending them double. [*Stf.*]

Drawing pains in the finger-joints.

1110. Drawing pains in the joints of the left fingers. [*Stf.*]

Tearing in the fingers. [*Ng.*]

Tearing in the left little finger, with cramp-pains. [*Ng.*]

Tearing in the joints of the right index, which are also painful when pressed. [*Ng.*]

Transient tearing in the left index.

1115. Tearing in the tips of all the fingers of the right and the left hands, with trembling of the hands.

Stitches in the little finger, which then extended upward, like stabs with a knife, with anxiety and aching about the heart (aft. 10 d.).

Contusive pain in the finger-tips, as if they would burst open, now in the one hand, now in the other (aft. 3 h.). [*Stf.*]

Contusive pain in the tip of the right little finger. [*Ng.*]

Throbbing pain as from an ulcer, in the posterior joint of the right thumb. [*Ng.*]

1120. Burning in the finger-tips.

Shooting burning pain in the joints of the fingers (aft. 32 h.). [*Hbg.*]

Tingling on the left ring-finger, with twitching on the inner side of the upper arm. [*Ng.*]

Numbness and insensibility of the fingers, with turgid fullness in them.

Dying off of the fingers; they become icy cold, white and insensible. [*Stf.*]

1125. Frequent dying off of the fingers, especially in the morning.

Itching between the fingers. [*Rl.*]

Itching on the posterior and middle joints of the fingers of the left hand. [*Fr.*]

Stinging itching in the index. [*Ng.*]

Itching of the left index, and, after scratching, a burning, itching nodule. [*Ng.*]

1130. A nodule on the right thumb, without sensation. [*Ng.*]

Itching tetter on the back of the ring-finger.

Ulceration of the tip of the thumb.

Under the nails of the fingers, pain on grasping anything.

Severe, burning, pressive pain under the finger-nails; but on grasping, pain as if festering underneath.

1135. The nates pain in sitting on them, as if from being beaten, or as if turgid.

Itching on the nates and on the posterior side of the thigh. [*Rl.*]

Stinging itching on the right natis. [*Ng.*]

Itching tetter on the nates (aft. 6 d.). [*Rl.*]

In the region of the hip, a violent cramp-pain.

1140. Pinching and squeezing in the region of the hips above the acetabulum, as if the muscles were seized with a pair of tongs, with a sensation of coldness, terminating in burning, even when at rest. [*Hbg.*]

Tension in the bend of the right thigh, in the morning, on rising, and on bending the knee. [*Ng.*]

Pressive pain above the acetabulum of the hip-joint, not aggravated by motion.

A drawing pressive pain in the hip, when sitting and when walking.

Tearing in the acetabulum of the hip-joint. [*Hrn.*]

1145. Tearing in the left hip, as if in the bone, both in rest and in motion; when pressed upon, pain as from a bruise. [*Ng.*]

Tearing in the hip-joint and down the whole limb, both sitting and walking (aft. 10. h.).

Stitches in the left hip, as if in the bone.

Dull stitches in the hip-joint, toward the abdomen, one every two minutes, for two hours (10th d.).

Frequently a stitch in the bend of the right thigh. [*Ng.*]

1150. Pain as from a sprain, or as if the foot had turned, or was strained, coming by jerks in the left hip-joint, so that he had to limp for several steps; coming and going suddenly. [*Stf.*]

Pricking, burning pain in the region of the hip. [*Hbg.*]

Itching in both hips. [*Fr.*]

Soreness in the upper part between the legs.

In the lower limbs, drawing pain, as if in the bones.

1155. Drawing in the right limb, with sore throat, in the evening.

Severe drawing and tearing, during a thunder storm, in both the lower limbs, from the toes up into the thighs.

Muscular twitching in both the lower limbs.

Acute, slow stitches in the lower limbs, first down from the hip-joint, then down from the knee-pan, more painful at rest than while walking (aft. 2 h.).

Slow tearing stitch in the lower limb, from the ankle to the knee and from there to the hip-joint, but not in the knee itself (aft. ¼ h.). [*Htm.*]

1160. **Pain, as from a bruise, in the thighs and legs, in the morning, in bed.**

Pain, as if twisted or paralyzed, in the muscles of the lower limbs, in the afternoon and evening.

Troublesome restlessness in both lower limbs, in the morning in bed, for several hours.

Restlessness in the left lower limb, at night; she knew not where to lay it.

Restlessness in the lower limbs, at evening, so severe she could not sit still.

1165. Severe formication in the thighs and legs, as well as in the foot.

The legs are apt to go to sleep.

Much painful heaviness in the lower limbs.

Lassitude in the lower limbs, especially in the legs and knees; he always wants to take a rest while walking. [*Ng.*]

Excessive weariness of the lower limbs, in the morning on awaking, in bed, vanishing after getting up

1170. Painful weakness of the lower limbs, both in the thighs and legs, when walking.

Trembling of the lower limbs, when beginning an ascent (*e.g.*, of a ladder); this ceases when he stands and continues to work.

Trembling and shaking of the lower limbs, as from a chill, in the open air, when walking and standing; it goes off in a room. [*Ng.*]

Distended veins (varices) on the lower limbs.

Itching on the lower limbs. [*Stf.*]

1175. Skin as if marbled, full of dark-red veinlets on the thighs and legs.

In the thighs, twitching pains, down from the nates (aft. 5 d.). [*Rl.*]

Muscular twitching in the left thigh, above the knee.

Tearing pain in the middle of the left thigh, vanishing on rising from the seat. [*Fr.*]

Scratching tearing in the left thigh.

1180. Paralytic tearing on the outer side of the right thigh. [*Ng.*]

Stitches in the left thigh (at once).

Stitches in the left thigh, extending into the chest, in the evening, in walking.

Violent needle-prick on the outer side of the right thigh, just above the knee. [*Ng.*]

Quick flush of heat on the inner side of the left thigh.

1185. Throbbing in the tendons of the left thigh, just above the knee. [*Ng.*]

Sensation of excessive weariness in the upper part of the thigh, toward the inner side, worst when the limb is at rest, when he is compelled to continually move the limb to and fro. [*Fr.*]

Weakness of the thighs, with lack of breath.

Feels as if paralyzed in the thighs, in sitting and in walking. [*Fr.*]

Trembling or quivering sensation, **like a painful sounding** vibration in the fleshy part of the thigh. [*Ng.*]

1190. Itching on the thighs.

Stinging itching on the thigh, on the outer side.. [*Fr.*]

Violently itching nettle-rash, especially on the thighs, just above the knee (12th d.).

Soreness, as if rubbed open, on the thigh, on the upper, inside part of the scrotum, with itching, and, when rubbing it, with excoriation (aft. 40 h.).

Painful soreness, on the upper, inner part of the female thighs, where they touch in walking.

1195. In the left knee, stiffness in walking.

Turgidity in the houghs in sitting, and when commencing to walk; better when continuing the walk.

Pain from stiffness in the patella, when rising up. [*Rl.*]

Tensive pain and stiffness in the hough, when walking. [*Rl.*]

Drawing pain in the knees, as if from fatigue in walking, more when stretching than when flexing the knees.

1200. Drawing pain, rather above the knees.

Drawing in the knee-joints. [*Rl.*]

Drawing and twitching pain in the left patella. [*Rl.*]

Twitching in the left knee, in the afternoon. [*Ng.*]

First a drawing pain then a twitching pain in the knee. [*Rl.*]

1205. Tearing on the outer side of the left knee. [*Ng.*]

Tearing in the right knee (aft. 48 h.)

Tearing in the left knee and from there downwards, even into the toes. [*Ng.*]

Drawing tearing in the knee and from there into the ankles, in the evening.

Tearing and shooting in the knee, so that he cannot tread on that foot, nor sleep for it at night.

1210. A stitch in the knee, while at work (aft. 10 d.).

Painful boring in the right knee, at times with pain as from a bruise when pressing upon it. [*Ng.*]

Pain as from soreness in the knee.

Ulcerative pain on the outer side of the knee, extending up to the thigh (aft. 14 d.).

Painful cracking in the knee, when walking, as if it was broken or sprained.

1215. Extraordinary weariness of the knee-joint and heaviness of the feet, after a walk. [*Fr.*]

Weariness of the knee-joints, more in going upstairs than while walking on a level. [*Fr.*]

Weakness in the knee, even so that it gives way.

The knees give way in walking.

Much itching on the patella.

1220. Itching, especially in the right hough (aft. 3 d.). [*Rl.*]

In the leg, a hard pressure down the tibia.

Tension in the right calf, as if some one forcibly drew together the skin, both in rest and in motion (in the evening). [*Ng.*]

Cramp in the calf, early in bed (aft. 20 h.).

Contraction of the right calf, both in rest and in motion. [*Ng.*]

1225. Cramp-like contraction down the whole of the outer side of the right leg, both sitting and standing. [*Tr.*]

Drawing pain in the leg.

Drawing in the calf, with the sensation as if the right leg was shorter, on rising from a seat, and in walking. [*Ng.*]

Tearing on the outer side of the left leg, from the knee down, when sitting; when rising from the seat it extends up into the hip-joint; when walking and when pressing on it, pain as from a bruise in the hip, not going off when sitting down. [*Ng.*]

Tearing downward in the left calf (aft. 1 h.). [*Ng.*]

1230. Tearing, from the outer surface of the right calf down to the outer edge of the foot, worse on moving the foot and the toes. [*Ng.*]

Violent tearing in the tendons below the right calf. [*Ng.*]

Tearing in the calf and in the dorsum of the foot. [*Ng.*]

Tearing in the left tendo-Achillis, when sitting. [*Ng.*]

Burning tearing on the tibia. [*Ng.*]

1235. Intermittent stitches in the left calf. [*Ng.*]

Pain as from a bruise on the right calf, extending into and around the knees, the whole forenoon. [*Ng.*]

Pain as from knocking against something, on the right shin bone. [*Ng.*]

Crawling and pricking in the left calf, as if it would go to sleep, at times extending into the hough. [*Ng.*]

Dull, tingling sensation of being asleep, in both the legs and knees, in the morning (4th d.).

1240. A red, painful spot on the shin, which extends in length, and itches when healing.

A blister on the calf, two and a half inches in diameter, almost without pain; water comes out for two days, and it heals without suppuration.

In the soles of the feet, aching, like nervous suffering.

Pressure on the dorsum of the foot. [*Ng.*]

Tension in the heel and the tendo-Achillis (aft. 20 d.).

1245. Cramp in the sole and the tendo-Achillis of the right foot, on stretching it.

Cramp in the feet (aft. 4th and 11th d.).

Cramp in the foot, on stretching it.

Stiffness in the ankle-joint.

Drawing in the ankle-joints (aft. 12 h.). [*Stf.*]

1250. Drawing pain in the ankle-joint, when sitting; accompanied with a sensation on treading with that foot, as if the leg would give way. [*Fr.*]

Drawing in the right foot, in the evening.

Drawing pain in the bend of the right foot, extending into the big toe, where it is only felt in motion. [*Ng.*]

Tearing in the inner border of the foot, also in the morning, in bed. [*Ng.*]

Tearing on the outer part of the ankle, in the evening. [*Ng.*]

1255. Tearing in the dorsum of the left foot.

Tearing in the ball of the foot, behind the big toe. [*Ng.*]

Sudden tearing in the right heel. [*Ng.*]

Pain as of a sprain in the ankle-joint, when she makes a misstep, or when the foot turns; the joint also then cracks.

Pain as of a sprain in the ankle-joint when walking, or as if it was being broken.

1260. Pain in the ankle-joint, as if crushed or fatigued, on sitting after walking; it vanishes as soon as she walks again.

Burning in the soles of the feet.

Swelling, especially of the front part of the foot, late in the evening, with heat, a burning sensation and interior itching, as if the foot had been frozen; it also pains on external pressure, as if festering internally.

Cold feet. [*Fr.*, *Hbg.*]

Always very cold feet.

1265. Formication and itching on the heel, as if it was going to sleep; it compels scratching and then goes off. [*Ng.*]

Formication in the soles of both the feet, as if something alive was in them.

A tingling, burning formication in the soles of the feet.

The feet go to sleep, while he is sitting and lying down. [*Ng.*]

Turgidity and numbness of the heel, when treading on it.

1270. Weariness of the feet in the morning, so that he could hardly stand. [*Ng.*]

Much itching on the dorsum of the foot.

Severe itching on the dorsum of the foot (aft. 16 d.).

Violent tickling on the dorsum of the right foot, so that she could not scratch enough. [*Ng.*]

Great blisters on the feet, from some rubbing.

1275. Corroding blister on the heel, which gradually disappears with much itching.

Ulcerated heel.

In the big toe, in the posterior joint, severe, pressive pain.

Tearing on the edge and on the outer side of the little toe. [*Ng.*]

Violent tearing in the big toe.

1280. Violent tearing in the left big toe, toward its tip. [*Ng.*]

Burning tearing in the toes and under their nails. [*Ng.*]

Fine stitches in the big toe.

A long stitch in the big toe. [*Rl.*]

Violent needle pricks in the ball of the big toe, both during motion and without.

1285. Violent burning stinging in the ball of the big toe, and under its nail. [*Ng.*]

Formicating burning on the ball of the big toe. [*Ng.*]

Pain in the big toe as if burnt.

Inflammatory pain behind the nail of the big toe. [*Ng.*]

Pain in the big toe, as if suppurated.

1290. Formication (and stinging) in the big toes, as if they would go to sleep. [*Ng.*]

Formication in the ball of the big toe. [*Ng.*]

Tickling in the toes, as if they had been frozen.

Voluptuous itching in the anterior joint of the big toe, both in motion and without

Paronychia, digging burning pain beside the nail of the left big toe, with proud flesh (3d d.).

1295. In the corn of the little toe, violent stitches.

Boring pain in the corn.

Burning pain in the corn.

Here and there in the body, cramp-like pain. [*Rl.*]

Muscular twitching in one part or another of the body.

1300. A little twitching here and there in the body.

Continual quivering on the right side of the body and on various other parts of the skin.

Pressive pains in the arms and thighs.

Drawing in the limbs, here and there. [*Stf.*]

Drawing in the fingers, the soles and toes of the feet.

1305. Drawing in various parts of the body, increasing to tearing.

Quickly passing drawing pain in the right index and the left second toe.

Gouty pains in all the limbs (aft. ½ h.).

Tearing in all the limbs, now in this, now in that, now more violent, then again more slight, but continual (aft. 1 h. and so for several days.)

Tearing, especially in the joints, and from them to the various bones of the body, also in several at the same time; the pain is not aggravated by external pressure.

1310. Tearing in various limbs of the body, worst in the joints, and from these it extends to the shafts of the long bones. [*Hrn.*]

Stinging pains in almost all parts of the body (the 1st days).

A sort of stinging pain in the joints, after a cold.

Transient stinging or contractive pains, now here, now there, in the body (after the cessation of the menses.)

Pain as from bruising, all over the body, especially in the arms, when sitting; going off when at work and in the open air (aft. 12 d.).

1315. Every part of the body which he touches, pains as if cudgeled. [*Rl.*]

Bruised feeling in all the right side of the body.

Stiff in all the joints, so that when she does not move for a quarter of an hour, while sitting or lying still, she has difficulty in getting about again.

Formication in the arms and legs, as if they would go to sleep (aft. 5 d.). [*Rl.*]

The whole left side of the body feels asleep and cold.

1320. Numbness and deadness of all the soft parts on the whole left side of the body, also in the foot and head, as if there was no blood in the skin.

The first effects seem to appear later in this antipsoric remedy than in others.

Coffee seems to aggravate the various symptoms. [*Ng.*]

The ailments seem to be aggravated while taking a walk **in the open air,** in the evening. [*Stf.*]

After walking a little in the open air, the blood rose to his head and face, and there was dimness like a mist before his eyes.

1325. After a slow walk in the open air, he is very much heated and excited.

After walking, flushes of heat and discomfort (aft. 4 h.).

On taking a walk in the open air, profuse sweat.

After a walk, sweat on the back and the abdomen, of long continuance.

While walking, sweat, with great lassitude, in the afternoon.

1330. After a short walk, lassitude, with indisposition for work (aft. 6 h.).

The ailments arising in the open air disappear in the room, excepting a pressive headache in the forehead. [*Fr.*]

Greater sensitiveness to the fresh air in May than in winter.

The open air affects her strongly. [*Ng.*]

Very sensitive to cold (aft. 10 d.).

1335. Very sensitive to draught; it is very disagreeable to him, and excites all his pressive pains [*Rl.*]

Great tendency to take cold after short exposure to a draught, at once chilliness all over the body.

Itching all over the body. [*Fr.*]

Itching all over the body, at night, with dry heat.

Itching on various parts of the body. [*Fr.*]

1340. Itching which goes off on scratching, in various parts of the body. [*Ng.*]

Itching, now here, now there, especially in the head and face. [*Ng.*]

A pricking itching over the skin.

A fine stinging itching, as from fleas, compelling to scratch, on the back, the shoulders, the arms, and the thighs, but especially on the backs of the fingers.

Creeping in the skin, as from ants.

1345. Whatever part she touches, burns.

Itching all over the body, with redness like scarlatina and with many vesicles; the itching does not vanish from scratching. [*Ng.*]

Eruptive pimples on various parts of the body, with gnawing erosive itching, that burns after scratching. [*Hrn.*]

Lumps under the skin, up to the size of a filbert, on the right side of the breast, the arm, the back, and the bend of the elbow, with stinging pain when touched, and pain as from a sore on pressing hard (aft. 24 d.); later, even when not touched, they have a stinging pain, not increased by touching.

Eruption, resembling chickenpox, in a suckling.

1350. Large blisters on chest and back, with oppression of the chest and a fever, which consists of chill, heat and sweat.

Large, painful blisters on the left side of the chest and back; they burst open; attended with feverish heat, sweat and anxious oppression.

An eruptive pimple (on the index) turns into a wart.

Eruptions of the size of a pin's head, with hollow tip; without moisture, on forehead, nape, scapulæ, arms, hypogastrium, especially on the thighs and in the houghs; they itch especially when warm, and especially in the warmth of the bed; when not warm, they, being white, are hardly visible in the skin; but when scratched, they come out quickly, and when scratched open, they leave red spots of larger size; for five days (aft. 16 d.).

Old, brown hepatic spots become elevated, causing an erosive itching. [*Stf.*]

1355. Lesions of the skin, already nearly healed, become sore again and fester.

An ulcer (on the leg) is surrounded with a red areola, which is hard and inflamed, and discharges more blood than pus; the discharge is very fetid and the pain makes the nights sleepless.

Much ebullition of the blood (1st d.).

Even the slightest pressure by the clothes on the stomach and the hips, is troublesome and intolerable to him.

Restlessness throughout the body, especially in the head, like a painless digging, for several days, at various times.

1360. Restlessness, on arising from a seat and in walking.

Intolerable restlessness in the limbs, in the evening.

Restlessness in the body, and oppression of the heart, when sitting; she has to rise and walk about.

With restlessness in the blood and anxiety of mind, she suddenly became so unwell and feeble, that she could neither stand nor walk; she had to lie down.

Weakness and trembling in all the limbs (18th d.).

1365. **Tremulous.** [*Rl.*]

General trembling.

Trembling all over the body, in the morning, on awaking.

Internal sensation of trembling.

Unsteadiness of the limbs, as in drunkenness; he staggers to and fro, and it seems to him that he reels even more than is actually the case; but without vertigo. [*Fr.*]

1370. Languid, broken down and as if bruised all over the body, especially in the evening, as if a severe illness were impending over him. [*Ng.*]

Sensation in all the limbs, as after a great effort, on rising from his seat.

Lassitude, with perspiration on walking (aft. 48 h.).

Lassitude with anxiety.

Very weakly, and at once exhausted by a little work.

1375. After a short walk, weariness, so that he could not drag his legs along. [*Rl.*]

Weakness in all the limbs, so that he could hardly walk, and had to leave his hands stretched out, while sitting. [*Hbg.*]

Sinking of strength, like fainting.

Fainting fit, after lying down in bed (aft. 12 h.).

Paralytic weakness of the limbs (aft. 3 h.).

1380. Attack of twitching of the limbs, in the evening.

Attack of spasms, in the morning, in bed, heat; after rising, a coolness darted into his arm; he first felt a jerk, with severe twitching in the upper part of the body, in the trunk and the arms, but with undiminished consciousness, only with anxiety (aft. 13 d.).

Attack of spasms: in slumber, in the evening in bed, he felt that he could not rightly move his tongue, he raised himself screaming, but fell back again, stretched out his arms and legs, then he moved them, contorted his eyes, gnashed his teeth; at the same time saliva flowed from his mouth and he was icy cold; after a quarter of an hour his consciousness returned, but with it, great anxiety; this recurred after three quarters of an hour; with flighty thoughts and a heavy tongue; all of this went off on drinking a mouthful of cold water.

An attack: in the evening in his room, his head involuntarily turned hither and thither; he felt at the same time dizzy and anxious, his sight was dim, and he felt heat all over his body; all of this vanished when he came into the open air (aft. 29 d.).

While walking in the open air, he suddenly fell down unconscious, but immediately rose again (aft. 1 h.).

1385. Attack (of uterine spasm): pains, now in the hypogastrium, then in the stomach, now in the chest, then again in the sacrum, which compelled her to bend double; she could not straighten herself without the most violent pains, could bear no clothes in the region of the stomach, and could not eat even things most easily digested, without getting the most violent pains in the abdomen and stomach; only warmed stones placed upon the parts gave her momentary relief; everything in her abdomen felt as if crammed full; as if it would burst open, with continual ineffectual effort to eructate (aft. some days).

Attack: first, pain in the back, like drawing and bruising, which thence passed into the sacrum and the abdomen, where much flatus accumulated, with severe pains; the flatus was discharged later on, with leucorrhœa (aft. 25 d.).

Very tired, he did not want to move a limb. [*Rl.*]

Great weariness about noon, which went off when taking a walk.

Weariness, in the morning in bed, as if he ought to go to sleep again; it goes off after rising.

1390. **Yawning, stretching and extending the limbs,** frequently [*Stf.*]

Stretching and extending the limbs, especially at night.

Violent yawning, the whole evening, without sleepiness (aft. 12 h.). [*Stf.*]

Frequent, violent yawning, often preceded by an abrupt hiccuping from 11 A. M. to 3 P. M. [*Br.*]

Frequent, repeated yawning, forenoon and afternoon. [*Ng.*]

1395. Lassitude and a drowsiness that can hardly be resisted. [*Hbg.*]

Very sleepy and weary by day.

Sleepiness, especially while sitting, but also while walking. [*Hbg.*]

Unusual sleepiness, in the afternoon. [*Stf.*]

Unusual inclination to sleep; she could sleep any hour, but sleep does not refresh her.

1400. **Great sleepiness, so that he** (even in company) **can hardly resist it and has to lie down.** [*Ng.*]

Drowsiness. [*Hbg.*]

She sleeps longer than usual, and can hardly be waked up in the morning (aft. 3 d.).

Very sleepy in the morning (aft. 9 d.).

Long morning-sleep. [*Rl.*]

1405. He goes to sleep after dinner, and gets sleepy early in the evening (aft. 3 d.). [*Rl.*]

After dinner, contrary to his custom, he has to lie down, and sleep. [*Ng.*]

He goes to sleep during a conversation. [*Ng.*]

In the evening, very tired, she has to lie down, and yet cannot go to sleep before 1 o'clock, from being so wide awake; her limbs were painful, as if too heavy.

Late in going to sleep in the evening, on account of great heat of body. [*Ng.*]

1410. **Insomnia, at night,** on account of dry heat.

At night, he can get no position in which he can rest quietly, and cannot lie still for a minute.

He can find no restful position; every part pains as if pressed upon.

Frequent awaking from sleep, without any known cause. [*Ng.*]

He sleeps till midnight, then he cannot go to sleep again, on account of pain of the whole body, as from being bruised; for three nights.

1415. He wakes up every night at 2 o'clock and can then not go to sleep again.

He wakes up every (winter) night at 4 A. M., and can then rarely go to sleep again.

At night, in bed, when rising and lying down again, vertigo.

The whole night, shooting headache, especially in the orbits, but not by day.

At night, the mouth is open, thence dryness of the mouth.

1420. Nocturnal dryness of the mouth (aft. 12 d.).

On awaking from the evening sleep, great nausea.

At night, when awaking with clear consciousness, pressure in the stomach, which she does not feel in the morning when fully awake.

At night, restlessness and twitching in the abdomen, which would not let him go to sleep before midnight.

At night, severe pain in the abdomen near the groin; the pains extended through the legs into the groin.

1425. At night, frequent urging to urinate, waking her from sleep. [*Ng.*]

At night, dry cough, which disturbs the sleep.

At night, drawing pain in the shafts of the bones of the arms, which does not permit sleep.

At night, before midnight, awaking with tendency to cramp in the arm and tingling in it from going to sleep. [*Ng.*]

At night, in the warmth of the bed, intolerable tearing in the upper arm, especially in the shoulder-joint.

1430. At night, she cannot move in bed, for lancinating pain in the **right upper** arm.

At night, the arms pain in the shoulder-joint and the elbow-joint, as if they were asleep, causing her to awake; the pain is worst in the morning, after awaking.

At night, the side, the hip and the thigh, on which he was lying, pained as if bruised, or squeezed, and he had to turn over frequently.

At night, painful heaviness in the lower limbs; this does not allow her to sleep (aft. 3 d.).

At night, in bed, sense of heaviness in the legs and feet.

1435. At night, tearing in the patella, so that he cannot sleep all night.

At night, cramp in the calves.

At night, with uneasy sleep, general sweat. [*Hbg.*]

At night, frequent awaking, with slight perspiration all over, increased while waking. [*Lgh.*]

He wakes up about 4 A. M., with profuse sweat all over the the body, without thirst, and twenty-four hours later, in the same way. [*Br.*]

1440. At night, she had to keep turning, and in the morning there was a light perspiration.

At night, on awaking from sleep, every time a shudder. [*Lgh.*]

At midnight, violent internal chill, especially in the arms and legs, with cutting pain in the back, then a general sweat, with tingling and heaviness in the head; he had to stay abed till noon (aft. 29 d.).

Toward morning, a chill in sleep.

Restlessness, at night in bed, with violent, very anxious weeping and indistinct speech.

1445. In the evening, before going to sleep, anguish; the boy could not go to sleep, because he had always to think about things causing fear; he could only with difficulty be induced to go to bed in the evening.

Every night, very restless; when she had slept a short time, she was waked up by great anguish and restlessness, which hardly allowed her to remain in one position for ten minutes; then she had to sit up, she tossed her head involuntarily from one side to the other, until being fatigued, she went to sleep again (aft. 12 d.).

At night, anguish and restlessness, which do not allow him to sleep (aft. 20 d.).

At night, in sleep, he makes many motions with his arms and legs.

She sleeps very uneasily for sixteen nights, and she weeps at times in her sleep.

1450. Loud laughing in sleep. [*Ng.*]

He laughs aloud in his dream.

He talks after midnight, moaning in his sleep: "Come here! Come here!" and breathed then so lightly that his breath could not be heard.

At first, merry dreams, then confused historical ones (1st d.). [*Ng.*]

Many dreams at night.

1455. Many confused dreams.

Lascivious dreams, with emission of semen. [*Ng.*]

Vexatious dreams.

Vexatious dreams, well remembered (aft. 5 d.). [*Rl.*]

Dreams full of quarrels, with restless sleep (1st night). [*Lgh.*]

1460. Sad dreams of deceased acquaintances. [*Ng.*]

Anxious dreams.

Frightful dream, from which she cannot, after awaking, recover herself for anxiety, and cannot go to sleep again (21st d.).

In sleep, she is often startled and screams.

Frightened starting on going to sleep.

1465. Repeated starting up from fright (4th and 5th night).

Frequent starting from sleep (1st night). [*Lgh.*]

Frequent, frightened starting up from sleep (aft. 3d and 12th d.).

In the morning, on awaking, anxiety.

In the morning, on rising, she is not cheerful, but fatigued; she has to sit down to dress herself; after some time she cheers up again.

1470. Chilliness in the open air, after dinner. [*Ng.*]

Painful coldness of the hand and of the sole of the foot.

Coldness of the hands and feet. [*Fr.*]

Coldness of the whole left side of the body.

Often internal coldness, with cold hands and feet.

1475. Shaking chill in the whole right side of the body.

Sensation as if a cold wind blew between the scapulæ, on the middle of the spine, which part remained cold, even by the warm stove.

Sensation as if cold water ran down from the right clavicle over the chest to the toes, along a narrow strip. [*Ng.*]

Chill over the whole body in the open air, which is not cold.

Much internal chill every day (1st week).

1480. Chill in different parts of the body. [*Fr.*]

Febrile rigor, at times with goose-skin, even in the warm room; or in the open air, and then going off in the room. [*Ng.*]

Chilliness and yawning. [*Ng.*]

Continual shaking chill on the back. [*Lgh.*]

Frequent shivering, now in this arm, now in that leg, then all over the body.

1485. Quick shudder from the face over the chest down to the knees. [*Fr.*]

Shivering from the face down the back, even to the knees. [*Fr.*]

Single fits of shaking chills in the back, extending almost all over the abdomen, without heat either afterwards or with it.

Shaking chill over the whole body, without thirst and without subsequent heat. [*Lgh.*]

Shudder in the whole body, as often as he puts down his left hand, after exercise. [*Ng.*]

1490. Shivering, with goose-skin all day, as often as she goes into the open air. [*Ng.*]

Sensation as if a shudder ran from the right temple through the forehead, where there is throbbing. [*Ng.*]

Shivering, with goose-skin and urging to stool, which is very soft, and accompanied by painful colic; then a general chill, with external coldness, which soon goes off in the room, where an internal feeling of warmth in the head is then experienced. [*Ng.*]

At 4 P. M., first, a chill, with shivering in the legs up into the back, with lassitude for three hours; then sweat without heat and without thirst.

He feels feverish, now chilliness, then heat in the face.

1495. Febrile rigor, lasting one hour, then heat in the forehead.

Chill, the first half of the night, then heat, and toward morning, a moist skin; only then some rest and sleep (aft. 3 d.).

He is always either chilly or in a sweat.

Every evening, heat for two hours, from 6 o'clock ownward (aft. 7 w.).

Heat over the whole body, without sweat and without thirst, then a gradual coolness, with yawning and stretching of the arms. [*Htm.*]

1500. Frequent attacks of sweat all over the body. [*Ng.*]

In the morning, he lay in a sweat.

Night-sweat, two nights in succession (aft. 36 h.).

Night-sweat, several nights in succession (aft. 11 d.).

Sour-smelling night-sweat, all over (aft. 26 d.).

1505. Night-sweat. [*Ng.*]

CLEMATIS ERECTA. VIRGIN'S BOWER.[1]

This perennial herb grows in hedges and by fences on hilly heights. It is gathered shortly before its time of blossoming, and the acrid juice is pressed out from its leaves. After being homœopathically prepared, it is used in its various degrees of potentized attenuation in small doses, to cure many ailments arising from the mercurial malady, complicated with psora. It has thus been found useful in severe eruptions on the head and the skin, in particular urinary troubles, stricture of the urethra, and peculiar varieties of very troublesome inflammations of the eyes. Medical Counselor Stapf has found this medicine serviceable in inflammations of the testes and indurated testicular swellings after badly treated gonorrhœa. In earlier times *A. von Stoerk** has praised its virtues from experience, even in cancerous ulcers of the lips and the breasts, in spongy

* *Libellus de Flammula Jovis*, *Viennae*, 1769, and in German: Leipzig, 1778.

[1] All these names, save Foissac's belong to a pathogenesis of *Clematis*, published (without information) in Vol. VII. of the Archiv (1828). *Foissac's* symptoms and those cited from *Stoerk* are the only additions made here.—*Hughes.*

excrescences, tophi, inveterate cutaneous eruptions, in especial kinds of long-continued headache and in melancholies.

Frequent smelling of camphor moderates its excessive action and the toothache caused by it is said to find its antidote in Bryonia.

The abbreviations of the names of my fellow-provers are: *Fr.*, *Dr. Franz; Gtn.*, dentist *Gutmann; Fr. H.*, *Dr. Friedrich Hahnemann; Lgh.*, *Dr. Langhammer; Stf.*, *Dr. Stapf; Fc.*, *Dr. Foissac* in Paris.[1]

CLEMATIS ERECTA.

Lost in sad thoughts, and in apprehensions of impending misfortunes. [*Lgh.*]

Sullen, without cause, and out of humor. [*Gtn.*]

Peevish, taciturn, he wishes that he need not go out at all. [*Gtn.*]

Indispositon to talk, which it goes off in the evening. [*Lgh.*]

5. Indifferent, quiet, almost without any thought. [*Kr.*]

He stares before him. [*Gtn.*]

Obtuseness and gloominess of the head, in the frontal region, with tendency to vertigo.

Gloomy and heavy in the head, at once in the morning, on rising. [*Gtn.*]

Pressive, tensive headache in the anterior part of the brain, more violent when walking than when sitting; with heaviness of the head (aft. 7½ h.). [*Gtn.*]

10. Pressive, tensive headache in all the right side of head, more in the bones than in the brain. [*Gtn.*]

Drawing headache, with some pressure, in the sides of the crown. [*Fr.*]

Drawing pain in the forehead, on the left side (aft. 2 h.). [*Lgh.*]

Boring pain in the left temple. [*Lgh.*]

Digging, pressive headache in the right half of the brain, in walking. [*Gtn.*]

15. Shocks in the brain, outward and from behind forward. [*Gtn.*]

Hammering in the head, in the evening, when lying down. [*Fr. H.*]

In the skin of the forehead, on the left side, a burning, cutting pain, most violent, when the skin is drawn smooth. [*Gtn.*]

Painful, eruptive pimples on the forehead. [*Fr.*]

Pain in the eyes, a pressure on the middle of the left eyeball. [*Kr.*]

20. Stitches in the inner canthus.

Stinging pain in the inner canthus of the left eye, as from a sharp and pointed body, for several minutes (aft. 13 h.). [*Gtn.*]

Smarting in the eyes, worse when he closed them; when he

[1] The symptoms marked *Kr.* were observed by *Dr. Kretschmar* cfr. GRAPHITES. *Transl.*

opened them again, after having closed them, they were very sensitive to the light. [*Fr.*]

Smarting pain in the eyes, especially on the edge of the lids.

Smarting in the eyes, almost as if sore, with redness of the veins there and lachrymation; on closing the eyes, the smarting became more violent, and the eyes were so sensitive to the air, that he did not again dare to open them; everything became black before them. [*Stf.*]

25. Burning pain in the upper lid of the right eye. [*Gtn.*]

Burning pain in the inner canthus of the left eye. [*Gtn.*]

Inflammation of the white of the eye, and lachrymation. [*Fr.*]

Inflammation of the inner canthi, and the eyes look weary. [*Gtn.*]

Otalgia, fine pecking stitches in the inside of the right ear. [*Gtn.*]

30. Burning pain in the external left ear. [*Gtn.*]

Ringing of bells before the ears. [*Gtn.*]

In the face, burning pain on the skin of the left cheek. [*Gtn.*]

Little eruptive pimples on the forehead (aft. 5 h.). [*Lgh.*].

Many little pimples, especially on the forehead, they come on with a fine stinging, and are somewhat painful to the touch. [*Kr.*]

35. Little pimples, painless in themselves, above the eyebrows, or the root of the nose, on the chin, on the tip of the nose; they contain pus, and are somewhat painful when touched. [*Kr.*]

Through the lower lip on the left side, a burning cutting stitch, as if it was being cut through (aft. 5 h.). [*Gtn.*]

An itching blister on the lower lip, just below the red part; water oozed from it, and then it became covered with a tough skin (aft. 3 d.). [*Fr. H.*]

In the upper jaw, on the left side, drawing stitches, upward, synchronous with the pulse. [*Kr.*]

On the upper lip, painful eruptive pimples. [*Fr.*]

40. The submaxillary glands are swollen, with hard nodules, which throb and are tense as if they would suppurate, are painful to the touch, and excite toothache. [*Kr.*]

Toothache in the last hollow molar, which ached, together with the upper teeth, even when they were painless; much aggravated by bread getting into it. [*Kr.*]

Toothache, bearable by day, but in a horizontal position in bed, it is increased even to desperation, and not to be relieved by any change of position or direction, but only gradually by lying still. [*Kr.*]

Toothache, violent even to despair, with tossing in bed, weakness of the limbs and anxious sweat; it cannot bear uncovering; the whole night. [*Kr.*]

Toothache spreads over the whole temporal region, even to the crown. [*Kr.*]

45. Toothache makes him incapable of any work, and most of all incapable of thinking. [*Kr.*]

Dull pain in a hollow tooth, only transiently appeased by cold water, also relieved by sucking out the air, when there was a stitch, as if something in the tooth was being lifted up. [*Kr.*]

A stitch in the tooth and upward from this, in all the left side of the face, a drawing twitching pain, synchronous with the pulse, with jerking straining in the ear, and painfulness of the eye, when moving. [*Kr.*]

Twitching shooting in the tooth, which passes as a drawing twitching over the cheekbone even into the ear, where there is a straining pain, and the eye, which is much affected, pains, and can bear neither motion nor light, with painfulness of the eyeball when touched. [*Kr.*]

Twitching, stinging, drawing toothache in the left side of the upper jaw, now in one, then in another undefined tooth of the whole row. [*Kr.*]

50. Twitching drawing toothache, by day, increased by smoking tobacco and only relieved for a few minutes by firmly pressing a cloth upon it. [*Kr.*]

The hollow tooth seems longer, and pains at the least touch; while much water runs from the mouth. [*Kr.*]

The gums of the left lower molars are painful as if sore, most violently while eating. [*Gtn.*]

In the root of the tongue, obtuse, boring stitches. [*Gtn.*]

Dry tongue, in the morning on awaking. [*Kr.*]

55. The saliva spit out, is mixed with blood. [*Gtn.*]

Long-continued satiety; he could, indeed, eat at meals, and had a relish for food; but he felt at once that it was too much for him, and that he had still no need of food. [*Htm.*]

After eating, nausea during the smoking of tobacco. [*Lgh.*]

After smoking tobacco, nausea, which caused a sensation of weakness in the lower limbs, so that they seemed to stagger, and he had to lie down. [*Fr.*]

Thrice in succession, eructation (at once). [*Kr.*]

60. The hepatic region is painful, when touched and in stooping, as if bruised, for about two weeks. [*Kr.*]

In the right side of the gastric and renal region, a contractive cutting pain, when walking. [*Fr.*]

Grumbling in the abdomen, as from emptiness (aft. 1 h.). [*Lgh.*]

In the abdominal ring, on the right side, a pain pressing outward, as if a hernia were being forced out or protruded already.

In the inguinal gland, a twitching pain.

65. Swelling of the inguinal gland (bubo). [ANTON V. STOERK, *Vom Brenn-Kraute*, Leipzig, 1787.[1]]

Frequent stool, which became thinner and thinner, without colic (aft. 3 d.). [*Gtn.*]

Urging to urinate, painless. [*Lgh.*]

Long-continued contraction and constriction of the urethra; the urine can only pass in drops, as in a spasmodic stricture.

He cannot pass the urine at one time; it was frequently interrupted in its stream before it was all discharged, then the rest kept dripping out involuntarily, and while the urine was interrupted, he felt, by jerks, a burning and tearing in the anterior part of the urethra. [*Htm.*]

---

[1] Symptoms appearing in patients taking the drug. In a syphilitic subject.—*Hughes.*

70. Repeated urination, but little at a time. [*Lgh.*]

Involuntary flow of urine. [STOERK, l. c.]

Urine reddish, discharged copiously and without pain (aft. 5 or 6 h.). [*Htm.*]

He urinates puriform matter. [STOERK, l. c.[1]]

When commencing to urinate, the smarting is worse; during urination, there are stitches out through the urethra, and afterwards it continues to burn and smart; while not urinating, there is tearing in the anterior part of the penis.

75. During micturition, painful drawing in the spermatic cord, extending up into the abdomen (aft. 24 h. and on 6th d.).

During micturition, shooting from the abdominal cavity up into the chest, more violent on inspiration. [*Gtn.*]

The urethra pains when touched.

The testicle pains when touched, as if bruised, with drawing and stretching in the inguinal region, the left thigh and the scrotum, which, when touched and in walking, pains as if squeezed. [*Htm.*]

Pain, drawing upward in the testicles and the spermatic cord.

80. Swelling of both testes.

Testicular swelling. [*Stf.*]

Painful sensitiveness of the testes (3d d.). [*Fc.*]

Swelling of the right half of the scrotum, which became thickened and descended, with the testes, low down; for twenty-four hours. [*Htm.*]

Excitation of the sexual instinct (1st, 2d d.). [*Fc.*]

85. Loathing of sexual intercourse by day, even during the erections, as if he had abundantly satisfied his sexual instinct. [*Htm.*]

Involuntary erections, by day. [*Htm.*]

Violent erections, lasting for several hours, with stitches in the urethra (3d d.). [*Fc.*]

Violent drawing pain in the left spermatic cord (3d d.). [*Fc.*]

Pollution in the night, after taking the drug, and next day, another during the noon siesta.

90. During the emission of semen in coitus, burning pain in the caput gallinaginis in the urethra.

Menses, eight days too soon, and more copious than formerly.

* * * * * * * *

Sneezing in the morning (aft 28 h.). [*Lgh.*]

Severe fluent coryza, during which a watery fluid sometimes rushed from his nose quite involuntarily. [*Fr.*]

Tussiculation, during his customary smoke. [*Lgh.*]

95. In the whole thoracic cavity, constant pressive pain, without reference to respiration (aft. 10 h.). [*Gtn.*]

Obtuse stitches in the chest, somewhat more violent during inspiration and expiration. [*Gtn.*]

Obtuse stitches in the right side of the chest, constant during inspiration and expiration. [*Gtn.*]

Obtusely shooting shocks, in all the left side of the chest and abdomen, so that he had to cry out aloud (aft. 15 d.). [*Gtn.*]

---

[1] In a case of gonorrhœal rheumatism. As this appeared, the arthritis departed.—*Hughes.*

Sharp stitches in the cardiac region, from within outward. [*Kr.*]

100. Externally on the chest, above the heart, tearing pain. [*Gtn.*]

An indurated gland below the nipple; it is painful when touched.

On the upper arm, a pressive pain (aft. 48 h.).

In the bend of the elbow, pressive pain on stretching out the upper arm.

In the left fore-arm, violent drawing stitches, in all positions of the limbs (aft. 1¼ h.). [*Lgh.*]

105. In the wrist, while taking a walk, sharp, violently drawing, shooting pains (aft. 11 h.). [*Lgh.*]

Fine, stinging pain in the whole surface of the hands (moistened with the juice), as soon as they are moistened with water and washed.

In the right thumb, a drawing tearing, both when at rest and in motion (aft. 9 h.). [*Lgh.*]

Pain in the hips, for three days (3d d.). [*Fr.*]

About the loins, an eruption of large pustules, very painful when touched.

110. Dull stitches in the right loin, only when not breathing. [*Gtn.*]

In the right thigh, drawing and stretching, which sometimes extend, in painful drawing, up close to the male organ (aft. 8 h.). [*Htm.*]

Tearing pain in the right thigh, when sitting and lying down. [*Fr. H.*]

A furuncle on the thigh.

In the knee, transient tearing.

115 After walking, there is a drawing in the knee and thigh, like tearing, but not felt in the joint.

The legs are heavy and tired, for two days. [*Fr. H.*]

Obtuse stitches in the left calf, in sitting. [*Lgh.*]

In the foot, on which there is an ulcer, drawing and tension, when walking.

Constant aching on the ball of the right heel, as if it had become turgid by jumping (aft. 6 h.). [*Lgh.*]

120. Crawling, anteriorly in the sole of the right foot, as from going to sleep. [*Kr.*]

On the toes, after lying down, violent itching, exciting to scratching, and between the toes, sweat. [*Lgh.*]

Violent pain, as from soreness, in the left big toe, toward the inner side, most violent when resting (aft. 8 h.). [*Lgh.*]

Muscular twitching, in almost all the fleshy parts of the body. [*Kr.*]

Lively, sensible pulsation through the whole body, especially in the heart. [*Kr.*]

125. Great desire for the open air. [*Htm.*]

Burning pain, or feeling of heat, in several parts of the body, without redness. [*Kr.*]

Pustules, like itch, all over the body. [STOERK, l. c.[1]]

---

[1] In subject of symptom 65.—*Hughes.*

In the wound, in the evening, after going to sleep, pulsating, shooting shocks; also at 3 A. M.

In the ulcers, a crawling and throbbing, stinging on their edges, when touched.

130. Throbbing pain in the ulcer, in the morning.

Burning pains in the ulcers. [STOERK, l. c.[1]]

Sensation in the body, in the morning, as after a pollution, or as if this had been suppressed. [*Kr.*]

Resounding throbbing through the whole body, after lying down, especially on the (right) side on which he lay. [*Kr.*]

Weariness in all the limbs, the knees have no steadiness, and give way easily; after a walk (aft. 3 h.). [*Kr.*]

135. Weariness and sleepiness after a meal, so that he had to lie down, with violent beating of the arteries; when he was awakened, he could not rouse himself, and fell down again into slumber. [*Kr.*]

Constant sleepiness and indisposition to work (aft. 4 h.). [*Gtn.*]

Sleepiness and yawning, when sitting (aft. 3 h.). [*Lgh.*]

In the evening, he cannot (according to his custom) go to sleep soon. [*Kr.*]

Though his eyes closed continually and he was very tired, he could not fall asleep all night; he felt internally as if there was a dry heat.

140. Uneasy sleep at night, with tossing about, turning over the coverlet, and dreams, which he could well remember in the morning. [*Fr.*]

In the morning, on awaking, he does not feel strengthened; he perspires somewhat, and only now, he wishes to sleep; at the same time, he cannot bear to be uncovered, owing to a disagreeable sensation of coldness. [*Kr.*]

In the morning, on awaking, drowsiness and weariness; he would like to rise, but feels too much fatigued. [*Fr.*]

Dreams of many kinds interrupt his sleep, and make it restless. [*Lgh.*]

Uneasy dreams at night.

145. Vivid, at times anxious, dreams. [*Kr.*]

Anxious dreams at night, *e. g.*, of conflagrations. [*Htm.*]

Dream, that he was innocently arrested on account of a crime of which he was accused. [*Stf.*]

Vivid, in part voluptuous, dreams. [*Lgh.*]

Shivering all over, when slightly uncovered, while the air is warm. [*Lgh.*]

150. Profuse night sweat. [STOERK, l. c.]

[1] In a putrid and fungous ulcer, prior to its improvement to a simple and clean one.—*Hughes.*

COLOCYNTHIS. BITTER CUCUMBER.

When preparing the medicine from the colocynthis, it is best to take a grain of the dried fruit of this cucumber-like plant (Cucumis colocynthis) and triturate it with sugar of milk for three hours, in the manner indicated at the end of volume I., so as to get the millionth potency; this is then dissolved and brought to the decillionth potency, so that we can use it in all its various grades of dynamization according to the nature of the circumstances of the disease. When well prepared it is of enormous virtue even in the smallest dose.

Camphor, causticum, crude coffee and staphisagria are used as antidotes of the bitter cucumber.

It has proved itself especially efficacious in the following ailments: Anxiety; lack of religious feeling; porrigo in the face; toothache; stomachache, also after eating; *violent colics*, especially after vexation; grumbling in the abdomen; inguinal hernia; long-continued diarrhœa; pain as from a bruise in the shoulder-joint after vexation; ill consequences and troubles springing from *indignation and embitterment, or internal, gnawing mortification over the unworthy treatment of himself or of other persons who excited his pity; e. g.*, cramp in the calves and the intestines; cramp-colic, bilious colic, bilious fever, insomnia, etc.; *pains in the hips*, where the hip-joint feels as if it were fastened to the pelvis and sacral region as if with iron clasps, attended with pains darting down periodically from the lumbar muscles into the thigh.

The chief characteristic of colocynthis is the excitation of cramp-pains in the internal and external parts, *i. e.*, tonic spasms, with squeezing pressive pains, and then staphisagria is the antidote. Also the drinking of coffee and camphor antidote its injurious action.

The abbreviations of the names of my fellow-provers are: *Aeg.*, *Dr. Aegidi; Fr. H., Dr. Friedrich Hahnemann; Hbg., Hornburg; Gtm., Gutmann; Lgh., Dr. Laughammer; Stf.*, Medical Counsellor, *Dr. Stapf; Rt., Dr. L. Rueckert.*

COLOCYNTHIS.

Dejected, joyless, indisposed to talk. [*Gtm.*]

Indisposed to speak, the whole day. [*Lgh.*]

Moroseness; he takes everything ill, and is unwilling to answer. [*Rt.*]

The proving of Colocynthis appears in the *Materia Medica Pura*, and 250 of the 283 symptoms recorded here belong thereto. The remainder are *Aegidi's* (from a patient, see note to Sympt. 144,) and Hahnemann's in his later manner.—*Hughes.*

Extreme peevishness; everything is amiss; he is extremely impatient; every word he has to answer, vexes him, and embarrasses him painfully; everything vexes him, even things the most harmless.

5. Uncomfortable; he wishes and desires many things. [*Rt.*]

Great anguish. [HOYER in *Misc. N. C. Dec. III., ann.* 7, 8. *Breslauer Sammlungen*, 1727, p. 48.[1]]

Obtuseness of the head, especially of the sinciput. [*Gtm.*]

Obtuseness and gloominess of the head. [ALIBERT in *Med. Nat. Zeit.*, 1799.[2]]

Gloomy and muddled in the head, as after a nocturnal drinking-bout. [*Hbg.*]

10. Stupidity and vertigo in the head, at the commencement of the colic. [*Fr. H.*]

Vertigo, on quickly turning the head, as if originating in the left temple, as if he should fall, with giving way in the knees. [*Stf.*]

Headache, very violent, as if from a draught, going off on taking a walk. [*Lgh.*]

Pressive impacts in the head, single, slight, now here, now there. [*Rt.*]

Pressive headache along the sagittal suture, more violent when moving and shaking the head, and when stooping. [*Stf.*]

15. **A pressive squeezing headache in the sinciput, most violent in stooping and when lying on the back,** for six hours. [*Gtm.*]

Pressive, cramp-pain in the upper part of the brain. [*Gtm.*]

Pressive, drawing pain in the left side of the forehead. [*Gtm.*]

Drawing, semi-lateral headache (aft. 1½ h.). [*Hbg.*]

Tearing headache in the whole of the brain, which in the forehead becomes pressive, as if it would press out the forehead, more violent on moving the eyelids. [*Gtm.*]

20. Boring stitches in the right temple, going off when touched. [*Lgh.*]

Painful pressive burrowing in the left temple. [*Gtm.*]

Painful tearing burrowing through the whole of the brain, aggravated by moving the upper eyelids to an unbearable degree (aft. 7 h.). [*Aeg.*]

Externally on the forehead, a dull lancinating pain, in the morning on rising (aft. ¼ h.). [*Lgh.*]

Burning pain in the skin of the forehead, above the eyebrows. [*Gtm.*]

25. Smarting burning on the left side of the hairy scalp. [*Gtm.*]

The roots of the hairs are painful.

Pain in the eyes; a sharp cutting in the right eyeball. [*Gtm.*]

Burning cutting in the right lower eyelid, when resting. [*Gtm.*]

Stitches as from knives, in the right eyeball, over into the root of the nose. [*Aeg.*]

30. Excoriative pain in the eyelids.

---

[1] Note to *Hoyer*, "From *decoction*," and to reference add O. 178. To *Bresl. Samml.* note: "Nothing about Colocynth is found here."—*Hughes.*

[2] Not accessible.—*Hughes.*

Burning sensation in the right upper eyelid (aft. 34 h.). [*Gtm.*]

Burning pain in the whole of the right eyeball. [*Gtm.*]

Pricking burning pain in the right inner canthus. [*Gtm.*]

Smarting burning pain under the upper eyelid.

35. Violent itching in the right eyeball, compelling rubbing. [*Gtm.*]

Obscuration of vision. [ORFILA, *Toxicologie* I., 567.[1]]

Sparks before the eyes. [SCHNEIDER in *Annal. d. Heilk.*, April, 1811.[2]]

Otalgia in the right ear, not going off on inserting the finger. [*Gtm.*]

Pressure behind the left ear. [*Hbg.*]

40. Painful drawing behind the left ear, long continuing. [*Hbg.*]

Crawling in the internal ear, going off on inserting the finger. [*Gtm.*]

Itching shooting deep in the ear, extending from the eustachian tube to the membrana tympana, and going off on introducing the finger (aft. 1½ h.). [*Stf.*]

Cutting, shooting pain in the lower cavity of the right auricle, going off on inserting the finger. [*Gtm.*]

Hardness of hearing. [ORFILA I., 567.]

45. **In the nose, throbbing and digging pain,** from the left side into the root. [*Gtm.*]

Violent itching in the left nostril, inciting to scratch, in the evening, with an irritation as from coryza (aft. 15 h.). [*Lgh.*]

The muscles of the face are relaxed and pale, and the eyes look sunken. [*Gtm.*]

Tearing and tension on the left side of the face, extending into the ear and the head.

Digging burning pain in the cheek, more when at rest than in motion. [*Gtm.*]

50. An eruptive pimple on the left cheek, which when touched pains and smarts, and after scratching exudes a watery moisture (aft. 4½ h.). [*Lgh.*]

White pimples in the face, chiefly between the eye and ear, on the forehead and on the chin, with some twitching, *per se*, and with smarting pain when touched (aft. 4 h.). [*Lgh.*]

In the corner of the mouth on the right side, burning pain. [*Gtm.*]

Pustule on the left corner of the mouth (aft. 2 h.). [*Lgh.*]

In the muscles of the chin, quivering, only when the parts are at rest. [*Gtm.*]

55. The teeth of the lower row ache as if the nerve was jerked and stretched. [*Hbg.*]

Shooting, throbbing pain in the right lower molars, as if struck with a metal wire. [*Stf.*]

Painful looseness of one of the lower incisors.

In the mouth, on the right cheek and on the side of the tongue, a smarting pain. [*Gtm.*]

---

1 From the apples taken for chronic gonorrhœa.—*Hughes.*

2 From colocynth given in apoplexy.—*Hughes.*

White tongue, with feeling of roughness upon it, as from too much smoking of tobacco. [*Lgh.*]

60. Rough tongue, as if sand had been strewn on it (aft. 36 h.). [*Fr. H.*]

On the palate, a scrapy feeling, also outside of coughing. [*Stf.*]

Fine stitches in the throat, as from the awn of an ear of wheat, on the upper part of the velum pendulum palati.

Fine smarting stitches in the fauces, not observed in deglutition. [*Gtm.*]

Saliva in the mouth, tasteless as water.

65. Metallic, astringent taste on the upper part of the tip of the tongue. [*Stf.*]

Loathsome, putrid taste, more so in the fauces than in the mouth. [*Gtm.*]

Bitterness in the mouth for four hours (at once). [*Fr. H.*]

Bitter taste in the mouth after drinking beer.

Lack of appetite. [ALIBERT, l. c.]

70. Diminished appetite, though the food tastes properly. [*Fr. H.*]

Feeling of thirst in the fauces. [*Rt.*]

Violent thirst. [HOFFMANN, l. c., *Bresl. Samml.*, l. c.[1]]

Much appetite for drinking, without thirst; the mouth is always watery, the liquid drunk tastes very good, but immediately after every drink a flat taste comes into the mouth.

Empty eructation. [*Hbg.*]

75. Empty eructation, causing palpitation of the heart and cramp in the fauces, and provokes a constant tendency to retching and vomiting. [*Aeg.*]

Belching up of a bilious fluid.

Frequent hiccup (aft. 1¼ h.). [*Lgh.*]

Nausea. [SCHNEIDER, l. c.]

Nausea for two hours (at once). [*Fr. H.*]

80. Nausea for six hours, till going to sleep at night; recurring in the morning on awaking. [*Fr. H.*]

Nausea for eight hours (aft. 5 min.). [*Fr. H.*]

Vomiting, very frequent. [HOFFMANN, *Ephem. N. Cent.* X., *obs.* 30.]

Vomiting twice, only of the food, without bad taste or nausea (aft. 10 m.). [*Fr. H.*]

In the stomach, a pressure as from a stone. [*Hbg.*]

85. Pressive stomachache.

Violent stomachache, precordial pressure (at once). [HOFFMANN, l. c.]

Sensation of pressure in the gastric region, especially after eating, with sensation of hunger, not relieved by repeated eating, every day. [*Rt.*]

Colic of the most violent kind. [HOFFMANN, l. c.]

Indescribable colic. [STALPAART VAN DER WIEL, *Cent.* I., *obs.* 41.[2]]

---

[1] After "HOFFMANN" for l. c. substitute "*Eph. Nat. Cur. Cent.* X., *O.* 30, and note: "Poisoning by a whole apple."—*Hughes.*

[2] Case of poisoning.—*Hughes.*

90. Excessive pain in the abdomen on a small spot below the navel, which after the night-sweat spreads through the whole abdomen. [*Fr. H.*]

Violent bellyache, alleviated by smoking tobacco, but leaving behind a long-continued sensation, as if he had taken cold. [*Fr. H.*]

Pain in the abdomen, as from catching cold, or from a variety of articles of incongruous food eaten together. [*Hbg*]

Colic, with restlessness of the whole body, while through both cheeks runs a shudder, ascending from the abdomen and disappearing at once after a more severe pain. [*Hbg.*]

Constant bellyache through all the intestines; this is composed of pain as from a bruise and from pressure.

95. Pressure in the bowels, which sometimes seems to come from emptiness, but is rather increased by eating, especially while bending forward when sitting, for six days in succession, particularly in the evening. [*Rt.*]

Pressure in the abdomen, as from fullness. [*Hbg.*]

Great distension of the abdomen from time to time.

Dull, tensive pain in the abdomen, going off by pressure. [*Gtm.*]

Distension of the abdomen, with passage of flatus and colicky pain of the abdomen. [*Stf.*]

100. Colic. [TULPIUS, *obs. lib.* 4, *Cap.* 25, ALIBERT, l. c [1]]

Cramp-like bellyache, so that he can neither sit still, nor lie, nor walk; with ineffectual urging and tenesmus to stool after eating. [*Hbg.*]

Squeezing in the abdomen, as if the bowels were squeezed between stones, and threatened to gush out, sometimes with a rush of blood to the head and face, with a breaking out of sweat on those parts; at the abatement of the pains, these parts felt as if blown upon by a cool breeze. [*Hbg.*]

Squeezing bellyache, as if the bowels were pressed in, with cutting toward the os pubis, with such violence below the navel that it distorted the facial muscles and closed the eyes; this pain was only allayed by pressing on the abdomen with the hand, and by the drawing in of the abdomen. [*Hbg.*]

Forcing together the abdominal intestines round about the region of the os pubis.

105. Constriction of the abdominal intestines, increasing in intensity every ten to twenty minutes, which goes off by a strong counter-pressure with the hands. [*Hbg.*]

Grasping in the bowels, as if the whole abdomen was griped together violently; he could neither lie down nor sit, and could only walk when bent double; the pains were not diminished by lying still, but by rapid motion or rolling around. [*Hbg.*]

Grasping and pinching in the abdomen (aft. 21 h.). [*Hbg.*]

Pinching pains in the abdomen, which terminated above the mons veneris. [*Hbg.*]

Pinching bellyache, without stool (aft. 34 h.). [*Gtm.*]

110. Cutting pains in the abdomen. [*Breslauer Samml.*, l. c.]

[1] Case of poisoning.—*Hughes.*

Cutting in the abdomen, with grumbling and creaking. [*Hbg.*]

Constant cutting in the hypogastrium, so that he had to walk bent forward, at the same time lassitude in the whole body, making walking a trouble, with dread of the work before him. [*Gtm.*]

Cutting in the epigastrium, quickly passing off. [*Rt.*]

Periodical attacks of fearful cutting in the abdomen, starting from the left renal region and spasmodically drawing the thigh toward the stomach, so that she had to bend double as far as possible. [*Aeg.*[1]]

115. Pressive cutting in the epigastrium, as from flatus, during inspiration [*Rt.*]

Sore cutting in the hypogastrium, which commenced when walking and increased in violence with every step (aft. 5 d.). [*Rt.*]

Stitches under the last ribs. [*Rt.*]

Shooting **pain in** a small spot of **the umbilical region,** which **compels him to bend double**, and is most aggravated by lifting anything (aft. ¾ h.). [*Fr. H.*]

Boring pain in the left iliac region, close to the bones of the pelvis. [*Gtm.*]

120. Digging, tearing pain in the umbilical region, more violent during expiration and when laughing aloud. [*Gtm.*]

Pain as from a bruising in the hypogastrial intestines, felt most while walking and while sitting bent forward.

Movement in the abdomen, as if he were still fasting in the afternoon (aft. 8 h.). [*Lgh*]

Emptiness in the abdomen, as if there was nothing in it. [*Hbg.*]

Emptiness in the abdomen, as after a severe diarrhœa. [*Stf.*]

125. Constant pressure in the region of the os pubis (aft. 8 and 10 h.). [*Hbg.*]

Tensive pain in the right inguinal region, more violent on pressure. [*Gtm.*]

In the inguinal region, pain as if a hernia was being forced out, and on pressure pain as if a hernia was being reduced, for half an hour in the afternoon, and recurring the next day at the same hour.

Forcing from both sides of the hypogastrium toward the middle of the pubic region, like flatus which will not pass off, exciting to seminal emission.

Very severe cuts and stitches in the intestines, from flatus which will not pass off; these even wakes person up at night.

130. Continual grumbling and croaking in the stomach, sounds as from frogs.

Obstructed flatus which remains behind. [*Hbg.*]

Abortive efforts to pass flatus; later on a violent discharge of flatus. [*Hbg.*]

Frequent noisy discharge of flatus. [*Lgh.*]

---

[1] This occurred twelve hours after a drop of Colocynth 3, in a patient already suffering several times a day from agonizing pain proceeding from the left kidney down the corresponding limb. Symptoms 22, 29, and 75 came on at the same time. [*Archiv.* VII., 3, 109.]—*Hughes.*

All the abdominal pains from colocynth passed away on drinking a cup of coffee, but he then had to go to stool at once. [*Hbg.*]

135. After eating a single potato, violent pain in the abdomen, and hurried stool. [*Fr. H.*]

Frequent urgent calls to stool, with sensation at the anus and in the lower part of the rectum as if these parts were weakened and had lost their tone by long continued diarrhœa. [*Hbg.*]

He had to keep back the stool by a great effort, in order that it should not be evacuated before reaching the night-chair. [*Hbg.*]

Violent urging to stool, which was copious, yellowish-brown, semi-liquid, as from a purgative, and of sourish, putrid smell; after this there was a temporary disappearance of the abdominal pains. [*Hbg.*]

But little fæces discharged, tough and mucous. [*Hbg.*]

140. Hard stool, with little straining (aft. 48 h.). [*Gtm.*]

Very hard stool, going off in lumps (aft. 5 and 6 d.) (after-effect?) [*Rt.*]

Diarrhœa, day and night, with nausea, without being able to vomit. [*Fr. H.*]

Diarrhœa, fifteen stools in eighteen hours, which causes the colic to be gradually relieved. [*Fr. H.*]

Greenish-yellow diarrhœic stools, with sensation as if he had taken cold. [*Fr. H.*]

145. Thin, foamy stool, yellow as tuemeric, of mouldy smell, almost as of burnt gray blotting-paper (aft. 12 h.). [*Hbg.*]

Stools first watery mucous, then bilious, and at last bloody. [HOFFMANN, l. c.]

Bloody stools. [HOYER, l. c., *Bresl. Samml.*, l. c.]

Dysentery. [ZACUT. LUSITANIUS in *Pharm.*, 208.[1]]

Flow of blood from the anus. [TULPIUS, l. c.]

150. Flow of blood from the anus several hours after death. [SCHENK, *obs. lib.*, 7.[2]]

Fatal dysentery. [PLAT., *obs. liber* 3, p. 858.[3]]

In the anus, a violent jerking stitch, outside of time for stool. [*Gtm.*]

Violently itching stitch in the rectum and anus (aft. 1 h.).

Pain at the lower part of the rectum from swollen varices, when sitting, walking and during stool.

155. Blind piles.

Retention of urine. [ORFILA I., 168.]

The urine seems to be secreted sparingly. [*Hbg.*]

Frequent strangury, with scanty discharge of urine (aft. 1 h.). [*Lgh.*]

Strangury with inability to pass urine; this generally passed very sparingly. [*Hbg.*]

160. Call to urinate, with pressure on the pubic region (aft. 8 h.). (*Hbg.*]

Urine at once of intolerable odor; in standing it immediately became thick, gelatinous, viscid, like coagulated albumen. [SCHNEIDER, l. c.[4]]

---

[1] Effect of an enema containing colocynth.—*Hughes.*
[2] Effect of an enema containing colocynth.—*Hughes.*
[3] Poisoning.—*Hughes.*
[4] This symptom not found.—*Hughes.*

Soon after urinating, a pressive pain at the end of the urethra, as if contused (aft. 14 h.).]*Lgh.*]

Tearing through the urethra, like a stitch.

Tearing pain in the glans.

165. In the right testicle, a painful twitch.

Painful drawing up of the testes. [ORFILA, l. c.]

Priapism. [ORFILA, l. c.]

Violent sexual instinct, with erections.

Complete impotence; the prepuce remained retracted behind the glans, though he was not deficient in sexual impulse.

* * * * * * *

170. Fluent coryza, in the morning, without sneezing. [*Lgh.*].

Tussiculation, while smoking tobacco, in the evening. [*Lgh.*]

Frequent titillating irritation to dry cough, in the larynx. [*Stf.*]

The spot in the larynx, where it scratches and tingles so as to cause coughing, becomes more scratchy on inspiration. [*Stf.*]

Breathing twice as short as usual, for several days, without asthma and without heat.

175. Fit of asthma, at night, with slow, heavy respiration, compelling him to cough.

Severe oppression of the chest as from a pressure from without, on inspiration, when there are also stitches in the chest. [*Rt.*]

Pressive tightness of the chest, everything seems too tight, with a compression on the sides, especially when sitting bent forward, and in the evening, for six days. [*Rt.*]

When inspiring, a wheezing on the chest, in the morning (in 1¾ h.). [*Lgh.*]

When inspiring, obtuse stitches, when expiring, a slight pressure on the chest, for six days. [*Rt.*]

180. Pressure in the middle of the sternum, as if something lay upon the lungs. [*Rt.*]

Pressive pain with dull stitches in the scrobiculus cordis, which compels to quick breathing, the lungs feel as if they could not properly expand, [*Rt.*]

Single stitches in the chest and under the ribs, here and there, every day. [*Rt.*]

Palpitation of the heart. [SCHNEIDER, l. c.]

Griping pain in the right costal muscles. [*Gtm.*]

185. Muscular twitching in the right costal muscles, going off when he raised himself up. [*Gtm.*]

Running and crawling, as of insects, on the skin of the left side of the chest and abdomen. [*Gtm.*]

Pain in the back, above the hips, with nausea and chill. [*Fr. H.*]

Tensive lancinating pain in the right loin, only perceived during inspiration, and most severe while lying on the back. [*Gtm.*]

Tensive lancinating pain between the scapulæ, chiefly when walking, so that for a time he had to walk bending forward.

190. Obtuse stitch under the right scapula, while inspiring. [*Rt.*]

Pressive pain as from a bruise in the lower part of the back, with severe pressure in the scrobiculus cordis, the same in rest and in motion.

Drawing pain, internally in the region of the right scapula, as if the nerves and vessels were stretched. [*Hbg.*]

Severe, drawing pain from the right side of the neck, extending down over the scapula, as if the nerves were forcibly opened out and jerked, or as if bruised. [*Hbg.*]

Pain of soreness in the left scapula, when at rest. [*Gtm.*]

195. In the left sterno-cleido-mastoid muscle, a drawing pain, like a violent contraction; on moving and walking it draws toward the back part and goes off entirely. [*Stf.*]

Stiffness of the left side of the neck, painful when moved. [*Hbg.*]

Severe, strongly drawing pain in the left cervical muscles, worse when moving. [*Hbg.*]

In the nape, a painful drawing, even when at rest, soon after, stiffness of the nape, painful, *per se*, and still more painful on moving the head. [*Hbg.*]

In the nape, toward the protuberance of the occipital bone, a sensation, as if a heavily pressing load lay across it, as sensible when at rest as when moving the head. [*Hbg.*]

200. Suppurating swelling of the glands of the axillæ. [KOELPIN in *Hufel. Journ.* III., *pp.* 5, 77.]

Sensation behind the right scapula, as if the arm were sprained, both when at rest and in motion. [*Hbg.*]

Pressive, drawing bone-pain in the shafts of the bones of the arm while at rest, especially under the head of the humerus and above the wrist-joint, where it also pains as if in the periosteum, on raising the arm.

Stitches in the arms, occasionally, now here, now there (aft. 4 h. [*Rt.*]

Paralytic pain in the arms, as from a bruise, from time to time (aft. 5 d.). [*Rt.*]

205. In the right upper arm, pricking, burning pain, when moving it. [*Gtm.*]

In the bend of the right elbow, fine itching stitch, when at rest. [*Gtm*]

In the fore-arm of the right sid , tensive pain (aft. 27 h.). [*Gtm.*]

In the palm, a spasmodic pain, so that he could only open the fingers with difficulty; the pain was more severe when at rest than when moving. [*Gtm.*]

In the thumb of the right hand, **violent drawing pains,** feeling as if in the tendons, beginning in the ball and terminating in the tip of the thumb (aft. 5 h.). [*Lgh.*]

210. Burning pain on a point of the right middle finger. [*Hbg.*]

In the gluteal muscles of the left side a tickling itching when sitting (aft ¼ h.). [*Hbg.*]

Pain in the right thigh, as if the psoas muscle that raises it was too short, only when walking. (aft. 32 h.). [*Gtm.*]

Drawing tension in the right thigh.

---

[1] **Critical phenomena in a rheumatic paralysis getting well under Colocynthis.—*Hughes.***

Shooting, tearing pain in the thighs, when sitting (and standing). [*Rt.*]

215. In the hough, only when moving, lancinating pains, as from needles, at length changing into itching pricking. [*Gtm.*]

Sensation of cold in the knees, although they are warm.

Paralytic pain in the knee, when walking, as if it was tied fast in the joint.

Violent itching in the left hough, inciting to scratch, with smarting after scratching (aft. 14 h.). [*Lgh.*]

On the leg, a tensive pressure on the tibia, even in sitting. [*Rt.*]

220. **Cramp in the legs.**

Cramp in the muscles beside the tibia, at night, toward morning, aggravated by bending the knee.

Violent cramp in the calf, especially after coitus.

Quivering in the right calf, when at rest, going off when moving. [*Gtm.*]

Tearing pains, at times in the calves, when sitting and standing. [*Rt.*]

225. Sharp cutting in the left calf, on the inside, when at rest. [*Gtm.*]

Itching stitch in the right tibia, most violent when at rest. [*Gtm.*]

Itching stitch in the right leg, also when moving. [*Gtm.*]

Itching stitch in the right calf, not going off when rubbing. [*Gtm.*]

Weakness of the legs, as from fatigue.

230. The varices of the legs, which hitherto were painless, begin to pain. [*Gtm.*]

In the ankle, pressing and tearing, while sitting. [*Rt.*]

Tearing in the sole of the right foot, most violent when at rest. [*Gtm.*]

Severe tearing on the dorsum of the left foot, upward. [*Lgh.*]

Tearing in the periosteum of the os calcaneum.

235. Itching, boring stitch on the dorsum of the right foot, most violent when at rest. [*Gtm.*]

The left foot goes to sleep, also when resting. [*Hbg.*, *Gtm.*]

Trembling of the feet, as after a violent fright, with shaking chill. [*Fr. H.*]

Under the nail of the left big toe, a tearing pain.

Inordinate tendency of the muscles of all parts of the body to contract painfully in a cramp.

240. Contraction of all the limbs, so that he becomes like a hedgehog. [STALPAART, l. c.]

Twitching of particular muscular parts of the limbs. [HOFFMANN, l. c.]

Tearing stitches lengthways on the whole body, on the head, the back, the abdomen, and the limbs. [*Lgh.*]

Itching, as after profuse sweat, in the morning, on awaking, and on rising, on the whole body, especially on the chest and abdomen (aft. 26 h.). [*Lgh.*]

Troublesome itching, in the afternoon and evening, followed by sweat. [HOFFMANN, l. c.[1]]

245. Smarting itching, here and there, in the evening, in bed, only removed for a time by scratching, and at last turning into restlessness, while he has continually to move the limbs, without being able to go to sleep (aft. 32 h.).

Eruption like itch. [KOELPIN, l. c.]

The skin of the whole body desquamates. [SALMUTH, *Obs. C.* III., *obs.* 2.[2]]

Total sinking of strength. [HOYER, l. c.]

Syncope. [VALENTINI, in *Eph. N. C., an.* III., *obs.* 78.[3]]

250. Syncope, with coldness of the external parts. [HOFFMANN, l. c.]

Fatal syncope. [HOYER, l. c.]

Lassitude in all the limbs, while taking a walk, as if he had made a long foot-tour, with great heaviness of the legs and trembling, especially of the right leg, so that sweat broke out over the whole body (aft. 11 h.). [*Lgh.*]

Sleepiness and indisposition to mental work. [*Gtm.*]

Invincible drowsiness and inclination to lie down, but when sleeping, constant restlessness in the limbs, but especially in the legs.

255. Restless sleep, he tosses from one side to the other. [*Hbg.*]

Sleeplessness the whole night; thoughts and reflections concerning the objects of life and its relations occupy him in a calm and impassionate manner.

About midnight, a sort of flatulent colic, from flatus suddenly arising here and there, painfully repelling one another (contending) and not discharged (2d n.).

When sleeping, he nearly always lies on his back, one hand under his occiput, the other arm above the head.

Sleep at night disturbed by many dreams. [*Lgh.*]

260. Very vivid, but not anxious, dreams, so much increasing in vivacity that he wakes up with them.

Vivid, anxious dreams.

Dreams full of troublesome meditation and mental exertion.

He dreams much, and about many different things. [*Hbg.*]

Lascivious dreams, with emission of semen, without erection, when lying on his back. [*Gtm.*]

265. Voluptuous dreams, without pollution, disturbing the sleep. [*Lgh.*]

Lascivious dreams, with uncontrollable erections, without pollution. [*Gtm.*]

Voluptuous dreams and seminal emission. [*Hbg.*]

Coldness of the whole body.

Ice-cold hands, in the evening, with warm feet.

270. Sensation of icy cold in the soles of the feet, though they are not cold.

Violent chill. [*Fr. H.*]

---

[1] For HOFFMANN read KOELPIN.—*Hughes*.

[2] Poisoning. Note, "During convalescence."—*Hughes*.

[3] No such observation found here.—*Hughes*.

Shivering through the whole of the body, in the morning, after rising, with cold hands, while the face and the rest of the body are hot, without thirst (aft. ½ h.). [*Lgh.*]

Warmth rapidly rushing over the whole body, without thirst. [*Rt.*]

Sensation of heat in the interior of the whole body, which is also externally warm when touched. [*Hbg.*]

275. Warmth in the face, in the morning, after rising, with icy coldness of the hands and finger-tips. [*Lgh.*]

Febrile heat.]HOFFMANN, l. c.]

Night-sweat. [*Fr. H.*]

At night, violent sweat on the head, hands, legs and feet, of a urinous smell.

Morning-sweat on the legs, on awaking. [*Lgh.*]

280. Slow, full pulse (the first 10 h.). [*Hbg.*]

Quick, full pulse. [SCHNEIDER, l. c.]

Palpitation of the heart. [SCHNEIDER, l. c.]

When he lies still, he feels his heart-beat, and the pulsation of the arteries all through the body. [*Rt.*]

CONIUM MACULATUM. HEMLOCK.

[The juice freshly pressed from the whole herb, just as it has begun to bloom, is mixed with an equal quantity of alcohol. As is done in Homœopathy with all the plant-juices which are preserved from corruption in this manner, two drops of this mixture are dropped into a vial which is filled two-thirds full with 100 drops of alcohol; it is well-stopped and shaken with ten strokes of the arm. One drop is then further diluted through twenty-nine other such vials (each containing 100 drops of alcohol), and each attenuation is thus potentized by ten successive strokes to the decillionth (X) dynamization. But instead of this we might also triturate two grains of the fresh leaves of this plant with sugar of milk to the millionth powder attenuation, within three hours, and then, dissolving this preparation, potentize it further.]

The considerable medicinal power of this plant may easily be concluded from what was published in the years 1700–1779, by *Stoerck* and his many imitators in numerous books, concerning the great results obtained from *Conium maculatum.* But frequently as its wonderful help was proved, at least in the beginning, by its use in the most horrible diseases, just as often, yea far oftener, its use in the favorite large doses, frequently repeated, has done harm, frequently irretrievable harm, and killed not a few men.

The riddle thus presented by so many startling experiences, sometimes so joyous, and then again so sad, with observers mostly honest, who nevertheless contradicted each other in such down-right fashion, could only be solved by Homœopathy in these latter days. For Homœopathy has first shown, that in order to use heroic medicines in a beneficent manner, and thus really to heal, we must not (as has hitherto been done) assault any *unknown* disease straightway with frequent doses as large as practicable of a violent unknown remedy, but "that after previously fully proving and investigating the peculiar virtues of a medicine on healthy men the remedy must then be used only in morbid states, the symptoms of which have great similarity with those of the medicine; and this must be done by means of the minutest doses of the higher and highest attenuations, prepared by appropriate dynamization."

This contrasts, indeed, greatly with the doses of that time which were increased even to 140 grains of the thickened juice (extract), or to a wine-glass full of the freshly expressed juice of the hemlock, given, perhaps, six times a day. But then no true Homœopath will miss applying it properly—nor will hundreds of patients be tortured to death with it, as in former days.

Those many, terrifying examples prevented me from recognizing sooner in this plant one of the most important antipsoric medicines; it is only within the last few years that I have given it its rightful place.

In order to act beneficially, this remedy must often be preceded by some other antipsoric medicines. It is given in the smallest doses.

More or less smelling of the sweet spirits of nitre, and in some cases also a drink of coffee, will moderate the excessive effects of this drug.

In healing the diseases for which this medicine is suitable, the following symptoms, more than others, were relieved or removed, even where the complaint appeared in separate paroxysms:

Sadness; hypochondria; anxiety; ill-humor and melancholy; dejection; irritability; timidity; inclination to peevishness; *indisposition to work;* forgetfulness and weakness of the head; vertigo, when looking around, as if the patient would fall to one side; heaviness of the head; fits of tearing headache, obliging one to lie down; stitches in the upper part of the head; long-continued lancinating headache; *falling out of the hair of the head;* itching below the eyes, and on rubbing, smarting, burning; feeling of coldness in the eyes, on taking a walk; stye on the eyelid; short-sightedness; far-sightedness; dark points and colored streaks before the eyes; in the room the eyes are dazzled by the daylight; stitches in the ear, when taking a walk; tearing, with stitches in and about the ears; drawing stitches in the ear outward; induration of the swollen parotid gland; accumulation of ear-wax; *roaring in the ears;* humming, hissing, sounding and *ringing in the ears;* flow of pus from the nose; itching in the face; itching pimples in the face; tetters in the face; eroding ulcers in the face; *heat of the face;* dryness and peeling off of the lips; drawing pain in sound teeth from taking a walk; shooting pain in the teeth;

involuntary deglutition; scraping in the throat; hawking; fullness in the pit of the neck, with abortive eructation; *frequent empty eructation, the whole day;* loud eructation, tasting of the ingesta; heart-burn rising up the throat; voracious hunger; bread will not go down, he has no relish for it; after meals, burning up the fauces; nausea with pregnant women; acidity of the stomach; pressure in the stomach, when eating; contractive pain in the stomach; cramp in the stomach; stitches in the left hypochondrium; fullness in the abdomen, in the morning, after awaking; squeezing contraction of the hypogastrium; writhing and digging in the umbilical region; sensation of soreness in the abdomen, when walking on a stone pavement; obstruction of the flatus; rumbling and growling in the abdomen; colic, with discharge of flatus; *constipation, with ineffectual call to stool; hard stool* only every other day; diarrhœa; stool coated with blood; the passage of urine stops suddenly and is only renewed after an interval; pressure on the bladder, as if the urine would be passed at once; whitish, turbid, *thick urine; during micturition, cutting in the urethra;* impotence and lack of erections; insufficient, transient erection; feeble coitus; lassitude after coitus; *uterine cramps*; uterine spasms, beginning above the pudenda, distending the whole abdomen, and comeing into the chest, with stitches of the left side; pinching and griping in the uterus; bearing down and stitches in the vagina; stitches in the labiæ; *itching on the pudenda* and inside; menses too scanty; during the menses, bearing down anu drawing in the thigh; vaginal flow; smarting, eroding leucorrhœa.

Excessive sneezing; stoppage of the nostrils; morning-stoppage of the nostrils; chronic stoppage of the nose for years; troublesome feeling of dryness of the nose; *cough*, especially with scrofulous patients; shortness of breath in walking; asthma, early on awaking; *morning-asthma;* stitches in the sternum; jerks in the chest; pressing and squeezing together over the hips; tension in the nape; pain as of soreness in the lowest cervical vertebræ; the top of the shoulders feel as if pressed sore; sweat of the palms; drawing pain in the hips; weariness in the knees; cramp in the calves; *coldness of the feet* and hands; the feet are apt to catch cold; restlessness in the lower limbs; itching of the skin; frequent red, itching spots on the body; brown spots on the body; nettle-rash from severe bodily exercise; inveterate, humid tetter; restlessness, especially in the lower limbs; hysterical and hypochondriac paroxysms; hypochondria from continence in unmarried men; an attack, where a pricking sensation comes from the stomach and shoots under the left ribs, extending to the back; stitches here and there, all over the body; *ailments and fatigue from taking a walk;* sudden lassitude while walking; bruisedness of the limbs; painfulness of the skin of the body; lassitude in the whole body, especially in lower limbs; lassitude in the morning in bed; feeling of illness in all the limbs, as from excessive fatigue; drowsiness in the daytime; drowsiness in the evening with closing of the eyelids; late in falling asleep, in the evening in bed; sleep full of phantasies; many dreams at night; unrefreshing sleep; nocturnal pains.

The abbreviations of the names of those who have furnished contributions to the symptoms subjoined are as follows: *Fr.*, *Dr. Franz; Gr.*, *Dr. Gross; Lgh.*, *Dr. Langhammer; Rl.*, *Dr. Rummel; Wl.*, *Dr. Wislicenus.*

CONIUM MACULATUM.

More inclined to be sad than cheerful.

She is easily affected by trifles and moved to tears.

Hypochondriac dejection and indifference when taking a walk. [*Fr.*]

Hysterical attack, with chill and a sort of spasmodic motions. [GREDING, *verm. Schrift.*, p. 118.[1]]

5. Hysterical anxiety. [*Medic. Obs. and Inq.* IV., 364.[2]]

Anxiety. [SCHMUCKER, *Chirurg. Wahrnehm.* II., 82–4.[3]]

Anxiety in the region of the scrobiculus cordis. [STOERK, *lib. de Cic.*, 2.[4]]

Lost in deep meditation, he anxiously thought over the present and the future, and sought solitude. [*Lgh.*]

Shyness at the approach of people, and yet also dread of being alone.

10. The propinquity and the talk of people passing by is very offensive to him, and he feels impelled to assault and maltreat them.

Superstitous thoughts.

Timid, lachrymose, despondent.

Fear of thieves.

He imagines that somebody has come in at the door by night.

15. Timidity.

Frequent thoughts of death.

Gloomy ill-humor (1st d.). [*Rl.*]

Very morose; every afternoon, from three to six o'clock, as if a great guilt weighed him down; at the same time a sensation of paralysis in all the limbs; indifferent and unsympathizing.

Extremely peevish and anxious thoughts after a meal, in the morning, with obtuseness in the forehead (aft. 29 h.). [*Fr.*]

Conium is one of the medicines of the *Materia Medica Pura*. Its pathogenesis there contains 89 symptoms from Hahnemann, 131 from Franz, Langhammer, and Wislicenus, and 155 from authors. A later list in the first edition of the *Chronic Diseases* adds observations from Hahnemann himself, from Gross and Rummel, swelling its number to 700, and in this second edition Hahnemann supplies 212 more.—*Hughes.*

[1] Observations on patients taking C. This symptom not found.—*Hughes.*

[2] After application of C. to cancerous breast. Patient had attacks of this with symptoms 232 and 563 till she died; there is no thought of ascribing them to the Conium.—*Hughes.*

[3] Observations on patients. This symptom not found.—*Hughes.*

[4] Observations on patients. This symptom, with 3, 210, 224, 318, 562, 870, and 909 arose from overloading the stomach; all disappeared after an emetic.—*Hughes.*

20. Peevish mood, he does not know what to do with himself, the time passes too slow for him (aft. 8 h.). [*Wl.*]

Moroseness; all his surroundings made a disagreeable impression on him. [*Lgh.*]

Great dissatisfaction.

Peevish and vexed about trifles.

Constant ill-humor and vexation.

25. He thinks of vexatious matters.

Readily moved to vexation and anger.

Indifference.

Lack of sympathy.

No agreeable affections in the mind.

30. Indisposed to work.

Cheerful mood and inclination to talk (curative effect.) [*Lgh.*]

Cheerful, open mood (aft. 3, 4 d.), (curative effect). [*Fr.*]

Cheerful, well and strong, in the morning (alternative curative effect aft. 24 h.). [*Fr.*]

Lack of memory.

35. Loss of memory. [W. ROWLAY, *seventy-four cases, London*, 1779.[1]]

Unable to recollect, on awaking from noon siesta.

Extraordinary inability to recollect.

He cannot well express himself in talking, nor can he rightly remember.

He offen utters the wrong words.

40. Dullness, difficult comprehension of what is read; obtuseness of the head.

Dullness, like stupefaction, it is hard for him to understand what he reads.

Dullness of the head, after drinking.

Obtuseness of all the senses. [SIM. PAULLI, *Quadripart. Bot.*[2]]

Insensibility and laziness. [SIM. PAULLI.]

45. He walks about as if half asleep.

Full of phantasies, in the morning (aft. 24 h.).

Hastiness.

Confusion of thoughts. [VAN EEMS in *Boerhave, praelect. de morb. nerv.* I., p. 97.[3]]

Delirium. [ANDRY, *Quaest. med.*[4]]

50. Insanity, deliriums. [CULLEN, *Mat. Med.*[5]]

Obtuseness of the head (aft. 1 h.).

Obtuseness of the left half of the head, as from coldness, or as if the brain did not fill out the skull.

Constant obtuseness of the sinciput, in the forehead, in the region of the eyebrows and the root of the nose (the 1st days).

Obtuseness and heaviness of the head, after awaking from a sound sleep.

55. Obtuseness and heaviness of the head (aft. 5 d.).

Heaviness of the head.

---

[1] Not accessible.—*Hughes.*
[2] No symptom mentioned in edition of 1667.—*Hughes.*
[3] Effects of cicuta aquatica.—*Hughes.*
[4] Not accessible.—*Hughes.*
[5] From gr. 30 of powder in an adult.—*Hughes.*

The head is heavy. [WATSON, philos. transact., 1744, p. 20.[1]]

Feeling of heaviness in the occiput, frequently passing away and recurring, comes from sitting bent double from time to time, and always goes off by raising the head. [*Wl.*]

Dizziness and whirling in the head, for two days.

60. Very dizzy while walking.

Intoxication. [BIERCHEN, *Tal om Kraftskador.*[2]]

The least spirituous liquor intoxicates him.

Even a mixture of water and wine affects his head.

Constant stupefaction of the head, with continual inclination to sleep.

65. Reeling. [VAN EEMS.]

Vertigo, whirling around, when he rises from his seat.

Vertigo, after stooping, when raising up again, as if the head would burst.

Vertigo, worse while lying down, as if the bed was whirling around in a circle.

Vertigo, early on rising from the bed.

70. Vertigo on going down stairs; she had to hold on to something, and for some moments she did not know where she was.

Vertigo, which fatigues the head. [FOTHERGILL, *Med. obs.* III., p. 400.[3]]

Vertigo, so that everything seems to whirl around. [BOERHAVE, *praelect. ad inst.* VI., p. 255.[4]]

Headache, simple pain; on taking a walk, he feels stupid; also in the morning till breakfast.

Headache on walking, she feels every step in her head.

75. Daily headache, owing to stools, which, though frequent, are too scant, connected with straining.

Headache with nausea and vomiting of mucus (3d d.). [*Rl.*]

Violent headache with vertigo, so that she spent three or four days sad and without speaking, sitting in one place. [LANGE, *dub. cic. vex. Helmst.*, 1774.[5]]

Stupefying, pressive headache, externally on the forehead. [*Lgh.*]

Headache in the morning, on awaking, as in epidemic fevers, as if the brain was torn, especially toward the occiput (aft. 10 h.).

80. Headache, as if the head was beaten to pieces, or as if it would go to pieces.

Semilateral, gradually increasing headache, as if the head was beaten to pieces, and like a downward pressure of something heavy, aggravated by turning the eyes to the affected side.

Headache, as if the head was too full, and would burst, in the morning, on awaking.

Feeling in the right half of the brain as if a large foreign body was in it.

Dull pressure in the head, on taking a walk; he has to rub his forehead.

[1] During convalescence.—*Hughes.*
[2] Observation.—*Hughes.*
[3] General statement from observations.—*Hughes.*
[4] Observations on self.—*Hughes.*
[5] Not accessible.—*Hughes.*

85. Pressive pain in the right hemisphere of the brain, posteriorly.

Pressure in both temples (aft. several h.). [*Rl.*]

Pressive headache above the eyes, from within outward. [*Wl.*]

Pressive headache, as from a stone on the top of the frontal bone (3d d.). [*Fr.*]

Tension in the head, and, as it were, a squeezing together from the two temples, after every meal; he has to rest the front part of his head on the table. [*Fr.*]

90. Headache, as from an external contraction on top of the frontal bone, which goes off on stooping and on laying his own hand upon it, with chilliness, vertigo, and a vexatious inability to recollect (aft. 1½ h.). [*Fr.*]

Drawing pain in the brain, in the middle, behind the forehead (the first days).

Drawing in the head, while the brain is asleep, diminished after eating. [*Fr.*]

Drawing pain in the temples, when touched. [*Fr.*]

Tearing in the right temple and the right ear.

95. Tearing headache in the occiput and the nape of the neck, and especially also in the orbits, with constant nausea; she had to lie abed.

Tearing pain through the temples, in the morning (4th d.). [*Fr.*]

Tearing headache in the temporal region, with pressure in the forehead, after eating (3d d.). [*Fr.*]

Tearing pain in the temples, during eating. [*Fr.*]

Slow tearing on the left side of the occiput, while walking (aft. ½ h.). [*Fr.*]

100. Tearing stitches from the left parietal bone down into the frontal region.

Stitches in the forehead.

Stitches outward in the forehead, after rising.

Shooting headache darting out through the forehead, with inclination to lie down, in the forenoon.

Shooting pain darting out through the forehead, at noon.

105. Shooting headache in the forehead, the whole day; but she did not have to lie down.

Shooting pain in the head, as from needles, for about an hour.

Shooting in the parietal bones of the head and in the forehead, with vertigo, so that he had to stand still and sit down; then also shooting in the cervical muscles.

Pain in the occiput, with every pulsation, as if pierced with a knife.

Throbbing in the forehead.

110. Sensation of heaviness and griping in the forehead, as if coming from the stomach, with so great a sensitiveness of the brain that it is even painfully shaken by a slight noise and by talking.

In shaking the head, headache from the forehead to the occiput, as if something was detached.

With every step in walking, a snapping sound in the vertex, without pain; not when sitting down.

Heat in the head.

Numbness and sensation of coldness, in one side of the head.

115. External pressure on the forehead. [*Lgh.*]

Sharp pressure on a small spot of the integuments of the head.

Drawing pain in the temporal bones.

Drawing pain in the forehead, above the eyebrows.

Much itching on the hairy scalp.

120. Several eruptive nodules above the forehead, of which one gets as large as a filbert in fifteen days, and pains when its tip is touched (aft. 24 d.).

Falling out of the hairs of the head.

The orbits pain, especially during the headache.

Pressure in the eyes, especially while reading.

Pressure in the outer canthus, as from a grain of sand.

125. Pressure in the eye, as from a grain of sand, especially in the forenoon, with inflammation and redness of the white of the eye, and smarting tears.

Painful pressure in the eyes, when she closes them to sleep, in the evening, in bed.

Drawing pain, with redness in the eyes.

Shooting in the inner canthus, while the lids are glued together there, in the morning.

Itching shooting in the inner canthi, not removed by rubbing (aft. 1½ h.). [*Wl.*]

130. Itching about the left eye.

Itching on the edge of the eyelids.

Smarting pain in the inner canthus, as if something caustic had gotten in, with lachrymation. [*Wl.*]

Heat in the eyes.

An almost burning heat quickly passes through the eye, in the forenoon and evening.

135. **Burning in the eyes.**

Burning on the inner surface of the eyelids.

Burning in the eyes, toward evening, with pressure in the orbits.

Red eyes. [BAYLIES, *Essays on Medical Subjects.*]

Inflamed eyelids, with incipient styes in several places; the boy often winks.

140. Yellowish color of the white of the eye (10th d.).

Languid appearance of the eyes. [*Gr.*]

Eye-gum in the eyes, in the morning.

Quivering of the upper eyelid.

Trembling look, as if the eye trembled.

145. Motion of the eyes, as if they were being pressed out. [FOTHERGILL'S Works (London, 1781), p. 315.[2]]

Protruding eyes.

Difficult opening of the eyelids in the morning, they feel as if drawn together. [*Rl.*]

Dilated pupil (aft. 1 h.). [*Fr.*]

[1] Not accessible.—*Hughes.*

[2] General statement from observation.—*Hughes.*

Contracted pupil (curative effect, aft 3¼ h.). [*Lgh.*]

150. Weakness of the vision. [GATAKER, *Essays on Med. Subj.*, *Introduct.*, p. 8.[1]]

Obscuration of the eyes. [BAYLIES, ANDRÉE.[2]]

Blindness, immediately after sleeping, in the heat of the sun. [AMAT. LUSITANIUS, *Cent.* V., *cur.* 93.[3]]

Blindness, in the afternoon, of short duration; after complaining of headache and eyeache, the child loses power of vision, and also later on, at times. [*Gr.*]

Obscurity before the eyes on taking a walk; in the room it seems brighter to him.

155. Far-sightedness (with a short-sighted person); he could distinguish pretty clearly remote objects (aft. 3½ h.). [*Lgh.*]

More short-sighted than formerly; he could only recognize subjects when very near to them (aft. 29 h.). [*Lgh.*]

He saw objects double and threefold, and nothing but arches before his eyes.

Before the right eye, a thread seems to float.

Clouds and light spots before the eyes.

160. Fiery zigzags crossing each other before the eyes, when he shuts them, at night.

Objects look red. [GREDING.[4]]

When looking at a closely held print, the lines seem to move up and down.

Fiery sparks before the eyes when walking in the open air.

Increased irritability of the eye (the 1st days).

165. Otalgia, as if the inner ear was pressed apart.

Sudden, sharp pressure in the ear, almost like straining in the ear.

Partly drawing, partly tearing pain in the external ear.

Drawing in the interior of the left ear.

Shooting pains in both ears.

170. Stitches behind both ears, especially in the mastoid process, and then a dull pain in the same place.

Pinching shooting in the ear, when drinking.

Sharp outward thrusts in the ears, especially and more violent when swallowing (aft. ¾ h.). [*Wl.*]

Throbbing of the blood in the ears.

Violent itching in the external ear.

175. Painful tension of the skin behind the ears and on the mastoid process; even when not moving (aft. 1½ h.). [*Wl.*]

Blood-red ear-wax.

Painful sensitiveness of the hearing, so that noise causes terror.

Noise is intolerable, and there is a longing for stillness and quiet (the 1st days).

He is startled at every sound.

180. On blowing the nose, her ear feels obstructed and as if stopped up.

---

[1] General statement from observation.—*Hughes.*
[2] In Andree's case, with giddiness.—*Hughes.*
[3] No such observation to be found.—*Hughes.*
[4] In a case of cataract which was improving under C.—*Hughes.*

Loud ringing in the ear.

Humming in the right ear.

Rushing sound in the left ear with hardness of hearing, aggravated during eating.

Rushing sound in the ears, as from a stormy wind, more after dinner, till going to bed and when making a mental effort while sitting, but most of all when lying in bed; also at night, on awaking.

185. Noise before the right ear, as from a waterfall (aft. 14 h.).

Noise in the ears, as if the blood was rushing through the brain.

Fluttering and humming in the right ear.

Fluttering and humming in both ears.

In the nose, twitching.

190. A momentary twitching in the root of the nose.

Frequent itching of the nose (aft. 2 d.).

Formication on the dorsum of the nose (aft. 1½ h.). [*Wl.*]

Itching formication in the nose. [*Wl.*]

Itching in the nose.

195. Stinging, itching irritation in the right side of the nose, as from a foreign body in it.

Itching formication on the tip of the nose and in the nostrils. [*Wl.*]

Burning about the nostrils.

Stinging pain as from soreness in the septum of the nose, when pressing on it, as if there was a pimple.

Pustule in the depression by the right ala nasi.

200. **Hemorrhage from the nose.** [EHRHARDT, *Diss. de Cic. Argent.*, 1763; LANGE, l. c.[1]]

Frequent epistaxis.

Epistaxis, when sneezing. [*Gr.*]

The sense of smell is excessively acute.

A sort of smell of tar, in the back of the nose, and he also seems to taste it.

205. From the posterior nares to the mouth, a taste as if from coryza.

Heat in the face, rush of blood to the head, and sensation of coryza in the nose (aft. 4 h.).

Complexion, sickly and pale (aft. 7 d.).

Face very pale, in the morning.

Blueness of the face. [SIM. PAULLI, *Quadrip. Botan. Cic. maj.*]

210. Bluish swollen face. [STOERK.[2]]

Swelling of the face. [LANDEUTTE, *Journal de Médec.* XV.[3]]

Swelling of the zygoma and the upper gums, with tensive pain (3d d.).

Prosopalgia, at night.

Pressive pain on the bones above the right eye, on the nose and in the zygoma, late in the evening, for ten minutes.

---

[1] (To EHRHARDT.) A list of symptoms from authors.—*Hughes.*

[2] See note to Sympt. 7.—*Hughes.*

[3] Symptoms observed in patients taking *C.* This occurred in a man convalescing from suppurative pneumonia, and treated by C. for splenic cancer, with S. 368, 542, 557, and 662, shortly before death.—*Hughes.*

215. Tearing, shooting pain in the face, close before the ear, on the cheek, in the evening.

Fine stitch through the right side of the face, beside the zygoma (aft. 2 h.). [*Wl.*]

Fine stitches through the right cheek, toward the corners of the mouth. [*Wl*]

Constant shooting itching down the cheek and face on the right side, only going off by repeated scratching. [*Fr.*]

Eroding itching on the forehead, only transiently relieved by rubbing. [*Wl.*]

220. Sensation of chapping in the face, as if the skin was rubbed off, after washing and drying the face.

On an old "liver-spot" on the cheek, a pimple appeared.

Eruptive pimple on the forehead, with tensive drawing pain. (4th d.). [*Fr.*]

Nodule on the forehead with tensive pain, which when touched and afterward, becomes a tearing pain all over it (aft. 2 or 3 d.). [*Fr.*]

Trembling of the lower lip. [STOERK.[1]]

225. Itching of the upper lip (aft. ½ h.). [*Wl.*]

Blisters on the upper lip, on the edge of the red part, with erosive pain.

Ulcers on the lips, after fever. [GREDING.[2]]

On the chin, slight stitches upward through the jaw. [*Wl.*]

Drawing from the jaw toward the ear and the head, not painful, soon after drinking.

230. Severe itching about the chin.

Spasm of the jaws. [EHRHARDT.]

Gnashing of teeth. [*Med. Observ. and Inq., London*, 1771.[3]]

Toothache (tearing?) toward the ear, eye and cheekbone, only while eating.

Pressive toothache.

235. **Drawing in a hollow tooth, when eating cold things, not when drinking cold drinks**, extending through the temples (aft. 3 h.). [*Fr.*]

Drawing pain from the lower teeth, on the right side, up into the zygoma.

Drawing and boring in the left molar.

Boring needle-pricks between the teeth-sockets, on the left side, on moving the lower jaw. [*Lgh.*]

Twitching and gnawing in the teeth.

240. Pain from looseness of the teeth, when chewing.

Looseness of the molars, as if they would fall out.

The gums ache and burn.

Swollen, bluish-red gums, as if suffused with blood.

Bleeding of the gums of the molars.

245. The gums bleed easily.

Pain of the tongue. [SIM. PAULI.]

Stiff, swollen, painful tongue. [STOERK.[4]]

---

[1] See note to S. 7.—*Hughes.*

[2] Literally "breaking out on the lips, following slight fever."—*Hughes.*

[3] See note to Sympt. 5.—*Hughes.*

[4] From touching the tongue with the juice of the root.—*Hughes.*

Heavy speech. [ANDRÉE.]

Speechlessness. [STOERK, EBERHARDT.[1]]

250. Sore throat, pain as from soreness, on deglutition (2d d).

Spasms in the fauces. [EHRHARDT.]

Difficult deglutition.

Impeded deglutition. [EHRHARDT.]

When she walks in the wind, she has to swallow frequently.

255. Dryness of the mouth. [STOERK.]

Dryness of the mouth, with sensation of acidity.

Dry tongue. [BAYLIES.]

Ptyalism. [BIERCHEN, l. c.[2]]

Violent ptyalism. [VALENT, in *Hufel. Journ.*, XXIX. III.]

260. Frequent hawking up of mucus.

Putrid taste in the mouth, when eating and swallowing.

The stomach is tormented with acidity, with insipid, somewhat putrid taste.

Sourish taste in the mouth.

Bitter, sourish taste, after breakfast.

265. Bitterness in the mouth and throat.

Bitterness in the throat.

Bitter taste at times in the throat, without cause. [*Fr.*]

Decrease of appetite (the first 4 d.).

Lack of appetite. [ANDRÉE, *Pharm. helv.;* LANG, LANDEUTTE.[3]]

270. Total lack of appetite and great weakness of the stomach. [LANGE.]

Appetite at once diminished, both for food and for smoking.

Thirst. [BAYLIES, FOTHERGILL.[4]]

Much thirst, every afternoon.

Violent thirst, the whole day (aft. 74 h.). [*Lgh.*]

275. Great desire for coffee.

Much appetite for sour things.

Much desire for salt and salty food.

After taking a little milk, rapid inflation of the abdomen.

After eating, bloatedness in the epigastrium, with pressure in the stomach, which causes an anxious interception of the breathing.

280. After eating, in the morning, aching in the abdomen, and the whole day, great fullness of the stomach and of the chest.

Immediately after eating, accumulation of flatus, which is then discharged in large quantities with noise, giving relief.

After a meal, nausea, with sensation of satiety.

After every meal, nausea and inclination to vomit.

After dinner, nausea, with pressive headache, in the nape, the crown and the forehead.

285. At the beginning of supper, hiccup.

After supper, bellyache in the umbilical region, as if the bowels were contused. [*Fr.*]

---

[1] In Stoerk's case as S. 249.—*Hughes.*

[2] In cases of cancrum oris.—*Hughes.*

[3] (To *Pharm. helv,*) General statement from experience.—*Hughes.*

[4] In Fothergill's case with S. 335 and 884.—*Hughes.*

Soon after a meal, drawing pain in the abdomen, in the umbilical region. [*Fr.*]

After dinner, drawing pain in the hypogastrium, when sitting. [*Fr.*]

When she has eaten anything, there comes, seemingly from the stomach, a sort of languid heat through the arms, even into the fingers, when the hands become pale and, as it were, become dead.

290. Chill at the conclusion of supper.

After eating, tightness, and hard pressure externally on the sternum.

During eating and drinking, sweat.

After breakfast, great lassitude and lack of tone in the abdominal muscles.

After a meal, great lassitude and lack of tone.

295. After eating, she has quite a sour taste in the mouth.

After eating, sour eructation.

After eating, regurgitation of a sour substance from the stomach.

After supper the whole mouth is full of sour water.

After breakfast, abortive eructation.

300. Frequent eructation.

Abortive eructation, causing pain in the stomach.

Frequent empty eructation, chiefly in the morning.

Eructation, chiefly toward evening.

Much empty eructation, without taste and smell.

305. Sour eructation in the evening.

Sourish eructation, with burning in the stomach.

Putrid eructation. [SCHMUCKER.[1]]

Eructation, with taste of the ingesta.

Eructation with taste of the ingesta, even six hours after a meal.

310. Eructation, with the taste of the ingesta, without inclination to vomit, with regurgitation.

Regurgitation of some food from the stomach, with the eructation.

Heartburn, in the evening.

Rancid heartburn.

Hiccup.

315. Frequent nausea and total lack of appetite. [LANGE.]

Nausea in the evening, with great lassitude, so that it is hard for her to speak.

Morning-nausea, going off after stool.

Nausea and inclination to vomit. [STOERK, FOTHERGILL.[2]]

Nausea and inclination to vomit, after every meal.

320. Inclination to vomit. [CULLEN.]

Inclination to vomit, with eructation and lassitude. [GREDING.]

Inclination to vomit after eating, and hiccup, but proper taste and good appetite.

---

[1] Not found.—*Hughes.*

[2] No such symptom found in Stoerk.—*Hughes.*

Frequent vomiting, with total lack of appetite. [LANGE.]

Violent vomiting. [EHRHARDT.]

325. Vomiting of mucus, in the afternoon, with headache, with nausea and subsequent frequent eructation. [*Rl.*]

The stomach is frequently distended with flatus.

Inflation of the stomach.

Pressure in the region of the scrobiculus cordis, as from fullness, intermixed with stitches, and aggravated by respiration and motion.

Pressure up from the scrobiculus cordis into the fauces, as if a round body was about to rise up (2d d.).

330. A pressure in the scrobiculous cordis, as if something was moving around in it, then some stitches in the side of the chest, also in the morning.

Drawing pain from the scrobiculus cordis up into the fauces, with short, difficult respiration, in the morning after rising and after the stool (11th d.).

Contractive pain in the stomach, with sensation of coldness in it and in the back, awaking her in the morning from sleep.

Cramplike pains in the stomach.

Spasms of the stomach. [*Pharm. helv.* l. c.]

335. Spasmodic pinching in the stomach. [FOTHERGILL.]

Pinching in the stomach, which contracts the chest, with grasping together of the back and much eructation, and wakes her from sleep.

Pinching in the stomach, which later in a dull form passes into the bowels.

Stitches in the gastric region, toward evening.

Fine stitches in the scrobiculus cordis. [*Wl.*]

340. Sensation of soreness and of rawness in the stomach.

Sensation of soreness in the scrobiculus cordis, as if festering underneath, in the morning when lying in bed and turning over, for three mornings (aft. 13 d.).

Tightness in the pit of the stomach when leaning backward, with interception of the breath and of speech.

Painful tension around the hypochondria, as from a constricting bandage.

In the liver, pressive pain, when walking.

345. Pressive pain in the right side of the abdomen and chest, aggravated by respiring.

Straining in the right side of the abdomen, when taking a deep breath.

Sharp drawing in the anterior lobe of the liver.

Sharp drawing jerks under the right ribs.

Painful tearing in the hepatic region.

350. Lancinating pain in the hepatic region, intermittingly (aft. 16 h.).

Stitches in the hepatic region.

Stitches in the hepatic region, intercepting the breathing.

In the left hypochondria, pressive tensive pain extending into the side of the hypogastrium.

Stitch in the left side of the abdomen (2d d.).

355. Lancinating pain in the left hypochondrium, in the morning, when lying in bed, with oppression of the breathing; it goes off on rising.

Shooting digging in the left side of the abdomen.

Pain in the abdomen above the hips, when walking.

Pain in the abdomen, when laughing.

Violent pains in the abdomen with chill. [STOERK.[1]]

360. Excessive pains in the abdomen. [KALTSCHMIDT, *Progr. de Cic. Jen* , 1778, p. 5.[2]]

Pressure in the hypogastrium and then fermentation in it.

Constant pressure in the hypogastrium, as from something heavy, when not eating.

Hard and severe inflation of the abdomen, in the evening, after a meal; the navel protrudes, making her sleep uneasy.

Inflation of the abdomen, after the noon-siesta.

365. Inflation and fullness of the abdomen, in the afternoon.

Distension of the abdomen, and twitching contraction up toward the chest, with pressive and pinching pain, for several minutes (2d d.).

Inflation of the abdomen, like flatulent-colic in the evening, with coldness of one foot.

Swelling of the abdomen. [LANDEUTTE, EHRHARDT.[3]]

Swelling of the mesenteric glands. [KALSCHMIDT.]

370. Very much contracted spot in the colon. [KALSCHMIDT.]

Compression in the abdomen.

Contractive pain in the hypogastrium, like after-pains, urging to stool.

Griping and forcing in the abdomen.

Cramp in the hypogastrium (6th d.).

375. Colic pain of the most violent kind. [STOERK, *lib. de Colchico.*[4]]

Pinching pain in the abdomen, but not just before, nor immediately after, the stool.

Pinching deep in the hypogastrium, after every meal, with good appetite.

Severe pinching in the abdomen, as if diarrhœa was coming.

Cutting colic, in the morning, after a few hours' chill, with headache and nausea. [*Kl.*]

380. Cutting in the left side of the abdomen, as if a tumor was forming.

Cutting colic, with diarrhœa (12th d.).

Cutting colic, deep in the abdomen, with good appetite and sleep at night.

Violent cutting in the abdomen, every day, especially in the right side.

Cutting stitches in the abdomen, as with a knife (4th d.). [*Rl.*]

385. Stabs in the abdomen, as with a knife.

---

[1] A patient under treatment by C. for a mammary scirrhus, had a chill in the street; got this and S. 428 and died with dysentery.—*Hughes.*

[2] Not accessible.—*Hughes.*

[3] See note to S. 211.—*Hughes.*

[4] A woman could not take more than four grains, without this.—*Hughes.*

Transient, lancinating pains in the abdomen (8th d.).

Shooting in the epigastrium, in the morning on awaking, worse on moving.

Drawing sensation in the abdomen, after drinking.

Drawing pain in the abdomen, on walking (aft. 3 h.) [*Fr.*]

390. Drawing pain in the abdomen, in the umbilical region, in the morning, after rising. [*Fr.*]

Drawing in the hypogastrium, and pressure toward the epigastrium, in the morning, when sitting.

Drawing pain, as from being bruised, in the intestines (aft. 9½ h.). [*Fr.*]

Tearing in the hypogastrium, above the pubes, extending to the abdominal ring.

Dull tearing, on a small spot just below the navel.

395. Tearing, as from a sore, intermittently from the gastric region into the side of the abdomen, as if everything in the abdomen was being torn out; for several mornings.

Several thrusts in the abdomen, outwardly toward the abdominal muscles, as in pregnancy from movements of the fœtus.

Itching in the abdomen.

In the abdominal muscles, above the navel, fine pinching, on bending the body forward. [*Wl.*]

Sharp stitches, darting upward, in the abdominal muscles, in short intermissions, on the left side below the navel. [*Wl.*]

400. In the groin, shooting pains, on rising from a seat.

Pain in the right groin, as from a swelling, and, on being touched, pain as if from festering within.

Pains, as if forcing a protrusion, in the place where the hernia is situated (2d d.).

Forcing outward, in the location of the hernia.

There is forcing toward the location of the former inguinal hernia, without the actual protrusion of the hernia.

405. Tearing in the mons veneris when sitting. [*Fr.*]

Growling and rumbling in the abdomen.

Swashing in the left side of the abdomen.

The flatus is discharged at once, easily.

A quantity of flatus is discharged (aft. 18 h.).

410. Discharge of fetid flatus.

Violent discharge of much flatus.

Discharge of cold flatus.

Before the discharge of flatus, cutting in the abdomen.

Constipation. [ANDREE.[1]]

415. **Frequent, ineffectual call to stool.**

Constant tenesmus.

Stool, only every two days, with straining.

Scanty stool.

Stool every two days, the first part always requires straining.

420. Daily, a repeated call to stool, every time only a little evacuation is passed.

---

[1] Literally, "irregular stools, attended with griping."—*Hughes.*

Constant call to stool, but he can only evacuate twice a day; and the motion is thin.

Frequent call to stool, but only a small quantity of soft fæces is discharged, and the abdomen becomes afterward continually more inflated.

Severe urging to stool, daily, with three diarrhœic stools.

Pappy stools, daily a couple of times, with burning in the rectum.

425. Liquid stool, mixed with hard pieces, discharged together with noisy flatus; at the same time, colic (7th d.).

Four liquid stools, with little hard clots (6th d.).

Diarrhœa. [LANDEUTTE, EHRHARDT.]

Weakening diarrhœa. [STOERK.[1]]

Frequent diarrhœic stools, like water, and much empty eructation, and copious passage of urine (aft. 24 h.).

430. Very frequent diarrhœic stools, like water and with it undigested food; with pinching in the stomach, spreading through the abdomen (4th d.).

Undigested stool (9th d.).

Undigested food is discharged with the stool.

Unconscious evacuation in sleep (2d d.).

Very fetid mucous discharge with the stool.

435. Flow of blood, with the morning-stool.

Before every stool, brief cutting pains in the abdomen.

During the stool, burning in the rectum.

During stool, much discharge of flatus, with straining, urging and cutting in the rectum.

With every stool, chilliness.

440. After every stool, palpitation of the heart, with intermission of the heart-beat.

After every stool, tremulous weakness; this goes off in the open air.

Forcing toward the anus and sacrum, in frequent paroxysms (the first days).

Drawing toward the anus and the hypogastrium.

Frequent stitches in the anus, unconnected with the stool (5th d.).

445. Itching of the anus.

Itching in the rectum, following after itching in the chest and abdomen.

Heat in the anus.

Heat in the lower part of the rectum (not in the anus).

Burning in the rectum and anus.

450. Suppression of urine; ischury. [BAYLIES.]

Strangury. [LANGE; EHRHARDT.]

Frequent urging to urinate every half hour, but little urine emitted at a time.

Very frequent micturition with incontinence of urine.

Involuntary flow of urine.[2] [BIERCHEN, GATAKER.]

455. Involuntary flow of urine[2] with great pains. [LANGE.]

[1] See note to S. 359.—*Hughes*.

[2] "*Harnfluss*" signifies either "involuntary discharge of urine" or "diabetes."—*Transl.*

At night, frequent micturition. (aft. 10 h.).

For several nights he has to get up at 2 A. M. to urinate.

Nocturnal wetting the bed.

Red urine. [BAYLIES.]

460. Hematuria. [HALLER, in *Gœtting. Anz.*, 1775, p. 523.[1]]

Frequent hematuria with asthma. [LANGE.]

Great pains in the urethra during the discharge of the urine, which always brings with it a viscid, turbid mucus. [LANGE.]

Cutting of the urine as it passes through the urethra.

During micturition, cutting in the orifice of the urethra (the first days).

465. During micturition, cutting drawing through the urethra.

During micturition, pressure on the uterus and cutting in the urethra.

During micturition, burning.

During micturition, burning in the urethra (11th d.).

Just after micturition in the morning, burning in the urethra, for half an hour.

470. After micturition, a smarting urging to urinate (aft. ½ h.). [*Fr.*]

Soon after micturition a cramplike pressure in the region of the neck of the bladder from without inward, with sharp stitches, lasting many hours, worse when walking than when sitting. [*Wl.*]

Sharp pressure on the bladder.

Violent stitch in the urethra, extending to its orifice.

Twitching stitches back into the urethra.

475. Burning in the urethra. [STOERK.]

Flow of mucus from the male urethra, also after urinating (4th, 5th, 6th d.).

Flow of pus from the urethra, after previous itching there.

Tearing through the penis, unconnected with micturition (4th d.). [*Fr.*]

Itching of the penis, the prepuce and the glans, not relieved by rubbing.

480. Inflammation of the prepuce.

Cutting pain in the glans.

In the testes, pain for several hours, chiefly after erections (the 1st days).

Pressive pain in the left testicle for several hours.

Drawing pain in the left testicle.

485. Pinching and tearing in the testes in the evening (4th d.).

Pain, as if a knife was cutting right through the middle of the scrotum, between the testes, up above the root of the penis, often returning for a short time. [*Wl.*]

Sweat in the perinæum.

The sexual desire is altogether lacking for several of the first days, despite the most inviting allurements.

Painful erections, in the evening before going to sleep.

490. Uncontrollable sexual desire. [LIMPRECHT, *Act. Nat. C.* I, *obs.* 52.[2]]

---

[1] In a gouty subject taking C.—*Hughes.*

[2] Poisoning by Cicuta root, but of what species is doubtful. Inordinate excitement was present, but nothing is said as to its being sexual.—*Hughes.*

Lewd lustfulness (aft. 12 h.).

Pollutions, three nights in succession, followed by awaking of sexual desire.

Pollution (the 1st n.).

Even while only fondling a female, the semen is emitted.

495. Prostatic juice is emitted, while straining for a stool.

With every emotion, prostatic juice is discharged, without voluptuous thoughts (with itching of the prepuce).

Severe itching of the female pudenda, also in the vagina, worst immediately after the menses; she has to rub them, and there ensues a pain liking bearing down of the uterus.

Violent itching deep in the vagina.

Severe stitches on the genitals.

500. Cutting between the labia, during micturition.

Large eruptive pimple on the mons veneris, painful when touched.

Supression of the menses. [ANDRY; ANDREE; GREDING.[1]]

Suppression of the menses which had just appeared, when there followed, by day and by night, a drawing pain down the back, extending to the sacrum.

Delay of the menses, for seven days.

505. The menses appear on the seventeenth day.

Brownish blood, instead of the menses (aft. 31 d.).

Before the menses appear, always a dry heat in the whole body, without thirst.

Before the menses, an anxious dream.

Before the menses, heaviness in all the limbs, with disposition to weep, restlessness and anxious solicitude about every trifle.

510. Before the menses set in, stitches in the hepatic region, mostly at night, when lying down, and chiefly when inspiring (aft. 23 d.):

After the appearance of the menses, contractive pain in the hypogastrium, going off in the open air.

Flow from the vagina (2d d.).

Copious leucorrhœa, followed by hoarseness, with cough and expectoration.

Leucorrhœa of white acrid mucus, causing burning. [BAYLIES.]

515. Thickish, milk-colored leucorrhœa, with pains in the abdomen, like labor-pains, contracting from both sides.

Bloody mucus, for ten days, instead of the leucorrhœa.

Leucorrhœa, for ten days after the menses, for several days, with much pain in the abdomen, before the flow.

Leucorrhœa, with weakness and paralytic sensation in the sacrum, before the flow, and consequent lassitude.

Before the passage of the leucorrhœa, pinching in the abdomen.

* * * * * * * *

520. Repeated sneezing, without coryza. [*Lgh.*]

Frequent sneezing.

---

[1] Checked while on, in Andrée's case; in Greding's case, delayed.—*Hughes.*

Frequent discharge of nasal mucus, for several days, as in coryza.

Water alone drips from the nose.

When blowing the nose, he blows out a watery fluid.

525. Violent catarrhal fever, with inflammation of the throat and lack of appetite. [*Gr.*]

Hoarseness.

Dryness of the chest. [STOERK.[1]]

Feeling of fullness in the chest; nothing is detached by coughing, which causes stitches on the sternum.

Rattling on the chest, in the evening, on lying down, and, when sitting up, much cough.

530. In the larynx a little dry spot, where it tingles, irritating to a dry almost constant cough.

Itching in the throat, with excitation to tussiculation.

Scratching and crawling up in the chest, exciting to a dry, almost constant, cough.

Cough, as from a titillation in the middle of the sternum, either with or without expectoration. [*Lgh.*]

Cough, easily excited by sour and salty food (without expectoration.)

535. Cough, almost only when he first lies down, in the day or the evening; he has to sit up to finish coughing, then he can rest.

Cough, increased by lying down, consisting in the beginning of a number of single impulses, almost causing vomiting.

In the evening, before going to bed, a continuous severe cough.

Nocturnal cough. [STOERK.[2]]

Short, shaking cough, caused by taking a deep breath.

540. Violent cough. [LANGE.]

Whooping cough and asthma. [LANGE.]

Nocturnal whooping cough. [LANDEUTTE.]

Whooping-cough, with expectoration of bloody mucus. [LANGE.[3]]

The most violent cough, while he has to keep his bed. [STOERK, *lib. de Stram. Hyosc. et Acon.*[4]]

545. Dry cough, with hoarseness.

Dry tussiculation. [STOERK.[5]]

Loose cough, but she cannot eject anything.

Cough, by which something is detached, which is not, however, ejected, until finally it comes out with a light cough, attended with coryza. [*Rl.*]

Yellowish expectoration, tasting like rotten eggs.

550. Expectoration of pus from the chest. [STOERK, *lib. de Cic.*[6]]

When coughing, something seems to dart into his head. [*Rl.*]

When coughing, lancinating pain in the head.

---

[1] In a case of mammary scirrhus, this and S. 546 coincided with the discharge becoming thin.—*Hughes.*

[2] Not found.—*Hughes.*

[3] Whooping-cough "keuchhusten" ought here to be rendered "urging cough;"—see also note to S. 211.—*Hughes.*

[4] This supervened in a case of tubercular breast, while taking C.—*Hughes.*

[5] See note to S. 527.—*Hughes.*

[6] In a case of mammary scirrhus, when the lungs were found cancerous after death.—*Hughes.*

When coughing, the child complains of pains in the abdomen.

From coughing, pain in both sides of the abdomen.

555. When coughing, shooting pains in the left mamma, for three hours; so that, being awakened by it, she sleeps uneasy.

Respiration, and chiefly inspiration, becomes hard for him, as if his chest could not be properly distended (aft. 4 h.). [*Fr.*]

Difficulty in breathing. [LANDEUTTE.[1]]

Difficult breathing, and violent pains in the chest. [LANGE.]

Difficult, slow inspiration, in the evening in bed. [*Fr.*]

560. Slow breathing.

Short breath, both in rest and in motion (7th d.).

Short, panting breath. [STOERK.[2]]

Asthma. [LANGE, *Med. ob. and Inquir.*[3]]

Frequent asthma. [LANGE.]

565. Frequent oppression in the upper right part of the chest, with a sensation as if it came from accumulated flatus.

Attack of suffocation, as if the throat was clogged with mucus. [*Rl.*]

Attack of suffocation, as if the upper part of the throat was clogged.

Very violent pains in the chest. [LANGE.]

Violent pains in the chest, with severe cough. [LANGE.]

570. Pain in the sternum, as if it was pressed inward.

Tension across the chest, and, in inspiration, pressure there.

Pressive pain on the sternum, the whole day, with a pain, now tearing, now lancinating, about the breasts and the nipples, with frequent tightness and with shortness of breath (4th d.). [*Fr.*]

Pressive pain on the sternum, in the morning, with difficult breathing when standing (3d d.). [*Fr.*]

Pressure at times in the cardiac region, as if it would be crushed, with dyspnœa (3d d.). [*Fr.*]

575. Cutting pressure in both sides of the chest, aggravated by inspiration (aft. 14 h.). [*Wl.*]

Fine, stitching pressure on both sides of the chest, most severe when leaning forward to rest on something. [*Wl.*]

Dull stitches over the heart, on taking a deep breath, and soon afterward on every movement of the body.

Stitches in the chest. (Pleuritic stitches.) [STOERK.[4]]

Severe stitches in the side, like stabs from a knife, causing loud moaning.

580. Fine stitches in the left side of the chest, under the axilla. [*Wl.*]

Stitches in the right side of the chest, as from needles, when taking a walk. [*Lgh.*]

Throbbing, lancinating pain in the upper part of the chest, more toward the middle.

Drawing and tearing through the whole chest, in the evening in bed, when lying on the side, with oppression of breathing, and

[1] Translate "laborious respiration," and see note to S. 211.—*Hughes.*
[2] See note to S. 7.—*Hughes.*
[3] Not found in *Med, Observ. and Inquiries.—Hughes.*
[4] In a case of caries of ribs. *Hughes.*

a hard pressure upon the sternum, which, on inspiring, takes away the breath (3d d.). [*Fr.*]

Tearing in the chest.

585 Cramp-like tearing on the right side of the chest. [*Lgh.*]

Pain, as from bruises, in the anterior part of the chest, and on the back.

Pain, as from bruising (on the inner surface), of the sternum.

Stiffness in the sternum, on moving the body.

Itching in the inside of the chest.

590. Burning in the region of the sternum. [STOERK.[1]]

Severe palpitation of the heart, after drinking.

On rising, palpitation of the heart.

Frequent, visible palpitation of heart. [*Gr.*]

Frequent thrusts against the heart.

595. Over the whole exterior chest, stinging itching, only transiently relieved by scratching (aft. 1 h.). [*Wl.*]

Eruptive pimples on the chest, which pain when touched.

Caries of the sternum. [KALTSCHMIDT.]

The mammæ are painful.

Agreeable, though violent, itching on both the nipples (aft. 4 h.).

600. Itching on both the mammæ; on rubbing, the skin becomes red and scaly, with a burning sensation.

Hardness of the right mamma, with pain when touched, and nocturnal stitches in it.

Inflammation of the scirrhus of the breast. [LANGE.]

Pains in the sacrum.

Pains in the sacrum, when bending backward.

605. Severe pains in the sacrum, after walking a little; then nausea and lassitude.

Stitches in the sacrum, with drawing through the lumbar vertebræ, when standing (aft. 3 h.). [*Fr.*]

Spasm in the back, with severe pressing and drawing.

Tensive pain in the back. [STOERK.[2]]

Painful tension in the muscles under both the scapulæ, when at rest, much aggravated by raising the arms. [*Wl.*]

610. Sharp pressure under the right scapula, at every motion of the arms.

Drawing through the lumbar vertebræ, when standing (aft. 1½ h.). [*Fr.*]

Drawing pain in the right scapula.

Obtuse stitches between the scapulae.

Pain, as from a sprain on the left side of the back (the first day).

615. Formication, as from going to sleep, in the spine.

Sensation of heat down the back, in the morning on awaking.

In the neck, a tensive pain when at rest, with sensation of dryness in the fauces.

Drawing in the neck, when taking a walk (aft. 1 h.). [*Fr.*]

Throbbing drawing in the neck, where it joins the right shoulder (aft. 8 h.) [*Fr.*]

---

[1] After injecting C. into a fistula in the neck.—*Hughes.*

[2] See Note to S. 590.—*Hughes.*

620. Itching shudder, from the nape toward the neck (4th d.).

In the neck, drawing down the right side, to the shoulder-joint, when at rest (3d d.). [*Fr.*]

Seeming thickening of the neck.

Increase of the goitre.

In the arm, drawing pain up and down, chiefly on moving it.

625. In the upper arm, paralytic drawing pain, when at rest (aft. 1½ h.). [*Fr.*]

Tearing through the upper arms, in the evening in bed (1st d.). [*Fr.*]

Tearing, alternating with stitches, in the upper arm, when at rest, only transiently relieved by motion. [*Fr.*]

In the elbow, a tearing pain, on walking in the open air.

Cutting pain in the bend of the left elbow, from within outward, when at rest (aft. 50 h.). [*Wl.*]

630. Heaviness in the joints of the elbow, with fine stitches.

Cracking in the elbow-joint, especially in the evening.

In the muscles of the forearm, cramp-like pain, especially when resting the arms on something (aft. ½ h.). [*Wl.*]

Dull drawing in the forearms, more severe when at rest than in motion (aft. 72 h.). [*Wl.*]

Pain as from a bruise, on the outer side of the left forearm, worse when touched (aft. 62 h.). [*Wl.*]

635. Itching formication in the forearm, only transiently going off by rubbing (aft. 1 h.). [*Wl.*]

In the wrist-joint, paralytic drawing pain, when at rest. [*Fr*].

Fine stitches in the wrist-joints (aft. 10 min.). [*Wl.*]

Shooting pain, as from a sprain, in the joint of the metacarpal bone of the left thumb with the wrist, especially when bending the thumb inward.

Cracking in the wrist-joint, especially in the evening.

640. Dying off[1] of the left hand, especially in the palm.

Sensitiveness of the skin on the back of the hand (the 1st d.).

Perspiring hands.

The fingers, while cutting with the scissors, become spasmodically rigid.

Sharp drawing in one or the other finger.

645. Sharp stitches in the middle joints of the fingers, when at rest (aft. 1½ h). [*Wl.*]

Stitches, as from needles, under the finger-nails (5th d.).

Cutting thrusts, in the lower joint of the thumb (aft. 48 h.). [*Wl.*]

Numbness of the fingers.

Itching on the dorsum of the fingers.

650. Burning pain on the flexing side of the index, and later a hard long-continuing lump there.

Yellow spots on the fingers (aft. 5 d.).

Yellow finger-nails (aft. 6 d.).

Paronychia with inflammation and throbbing, festering, burning pain.

Between the nates in the fold, excessive itching.

[1] Or "numbness."—*Transl.*

655. The ischiatic bones are painful, when rising from a seat, but not when sitting.

Long continued deep stitch, superiorly at the insertion of the gluteus maximus (aft. 3½ h.). [*Fr.*]

The right hip is painful in the evening; when walking, it feels sprained.

Dull stitches in the region of the hip, near the trochanter of the thigh, when sitting; they do not interfere with walking (aft. ¼ h.). [*Wl.*]

In the lower limbs, a humming and tingling.

660. Drawing and tearing in the left limb, with great restlessness, so that she could not keep it still a minute.

The lower limbs go to sleep, when sitting.

Swelling of the thighs. [LANDEUTTE.[1]]

In the right thigh, cramp-pains in the anterior muscles, when walking in the open air (aft. 13 h.). [*Lgh.*]

Sensation of weakness, even to trembling, in the right thigh, when walking.

665. Fine clawing sensation on the posterior side of the thigh. [*Wl.*]

Dull drawing in the right thigh when at rest, relieved by motion (aft. 1½ h.). [*Wl.*]

Dull tearing, anteriorly in both thighs, when walking.

Pricks in the muscles of the left thigh, as from needles, when sitting. [*Lgh.*]

Itching needle-pricks on the posterior side of the thigh, most severe while sitting. [*Wl.*]

670. In the knee, dull pain when treading.

Dull pain in the left knee, when treading. [*Rl.*]

Gouty pain in the knee, the whole day (aft. 15 d.).

Tearing pain around the knee-joint.

Tearing around the patella, when sitting. [*Fr.*]

675. Stitches on the outer tendon of the flexor muscle in the hough, when walking in the open air. [*Fr.*]

Pain as from a bruise, or as if the patella was broken, causing one to cry out; all the left knee thus pains, when walking and standing in the open air, with an anxious heat all over, when making an effort in walking. [*Lgh.*]

Pain as from a sprain, in the right knee.

Paralytic pain in the hough, as in dropsy of the knee-joint.

Pain as from weariness around the knee, for one-half hour.

680. Cracking of the knee (in the patella?) when straightening oneself up.

In the leg, a clucking pressure on the tibia, when stretching the limb, when sitting. [*Fr.*]

Twitching and restlessness in the legs at night, followed every time by a shudder.

Tensive stiff pain in the calves.

Drawing on the inner side of the left calf, and on the dorsum of the right foot. [*Fr.*]

685. Tearing on the tibia, in the evening, in bed (1st d.). [*Fr.*]

[1] See Note to S. 211.—*Hughes.*

Tearing, extending up the leg from the inner side of the foot, in the open air.

Dull tearing, extending up the leg from the external ankle, in the open air.

Cramplike tearing on the tibia, when taking a walk. [*Lgh.*]

Pain in the tibia, as if bruised. [*Fr.*]

690. A spot on the leg that had been injured (twelve days before by a blow) and was painful all the way down, becomes blue and spotted, and pains at the least motion, like thrusts from a knife, but when walking and when touched, it pains as if bruised.

In the ankle-joint, a dull pain. [*Rl.*]

Tearing in the ankle-joint, from noon till evening, worse when sitting than when walking.

Burning and throbbing stitches in the bend of the foot.

Tearing in the dorsum of the foot, in the evening in bed (1st d.). [*Fr.*]

695. Tearing in the soles of the feet, when walking.

Sharp drawing under the heel.

Shooting on both ankles of the right foot, first fine, then sharp, for two days; they wake him from sleep at night, extending at last into the calf; when sitting the stitches were slower, when walking, more frequent and severe.

Formicating pain in the soles of the feet, when treading; but when walking, there are stitches in them.

Numbness and insensibility of the feet.

700. Trembling of the feet, in the morning, on rising.

Acute burning pain under the heel, when treading, with redness and swelling of the spot.

Swelling of the whole foot, with burning pain.

The swelling of the feet is painful, and does not go off even in sleep.

Severe itching and a little itching pimple on the soles of the feet.

705. Little pustules on the feet.

The tips of the toes pain, as if festering underneath.

Throbbing stitches in the little toe, which also pains when walking.

Tearing in the ball of the big toe, in the morning, when standing and sitting. [*Fr.*]

Burning tearing on the posterior joint of the big toe, when waking up from sleep, while lying down.

710. Burning pain under the toes, when sitting.

It excites the podagra [CLARK in *Essays and obs. phys. and liter.* III, *Edinb.*, 1771.[1]]

Sensation as if the bones of the legs and arms were firmly clasped, causing weariness.

Spasmodic, cramp-like pains in various parts, as in the chest, the jaws, etc.

Throbbing twitches in the abdomen and in the sacrum.

715. A sort of stiffness of the body; the movement of the limbs, the neck, etc., excites a disagreeable sensation.

---

[1] Add "p. 434."—Observation in gouty subjects.—*Hughes.*

Tearing through various parts of the body (4th d.). [*Fr.*]

Tearing in all the limbs, almost as if from a sprain.

Erratic tearing in the arms and legs, as also in the teeth (the first days).

Tearing stitches, now here, now there, very penetrating as if they reached the bones.

720. Burning on the tongue and in the hands.

Sensation as of bruising in all the joints, when at rest; little or not at all, in motion.

Severe pain as from bruises, in all the limbs.

Pain, as if from fatigue, in all the joints.

Tendency to strains.

725. The limbs go to sleep.

Numbness and coldness of the fingers and toes.

The pains mostly begin when at rest; only in rare alternative action, while moving, [*Fr.*]

The ailments come most severely at night, waking from sleep.

• Walking in the open air fatigues her, and the air fatigues her.

730. On returning from walking in the open air, headache with pressure on the right eye.

When walking, itching on the scrobiculus cordis.

Constant lack of vital warmth, and continual chilliness.

Little vital warmth, after the noon-siesta, and chilliness.

Sensation of lack of vital warmth, with sadness.

735. **Great tendency to catch cold,** even in the room, after a walk, in which he perspired, while sitting down.

Excessively heightened susceptibility to colds.

From taking a cold, he wakes up at 4 A. M. with pain in the head and the scapula; when turning the body, it feels bruised, with pain of the abdominal muscles in the region of the stomach, when taking a deep breath, thus arresting the breathing.

The skin of the body seems to him hotter than it really is.

Itching of the limbs. [STOERK.]

740. Itching of the thighs and arms.

Transient itching, now here, now there, in all parts of the body.

Eroding itching, always commencing with a stitch, in the evening in bed, confined to the right half of the body, chiefly when he lies on it, with restlessness in all the limbs, easily assuaged by scratching, but always reappearing in another spot.

Stinging sensation all over the body.

Itching stitches as from fleas, in close succession, here and there all over the body, but singly, never two at a time.

745. Slow, itching, smarting, burning stitches, here and there over the body.

Inflammation of the skin of the whole body, with burning pain. [BAYLIES.]

Fine, scarcely visible eruption in the face, on the back and the rest of the body, itching, like a thrill running under the skin.

Eruption of white, transparent pimples, which, filled with an acrid humor, turn into scurf, like that formed by itch; with this there is a local, fetid, smarting sweat. [STOERK.[1]]

A spot, which had a lesion many years before, begins to pain frequently.

750. Increased, intolerable pains in the affected parts. [LANGE.]

Formication in the affected part. [COLLIN, *Annot. med.* III. 104.[2]]

Pain from coughing darts into the ulcers. [STOERK.]

Increased pain in the ulcer. [STOERK.[3]]

Tensive pain in the ulcer. [STOERK.[3]]

755. Bleeding of the ulcers. [GREDING.[4]]

The edges of the ulcer turn black discharging a fetid ichor. [STOERK.[3]]

Fetid ichor from an ulcer. [STOERK.[3]]

Gangrene of a part of an ulcer. [GREDING.[5]]

Petechiæ. [SIM. PAULLI.]

760. Blueness of the whole body. [EHRHARDT.]

In an old wart on the upper lip, a drawing pain.

In the bones, especially in the middle of the shafts, concealed caries, with a burning, gnawing pain. [STOERK.[6]]

The glands become painful in the evening. [STOERK.[7]]

Formication and agreeable itching in the glands. [STOERK.[8]]

765. Lancinating pains in the swelling of the glands.

Stinging pain around the grandular swelling, as if excoriated.

Free cutting around the glands.

Orgasm in the body (at once).

Severe, continued ebullition of blood, mixed with twitches around the heart.

770. He feels his blood all through the body to be in an excited state.

Quivering sensation and trembling of the body, especially severe in the arms (5th d.).

Trembling. [BAYLIES, CULLEN, EHRHARDT.]

Trembling of all the limbs. [FOTHERGILL, SCHMUCKER.[9]]

Continual trembling. [ANDRY.]

775. Subsultus of the tendons. [EHRHARDT.]

Convulsions. [ANDRY, WATSON, CULLEN.[10]]

Convulsions of the affected part and of the whole body, with danger of suffocating. [LANGES.]

Ill and fatigued, in the morning in bed, with ill-humor, drowsiness, and pains in the stomach (2d d.).

Chaotic sensation in the whole body, in the morning, fasting, as after a severe illness, with lack of appetite, as if one had eaten too much, and loathing for food.

---

1 Critical, with S. 906 in a gouty patient.—*Hughes.*

2 Symptoms observed on patients taking C.—*Hughes.*

3 Symptoms 753, 754, 756 and 757 occurred in an open cancer, while patient was taking C. —*Hughes.*

4 In mammary cancer.—*Hughes.*

5 Not found.—*Hughes.*

6 Not found.—*Hughes.*

7 In a case of mammary scirrhus.—*Hughes.*

8 Not found.—*Hughes.*

9 Not found in Schmucker.—*Hughes.*

10 To WATSON add "Phil. Trans." No. 473, 1744. Note, "As a consequence of poisoning." To CULLEN add "Mat. Med." and note "From thirty grains of powdered leaves in an adult." —*Hughes.*

780. Everything feels squeezed full, the chest, the head and the hypochondria, for ten minutes, on several mornings, on awaking.

Heaviness and qualmishness in the whole body, in the afternoon.

Contractive sensation in the interior of the body, while saliva collects in her mouth.

Illusion of sensation; when walking, he feels as if something checked his steps, and yet he walked very fast. [*Fr.*]

Attack: Being alone at home, she felt an inclination to weep, which, when she gave way to it, degenerated into loud sobbing, then flickering before the eyes and indistinct vision, so that in walking she has to hold on to something; then lack of tone in all the limbs and dull headache.

785. Attacks, usually after a meal, beginning with yawning, shooting pains in the sternum and pressure in the scrobiculus cordis, even when touched, when it passes into the back, where there are lancinations in the renal region.

Attacks of weariness and chilliness, so that he has to lie down, then next day, headache and palpitation of the heart in the highest degree; with every pulsation, it seemed to him as if the occiput was pierced with a knife, and the heart now seemed to throb strongly, at the same time in a hurrying, then in a rocking manner.

Great lassitude.

Startling lassitude in the whole body, in the evening and morning.

Lassitude in the morning, after awaking, as after a fever.

790. Lassitude in the morning on awaking; it goes off after rising.

Lack of tone in mind and body (4th d.).

General feeling of being worn out.

The clothes lie on the chest and shoulders like a load.

Weakness of the whole body. [WHYTT, *On Nervous Disorders.*[1]]

795. Sinking of all the strength. [STOERK.[2]]

Nervous asthma. [SCHMUCKER.[3]]

Lack of strength, and heaviness in the lower limbs, especially in the knees, as if they would give way; they tremble.

Lack of strength on awaking from the noon-siesta, the arms and legs feel bruised all over.

Very much exhausted, languid, and as it were paralyzed, after a short walk; mood, peevish and hypochondriac. [*Fr.*]

800. On returning from his walk, every step he makes is fatiguing, and he can hardly wait in his ill-humor and impatience, until he may rest in solitude.

Standing is a great exertion for him.

So weak that she has to lie down.

He has to keep his bed from lassitude and chilliness, accompanied by headache and palpitation.

The strongest and most active persons lost all their strength, and had to keep their bed. [LANGE, l. c.]

---

[1] Oserved on self; with dazzling of sight and giddiness.—*Hughes.*

[2] In case of S. 527. This and S. 874 supervened until a purulent discharge set in, and they were removed by bark.—*Hughes.*

[3] After taking C. for seven months.—*Hughes.*

805. He cannot recruit himself in any position.
Loss of all strength, even to death. [LANGE.]
With all his lack of vital force, there is inclination to laugh.
During his lack of tone, there is excitation to laughter as if starting from the right hypochondrium and stomach.
Fainting fits. [LANGE, *Pharm. helv.*]
810. **Consumption.** [REISMANN, COLLIN.[1]]
Dropsy. [TARTREUX, *Epist. apol.*, p. 51.[2]]
Apoplexy. [LANGE.]
Dropsical apoplexy. [COLLIN.[3]]
Paralyses. [ANDRY, ANDRÉE.]
815. Putrid disintegration of the humors. [REISMANN.]
Repeated yawning, as if from not having slept enough. [*Lgh.*]
Very sleepy and tired in the morning, for the first two hours on awaking.
Sleepy in the morning, on rising.
Feels as if he had not slept enough, in the morning.
820. He cannot shake himself free from sleep at his usual hour of rising, and continues half asleep for some time.
In the morning, a pressive pain in the humerus and the femur compels him to sleep.
Drowsy during the day, without being able to sleep.
Drowsiness by day, he cannot keep awake while reading (aft. 3 to 8 h.). [*Col.*]
Somnolence. [WATSON, *Sim. Paulli.*[4]]
825. Somnolence, even while taking a walk.[4]
Slumbering all day, with great decrepitude.
Somnolence in the afternoon; despite of all his efforts, he had to lie down and sleep. [*Lgh.*]
In the evening, great drowsiness and indisposition to anything. [*Fr.*]
Late in falling asleep, not till after midnight.
830. **Insomnia.** [REIMANN, LANGE.[5]]
Sleeplessness, from restlessness and heat; he tosses about in his bed.
Stupid sleep, all too deep, after which the headache, hardly perceptible before, becomes ever stronger.
Quiet sleep, especially very sound and longer in the morning (partially curative effect.). [*Fr.*]
From a sound sleep, an anxious half-awaking.
835. Interrupted sleep.
Earlier awaking, in the morning.
In the evening in bed, throbbing in the right side of the head.
At night in bed, headache with nausea
At night, boring pain in the tongue (2d n.).

---

[1] In Collin's case this was the end of Mesenteric disease, for which C. had been taken There being no reference in the case of Reismann, his observation cannot be traced.—*Hughes.*

[2] Observations on patients. This was the end of a case of mammary cancer.—*Hughes.*

[3] In an old woman of 80, ten days after leaving off C.—*Hughes.*

[4] "Coma" is Watson's word, and "Schlummersucht" somnolence, might be so rendered here, and "sopor" in the next symptom.—*Hughes.*

[5] See note to S. 7.—*Hughes.*

840. At night, between 1 and 2 o'clock, cramp in the stomach. like griping and contraction.

At night, scraping in the throat, with coughing.

At night, epistaxis and then in the morning on rising, vertigo.

At night, when going to sleep from vexation, twitches in the arms and hands during sleep, the eyes open staringly, and roll to and fro.

He uncovers his arms, when sleeping.

845. At night in bed, he feels too warm; he has to rise and spend the night on the sofa.

At midnight, he wakes up in a sweat.

At night, severe itching on the anus, the nates, the perinæum and beside the scrotum, so that he had to rise repeatedly.

In the evening in bed, tearing, now in this limb, then in the other. [*Fr.*]

At night, during sleep, violent weeping with a flow of tears.

850. At night, he growls in his sleep.

At night, she is awakened by anxiety, which long kept her from sleeping.

At night, nightmare.

After midnight, seemingly only half awake, very anxious thoughts, almost rising to a deadly anguish.

Bad dreams frequently interrupt the sleep (the first days).

855. Anxious, frightful, well-remembered dreams.

Anxious, hostile dreams.

Anxious, vivid dreams. [*Lgh.*]

Anxious dreams, full of threatening danger.

Many frightful dreams, at night and toward morning. [*Fr.*]

860. On awaking, at night, fearful thoughts.

Frightening dreams.

Dreams of lamentable diseases.

Dreams of bodily mutilation.

Many dreams of the dead, and of living persons who seem to have died.

865. Dreams, full of shame.

Dreams, full of vexation and scuffling.

Vivid, voluptuous dreams. [*Lgh.*]

Confused dreams, in an uneasy sleep.

Shudder (at once).

870. Shudder. [STOERK.]

Shudder on moving.

Shudder all over the body. [*Lgh.*]

Shuddering for one and a half hours, for several mornings in succession, at 8 o'clock.

Shudder over the whole body, from time to time, and then quick pulse, with heat and thirst. [STOERK.[1]]

875. Shuddering and coldness in the afternoon; then, after five to six hours, a flush of glowing heat over all the limbs, whereupon the numbness in the head and the indifferent sadness vanish and the liveliest interest in everything takes its place (aft. 7, 8 h.). [*Fr.*]

---

[1] See note to S. 795.

Coldness and chilliness, in the morning, with giddy constriction of the brain, and an indifferent dejection. [*Fr.*]

Chill in the morning for two hours, with headache and nausea (3d d.).

Rigor, with trembling in all the limbs, so that he has always to be in the sun.

Rigor, with cold hands and hot face, with nausea.

880. Chilliness in the afternoon, from 3 to 5 o'clock.

He awakes with internal chilliness at 5 A. M. (almost without thirst), the hands and the soles of the feet are cold, and the face hot for eight hours; then more severe heat in the face and lassitude (aft. 24 h.).

Sensation of heat in the whole body, greater heat of the skin, also observable externally, with dry, sticky lips, without thirst, and even with aversion to any beverage, and insipid saliva in the mouth; noise and bright looking objects tire him, as well as every movement; he wishes to sit by himself with closed eyes.

Flushes of heat, in the afternoon, without thirst. [*Fr.*]

Heat. [BAYLIES; FOTHERGILL.]

885. Internal heat, especially in the face, with redness of the same, without thirst. [*Wl.*]

Sensation of internal and external heat, after sleep.

Constant heat.

Excessive heat. [BAYLIES.]

Hot (deadly) fever. [LANGE.]

890. Severe febrile heat, with great sweat and thirst, with lack of appetite, diarrhœa and vomiting. [GREDING.]

Fever. [ANDRÉE; COLLIN.]

Quotidian fever. [LANDEUTTE, l. c.]

Various attacks of fever. [TARTREUX.[1]]

Slow fever, with complete loss of appetite. [LANGE.]

895. Perspiration. [GATAKER.[2]]

Sweat all over, especially on the forehead, with redness of the face and the whole body, without any particular heat.

In the evening, profuse sweat, when sitting, with heat in the face.

Only while going to sleep, as soon as she shuts her eyes, some perspiration; even by day, while slumbering, sitting in a chair.

The child demanded to go to bed early in the evening, is then very hot and perspires all over, with uneasy sleep, strong trembling and short, rattling moaning respiration. [*Gr.*]

900. At night, slight perspiration only on the lower limbs.

Night-sweat.

Sweat about midnight.

After midnight, profuse sweat.

In the morning, on awaking from sleep, slight perspiration all over the body. [*Lgh.*]

905. In the morning, on awaking and afterward, tendency to perspire, even on the cold lower limbs.

---

[1] See note to S. 811. After these, patient died dropsical.—*Hughes.*

[2] Note "slight" perspiration.—*Hughes.*

Local, fetid, smarting sweat. [STOERK.[1]]

He feels the pulsations all over the body.

Quick pulse. [EHRHARDT.]

Pulse unequal as to strength and rapidity. [STOERK.[2]]

910. Large, slow pulse; between these pulsations there are several small, quick pulsations without regularity.

Slow, weak pulse. [SIM. PAULLI.]

Collapse of pulse. [SIM. PAULLI.]

CUPRUM. COPPER.

A piece of pure metallic copper is rubbed upon a hard, fine whetstone under distilled water in a porcelain bowl. The fine powder that sinks to the bottom is dried, and then like other metallic powders, it is raised by three hours' trituration with sugar of milk to the millionth potency, then by the attenuation and potentizing succession of the solution of one grain of this powder, it is brought to the decillionth dynamical development. One or two fine pellets, moistened with the medicinal fluid of one of these degrees of potency, according to the circumstances of the invalid, are used as a dose.

Physicians have always been deterred from the internal use of this medicine in diseases, owing to the not infrequent accidental cases of poisoning by means of this metal and its solutions, and the consequences, fearful, if not fatal, arising from its use.

F. G. VOIGTEL in his Materia Medica adduces the following effects of copper: "Loathing, nausea, anxieties and vomiting, even after a few minutes, disagreeable burning in the mouth, ineffectual retching, violent pains in the stomach after several hours, obstruction to the intestinal evacuations, or excessively violent discharges, then also bloody diarrhœa, constant restlessness, insomnia, exhaustion, weak and small pulse, cold sweat, paleness of the face, pains in the whole body or in particular parts, pain in the thyroid cartilage, pain in the hypochondria, formicating sensation in the vertex, palpitation of the heart, vertigo, painful constriction of the chest, cough with interrupted, almost suppressed respiration, excessively hurried breathing, spitting of blood, hiccup, unconsciousness, eyes with a wandering look—also at times convulsions, ravings, apoplexy, paralysis and death."

Only Homœopathy, owing to her peculiar method of preparing medicines, and the greatly diminished size of her doses, is able to

[1] See note to S. 748.—*Hughes.*
[2] See note to S. 7.—*Hughes.*

use in healing even those natural substances which have shown themselves as invincibly harmful, even in small quantities.

Most of the violent symptoms with those poisoned with copper, are wont to appear in groups, lasting for a half or a whole hour, and they are apt to recur from time to time in renewed attacks with an almost identical composition of the symptoms, *e.g.*: Palpitation, vertigo, coughing, hemoptysis, painful constriction of the chest, suppressed respiration—or again: pressive pain on the chest, weariness, vacillation of sight, closing of the eyes, unconsciousness, rapid, moaning respiration, tossing about, cold feet, hiccough, tussiculation, checking the respiration, etc. Copper is, therefore, all the more homœopathically indicated in diseases that show themselves in such irregular attacks of similar groups of symptoms, as is the case with copper.

The chief sphere of the appropriate application of copper seems, therefore, to lie in various kinds of partial or general clonic spasms, some kinds of St. Vitus' dance (*Niemann*), epilepsis, (*Aretæus, Duncan, Kœchlin*), whooping-cough, cutaneous eruptions, old ulcers, and especially also spasmodic affections, accompanied with too sensitive and acute senses; it has also proved itself indispensable for the prevention of the murderous cholera, or for its cure where it had been already developed.

The antidotes, where copper articles have been swallowed, are solutions of (potash-soaps and) hepar sulphuris calcareum, as well as the white of eggs, highly praised from his own experience by *Orfila*. Dynamic ailments, resulting from the excessive effects of copper-medicine, may be mostly removed by repeated smelling of camphor dissolved in alcohol; but we also count among its antidotes, Bell., Chin., Cocc., Dulc., Hep. sulph., Ip., Merc., and Nux vomica.

The action of the copper-medicine seems to extend over only a few days.

As an antipsoric remedy, copper has among others removed also the following symptoms:

Discouragement; headache after epileptic attacks; pains in the head, as if it were hollow; pressive pain in the eyes; tearing, extending from the teeth into the temples; water-brash, after drinking milk; nocturnal micturition; stoppage of the nose; some kinds of whooping-cough; burning in the soles of the feet; sweating of the feet; suppressed sweat of the feet; old ulcers; long continued lassitude; nervous disorders with too great subtlety and acuteness of the senses; some kinds of epilepsy; jerking in sleep; chills after epileptic attacks.

The abbreviations of the names of my fellow-provers are as follows: *Fr.*, *Franz*, *Fr. H.*, *Frederick Hahnemann; Hrm.*, *Herrmann; Rkt.*, *Ruckert.*

CUPRUM.

Melancholy; she shuns the sight of men, seeks and loves solitude, and troubles herself about her imminent death, which she supposes to be unavoidable.

Anxiety of heart. [WILLICH, in *Pyl's Magaz.* I., *St.* 4, p. 667.[1]]

Anguish.

Short attacks of deadly anguish, without heat.

5. A kind of timidity; he felt as if he had to step softly, in order not to hurt himself, nor to disturb his room-mates.

Restless tossing, and constant uneasiness.

Irresolute and dissatisfied with everything, but only so long as he is peevish. [*Hrm.*]

Peevishness, he himself does not know what he wants, he wishes to be alone; after a time, indeed, this is changed to cheerfulness, but it soon returns. [*Hrm.*]

Indisposed for everything. [*Fr. H.*]

10. Indisposition to work, and yet idleness is a burden to him. [*Hrm.*]

Thoughtlessness, weakness of memory (aft. 2 h.). [*Hrm.*]

Stupidity and headache. [RAMSEY, in *Med. Obs. and Inq.*[2]]

He becomes unconscious.

Inability to recollect, as if he were half dreaming. [*Rkt.*]

15. She at once lost her senses and thoughts, for a short time. [GREDING, in *Advers. med. pr.;* LUDVIG I., p. 635.[3]]

Insensible and stupid, he mopes in a corner. [RAMSAY.]

Exaltation, ecstasy. [PFUENDEL, in *Hufel. Jour.* II., p. 274.[4]]

Startling laughter in the evening.

Convulsive laughter.

20. **Delirium.** [RAMSAY.]

Incoherent, delirious talk. [RAMSAY.]

Frightened confusion of mind, he seeks to escape. [COSMIER, *Recueil period d'observation*, 1775, Vol. III., p. 202.[5]]

Fits of Insanity, imagining he is a military commander. [RAMSAY.]

Fits of insanity, he imagines he has green herbs for sale. [RAMSAY.]

The four names given here are of disciples who co-operated with Hahnemann in proving the acetate—doubtless in his earlier manner, as the results were published in Vol. III of the *Archiv* (1824). The present pathogenesis includes, besides the symptoms there given, and 154 from others, those contained in the *Fragmenta de Viribus* as effects of the sulphate.—*Hughes.*

1 Not accessible.—*Hughes.*

2 From verdigris in food.—*Hughes.*

3 Effect of grain doses of the sulphate in epileptics.—*Hughes.*

4 From Cuprum ammoniatum given to epileptics.—*Hughes.*

5 Not to be found here or traced elsewhere.—*Hughes.*

25. Fits of insanity, he imagines he is repairing old chairs. [RAMSAY.]

Fits of insanity, with merry singing. [RAMSAY.]

Fits of insanity, he spits into people's faces, and laughs heartily over it. [RAMSAY.]

Fits of morose, malignant insanity. [RAMSAY.[1]]

Those attacked by insanity had a full, quick, strong pulse, accompanied with red, inflamed eyes and wild looks, talking without coherence, all ending in a sweat [RAMSAY.]

30. Attacks of fury, oft-recurring; they snapped at the bystanders. [RAMSAY.]

Attacks of vertigo.

Vertigo. [HEYSHAM, in *Edinb. Med. Comment.* 7; F. HORSTIUS, in *Schenck*, *lib.* VII., *obs.* 223; PILARGUS, *obs. T.* II., p. 381; WILLICH.[2]]

Vertigo on looking upward, with loss of sight, as if from a gauze over the eyes.

Vertigo when reading, he had to turn his eyes from the book for awhile. [*Fr. H.*]

35. Vertigo, with lassitude, his head will bend forward; worse when moving, diminished by lying down. [*Hrm.*]

Vertigo, at once, and continuing during all the ailments, as if things whirled about in his head, and as if his head would sink down. [*Hrm.*]

Pains in the head, of the most violent kind. [HORST.]

Headache in the parietal bone (especially on grasping it) causing him to cry out. [*Fr. H.*]

Tingling sensation in the crown. [VOIGTEL, *Arzneimittellehre.*[3]]

40. Formicating, dull sensation in the vertex of the head, as from its going to sleep, with a pressing-down feeling and some stupefaction (aft. 1 h.).

Pain, as from bruising, in the brain, as well as in the orbits, when turning the eyes.

Feeling of heaviness in the head. [WILLICH.]

Feeling of heaviness in the head, with a fine stitch in the left shoulder, when he moves the head from one side to the other. [*Rkt.*]

Pressing down sensation in the vertex of the head.

45. Pressive pain, first on the right, then on the left side of the head.

Hard pressure on the right temple, more violent on motion. [*Hrm.*]

Hard pressure on the temples, the eminences of the forehead, the occiput, and at the same time internally in the brain, with vertigo; increased by motion and by touching. [*Hrm.*]

Tearing pressure in both temples, more violent on touching them. [*Hrm.*]

---

[1] More literally "surly and ill-natured."—*Hughes.*

[2] (To HEYSHAM) From C. ammoniatum. (To HORSTIUS) Not found. (To PELARGUS) from inhaling vapor.—*Hughes.*

[3] General statement from authors.—*Hughes.*

Pain, like pressure of the brain outward, in the sinciput, especially on stooping forward, with obtuseness of the head, like stupidity. [*Rkt.*]

50. Drawing pain in several places of the head, with whirling vertigo, only diminished by lying down; with it all, qualmishness; he does not know himself, how he feels. [*Hrm.*]

Pressive drawing pain in the left temple, more violent on touching it. [*Hrm.*]

Cutting jerk in the left side of the head (2d d.).

Inflammation of the brain (Phrenitis). [*Horst.*]

On the left side of the forehead, sharp, burning stitches (aft. 60 h.). [*Fr. H.*]

55. Sharp, burning stitches on the left temple and on the vertex (aft. 54 h.). [*Hrm.*]

Burning tearing on the occiput, at the insertion of the muscles of the nape of the neck, when he moves the head forward. [*Rkt.*]

If he moves the head backward, there is felt an opposing straining pain in the muscles, where the neck and back are united. [*Rkt.*]

The head is drawn backward. [ORFILA, *Toxicologie, sub voce,* 427.[1]]

The head is twisted crooked. [RAMSAY.]

60 Swelling of the head, with very red face. [PFUENDEL.]

The orbits are painful, as if bruised, on turning the eyes.

Pressive pain in both eyes, as if there had been no rest at night. [*Rkt.*]

Pressure in the eyelids, as well with open as with closed eyes, worse when touched. [*Hrm.*]

Itching in the eyeballs.

65. **Severe itching in the eyes,** toward evening.

Burning, pressive pain in the eyes.

Burning pain as from a sore, now in the one eye, then in the other.

Red, inflamed eyes, with a wild look (in the fits of insanity). [RAMSAY.]

Dim eyes, they tend to close from lassitude. [*Hrm.*]

70. Quivering, closed eyelids (at once).

The power of opening returned more slowly than consciousness (patients lie there conscious, but unable to open the eyes).

Eyes wavering, moving to and fro.

Eyes wandering. [VOIGTEL.]

Fixed eyes. [RAMSAY.]

75. Staring, sunken eyes.

Protruding, glistening eyes. [COSMIER l. c.]

The pupils are less movable, contract but little in the light, and dilate but little in the dark. [*Rkt.*]

Dilated pupils.

Obscuration of the sight. [PFUENDEL.]

80. Otalgia, pressive tearing in the interior of the right ear (aft. 7 h.). [*Hrm.*]

[1] Cases of poisoning by verdigris.—*Hughes.*

Pressure in the right concha, as from something hard. [*Hrm.*]

Fine tearing in the cartilage of the left ear (aft. 2 h.). [*Hrm.*]

Stinging pain in the right ear.

Boring pain in and behind the ear.

85. Frequent itching in the ear.

Fluttering in the left ear (aft. ¼ h.). [*Hrm.*]

Sense of distant drumming in the ear, on which he is lying, in the morning, in bed, going off every time on raising up.

Deafness. [ORFILA.[1]]

The nose itches internally.

90. **Sensation of violent rush of blood to the nose.**

The complexion becomes pale.

Paleness of the face. [PELARGUS; VOIGTEL.]

Pale, cachectic complexion. [VOIGTEL.[2]]

Bluish face, with bluish eyes.

95. Sunken, deep-set eyes, with blue borders. [ORFILA.]

Features changed, full of anguish. [ORFILA.]

Sad, dejected features. [ORFILA.]

Spasmodic contortion of the features. [RAMSAY.]

Pain as from a thrust, in the left side of the face.

100. Pressive pain in the face, before the ear.

Stitches in the right side of the face.

Hot face, without sensation of heat (aft. 2 h.). [*Hrm.*]

Soreness on the inner side of the upper lip.

On the lower jaw, on the right side, drawing pressure, becoming more violent when touched. [*Hrm.*]

105. Hard pressure in the left ramus of the lower jaw, more violent when touched. [*Hrm.*]

Drawing under the chin, inward, more violent when touched. [*Hrm.*]

Obtuse shooting pain on the left side of the lower jaw, inward, and at the same time in the left tonsil, both during deglutition and at other times more violent on being touched from without. [*Hrm.*]

Spasmodic contraction of the jaws. [ORFILA.]

He lost his speech.

110. The ability to talk returns later than consciousness; patients lie there conscious, but without being able to speak.

Inability to speak, owing to spasm in the throat. [ORFILA.]

Screaming, like a child. [RAMSAY.]

Crying, like the croaking of frogs. [COSMIER.]

The water collects in his mouth (at once). [*Rkt.*]

115. Foam at the mouth.

Accumulation of mucus in the mouth, in the morning.

White furred tongue. [PERCIVAL in *Med. transact. of Coll. of Phys.*, Vol. III., p. 8.[3]]

In the throat, fine stinging pain (aft. 22 h.).

---

[1] Slight.—*Hughes.*

[2] Effect of continued small doses.—*Hughes.*

[3] From eating coppery pickles.—*Hughes.*

Inflammation of the fauces, with obstructed deglutition. [ORFILA.]

120. When drinking, the liquid audibly gurgles down the gullet.

Dryness in the throat, with thirst. [DR. LANZONUS, *Misc. Nat. Cur. Dec.* III, *ann.* 7-8.[1]]

Extremely violent thirst. [ORFILA.]

Bitterness in the mouth. [GREDING.]

Sweet taste in the mouth (aft. 6 h.).

125. Sourish taste in the mouth all the afternoon, as if the tongue was held against iron.

Salty-sour taste in the mouth, in the morning.

Coppery taste, and troublesome burning in the mouth. [VOIGTEL.]

The food tastes like nothing but water. [*Fr. H.*]

Lack of appetite, for two days. [GREDING.]

130. No appetite in the evening, eight hours after dinner.

More appetite for cold food than for warm. [*Hrm.*]

He eats very hurridly.

Continual eructation. [PERCIVAL; VOIGTEL.[2]]

Eructations all the afternoon and evening.

135. Usually in the afternoon, heartburn, and then bitter mucus in the throat.

Hiccup. [VOIGTEL.]

Frequent hiccup.

Nausea. [HAYSHAM.]

Nausea (at once). [*Fr. H.*]

140. Nausea, repeatedly. [KLINGLAKE in *London Med. and Phys. Journ.* V, 438.[3]]

Violent Nausea. [GREDING; VOIGTEL.]

Nausea and loathing, for one-quarter hour (at once).

Nausea in almost the whole of the hypogastrium, drawing up into the throat and most violent in the scrobiculus cordis: attended with putrid taste in the mouth, and a sensation as if he should vomit at once. [*Hrm.*]

Nausea, with inclination to vomit.

145. Inclination to vomit, as if connected with intoxication.

Tendency, in the abdomen toward water-brash.

Inclination to vomit, with spasmodic pain in the abdomen. [PFUENDEL.]

Vomiting. [LANZONUS; GREDING; VOIGTEL.]

Constant vomiting. [FABAS in *Jour. d. méd. et d. chir.* 1782, *Tom.* XVI, p. 228.[4]]

150. **Violent** vomiting. [HORST.; LANZONUS.]

Violent vomiting, recurring from time to time.

Violent vomiting, with nausea and diarrhæa. [WILLICK.]

Continual vomiting, with the most terrible colic. [PYL. *Samml.* VIII., p. 90.[5]]

---

1 Poisoning with verdigris.—*Hughes.*

2 In Percival's case, these were rather hiccups.—*Hughes.*

3 Note from *C. sulph.* given for epilepsy. He says "Occasional" rather than "frequent." —*Hughes.*

4 Poisoning by verdigris.—*Hughes.*

5 Poisoning by verdigris.—*Hughes.*

Excessive vomiting, with continual stomachache and tenesmus. [ORFILA.]

155. Excessive vomiting, with colic and diarrhœa. [WEIGEL in *Pyl's Magaz. Tom.* I., St. I.[1]]

Frequent vomiting, with colic and diarrhœa; like cholera. SICELIUS, *Dec. obs.* IV., cas. 8.[2]]

Ill-smelling vomiting, tasting of copper, always preceded by hiccups. [PERCIVAL.]

Vomiting of water, after slight nausea, while much water flows from the eyes. [*Rkt.*]

Mucous vomiting. [GREDING.]

160. Vomiting of greenish, bitter mucus, after nausea in the upper part of the throat, with pressive stomachache (aft. sev. h.). [*Hrm.*]

Frequent vomiting of mere bile (aft. 1/4 h.). [PFUENDEL.]

Hematemesis without cough, with deep stitches in the left side of the chest (aft. 3 d.)

The vomiting was suppressed by drinking cold water.

Weakness of the stomach. [COSMIER.]

165. **Stomachache.** [HEYSHAM; PERCIVAL; VOIGTEL.]

Excessive, fierce pains in the stomach and in the gastric region. [COSMIER; HORST.]

Cramps in the stomach. [LANZONUS.[3]]

Cramps in the stomach and colic, without stool. [SICELIUS.]

Pressure in the scrobiculus cordis.

170. Pressure in the scrobiculus cordis, as from something hard, *per se*, but more violent when touched. [*Hrm.*]

Sensation in the stomach, as of something bitter in it.

Eroding, finely stinging pain in the stomach, as if pricked with needles (when consciousness returned). [HORST.]

Dull stitches on the left side, beside the scrobiculus cordis, without respect to respiration. [*Hrm.*]

Peculiar, anxious oppression in the scrobiculus cordis. [ORFILA.[4]]

175. The hypochondria are painful. [VOIGTEL.]

Bellyache. [LANZONUS; COSMIER; RAMSAY; FABAS.]

Anxious pains in the abdomen. [WILLICH.]

Bearing down in the hypogastrium, as from a stone. [*Rkt.*]

Pressive pain in the stomach, as from something hard; more violent on touching it. [*Hrm.*]

180. A drawing pressure in the hypogastrium, as from something hard; aggravated by touching. [*Hrm.*]

Pressive pain on the left side, near the navel.

Inflated abdomen. [SICELIUS.]

Distension of the abdomen. [ORFILA.[5]]

185. The abdomen is drawn in. [ORFILA.]

Hardness of the abdomen, with great painfulness when touched. [ORFILA.]

---

[1] Not accessible.—*Hughes.*
[2] Not accessible.—*Hughes.*
[3] Should be "cardialgia."—*Hughes.*
[4] In the original, "That *anxietas* which is peculiar to pain in the stomach."—*Hughes.*
[5] Coming on rapidly.—*Hughes.*

Squeezing together of the intestines, and sensation of a heavy pressure from behind and above to the left and downwards; aggravated by walking and by external pressure; pain not relieved by stool and recurring every forenoon. [*Rkt.*]

Spasmodic motion of the abdominal muscles.

Violent, spasmodic movements in the intestines and in the stomach. [LANZONUS.]

Violent cramps in the abdomen, and in the upper and lower limbs, with piercing, torturing screams. [COSMIER.]

190. Pinching, like colic, in the abdomen, as soon as he walks about after eating (a green vegetable), it goes off by lying down and resting, but leaves a great weakness behind.

Pinching in the abdomen, after drinking the warm milk in the morning.

Pinching in the left side of the abdomen.

Pinching pain, extending from the left hypochondrium to the hip.

Cutting and tearing in the intestines. [ORFILA.]

195. **Drawing pain, extending from the left hypochondrium to the hip.**

Sharp drawing, in the right side of the abdomen.

Eroding stitches and internal ulcers in the bowels. [PET. DE APONO, *de venen.* c. 14.[1]]

Sensation in the left side of the abdomen, as if blisters were forming, which also burst open again, without pain.

Constipation, with great heat of the body. [GREDING.[2]]

200. **Constipation for several days.** [GREDING; PERCIVAL.]

Obstruction of the intestinal canal, or else violent evacuation. [VOIGTEL.]

A sort of diarrhœa, the fæces not being altogether thin. [*Hrm.*]

Diarrhœa. [LANZONUS; GREDING.]

Violent darrhœa. [LANZONUS; HORST.]

205. Bloody diarrhœa. [VOIGTEL.]

In the rectum, tickling, as from ascarides.

Sharp stinging, close above the anus.

Flow of blood from the hemorrhoidal vein, for four days. [GREDING.[3]]

Urging to micturition, with scanty discharge, burning, stinging or cutting, chiefly at the orifice of the urethra. [*Hrm.*]

210. Rare micturition, and more scanty discharge than usual. [*Hrm.*]

Enuresis. [PFUENDEL.]

Frequent emission of an ill-smelling, tenacious urine, without sediment. [PFUENDEL.]

Dark-red, turbid urine, with yellowish sediment. [ORFILA.]

At the orifice of the urethra, burning stinging pain, during micturition and at other times. [*Hrm.*]

215. The glans is inflamed, the penis swollen. [*Hrm.*]

* * * * * * * * *

---

1 Effects of verdigris.—*Hughes.*

2 No unwonted occurrence G. says.—*Hughes.*

3 Repudiated by G. as effect of C.—*Hughes.*

Very frequent sneezing.

The limbs feel heavy, as if a cold was coming on.

Coryza and stuffed coryza, with sleepy yawning.

Profusely fluent coryza. [*Fr. H.*]

220. Hoarseness, as soon as he breathes dry, cold air.

Constant hoarseness, so that he cannot speak a word, with inclination to lie down.

Spasm in the throat, impeding speech. [ORFILA.]

Cough, continuing uninterruptedly for a half hour or a whole hour and even two hours (early in the morning).

Dry cough, without intermission, not allowing him to speak (at once). [PELARGUS.]

225. Very fatiguing cough, with expulsion of blood, when he blows his nose.

Dry cough. [RAMAZZINI, *Krankh. d. Handw. u. Kuenstler.*[1]]

Tussiculation, arresting the breathing (after the return of consciousness).

Cough, interrupting and almost suppressing the respiration. [VOIGTEL.]

Nocturnal, very violent cough, followed by severe hoarseness, and chilliness from morning to evening

230. Cough, with expectoration of putrid taste, in the morning.

Cough, with bloody expectoration.

Coughing up of blood. [VOIGTEL.]

Quick respiration, with moaning.

Very quick respiration. [VOIGTEL.]

235. Very quick breathing, with slight rattling in the bronchial branches, as if they were full of mucus.

Rattling on the chest, while awake.

Rattling in the chest, with flow of bloody mucus from the nose and the mouth (which was relieved during epilepsy).

Asthma. [RAMAZZ. PELARG.]

Spasmodic attacks of asthma; the chest feels contracted, the respiration difficult, even to suffocation, and, when these cramps abate, a spasmodic vomiting, after which the attack subsided for half an hour.

240. Constriction of the chest. [VOIGTEL.]

Painful contraction of the chest, chiefly after drinking.

Suffocating obstruction of breathing. [PET. DE APONO.]

During respiration, tearing pain in the hypochondria, which pain, as if bruised, when touched.

On the chest, a pressive pain.

245. Pressive pain in the right side of the chest.

Pressure as of something hard on the cartilage of the third rib, more violent when touched. [*Hrm.*]

Shooting pain in the side, with a scream before or afterward, interrupting the sleep.

Sharp stitches, just below the heart, in the left side of the chest.

Sharp drawing pain, independent of the touch, on the cartilage of the sixth rib (aft. 11 h.). [*Hrm.*]

[1] Observations on workers in copper. Effect of inhaling the pulverized metal.—*Hughes.*

250. Pinching pain in the left side of the chest, extending to the hip.

Boring pain in the cardiac region.

Sensation of excessive accumulation of blood in the chest, without any palpitation.

Very quick pulsation of the heart, for one-fourth hour, soon after a (light) supper.

Palpitation of the heart. [VOIGTEL.]

255. Severe palpitation.

Stitch, transversely through the sacrum.

In the back, a severe pressive pain under the right scapula, which at inspiration changes into a lancinating pain.

Sharp, cutting drawing in the left side of the back.

Broad stitches, as if from a knife, under the scapula, on the left side near the spine; independent of respiration. [*Hrm.*]

260. In the nape of the neck, tensive pain.

In the cervical muscles, an intermittent, stinging tearing. [*Hrm.*]

The glands of the right side of the neck are swollen, and painful when touched.

Pain in the thyroid cartilage. [VOIGTEL.]

In the gland of the axilla, heaviness. [SIMMONS, in *Med. and Philos. Comment.*, *Edinb.* 4, 33.[1]]

265. In the shoulder, a drawing pain.

The arms are painful, chiefly the right one, when held quiet. [*Fr. H.*]

Twitching in the arms and hands.

Red, not sharply circumscribed, spots on the arms, with burning itching, chiefly at night.

In the upper arm, pain, as if broken or contused.

270. A blow or jerk in the upper arm.

Pressive pain in the upper arm.

Sensation in the upper arm, as if bubbles of air were pressing out.

In the bend of the elbow, a tetter, forming yellow scales, and itching violently, chiefly in the evening.

In the fore-arm, a twitching tearing in the shaft of the elbow. [*Hrm.*]

275. Tearing in the shaft of the elbow, chiefly in the region of the carpus, aggravated by touching it. [*Hrm.*]

Drawing pain, first in the right, then in the left fore-arm, toward the thumb.

Pain, as if something was broken in two, in the left fore-arm, below the elbow-joint.

In the hands, twitching, in the morning after rising.

A hard pressure in the metacarpus of both hands, aggravated by touching. [*Hrm.*]

280. Twitching tearing on the metacarpal bones of the thumb and of its posterior joint, worse when touched. [*Hrm.*]

Pain in the ball of the hand, as if something was about to pierce through there.

---

[1] From touching wound in hand with sulphate. "Weight" should be "pain."—*Hughes*.

Cold hands.

Weakness and paralysis of the hand. [FALCONER, *on Bath Waters.*[1]]

Inflammation of a lymphatic vessel, from the hand to the shoulder, with severe swelling of the hands. [SIMMONS.]

285. In the finger-tips, fine tearing. [*Hrm.*]

Tensive pain in the balls of both thumbs.

Pain, as from a sprain, in the joint of the thumb.

Pain, as after a knock, below the joint of the thumb.

Numbness and shriveling of the fingers.

290. Vesicles on the finger-tips, exuding water.

In the nates, a pressive, drawing pain.

The lower limbs ache very much. [*Fr. H.*]

Excessive weakness in the lower limbs. [ORFILA.[2]]

In the muscles of the thighs, obtuse pain, on the anterior side. [ORFILA.]

295. Drawing pain in the right thigh.

Pain in the thigh, just above the knee, as if broken or contused.

The knee-joint pains, as if broken.

Lassitude of the knee-joint, with painful drawing, when walking and standing, which is very troublesome to him; the knees will give way. [*Hrm.*]

On the leg, cramp, from the ankle to the calf. [*Rkt.*]

300. Pain, as from a jerk or blow, below the calf.

Cramps in the calves. [ORFILA.]

Cramp in the calves.

Tensive, drawing, cramp-pain in the calves.

Drawing pain below the calves.

305. Digging pain in and below the calf.

The calves pain, chiefly when kept still. [*Fr. H.*]

Tearing pressure in the leg, just below the knee-joint. [*Hrm.*]

The leg, up to the knee, goes to sleep and feels very heavy.

In the ankle-joint, painful heaviness.

310. Violent, pressive pain on the inner edge of the sole of the left foot.

Hard pressure on the metatarsal bone; aggravated by touching. [*Hrm.*]

Drawing pain in the metatarsal bone, where the great toe is joined to it, independent of motion and touch. [*Hrm.*]

Drawing pain on the sole of the left foot, worse when walking. [*Hrm.*]

Twitching tearing on the sole of the foot and its dorsum. [*Hrm.*]

315. Pain, as from a misstep, in the sole of the left foot.

Severe itching on the sole of the foot.

On the toes, a pressive pain.

Sensation of blowing on the toes, as if a wind were blowing out of them.

---

[1] Note, "Observations on workers in copper."—*Hughes.*

[2] See S. 352.—*Hughes.*

Pain between the scapulæ, in the knee-joint and elbow-joint. [COSMIER.]

320. Rheumatic pains. [WEIGEL.]

Shooting pains darting through the whole body, especially on the right side. [PERCIVAL.]

Painful jerks or shocks in diverse parts of the body.

Pains in the bones, in the morning, with headache and nausea. [RAMSAY.]

Pains in the bones and headache, in the intervals which are free from frenzy and convulsions. [RAMSAY.]

325. **Cutaneous eruptions.** [*Hamb. Magaz.*, *Bd.* 8, p. 442.[1]]

Rash on the chest and the hands. [PERCIVAL.]

A sort of a dry itch. [GREDING.[2]]

Eruption resembling leprosy. [VOIGTEL.[3]]

Contraction of the skin on all the limbs. [ORFILA.]

330. Restlessness in the body, with twitching in the limbs.

He is very restless and utters from time to time a piercing cry [ORFILA.]

Trembling. [WEIGEL.]

Trembling in all the limbs. [ORFILA.]

Convulsive movements of the limbs. [ORFILA.]

335. Convulsive movements and contortions of the limbs. [FABAS.]

General convulsions. [RAMSAY; FONDI, *Instit. d. chim. Napoli.*, 1778.[4]]

Convulsions so severe, that two men could scarcely hold the boy. [RAMSAY.]

Convulsions, so that six men had to hold him. [RAMSAY.]

Convulsions, with the constant vomiting and the violent pains of the abdomen, which gradually passed into paralysis. [PYL.]

340. Convulsive attacks in sleep, twitching with the fingers, the arms and hands, backward and also toward the body, the feet were also drawn back; now she would open her eyes and turn them about, then again, she would close them, and distort her mouth.

With sudden convulsions, he would fall down unconscious. [RAMSAY.]

Epileptic convulsions, he trembled, reeled and fell down unconscious, without a cry.

Fits of epilepsy, recurring at short intervals. [LAZORME, *de morb. capit.* p. 253.[5]]

Epileptic fits, with foaming at the mouth, the trunk bent outward, and the limbs spread out on the sides, with open mouth.

345. The child lies on his belly and raises up the nates spasmodically.

Spasms in the limbs. [ORFILA.]

The limbs and the trunk became stiff and the jaws shut up. [ORFILA.]

Lassitude of the limbs. [PELARGUS; VOIGTEL.]

Lack of tone of the whole body. [*Hrm.*]

---

[1] Effect of verdigris.—*Hughes.*
[2] Not ascribed to C.—*Hughes.*
[3] Effect of continued small doses.—*Hughes.*
[4] Not accessible.—*Hughes.*
[5] Not accessible.—*Hughes.*

350. Great lassitude of the body, especially of the knee-joints, which threaten to give way; it is almost impossible for him to stand and to walk, as after a long foot-tour. [*Hrm.*]

Great weariness after a walk, so that all the limbs seem to tremble.

Excessive weakness in the whole body. [ORFILA.[1]]

He cannot stay up, but has to lie abed for two and one-half days without getting up. [*Fr.*, *H.*]

Repeated fainting fits. [ORFILA.[2]]

355. Jaundice, with an expression of rest. [ORFILA.]

Marasmus. [VOIGTEL; ZWINGER, *act. helvet.* V. p. 252.[3]]

Consumption. [RAMAZZINI.[4]]

Apoplexy. [VOIGTEL.]

Paralyses. [VOIGTEL; PYL.]

360. Frequent yawning, without sleepiness. [*Hrm.*]

Much yawning, in the evening.

Sleepiness and lassitude.

After lassitude, a deep sleep of two to three hours. [WIENHOLD, *Heilkr. d. thier. Magn. Th.* II., p. 484.[5]]

Deep sleep, on the cessation of the pains in the abdomen. [SICELIUS.]

365. Lethargic sleep, after the vomiting. [ORFILA.]

Deep sleep for several hours, with twitching of the limbs.

At night (in sleep) frequent twitches. [RAMSAY.]

During sleep, constant grumbling in the abdomen.

Insomnia. [VOIGTEL.]

370. Difficulty in getting to sleep, and the sleep is full of dreams with frequent awakings.

Feverish movements. [WEIGEL.]

Violent fever. [LANZONUS.[6]]

Wasting fever. [VOIGTEL.]

Chilliness (aft. 4 h.). [*Rkt.*]

375. Chill, especially on the hands and feet.

Chill and chattering of teeth. [GREDING.[7]]

Shaking chill over the whole body (at once).

Febrile heat, for several days. [SICELIUS.]

Flush of heat. [HEYSHAM.[8]]

380. Full pulse, but of normal quickness. [PFUENDEL.]

Accelerated pulse. [PFUENDEL.]

Softer, slower pulse. [PFUENDEL.]

Slow pulse, twenty-four beats a minute. [ORFILA.]

Weak and small pulse. [VOIGTEL.]

385. Moist skin. [PFUENDEL.]

Cold sweat, for several hours. [HEYSHAM.[9]]

At night, profuse sweat.

---

[1] See S. 293.—*Hughes.*
[2] When fatigued by much vomiting.—*Hughes.*
[3] Not accessible.—*Hughes.*
[4] Not found.—*Hughes.*
[5] Not accessible.—*Hughes.*
[6] Not found.—*Hughes.*
[7] In association with slight epileptic manifestations.—*Hughes.*
[8] Not found.—*Hughes.*
[9] Sweat is not described as cold, and lasted nearly an hour, instead of several hours.—*Hughes.*

DIGITALIS PURPUREA. FOXGLOVE.

This plant, which grows wild on open mountainous plateaux, is one of the most powerful medicinal substances of the vegetable kingdom; it has been frequently abused by the physicians of the old school, who sought to gain consideration through violent action on the patient, without considering of what nature this action might be; for they had not knowledge sufficient to apply this remedy to the various diseases for which it is suitable. Countless murders have thus been committed by men who were not conversant with its pure effects. In extremely rare instances, when they unconsciously used it in cases where the disease-symptoms had a striking similarity to those produced by foxglove, they produced wonders by rapid cures. The true Homœopath will never use it injuriously, but always for the salvation of his patients; he will not consider it indicated by a quick pulse, as has been customary in the old school; for though in its first effects it greatly retards the pulse, in its after effects it causes so much greater an acceleration through the counter effects of the vital force.

The homœopathic medicine is prepared from this plant by dynamizing one drop of its freshly expressed juice, mixed with ninety-nine drops of alcohol, by ten strong succussive strokes, which is then repeated in twenty-nine other vials, as has been taught at the conclusion of Part I. of the Chronic Diseases as to the second method. Instead of this we can triturate two grains of the fresh herb with one hundred grains of sugar of milk, and then develop it to the thirtieth potency of its medicinal powers, as is usually done with dry medicinal substances.

In its homœopathic use, this medicine need only be given in the smallest dose, and if even such a dose should produce too violent effects, repeated smelling of a solution of Camphor will serve to moderate its action. Nux vomica and Opium are also said to have been found useful as antidotes. A cautious physician, however, will hardly ever need antidotes. By spirits of nitre the action of digitalis is immensely increased. Digitalis has a long period of action.

The abbreviations of the names of my fellow-provers are: *Bchr.*, *Becher; Fr.*, *Dr. Franz; Gr.*, *Dr. Gross; Hbg.*, *Hornburg; Jr.*,

Of these thirteen fellow-observers, ten belong to the pathogenesis of *Materia Medica Pura*. The remaining three, *Jahr* and *Piepers* contribute here for the first time. The two symptoms belonging to *Trinks* are from the list given in his own and Hartlaub's *Arzneimittlehre*, Vol. III.—*Hughes*.

Jahr.; Lgh., Dr. Langhammer; J. Lh., J. Lehmann; Myr., Meyer; Pp., Piepers; Rkt., Dr. Rueckert; Stf., Medical Counselor Dr. Stapf; Tth., Teuthorn; Trs., Dr. Trinks.

DIGITALIS.

Dejection and anxiety. [WITHERING, *Abhandl. ueb. d. Fingerh*, Leipzig, 1786.[1]]

Sadness, with a sensation of being quite sick; all objects seem to him as in the changed visual sensation of fever.

Great sadness and dejection, the whole time. [*Jr.*]

Tearful sorrow over many things which have failed with him.

5. Anxiety, as if originating in the epigastrium. [*Jr.*]

Anxiousness, with many sighs, during the whole time. [*Jr.*]

Anxiousness, with great apprehension of the future, most intense every evening at 6 o'clock, with sadness and weeping, which give relief. [*Jr.*]

Anxiety, as if he had done wrong. [*Lhm.*]

Internal anguish, like anguish of conscience, as if he had committed a crime, or had to expect reproaches (continuing for more than three months). [*Jr.*]

10. Great anguish. [KRAUSE, in *Hufel. Journ.*, 5th *Bd.*, 3d *St.*, p. 684.[2]]

Anxious apprehension of a sad kind, with great dejection, extremely aggravated by music. [*Pp.*]

Despondency. [PENKIVIL, *Med. and Phys. Journ.* III., p. 315.[3]]

Fear of death.

Great excitability; he is very much affected by everything, but especially by sad things, and the least trifle can throw him into disconsolate despair (continuing over three months). [*Jr.*]

15. Great inclination to solitude. [*Pp.*]

Indisposed to talk. [*Hbg.*]

Gloominess and peevishness. [*Hbg.*]

Gloomy, morose humor, he scolds about everything. [*Rkt.*]

Indifference and lack of interest. [GUIBERT, in *Gazette de Santé*, 1826, No. 24.[4]]

20. Very indifferent to everything, for several days. [*Pp.*]

Indifferent mood, looking down before him, as if he had not finished his sleep, but without drowsiness. [*Tth.*]

Well disposed for mental work and all business. (Curative effect.) [*Hbg.*]

Violent desire for work (aft. 1½ h.).

Peaceable, tranquil mood. (After-effect.) [*Fr.*]

25. Many vivid fancies. [*Fr.*]

Delirious talk and restlessness, at night. [KRAUS, l. c.]

---

[1] Effects of D. on patients. (The symptoms have been revised from the original English edition.) This symptom not found.—*Hughes.*

[2] Read "*Knaus.*" Effects of D. in a case of anasarca.—*Hughes.*

[3] Effects of D. in phthisis. This discouragement was on account of the apparent inefficiency of the medicine. *Hughes.*

[4] Effects of D. in a case of enlarged heart.—*Hughes.*

Secret insanity, with disobedience and obstinacy; he tries to run away.

Weakness of memory. [LETTSOM, *Mem. of the Med. Soc. of Lond.*, Vol. II., Art. 16.[1]]

Thinking requires an effort, and he would at once forget everything again, with internal and external heat in the head. [*Myr.*]

30. The head is affected. [WITHERING.[2]]

Gloominess of spirit, with indifference, mostly in the evening. [*Pp.*]

Gloomy in mind, as if hypochondriac.

Obtuseness of the head.

Dizziness of the head, with inability to recollect. [*Fr.*]

35. Obtuseness of the head, with very limited power of thinking. [JOERG, *Mater. z. e. Kuenft. Heilm. Lehre.*[3].]

Head muddled, as from intoxication, with increased cerebral activity. [JOERG.]

Vertigo. [QUARIN, Animadvers. pract.; MACLEAN, in *Med. and Phys. Journ.* II., 91; JOERG; PENKIVIL; LETTSOM.[4]]

Vertigo, frequently, after rising from sitting or lying down. [*Pp.*]

Vertigo, so that she fell down on going up stairs. [PENKIVIL.]

40. Vertigo and trembling. [DRAKE, in *Med. and Phys. Journ.* IV., 521.[5]]

Headache. [QUARIN; LETTSOM.]

Headache for several days. [SCHIEMANN, *diss. de dig. purp. Goett.*, 1786.]

Headache, with obtuseness of the head. [*Stf.*]

Headache in the frontal region. [JOERG.]

45. Headache on stooping, at once in the morning, after rising. [*Pp.*]

Headache, pressure and heaviness as from a rush of blood to the head.

Pressive headache, with slight obtuseness. [JOERG.]

Pressive headache in the occiput, or starting from the vertex and extending all over the head, arising from original feeling of obtuseness. [JOERG.]

Pressure in the forehead, the region of the vertex and the occiput. [JOERG, l. c.]

50. Pressure in the occiput, from the right to the left side and then spreading toward the vertex. [JOERG.]

Pressive, very acute headache, after awaking in the morning, all the forenoon. [JOERG.]

Pressive pains in the head, so much aggravated in the afternoon and especially in the evening, that he has to lie down before his customary time; during the day the pain made work impossible. [JOERG.]

---

[1] Effects of D. when given to dropsical patients.—*Hughes.*

[2] Not found.—*Hughes.*

[3] Provings on the healthy with one-third grain doses of the powdered leaves.—*Hughes.*

[4] Nothing about D. mentioned by Quarin here, but most of Quarin's symptoms are cited in *Bayle's Bibl. de Therap.* III., 320, as effects of the drug in scrofula. Maclean gives "Effects on patients."—*Hughes.*

[5] Effects of D. in phthisis.—*Hughes.*

Pressure as from a heavy load, in the middle of the upper part of the forehead, on exerting the thoughts. [*Fr.*]

Sharp pressive pain in the forehead, on a small spot above the eye. [*Stf.*]

55. Pressure and stretching in the sides of the head (soon). [*Gr.*]

Muddling, tensive pressure in the head, chiefly in the forehead and left temple, in the evening (aft. 3, 12 d.). [*Jr.*]

Tensive pressure anteriorly in the forehead. [*Hbg.*]

Contractive pressure anteriorly in the forehead and temples, increased by reflecting. [*Fr.*]

Jerking pressure on the right side of the head (7th. d.). [*Jr.*]

60. Pressure by jerks, now in the temples, now in the whole head. [*Rkt.*]

Tensive sensation in the sinciput, when turning the eyes to the side. [*Bchr.*]

Stitchlike tension on a small spot in the side of the brain, every time he stooped forward; there was a drawing sensation in an upper tooth on the left hand side; this went off every time he raised himself up. [*Stf.*]

Drawing in the side of the head, which made him giddy [*Gr.*]

Tearing in the left side of the head. [*Gr.*]

65. Tearing in the right temporal region, close to the ear. [*Gr.*]

Shooting, now in the right, now in the left temporal region. [*Myr.*]

Single obtuse stitches in the left temple, darting through the whole brain, in the evening, and at night when sleeping.

Violently shooting pains in the head, especially in the occiput and the crown. [JOERG.]

Throbbing headache in the forehead or in the fundus of the orbits. [MACLEAN.]

70. Headache, coming with an ebullition, beating like waves toward both sides, in the interior of the head, aggravated by standing and by bending backward, diminished by lying down and by bending forward. [*Tth.*]

Pulsating sensation as if the brain, like water, was beating against both sides of the skull, and would burst it, with obtuseness. [*Tth.*]

Frequent sensation on bending the head forward, as if something fell forward in it. [*Rkt.*]

Sudden cracking knack in the head, during the noon-siesta, with frightened starting up. [*Jr.*]

Semilateral headache, as if from an internal itching. [*J. Lh.*]

75. At the occipital protuberance, a pressive pain as from a knock or a fall. [*Hbg.*]

Pressive stitches externally on the left side of the forehead. [*Lgh.*]

Tearing stitches in the left temple. [*Lgh.*]

Single stitches in the left frontal region. [*Lgh.*]

Heat, on and in the whole head. [*Myr.*]

80. Swelling of the head. [QUARIN.[1]]

The head always falls backwards, when sitting and in walking, as if the anterior cervical muscles had no strength, as if they were paralyzed. [*Tth.*]

Pain of the eyes, excessive aching in the eyeball, when touched.

Pressive pain in the eyeballs.

Pressure in the right eyeball, rapidly coming and vanishing. [*Stf.*]

85. Pressive pain in the right eyebrow, toward the external canthus. [*Lgh.*]

Painful scratching in the inner canthus, as from coarse dust. [*Hbg.*]

Pain of the edges of the eyelids as if sore, when closing the eyes, in the evening in bed. [*Rkt.*]

Throbbing pains in the orbits. [MACLEAN.]

Burning pain in the arch of the right eyebrow, with dimness of vision as through a gauze. [*Myr.*]

90. Eroding burning in the outer canthi. [*Jr.*]

Reddened eyes, with painfulness, especially in the evening, for five days. [*Pp.*]

Inflammation of the Meibomian glands on the edges of the eyelids.

Violent inflammation of the eyes.

Swelling of the lower eyelid, troublesome on looking downward.

95. Watery discharge from the eyes. [WITHERING.]

The eyes become full of water, more in the room than in the open air; they are dim, hot, full of red blood-vessels, with pressive pain and eye-gum in the canthi. [*Stf.*]

Eyes glued together in the morning, and then weakness in the eyes. [*Pp.*]

Smarting tears.

Heaviness of the eyelids in the evening, with inability to keep them open. [*Pp.*]

100. Tendency of both eyes to turn toward the left, with pain when he turned them to the right side, on which he then sees all things double and threefold; at the same time the face is puffed up. [*Bchr.*]

Pupils strongly contracted (aft. ½ h.). [*Stf.*]

Great dilatation of the pupils (aft. 1 h.). [*Tth.*]

Dilated, insensible pupils. [*Journ. d. Chim. méd.* 1827, Dec., p. 593.[2]]

Pupil has but little irritability. [TROSCHEL in *Hufel. Journ.* 1828, Sep.—GUIBERT.[3]]

105. Obscuration of the eyes. [QUARIN.]

Slight obscuration of the vision. [MOSSMANN, *Essay to elucid. the scrofula*, Lond., 1800.[4]]

He sees objects only darkily. [WITHERING.]

---

[1] This was only a sensation as of swelling.—*Hughes.*

[2] From an overdose. With S. 592.—*Hughes.*

[3] Troschel's is simply a translation of Guibert's case. (See S. 19.)—*Hughes.*

[4] Not accessible.—*Hughes.*

Weak sight, imperfect vision. [PENKIVIL.]

Dimness of vision. [WITHERING.]

110. Dim, weak vision, for forty-eight hours. [*Trs.*]

Dimmed, diminished vision. [JOERG.]

Imperfect vision, as if a cloud or a mist was passing before the eyes. [MACLEAN.]

Blindness. [LETTSOM.[1]]

Blindness, amaurosis, for three days. [REMER, *Annal. d. Kl. Anst.*, *Bd.* I.[2]]

115. Double vision. [JOERG.]

External objects present themselves in a false semblance and not in their true light. [JOERG.]

Various appearances before the eyes. [LETTSOM.[3]]

All sorts of figures hover before the eyes. [PENKIVIL.]

Muscae volitantes float before his eyes, when he wishes to look at distant objects. [BAKER, in *Arzneik, Abhandl. d. Kolleg. d. Aerzte in London*, Th. III, Art. 17.[4]]

120. Bright bodies seem to dance before his eyes, when he covers his eyes. [BAKER.[5]]

All objects seem as if covered with snow, in the morning on awaking. [MOSSMANN in *Med. and Phys. Journ.* III, 13.[6]]

The face of persons coming into the room, seemed to him deadly pale. [BAKER.]

Color appearances before the eyes, red, green and yellow, like flickering light; in the dusk. [*J. Lh.*]

Objects appear green or yellow. [WITHERING.]

125. Objects appear to him yellow, even silver. [PENKIVIL.]

The flame of the candle appears to him larger and brighter than usual. [BAKER.]

Flickering before the eyes. [JOERG.]

The eyes are dazzled, as from the sudden transition from darkness into bright light; then sparks appear before the eyes with vertigo, for a quarter of an hour, after dinner. [JOERG.]

Otalgia, as if the ears were internally constricted; he hears the pulsation in the ear. [*Fr.*].

130. Tensive pressure in the left ear. [*Stf.*]

Twitching in the external and internal ear.

Drawing pain in the muscles under the mastoid process. [*Fr.*]

Drawing pain under the right mastoid process, it goes off when pressing upon it. [*Fr.*]

Single stitches behind the ear. [*Tth.*]

135. The glands by and behind the ear are painfully swollen. [*Pp.*]

His hearing is suddenly obstructed, with ringing in the ear. [*Jr.*]

---

[1] This lasted for a month after omitting the medicine, with throbbing pains and sense of fullness and enlargement in the eyeballs.—*Hughes.*

[2] Not accessible.—*Hughes.*

[3] With S. 41.—*Hughes.*

[4] Effects of D. in a case of anasarca.—*Hughes.*

[5] The muscae of S. 119 became these when the eyes were covered *and pressed upon.*—*Hughes.*

[6] Effects of D. in pneumonia.—*Hughes.*

Hissing before both ears, like boiling water.* [*Tth.*]

Pain above the root of the nose. [NEUMANN, in *Hufel. Journ.* LV., 78.[1]]

Epistaxis from both nostrils, bright blood (aft. 1 h.). [*Tth.*]

140. Paleness of the face. [WITHERING, l. c.[2]]

Cramp under the right zygomatic arch on moving the lower jaw, which, when he bites, is drawn together spasmodically. [*Fr.*]

Paralytic drawing, below the left zygomatic arch, going off when it is pressed upon. [*Gr.*]

Cramp-like drawing pain on the zygomatic arch, before the ear. [*Fr.*]

Convulsions on the left side of the face. [MOSSMANN.]

145. Swelling of the cheek, extending from the ear to the corner of the mouth, with pain when touched, and with eruption. [*Pp.*]

Erosion and itching on the cheek and chin, worse at night.

Itching eruption on the cheek and chin, which forms a scab and leaves red spots behind. [*Pp.*]

Large pimple, with smarting pain, under the left nostril.

Red nodule, with burning, smarting pain, increased by touching, on the middle of the forehead. [*Hbg.*]

150. Black perspiration-pores on the skin of the face, which fester and suppurate. [*Pp.*]

Swelling of the lips. [HENRY in *Ebinb. Med. and Surg. Journ.* VII., 148.[3]]

Swelling on the inner side of the lower lip, without any pain.

Eruption on the upper lid.

In the lower jaw, stitches.

155. The teeth in the front row are painful. [*Stf.*

Fetor of the mouth.

Swelling of the tongue. [HENRY.]

Tongue coated, for several days.

Tongue coated white, in the morning. [*Lgh.*]

160. Collection of saliva in the mouth, with spitting of it out, and great nausea on swallowing it down. [*Bchr.*]

Accumulation of saliva, as after vinegar. [*Hbg.*]

Collection of watery saliva in the mouth, first tasting sweet, but later on very salty, frequently recurring. [*Stf.*]

Collection of very sweet saliva. [SCHIEMANN.]

Flow of saliva. [LENTIN, *Beobacht. ein. krankh.*, 1774, p. 167; WITHERING; GREMLER, in *Rust's Magazin.* XXV., 578.[4]]

165. **Flow of saliva.**

Copious flow of saliva of fetid smell. [HENRY.[5]]

Flow of saliva, with soreness in the mouth, on the tongue and

* Digitalis has not unfrequently cured deafness attended with a noise in the ear as of boiling water, in cases where it was otherwise homœopathically appropriate.

[1] Effects of D. in phthisis. With vertigo.—*Hughes.*
[2] With S. 344. - *Hughes.*
[3] From overdosing an ascitic patient with D.—*Hughes.*
[4] Effect of overdosing with D.—*Hughes.*
[5] Henry states saliva to have been of viscid consistence, but says nothing about "stinking odor."—*Hughes*

in the gums for three days. [BAYLIES, *Pract. Essays on Med. Subj.*, *Lond.*, 1773.[1]]

Dryness in the throat. [NEUMANN.]

Roughness and softness in the mouth, as if it was covered with velvet. [*Tth.*]

170. Roughness of the palate, as after smoking too much tobacco. [*Fr.*]

Scrapy, rough feeling in the palate. [*Stf.*]

Scraping and burning in the fauces and the œsophagus, after dinner and in the evening. [JOERG.]

Sensation in the fauces, as if the walls of the pharynx were swollen or pressed together by a swelling of the tonsils. [JOERG.]

Shooting sore throat, even when not swallowing.

175. Stitches in the posterior part of the palate and in the commencement of the gullet, not observable when swallowing. [*Rkt.*]

Pain as of soreness in the throat, when swallowing. [*Jr.*]

Soreness of the fauces and of the posterior nares, chiefly painful in the morning and evening, for several days. [*Jr.*]

Soreness of the mouth, the fauces and the œsophagus. [BOERHAVE, *hortus*, *Lugd. Batav.*, p. 301.[2]]

Flat, slimy taste. [*Tth.*]

180. Taste as of sweet almonds, after smoking tobacco. [*Fr.*]

Little appetite, he feels sated at once. [*Stf.*]

Lack of appetite, with clean tongue. [PENKIVIL.]

Anorexia, with great emptiness in the stomach. [KINGLAKE in *Beddoes*, in *Med. Facts and Obs.*, Vol. V., Lond., 1797.[3]]

Loss of appetite. [MUELLER in *Wasse's Zeitschrift fuer Anthropologie.*[4]]

185. Total anorexia, in the morning and evening. [JOERG.]

Violent hunger, also in the afternoon. [JOERG.]

Thirst. [NEUMANN.]

Thirst for acid drinks. [*Tth.*]

Desire for bitter food. [*Bchr.*]

190. Bread tastes bitter, with good appetite. [*Tth.*]

After a meal, the food presses into the scrobiculus cordis, while sitting, not while standing. [*Fr.*]

After dinner, great drowsiness, with frequent yawning, for many days.

After a meal, the stomach and epigastrium are always full and inflated, with clumsiness and distaste to work. [*Jr.*]

Sour eructation after a meal. [*Tth.*]

195. Regurgitation of a sourish fluid. [*Pp.*]

Regurgitation of an acrid fluid and then of acidity in the mouth, like vinegar. [*Pp.*]

Regurgitation of a tasteless fluid. [*Pp.*]

Heartburn, in the afternoon and toward evening. [JOERG.]

A somewhat sharp burning, extending from the stomach up the œsophagus. [JOERG.[5]]

---

[1] Not accessible.—*Hughes.*

[2] Observed effects of D. This symptom is ascribed by the author to the acrimony of the plant.—*Hughes.*

[3] Nothing from Kinglake found here.—*Hughes.*

[4] Not accessible.—*Hughes.*

[5] The original numbering of symptoms leaps here from 199 to 300.—*Transl.*

300. Hiccup. [LENTIN.]

Hiccup, which does not rise quite up into the throat, six or seven times. [*Bchr.*]

Repeated hiccup. [*Pp.*]

Loathing. [NEUMANN.]

Qualmishness, almost bordering on nausea. [JOERG.]

305. **Nausea.** [BAYLIES.]

Nausea in the gastric region, with little appetite. [*Bchr.*]

Nausea after eating. [*J. Lh.*]

Nausea for three days. without cessation. [MACLEAN.]

Deadly nausea. [WARREN, in *London Med. Journ.* VI. 2, 145.[1]]

310. Deadly nausea, as if he should vomit, in recurring fits, with extreme depression of the spirits and anxious oppression. [WITHERING.[2]]

Inclination to vomit. [GUIBERT, TROSCHEL.]

Retching. [KRAUS.]

Almost convulsive effort to vomit. [GUIBERT.]

Vomiting. [*Journ d. Chim.*]

315. Vomiting, through the day and night. [GUIBERT.]

Morning vomiting. [MOSSMANN, PENKIVIL.]

Vomiting in the night. [PENKIVIL.]

Long-continued vomiting. [WITHERING.]

Vomiting for six days, uncontrollable until death ensued. [*Edinb. Med. Comment.* B. X., 358.[3]]

320. Violent vomiting for four hours. [BAYLIES.]

Excessive vomiting. [LENTIN.[4]]

Vomiting with nausea. [NEUMANN.]

Vomiting with severe, violent nausea. [MACLEAN.]

Excessive vomiting, with inordinate nausea, coldness of the limbs and cold sweat, for two days. [BAKER.]

325. Retching vomiting, with violent nausea, with great anguish in the scrobiculus cordis, with external heat intermixed with chilly shudders, and subsequent sweat with chill, several days successively, at 5 to 6 P. M. [*Pp.*]

Vomiting of the food eaten, which was enveloped in tasteless mucus, with increased nausea and diminution of the bellyache. [*Bchr.*]

Vomiting of a green liquid, like an infusion of herbs, in repeated attacks, with an abatement of the ailments. [GUIBERT.]

Vomiting of green bile, with inordinate nausea. [BAKER.]

Bilious vomiting, for several days. [BEDDOES, in *Med. facts and obs.* V., Lond., 1794, Art. 2.[5]]

330. **Stomachache.** [GUIBERT; KRAUS; TROSCHEL.]

Disagreeable sensation in the gastric region. [MOSSMANN.]

The stomach is weak in digesting food for a long time. [*Pp.*]

Weakness of the stomach, like a sinking down, as if life

---

[1] Effect of overdose.—*Hughes.*
[2] Not found.—*Hughes.*
[3] From overdosing.—*Hughes.*
[4] Not found.—*Hughes.*
[5] From an overdose.—*Hughes.*

were being extinguished, with all the patients in the same manner. [MACLEAN.[1]]

Heaviness in the stomach. [PENKIVIL.]

335. Heaviness in the stomach, alternating with lassitude. [MOSSMANN.]

Pressure, repeatedly in the stomach and in the epigastrium. [*Jr.*]

Pressure in the scrobiculus cordis, as from a hard load, on raising the body. [*Fr*]

Cutting pressure in the scrobiculus cordis, with nausea there. [*Gr.*]

Constriction over the gastric region, toward the liver. [*Hbg.*]

340. Cramplike pains about the stomach (7th d.). [*Jr.*]

Spasms of the stomach. [WITHERING.]

Cutting in the stomach. [JOERG.]

Squeezing stitches in the scrobiculus cordis, unchanged by respiration and increased by touching, only when standing, not when sitting. [*Gr.*]

Great heat in the stomach, with painfulness of the same. [WITHERING.]

345. Burning in the stomach, extending up into the œsophagus. [JOERG.]

Burning and pressure, in the gastric region. [HORN, *Neues Archiv Y.*, I., p. 504.[2]]

In the hypochondria, anxious tension and constriction.

Pressure in the left hypochondrium. [*Jr*]

Continuous stitch in the left hypochondrium, with feeling as if the parts around it had gone to sleep. [*Fr.*]

350. Pain, as if all things within were torn, on a spot below the third false rib on the left side. [*Fr.*]

Bellyache, of a violent and constant kind. [*Journ. d. Chim.*]

Fullness in the abdomen, at noon, with good appetite. [JOERG.]

Pressive colic in the epigastrium, by jerks and, as it were, spasmodic. [*Jr.*]

Contractive pain in the abdomen, for a quarter of an hour. [JOERG.]

355. Sensation of twisting in the bowels and as if the gastric region was drawn in. [DRAKE.[3]]

Pinching contraction in the abdomen, as from taking a violent cold, when sitting, not when walking (aft. 3 or 4 days). [*Fr.*]

Pains in the abdomen, like colic, with growling and rumbling, for half an hour.

Pinching in the belly (almost at once).

Pinching in the hypogastrium, as from a purgative. [*Myr.*]

360. Pinching in the belly, with single stitches and transient fits of nausea. [*Rkt.*]

Cutting all over the epigastrium and hypogastrium. [*Gr.*]

---

[1] The original is "A faintness or sinking at the stomach, as if life were going from them. –*Hughes.*

[2] Nothing about D. here.—*Hughes.*

[3] Original is "Sensation of twisting in the bowels after each dose, and of much sinking the pit of the stomach."—*Hughes.*

Cutting in the abdomen, with urging to stool. [JOERG.]

Cutting in the abdomen, extending to the lowest part of the belly in the region of the os pubis, where it presses and bears downward through the pelvic cavity to the testes; the cutting arose from previous increased movements in the abdomen. [JOERG.]

Shooting pains in the renal region. [JOERG.]

365. Fine stitches in the left renal region, when sitting. [*Hbg.*]

Stitches, also single fine stitches in the left side of the abdomen, in rest (and in motion) and especially on expiration. [*Lgh.*]

Fine stitches on the right side of the abdomen, on expiration, when standing and walking (aft. 50 h.). [*Lgh.*]

Flying needle-pricks in the whole abdomen. [*Gr.*]

Sharp stitches in navel. [*Gr.*]

370. Obtuse, almost pinching stitches, on the right side over the navel, when eating. [*Gr.*]

Tearing pains in the navel, in the morning.

Tearing rather than shooting pains in the abdomen, in the morning in bed, with subsequent diarrhœa, followed by tenesmus

Single, cutting, tearing pains in the umbilical region when walking. [*Fr.*]

Single cutting, tearing pains in the abdomen, in the evening, as if from a cold, especially when rising up from a seat, with pressive headache in the vertex. [*Fr.*]

375. Burrowing, pressing and shooting in the abdomen, just above the umbilical region. [*Gr.*]

Boring and pressing down, anteriorly, in the left side of the abdomen. [*Fr.*]

Sensation in the left side of the abdomen, as if something was forcing itself through. [*Fr.*]

The abdomen pains on motion, as if ulcerated, but not so when touched. [*Fr.*]

Tension of the skin on the abdomen, when he raises himself up. [*Fr.*]

380. In the bend of the groin there is, almost only when walking, a pressive tension in the tendon of the psoas muscle, that becomes prominent on moving; when pressed on, it is painful, as if there was a pressure from a hard body under the skin. [*Fr.*]

Drawing cramp, anteriorly in the bend of the right groin, which is aggravated on moving the psoas muscle, and became, as it were, clucking, and then even continues when sitting. [*Fr.*]

Twitching tearing, extending from the mons veneris to the left groin, on bending the body backward. [*Fr.*]

Shooting pain in the bend of the groin, when walking. [*Fr.*]

Pain, as from excoriation, in the left inguinal ring, as if a hernia would protrude.

385. Many ailments from flatus. [*Jr.*]

The flatus moves about audibly in the abdomen, with growling and grumbling and a sensation as if bubbles of air moved about in the large intestines. [*Jr.*]

Movements of flatus, with clucking and pressure in the hypogastrium. [*Gr.*]

Noises in the abdomen, without sensation of flatulence, or discharge of flatus. [*Bchr.*]

Much rumbling in the bowels. [JOERG.]

390. Flatulence and discharge of flatus. [*Rkt.*]

Discharge of much flatus, in the afternoon. [JOERG.]

Constipation, almost the whole time. [*Pp.*]

Call to stool. [*Hbg.*]

Several stools during the day. [*Journ. d. Chim.*]

395. Stool, two or three times a day, for several days. [*Lgh.*]

Soft, liquid, frequent stool (aft, 72 h.). [*Fr.*]

Thin stool. [*Hbg*]

Thin evacuation. [JOERG.]

Thin stool, two or three times a day, and on the following morning, constipation (aft. 24 h.). [*Stf.*]

400. Diarrhœa. [WITHERING.]

Violent diarrhœa. [LENTIN, BAYLIES.]

Diarrhœa, with subsequent urging to stool, in the rectum.

Painful diarrhœas for three or four days. [WITHERING.[1]]

Diarrhœas with colic during and before the stool. [*Bchr.*]

405. Diarrhœa of fæces mixed with mucus, preceded by bellyache, sometimes pressive, sometimes cutting, which went off each time he went to stool (aft. 6 to 8 h.). [*Bchr.*]

Yellow, white stool, without any trouble after constipation for forty-eight hours. [*Fr.*]

Ash-colored diarrhœa, as with one having jaundice. [SCHIEMANN.]

Ash-colored, pappy diarrhœa, as in jaundice, after previously vomiting four times, followed by fainting. [MEYER in *Richter's Chir. Bibl.* V., p. 532.]

Almost incurable dysenteries. [BOERHAVE, *Rar. Morb. Hist. Jen.*, 1771.[2]]

410. Involuntary evacuation of stool.

Many ascarides in the stool, in the evening. [*Stf.*]

Before the diarrhœic stool, in the morning in bed, bellyache, more tearing than shooting.

Before the stool, chill.

After the stool, pressure on both sides of the spine in the lumbar region. [*Jr.*]

415. Suppression of urine. [HENRY.[3]]

Forcing pressure on the bladder, with sensation as if this was too full, this sensation did not disappear on urinating. [JOERG.[4]]

Urging to urinate. [*Hbg.*]

Constant urging to urinate, even after micturition. [*Joerg.*]

420. Violent ineffectual urging to urinate. [MANGOLD, in *Horn's Archiv.* III , 1, p. 141.[5]]

Incessant urging to urinate, with scanty discharge each time. [JOERG.]

Uninterrupted urging to urinate, and every time only a

---

[1] Not found.—*Hughes.*
[2] As with S. 178, q. v.—*Hughes.*
[3] For nearly three days.—*Hughes.*
[4] The omission of one number between 415 and 420 occurs in the original text.—*Transl.*
[5] Not accessible—*Hughes.*

few drops of dark-brown, hot urine, scalding while discharged, are emitted (aft. 9 d.). [*Jr.*]

Frequent urging to urinate, while the red urine only passes in drops, with burning in the urethra and glans. [*Myr.*]

Frequent discharge of water colored urine, in small quantity. [JOERG.]

425. Constant urging to urinate at night, and when he arose for the purpose, dizziness and vertigo. [*Myr.*]

She has to rise every night to pass water.

Rare micturition, only twice a day and a little at a time, but without trouble; but after forty-eight hours more copious urine, with cutting drawing in the bladder. [*Fr.*]

Urging to urinate, with much urine of normal color (aft. 8, 9, 10 h.). [*Bchr.*]

Urging to urinate, with copious discharge of ordinary urine. [JOERG.]

430. Inordinately increased secretion of urine, day and night, for forty-eight hours, with much exhaustion (aft. 2 h.). [*Trs.*]

Diuresis.

Increased discharge of urine, with increased urging thereto, and inabilty to retain it. [WITHERING.]

Inability to retain the urine. [WITHERING.]

Involuntary discharge of urine.

435. Frequent copious discharge of pale yellow, watery urine. [JOERG.]

Frequent passing of watery urine. [*Stf.*]

Frequent and copious passing of dark urine. [JOERG.]

Dark colored urine. [JOERG.]

Dark urine, without urging, in standing, this became more red and also turbid (aft. 14 h.). [*Bchr.*]

440. Acrid urine. [WITHERING.[1]]

Thin, brownish sediment in the urine, when it has stood several hours. [JOERG.]

During urination, a contractive pain in the urinary bladder, with difficult passage of the urine. [*J. Lh.*]

While urinating, a pressing burning in the middle of the urethra, as if this was too narrow, but this diminishes during the continuance of micturition.

During the diuresis and diarrhœa, small, quick pulse, while the hands and feet are cold. [WITHERING.]

445. **After the diuresis,** retention of urine, then **nausea,** vomiting and diarrhœa.* [WITHERING.]

---

* A very rare alternating action of foxglove, and only when given in a dose too large. Usually the first effect of this medicine is to produce difficulty in urination. By means of this action, it frequently has been of great use in diseases involving swellings, which were attended with similar difficulty in the secretion of urine and with other symptoms found among the pure primary effects of digitalis. The copious, often involuntary, flow of urine, or diuresis, resulting from the use of digitalis, is merely a counter effect of the organism, in answer to the above mentioned primary effect of the drug.

---

[1] Not found.—*Hughes.*

Inflammation of the neck of the bladder. [DON MONRO, in *Samml. f. pr. Aerzte* XIII., p. 288.[1]]

In the glans, an itching irritation. [JOERG.]

In the right testicle, pain as from a contusion.

Excitation of sexual desire. [JOERG.]

450. Excited sexual organs, with repeated, painful erections, disturbing the night's sleep. [JOERG.]

Excited sexual desire, with frequent erections, by day. [*Jr.*]

Fancy very much excited voluptuously, with lascivious images by day and night, and frequent erections. [*Pp.*]

Pollutions, almost every fourth night, always with lewd dreams. [*Jr.*]

Pollutions, with subsequent pain in penis. [*Pp.*]

455. Frequent sensation at night, as if pollutions were coming, without emission of semen; in the morning, a viscid fluid at the orifice of the urethra.

* * * * * * * *

Much sneezing, without a cold, during the first days. [*Jr.*]

Coryza in the morning, with stoppage of the nose. [*Lgh.*]

Fluent coryza, with much sneezing, followed by stoppage of the nose. [*Pp.*]

Stuffed coryza, in the night and evening, but fluent coryza by day (aft. 20 d.). [*Jr.*]

460. Roughness in the windpipe. [JOERG.]

Hoarseness in the morning.

Great hoarseness in the morning, after a night-sweat, so that he could not speak.

Hoarseness, in the morning, on awaking. [*Pp.*]

Frequent painless hoarseness. [*Jr.*]

465. Adhesive phlegm in the throat, detached by coughing. [*Pp.*]

Adhesive mucus in the larynx, detached by a hacking cough. [*Jr.*]

Expectoration in the morning, by involuntary retching. [*Lgh.*]

Mucus in the throat in the morning, which is easily detached, but when he wishes to cough it up, it generally gets into the fauces, so that he has to swallow it. [*Gr.*]

Cough and coryza, so that he can hardly talk.

470. The irritation to cough extends to the top of the palate.

Cough, short and dry, caused by an itching irritation in the larynx. [*Jr.*]

Dull cough, as from a titillation in the windpipe, without expectoration. [*Stf.*]

After much speaking, dry, spasmodic cough.

After eating, a cough so severe that he vomits up the food.

475. At twelve o'clock at night, cough, with sweat.

In the morning, on rising, dry cough, with asthma. [*Hbg.*]

Dry cough, with tensive, pressive pain in the arm and shoulder. [*Stf.*]

---

[1] Effects of D. given for dropsy. Literally, it is "urging to urinate, even to inflammation of the bladder."—*Hughes.*

Coughing is rendered difficult by a pain in the chest. [BRANDIS, in *Schiemann*, p. 61.]

Expectoration from the chest, colored with blood. [PENKIVIL.[1]]

480. **Hemoptysis.**

Breathing, heavy, and slowly drawn from deep down in the chest. [*Rkt.*]

Short breathing and not enough of it; he cannot hold his breath long, but must quickly breathe anew. [*Fr.*]

Painful asthma for many days; he had often to draw a deep breath; and yet he felt as if air failed him, especially when sitting. [*Stf.*]

Spasmodic constriction of the throat. [LENTIN.[2]]

485. Suffocating, painful constriction of the chest, as if the interior parts were grown together, especially in the morning, on awaking, he has quickly to sit up.

With every respiration, a sensation as if he was being electrified. [SACKREUTER, in *Annalen der Heilkunde*, 1811; Maerz.[3]]

Pain in the chest, pressure on the lower part of the chest when sitting bent forward, with shortness of the breath. [*Fr.*]

Tension on the chest, and pressure in the scrobiculus cordis, often forcing him to take a deep inspiration. [*Rkt.*]

When raising up the body, tension on the left side of the chest, as if those parts were contracted. [*Fr.*]

490. Contractive pains in the sternum, increased by bending forward the head and the upper part of the body. [*Bchr.*]

Drawing pain in the middle of the sternum, when walking. [*Fr.*]

Pressive drawing on the chest, when coughing. [*Fr.*]

Sharp stitches on the chest, on the right side, above the scrobiculus cordis. [*Gr.*]

Fine, eroding, itching shooting, synchronous with the pulse, in the left side, opposite the scrobiculus cordis. [*Gr.*]

495. Dull, pinching stitches under the ribs, below the right axilla. [*Jr.*]

Feeling of rawness and stitches in the chest.

Strongly perceptible beating, as from a large artery, in the right side of the chest. [*Hbg.*]

Stronger heart-beats, almost audible, with anxiety and contractive pains under the sternum. [*Bchr.*]

Pressing, squeezing, contractive heart-beats, with anxiety and spasmodic pains in the sternum and under the ribs. [*Bchr.*]

500. Heart-beats, hardly perceptible. [TROSCHEL; GUIBERT.]

Great heat externally on the chest, as if he stood undressed before a warm stove, soon followed by coolness about the chest. [*Hbg*]

From violent exertion of the arm, he at once feels a cutting pressure on the opposite side of the chest, anteriorly in the region of the third rib, externally. [*Fr.*]

---

[1] A standing symptom with the patient.—*Hughes.*
[2] Not found.—*Hughes.*
[3] Not accessible.—*Hughes.*

Pain in the sacrum, when stooping.

Pain in the sacrum as if bruised, when starting to move after lying down.

505. Pain as from bruising in the sacrum, when blowing the nose.

Tearing and sharp shooting in the sacrum, on moving. [*Jr.*]

Pain in the back, on the left side in the region of the lumbar vertebræ, a drawing cutting, diminished by pressing on it with the hand. [*Fr.*]

Tearing, below the right scapula. [*Gr.*]

Obtuse stitches between the scapulæ.

510. Sensation as if from a knock, in the first dorsal vertebra. [*Hbg.*]

Erosive itching on the left side of the loin, inciting him to scratch. [*Gr.*]

Eruption of pimples on the back.

In the nape, a pressive drawing in the occiput, where the cervical muscles are inserted, when bending the head backward. [*Fr.*]

Pain as if excoriated, in the articulation of the first dorsal and the last cervical vertebræ, on bending the neck forward, but not on touching it. [*Fr.*]

515. Cutting pain, with sensation of numbness in the nape, compelling him to draw the head backward, which seems, however, to be prevented by a soft dead part, jammed in between the joint. [*Fr.*]

Tearing and sharp shooting, in the neck, when moving it. [*Jr.*]

Pressive pain in the cervical muscles, as if they were pressed by a bandage.

Stiffness on the nape and the sides of the neck, with a pain pressive by jerks. [*Hbg.*]

Painful stiffness and tension in the neck and the nape, chiefly when moving it. [*Stf.*]

520. Shooting pains in the muscles of the neck, when moving it. [*Bchr.*]

In the axilla, voluptuous itching. [*Fr.*]

The muscles of the arm and shoulder ache with a tensive pressive pain, on moving the arms. [*Stf.*]

Burning on the right arm, as if from excoriation.

Heaviness in the left arm, observable also when at rest.

525. Paralytic weakness in the left arm; he could hardly raise it, nor double up the fist, without pain. [*Hbg.*]

On the upper arm, in its lower part, needle-pricks, continuing even when moving it. [*Rkt.*]

Tearing stitches on the right upper arm, when walking. [*Lgh.*]

Burning shooting in the left arm. [*Hbg.*]

Painfully itching throbbing in the muscles of the upper arm.

530. In the elbow-joint, a tingling sensation, as if the nerve was squeezed together, or as if the arm would go to sleep, also observable when touching the spot. [*Rkt.*]

On the fore-arm, a paralytic pain in the middle of the shaft of the ulna, on extending the arm or when it lies outstretched. [*Fz.*]

Pinching, and sharp, shooting squeezing on the back of the ulna, above the wrist. [*Gr.*]

Severe tearing on the right fore-arm, both at rest and in motion. [*Lgh.*]

Severe stitches in the muscles of the right fore-arm. [*Lgh.*]

535. In the wrist-bones, a paralytic tearing. [*Gr.*]

Paralytic tearing in the right metacarpal bones. [*Gr.*]

Swelling of the right hand and fingers, for three hours at night. [*Myr.*]

Itching on the back of the hand, chiefly at night.

Rash on the dorsum of the hand, without sensation.

540. The fingers frequently become suddenly stiff. [*Jr.*]

Involuntary twitching and drawing outward of the left index. [*Fr.*]

Twitching, paralytic tearing in the right index. [*Gr.*]

Paralytic tearing in the finger-joints, both at rest and in motion. [*Gr.*]

Spasmodic stitches in the ball of the left thumb, both at rest and in motion. [*Lgh.*]

545. Burning shooting in the left thumb, just above the nail, aggravated by pressing upon it. [*Fr.*]

Numbness and insensibility of the last three fingers and half of the ball of the right hand (aft. sev. weeks). [*Jr.*]

The fingers tend to go to sleep frequently. [*Jr.*]

The nates go to sleep in the evening, in sitting, and become as if dead. [*Fr.*]

Slow drawing above the nates. [*Fr.*]

550. The lower limbs ache, on starting to move after lying down, as if bruised, both in the thighs and legs.

Great stiffness in the joints of the lower limbs, after sitting in a carriage, it goes off through walking.

Weakness and lassitude of the lower limbs, with trembling. [*Rkt.*]

Asthenia and paralyzed weakness of the lower limbs. [*Hbg.*]

In the thigh on the anterior side, a pain more pressive than drawing, which gradually increased and again diminished. [*Hbg.*]

555. Drawing on the inner side of the thigh, when sitting. [*Fr.*]

Pressive drawing in the anterior muscles of the thigh. [*Fr.*]

Cramplike drawing in the muscles of the thigh above the hough, when sitting, it goes off after some walking. [*Fr.*]

Cutting in the thigh, on crossing the legs; it goes off in uncrossing them. [*Fr.*]

Sharp stitches on the thigh, somewhat above the left knee, on the outer side. [*Gr.*]

560. Painful itching throbbing in the muscles of the thigh.

Eroding itching on the upper and interior part of the thigh. [*Gr.*]

In the knees, sensation as of great weariness, in going upstairs. [*Bchr.*]

Painless stiffness on the outer condyle of the knee-joint, as from an internal swelling, with sensation of coldness. [*Fr*]

Tension in the houghs; which prevents their being straightened. [*Fr.*]

565. The legs are tired, and he has to stretch them continually. [*Hbg.*]

Sore pain in left leg, when standing, as if it was shattered. [*Fr.*]

Pain as from weariness in the tibiæ and knees, as after a long foot-tour, when walking. [*Bchr.*]

Heaviness in the left leg, as it were in the shaft of the tibia, interfering with walking.

Drawing on the shaft of the left tibia, as if a part of it was torn out. [*Fr.*]

570. Twitching of the muscles under the left hough, synchronous with the pulse, going off when touched. [*Fr.*]

Sharp stitches on the outer side of the tibia, below the knee, both at rest and in motion. [*Gr.*]

Burning in the right calf, when he lays it over the other leg. [*Fr.*]

Eroding itching on the leg above the outer ankle of the foot. [*Gr.*]

The ankle-joint pains when extended, as if strained. [*Fr.*]

575. Sharp stitches in the sole of the right foot, so acute, that the whole limb twitches, in the evening. [*Fr.*]

Itching on the dorsum of the right foot, chiefly at night.

The trunk and the limbs, but especially the thighs, are painfully stiff (10th d.). [*Jr.*]

General soreness of the whole body. [PENKIVIL.]

Piercing pain in the joints.

580. Pain of all the joints, as if broken on the wheel, after the noon-siesta.

Drawing in the back, the upper and lower limbs, and the fingers, as after a cold [*Rkt.*]

The ailments seem aggravated in the warm room. [*Stf.*]

Eroding itching on various parts of the body, recurring soon after scratching. [*Gr.*]

The eroding itching becomes even worse, if he does not scratch the parts, and is finally heightened into unbearable, burning needle-pricking, which occasionally diminishes, but soon returns worse. [*Gr.*]

585. Tearing, burning and somewhat itching needle-pricks in various parts.

Peeling off of the skin of the whole body. [V. HALLER, in *Vicat.*, *mat. med.* I, p. 112.[1]]

Tickling of the affected part. [QUARIN.]

Tight, white swelling of the whole body, with great painfulness at every touch; after many weeks it goes off, becoming soft and passing into anasarca. [KURTZ, in *Jahn's med. Convers.*, *Bl.*, 1830.[2]]

---

1 Statement.—*Hughes.*

2 Not found.—*Hughes.*

Tight, painful swelling, first of the legs, and then also of the hands and fore-arms, only passing off slowly after several months, while the pulse is in no way retarded, and without increased flow of urine. [KURTZ.]

590. General paleness of the skin. [GUIBERT.]

Jaundice. [WITHERING.[1]]

Convulsions of a violent kind. [*Journ. d. Chim.*]

Convulsions. [WITHERING.]

Epileptic fits. [REMER.]

595. Nervous symptoms of every kind, and great debility. [PERCIVAL, *med. facts and exper.*, Vol. I., Lond., 1791, p. 113.[2]]

Emaciation of the body, in proportion as the intellectual activity increases. [MUELLER.]

Feeling of great tightness in the body. [*Fr.*]

Awkwardness and clumsiness of the limbs. [*Pp.*]

Heaviness and indolence of the limbs. [MOSSMANN.]

600. Lazy and weary, in the morning, on rising from bed. [*J. Lhm.*]

Lack of tone of all the muscles, with a sensation as if he had not slept enough. [*Fr.*]

Lassitude, unbending and weariness, in bodily and in mental respects. [JOERG.]

Great lassitude in the arms and legs. [*Jr.*]

Frequent lassitude; she has to lie abed, because sitting up tires her. [PENKIVIL.]

605. Extreme languor. [MACLEAN.]

Considerable degree of languor, with vertigo and intermitting pulse. [DRAKE.]

Sinking of the vital powers.

Weakness, sinking of the strength. [WITHERING.]

General weakness. [TROSCHEL; LETTSOM.]

610. General weakness, as if all parts of the body were tired out (aft. 2 h.). [*Hbg.*]

Great weakness. [NEUMANN; PERCIVAL.]

Extreme weakness. [GUIBERT.]

Extreme weakness and lassitude, which the patient thinks he cannot bear without dying. [DRAKE.[3]]

Weakness, as if to death. [MACLEAN.]

615. Sudden sinking of the strength, with general sweat, and a few hours later, cough.

Sudden, extreme weakness, as if he would lose his consciousness, with general heat and sweat, without thirst (after dinner).

Relaxation of the vital powers and tendency to fainting. [DRAKE.]

Tendency to syncopes. [NEUMANN.]

Great tendency to syncopes. [DRAKE.]

620. Constant tendency to fainting fits. [MACLEAN.]

Syncopes. [GUIBERT; TROSCHEL.]

---

[1] This occurred in several of Withering's patients, but always in the natural sequence of their maladies and never as traceable to D.—*Hughes.*

[2] Effects of D. in hydrocephalus.—*Hughes.*

[3] The original has: "Much languor and sense of faintness; the patient says, he would rather die than endure it.—*Hughes*

Syncopes, between the attacks of nausea. [WITHERING.]

Deadly apoplexy. [SCHERWEN, in *Med. and Phys. Journ.* III., 207.[1]]

Death after twenty-two hours. [*Journ. d. Chim.*]

625. Frequent yawning and stretching, with chilliness. [*Stf.*]

Drowsy weariness; slumber.

Frequent drowsiness. [DRAKE.]

Frequent great drowsiness. [MACLEAN.]

Coma. [GUIBERT; *Journ. d. Chim.*]

630. Somnolence, interrupted by violent, convulsive fits of vomiting. [TROSCHEL.]

Early drowsiness in the evening, with indolence and stupor of the spirit, for several days. [*Pp.*]

A deep sleep. [MACLEAN.[2]]

Deep sleep from noon till midnight. [*Journ. d. Chim.*]

Difficult going to sleep (6th, 7th d.). [*Jr.*]

635. Before going to sleep, frequently a sensation of great emptiness in the stomach. [*Jr.*]

Uneasy sleep. [JOERG.]

Uneasy, unrefreshing sleep. [JOERG.]

At night, merely slumber, instead of sleep, with clear consciousness, without being able to sleep soundly.

Restless sleep, with tossing about and waking up half conscious. [*Rkt.*]

640. Restless sleep, he could not lie on any other spot but on his back. [*J. Lh.*]

At night, violent pain in the left shoulder-joint and the elbow-joint; in a half-conscious sleep, lying on his back, the left arm over his head. [*Rkt.*]

At night, tossing about with frequent awaking, at the same time, he always lies on his back, with frequent pollutions. [*Pp.*]

At night, restless sleep, owing to constant urging to urinate. [*Myr.*]

Restless sleep, with tossing to and fro in bed, with merry dreams. [*Hbg.*]

645. Many, not disagreeable dreams. [*Hbg.*]

Many confused, vivid dreams. [*Pp.*]

Disagreeable dreams of many miscarried projects, disturb his sleep. [*Lgh.*]

Anxious, confused dreams. [*Jr.*]

Frequent awaking, as from anxiety, and impression that it was already time to get up.

650. **Frequent waking in a fright at night**, owing to his dreaming, that he was falling down from a height or falling into water. [*Lgh.*]

Febrile state. [QUARIN.[3]]

Small, quick, hard pulse.

---

[1] From an overdose. The reporter writes: "He was suddenly and unexpectedly carried off, with all the dreadful distress and jactitation which an overdose of D. sometimes produces. His death was pretty generally ascribed to apoplexy, and was indeed truly apopletic." —*Hughes.*

[2] Curative effect.—*Hughes.*

[3] Not found.—*Hughes.*

Small, soft pulse. [JOERG.]

Irritated pulse. [KRAUS.]

655. Quick pulse, of one hundred beats, before his death. [WITHERING.[1]]

Quickened pulse (aft. 1 h.). [JOERG.]

First quickened, then retarded pulse. [JOERG.]

Irregular, small pulse. [GUIBERT; TROSCHEL.]

Irregular pulse; unequal distension of the arteries. [JOERG; NEUMANN.]

660. Irregular, weak pulse. [*Journ. d. Chim.*]

Irregular and slow pulse. [NEUMANN.[2]]

Slow pulse of fifty beats, which were quite irregular, always between three or four soft beats, one full and hard beat, on the first day; on the third, seventy-five beats. [*Fr.*]

The slow, small pulse frequently makes shorter or longer pauses. [*Bchr.*]

The pulse is at first slow, then suddenly commences to make a couple of beats, or it now and then loses a whole beat. [MACLEAN.]

665. Slow, irregular pulse, from forty to fifty-eight beats. [BAKER.[3]]

Slow pulse. [LENTIN.[4]]

Extremely slow pulse the first forty-eight hours; but then the more accelerated and suppressed. [LETTSOM *[5]]

Slower, but stronger pulse. [*Hbg.*]

Retardation of the pulse from one hundred to forty beats. [MOSSMANN.]

670. Retarded pulse of forty beats. [WITHERING.]

Retardation of the pulse from eighty-two to thirty-nine beats, with weakness and laziness of the body. [*Bchr.*]

Slow pulse, sunk to fifty and then to thirty-five beats. [WITHERING.]

Retardation of the pulse by one-half, for several days.

Retardation of the pulse beats to almost half their number. [BAKER.]

675. When the pulse has become slow, it is accelerated by the slightest bodily exertion. [MACLEAN.]

The pulse is retarded little when standing and sitting, but chiefly when lying, when it sinks down to sixty, while it is one hundred when he stands. [BAIDON, in *Edinb. Med. Journ.* III., 11, No. 4, p. 271.[6]]

*The most usual and assured phenomenon from foxglove is, that after the preliminary slowness of the pulse (primary action), after some days the reverse (reaction or secondary action), a much quicker and smaller pulse, is permanently induced by the vital force. This shows how much the physicians of the old school are at fault, who endeavor to produce a permanently slower pulse by foxglove, and thus frequently kill.

[1] Subsequent to S. 672.—*Hughes.*

[2] The original has: "Pulse suddenly quickened for a few beats, then slow again; or it loses a whole beat."—*Hughes.*

[3] The original instead of "40 to 58" has "48 to 56" beats.—*Hughes.*

[4] Not found.—*Hughes.*

[5] Instead of "*unterdrueckt* (suppressed)" the original has "quicker and proportionately weaker."—*Hughes.*

[6] Statement from observation.—*Hughes.*

Chilliness. [*Stf.*]

Excessive sensitiveness to cold. [*Pp.*]

Constant chilliness, chiefly in the back. [*Rkt.*]

680. **Coldness of the limbs.** [GUIBERT; TROSCHEL.]

Internal coldness in the whole body. [*Gr.*]

Coldness, first of the fingers, then of the palms and the soles of the feet, then of the whole body, and especially of the limbs.

Coldness, first in the arms and hands, then in the whole body. [*Bchr.*]

Coldness of the body, with clammy sweat. [WITHERING.[1]]

685. Coldness in the whole body, also observable externally, with warm face. [*Bchr.*]

Coldness of one hand, with warmth of the other. [*J. Lh.*]

Coldness and chill, internally and externally, in the whole body. [*Gr.*]

Internal chill by day; he could not get warmed by walking.

Chilliness in the back. [*Bchr.*]

690. Internal chilliness in the whole body, while the heat externally observable is increased. [*Gr.*]

Shivering over the back. [*Myr.*]

Shivering, three or four times in the afternoon; the following night, sweat, even on the head and on the hair.

Increased warmth in the face. [JOERG.]

Increased warmth all over the body. [JOERG.]

695. Sudden warmth all over the body, which quickly vanished, leaving behind a weakness of all the parts. [*Bchr.*]

Frequent warmth all over the body, with cold sweat on the forehead; thirteen or fourteen hours after the coldness. [*Bchr.*]

Fever: first shivering, then heat, then profuse perspiration. [MOSSMANN.]

With slight chilliness of the back, there is burning of the head, the face and the ears, with redness of the cheeks; at the same time the left eye is much smaller (after a meal, in the room). [*Stf.*]

Chill all over the body, with heat and redness of the face. [*Tth.*]

700. The palms are warm and perspire. [*Hbg.*]

Night-sweat during sleep.

In the morning, on waking, a slight general perspiration [*Lgh.*]

[1] Not found.—*Hughes.*

DULCAMARA. SOLANUM DULCAMARA.

(BITTERSWEET.)

This medicine has a long duration of action, and its excessive action is moderated by camphor.

It is said to have shown itself useful thus far in diseases in which the following were some of the ailments: Boring and burning in the forehead; sensation as if there was a board before the forehead; scrofulous inflammation of the eyes; incipient amaurosis; crusta lactea; cough with hoarseness; catarrh of the bladder, with urinary troubles; a sort of whooping cough, after taking a cold; tearing pains in the limbs after a cold; humid, suppurating herpes; herpetic eruption, with glandular swellings, etc.

It will be found sp cific in some epidemic fevers, also in various acute diseases brought on by cold.

The abbreviations of the names of my fellow provers are: *Ar.*, *Ahner; Cbz.*, *Cubitz; Gr.*, *Gross; Mr.*, *Mueller* from *Treuen; Ng.*, Anonymous prover in *Hartlaub* and *Trinks' Reine Arzneimittellehre;* and that work itself: *Htb. und Tr.; Rkt.*, *Rueckert* the elder; *Stf.*, *Stapf; Wr.*, *Gust. Wagner; Whl.*, *Wilh. Wahle.*

DULCAMARA.

Very ill-humored, not disposed to do anything for several days. [*Ng.*]

Quarrelsome disposition, in the afternoon, without getting vexed. [*Ng.*]

Impatient, in the morning, he stamped his feet, wanted to throw everything away, began to be delirious, and at last to weep [STARK in *Carrere, ueber d. Bittersuess. Jen.*, 1782.[1]]

Restlessness. [CARRERE, l. c.[2]]

5. Delirious talk. [DE HAEN, *rat. med.* IV., p. 288.]

Delirium, at night, with increased pains. [CARRERE.[3]]

Insane phantasies and delirium. [STARK.]

Save for eight additional symptoms this pathogenesis is identical with that given in Vol. I of the *Materia Medica Pura* (3d ed., 1830); and the latter, save for the fifty-two symptoms by which it exceeds the symptom-list of 1822, and which are mainly Nenning's (obtained as already described under Agaricus), belongs to Hahnemann's earlier manner of working.—*Hughes.*

[1] This is Carrere's German translator. His work is not accessible, but Roth says that his symptoms are of the same kind as Carrere's own (see below).—*Hughes.*

[2] Carrere's original work is "*Traite des propriete's, usages, et effects de la Douce-amere, Paris*, 1789." The citations have been corrected from this treatise. They consist of the effects of D. when given for chronic rheumatism, suppressed secretions and cutaneous diseases. The author says that he has, after seventeen years' experience with the medicine, seen no inconvenience result from full doses, save those described in S. 70, 96 and 297, S. 216, S. 4, 376 (sometimes the precursor of a new eruption, and then associated with 359 and 360); S. 30 and 71; and S. 109.—For this symptom see note to S. 361.—*Hughes.*

[3] Not found—*Hughes.*

Stupid feeling in the head, as after intoxication; it goes off in the open air. [*Wr.*]

Stupid and chaotic feeling in the head, in the evening. [*Ng.*]

10. Stupid feeling in the head, with drawing, in the protuberance of the forehead. [*Ng.*]

Stupid feeling and painful stupefaction of the head.

Stupefaction of the head. [CARRERE.]

Violent stupefaction. [STARK.]

Tipsiness in the head, with warmth rising up in the whole face. [*Ng.*]

15. Vertigo. [ALTHOF in *Murray*, *Appar. Med.* I., 621.[1]]

Momentary vertigo. [PIQUOT, *Samml. br. Abhandl.*[2]]

Slight, quickly transient vertigo. [*Ng.*]

Vertigo, in the morning, on rising from bed, so that he almost fell, with trembling of the whole body and general weakness. [*Mr.*]

Vertigo while walking, at noon, before dinner, as if all objects stood still before him, and things turned black before his eyes.

20. Headache, in the morning in bed, aggravated by rising. [*Mr.*]

Headache in the occiput, in the evening in bed. [*Whl.*]

Headache, with laziness, icy coldness of the whole body and inclination to vomit. [*Mr.*]

Obtuse headache in the forehead and the root of the nose, as if he had a board before his head. [*Gr.*]

Obtuse headache, chiefly in the left frontal protuberance. [*Ng.*]

25. The dull, pressive headache becomes worse in the evening, with increasing coryza. [*Ng.*]

Stupefying pain in the head, just above the left ear, as if somebody pressed with a blunt instrument into the head. [*Gr.*]

Stupefying, pressive pain in the occiput, upward from the nape. [*Rkt.*]

Stupefying, pressive pain in the left upper part of the head. [*Ng.*]

Stupefying headache for ten days. [*Ng.*]

30. Heaviness of the head. [CARRERE.]

Heaviness in the forehead (aft. 12 h.). [*Whl.*]

Heaviness in the forehead, for several days, with stitches in the temporal region, from within outward. [*Whl.*]

Heaviness in the occiput, for three days. [*Whl.*]

Heaviness of the whole head, throughout the day, as if the integuments of the head were stretched, especially in the nape, where the sensation turns into formication. [*Whl.*]

35. Heaviness of the head, with pain boring outward in the temple and forehead, as after a nocturnal spree. [*Wr.*]

Pressure, as with a peg (a blunt instrument), in the temples, now on the right, then on the left side. [*Gr.*]

Pressure, as with a blunt instrument, always on various small spots on the head. [*Gr.*]

---

[1] Statement from observation.—*Hughes.*
[2] Statement from observation.—*Hughes.*

Intermitting pressure on the left of the crown, as with a blunt instrument, from without inward. [*Gr.*]

Pressive pain in the left part of the occipital bone. [*Whl.*]

40. Headache, pressing outward, while taking a walk, toward evening. [*Whl.*]

Pain in the left frontal protuberance, pressing outward, quite late in the evening. [*Ng.*]

Pressing outward, by jerks, in the sinciput, worse on moving. [*Ng.*]

Tearing compression in the upper part of the head. [*Gr.*]

Pressive, tensive pain in the head, above the right eye (aft. 3 h.). [*Wr.*]

45. Drawing in the head, from both temples inward. [*Whl.*]

Drawing pain on the vertex down into the nasal bones, where it becomes contractive, when eating in the evening. [*Whl.*]

Drawing downward, in quick, twitching jerks, from the frontal protuberance into the tip of the nose. [*Gr.*]

Drawing, in the left frontal protuberance, especially when stooping forward. [*Ng.*]

Slow, drawing pain through the whole brain, especially in the evening (aft. ¼ h.).

50. Pressive drawing in the left frontal protuberance. [*Ng.*]

Pressive drawing in the left temporal region, in the afternoon. [*Ng.*]

Tearing in the left temple, intermitting. [*Gr.*]

Intermitting, pressive tearing in the temples. [*Gr.*]

Stitches in the head, so as to make her angry, chiefly in the evening; relieved by lying down.

55. Violent shooting in the sinciput, deep in the brain, with nausea. [*Mr.*]

Slow pricking in the occiput, as from a needle, that was always drawn back again. [*Whl.*]

Digging headache, deep in the sinciput, with gloominess and sensation of inflation in the brain; at once in bed in the morning, and worse after rising. [*Mr.*]

Digging and pressing in the whole extent of the forehead. [*Gr.*]

Boring headache in the right temple. [*Whl.*]

60. Boring headache, from within outward, before midnight. [*Whl.*]

Boring headache, from within outward, now in the forehead, then in the temples. [*Wr.*]

Boring pain, from within outward, in the right half of the forehead, above the arch of the eyebrow. [*Whl*]

Heat in the head. [CARRERE.]

A painful, pressive throbbing in the left side of the forehead, with a whirling feeling. [*Ng.*]

65. Sensation as if the occiput had enlarged. [*Whl.*]

On the margin of the orbit, a contractive pain. [*Gr.*]

Pressure in the eyes, much aggravated by reading. [*Rkt.*]

Inflammation of the eyes. [TODE; STARK.[1]]

[1] No reference given for Tode and he cannot be traced.—*Hughes.*

A sort of paralysis of the upper eyelid, as if it would close down. [*Mr.*]

70. Twitching of the eyelids, in the cold air. [CARRERE.]

Dimness of vision. [CARRERE.[1]]

Incipient amaurosis, and such dim-sightedness, that he saw all things as through a veil. [*Mr.*]

Sparks before the eyes. [PIQUOT.]

Sensation as if fire darted from the eyes, when walking in the sun and in the room.

75. Otalgia all night, so that he could not sleep; in the morning the pain ceased suddenly, except some rushing sound, which still continued. [*Htb. u. Trs.*]

Straining pain in the left ear; with great nausea. [*Htb. u. Trs.*]

Straining in the right ear, with little stitches. [*Whl.*]

Tearing in the left ear, with stitches from within outward; with a drumming and bubbling before the ear, so that he cannot hear well; on opening the mouth, there is crepitation as if something was broken. [*Htb. u. Trs.*]

Transient drawing, in the external meatus. [*Gr.*]

80. Pricks in the meatus auditorius and in the parotid gland. [*Rkt.*]

Pinching stitch in the left ear, toward the membrana tympani. [*Whl.*]

Pricking in the ears, as if cold air had gotten into it. [*Whl.*]

Ringing in the ears.

Ringing in the ears. [*Rkt.*]

85. Clear ringing in the ears (aft. 4 to 8 d.). [*Stf.*]

Pimples in the angles of the nose.

In the inner side of the left ala nasi, a pimple with ulcerative pain. [*Whl.*]

Epistaxis. [STARK.]

Bleeding of the nose, with a strong flow of bright-red, very warm blood, with a pressure in the region of the longitudinal sinus, which pressure also continued even after the bleeding. [*Ng.*]

90. Spasmodic contraction in the face, below the left ear, toward the ramus of the lower jaw. [*Jr.*]

Painless pressure on the left zygoma (at once). [*Gr.*]

Drawing and tearing in the whole cheek.

Itching on the cheek, close by the alæ nasi.

Humid eruption on the cheek. [CARRERE.[2]]

95. Lumps and blotches on the forehead, with stinging pain when touched.

In the lips, twitching movements, in the cold air. [CARRERE.]

Pimples and ulcers about the mouth, with tearing pains on moving the parts.

On the lower part of the chin in a small spot, pinching pain. [*Gr.*]

Itching pimples about the chin.

---

[1] With S. 30.—*Hughes.*

[2] Not found.—*Hughes.*

100. The teeth are dull and as if without sensation. [*Mr.*]

The gums are loose and spongy.

In the mouth, on the inside of the upper lip, on the anterior part of the palate, pimples and small ulcers, which on moving the parts give rise to tearing pains.

Itching tingling on the tip of the tongue. [*Whl.*]

Dry tongue. [CARRERE.]

105. Dry, rough tongue. [CARRERE.[1]]

Paralysis of the tongue. [GOUAN, *Mém. d. l. Soc. d. Montpell.*[2]]

Paralysis of the tongue, after taking it for a long time. [LINNÆUS, *diss. de Dulcamara.*[3]]

Paralysis of the tongue interfering with speaking (in cold damp weather). [CARRERE.]

Pains in the throat. [CARRERE.]

110. Pressure in the throat, as if the uvula was too long.

Sensation of increased warmth in the fauces. [*Rkt.*]

Flow of saliva. [CARRERE.[4]]

Flow of saliva, with loose, spongy gums. [STARK.]

Flow of much viscid, soapy saliva. [STARK.]

115. Constant hawking up of very viscid mucus, with much scraping in the fauces. [*Ng.*]

Insipid, soapy taste in the mouth, with lack of appetite. [STARK.]

Hunger, with aversion to every kind of food.

Good appetite, and the food tastes good, but he is at once satiated and full, with much rolling and rumbling in the abdomen. [*Gr.*]

When eating, inflation of the stomach and repeated pinching in the abdomen. [*Gr.*]

120. After a moderate meal, at once inflation of the abdomen.

Repeated eructation while eating, so that the soup he has swallowed at once comes back up his throat. [*Gr.*]

Empty eructation, with shuddering, as if from loathing. [*Ng.*]

Frequent empty eructation. [*Gr.*]

Frequent eructation, with scraping in the œsophagus and heartburn. [*Ng.*]

125. Much eructation. [*Mr.*]

Eructation combined with hiccup. [*Gr.*]

Nausea. [ALTHOF; LINNÆUS.]

Nausea and loathing. [CARRERE.]

Loathing, with shuddering, as if vomiting would come. [*Ng.*]

130. Great nausea, as if he would vomit, with chilliness. [*Htb. u. Trs.*]

Retching. [ALTHOF.]

Waterbrash.

Vomiting. [LINNÆUS.]

Vomiting, with nausea, heat and anguish. [STARK.]

---

[1] See note to S. 361.—*Hughes.*

[2] Not accessible.—*Hughes.*

[3] Not accessible. According to Murray this is only a citation of Gouan (S. 106) not an independent observation.—*Hughes.*

[4] Not found.—*Hughes.*

135. Vomiting of mucus, in the morning, after previous warm rising in the fauces.

Vomiting of mere viscid mucus. [*Ng.*]

In the region of the stomach, a constant pinching, in the evening, after lying down, till going to sleep. [*Ng.*]

Pressure in the stomach, extending up into the chest.

Painful, pressive aching in the scrobiculus cordis, as from a blow, worse when pressing upon it. [*Ahr.*]

140. Sensation of inflation in the scrobiculus cordis, with a disagreeable sensation of emptiness in the stomach. [*Ng.*]

Tensive pain on the right, near the scrobiculus cordis, as if he had strained or otherwise injured himself. [*Whl.*]

The stomach is squeezed together, so as to intercept respiration.

Shooting pain in the scrobiculus cordis. [*Ahr.*]

Obtuse stitch on the left side, near the scrobiculus cordis. [*Ahr.*]

145. Pain in the abdomen (at once).

Sensation of distention and restlessness in the abdomen, with frequent eructation of air. [*Ng.*]

Distention of the abdomen after a moderate meal, as if it would burst. [*Gr.*]

Sudden, cutting contraction in the left side of the abdomen. [*Gr.*]

Pinching pain in the abdomen, close below the navel, on sitting bent forward; on stretching himself, this diminishes and ceases. [*Ahr.*]

150. Pinching pain about the umbilical region, as if he must go to stool, but without any urging. [*Ahr.*]

Pinching pain in the umbilical region and above the left hip, that compels him to go to stool; after the passage of some flatus, and with a diminution of the pains, only a little hard fæces is passed with straining. [*Ahr.*]

Pinching in the evening in the whole hypogastrium, with call to stool. [*Gr.*]

Obtuse pinching in the abdomen, as if diarrhœa was coming on. [*Ng.*[1]]

155. Fine pinching in the abdomen on a small spot, to the left above the navel. [*Gr.*]

Violent pinching in the abdomen, as if a long worm was crawling up and down it, and gnawed and pinched it. [*Ahr*]

Transient pinching and cutting in the abdomen and chest; as from accumulated flatus. [*Gr.*]

Transient pinching and cutting in the abdomen, with distention there, at once in the morning, while fasting. [*Gr.*]

Transient pinching and twitching cutting, here and there, in the abdomen. [*Gr.*]

60. Digging, pinching, cutting and moving about in the abdomen, as if diarrhœa was coming on. [*Gr.*]

Writhing, digging and pinching about the umbilical region (aft. 10 h.). [*Ahr.*]

[1] One number between 150 and 155 omitted in the original. - *Translator.*

Gnawing, throbbing close above the navel. [*Gr.*]

Shooting pain in the umbilical region (aft. 1 h.). [*Ahr.*]

A pinching, lancinating pain in the right side, beside the navel (aft. 4 d.). [*Ahr.*]

165. Obtuse stitches, outward, in quick succession, on a small spot to the left in the abdomen, taking away the breath, with a sensation as if something was forcing its way out; on pressing on it the spot aches. [*Gr.*]

Dull stitches in the right side of the abdomen, below the ribs, taking away the breath. [*Gr.*]

Obtuse, intermitting stitches in the left side of the abdomen, increased by pressing with the finger on the painful spot. [*Gr.*]

Obtuse, short stitches, to the left, beside the navel, in the evening. [*Ng.*]

Single, throbbing stitches, on the left side, below the short ribs, when sitting; it goes off by rising. [*Ahr.*]

170. Pain forcing outward below the navel, to the left, as if a hernia was forming. [*Stf.*]

Sensation of emptiness in the abdomen.

Pains in the abdomen, as from a cold.

Pains in the abdomen, as if he had taken a cold. [*Whl.*]

Pains in the abdomen, as are wont to come in cold, damp weather. [*Whl.*]

175. **Bellyache, as if diarrhœa was coming on.**

Bellyache, as from a coming diarrhœa; it goes off on discharge of flatus. [*Whl.*]

Bellyache, as after a purgative, with a gushing about in the bowels every time he stoops forward. [*Ng.*]

Bellyache, as if a stool was coming, with rumbling and pain in the sacrum. [*Ng.*]

Tension in the groin, in the region of the os pubis, on rising from the seat.

180. In the inguinal glands, a pressive pain, now in the left, now in the right side.

Swelling of the left inguinal gland as large as a walnut.

Swelling of the glands of the groin. [CARRERE.[1]]

The inguinal glands are swollen hard, of the size of a white bean, but painless. [*Whl.*]

Severe burning (and some shooting) in the bubo at the least motion, and on touching it.

185. Growling in the abdomen (at once).

Growling in the abdomen, as if a stool was coming, with some pain in the sacrum. [*Ng.*]

Growling in the abdomen, pain in the left groin, and feeling of coldness in the back. [*Ng.*]

Growling in the abdomen, with call to stool.

Much discharge of flatus. [*Whl.*]

Flatus smelling of asafœtida. [*Mr.*]

Call to stool in the evening, with pinching in the whole hypogastrium, and then a large moist, and lastly quite thin, sour-smelling

[1] During treatment of scrofula with D., there supervened S. 395 going on to 398, and followed by swelling of the inguinal glands, and also those of the neck and axillæ. The continued use of D. removed them all.—*Hughes.*

[2] 194, 195, 196 critical.—*Hughes.*

ing stool, whereupon he felt relieved but exhausted; during the afternoon, he had had his usual stool, but very hard and difficult. [*Gr.*]

Soft stool (at once).

Soft stool in small lumps. [*Whl.*]

Slimy stool with lassitude. [CARRERE.[1]]

195. White, slimy, diarrhœic stool. [CARRERE.[1]]

Slimy diarrhœic stools, alternately yellow and green. [CARRERE.[1]]

Several successive afternoons, thin evacuations with flatus (aft. 3 d.).

Normal stool, but with some straining (aft. ¾ h.). [*Ng.*]

Hurried call to stool, which he could hardly hold back, although only little and hard fæces came away (aft. ½ h.). [*Ahr.*]

200. Suddenly an immense pressure on the rectum, so that he can scarcely keep back the motion; and yet after sitting down, the very hard fæces come away only after a while, with severe straining, with transient pinching and cutting here and there in the abdomen. [*Gr.*]

Ineffectual call to stool, the whole day, with nausea (aft. ½ h.). [*Mr.*]

Tenesmus with colic; but he is quite costive, and only discharges a little stool, with severe straining (aft. 8 h.). [*Ahr.*]

Difficult, dry, rare stools. [CARRERE.]

Rare, slow and hard stool; even when there is a call to stool, there is no urging in the rectum, and it is only by a great effort that a very large hard motion comes slowly away. [*Gr.*]

205. Before and after the stool, pressive bellyache with rumbling. [*Rkt.*]

Urine, turbid and whitish. [CARRERE.[2]]

Copious discharge of urine, at first viscid and clear, then thick and milk-white. [CARRERE[3]]

Urine at first clear and viscid, then white, then turbid, then clear with white, sticky sediment. [CARRERE.[4]]

Turbid, ill-smelling urine and fetid sweat. [CARRERE.[4]]

210. **Turbid urine.** [CARRERE.[4]]

Reddish, scalding urine. [CARRERE.[5]]

Mucous sediment, now red, now white, in the urine. [CARRERE.[6]]

Pulsating (stitches?) in the urethra outward. [*Whl.*]

Strangury, painful micturition. [STARK.]

215. During micturition, burning in the orifice of the urethra.

On the genitals, heat and itching and excitation to coitus. [CARRERE.]

Tetter-like rash on the labia majora. [CARRERE.[7]]

Increase and anticipation of the menses. [CARRERE.[8]]

---

[1] 194, 195, 196 critical.—*Hughes.*
[2] Critical.—*Hughes.*
[3] Critical. For "viscid" the original "limpid."—*Hughes.*
[4] Critical.—*Hughes.*
[5] Critical. See note to S. 361.—*Hughes.*
[6] Critical.—*Hughes.*
[7] During treatment of "dartrous" vagina and uterus by D.—*Hughes.*
[8] Curative effect.—*Hughes.*

Increased menstrual flux. [CARRERE.]

220. Diminished menstruation. [CARRERE.[1]]

Menstruation delayed, even as many as twenty-five days. [CARRERE.[1]]

* * * * * * * *

Sneezing. [*Whl.*]

Very dry nose, in the evening. [*Ng.*]

Stuffed coryza, with obtuseness of the head and sneezing. [*Ng.*]

225. Short, hacking cough, seemingly excited by taking a deep breath. [*Gr.*]

Cough, with expectoration of tenacious mucus, with shooting in the sides of the chest. [*Mr.*]

Hemoptysis. [CARRERE.[2]]

Oppression of the chest, as after sitting bent forward. [*Whl.*]

Oppression on the chest. [*Whl.*]

230. Severe, oppressive pain in the whole chest, chiefly on respiring. [*Ahr.*]

Intermitting pressure under the whole extent of the sternum. [*Gr.*]

Obtuse, painful pressure, with long intermissions, like shocks, penetrating deep into the chest to the left above the xiphoid cartilage, when sitting bent forward, afterward also in erect posture. [*Gr.*]

Intermittent pain in both sides of the chest below the top of the shoulders, as though violent blows with the fists were delivered there. [*Gr.*]

Intermitting squeezing on a small spot below the upper part of the sternum. [*Gr.*]

235. Tension on the chest, when breathing deeply. [*Whl.*]

He feels as if something was forcing its way out of the chest on the left side, [*Gr.*]

Pinching pain in the chest increased on inspiring. [*Ahr.*]

Undulatory, tearing, pressive pain darts intermittingly through all the left side of the chest. [*Gr.*]

Twitching and drawing under the sternum. [*Gr.*]

240. External tension and drawing on the front of the chest. [*Ng.*]

Twitching pain in the right axilla. [*Ahr.*]

A pulsating pain in the left axilla, going off by movement. [*Ahr.*]

Shooting pain on the sternum. [*Ahr.*]

Painful stab in the left side of the chest, as from a blunt knife, in the region of the fifth and sixth ribs. [*Ahr.*]

245. Painful stitches in the right side of the chest, coming and going quickly. [*Ahr.*]

Dull, slowly intermittent stitches in the left side of the ribs. [*Gr.*]

Dull, shooting pain in the right side of the chest, in the region

---

[1] 220 and 221 ascribed to abundant evacuations.—*Hughes.*

[2] Not found.—*Hughes.*

of the third rib, especially when pressing upon it, thence it spread into the sacrum and up to between the shoulders, where there was a stitch on the border of the left shoulder-blade on inspiring. [*Htb. u. Trs.*]

Obtuse stitch, like a thrust, on the sternum. [*Ahr.*]

Obtuse, stupefying stitch into the chest, under the right clavicle. [*Gr.*]

250. Shooting tearing pain from the middle of the sternum to the spine, when sitting; it went off on rising. [*Ahr.*]

Deeply cutting pain in the left side of the chest, close under the clavicle, going off by pressing on it. [*Ahr.*]

Transient cutting and pinching in the chest, as from accumulated flatus. [*Gr.*]

Digging pain on the right side of the chest, going off by pressing on it. [*Ahr.*]

Digging pain in the chest, or as if he had strained himself in lifting. [*Gr.*]

255. Palpitation, especially at night, violent and observable externally.

Violent palpitation of the heart, it seemed as if he felt the heart beating outside of the thoracic cavity. [*Stf.*]

Pains in the sacrum, as after long stooping. [*Whl.*]

Digging, shooting pain on the left side, near the sacrum. [*Ahr.*]

Under the left crest of the ilium, a digging pain; it went off by pressing on it. [*Ahr.*]

260. Obtuse stitch outward, a kind of forcing out, in both loins, at every inspiration, while sitting bent forward (after a short walk). [*Gr.*]

Pain, as after a blow had been received, above the left hip, close by the lumbar vertebræ (aft. ½ h.). [*Ahr.*]

Deep cutting pain in the right loin, only transiently relieved by pressing on it; later it goes off of itself. [*Ahr.*]

Pain, as if the body should be cut off above the hips, forcing him to move to and fro, without any relief. [*Gr.*]

Digging stitches in the left loin, disappearing when walking, but recurring when sitting. [*Ahr.*]

265. Severe single stabs, in jerks, as with a fork, close above the right hip, beside the lumbar vertebræ. [*Ahr.*]

Dull stitch outward in the left loin, close above the hip, at every breath. [*Gr.*]

Painful stitches in the middle of the spine, when respiring. [*Ahr.*]

Dull, throbbing, intermitting stitches, on the left, beside the spine. [*Gr.*]

Intermittent pressure on the upper part of the nape, to the left by the spine, while lying on the back, in the morning, in bed. [*Gr.*]

270. Agreeable titillation on the outer border of the right scapula. [*Ahr.*]

Tickling stitch in the middle of the right scapula. [*Ahr.*]

Drawing tearing on the outer border of the right scapula (aft. 6 d.). [*Ahr.*]

Intermitting tearing shocks on the outer side of the right scapula. [*Gr.*]

Pain causing stiffness in the muscles of the nape, on turning the head sideways. [*Gr.*]

275. Stiffness in the muscles of the nape. [*Rkt.*]

Pain in the nape, as if the head had lain in a wrong position. [*Whl.*]

Constrictive pain in the muscles of the nape, as if his neck was twisted round. [*Gr.*]

Drawing pain in the muscles on the right side of the neck. [*Mr.*]

Drawing tearing in the right shoulder, above the right hip-joint and above and below the right knee-joint. [*Htb. u. Ts.*]

280. Dull violent pain in the whole of the right arm, as from an apoplectic stroke, it feels heavy like lead, immovable, the muscles are tense and the whole arm cold as if paralyzed; on endeavoring to bend it, and also on touching it, pain in the elbow-joint as if it were bruised; the icy coldness of the arm returned the following morning after twenty-four hours (aft. ½ h.). [*Mr.*]

She could not bring her arms forward or backward, as these movements brought on jerks in the arms.

Twitching in the upper arm, when she bent it and moved it backward; in stretching it, it did not twitch, but the fingers became stiff, so that she could not close them.

The left arm pains as if paralyzed and contused, almost only when at rest, it pains less when in motion, and not at all when touched; but the arm has its proper strength.

Paralytic sensation in the right upper arm; it goes off on violent motion. [*Ahr.*]

285. Pain in the upper arm, in the evening in bed, and in the morning, after rising.

Burning itching, externally on the right upper arm, exciting him to scratch it; the place was red and there was a burning pimple on it. [*Whl.*]

Eroding gnawing on the outer side of the elbow, with brief intermissions. [*Gr.*]

Red pimples in the bend of the elbow, visible in the morning and evening in the warmth of the room, with fine smarting itching, and burning after scratching; for twelve days.

In the right fore-arm, a drawing pain (aft. 3 d.). [*Ahr.*]

290. Obtuse drawing from the left elbow to the wrist, especially observable when bending it. [*Ng.*]

Painful drawing in the shaft of the left ulna, frequently recurring. [*Gr.*]

Suddenly jerking pinching tearing in the middle of the left fore-arm (aft. 12 d.). [*Ahr.*]

A twisting boring, slowly drawing down from the elbow-joint toward the wrist; it goes off by moving the arm, but recurs at once when at rest. [*Ahr.*]

Lack of strength in the left fore-arm, with paralytic sensation, chiefly in the elbow-joint. [*Whl.*]

295. Disagreeable itching on the middle of the right fore-arm, soon recurring after scratching it, to which it compelled. [*Ahr.*]

On the right wrist, a dull stitch, which goes off on motion. [*Ahr.*]

Trembling of the hands (in damp cold weather). [CARRERE.]

Tetter-like eruption, especially on the hands. [CARRERE.[1]]

Much sweat on the palms. [*Whl.*]

300. Warts cover the hands. [*Stf.*]

Redness on the back of the hand, with burning pain, when he gets warm on taking a walk.

Cramplike drawing in the ball of the left thumb, so that he dares not move his thumb. [*Gr.*]

Cramplike twitching in the first phalanx of the right middle finger. [*Gr.*]

On the right buttock, single small stitches. [*Ahr.*]

305. Drawing tearing in the left hip. [*Ahr.*]

Drawing pinching in the right hip (aft. 6 h.). [*Ahr.*]

Drawing shooting in the left hip-joint, extending to the groin, only when walking; at every step, a sensation as if the head of the hip-bone would be dislocated; stretching it out forcibly diminished the pain and causes a sensation as if the femur was thereby restored to its place; but a bruised pain remained for some time, which made him limp (for 14 days). [*Cbz.*]

Falling asleep and weakness of the lower limbs. [CARRERE.]

Twitching of the lower limbs. [CARRERE.[2]]

310. Pain in the thighs.

Shooting tearing in the whole thigh, not going off by pressure. [*Ahr.*]

Pricking as with needles, on the posterior side of the left thigh, close to the knee. [*Ahr.*]

Drawing tearing pain or constant **pain**, now shooting, now pinching, **in both thighs, which vanished in walking**, then changed into weariness and **at once returned on sitting down.** [*Ahr.*]

Drawing in the muscles of the thighs, here and there, with sensitiveness to the touch. [*Ng.*]

315. Drawing pain on the anterior side of the right thigh. [*Ahr.*]

Drawing tearing from the middle of the posterior side of the thigh to the knee-joint. [*Ahr.*]

Drawing paralytic sensation on the front side of the right thigh. [*Ahr.*]

Shooting tearing, extending from the knee-joint up on the thighs, when taking a walk. [*Rkt.*]

Burning itching on the thighs; he has to scratch. [*Whl.*]

320. Knees feel tired out, as after a long foot-tour. [*Ng.*]

Tearing in the knee-joint, when sitting. [*Rkt.*]

On the inner side of the knee, a rhythmical, undulatory pressure. [*Gr.*]

[1] Critical.—*Hughes.*
[2] Not found.—*Hughes.*

On the outer side of the right leg, itching, ending with an itching lancination. [*Whl.*]

Itching on the outer side of the left leg, recurring after scratching. [*Whl.*]

325. Cramp-like, almost cutting drawing, extending down through the left leg. [*Gr.*]

Distention and swelling of the leg and the calf (but not of the foot) with tensive pain and sensation of great weariness toward evening.

Tearing, extending up the right tibia, in the morning. [*Ng.*]

Pain as of weariness in the tibia, as after a brisk walk. [*Whl.*]

A ripping pain draws down the left calf on the posterior side. [*Ahr.*]

330. Tearing pain on the back of the left calf; it went off on moving the foot. [*Ahr.*]

Sudden pricking as of needles in the left calf, and then sensation as if warm blood or water flowed down from that place. [*Ahr.*]

Sensation of numbness in the calf, in the afternoon and evening.

Painful cramp in the left calf, when walking. [*Whl.*]

Burning in the feet.

335. Severe cramp on the inner ankle of the right foot wakes him up at night; he had to walk about, and it then went off.

Drawing tearing, beside the inner ankle of the right foot. [*Ng.*]

Tearing from the outer ankle toward the front of the foot. [*Ng.*]

Cutting pain in the sole of the right foot, not going off by treading. [*Ahr.*]

Pulsating tearing in the left big toe and second toe. [*Whl.*]

340. Intermitting, shooting burning on the toes. [*Gr.*]

Slight twitchings on hands and feet. [CARRERE.]

Convulsions, first in the muscles of the face, then in the whole body. [FRITZE, *Annal. des Klin. Inst.*, in Berlin, III., p. 45.[1]]

Cramp-pain here and there in the limbs, especially in the fingers. [*Gr.*]

Pain in the limbs.

345. Pains, as if from a cold, in various parts of the body. [*Whl.*]

Dull stitches here and there in the limbs and other parts of the body, mostly outward. [*Gr.*]

Violent trembling of the limbs. [CARRERE.[2]]

The symptoms seem by preference to appear in the evening. [*Ng.*]

Violent itching on the whole body. [CARRERE.[3]]

350. Shooting itching on various parts of the body. [CARRERE.]

Itching, pinching stitches on various parts of the body. [*Whl.*]

Burning itching here and there, running quickly to and fro,

---

[1] Statement from observation.—*Hughes.*

[2] Not found.—*Hughes.*

[3] See note to S. 361.—*Hughes.*

like vermin; he has to scratch violently, when it at first increased and then declined; it itches but little by day, only by night, and chiefly from twelve to three o'clock; it causes him to wake up after a short sleep (aft. 14 d.). [*Stf.*]

Severely itching eruption of red spots with white vesicles. [CARRERE.[1]]

Eruption of white nodules (blotches) with red areola, with stinging itching, and with burning after rubbing, on the arms and thighs.

355. Little pimples, itching moderately, on the chest and abdomen. [*Stf.*]

A tetter-like scurf all over the body. [CARRERE.[2]]

Light-red pointed papules on the skin, which after some days filled with pus. [STARKE.]

Red, elevated spots, as from nettles. [CARRERE.[3]]

Red spots on the body. [CARRERE.]

360. Red spots as from flea-bites. [CARRERE.]

Dryness, heat and burning of the skin. [CARRERE.[4]]

Dryness and heat of the skin, constipation and painful retention of urine, with soft, full, slow, and leaping pulse. [CARRERE.[5]]

Sudden swelling of the body and bloatedness of the limbs; at times painful or accompanied by a sensation of falling asleep. [STARKE.]

Emaciation.

365. Laziness; he avoids motion.

Weariness.

Indolence, heaviness and weariness of all the limbs, compelling him to sit or lie down. [*Whl.*]

Sensation of severe bruising in all the limbs, the whole day [*Ahr.*]

Heaviness in the thighs and arms. [*Rkt.*]

370. Great, continuing weakness. [CARRERE.[6]]

Fits of sudden weakness, like fainting fits.

He has to lie down.

Sleepy the whole day, with much yawning. [*Ahr.*]

Great sleepiness, laziness, and yawning. [*Mr.*]

375. Frequent great yawning. [*Gr.*]

Insomnia, restlessness, and twitching. [CARRERE.]

Sleeplessness, ebullition of blood, stinging, and itching of the skin. [CARRERE.]

Restless sleep, with frequent respiration, and interrupted by confused dreams. [*Whl.*]

Restless, interrupted, anxious sleep, full of heavy dreams. [STARKE.]

380. In the evening, on going to sleep, he started up, as if from terror. [*Gr.*]

---

1 On parts affected by *dartres.—Hughes.*

2 Critical. See note to 361.—*Hughes.*

3 On seat of vanished *dartres.—Hughes.*

4 A youth hereditarily dartrous, and in bad health, after taking D. had S. 4, 349, 211, and 105, with hard and tense pulse. Then came S. 356, with relief to all symptoms. D. was continued and he got well.—*Hughes.*

5 Not found.—*Hughes.*

6 After much sweating. *Hughes.*

Violent snoring in sleep, with open mouth (at once).

After midnight, fear and anxiety of the future.

Frightful dreams, which compel him to jump out of his bed (1st n.). [*Whl.*]

Restless sleep after four A. M., no matter how he would lie. [*Ahr*]

385. Tossing about in bed the whole night, with stupid feeling in the head. [*Whl.*]

Restless sleep, he tossed about uncomfortably. [*Stf.*]

Awaking early, he could not go to sleep again; he stretched himself, full of weariness, and lay first on one side, then on the other, because the muscles of the back of the head were as if paralyzed, and he could not lie on them. [*Whl.*]

She wakes up early, as if she had been called, and sees a ghostly figure that seems continually to enlarge and to vanish upward.

Toward morning, a sort of wakefulness, with closed eyes. [*Whl.*]

390. Toward morning, no sleep, and yet fatigued, and, as it were, paralyzed in all the limbs, as after enduring a great heat. [*Whl.*]

At night, no sleep, on account of itching, like flea-bites, on the anterior part of the body and the thighs; with this there is heat and ill-smelling transpiration, without being wet.

Shivering, as from nausea and chilliness, with coldness and sensation of coldness all over the body, so that he could not get warm by the hot stove; with this, shivering from time to time (at once). [*Mr.*]

Double tertian fever. [CARRERE.[1]]

Chill and discomfort in all the limbs. [*Whl.*]

395. Frequent chilliness, heaviness of the head, and general lassitude (after a cold). [CARRERE.[1]]

Chilliness on the back, without thirst, in the open air, especially in a draught. [*Ng.*]

Chilliness over the back, nape and occiput, toward evening (with a sensation like horripilation), for ten days. [*Ng.*]

Dry heat at night. [*Ng.*]

Hot, dry skin with ebullition of blood. [CARRERE.[2]]

400. Burning on the skin of the whole back, as if he was sitting by the hot stove, with sweat in the face and moderate heat. [*Whl.*]

Heat and restlessness. [CARRERE[3].]

Violent fever with violent heat, dryness of the skin and delirium, every day, recurring every fifteen, sixteen hours. [CARRERE.[4]]

Heat and sensation of heat all over the body, especially in the hands, with thirst, and equable, slow, full pulse; then chilliness.

Heat of the body, burning of the face and constipation. [CARRERE.[5]]

---

[1] See note to S. 182.—*Hughes.*
[2] Not found.—*Hughes.*
[3] Not found.—*Hughes.*
[4] Critical.—*Hughes.*
[5] Not found.—*Hughes.*

405. **Sweat for five days and more.** [CARRERE.[1]]

General sweat, especially in the back.

Sweat, at night all over, by day in the axillæ and palms. [CARRERE.[2]]

Profuse morning-sweat all over, but chiefly on the whole head (aft. 20 h.).

Ill smelling sweat, and at the same time copious discharge of clear urine. [CARRERE.[3]]

EUPHORBIUM.

This gum-resin contains about two-fifth of genuine resin. It is the juice of a thick-stemmed perennial plant which exude, swhen the plant is ripped open. Formerly it was chiefly obtained from the *Euphorbia officinarum* growing in the hottest part of Africa, now it is brought to us more frequently from the Canary Isles, being gathered from the *Euphorbia canariensis.*

When chewed, it first appears to be tasteless, but afterwards causes an extremely caustic burning, which is long continued, and can only be removed by rinsing the mouth with oil. The many species of Euphorbium seem to resemble each other closely as to their medicinal virtues.

Euphorbium has been much abused by surgeons of old, being sprinkled on in cases of caries of the bones and in other inactive cutaneous ulcers; it is also still misused to torment men as an ingredient of the continually used vesicatories. It promises, however, to become extremely useful, when internally applied, after having been prepared like other dry drugs in the manner peculiar to Homœopathy. When used in high potencies and in minimal doses, it will accomplish much; as may be seen from the pure symptoms as observed in healthy persons. It seems to deserve additional provings as to its pure symptoms.

Its action continues for several weeks, and its antidote is camphor. Whether lemon juice may be of use in counteracting some of its troublesome symptoms, is yet uncertain.

The abbreviations of the names of my fellow-provers are as follows: *Lgh., Dr. Langhammer; Wl., Dr. Wislicenus; Htb., u. Tr.,* the *Doctors Hartlaub* and *Trinks* in their *Reine Arzneimittellehre.*

The contributors to this pathogenesis—besides the authors cited—are really four in number, Hahnemann himself, Langhammer, Wislicenus and Nenning. The symptoms referred to Hartlaub and Trinks, belong to the last named; those of the three former come from a pathogenesis published in Vol. VI. of the *Archiv* (1826).—*Hughes.*

[1] Critical; in rheumatism.—*Hughes.*

[2] Not found.—*Hughes.*

[3] Not found.—*Hughes.*

EUPHORBIUM.

Melancholy. [TRAGUS, *hist. des Plantes.*]

Anguish, as if he had swallowed poison. [*Wl.*]

Attacks of anxiety. [EHRHARDT, *Pflanzen-Hist.* VII.[1]]

Anxious, apprehensive mood, but not indisposed to work. [*Lgh.*]

5. Serious and quiet, even in company. [*Lgh.*]

Taciturn, introverted, he seeks tranquility, but is disposed to work. [*Lgh.*]

Vertigo, while standing, everything turned around; he felt as if he should fall to the right side. [*Wl.*]

Violent attack of vertigo, when taking a walk; he came near falling to the left side. [*Lgh.*]

Headaches, as if from a spoiled stomach.

10. Stupefying aching in the right half of the head, which then spreads into the forehead. [*Htb. u. Tr.*]

Dull, stupefying, pressive pain in the forehead. [*Htb. u. Tr.*]

Pressive pain in the forehead (aft. 24 h.). [*Wl.*]

Pressure in the right side of the forehead. [*Lgh.*]

Pressure in the left half of the brain.

15. Pressive pain in the occiput. [*Wl.*]

Dull pressure in the forehead, above the left orbit. [*Htb. u. Tr.*]

Pressive, shooting pains below the right parietal bone. [*Wl.*]

Stitch-like headache, especially in the forehead. [*Lgh.*]

Headache, as if the head would be pressed asunder. [*Wl.*]

20. External pressive pain on the forehead, above the left eye, with lachrymation and inability to open the eye for pain. [*Lgh.*]

Tensive pressure in the head, especially on the forehead and in the nape; in every position of the body. [*Lgh.*]

The whole brain and also the zygoma feel as if screwed in a vise, during toothache.

Tearing, resembling vertigo, on the left side of the forehead, on moving the head. [*Lgh.*]

Stitch-like pain on the left side of the forehead. [*Lgh.*]

25. Pressive stitch-pain, externally on the temples. [*Lgh.*]

Pain, as from a bruise, on the left occiput; he could not lie on it. [*Lgh.*]

Little pimples above the right eyebrow, itching, exciting to scratching, with a tip filled with pus and exuding bloody water after scratching. [*Lgh.*]

In the eye, pressure as from sand. [*Htb. u. Tr.*]

Pinching in the left outer canthus. [*Wl.*]

30. Itching in the left outer canthus, it goes off by rubbing. [*Wl.*]

Violent itching on the left lower eyelid, forcing him to rub it. [*Lgh.*]

Smarting in the eyes, with lachrymation.

---

[1] General summary from authors.—*Hughes.*

Pale-red inflammation of the eyelids, with nocturnal secretion of pus, causing them to be glued together. [*Htb. u. Tr.*]

Swelling of the eyelids, with tearing above the eyebrow, on opening the eye. [*Lgh.*]

35. Feeling of dryness in the eyelids, they press upon the eye. [*Wl.*]

Sticky feeling in the right eye, as if it was full of pus. [*Lgh.*]

Eye-gum in the right external canthus. [*Lgh.*]

The right eye is closed by suppuration, in the morning on awaking, so that he can only open it with difficulty. [*Lgh.*]

Heaviness of the eyelids, they tend to close, with reeling sensation in the head. [*Wl.*]

40. Dilated pupil (aft. 6 h.). [*Lgh.*]

Short-sightedness and dim-sightedness, so that he could only recognize the persons he knew, when they were quite near, and then only as if through a veil.

Seeing double; when he sees a man walking, it seems to him as if the same man was walking close behind the first. [*Wl.*]

All objects appear to him in variegated colors. [*Htb. u. Tr.*]

Everything appears to him too large, so that he also in walking lifts his feet up high, as if he had to step over mountains. [*Htb. u. Tr.*]

45. Otalgia in the open air. [*Wl.*]

Ringing in the ears, also when sneezing. [*Lgh.*]

Rushing sound in the ears, at night.

Chirping in the right ear, as from crickets. [*Lgh.*]

Paleness of the face, sallow appearance. [*Wl.*]

50. Jerking tearing in the muscles of the left cheek, almost as in toothache. [*Lgh.*]

Tensive pain in the cheek, as if it were swollen. [*Lgh.*]

Violent burning in the face (from rubbing it with the juice). [*Rust's Magaz.*, XIX., 3, p. 498.[1]]

Erysipelatous inflammation in the face and external head. [SPIELMANN, *Inst. Mat. Med.*, p. 483.[2]]

Red, inflamed swelling of the cheek, with boring, gnawing, and digging from the gums to the ear, and with itching and tingling in the cheek, when the pain is remitted. [*Lgh.*]

55. Red, enormous swelling of the cheeks, with many yellowish blisters thereon, which break open, exuding a yellowish humor (caused by rubbing the juice on it). [*Stf.*]

Erysipelatous, inflammatory swelling of the cheeks, with blisters of the size of peas, containing a yellowish humor (from rubbing the juice on the parts). [RUST.]

Swelling, even of those parts of the face on which the juice had not been rubbed. [RUST.]

Swelling of the left cheek, with tensive pain *per se*, and pain as from a blow when pressing on it. [*Wl.*]

White swelling of the cheeks, œdematous to the touch, for four days. [*Wl.*]

---

[1] From application of Euphorbium peplus to face for freckles.—*Hughes.*
[2] Observations. From local application.—*Hughes.*

60. On the lower lip, pain as from excoriation, on the red part, as if he had bitten on it. [*Lgh.*]

On the chin, a reddish nodule, which, when touched, pains as if pressive, and like a furuncle. [*Lgh.*]

Toothache, aggravated by touching and by chewing, in the left molar of the upper row, next to the last. [*Lgh.*]

Pain as from a boil, in the tooth, when grasping it.

Toothache, when beginning to eat, with chill; a gnawing tearing, at the same time headache as if the head was shattered from toothache, and as if the brain and the zygomata were screwed together as in a vise.

65. Toothache, as if in a vise, in a hollow tooth, with jerks as if it was being torn out. [*Lgh.*]

Pressive toothache in the posterior lower molar of the left jaw, which goes off on biting the teeth together. [*Wl.*]

Dull pressive pain in the second back molar of the left upper row. [*Wl.*]

Shooting pain in the first molar of the left lower jaw. [*Wl.*]

Dull, shooting pain in the posterior molar of the left upper jaw. [*Wl.*]

70. Sensation of dryness in the mouth, without thirst. [*Wl.*]

Much collection of saliva in the mouth. [*Lgh.*]

Collection of saliva, after repeated shiverings of the skin. [*Wl.*]

Collection of saliva, with nausea and shuddering. [*Wl.*]

Excessive gathering of saliva, with salty taste of the saliva on the left side of the tongue. [*Wl.*]

75. Much tenacious mucus in the mouth, after the noon siesta. [*Htb. u. Tr.*]

On the upper part of the palate, a little membrane is detached. [*Lgh.*]

Burning on the palate, as from glowing coals (aft. 5 min.). [*Wl.*]

In the throat, scrapy and rough sensation all the day. [*Wl.*]

Burning in the throat. [ALSTON, *Mat. Med.* II., 431.[1]]

80. Burning in the fauces, extending into the stomach, as if from red pepper, with gathering of saliva in the mouth. [*Wl.*]

Burning in the throat and stomach, as if a flame was streaming out; he had to open the mouth. [*Wl.*]

Burning in the throat, extending to the stomach, with tremulous anxiety, and heat in the whole of the trunk; attended with nausea and running of water from the mouth, with dryness in the cheeks. [*Wl.*]

Inflammation of the œsophagus. [EHRHARDT, *Pflauzen Hist.* VII., p. 293.]

Taste in the mouth as if it was covered inside with a rancid fat. [*Lgh.* [

85. Insipid taste in the mouth, after breakfast, with white-coated tongue. [*Wl.*]

Bitter, astringent taste in the mouth. [*Lgh.*]

---

[1] Local effects of Euphorbium cyparissias.—*Hughes.*

Very bitter taste.

Putrid, bitter taste in the mouth, after drinking beer, which he relished; especially on the back of the tongue. [*Wl.*]

Thirst for cold drinks. [*Lgh.*]

90. Great hunger, while the stomach hangs down relaxed and the abdomen seems collapsed; he ate much and with the greatest appetite (aft. 2 h.). [*Wl.*]

After dinner, great somnolence. [*Htb. u. Tr.*]

Incessant eructation.

Empty eructation. [*Htb. u. Tr.*]

Severe empty eructations.

95. Frequent empty eructation. [*Lgh.*]

Frequent hiccups. [*Lgh.*]

Nausea with shuddering (soon). [*Htb. u. Tr.*]

Nausea in the morning (aft. 24 h.). [*Wl.*]

Vomiting. [MAYERNE, *Syntagma Prax.*[1]]

100. Vomiting and diarrhœa. [EHRHARDT.]

The stomach pains when touched, as if he had received a blow on it. [*Wl.*]

Pressure on the left side of the stomach. [*Wl.*]

Spasmodic pain in the stomach. [*Wl.*]

Spasmodic contraction of the stomach, with eructation of air. [*Wl.*]

105. Contractions of the stomach from all sides toward the middle, as if constricted, with gathering of the saliva in the mouth and nausea. [*Wl.*]

Griping and grasping in the left side of the stomach, with subsequent constriction of the orifice of the stomach, with increased secretion of salty saliva and with shuddering of the skin. [*Wl.*]

Painful griping in the stomach, as if it was being compressed, with subsequent flow of saliva and nausea. [*Wl.*]

Agreeable feeling of warmth in the stomach, as after spirituous liquors (aft. ¾ h.) [*Wl.*]

Burning in the stomach as from red-hot coals. [*Wl.*]

110. Burning in the stomach, as from swallowing pepper. [*Wl.*]

Burning sensation in the scrobiculus cordis, after eating, attended with pressure.

Inflammation of the stomach. [EHRHARDT.]

Relaxation of the stomach; it hangs down relaxed. [*Wl.*]

Bellyache of an extremely violent kind. [EHRHARDT.]

115. Excessive bellyache and inflation. [EHRHARDT.]

Anxious aching as from excoriation in the hypogastrium. [*Htb. u. Tr.*]

Restlessness and heat in the abdomen. [*Htb. u. Tr.*]

Agreeable sensation of heat through the whole intestinal canal, as from spirituous liquors. [*Wl.*]

Sensation of emptiness in the abdomen, as after an emetic, in the morning. [*Wl.*]

120. The abdomen is sunken in, as if he had none, with great hunger. [*Wl.*]

---

[1] Observations.—*Hughes*

Spasmodic flatulent colic, in the morning in bed; the flatus presses against the hypochondria and the thoracic cavity, and causes a spasmodic pressing apart and constriction, which is diminished by turning over, but at once recurred on lying still. [*Wl.*]

The flatulent colic is not relieved until he rests his head on his elbow and knee, after which some flatus is discharged. [*Wl.*]

Pinching pain on the posterior surface of the ilium.

Writhing, twisting through the whole intestinal canal; then a thin stool, with burning itching around the rectum. [*Wl.*]

125. Growling and moving of flatus in the abdomen. [*Htb. u. Tr.*]

Loud rumbling in the left side of the abdomen, as from incarcerated flatus and then passage of flatus. [*Lgh.*]

Much discharge of flatus. [*Htb. u. Tr.*]

In the inguinal region, pressive pain. [*Wl.*]

Tearing pain in the left groin, as from a strain, when standing. [*Lgh.*]

130. Violent pain as from a dislocation or from paralysis in the left groin, extending into the thigh, when stretching the limb after sitting down. [*Htb. u. Tr.*]

Pressing from within ontward in the left flank, with pain as from excoriation, and after urination, it comes also in the right side. [*Htb. u. Tr.*]

Constipation for two days (after-effects).

Hard, difficult stool.

Stool, first natural, then as if fermented and thin, like water. [*Wl*]

135. Soft, scanty stool mixed with little lumps, and fifteen hours later than usual. [*Wl.*]

Pappy stool (aft. 3, 10, 23 h.). [*Lgh.*]

Pappy, yellowish stool. [*Wl.*]

Gluey stool, after previous itching in the rectum, during the urging thereto. [*Wl.*]

Thin stool, after some straining, and at last three hard lumps, discharged without trouble. [*Wl.*]

140. Diarrhœic, profuse stool, after previous itching around the rectum, during call to stool. [*Wl.*]

Diarrhœa, several times a day, with burning at the anus, inflation of the abdomen, and pain in the abdomen, as if from internal excoriation.

Fatal dysentery. [ALEX. BENEDICTUS, Pract. 12, 117.[1]]

In the rectum, severe itching during the call to stool, and after stool (which came five hours too early). [*Wl.*]

Burning pain, as from excoriation, around the rectum. [*Wl.*]

145. Urging to urinate; the urine came by drops, with stitches in the glans, followed by the customary discharge. [*Wl.*]

Strangury. [SPIELMANN.]

Frequent urging to urinate, with slight discharge of urine. [*Lgh.*]

Much white sediment in the urine. [*Wl.*]

---

[1] Poisoning—*Hughes.*

In the urethra, anteriorly, an itching stitch, when not urinating. [*Wl.*]

150. On the tip of the glans, remitting, sharp-cutting stitches, when standing. [*Lgh.*]

On the prepuce, a voluptuous itching, forcing him to rub it, with emission of prostatic juice. [*Lgh.*]

In the testicle, tearing pain.

On the scrotum, a pinching burning pain on the left side.

Erection, while sitting, without cause (aft. 1½ h.). [*Lgh.*]

155. Nocturnal, constant erections, without pollutions, and without lewd dreams. [*Lgh.*]

Emission of prostatic juice from the relaxed penis. [*Lgh.*]

Violent, abortive incitation to sneezing in the left nostril.

Sneezing.

Sneezing on smelling the powder of E. [*Wl.*]

160. Frequent sneezing, without coryza. [*Lgh.*]

Increased flow of mucus from the nose, without any trace of coryza. [*Wl.*]

Fluent coryza, without sneezing. [*Lgh.*]

Fluent coryza, without sneezing. [*Htb. u. Tr*]

Much flow of mucus from the posterior nares. [*Htb. u. Tr.*]

165. Profuse flow of mucus from the nose, without sneezing, with suffocative smarting, extending up into the cavity of the forehead, so that she cannot get any air.

Tussiculation, excited by even a slight tingling in the throat. [*Wl.*]

Violent excitation to short cough, in the upper part of the windpipe. [*Lgh.*]

Cough, rising from a burning tickling in the upper part of the windpipe. [*Wl.*]

Cough, day and night, as from asthma and shortness of breath, followed in the morning by much expectoration.

170. Dry, hollow cough, as if caused by a tickling in the middle of the chest, when at rest. [*Wl.*]

Almost incessant dry cough.

Asthma, as if the chest were not wide enough, with tensive pain in the muscles of the right side of the chest; especially when turning the body to the right, for ten hours. [*Wl.*]

Obstruction to deep breathing, by a sensation as if the left lobe of the lung had become attached. [*Wl.*]

Tensive pain on the left side of the chest, especially when turning the upper part of the body to the right (aft. 2 d.). [*Wl.*]

175. Spasmodic pressing apart of the lower part of the chest. [*Wl.*]

Shooting pressure on the sternum, when sitting and standing. [*Lgh.*]

Shooting in the left side of the chest, when standing and sitting. [*Lgh.*]

Shooting pain in the left side of the chest, when taking a walk, so that he has to stand still. [*Lgh.*]

Continual shooting in the left side of the chest, when sitting; it went off in walking. [*Lgh.*]

180. Intermitting, fine shooting in the left side of the chest, when reading. [*Lgh.*]

Feeling of warmth in the middle of the chest, as if he had swallowed hot food. [*Wl.*]

Pressive pain in the sacrum, while at rest. [*Wl.*]

Jerking, shooting pain in the sacrum. [*Wl.*]

Pain in the back, a pressure in the muscles. [*Wl.*]

185. Spasmodic pain in the dorsal vertebræ, in the morning in bed, while lying on the back. [*Wl.*]

Pinching pain in the left scapula. [*Wl.*]

Intermitting, severe stitches, always in one spot in the middle of the back, when sitting. [*Lgh.*]

In the shoulder-joint, tension, like paralysis, in the morning, after rising, aggravated by motion. [*Wl.*]

Tensive pains in the right shoulder do not allow him to easily raise his arm upward. [*Wl.*]

190. The tensive pains in the right shoulder diminish in walking, but when at rest they at once become again more violent (aft. 3 d.). [*Wl.*]

Pain with stiffness in the right shoulder, especially when stretching toward the left side. [*Wl.*]

Painful drawing in the right shoulder. [*Htb. u. Tr.*]

In the arm, an internal, very painful drawing; as if connected with weakness, especially in the radius, the humerus and in the wrist bones. [*Htb. u. Tr.*]

In the upper arm, a pressive pain on the outer side, above the elbow-joint, in the morning, in bed. [*Wl.*]

195. Pain as from a sprain in the right upper arm, near the elbow-joint, on moving the arm. [*Lgh.*]

Shooting itching on the upper arm, near the elbow. [*Lgh.*]

On the fore-arm, a very painful drawing pain in the shaft of the ulna. [*Htb. u. Tr.*]

Burning itching on the outer side of the left fore-arm. [*Wl.*]

Scarlet-red streaks on the left fore-arm, which itch on being touched with the finger, but when stroked with the finger, they disappear; with a sensation as if a thin string lay under the skin; for several days (aft. 7 d.). [*Wl.*]

200. In the wrist, paralytic pain on moving it. [*Lgh.*]

Intermitting tearing in the muscles of the left hand. [*Lgh.*]

Cramp pain in the muscles of the right hand, near the wrist, especially when this is moved. [*Lgh.*]

Cramp-like drawing in the right hand, when writing. [*Wl.*]

Fine itching on the dorsum of the left hand, forcing him to rub it. [*Lgh.*]

205. Burning itching as from nettles, on the knuckle of the middle joint of the index, with excitation to rubbing. [*Lgh.*]

Pressive pain in the ball of the right thumb, relieved by touch and motion. [*Lgh.*]

The gluteal muscles of the left side are painful when moved, as from a blow. [*Wl.*]

Nocturnal pains in the os ischium.

In the right hip-joint, paralytic pain, when treading on that foot. [*Htb. u. Tr.*]

210. Pain as from contusion, on the anterior part of the hip, only when moving the body while sitting, not when sitting quiet, nor in walking, nor when touched. [*Lgh.*]

Pain as from a sprain, in the hip-joint, on both sides.

Pressive pain in the muscles around the left hip. [*Lgh.*]

Pressive tearing in the muscles of the left hip. [*Lgh.*]

Painful tearing in the muscles around the right hip-joint, when sitting. [*Lgh.*]

215. Intermitting shooting tearing in the muscles of the left hip, when sitting. [*Lgh.*]

Burning pain at night in the bones of the hip and **the thigh**, so that he was often waked up by it, several nights in succession.

The lower limbs often go to sleep, even above the knee, with painful formication therein, and inabilty to move them. [*Htb. u. Tr.*]

Sensation of drying off and of coldness in the left lower limb, as if it was going to sleep, while sitting; it was not improved by motion, and while walking, there remained a continual painful feeling of coldness internally in the limb, and especially in the leg and foot. [*Htb. u. Tr.*]

In the thigh, when stepping forward, a tensive pain from the left gluteal muscles even into the hough, as if the tendons were too short. [*Wl.*]

220. Tearing pains in the anterior muscles in the left thigh (when sitting). [*Lgh.*]

Painful tearing in the muscles of the right thigh, when standing and sitting. [*Lgh.*]

Intermitting tearing in the muscles of the outer side of the right thigh, when sitting; not diminished by standing, but by walking [*Lgh.*]

Pain as from a sprain in the left thigh, in the upper part near the groin, while taking a walk; it goes off when he stands still. [*Lgh.*]

Eroding itching on the left thigh. [*Lgh.*]

225. Eroding itching, exciting him to scratch, on the right thigh, close to the hip. [*Lgh.*]

On the knee, on the outer side, a tearing.

Shooting pain on the inner side of the knee, when sitting. [*Lgh.*]

In the right leg, a shooting pressure. [*Lgh.*]

Tearing, anteriorly, in the left leg, when sitting; it vanishes at once during standing and walking. [*Lgh.*]

230. Tearing in the muscles of the right leg; when taking a walk. [*Lgh.*]

Tearing in the upper part of the left tibia, close below the knee, when sitting. [*Lgh.*]

Violent, gnawing tearing in the right calf, when sitting and standing. [*Lgh.*]

Violent shooting tearing in the muscles of the legs, near the ankle, when sitting. [*Lgh.*]

Painful hot stitch, as with a knife, in the left calf. [*Htb. u. Tr.*]

235. Pain, as from a blow, on the outer side of the left calf. [*Wl.*]

Cold sweat on the legs, in the morning.

Great weakness of the legs up to the knee, as if they would give way and could not support the body.

Eroding itching near the knee on the left leg, forcing him to scratch, in the morning. [*Lgh.*]

On the foot, cramp-pain, more on the external ankle, when sitting and standing; it goes off when he walks. [*Lgh.*]

240. Cramp of the metatarsus, drawing the toes crooked, for half an hour.

Tearing burning pain about the ankles, so that he almost screamed out; for two hours, with heat of the parts.

Sore pain on the right heel, as if from an internal festering, when walking in the open air. [*Lgh.*]

Violent pain, as from a sprain, in the left heel, continuing for several days uninterruptedly, and then appearing at times; worst when walking. [*Htb. u. Tr.*]

The feet frequently go to sleep, when sitting, with inability then of moving them, and with painful formication therein. [*Htb. u. Tr.*]

245. Tickling itching on the sole of the right foot, exciting to scratch. [*Lgh.*]

Rheumatic pains of the limbs. [PYL, *Aufsaetze u. s. w.*[1]]

The effects of Euphorbium seem mostly to appear after the lapse of some time. [*Htb. u. Tr.*]

Inflammations of external parts. [SCOPOLI, *flor. Carn.*[2]]

Gangrene. [SCOPOLI.[3]]

250. General swelling, inflammation, gangrene, death. [SIEGESBECK, in *Bresl. Samml.*, 1792, II., p. 192.[4]]

Languid and weary all over the body. [*Wl.*]

Lassitude in the limbs, when taking a walk; walking is hard for him. [*Lgh.*]

Frequent yawning, as if he had not slept enough. [*Lgh.*]

Great drowsiness after dinner [*Htb. u. Tr.*]

255. He cannot keep off sleep during the day.

Stupefied sleep in the afternoon; he cannot rouse himself, and would like to slumber on.

He sleeps at night with his arms extended high above his head. [*Wl.*]

Insomnia and tremulous tossing about in bed before midnight, with roaring before the ears; he could not shut his eyes.

He easily and frequently wakes up from sleep.

260. He often woke up at night, but went to sleep right away again. [*Lgh.*]

---

[1] Effect of application to abdomen.—*Hughes.*
[2] From local application.—*Hughes.*
[3] The original has "caries."—*Hughes.*
[4] Not found.—*Hughes.*

At night, while lying awake in bed, he is suddenly startled, as if by an electric shock. [*Lgh.*]

Anxious, confused dream, without any ending.

Anxious, vivid dreams, at night, which force him to scream, so that he wakes up. [*Lgh.*]

Vivid, lascivious dreams, with emission of semen. [*Lgh.*]

265. Dream about things transacted two days before, after 3 A. M. [*Wl.*]

Sensation as if he lacked warmth, and had not slept all night, and had been on a big spree; while all the veins on his hands were invisible. [*Wl.*]

Chilly all over the body, in the morning. [*Wl.*]

Chill, when walking in the warm, open air.

Continual chilliness, with constant perspiration.

270. Shivering. [EHRHARDT.]

Shivers, all over the upper part of the body. [*Wl.*]

Shivering all over the back, with red cheeks and cold hands. [*Lgh.*]

Heat (after effect?). [EHRHARDT.]

Great heat, the whole day; all his clothes seem a burden to him, as also his whole body felt heavy, as if he was carrying a heavy burden.

275. Sensation of heat over the whole face, with warm forehead and cold hands, without thirst. [*Lgh.*]

Fever. [RUST, l. c.]

Thirst for cold drinks. [*Lgh.*]

Perspiration on the neck, every morning in bed, and on rising.

Morning perspiration, extending from the feet all over the body, with great heat, but with no especial thirst.

280. Perspiration in the morning on the thighs and legs, but not on the feet.

In the morning, cold sweat on the legs.

GRAPHITES. PLUMBAGO.

A grain of the purest plumbago from an English lead pencil of the best quality is pulverized, and according to the direction for preparing antipsoric medicines, as given at the end of the first volume, it is first triturated up to the one millionth powder-attenuation. Then, according to the direction there given, the solution of one grain of this preparation in a mixture of fifty drops of water and fifty drops of alcohol, after being shaken up ten times, is further diluted in pure alcohol to the billionth (II.), quadrillionth (IV.), sextillionth (VI.), octillionth (VIII.), and decillionth (X.) degree, and every time potentized with ten strokes of the arm. In these forms and degrees of potency, this medicine is then applied to its homœopathic antipsoric use, taking one or two small pellets moistened with the medicine, for a dose.

The purest plumbago is a sort of mineral carbon, and the small contents of iron are probably to be viewed merely as an admixture not essential to the nature of plumbago, which is further confirmed by the fact, that *Davy* has fully proved the actual transition of diamond into plumbago by treating the same with metallic potassium.

The first thought of the medicinal use of plumbago was given to *Dr. Weinhold* by the fact, that during his journey in Italy he saw workmen in a mirror factory in Venice use it externally for driving away herpes. He imitated them, and described the result in a little work: *Der Graphit als Heilmittel gegen Flechten* (Plumbago as a remedy for herpes), (2d ed., Meissen, 1812). He prescribed its external application either with saliva or with some fat, or he rubbed in the ointment, or applied a plaster of plumbago. He also administered it in several cases internally, as a confection or in pills, not without success.

We go somewhat further, and administer graphites as a very serviceable antipsoric remedy, and this, whether herpes be present in the (non-venereal) chronic disease or not, provided that the present (and previous) symptoms of the patient are found to be homœopathically as similar as possible to the pure symptoms below adduced, which are peculiar to graphites, and caused by it in the healthy body. Graphites has a lengthy period of action.

Graphites has proved itself especially useful, in chronic diseases where it is otherwise appropriate, in curing the following symptoms:

Feeling unhappy; apprehension in the morning; anxiety; *anxiety during sedentary work;* peevishness; dislike of work; feels as if intoxicated on rising from bed; chaotic feeling in the head; fatigued by scientific work; buzzing in the head; tearing pain in the side of the head, the teeth and the glands of the neck; *the falling out of hair, even on the sides of the head;* itching on the head; scab-head; perspiration of the head when in the open air; *pressive pain in the eyelids*, as from a grain of sand; pressing, shooting and lachrymation of the eyes; dry pus on the eyelids and eyelashes; everything becomes black before the eyes on stooping; the letters in reading run together; *flickering before the eyes;* the eyes fear the daylight; dryness of the internal ear; flow of pus from the ear; bad smell from the ear; porrigo behind the ears; *hardness of hearing;* singing and ringing in the ears; humming in the ears; thundering rumbling before the ears; hissing in the ears; bad smell from the nose; dry scabs in the nose; swelling of the nose; *flying heat in the face;* semi-lateral paralysis of the face; freckles in the face; humid, *eruptive pimples* in the face; falling out of the hair of the beard; ulcerated corners of the mouth; ulcers on the inner side of the lips; nocturnal toothache; shooting toothache after drinking something cold; swelling of the gums; dryness of the mouth in the morning; hawking up of mucus; sensitiveness of the throat, in the region of the larynx; almost constant sore throat, during deglutition; nocturnal pain in the throat, as if a plug were lodged in the throat, or as if the food filled the gullet all the way up; painful lumps on the lower jaw; repugnance to cooked food; *voracious hunger; eructation; nausea in the morning;* nausea after every meal; weakness of the stomach; pressure in the stomach; nocturnal pinching in the stomach and digging in the chest; *heaviness in the abdomen;* hardness in the hypogastrium; tapeworm; painfulness in the groin; inflation of the abdomen; inflation after meals; *accumulation of flatus;* obstruction of flatus; *excessive discharge of flatus;* chronic constipation, with *costiveness* and hardness of the hepatic region; insufficient stools; long-continued, excessive softness of stools; discharge of mucus from the rectum; *pains in the varices of the anus;* pains as from excoriation of the varices of the anus after stool; burning, painful fissure between the varices of the anus; large varices of the anus; micturition at night; quiescent sexual desire; uncontrollable sexual desire; *lack of morning erections; almost involuntary emission of semen, without erection;* too scanty voluptuous sensation in coitus; excoriation between the lower limbs, on the pudenda; delayed menses; *menses retarded*, with severe colic; *menses too scanty* and too pale; pains during the menses; cramps in the abdomen, with the menses; pain in the chest, with the menses; weakness, during the menses; *leucorrhœa*, like water; profuse leucorrhœa, before and after the menses.

Stoppage of the nose; troublesome dryness of the nose; flow of mucus from the nose; daily coryza, when becoming cold; the voice in singing is not clear; scraping in the throat; cough; nocturnal cough; asthma; *oppression of the chest;* spasm of the chest; pain in the sacrum as if it was bruised or broken; contractive pains in the back; *pain in the nape;* cramp in the hand; horny callosities in the palms; knotty, arthritic fingers; constant excoriation between the fingers; pain as from a sprain, in the joint of the thumb; excoriation between the legs; restlessness in the lower limbs; numbness of the thigh; herpes on the thigh; herpes on the houghs; stitches in the heel when treading; *coldness of the feet in the evening in bed;* burning of the feet; swelling of the feet; horny skin on the toes; eroding blisters on the toes; suppurating toes; thick, crippled toe-nails; cramp in many places, *e. g.*, on the nates, the calves, etc.; drawing in the limbs; *tendency to strains;* the outside of the chest, the arms and the legs *go to sleep; tendency to take colds;* chronic lack of bodily perspiration; perspiration on slight exertion; excoriation of the skin on the bodies of children; the skin does not heal easily, is apt to ulcerate; *herpes;* difficulty in falling asleep; when going to sleep, suffocating tightness of the chest; light slumber at night; starting from sleep; nocturnal pains, sensible while asleep; *sleep full of ravings;* drowsy slumber in the morning; anxious, frightful dreams; anxiousness at night, forcing him to get up; night-sweat.

Where chronic constipation and menses, delaying several days, cause trouble, graphites is often indispensable. It is not often repeated to advantage, even after intervening remedies. Smelling of Arsenicum X^0 seems to be an antidote, especially to desperate grief caused by graphites. A very small dose of nux vomica antidotes several troublesome symptoms from graphites.

The symptoms marked *Htb.* were observed by *Dr. Hartlaub*, those marked *Ng.* by an anonymous observer in the pure *Arzneimittellehre* of the *Drs. Hartlaub and Trinks; Rl.*, *Dr. Rummel; Kr.*. *Dr. Kretschmar.*

GRAPHITES.

Dejection, gloomy mood (aft. 72 h.).

Dejection, with great heaviness of the feet.

Sad mood (aft. 4 d.).

Troubled mood.

5. Quite despondent in mood, and full of anxiety, till evening when he lies down.

Grief even to despair, about the most trifling matters.

Very much disposed to grieve and to weep, in the evening; while in the morning, contrary to her wont, she laughs at every trifle.

Mournfulness, with nothing but thoughts of death (aft. 11 d.)

Sad, melancholy, she has to weep.

10. She has to weep over music.

He has to weep in the evening, without provocation.

The child weeps and is peevish. [*Htb.*]

Oppression with inclination to weep, in frequent fits. [*Ng.*]

Extraordinary apprehensiveness, so that she cannot compose herself; it goes off on weeping. [*Ng.*]

15. **Anxious oppression.**

Oppression and anguish, with very disagreeable sensation in the stomach.

Great anguish, so that she trembles all over, for several minutes.

A pathogenesis appeared in the first edition of this work, containing 590 symptoms of Hahnemann's own, obtained in the manner we have described. It was then proved by Nenning in his usual way, and by Hartlaub. The 200 symptoms thus obtained are incorporated here with the original stock (which has been largely augmented), and with a few from Rummel and Kretschmar, resulting from provings of the 30th dilution.--*Hughes.*

Anguish with headache, vertigo and ill-humor.

Great anguish in the evening, as if a misfortune had happened, with heat in the face and coldness of the hands and feet.

20. He often feels as if his end was near, or as if the greatest misfortune impended over him.

Anguish, so that she cannot sit still, with perspiration and nausea.

Anguish and hurry chase him about, like a criminal.

Restless and unsettled, he cannot fix his thoughts on his work, has no pleasure in anything; better after taking a walk.

Slow to determine and to recollect.

25. Though usually quick to decide, she, soon after taking the medicine, becomes slow of recollection and resolution.

Extreme scrupulousness; she cannot take anything lightly.

Timidity.

Easily affected and frightened.

Easily frightened (aft. 6 h.).

30. Irritable and passionate, in the morning; in the afternoon, hypochondriac.

Very easily excited; even from speaking, the hands get hot.

Irritable and restless.

Peevish.

Peevish and hypochondriac, without particular cause.

35. Very peevish; everything vexes him and makes him indignant.

He would like to be alone, every disturbance vexes him.

Peevish (aft. 3 h.).

Very peevish and passionate.

She gets vexed readily, but she can also easily dismiss it again from her mind.

40. Lack of disposition to work.

In the morning cheerful, in the evening dejected.

Distracted.

Apt to make mistakes in speaking and in writing.

Continual forgetfulness.

45. Extreme forgetfulness (aft. 8 d.). [*Rl.*]

Only obscure remembrance, even of what has just passed.

Stupid feeling in the head, in the morning, for three days in succession.

Unfit for mental work after the noon-siesta, for four hours.

Great and painful obtuseness of the head, in the morning, for one hour (aft. 4 d.).

50. Obtuseness of the head, at once in the morning, with nausea and sour vomiting.

Pressive obtuseness of the head, chiefly in the morning.

Gloominess in the forehead, with a contractive sensation.

Feels intoxicated in the head.

Reeling and whirling around, in the evening, while taking a walk.

55. Staggering, and tendency to vertigo, with unconsciousness, shivering and a chill.

Giddy and dizzy in the whole head. [*Ng.*]

Fits of vertigo, with tendency to fall forward. [*Ng.*]

Vertigo in the morning, on awaking.

Vertigo in the morning, on awaking (aft. 7 d.).

60. Severe vertigo, in the morning, after a sound sleep (aft. 15 d.).

Vertigo, in the evening, with stupefaction; she had to lie down.

Vertigo, when looking upward.

Vertigo, when stooping and afterward, for several minutes, a tendency to fall forward, with nausea.

Headache, early on awaking, every morning, for half an hour.

65. Headache in the morning, as if she had not done sleeping (aft. 9 d.).

Semilateral headache, in the morning in bed, with inclination to vomit; this goes off on rising.

Severe headache in the morning, on awaking, with nausea, diarrhœa and icy cold sweat, even to fainting; then she had to keep her bed for two days, with constant alternation of chill and heat.

Dull headache in the forehead and the crown, early in bed, while still half asleep; when fully awake, it was gone (aft. 9 d.). [*Rl.*]

Headache, at night, in that side of the head on which he was not lying.

70. Headache, on turning the head, for two days.

Headache on moving the head; she is afraid to move it.

Headache, while out driving.

Headache, during and after the meal.

Headache, with nausea, as if rising from the abdomen, a very disagreeable sensation.

75. Pain, as if the head was numb and turgid. [*Htb.*]

Pain, as if bruised in the head, with general ill-feeling, in the evening.

Pain, as if the sinciput was torn to pieces, from the morning after rising till toward noon. [*Ng.*]

Pressive headache, now here, now there, in the brain, lastly behind the left ear (aft. 24 h.).

Pressure, extending from the forehead deep into the head (aft. 30 d.). [*Ng.*]

80. Pressure outward at the forehead, for two hours after the meal.

Dull pressure in the forehead, in the morning, after rising, worse on moving.

Pressive pain in the left temple, for one minute.

Sharp pressive pain in the temple, on which he was not lying, in the morning in bed.

Pressive pain on the head (aft. 24 d.).

85. **Pressive headache in the occiput.**

Much pressure in the occiput and nape.

Headache, as if the forehead would burst, after a meal. [*Ng.*]

Sensation as if all within the head was screwed in a vice and filled up.

Pain as if constricted, especially in the occiput toward

the nape, which on looking upwards, pains as if broken, at noon; later the pain draws down the back and forward into the chest.

90. Tensive, severe headache, on awaking from sleep; this occupies the whole head, more on the surface of the brain and most in the occiput, without impeding thought, with painful stiffness of the nape; the more he tries to sleep more soundly, the worse the pain becomes (aft. 24 h.).

Sharply drawing tension of the nerves of the brain.

Drawing headache in the forehead, with pain in the nape of the neck, as if stiff.

Drawing in the forehead, for half an hour, recurring for several days successively.

Drawing, first in the sinciput, then in the occiput, in the evening.

95. Drawing pain on (in) the head, down the face, extending to the neck.

Twitching pain in the right side of the head.

Tearing headache in the forehead, in the morning on awaking, for one hour.

Tearing in the forehead, with internal sensation of heat, in the afternoon. [*Ng.*]

Violent tearing in the right side of the head, in the evening (1st d.). [*Ng.*]

100. Shooting pains, from both sides of the crown toward the middle, as if the head would burst, from the morning till 3 P. M., when the pain went off, during a profuse sweat in the heat of the sun. [*Ng.*]

Flying stitches in the left temple (aft. 11 d.).

Ebullition of blood and sensation of heat in the head, repeatedly during the day, with sweat. [*Ng.*]

Ebullition in the head, with compressive pain in the crown, in the afternoon. [*Ng.*]

Throbbing in the forehead. [*Ng.*]

105. Throbbing in the right side of the head, in the afternoon; recurring for several days. [*Ng.*]

Painful blows on the right side of the head. [*Ng.*]

Sensation of looseness of the whole brain. [*Ng.*]

Disagreeable warmth in the whole head (after dinner). [*Ng.*]

Burning on the crown, in a small spot. [*Ng.*]

110. Rushing sound in the head (aft. 3 d.).

Weakness of the head, extending down to the neck.

Coldness and cramp-like contraction of the skin of the head.

Sensation as if the forehead was wrinkling.

Pain in the forehead as if excoriated, when touched.

115 Pain on the head, as if from excoriation.

Tearing on the head, as from rheum, in the morning.

Itching on the hairy scalp.

Much dandruff on the head, causing a very troublesome itching, and causing scabs, which go off when the head is washed, and leave the parts humid.

Eruption on the crown, which pains and becomes moist when touched.

120. **Humid eruption on the head, which does not itch, but only aches when touched, as if festering underneath.**

Scurfy spot on the crown, with violent pain as from excoriation, when touched.

Painfulness and moistness under the scurfy spots on the head. [*Htb.*]

The old scurfs on the hairy scalp become detached and begin to emit a fetid smell. [*Htb.*]

Single hairs turn gray.

125. **Falling out of the hair of the head** (aft. 36 h. and aft. 16 d.).

Pains of the eyes, on opening them, as if strained by reading.

Pressure on the right eyebrow, and from there through the whole eye.

Pressive pain in the eyes, every morning, also in the evening.

Heaviness of the eyelids.

130. Paralytic pain of the eyelids.

Drawing pain in the eyes.

Violent stitch into the right eye. [*Ng.*]

Itching in the inner canthus.

Smarting and heat **in the eyes.**

135. Smarting in the eyes, as if something acrid had gotten in.

Smarting pain in the eyes, as if from something acrid. [*Ng.*]

Burning smarting in the inner canthus.]*Ng.*]

Coldness above the eyes.

Heat in the eyes; he could not see clearly.

140. Heat about the eyelids.

Heat in the eyes, and some pus in the canthi.

Burning in the eyes, by candle-light and in the evening (aft. 30 d.). [*Ng.*]

Burning about the eyes.

Severe burning of the eyes, in the morning.

145. Burning and dryness of the eyelids, in the evening when reading, and in the morning.

Burning and lachrymation of the eyes, in the open air.

Redness of the white of the eye, with lachrymation and photophobia. [*Htb.*]

Redness and painful inflammation of the lower eyelid and the inner canthus.

Redness and inflammation of the eyes, with drawing and pressive pain; then smarting lachrymation of the eyes.

150. Inflammation of the outer canthus.

Severe inflammation of the edges of the eyelids.

A stye on the lower eyelids, with drawing pain before the discharge of the pus.

Swelling of the eyelids and of the lachrymal gland.

Suppuration of the eyes, with pressure therein and drawing pain up into the head.

155. **Lassitude of the eyes.**

Weakness and reddish appearance of the eyes.

Sensation of dryness in the eyelids and pressure.

Frequent lachrymation of the eyes and pressure therein.
Much eye-gum in the eyes.

160. Dry eye-gum in the eyelashes.
Agglutination of the eyes, in the morning. [*Ng.*]
Quivering below the eyes.
Tendency of the eyes to contract in the outer canthi.
She sees everything as through a mist. [*Ng.*]

165. Short-sightedness; he cannot recognize anyone ten paces off (aft. 13 d.).
In writing he sees letters double, while his eyes burn. [*Ng.*]
Great sensitiveness of the eyes to daylight, for several days.
Light is intolerable to him; he cannot look into the brightness; the white also of the eyes is red.
Light dazzles the eyes.

170. In the evening, he sees with open eyes, fiery zigzags all around, outside of the field of vision.
The eyes are sensitive to the sunlight, it causes them to water. [*Ng.*]
If he looks at anything white, his eyes are dazzled and they water.
When he looks sharply at anything white or red, or into the sun, there arise stitches from the temple through the eye into the inner canthus.
Only the daylight affects her eyes, not the candle-light; she can read well and without trouble by the latter.

175. Pain in the ear, a painful pressure in the internal ear like straining.
Sensation of tightness about the left ear (aft. 30 h.).
Tearing in the right ear.
Shooting in the ears.
Stitches in the ear. [*Ng.*]

180. Shooting pains in the left ear, in the evening after supper.
Pain, as from ulceration, in the left ear, frequently renewed.
Throbbing, like pulsation in the ears, especially on stooping and after a meal.
Throbbing in the ear, slower than the pulse, in the morning after awaking, for one hour.
Sensation in the right ear, at every step, as if a valve were opening and shutting in it. [*Ng.*]

185. Fanning in the ear, at every eructation, as if air entered through the Eustachian tube.
Sensation in the left ear, as if it was filled with water.
Red, hot ears.
Swelling of the interior of the left ear (12th d.).
Swelling of the right parotid gland.

190. Itching behind the ears.
Itching in the left ear, in the evening, for a quarter of an hour.
Itching of the lobule and on the cheek; after scratching, a lymph exudes, which hardens on the spots.
Hard lump behind the right ear, painful when touched, for many days. [*Htb.*]

The herpes behind the ears scales off and improves. [*Htb.*]

195. Moisture on the ears. [*Htb.*]

Humidity and excoriated spots behind both ears.

Ulcerated condition of the left helix. [*Rl.*]

Bloody discharge from the ear, for thirty-six hours.

Being hard of hearing, she hears better while riding in a wagon.

200. First, ringing, then a rushing sound in the left ear (aft. 2 h.).

Humming before the ears.

Roaring sound in the ears, during coitus.

Violent roaring and rushing sound in the ears (aft. 14 d.).

Roaring in the head, then explosion in the ear, then better hearing.

205. **Violent roaring in the ears at night**, with obstruction of the ears at times (during full moon).

Thundering pealing before the ears.

Reverberation in the ear.

Roaring sound in the ears, in the evening in bed, darting through all the limbs (aft 7 d.). [*Rl.*]

Hissing in the ear, the whole day.

210. Sound of gnawing in the ears, on moving the head.

Clucking sound in the ears on stooping, with heaviness of the head; on straightening himself again and leaning backward, there is again the clucking sound; just as if something fell forward and back again.

Cracking sound in the ear, when eating, in the evening.

Cracking sound in the ear, on moving the jaws, but only in the morning, while lying in bed.

Repeated sensation and noise in the ear, as if a blister burst open (2d d.).

215. Detonation and explosion in the left ear; when swallowing. [*Ng.*]

The nose is painful internally.

In the inside of the nose, a sensation of tension. [*Ng.*]

Sensation of excoriation in the nose, when blowing it.

Ulcerated pain in the right nostril. [*Ng.*]

220. Itching in the nose

Sudden burning on a small spot, on the left side of the nose. [*Ng.*]

Redness of the nose.

Black pores on the nose (comedones).

Eruptional pimples in the left nostril, which first itch then burn.

225. Large humid pimple on the nose.

Painful scabs inside of the nose.

Blowing out bloody mucus from the nose.

Blowing out blood from the nose, **for several days in succession.**

Epistaxis (also aft. 15 d.).

230. Epistaxis, in the morning.

Epistaxis, two evenings in succession, with palpitation of the heart, heat and pain in the back (aft. 3 d.).

Epistaxis in the evening at ten o'clock; the afternoon preceding it, rush of blood to the head, with heat of the face.

Olfaction too sensitive; she cannot bear any flowers.

Smell in the nose as from an inveterate coryza.

235. Smell at night, as of burned hair mixed with fumes of sulphur.

Smell in the nose as of burned soot, in the morning.

Paleness of the face.

Sudden paleness of the face from light mental occupation, *e. g.*, reading.

Paleness of the face, with blue rims around the eyes.

240. Yellowness of the face, with weary eyes, as if worn out (aft. 24 h.).

Erysipelas on both sides of the face, with burning shooting pain, then coryza for one day, with shooting in the gums (aft. 7 and 14 d.).

Swelling of the left side of the face, in the morning after rising.

Incipient paralysis of the left side of the face, after there had been some swelling of it, with some toothache; the muscles on the right side of the face are suddenly distorted, the mouth drawn to the right, and its motion, as well as speech, become difficult; the left eye often closes involuntarily, while the right cannot be fully closed, but often remains open, even in the dazzling light, in wind, and dust (aft. 18 d.).

Constant sensation as from cobwebs in the face. [*Ng.*]

245. Pain, alternating in all the bones of the face.

Drawing pain in the left upper jaw.

Very painful tearing in the left zygoma, which almost made her scream, in the evening, in bed. [*Ng.*]

Spasmodic contraction of the muscles of mastication.

He cannot open his jaws when eating, owing to pain in the masticating muscles; it is as if they were paralyzed.

250. Itching in the right temples, very violent, with burning after scratching. [*Htb.*]

Itching pimple in the face, humid after scratching.

A sort of encysted tumor on the cheek. [*Kr.*]

The lips are dry.

Quivering on the upper lip.

255. Shooting in the upper lip, as if a needle and thread were drawn through it, in the evening. [*Ng.*]

Burning and feeling of heaviness in the lower lip. [*Ng.*]

Sore pain, as from excoriation, in the left corner of the mouth.

Soreness and chapping of the lips and nostrils, as from a chill.

Chapped lower lip.

260. Eruption in the corner of the mouth.

Eruptions on the lip.

Eruptive pimple on the upper lip, which first itches and then burns.

Small, white tubercles on the upper lip.

Thick-set, whitish pimples on a red base, and itching somewhat, on both corners of the mouth, below the lips.

265. A blister on the upper lip, with cutting pain.

The left corner of the mouth is ulcerated.

Scurfy, painless ulcers on both corners of the mouth.

Chin, full of eruption.

In the lower jaw on the left side, shooting tearing. [*Ng.*]

270. In the sub-maxillary glands, pressive pain.

Inflammation and swelling of the right sub-maxillary gland, which after some days becomes indurated and scales off.

Swelling of the sub-maxillary glands.

Swelling of the sub-maxillary glands, painful when touched, with stiffness of the neck.

Swelling of the parotid gland, with tensive pain.

275. Toothache of the right molars, when biting firmly.

Toothache, especially at night, with heat in the face, or in the evening, with pain as of excoriation on the palate and on the swelling of the cheeks.

Shooting pain, darting about in the teeth. [*Ng.*]

Pain, as of soreness of the teeth, while eating, increased after eating.

Pressive pain in all the teeth and in the jaws, at night, for two hours, and renewed in daytime by chewiug and biting.

280. Painful pressure in all the teeth, aggravated by touching them.

Drawing toothache.

Drawing pain in a hollow tooth.

Drawing pain in the molars, when walking in the wind.

Tearing in the root of the tooth. [*Ng.*]

285. Tearing pain in all the teeth, aggravated by warmth, renewed on lying down in bed, and thus destroying the night's rest before midnight.

Shooting toothache (aft. 6 d.).

Dull, jerking stitches in a tooth.

Dull, jerking stitches in a hollow molar, on taking a walk (aft. 4 h.).

Single, burning stitches in a left upper molar, after a meal.

290. Tingling toothache, and when she takes cold water in her mouth, stitches in the tooth.

Gnawing in the sockets.

Burning toothache, as from looseness of the teeth, now in one tooth, now in another, mostly at night in bed, or in the evening, when sitting and leaning back, with collection of saliva in the mouth; pain aggravated by chewing.

Pain of the lower teeth, as from looseness, when masticating.

Black, sour blood often flows from the hollow teeth. [*Ng.*]

95. The gums are painful, with a sensation of excoriation on the palate and flow of water from the mouth.

Pain, as from excoriation of the gums, on the inner side of the teeth, as after eating hot things (aft. 10 d.).

Pain, as from excoriation of the gums of the upper incisors, on touching them with the tongue.

Ulcerative pain of the gums.

Itching gnawing in the gums.

300. Rush of blood to the gums, so that she feels like cutting into them.

Swelling of the gums and dryness in the mouth.

Swelling of the gums, in the evening.

Acutely painful swelling of the gums. [*Ng.*]

Painful swelling of the gums, with swelling of the cheeks and lassitude in the whole body.

305. Painful swelling of the gums on the teeth of the upper jaw, as if excoriated, even while touching the cheek, with pain in the molar belonging to it, as if a swollen cheek would ensue.

The gums bleed easily on being touched.

Putrid smell from the gums and the mouth.

Sourish putrid smell from the mouth.

Urinous smell and breath from the mouth and through the nose.

310. Bad smell from the mouth. [*Htb.*]

The tongue after a meal feels raw, rough and scrapy, and the papulæ are too sensitive, as if they rubbed against the teeth.

Pain on the left side of the tongue, as from excoriation, when moving and stretching the tongue.

White tongue.

Burning vesicles on the lower surface and the tip of the tongue. [*Ng.*]

315. Painful nodules and blisters posteriorly on the tongue, which are most painful while eating and spitting, and sometimes bleed.

Whitish, painful ulcer on the lower surface of the tongue.

Sore throat in the morning, on rising, with both pressing and shooting pain.

Sore throat, as from a glandular swelling.

Pressure in the region of the pit of the throat, as if he was over-sated, or had swallowed too large a morsel.

320. Sensation in the throat as if there was an excrescence in it or adhesive mucus, so that if he tries to swallow even a little thing (a crumb) it lodges in that place.

Sensation in the left side of the throat, as if he had to swallow over a lump, with scraping in it; not worse when swallowing food than in empty deglutition.

Sensation in the throat, when swallowing, as if there was a lump in it, and especially in empty deglutition there is a contracting choking from the œsophagus to the larynx.

Spasm in the throat, with nausea (aft. 3 d.).

Constant spasm in the throat, compelling him to swallow with a choking sensation, as if the food he is eating would not go down (aft. 24 h.).

325. Sensation in the throat as if it was sewed up, with constant scraping therein.

Scraping in the throat (aft. 24 h.)

Intolerable scraping and scratching in the throat.

Scraping in the throat, with a sensation in the fauces, behind the velum pendulum palati, as if it was parched; this only diminishes after detaching some tenacious phlegm; several days in succession, in the morning, on awaking. [*Rl.*]

Scraping in the throat (after a meal), with rawness and roughness.

330. Roughness in the throat, only sensible when speaking. [*Ng.*]

Roughness and scraping excoriation in the throat.

Shooting in the throat, even when not swallowing. [*Ng.*]

Shooting and choking in the throat in deglutition, with dryness posteriorly in the left side of the throat, in the palate.

Severe shooting in the throat, on swallowing, with ulcerative pain and choking. [*Ng.*]

335. Quickly appearing twitching stitches, in a point deep within the throat on the right side, merely on moving the neck, on talking, stooping, and rising again, not when swallowing.

Pinching pain in the throat (aft. 5 d.).

Swelling of the tonsils in the throat, with pain on deglutition.

Flow of water from the mouth, with swelling of the upper lip, with a painful pimple on it, with painful gums and excoriated palate.

Much spitting of saliva (aft. 2 d.).

340. **The saliva runs from his mouth, in the morning, when stooping.**

Mucus in the mouth, in the morning; the mouth is so glued together thereby, that he could hardly open it. [*Ng.*]

Salty, burning mucus in the mouth, in the morning, on awaking.

Much mucus, deep down in the throat.

Much mucus in the fauces, for several days; he has to eject it by hawking.

345. Hawking up of mucus, with dryness in the palate from talking.

Spitting of blood, with great sensitiveness of the palate and the tongue. [*Ng.*]

Salty taste in the mouth.

Bitterish taste in the mouth, in the afternoon (aft. 7 d.).

Bitterish taste in the mouth, with heavily coated tongue (aft. 28 h.).

350. Bitter taste on the tongue, with sour eructation.

Bitter taste of food.

Acidity in the mouth, after breakfast.

Sour taste frequently, especially after eating and drinking.

Sour taste in the mouth, and no appetite for drinking.

355. Acidity in the stomach, with voracious hunger.

Taste of rotten eggs in the mouth, in the morning, after rising. [*Ng.*]

The appetite is increased. [*Ng.*]

Voracious hunger, but after eating nausea and vertigo (aft. 3 d.).

No appetite, in the evening.

360. He loathes the food.

Little appetite for warm food.

Repugnance to salty food.

Liquids are repugnant and loathsome to her.

Meat and fish are repugnant to her.

365. Repugnance to meats, when thinking of them; though she has a tolerable relish for them when eating them; still, she prefers bread.

Good appetite for meat at supper, when he at other times had no desire for meat.

Unusual thirst in the morning, for several days successively.

Violent thirst, at once, in the morning. [*Ng.*]

Much thirst, after eating (aft. 13 d.).

370. Much craving for beer, without actual thirst, only to get cooled off internally.

While eating, perspiration.

During and after eating, a pressive headache.

After dinner, chaotic feeling in the head.

After a meal, rancid heartburn.

375. After a meal, pain in the stomach, relieved by drinking something.

After a meal, pressure like cramp in the stomach, from the fauces to the navel (aft. 24 d.).

After a meal, grasping pain in the stomach.

Soon after a meal, burning in the stomach, with heaviness in the body and ill-humor.

Immediately after eating, colic.

380. Just after eating, feeling of fullness, and for several hours, a sourish, contractive taste, as if arising from the stomach.

An hour after a meal, fullness in the abdomen, as if he had eaten too much.

When she eats anything, it inflates her abdomen.

After a meal, she cannot bear anything tight about her abdomen.

After a meal, great stiffness, pressure and shooting in the sore foot (aft. 5 d.).

385. **After dinner, drowsiness.**

After a meal, he is weary and falls asleep.

After dinner, shivering on the lower limb on the right side.

After breakfast, coldness and shivering through the whole body.

Abortive eructation; eructations would constantly arise, but they cannot.

390. Continual eructation, with nausea and lack of appetite all the day (at once).

Much eructation, with the taste of the ingesta (aft. 4 d.).

Sour eructation, with bitter taste in the mouth.

Sour regurgitation of food.

Green, bitter water rises in her mouth, in the morning, on drinking or just after eating, for four days in succession.

395. Heartburn.

Rancid heartburn.

Hiccup, in the morning after rising and after dinner. [*Ng.*]

Hiccup after a meal, with dullness in the head or drowsiness.

Hiccups after every meal, whether hot or cold.

400. Hiccup in the evening for an hour (aft. 4 d.).

Qualmishness in the stomach, after dinner. [*Rl.*]

Great qualmishness and nausea before supper, without any inclination to vomit.

Qualmishness, as if arising from the abdomen, with contractive pain below the navel and much mucus in the throat, chiefly in the morning and several hours after a meal.

Nausea, for several hours (at once).

405. Nausea, at noon, with loathing of beef-tea, several days in succession.

Nausea, like fainting, as if coming from the left hypochondrium.

Nausea, with inclination to vomit, the whole day (at once). [*Ng.*]

Nausea, with inclination to vomit, in the region of the stomach, for two minutes in the morning, just after rising (the first 8 d.).

Nausea, with inclination to vomit, in the morning, after rising, with dizziness, as if owing to darkness before the eyes, he imagined he would fall over in walking; at the same time, paleness of the face, for two weeks.

410. Inclination to vomit, in the afternoon, with flow of water from the mouth (2d d.).

Severe inclination to vomit, with pretty good appetite, both when fasting, and also during, before and after eating; then vomiting of water (not of food), with much secretion of saliva (aft. sev. d.).

Waterbrash.

Retching up of much mucus, in the morning, with normal appetite and stool.

Vomiting, brought on at every slight qualmishness, with flow of much water from the mouth.

415. Vomiting in the afternoon, after a two hours' walk, with great nausea; sudden weariness and a severe chill for several hours.

Vomiting, with nausea and colic, the whole day, without diarrhœa.

Vomiting, with nausea and colic, for two days in succession (aft. sever. h.).

Vomiting of all the ingesta, with nausea.

She immediately vomits her dinner up again, without nausea, but with a sickly aching in the scrobiculus cordis (aft. 10 d.).

420. Stomachache, like voracious hunger, from morning till in the afternoon. [*Ng.*]

Insipidity, and sensation, as if the stomach was spoiled, while the appetite is good.

Pain in the stomach, with oppression and anguish.

Pains on the right side of the stomach, which always go off on eructation.

Pressure in the stomach all day, only relieved by lying down and by the warmth of the bed, but it recurs at once when rising again from bed.

425. She has to vomit owing to the pressure on her stomach.

Pressure in the region of the scrobiculus cordis, the whole forenoon, relieved by eructation. [*Ng.*]

Griping in the stomach, with nausea, she had to spit continually, almost like waterbrash.

Griping pain in the stomach in the forenoon, going off during and after the dinner.

Gnawing clawing in the stomach, before dinner.

430. Contractive pain in the stomach (aft 6 d.).

Stitches, frequently in the stomach and in the belly.

Shooting and throbbing in the scrobiculus cordis. [*Ng.*]

Feeling of coldness and great emptiness of the stomach. [*Ng.*]

Burning in the stomach, when fasting and before a meal, forcing him to eat.

435. Burning in the stomach, then heat in the whole body and then sweat. [*Ng.*]

Fermentation in the stomach, followed by discharge of flatus; then alternately in the body, a dull pressure, drawing and shooting; then weariness in the eyes.

In the hypochondria, tension as from a tight bandage, with oppression of the chest.

Shooting in both hypochondria, forcing the person to lie down (3d d.).

Throbbing under the short ribs, at night, on awaking.

440. In the region of the liver, immediately after breakfast, such acute pains, that she had to lie down again.

Stitches in the right hypochondrium, in the morning, just after rising.

Acutely painful stitches in the hepatic region, so that she had to grit her teeth together.

In the splenic region, a pressive pain.

Shooting in the right hypochondrium, toward the back, like splenetic stitches.

445. Stitches in the left hypochondrium, on moving the body,

Burning in the left hypochondriac region, when sitting; going off by motion; frequently recurring. [*Ng.*]

Pain in the stomach, going off by pressing on it.

Pain to the right in the hypogastrium, more violent at every step and every breath.

Violent colic in the morning, for several seconds; then a diarrhœic and afterward a firm stool (aft. 6 d.). [*Rl.*]

450. Hard, tensive pressure in the abdomen, extending from the hypochondria deep into the hypogastrium, both at rest and in motion, and without any trace of flatulence; nor does the discharge of flatus give any relief.

Heaviness in the hypogastrium, with urging. [*Ng.*]

Fullness and heaviness of the abdomen.

Fullness in the abdomen and stomach, with loss of appetite, with constipation for four days (aft. 12 d.).

Fullness and hardness of the hypogastrium, with sensation as from incarcerated flatus, chiefly in the evening and at night.

455. Inflation of the abdomen, chiefly after eating, with painful sensitiveness when pressed upon.

Inflation of the abdomen, with rush of blood to the head, heaviness in the head, vertigo and dizziness (aft. 4 d.).

Severe inflation of the belly, with dullness and heaviness in the head.

Abdomen thick, as if from accumulated and obstructed flatus; she cannot put on anything that presses on the hypochondria.

Distended abdomen (aft. 6 d.).

460. Distended abdomen, with diarrhœic stool.

Griping in the belly, by jerks, both when at rest and in motion; attended with much thirst, without appetite.

Spasmodic colic, at night; an excessive cramp-pain of all the intestines, alike unbearable at rest and in motion, without any trace of flatulence; at the same time deficient secretion of urine.

Contraction, pinching and cutting about the navel; soon after, a natural stool (soon after taking the medicine). [*Ng.*]

Pinching in the abdomen, especially in the region of the caecum (immediately).

465. Cutting colic, on taking a walk.

Cutting colic, in the morning, with repeated, but not diarrhœic stool.

Dull shooting in the left side of the abdomen.

Cramp-like shooting in the hypogastrium (17th d.).

Drawing pain in the abdomen, at night, with urging to stool, but without diarrhœa.

470. Twitches in the abdomen (aft. 1 h.).

Twitches in the side of the abdomen.

Digging pain in the abdomen.

Qualmishness in the hypogastrium. [*Rl.*]

Burning on (in) the left side of the abdomen.

475. Burning on a small spot in the left side of the abdomen. [*Ng.*]

Burning and cutting in the abdomen.

Tension in the groins, when walking. [*Ng.*]

Violent pains in the right inguinal region, a burning and urging, as if the intestines would be forced out there, and these seemed to be moving; worse on stretching the body, relieved on stooping. [*Ng.*]

Stitches in the groin.

480. The glands in the left groin are painful as if swollen.

Sensation of swelling in the left inguinal glands, so that he cannot make a sufficiently long step in walking; and yet they are not swollen, and do not pain when touched.

Swollen glands in the right groin (9th d.).

Swelling and great sensitiveness of one of the inguinal glands.

An inflamed glandular lump in the right groin.

485. Flatulence arises suddenly, and presses painfully toward the abdominal ring (aft. 3 h.).

Flatulent colic when taking a walk.

Much flatulence, arising with griping in the stomach and loud rumbling; the flatus passed off with much violence upward and downward, without relieving.

Incarceration of the flatus in the hypogastrium, especially in its side, with growling.

Growling in the abdomen, in the morning, in the bed and for some time after rising.

490. **Rumbling in the abdomen**, during dinner.

Rumbling in the abdomen, after drinking.

Continual rumbling in the abdomen, as if diarrhœa was setting in.

Loud rumbling in the abdomen.

Clucking in the right side of the abdomen, down into the lower limb, as from softly falling drops.

495. Croaking as from frogs, in the abdomen.

Almost involuntary discharge of flatus; he can hardly restrain it.

Frequent discharge of fetid flatus, with occasional inflation of the abdomen. [*Ng.*]

Discharge of much fetid flatus, which is constantly generated anew. [*Ng.*]

Before every discharge of flatus, there is **colic.**

500. After the discharge of flatus, bellyache.

After the stool, distension, restlessness and pinching in the abdomen.

No urging, nor call to stool.

Frequent intermission of the stool. [*Ng.*]

Much tendency to stool, which, though not hard, required much straining for its evacuation, on account of the total inaction of the rectum.

505. Urging to stool, without any need of it.

Hard stool, with much urging and shooting in the anus. [*Ng.*]

Hard, knotty stool. [*Ng.*]

Knotty stool (aft. 2 d.).

Knotty stool, wound around with a mucous thread, and after it, there is still mucus on the anus.

510. **Stool of very thin formation, like a lumbrical worm.**

It gradually secures a daily stool, while before, he was constipated.

Repeated stool, daily for several days, the first, very hard and formed too thick, the others, soft.

Three stools a day, for the first five days, then for several days, two, the last days, only one.

In time, the stool, which was formerly diarrhœic, becomes firmer.

515. Three times, a soft stool, at night, with pains in the abdomen. [*Ng.*]

Diarrhœa, almost without pain in the abdomen, for twenty hours, then great lassitude of short duration.

Three diarrhœic stools, with burning in the anus (17th d.). [*Ng.*]

Repeated liquid diarrhœic stool, with discharge of mucus for three days. [*Ng.*]

Sudden mucous diarrhœic stool, with sensation as if flatus would be discharged, after previous qualmishness and sensation of having taken a cold in the abdomen. [*Rl.*]

520. Much white mucus is discharged with the stool.

Reddish mucus is discharged with the stool

Sour-smelling stool, with burning in the rectum.

Sourish, putrid-smelling, soft stools.

Dark-colored, only half-digested stool, of intolerable fetor.

525. **Blood in the stool** (aft. several h.).

Blood is discharged with a soft stool.

Some blood with the stool, every day, on the cessation of the menses, with pain in the rectum as from excoriation, for seven days (aft. 42 d.).

Lumbrici are discharged with the stool. [*Ng.*]

Discharge of ascarides, with itching in the rectum.

530. Tenesmus during the stool (aft. 21 h.).

During the stool, burning in the anus.

In the rectum, pressure and straining, without stool.

Violent straining in the rectum, as in piles.

Straining and burning in the rectum and anus.

535. Stitches in the rectum (aft. 2 h.).

Shooting pain in the rectum, as if everything there was indurated.

Single stitches in the anus. [*Ng.*]

Obtuse, tearing stitch from the anus up into the rectum

Cutting in the anus (rectum?), in the morning, in bed

540. **Itching of the anus** (aft. 2 h.).

Itching and sensation of excoriation on the anus.

Pain as from excoriative soreness in the anus, when wiping it.

Sense of swelling on the anus, but without pain.

Swelling of the anus, all around.

545. The veins around the anus are severely swollen..

A thin cord, like a swollen vein, extends from the anus toward the nates, not painful to the touch.

Varices on the anus, causing burning.

Discharge of blood from the rectum, with violent shooting in it.

Prolapsus recti (with its varices) even without tenesmus, as if the anus had lost its contractible power and was paralyzed.

550. Anxious straining and pressure to urinate at night, with cutting in the abdomen; she had often to get up for it, but only a little water passed, with a cutting pain, for two days.

Painful urging to urinate, in the morning in bed, and yet only a few drops were passed, attended with cutting in the urethra (aft 5 d.).

The stream of urine is quite thin, as if the urethra was too narrow.

Hurried urging to urinate, and but little urine.

Frequent micturition.

555. She has to urinate very frequently.

There is an urging to urinate, quite early in the morning.

More frequent, profuse micturition than usual, she has also to get up at night for the purpose (the first days). [*Ng.*]

Nocturnal urging to urinate.

He has to get up at night to urinate, contrary to his custom. [*Htb*]

560. **Wetting the bed at night.**

Involuntary micturition.

Urging to urinate, and dropping of the urine after the customary micturition (1st d.). [*Ng.*]

Sharp, sourish smell of the urine.

Very dark brown urine, during its discharge there is a slight stitch in the urethra.

565. Dark colored urine, which, in two hours, deposits a reddish sediment.

The urine grows very turbid, after two hours, with a reddish sediment; while being passed, the urine caused the urethra to smart.

The urine grows turbid and deposits a white sediment.

Before urination, cutting urging down from both the kidneys (the 1st days). [*Ng.*]

During micturition, titillation in the urethra.

570. During micturition, pain in the coccyx.

After micturition, burning at the orifice of the urethra. [*Ng.*]

Rough pressure in the root of the urethra, with urging to urinate.

Burning in the urethra, even when not urinating.

In the genitals, tension and a disagreeable sensation, when walking or at the least touch of the clothes.

575. Cramp pain in the penis.

Twitching pain in the penis, for several minutes. [*Rl.*]

Eruptions on the penis.

The glans is coated with a thick mucus, although he washes it off every two or three days.

Drawing pain in the glans.

580. The prepuce swells up, forming a large watery blister, without pain.

Eruptive vesicles on the prepuce.

The right testicle seems swollen.

Drawing sensation in both testes.

Shooting pain, occasionally, in the right testicle.

585. Swelling in the scrotum (in the tunica vaginalis testis? hydrocele?)

Itching, inside of the scrotum.

Itching on the scrotum.

Itching, and moist eruption on the scrotum.

In the left spermatic cord, twitching pain.

590. **Excitation of the sexual desire and of sexual fancies.**

Extremely voluptuous thoughts, which torment him, so that he is afraid of becoming insane, and runs about restlessly; with heaviness in the perinæum and tensive pain in the penis, without erection.

Voluptuous excitation in the genitals.

His sexual desire, which was habitually very excited and even almost excessive, at once became totally quiescent for several days.

He gradually loses all desire for coitus.

595. No desire for coitus at all, during the first thirty days after taking graphites; also his fancy, which at other times was very active, was cold, and there was no tendency to erections at all; but at the end of this time all these awakened in so high a degree, that on touching a woman, he felt a voluptuous thrill and trembled in all his limbs.

His fancy was quite cold with regard to coitus.

Very indifferent with respect to coitus, and little excitation during it.

Erection, without voluptuous thoughts.

Intense erection (aft. 48 h.).

600. Violent erection (aft. 8 d.). [*Ng.*]

During erections, clucking of the penis.

Pollutions, almost every night.

Pollution, almost every night (the first 7 d.).

The pollutions seem to cease (aft. 20 d.).

605. While the sexual organs are excited, there is flatulent colic, which prevents coitus.

In the beginning of the coitus, very painful cramp of the calves, which makes a continuation impossible.

During the coitus, despite of every effort, there is on emission of semen.

After coitus, there is at once renewed erection (aft. 27 d.).

After coitus, the legs quickly become cold.

610. After coitus, lassitude (aft. 14 d.).

Immediately after coitus, his whole body becomes burning hot, and he perspires all over.

Painful pressure toward the genitals.

Straining toward the genitals, occasionally, while standing.

Smarting in the vagina.

615. Repeated shooting pains in the labia majora. [*Ng.*]

Vesicle on the labia, with itching smarting pain.

Eruption of pimples on the pudenda, with some itching.

Itching on the pudenda, before the menses.

Painless pimple on the inside of the labia.

620. Excoriation of the pudenda.

Painful excoriation between the pudenda and the thigh, covered with pimples, vesicles and ulcers.

The left, indurated ovary swells up and becomes as hard as a stone, with violent pain when touched, and even while inspiring or hawking, when the most violent stitches dart there, so that she almost gets beside herself, with a profuse general sweat, and continued sleeplessness.

The menses at first seem to appear tardily.

It retards the menses by three days, in its primary effect (aft. 4 d.).

625. The menses appear seven days too late (aft. 29 d.).

The menses appear nine days too late, with heaviness in the

abdomen and a dull feeling in the head, on the first day of the menses. [*Htb.*]

The menses are retarded by eleven days.

The menses do not appear at the regular time, the delay causing no trouble. [*Ng.*]

Suppression of the menses, with heaviness of the arms and legs.

630. The menses appear three days earlier, as an after-effect (aft. 29 d.).

Menses two days too early, very thin, of short duration and with violent, unusual pains in the sacrum, which went off during exercise. [*Ng.*]

Several days before the menses, violent itching on the pudenda.

A day before the menses, and two days during their flow, a violent pressive pain in the abdomen, with sensation of heat in the belly.

Before and during the menses, a cough, fatiguing the chest, in the morning and by day, but not at night.

635. During the menses, violent headache, with eructation and nausea (aft. 5 d.).

During the menses, violent headache, chiefly in the evening.

During the menses, nausea in the morning, with weakness and trembling by day.

During the menses, pain in the epigastrium, as if everything would be torn asunder.

During the menses, pain in the abdomen, straining and pressure, like labor pains, pain in the back, anxious pain in the sacrum commencing with tickling; attended with eructation, and toothache, shooting and twitching upward.

640. During the menses, excoriation between the thighs near the pudenda (aft. 28 d.).

During the menses, hoarseness, severe coryza and catarrhal fever (aft. 20 d.).

During the menses, dry cough and profuse perspiration.

During the menses, swelling of the feet, and painless swelling of the cheek.

During the menses, pain in the varices.

645. During the menses, her sight fails her, it becomes black before her eyes, the left hand becomes numb and dies off, with formication in it, extending up into the arm, and there is also tingling in the lips.

During the menses, a chill.

Just after the menses, a chill, colic and then diarrhœa.

Leucorrhœa (aft. 3 d.).

Leucorrhœa. [*Ng.*]

650. **Profuse leucorrhœa** (5th d.).

Severe vaginal discharge of mucus, quite white (aft. 7 d.).

Profuse vaginal discharge, with weakness in the back and sacrum, when walking and sitting (aft. sev. h.).

Leucorrhœal discharge, about an ounce during a day and

night, for eight days, chiefly in the morning, after rising from bed.

Thin leucorrhœa, with distended abdomen (aft. 8 d.).

* * * * * * * *

655. Sneezing, with very dry nose.

Catarrhal, contractive and stuffed sensation in the nasal cavity.

Stoppage of the nose, but nevertheless clear water flows out. [*Ng.*]

Coryza with sneezing and dull feeling in the head. [*Ng.*]

Stuffed coryza, with obtuseness of the head, oppression of the chest, heat in the sinciput and face, especially about the nose, and loss of smell (the first 4 d.).

660. **Severe stuffed coryza, with great nausea and headache, without vomiting; he had to lie down** (aft. 48 h.).

Coryza (aft. 4, 5 d.).

Severe coryza (aft. 8 d. and the first days).

A severe coryza, which he had not had for years.

Coryza with headache, and alternation of chill and heat.

665. Fluent coryza of short duration, with frequent sneezing (aft. 3 h.).

Constant fluent coryza, which had not come to an outbreak for years, though it had showed itself very frequently for an hour at a time; with much sneezing.

Fluent coryza with headache, chilliness and internal dry heat with thirst (aft. 48 h.).

Fluent coryza, with epistaxis (aft. 11 d.).

Fluent coryza, with catarrh and frequent sneezing, and with pressive pain in a submaxillary gland; he was sensitive to the air in any uncovered part of the body, as if he could easily catch a cold there (aft. 2 h.).

670. Profusely fluent coryza with catarrh; the chest feels heavily oppressed, the head is muddled and very hot; but little air passes through the nose (aft. 16 d.).

Frequent secretion of mucus from the nose, sometimes thin, sometimes thick and yellowish, for eight days. [*Ng.*]

Tenacious white mucus, only in the left nostril, detached with difficulty the first day, more easily the second. [*Htb.*]

Putrid smelling nasal mucus.

Fetid purulent discharge from the nose. [*Ng.*]

675. Sensation in the throat, as if a catarrh or cold was coming.

Catarrhal roughness, with mucus on the chest and windpipe.

Catarrh and coryza, with roughness, continually exciting to cough by its titillation, with lassitude and headache (quickly wiped out by Aconite).

Pain from rawness in the chest, like raw flesh.

Scrapy feeling in the windpipe.

680. Rough throat (aft. 6 d.).

Hoarseness, every evening.

She could not speak loud, for burning in her throat, as if everything was excoriated.

Mucus on the chest (aft. 20 d.).

Scraping in the throat, exciting a dry cough.

685. Frequent tickling in the throat, exciting to retching and a short cough, chiefly in the evening, in bed.

Tickling, deep in the chest, with loose cough and salty expectoration. [*Ng.*]

Cough, with coryza and catarrh and with heat in the head (aft. 8 d.).

Cough which tires the chest, with pain deep in the chest.

Dry tussiculation wakes him at night from sleep and continues the whole of the following day (aft. 5 d.). [*Ng.*]

690. Cough with much expectoration, in the evening, when lying down.

Dyspnœa (aft. 20 d.).

Oppression of the respiration, from tightness of the chest.

Asthma, in the evening, when lying in bed; the cough is excited when taking a deep breath.

Sudden asthma, with difficult, shortened respiration (aft. 3 h.).

695. Severe asthma, as if she should suffocate every moment, when taking a walk.

Tightness of the chest (aft. several h.).

Tightness of the chest, especially on inspiring, in the morning on rising (aft. 21 d.).

Tightness of the left part of the chest and of the heart, in the morning, for several hours.

On taking breath, a pressure in the region of the heart.

700. On inspiring, there is at times a wheezing in the windpipe.

Pains in the chest, from constant sitting (aft. 7 d.). [*Rl.*]

Pain of the right ribs of the chest, when touched.

The lower ribs near the sternum are painful when touched (aft. 21 d.).

Pain in the upper part of the chest, when yawning, or when touching it, or when riding.

705. Pain in the chest, when ascending an elevation.

Everything presses upon her chest; she cannot endure anything tight on it.

Pressive pain, passing from the left into the right side of the chest (aft. 24 d.). [*Ng.*]

Pressure on the left side of the chest, which increases to squeezing and an almost unbearable straining, but only while sitting; it goes off while standing, but returns when sitting, and quite vanishes when lying down in bed.

Squeezing pressure on the chest, which compels him to stretch and extend his limbs, in the evening, for half an hour.

710. Squeezing pressure on the chest, when taking a longer walk.

Squeezing pain in the chest.

Violent tearing in the whole right side of the chest. [*Ng.*]

Shooting in the middle of the chest, with oppression of the chest, when going up stairs. [*Ng.*]

Painful stitches, anteriorly on the left side of the chest, so that she was startled by it in the evening. [*Ng.*]

715. Severe stitches in the left side of the chest, so that she thought she could hardly stand it (aft. 11 d.). [*Ng.*]

Shooting in the sternum, between the two breasts (aft. 4 d.).

Violent shooting in the right side, every stitch arresting the breath (aft. 8 d.).

Violent stitches in the right side of the chest, when catching breath, she has to press on her chest with her hand, to alleviate it (for several days).

Pleuritic stitch in the side, with every least motion (aft. 6 d.).

720. Shooting pain in the cardiac region.

Throbbing in the cardiac region, in the evening, after lying down, when lying on the left side; this was so violent that it caused the coverlet to move; attended with anxiety; it went off on turning over. [*Ng.*]

Strong pulsation of the blood about the heart and the rest of the body, at every slight motion.

Strong pulsation of the heart, causing the arm and the hand to move, and making him anxious.

Strong palpitation of the heart.

725. Violent palpitation, several times, darting in a moment like an electric shock from the heart toward the neck.

(Continual emptiness and coldness about the heart and in the chest, with sadness.)

Externally, on the right side of the chest, a shooting pain, near the sternum, particularly severe when lying on that side.

Burning pressure on the left side of the chest under the axilla. [*Ng.*]

Burning throbbing, externally on the left side of the chest, aggravated by inspiration. [*Ng.*]

730. Burning and tensive sensation in the middle of the chest, when inspiring, with sensitiveness of that spot. [*Ng.*]

Perspiration on the sternum, every morning.

The nipples of the breast are painful.

In the coccyx, a dull drawing, in the evening.

Severe itching on the coccyx, above the anus, with moisture and scurfy formation.

735. Pains in the sacrum, very violent, for two hours. [*Ng.*]

Severe pain in the sacrum, in the morning on rising, going off on motion.

Violent pain in the sacrum, as after long stooping (5th, 6th d.). [*Ng.*]

Pain as from a bruise in the sacrum.

Violent pain as from a bruise, in the sacrum, particularly when touched. [*Ng.*]

740. Pressure in the sacrum.

Severe griping and twisting in the sacrum, as with a pair of tongs, and then also pain in the arms and feet, as if it would turn them outward.

Shooting pain in the sacrum (aft. sev. h.).

Throbbing in the sacrum.

Pain in the back; pressure by the side of the spine.

745. Pressure in the back, between the scapulæ.

Violent drawing in the back.

Contractive pain between the scapulæ, day and night. [*Ng.*]

Rheumatic pain in the left scapula, for several days. [*Ng.*]

Stitches and pains in the left scapula.

750. Pain, as from bruising, in the scapulæ.

Crawling on the back, as from ants.

The nape and the shoulders are painful on lying on them and on turning over, (owing to the glandular swellings on the side of the neck, and yet these themselves are not painful).

Pain, so that she would like to scream, in the neck and on both shoulders, on bending the head forward; she cannot raise either of her arms to her head for pain.

Violent pains in the nape of the neck.

755. **Stiffness of the nape.**

Stiffness and shooting pain in the neck. [*Htb.*]

Tearing stitches in the nape, frequently (aft. 21 d.). [*Ng.*]

Rheumatic pain in the nape (aft. 12 d.).

Excoriative, cutting pain, as from an ulcer, on the seventh cervical vertebra.

760. Painful tension in the nape and on the right side of the neck, on moving the head. [*Ng.*]

Sensation on turning the head to the left side, as if there was a hard body of the size of an egg behind the ear (9th d.). [*Ng.*]

Stitches on both sides of the neck, when moving the head. [*Ng.*]

Many lumps about the neck, which disfigure it, like a large goitre, but after a few days, they pass away entirely.

The glands on the side of the neck, down toward the shoulder, are swollen and painful when the neck is bent sideways, and when lying on it, as if tense and stiff.

765. The axillæ are painful, for two days (aft. 26 d.).

Pinching and shooting in the right axilla (12th d.). [*Ng.*]

In the left shoulder, rheumatic pain

Tearing in the left shoulder-joint, on moving the arm. [*Ng.*]

Violent tearing in the right shoulder at night; it goes off through external warmth. [*Ng.*]

770. Shooting in the shoulder-joint and elbow-joint, also when at rest; worst at night.

Severe shooting in the left shoulder, arresting the breath, for three days (aft. 4 d.).

Burning stitch, frequently on the left shoulder. [*Ng.*]

Burning in the shoulder-joint (aft. 14 d.). [*Ng.*]

In the arm, a drawing.

775. Shooting consisting of two or three stitches in the upper arm, the fore-arm and the hand.

Twitching in the muscles of the arm.

Cramp pain in the left arm, with sensation of heat therein.

The right arm goes to sleep.

The arm goes to sleep, when lying on it.

780. The arm and the hand go to sleep, when sitting down (3d d.).

On the upper arm, sense of excoriation (aft. 7 d.).

Sudden burning on a small spot of the right upper arm, with simultaneous feeling of coldness therein (10th d.). [*Ng.*]

The olecranon processes of the elbows are painful when touched.

Pain in the bend of the elbow, so that he cannot straighten out his arm. [*Rl.*]

785. Pain in the bend of the elbow, on stretching out the arm, as if something was too short.

Muscular twitching in the elbow-joint.

Paralytic pressure in the left elbow-joint and forearm after the noon-siesta.

Drawing in the elbow-joint, when at rest, and tearing in it, when raising the arm, with a sensation as if cold water ran through its shaft bones.

Sharp cutting drawing in the right elbow-joint, whereby the arm became momentarily, as it were, paralyzed and useless.

790. In the forearm, a drawing cramp-like tension in a muscle.

Severe tearing in the left forearm, near the wrist. [*Ng.*]

Gnawing pain in the bones of the right forearm. [*Ng.*]

Burning pain, like fire, in the right forearm on which he lay at night, with sensation in the elbow as if asleep. [*Ng.*]

Sudden burning on a small spot of the forearm. [*Ng.*]

795. **In the hands, tearing,** like rheumatism (aft. 24 d.).

Tearing in the hand, in the phalangeal bone behind the last joint of the thumb. [*Ng.*]

Severe tearing in the right hand. [*Ng.*]

Violent dull shooting through the right wrist-joint. [*Ng.*]

Pain as from a blow, on the back of the left hand, worse when pressed upon. [*Ng.*]

800. Pain as from a sprain, in the right wrist-joint.

Shooting burning pain in the left palm, which soon passes over into the thumb, in the evening in bed. [*Htb.*]

The right hand goes to sleep (aft. 19 d.).

The hand goes to sleep, when sitting (3d d.).

Numbness and sensation as of being asleep, in the hand, after straining it in working for several hours.

805. The hands become emaciated.

Itching in the ball of the left hand.

Erysipelas on the hands.

The skin of the hands is parched, being chapped in several places.

Painful chapping everywhere on the hands; on moving the fingers, the skin tears open.

810. The fingers at times cross spasmodically over each other, without pain, and when she strikes on them, they separate again in the same way.

Sensation, as if her thumb would be drawn inward, when holding something in her hand. [*Ng.*]

The left index is spasmodically drawn inward.

Cramp-like drawing together of the fingers.

After grasping anything, the fingers still remain for some time bent and stiff.

815. A stitch in the ball of the thumb. [*Ng.*]

Violent stitch in the tip of the right thumb, under the nail. [*Ng.*]

Shooting and ulcerative pain in the finger-tips of the right hand. [*Ng.*]

Gouty, pressive tearing on the posterior joint of the right thumb, more when at rest than when in motion.

Tingling and sensation of numbness in the tip of the index. [*Ng.*]

820. Swelling and lack of flexibility of the middle joint on the middle finger, for several days.

Miliary eruption on the fingers.

Eroding vesicle on the little finger; it itched, festered and poured out much pus with burning and shooting; this continued for a long while, as well as the suppuration.

The finger-nails grow thicker.

In the muscles of the pelvis, dull stitching; very painful jerks about the right hip-joint, when sitting.

825. On one of the nates there is a furuncle (aft. 4 d.).

Eruptive pimples on the nates, which pain when touched.

Excoriative soreness, between the nates.

Soreness between the thighs, at the top, when taking a walk and afterwards (aft. 10 d.).

Painful soreness between the thighs, near the genitals.

830. In the hips, arthritic tearing.

Shooting in the left hip (3d d.).

In the lower limbs, a drawing downward.

Cramp-pain in the varices, when stretching the legs.

Cramp-pain and feeling of heat, here and there on the lower limb.

835. Rheumatic pain in the lower limbs.

Arthritic tearing in both the lower limbs and in the left hip.

Shooting in some parts of the thighs and legs.

Great restlessness in one of the lower limbs in the evening; he could not let it lie still for a minute.

Heaviness of the lower limbs.

840. Great heaviness in the right lower limb, so that he can hardly lift it. [*Ng.*]

Great heaviness and fatigue of the lower limbs. [*Ng.*]

The lower limbs go to sleep (aft. 24 d.).

The lower limbs go to sleep and feel dead, while taking a walk.

In the thighs, a drawing pain, seemingly in the bones.

845. Twitching drawing pain in the thigh, toward the groin, chiefly on rising from a seat.

Twitching sensation in the muscles of the thighs.

Tearing on the posterior side of the thigh, in the morning.

Tearing, now in the right thigh, now in the left, up into the hip, from the afternoon to the evening. [*Ng.*]

Stiffness of the right thigh, when walking, with a sensation as if it was bandaged above the knee.

850. Partly shooting, partly burning in the thigh at night, disturbing the sleep.

Pain as from a bruise, in the shaft of the femur.

Pain as from a bruise, in the middle of the thigh.

Much weariness in the thighs; he could hardly walk (aft. 5 d.).

Sensation of numbness and heat in the thigh, especially after sitting down.

855. Shooting itching on the thigh, as if an eruption would break out, where there was formerly a furuncle.

Red spot on the thigh, without any pain.

Red rough spot, like a tetter, on the upper part of the thigh, opposite the scrotum, usually itching a little in the morning.

Numberless red dots on the thighs; only a few of them, however, itch.

In the swelling above the knee, severe cutting, as from a knife.

860. In the houghs, a tension so that he could not straighten his limbs, the whole day (aft. 13 d.). [*Ng.*]

Pain in the hough, as if too short, with tension in the tendo Achillis, so that she cannot tread.

Sensation of stiffness in the houghs, in sitting, as if she was held fast there with hands. [*Ng.*]

Painful stiffness of the knees, when bending them.

Drawing pain in the knees.

865. Drawing and twitching in the left knee.

Shooting in the left knee.

Stitches in the patella.

Pain as from a strain in the left knee-joint, when walking. [*Ng.*]

Pain as from a bruise in the knees, at night.

870. Pain as from bruising in the knees, in bed in the morning; it goes off after rising. [*Ng.*]

Pain as from weariness, particularly in the knee-joints, in stooping and in sitting down, so that she cannot rise again when she sits down.

Weariness and heaviness in the left knee.

Numbness in the knee, causing him to wake up at night.

The legs are tense in walking, and pain as if bruised.

875. Straining and tension in the leg, where some of the veins are swollen, attended with stitches in them.

Cramp in the calves, the whole day.

Cramp in the calves, in the morning, in bed.

Cramp in the calves, from carrying something, with trembling of the lower limbs.

Cramp-like drawing in the calves, when rising.

880. Cramp-like drawing in the calves, at night, when stretching.

Cramp-like drawing in the legs, extending from the toes, which are drawn inward, to the knees.

Twitching in the calf.

Twitching of the muscles in the left calf.

Drawing pain on the tibia.

885. Drawing pain in the tendo Achillis (8th d.).

Tearing in the tibiæ. [*Ng.*]

Shooting in the calves, when pulling on the boots.

Stitches in the right leg, when blowing the nose.

Pain in the tibiæ, as from bruising, as if he had knocked against them.

890. Pain in the tibia, as if broken and shattered.

Pain in the calf, as from a misstep in jumping.

Throbbing on the outer side of the calf, for four days in succession, every hour, lasting for about fifteen minutes.

Severe shooting, burning pain on the leg, on a small spot above the ankle, so that she could not stand up straight; she had to lay her limb high, for when she let it hang down, the blood accumulated in it and it burned and stung.

In the swollen varices on the leg, a shooting pain.

895. **Swelling of the leg**, even when lying in bed.

Hard swelling of the leg, with lancinating pain (aft. 13 d.)

Great heaviness of the legs (4th d.).

Tingling of the legs, as if going to sleep.

Sensation of numbness in the bones of the right leg, but without pain.

900. Itching on the leg, where the veins are distended.

A tetter on the tibia vanishes. [*Htb.*]

Scurfy ulcer on the tibia, with a red, inflamed border, and swelling around it, which is so sensitive, that at night he cannot bear the coverlet upon it.

The ankles pain when touched.

Pain around the ankles (aft. 5 d.).

905. Pressive pain in the right ankle.

Pressure in the soles of the feet, under the balls of the toes, so that he had to limp.

Pressure and shooting in the heel (aft. 6 d.).

Pressive constriction in the ankle-joint.

Stiffness of the ankle-joint.

910. Severe twitching in the soles of the feet (aft. 24 d.).

Tearing in the heel.

Tearing in both edges of the foot. [*Ng.*]

Tearing in the ball of the foot, when walking. [*Ng.*]

Tearing in the sole of the right foot, with tickling. [*Ng.*]

915. Violent tearing in the dorsum of the foot. [*Ng.*]

Gouty tearing in the feet and toes.

Gnawing pain in the ankles and heels.

Very violent shooting in the heels, causing him to start, even when sitting.

Excessive pain in the malleoli of the right foot, as if they were broken, and at every step, a stitch in it, extending into the big toe; so that he had to hold on to something, else he would have fallen, especially during the first hour after rising in the morning.

920. Pain in the heel, as from a festering within.

Ulcerative pains in the soles of the feet. [*Ng.*]

The blood shoots into the sore foot, when standing.

Burning of the feet, for several days.

Burning in the sole of the left foot.

925. Burning of the soles of the feet, worse when walking. [*Ng.*]

Burning in the heels, with formication, chiefly in the morning in bed. [*Ng.*]

Sweating of the feet in the evening, with tearing in the feet and hands (aft. 12 h.).

Sweating of the feet, most profuse in the afternoon and evening.

Profuse sweating of the feet, they begin to smell.

930. Profuse sweating of the feet, on walking a short distance, causing the toes to be excoriated.

Profuse sweating of the feet, which become excoriated between the toes from walking, so that frequently he does not know what to do because of the pain.

Swelling of the sore foot.

Heaviness and lassitude of the feet, while the other parts of the body feel light (aft. 6 d.).

Tingling in the feet, toward the toes, like a slight tearing (aft. 5 d.).

935. The left foot goes to sleep, in the evening, when sitting. [*Ng.*]

Numbness and increased cold in the dorsum of the foot, when taking a walk (in June).

Cold feet (aft. several h.).

Ice-cold feet, all the morning.

Eruption of blisters below the ankles.

940. The toes are drawn inward (aft. 3 d.).

Constriction of the ball of the big toe, as if held with iron pincers.

Severe pressive pain in the right big toe.

Frequent tearing in the little toe, as if it would be drawn to one side. [*Ng.*]

Tearing in the left big toe, so that he could hardly stand it (1st d.). [*Ng.*]

945. Arthritic tearing in the toes.

Violent stitch in the left big toe, when sitting. [*Ng.*]

Swelling of the toes and the balls of the toes.

Itching on all the toes.

Shooting itching in the right big toe. [*Ng.*]

950. Soreness between the toes, with violent itching, for many days. [*Ng.*]

White blisters on one of the toes.

Large blisters with pus, with shooting pain, on each one of the little toes.

Ulcer on the fourth toe.

Suppuration of the edges of both the big toes

955. Pain on the nail of the big toe.

In the corn, pressive, burning pain. [*Htb.*]

Pain, as from excoriation of the corns, with hardly any pressure from without (aft. 2 d.).

Occasionally here and there a momentary pain, and then that part is also painful when touched.

Cramplike sensation occasionally on various parts of the body, on the arms, the neck, the fingers and the feet; the parts then swell up for a few days, become reddish, are indurated and sensitive to external touch.

960. Stiffness of the arm-joints and knees.

Stiffness of the limbs.

Painfully drawing tension all over the body, both at rest and in motion, particularly on the arms and the trunk.

Drawing in the whole body, as in intermittent fever, in the morning after rising.

Pain in the periosteum of all the bones, more a pressive than a drawing pain, only momentary, now here, now there, when at rest, especially when falling asleep.

965. Violent twitching in all the limbs, now in one, then in another, also in the shoulder and in the scrotum (aft. 10 d.).

Twitching here and there in the arms, in the evening in bed. [*Ng.*]

Stitches dart like lightning, from top to toe, through the body.

Pricks, as from needles, now here, now there, all over the body.

Pain, as from bruising, of the lower limb and of the scapula on which he is lying.

970. Pain, as from bruising, in all the limbs.

Pain, as from bruising, of the whole side of the body on which he lay during his noon-nap, and the arm is asleep.

Pain of the joints, as from weariness, when stooping and sitting down, so that she cannot rise again from her seat.

The arms and legs go to sleep.

The arms and legs go to sleep when sitting; when walking, there is formication in them, in the evening (8th and 9th d.). [*Ng.*]

975. The troubles present disappear when walking in the open air.

When starting on his walk, the pains recur.

On walking in the open air, the eyes began to run and they closed, as from drowsiness.

On taking a walk, pain in the left ankle-joint, as if strained, this goes off in the room.

On walking in the open air, very weary.

980. While walking in the open air and afterwards, weariness, so that he is ready to sink down, with choking and nausea.

While taking a walk, faint-like lassitude, as if coming from the abdomen.

Dislike of the open air, in the morning.

Sensitiveness to every draught, with hoarseness, chilliness, dryness of the nose, and anxiety in the evening.

Tendency to take cold; he has to avoid draughts.

985. Tendency to take cold, and consequent headache (aft. 3 d.).

Itching by day, on the back and the arms.

The itching becomes general and much excited; also in the face and on the genitals.

Momentary eroding itching, now here, now there, exciting to scratch.

Itching over the whole body, and after scratching, little pimples, containing water appear (aft. 17 d.). [*Ng.*]

990. Small pustules on the chin and on the chest. [*Ng.*]

Itching nodules full of smarting water, in various parts of the body, for twelve hours. [*Ng.*]

Little nodules, without sensation, spring up at night over the whole body, and go off in the morning. [*Ng.*]

Many small, red, itching pimples, with pus in their tips, burning after scratching; they vanish on the following day. [*Ng.*]

Spots, like flea-bites, here and there, on the body.

995. Many red, itching spots all over the body, especially on the calves, for seven days (aft. 25 d.). [*Ng.*]

The tetter turns into an inflammatory swelling, for four days.

The skin chaps on the limbs covered with herpes.

Unhealthy skin, every little lesion goes into suppuration.

Several small furuncles on the neck, on the back and on the arms.

1000. The ulcer becomes very painful.

The limb on which the ulcer had healed entirely, begins to pain occasionally, with drawing and tearing, particularly in the open air.

The limb on which there is an ulcer, begins, even in the parts at a distance from the ulcer, to pain violently, when touched or when moving slightly, as if the bone was shattered.

Itching pressure in the ulcer (aft. 5 d.).

Pressure and shooting in the ulcer (aft. 3 d.).

1005. Tearing in the ulcer (aft. 5 d.)

Burning pain in the cicatrix of an old ulcer.

Fetor of the ulcer (aft. 20 d.).

The scurf of the ulcer smells like herring-pickle.

Proud flesh in the ulcers.

1010. On the cicatrix of a wart, frequent shooting itching, like flea-bites, only transiently going off by rubbing.

In the varices, shooting and straining.

Itching on the swollen varices of the lower limbs.

Strong pulsation of the blood in the whole body, but especially about the heart, increased at every motion.

Pulsation for several minutes, in the heart, the trunk and the head, without anxiety, in the morning in bed.

1015. **Tremulous sensation throughout the whole body.**

Tremulous, in the morning.

Trembling and quivering about the head, neck and right arm.

Shocks, occasionally, throughout the whole body, as from fright, or from an electric shock, both in rest and in motion.

Twitching of the limbs in the evening, or at least tendency that way, almost every day.

1020. Frequent starts in the hands and feet (aft. 30 d.). [*Ng.*]

Involuntary twisting outward of the limbs, late in the evening, but while still conscious.

Heaviness in all the limbs, with gloominess.

Great indolence in the whole body; it went off on taking a long walk.

Fatigued and feels sick; he has to groan, without knowing for what pain.

1025. Feels broken down, but the head feels light.

Lassitude of all the limbs (aft. 3 or 4 d.).

Weary lack of tone in the whole body, as if from a cold.

Great lassitude in all the limbs (aft. 24 h.).

Great lassitude, especially in the lower limbs, which he can hardly drag along, with continual weariness.

1030. Sudden sinking of the strength.

Emaciation.

Fits of fainting (aft. 8 d.).

Paralytic sensation in all the joints.

Stretching of the limbs, with lassitude.

1035. Very much inclined to extend and stretch the limbs, without being able to stretch sufficiently (aft. 2 d.).

Frequent yawning (aft. 1 h.).

Feels in the morning as if she had not slept enough, it is hard for her to get out of bed.

Great weariness and sleepiness, in the forenoon and toward evening, with much yawning.

Incredibly tired and drowsy (aft. several h.).

1040. Drowsiness by day and great weariness (aft. 11 d.).

Great drowsiness during the day, so that she has to lie down.

Somnolence.

Very drowsy toward noon.

Falls aleep too early in the evening, with great weariness.

1045. She cannot go to sleep before 2 A. M.

Restless nights, with heat in the whole body (the first w.). [*Ng.*]

Restless nights, with heat (aft. 12 d.).

She cannot go to sleep before 12 at night, for heat and anguish.

She could not sleep all night, owing to restlessness in her lower limbs, which she could not keep still.

1050. Constant tossing about during the night, without weariness.

Restless nights, she always awakes about midnight, and cannot go to sleep again before 2 A. M. [*Ng.*]

Waking up too early.

Frequent awaking at night, as if in a slumber (aft. 15 d.).

Frequent awaking at night. [*Ng.*]

1055. Waking up in the morning at 2 o'clock, for several nights, with great restlessness.

She awakes at 3 A. M. and cannot go to sleep for several hours, and wakes up at 7, dizzy and fatigued.

Frequent awaking, as if frightened.

Frequent starting up in sleep. [*Ng.*]

Sleep, troubled with dreams.

1060. Nights constantly full of dreams. [*Ng.*]

Voluptuous dreams (aft. 3 d.). [*Ng.*]

Very vivid dreams.

Vivid dreams, long-remembered.

Very vivid, anxious dreams.

1065. **Anxious dreams**, so that on awaking she is quite beside herself.

Anxious dreams, from which she wakes up with anguish or fear. [*Ng.*]

Dreams about disagreeable things, which she heard of during the day, from which she awakes with anxiety.

Anxious dreams about drowsiness and unconsciousness; then very difficult awaking from a deep sleep, with stiffness in the muscles of the neck.

Anxious dreams, taking away her breath; she screamed and lay in a perspiration.

1070. Anxious talking in sleep.

Anxious, fearful dreams.

Fearful dream of danger threatening from water. [*Ng.*]

Terrible dreams (aft. 5 d.).

Dreams about the dead (2d night).

1075. Dreams about the dead (aft. 29 d.). [*Ng.*]

Dream about fire.

Vexatious dreams.

Vexatious, anxious dreams.

Vexatious dreams, with groaning and moaning in sleep.

1080. Dreams, straining the head.

She dreams only what she had seen and thought about during the day.

Troublesome dreams.

Many dreams, with distorted images, with reference to everything that happened the last two days.

All kinds of images before the eyes as soon as she has closed them at night.

1085. Fanciful ravings at night.

At night, continual anxiety, so that he could not stay in bed; he also talked in his sleep continually (aft. 12 h.).

In the night, after lying down, solicitous thoughts, which she cannot get rid of, and which become so tormenting and disquieting, that the blood came into ebullition and she could not sleep all night (5th d.).

He awakes at 2 A. M., restless in mind; he thought of everything that could distress him, and this disquieted him, so that he often did not know where to turn, for seven nights (aft. 12 h.).

She had to think at night about many things, so that she could not sleep all night.

1090. A fixed idea did not allow him to go to sleep before midnight.

At night, restlessness, with anxious warmth and disquieting dreams.

At night he could not stay under cover for heat (aft. 5 d.).

Heat at night, and in the morning, on awaking, ebullition of blood.

In the first sleep, at night, twitches in the arms, frequently in succession.

1095. At night, while asleep, slight twitches.

On going to sleep, sweat on the head.

At night, epistaxis comes on.

At night, toothache, till morning.

At night, great dryness in the mouth and throat.

1100. In the evening, in bed, nausea like a fainting fit, which kept him from sleeping for two hours.

At night, inclination to vomit, with swoon-like weakness.

At night, eructations, still tasting of the soup at dinner (aft. 7 d.).

At night, in bed, waterbrash.

At night and in the morning, pressure in the scrobiculus cordis (aft. 9 d.).

1105. **At night, frequent micturition**, hypochondriac restlessness, despondency, sweat of anguish, insomina.

At night, wetting the bed, while asleep.

At night, suffocating fit, causing her to wake up; she could not get her breath.

At night, the lower limb tends to go to sleep, attended with great peevishness.

At night, chill and drawing pain in the limbs, causing him to awake; then shooting pain in the fleshy part of the chest and in the left side, at every breath.

1110. Much sensation of chilliness, with cold hands and feet. [*Rl.*]

Chilliness, in the morning in bed, in the morning.

Chilly feeling in the morning in bed, for many mornings in succession.

Chill during the day, when lying down to sleep.

Chill from 4 P. M. till in the evening after going to sleep (aft. 24 d.). [*Ng.*]

1115. Chilliness for several days, before dinner.

Chilliness the whole day and the night; no sleep on account of chill.

Chill in the evening before going to sleep, then itching.

Sensation of coldness, as from lack of blood.

Sensation of cold and chilliness, with ringing in the ears (aft. ¼ h.).

1120. Sudden coldness all over.

Every evening, the child complains of coldness for half an hour.

Coldness in the whole body, commencing at 5 P. M. with icy cold feet.

Much coldness and shivering, especially coldness of the hands and feet.

Cold hands and feet, the whole day, in balmy weather. [*Rl.*]

1125. Cold hands and feet in the evening, with heat in the face (aft. 6 d.). [*Rl.*]

Shivering in the back, in the forenoon, with frequent yawning and inclination to sleep.

Febrile rigor in the back for several evenings.

Cold shiver before and after a meal, then in the evening for one and one-half hours, heat with anxiety.

Violent fever; he could not get warm, not even in the evening in the warmed bed; the whole evening and the whole night, violent thirst; after midnight, violent sweat till morning; in the evening, during the chill, headache and tearing in all the limbs, with coated tongue (aft. 36 h.).

1130. Febrile rigor, in the evening, with stitching pain in the temples, the left ear and the teeth; in the night following, sweat.

Severe febrile rigor, in the morning and evening; then heat, followed by sweat.

Intermittent fever, every day; in the evening a shaking, chill, an hour later, heat in the face and cold feet, without subsequent sweat.

Heat, when sitting down, often coming on suddenly, at times with anxieties (aft. 17 d.).

Heated, from driving in a carriage.

1135. Dry heat in the whole body, in the evening, for one-quarter hour. [*Ng.*]

Dry heat, every evening and through the night till morning, with headache in the crown and the nape, lasting till noon (aft. 17 d.).

Hot hands, and heat and burning in the soles of the feet, so that she can hardly tread (at once).

Perspiration even at the slightest motion, in a woman who else was not given to perspiring (aft. 4 d.).

Perspiration, coloring the linen yellow, even after a short walk, with fatigue.

1140. Perspiration all over, from a serious conversation (aft. 7 d.).

Night-sweat, for several nights (cured by wine).

For several mornings, in bed, perspiration.

Very fetid transpiration of the body.

Sour smelling perspiration.

GUAJACUM. JUIAC.

The sap which flows from the West Indian tree *Guajacum officinale*, which when inspissated is called *Gummi Guajaci*, consists in great part of a peculiar kind of resin. For homœopathic use this is triturated dry with sugar of milk for three hours to the one millionth attenuation, and then dissolved and raised to the thirtieth potency. The homœopathic physician will not allow himself to be led astray by the indefinite and delusive recommendation of the old Materia Medica to use Guajacum for gout and rheumatism. He will not look to fictitious names of diseases, but he will look to the similarity of the symptoms existing on the one side in the disease to be healed, and on the other in the symptoms excited by the remedy.

The whole of this pathogenesis, save for fifteen symptoms of Hahnemann's, appeared in Vol. IV. of the *Materia Medica Pura;* it belongs accordingly to his earlier manner.—*Hughes.*

In diseases for which it is homœopathically appropriate it has shown itself serviceable especially where the following ailments were present: Attacks of cephalagra; swelling of the eyes; painful straining in the ears; sensation of mucus in the throat, causing nausea· repugnance to milk; constipation; stitches in the chest; arthritic lancination in the limbs, especially contractions produced by tearing, lancinating pains in the limbs, where the pains are produced by the slightest motion and are combined with heat in the painful parts, especially after previous misuse of mercury; pulmonary consumption, with fetid pus, etc.

The abbreviations of the names of my fellow-provers are: *Htn.*, *Dr. Hartman; Lgh.*, *Dr. Langhammer; Tth.*, *Teuthorn.*

GUAJACUM.

Morose mood; he speaks but little.

Great peevishness.

Contemptuous humor.

Obstinacy.

5. Indisposed to work. [*Htn.*]

Weakness of memory.

Weak memory; he forgets what he has just now read, and old names he does not remember at all.

Without thinking, he stands in one place, and looks right in front of him without thought; in the morning (at breakfast) when standing. [*Tth.*]

Headache, at night, like a pressure from below upward in the brain.

10. Pressive pain in the right temple, as with something broad. [*Htn.*]

Painless pressure in the left temple.

Pressive headache across the forehead. [*Lgh.*]

Pressing and squeezing in the anterior part of the forehead. [*Htn.*]

Dull, pressive pain in the head, terminating with a sharp stitch in the right frontal protuberance. [*Htn.*]

15. Dull, pressive pain, going up obliquely from the left side of the nape to a point over the vertex, and terminating at the top with a stitch. [*Htn.*]

Dull, stitch-like pain in the right frontal eminence. [*Htn.*]

Drawing pain from the middle of the frontal bone down into the nasal bones. [*Htn.*]

Tearing in the whole of the left side of the head. [*Htn.*]

Tearing in the right side of the occiput. [*Htn.*]

20. Drawing tearing in the anterior part of the forehead. [*Htn.*]

Drawing tearing in the occiput and the forehead. [*Htn.*]

Violent, coarse stitches in the brain, upward.

Dull, drawing stitches from the left parietal bone into the frontal eminence, where they all terminate in a single stitch. [*Htn.*]

Pressive, drawing, tearing stitch in the right side of the head, toward the frontal bone. [*Htn.*]

25. Sensation as if the brain was detached and loose, and moved at every step, in the morning.

A tearing, externally, on the left temple. [*Htn.*]

A tearing, externally, from the left side of the frontal bone downward into the muscles of the cheeks. [*Htn.*]

Lively stitches on the left side of the head, at the junction of the parietal and the frontal bones. [*Htn.*]

Dull, painful stitches on the left side of the occiput. [*Htn.*]

30. An external headache, as if there were too much blood in the integuments of the head, and as if the head were swollen, when sitting. [*Tth.*]

External pulse-like throbbing headache, with stitches in the temples, only transiently removed by external pressure, relieved by walking, but aggravated by sitting and standing (aft. 3 h.). [*Tth.*]

In the right eyebrow, a hard pimple, with a white apex and severe pain, as if wounded, when touched.

Sensation of swelling of the eyes and as if they protruded; the eyelids seemed too short to cover the eyes: at the same time, he felt all day as if he had not slept enough, with yawning and stretching. [*Tth.*]

Eye-gum in both the canthi of the right eye (aft. 1 h.). [*Lgh.*]

35. Dilatation of the pupils (aft. 3 h.). [*Tth.*]

Amaurosis for some days. [WHITE, in *Edinb. Med. Comment.* IV., p. 327.[1]]

Straining earache in the left ear. [*Htn.*]

Tearing in the left ear. [*Htn.*]

Tearing in the outer border of the cartilage of the left ear. [*Htn.*]

40. In the nose, a pimple, with pain as from excoriation.

The face is red and painfully swollen for some days. [BANG. *Tageb.* d. Krank. Haus., 1784.[2]]

Dull, spasmodic drawing in the muscles of the right cheek, in the morning on rising.

Single stitches in the right zygoma. [*Htn.*]

Stitches, as from a knife in the right cheek (aft. 1 h.). [*Lgh.*]

45. In the lower jaw, on the left side, a dull, pressive pain. [*Htn.*]

On the left side of the lower jaw, a drawing pain, terminating in a stitch. [*Htn.*]

Toothache, a pressive pain in the left upper molars, on biting. [*Htn.*]

Tearing in the upper molars of the left side.

Flat taste in the mouth. [*Tth.*]

50. Lack of appetite, and loathing of everything. [*Tth.*]

---

[1] In a hysterical subject. The writer states that any sudden surprise will make her speechless for an hour or so, and that G. always makes her lose her sight for some hours.—*Hughes.*

[2] Not accessible.—*Hughes.*

Great hunger, in the afternoon and evening (aft. 7, 9 h.). [*Lgh.*]

Much thirst.

Eructation (immediately). [*Htn.*]

Empty eructation.

55. Empty eructation of mere air. [*Tth.*]

In the scrobiculus cordis, a frequently recurring pressure, with impeded breathing, and with oppression and anguish (aft. 1 h.). [*Htn.*]

Constrictive sensation in the gastric region, with anguish and impeded breathing (aft. 19 h.). [*Htn.*]

Pain in the abdomen, pinching on the left side of the navel, on a small spot (aft. 3½ h.). [*Htn.*]

Pinching in the abdomen, as from incarcerated flatulence, which continually extended further backwards, whereupon flatus was discharged. [*Htn.*]

60. Dull pinching in the hypogastrium, that always sinks deeper backward. [*Htn.*]

Pinching cutting, transversely through the abdomen, during inspiring. [*Htn.*]

Stitches in the left subcostal region. [*Htn.*]

Dull stitches in the left epigastrial region. [*Htn.*]

A constant quivering in the inner abdominal muscles on the right side, close to the os ilii. [*Htn.*]

65. Pain in the groin, as from an inguinal hernia.

Rumbling in the abdomen (aft. 10 h.).

Rumbling in the abdomen, with dull pinching, which extends ever further backward, whereupon flatus is discharged (aft. 1 h.). [*Htn.*]

Growling in the abdomen, as from emptiness (aft. 5 h.) [*Lgh.*]

Constipation (1st d.). [*Tth.*]

70. Costiveness (2d, 3d d.). [*Tth.*]

Soft, broken up stool. [*Htn.*]

Thin, slimy stool, after previous pinching in the abdomen. [*Htn.*]

Frequent urging to urinate, even immediately after doing so. [*Tth.*]

Frequent urgent desire to urinate, with scanty discharge (aft. 5 h.). [*Lgh.*]

75. He has to pass water every half hour, and much at a time; when he has passed it, he has again urging to urinate for about a minute, whereby only a few drops come away. [*Tth.*]

Constant urging to urinate, and every time he passes much urine. [*Htn.*]

Cutting during micturition, as if something acrid was discharged.

After micturition, stitches in the neck of the bladder. [*Tth.*]

Emission of semen, at night, without lascivious dreams. [*Lgh.*]

80. Increased flow from the vagina.

* * * * * * * *

Frequent discharge of a watery fluid from the nose, for one month. [BANG.]

Expectoration of mucus by hawking, and by hacking cough. [*Tth.*]

Sudden sensation of stoppage or stagnation on the chest, in the region of the scrobiculus cordis, like obstruction of breath; this often seizes upon her suddenly even at night in sleep, and compels her to an almost dry cough, which recurs until there is some expectoration.

Pain in the chest, stitches in the left side under the true ribs, more toward the back. [*Htn.*]

85. A crawling in the chest.

Shudder in the breast.

Pain in the back, with contractive sensation, between the scapulæ. [*Htn.*]

Rheumatic stiffness in the whole left side of the back, from the nape down into the sacrum, with unbearable pain at the least motion and turning of the parts; this was not felt when at rest or when the parts were touched.

Drawing and tearing, down along the right side of the spine, from the axilla to the last rib. [*Htn.*]

90. Tearing stitches on the posterior border of the right scapula (aft. 10 h.). [*Htn.*]

Tearing stitches on the border of both scapulæ, followed by a constriction in the dorsal muscles (aft. 3 h.). [*Htn.*]

Constant stitches, which seemed at last to change into a single continuous stitch, close under the right scapula, seemingly coming from the middle of the right side of the thoracic cavity, aggravated by inspiration. [*Htn.*]

Eroding itching in the back by day.

Pressive pain in the neck, on the right and left sides of the cervical vertebræ (aft. 4 h.). [*Htn.*]

95. Constant frequent stitches, on the left side of the neck, from the scapula even to the occiput, when moving; also when the head is held still. [*Htn.*]

Violent, continued stitches in the neck, from the larynx to the left clavicle (aft. 9 h.). [*Htn.*]

Sharp stitches on the top of the right shoulder, frequently recurring. [*Htn.*]

Painful drawing tearing in the left arm, from the upper arm even into the fingers, but particularly continued in the wrist. [*Htn.*]

Severe painful stitches in the right upper arm, chiefly in its middle. [*Htn.*]

100. Lassitude of the upper arms, as after hard work. [*Tth.*]

In the right fore-arm, tearing, down into the wrist-joint. [*Htn.*]

Frequent drawing tearing stitches, from the left elbow into the wrist-joint. [*Htn.*]

Pressive-like tearing in the left wrist-joint. [*Htn.*]

Continuous drawing tearing in the left wrist-joint (aft. 2 h.). [*Htn.*]

105. Single, violent stitches in the right thumb (aft. 1 h.). [*Htn.*]

In the nates, needle pricks when walking, but more yet when sitting down; she feels as if she sat on needles.

The lower limbs, especially the thighs, are fatigued, as if after a long walk on the previous day. [*Tth.*]

Formication in the thighs and legs, extending to the toes, as if the limbs would go to sleep while sitting.

In the right thigh, from the middle to the knee, a formicating pressive pain in the bones, while sitting still (aft. ¼ h.). [*Htn.*]

110. Pain, like growing pains, in the right thigh. [*Htn.*]

Tension in the thighs, especially in the right thigh. when walking, as if the muscles were too short, attended with weariness; aggravated by touching it, allayed when sitting. [*Tth.*]

An aching drawing pain from the middle of the right thigh to the knee, when extending the right leg; on drawing up and flexing it, the pain goes off. [*Htn*]

Drawing tearing from the middle of the left thigh to the knee. [*Htn.*]

Twitching tearing, from the middle of the right thigh to the knee (aft. ½ h.). [*Htn.*]

115. Dull stitches in the thigh, above the right knee. [*Htn.*]

Single stitches on the left thigh, above the knee, from both sides, meeting in the middle (aft. 3 h.).

Bruised pain in the left thigh, when walking in the open air. [*Lgh.*]

Single itching stitches, like flea-bites, in the skin of the thighs, particularly on both sides of the hough; removed by scratching. [*Tth.*]

Drawing pain in the knee, ending in a stitch. [*Htn.*]

120. On the leg, a painless contraction in the right calf (aft. ½ h.). [*Htn.*]

Violent twitching stitches on the outer side of the calf.

Drawing stitches in the leg, from the right ankle-joint to the middle of the tibia (aft. 3 h.). [*Htn.*]

Tearing obtuse stitches, from the middle of the left tibia to the toes. [*Htn.*]

Tearing stitches between the tibia and fibula, up into the patella, so violent that it made him jump up high.

125. Tearing drawing stitches, from the middle of the right tibia to the knee (aft. 14 h.). [*Htn.*]

Long drawing, tearing stitches in the leg, from the right ankle into the knee. [*Htn.*]

After walking, the legs feel bruised, as if they were brittle.

Tingling in the skin of the whole leg, with sensation of heat in it.

In the ankle-joint, on the right side, single sharp stitches, when sitting. [*Htn.*]

130. Pain terminating in a sharp stitch, on a small spot on the dorsum of the right foot, going off by motion. [*Htn.*]

The symptoms almost all occur when sitting, most of them in the morning immediately after rising, or in the evening shortly before going to sleep; some from 9 A. M. till 12. [*Htn.*]

Burning itching of the skin, increased by scratching.

General discomfort in the whole body (aft. 7 h.). [*Htn.*]

Weariness, especially in the thighs and upper arms, as after great exertions. [*Tth.*]

135. Marasmus and hectic fever, with persons of a dry habit of body. [MATTHIOLI, *d. morb. Gall.*, p. 63, 1537.[1]]

Indolence and indisposition to move.

Yawning and stretching of the limbs, with comfortable feeling (aft. ½ h.). [*Htn.*]

Stretching of the upper extremities, with yawning. [*Htn.*]

Yawning and stretching of the limbs, with a sensation during the whole day of not having slept enough. [*Tth.*]

140. Great drowsiness in the afternoon. [*Lgh.*]

Later in falling asleep in the evening, and earlier than usual in waking up. [*Tth.*]

In the evening, in bed, he cannot fall asleep for two hours, and tosses about in his bed. [*Tth.*]

He wakes up in the morning unrefreshed, as if he had not slept at all. [*Tth.*]

On awaking too early, everything feels too tight, and he tosses about in bed. [*Tth.*]

145. Sleep full of dreams. [*Tth.*]

Vivid dream about scientific subjects. [*Lgh.*]

Dreams of fighting.

Dreams, as if she should be killed by being stabbed with knives.

Nightmare, while lying on his back, awaking with a scream. [*Tth.*]

150. Frequent waking out of sleep, as from fright; or as if he were falling. [*Lgh.*]

When going to sleep in the evening, he felt as if some one threw a cloth in his face, at which he was much frightened. [*Tth.*]

Shivering in the back, in the afternoon. [*Lgh.*]

Febrile chill in the back, in the afternoon (aft. 8 h.). [*Lgh.*]

Chilliness, even behind the warm stove. [*Htn.*]

155. In the forenoon, a chill for two hours, and in the evening a chill before going to sleep; this continued also in bed; in the morning some perspiration.

Internal chill in the whole body, immediately followed by heat, especially in the face, without thirst, toward evening. [*Tth.*]

Heat in the whole face, with thirst, without redness and without perspiration. [*Htn.*]

When walking in the open air, much perspiration, particularly on the head; on the forehead, beads of sweat.

Profuse perspiration at night, in the back.

160. Every morning some perspiration.

---

[1] Observation.—*Hughes.*

HEPAR SULPHURIS CALCAREUM.

A mixture of equal parts of finely powdered, clean oyster shells and quite pure flowers of sulphur is kept for ten minutes at a white heat in a hermetically closed crucible and afterwards stored up in a well-corked bottle. To develop its powers, it is treated like other dry drugs in order to potentize it to the higher degrees, according to the directions at the end of the first volume.

Besides belladonna, chamomilla is an antidote to the colic and diarrhœa.

Hepar sulphuris has proved itself particularly useful, when having been selected according to the similarity of symptoms, there were besides present one or more of the following symptoms:

Boring headache in the root of the nose, every morning from seven to twelve o'clock; ulcerative pain just above the eye every evening; shooting pains in the eyes; photophobia; flow of fetid pus from the ear; erysipelas in the face with prickling turgidity; dryness of the throat; scrapy sore throat, interfering with speaking, but not with deglutition; a plug in the throat; voracious hunger; eructation; fits of nausea, with coldness and paleness; swelling and pressure in the gastric region; frequent and too easy derangement of the stomach; contractive pain in the abdomen; stitches in the left side of the abdomen; incarceration of flatus; difficult discharge of flatus in the morning; nocturnal passage of urine during sleep; flow of mucus from the urethra; lack of sexual desire; lack of erections; weak erections during coitus; *emission of prostatic juice after micturition*, during a hard stool and *per se;* retarded menses; leucorrhœa, with excoriation on the pudenda; cough; severe cough in the evening, when lying abed; spasmodic contraction of the chest, after speaking; cancerous ulcers on the chest, with shooting, burning pain on its edges and fetor as of old cheese; tearing in the arm toward the ulcer in the chest; drawing in the back between the scapulæ; fetid sweat of the axillæ; encysted tumor on the point of the elbow; dying-off of the fingers; drawing pain in the limbs, chiefly in the morning on awaking; trembling weariness after smoking tobacco; yawning; tendency to perspire by day; flying heat, with perspiration.

The symptoms marked *Fr. H.* are from *Dr. Friedrich Hahnemann;* those marked *Stf.*, from Medical Counselor *Dr. Stapf.*

A pathogenesis of Hepar sulphuris appeared in Vol. IV. of the *Mat. Med. Pura*, containing 282 symptoms from Hahneman, and 16 from the two fellow-observers mentioned above. The additional ones in the present work are all from himself and belong to his later manner.—*Hughes.*

HEPAR SULPHURIS CALCAREUM.

Sad mood, for many hours; she had to weep violently.

Very hypochondriac.

Dejected, sad and apprehensive.

Fearful anguish, in the evening, for two hours; he thought he had to perish, and was sad even so that he could have committed suicide.

5. Fears about the illness of his family, especially while walking in the open air.

Ill-humored, in the morning after rising, is unwilling to speak, but cheerful while in bed.

Contrary mood; he does not like to look at his folks.

Very discontented and peevish over his pains, and discouraged.

Irritable mood; whatever she started to do, was not satisfactory, she wished to be alone (1st d.).

10. No pleasure in anything.

Dissatisfied with oneself.

She thinks about everything disagreeable that happened to her in her lifetime.

Whatever she thought about was unsatisfactory and did not suit her.

Peevishness and impatience.

15. Extremely peevish and obstinate.

Vexed about trifles.

Very peevish; every trifle vexed her.

The least thing put him into a violent passion, he could have murdered anyone without hesitation.

Great weakness of memory during his peevishness; he had to think quite a while before he could remember anything.

20. Visionary appearance of a deceased person, in the morning in bed, after becoming awake and conscious; this frightened him; he also imagined he saw a neighboring house in flames, which terrified him also.

Vertigo, with nausea, in the evening.

In the morning, an hour after rising, violent vertigo.

Everything seems to turn around with her, when she closes the eyes for the noon nap.

Vertigo at dinner, with eructation; everything became black before her eyes, as in a swoon; but it only lasted a short time.

25. Fainting vertigo with staring of the eyes, or failing of sight, as if he sat wrapped in thoughts.

Vertigo, while riding in a carriage; this was so violent that on getting out she could not stand alone.

Frequent brief fits of inability to recollect while walking in the open air.

He became quite sad from stretching himself on the sofa.

While at work, his thoughts all at once were quite gone.

30. He was quite stupid and could neither comprehend nor remember anything.

She easily makes slips in speaking and in writing.

Stupefaction and heaviness in the sinciput.

Dizziness and heaviness in the head.

Headache when shaking the head, with vertigo.

35. Aching in the head, every morning, at every concussion.

Dull headache, in the morning, in bed, diminished after rising. [*Stf.*]

Headache in the forehead, as if bruised, in the morning, on awaking; this lasts till some time after rising; at the same time a similar quiet but very disagreeable aching in the abdomen; the headache is aggravated by moving the eyes.

From midnight onwards, while in bed, headache, as from a boil in the forehead; when stooping and coughing, pricking as from needles; also externally when touched, the forehead was painful as from a furuncle and like needle-pricks; for several mornings.

Pressive headache in the morning, on awaking.

40. Pressure in the right half of the brain, now sharper, then again duller, from time to time.

Pressive pain, with heat on the crown.

Sensation of severe heat in the forehead.

Pressive pain in the crown, with palpitation, in the evening (3d d.).

Pressure and drawing in the temples by day.

45. Constant pressive pain in one-half of the brain, as from a peg or nail.

Tensive headache, above the nose.

Contractive headache, also resounding while walking, and pressing on the skull from within; this becomes very violent in the open air, but passes away in the room.

At night, violent headache, as if the forehead would be torn out, with general heat without thirst.

Stitches in the head and severe sensation of obtuseness as if the skull would burst; it wakes him up at night.

50. Stitches in the head when stooping, with a sensation as if the head would burst; the eyes close from pain.

After a deep sleep, in the morning, a shooting headache, which goes off on taking a walk (4th d.).

Shooting headache.

Shooting headache in the forehead, as from needle-pricks.

On rising up again after stooping, and on every movement, stitches in the head, particularly after taking a walk.

55. Shooting pain, like pulsation, in the occiput and in its lower part.

A boring pain on a small spot in the side of the head.

Boring pain in the right temple, extending into the upper part of the head.

Burrowing headache with nausea, at once while in bed, for four mornings in succession; it goes off by tying a bandage tightly around the head.

Painful beating in the right temple.

60. Hammering in the head.

Swashing in the head.

Externally on the right side of the occiput, a pressive pain, which gradually passes into the nape, the neck and the scapulæ.

In the afternoon, on lying down, a spasmodic twitching in the frontal muscles; it only went off on getting up.

Eruption of pimples, like blotches, on the hairy scalp and in the nape, which feel sore when touched, but not when let alone.

65. Eruption of many pimples on the side of the forehead, which feel worst in the room, but which soon get better in the open air.

Two painless swollen elevations on the forehead.

The forehead is painful from the hat.

The hair falls out very much (aft. 5 d.).

The hair falls out and bald spots are formed on several parts of the head.

70. Rings below the eyes, very blue.

At every step, his eyes ache.

The eyes pain violently, as if they were drawn into the head.

Pressive pain in the eyeballs, and bruised feeling when touched.

Pressure in the eyes, especially on moving them, with redness of the same.

75. Pressure in the eyes, in frequent fits during the day, followed by lachrymation.

Obtuse stitch in the eyes.

Boring pain in the upper bones of the orbit.

Cutting pain in the outer canthus.

Pain as from excoriation in the outer canthus with accumulation of eye-gum.

80. Pressure in the eyelids, as if from sleepiness; they are reddened.

Redness, inflammation and swelling of the upper eyelid with a pain more pressive than shooting.

Inflammation and swelling of the eye, with redness of the white part.

The white of the eye turns reddish.

Sore eyes, closed at night by suppuration; eye-gum is secreted, the eyes become dim, and he cannot see well by candle-light.

85. Eruption of pimples on the upper eyelids, and below the eyes.

On waking in the morning, the eyelids are closed, so that she is unable to open them for a long time.

After writing, she has to wink with her eyes.

The eyes are obscured while reading.

On rising and standing up, after sitting while stooping forward, his eyes seem blinded.

90. Flickering before the eyes; whatever she looked at, seemed dark; then great lassitude.

Flickering and sensation as of a veil before the eyes, he could not recognize any object.

Daylight causes the eyes to be painful.

His eyes are painful in bright daylight, when he wishes to move them.

The ear pains externally at night, when lying on it.

95. Twitches of pain through the ear.

Violent stitches in the ear, when blowing the nose.

Itching in the ears.

Heat, redness and itching of the external ears, for six days.

Increase of the ear-wax.

100. Flow of pus from the ear.

Rushing sound in the ear.

Hissing in the left ear.

Hissing and throbbing before the ears, in the evening on lying down, till the person falls asleep.

Crepitation in the ears, as from electric sparks.

105. Whistling in the ears, when blowing the nose.

When blowing the nose, there is a whistling sound in the right ear.

Explosion in the ear, when blowing the nose.

A cracking sound in the head on the right side, after violently blowing the nose; after this the roaring in the ear of the (deaf) person ceased and he heard again a little (curative effect).

The bones of the nose pain on being touched.

110. Drawing pain in the nose, which pain then passes into the eyes, and becomes a smarting, in the morning.

Sensation of contraction in the nose.

Itching in the nose.

When blowing the nose, a disagreeable formication in the left nostril as from a foreign body within it.

Redness and heat internally and externally on the nose, with swelling of the same.

115. Burning in the nose, lasting into the night.

Bruised pain in the tip of the nose.

Pain as from soreness, on the back of the nose,, when touched.

Pain as from ulceration in the nostrils.

Scabs in the right side of the nose.

120. Yellowish water, very glutinous, drips from the one nostril.

Rush of blood to the nose (at once).

Coagulated blood is blown from the nose.

Epistaxis, two days in succession.

Epistaxis after singing.

125. The mucus from the posterior nares was mixed with much blood.

Every morning some drops of blood come from the nose (also after ¼ h.).

Very sensitive olfaction.

Very acute smell.

Loss of the sense of smell.

130. The complexion is yellow, there are blue rings around the eyes.

Yellowish color of the face and skin.

Excessive paleness of the face, when she grows heated from exercise.

Heat in the face, in the evening at seven o'clock.

Heat in the face, at night and in the morning, on awaking.

135. Much flying heat in the **face and** in the head.

Redness of the cheeks, sensible and visible, during the whole day, without thirst and without shuddering, for several days.

Cheeks fiery red, in the morning.

Cheeks fiery red and burning in the evening.

Erysipelatous swelling of the cheeks, in the morning.

140. Swelling of the left cheek, for two days. [*Fr. H.*]

Pain of the bones of the face, on being touched.

Itching on both the zygomata.

Miliary eruption in the face.

Pain of the lips, tension in the middle of the upper lip.

145. Chapped lips and pimples in the red of the lower lip, with a burning pain.

The lower lip is cracked in the middle.

Great swelling of the upper lip which is very painful when touched, but at other times is only tense; for three days. [*Fr. H.*]

Itching about the mouth.

Eruption in the corner of the mouth, with sensation of heat therein.

150. A severe scurfy eruption without sensation, below the left corner of the mouth.

Twitching and trembling on the left side of the upper lip.

A red itching spot below the lower lip; this spot is soon covered with a number of yellow vesicles, which pass into scabs.

A pimple, paining as if excoriated, in the red of the upper lip.

An ulcer in the corner of the mouth (removed by Belladonna).

155. Eruption of pimples on the chin, above and below the lips, and on the neck; they are like wheals, and pain as if excoriated when touched, but not when let alone.

Itching pimples on the chin (2d d.).

On the right side of the chin, toward the lower lip, vesicles and ulcers with sensation of burning.

Toothache. [*Fr. H.*]

Toothache, particularly while eating.

160. Drawing toothache, in the evening, in a hollow tooth, as if too much blood pressed upon the nerve.

After drinking anything cold, and after opening the mouth, toothache at once in all the teeth.

Drawing toothache in a tooth, which begins to waggle, worse in the warm room, relieved by the open air, and only *aggravated by biting*, when there is jerking in the tooth; in the evening.

Jerking pains in the teeth, extending into the ears.

Stitches in the teeth.

165. Looseness of the teeth.

A hollow tooth becomes loose, attended with pain when biting on it.

The hollow tooth is too long and is painful.

The gums bleed easily.

Jerking in the gums.

170. Inflammation and swelling of the inner side of the gums in front.

Swelling of the gums at the back molars, with a pain pressing outward, as if a new tooth were about to come there; the pain is worse when touching or biting on the teeth.

Ulcer on the gums.

Burning pain on the tip of the tongue, even waking him up at night.

The tip of the tongue is very sensitive, as if excoriated.

175. Sensation in the neck as from a plug of mucus, or from an internal swelling in the pharynx, in the morning.

On swallowing, a feeling in the throat, as if there were a swelling, over which he has to swallow.

Bruised pain of the external cervical muscles, with pain in the throat on swallowing, as from an internal swelling.

Pressure below the larynx, immediately after supper, as if something was lodged in the throat.

Severe pressure in the throat, so that she imagined it was quite constricted, and she would suffocate, toward evening.

180. Deglutition of food difficult, requiring great effort, without any soreness of the throat.

Scratching and roughness as if from excoriation in the throat, most severe when swallowing solid food.

Scrapy and choking sensation in the throat as from burned lard, in the morning.

Scraping in the throat for three days. [*Fr. H.*]

Scraping in the throat; it is always so full of water that she has to spit continually.

185. Water gathers in the mouth.

Stitches in the throat, when taking a deep breath.

Stitches in the throat as from a splinter, when swallowing; on yawning, the stitches extend to the ear.

Shooting pain and dryness in the throat, every morning, for several hours.

Shooting pain in the throat, extending to the ear, when turning the head.

190. The mucus hawked up is mixed with blood.

Much hawking up of mucus from the throat, in the evening, after eating.

Much mucus in the mouth.

Salivation (collection of saliva) on the right side of the mouth.

Doughy taste in the mouth, in the morning (5th d.).

195. Bad smell in the mouth, as from a spoiled stomach; this he perceives himself.

Loss of the sense of taste.

Bitter, slimy taste in the mouth, in the morning.

Bitter taste in the mouth, and also of the food.

Bitter taste in the posterior part of the throat, while food tastes normally.

200. Earthy taste in the throat, while food tastes all right.

Putrid taste and like that of rotten eggs in the mouth.

Metallic taste in the mouth.

Sourish metallic taste in the mouth.

No appetite for eating, while there is a feeling of emptiness in the abdomen.

205. Unusual hunger in the forenoon.

Loathing for everything, especially for fat.

There is sometimes appetite for something, but when he gets it, he does not want it.

Appetite only for sour and strong tasting, piquant things.

Much appetite for vinegar.

210. Inordinate desire for wine, only temporarily satisfied by wine and water. [*Stf.*]

More thirst than hunger.

Thirst; but she cannot drink much, else the abdomen is inflated.

Uncommonly great thirst, from morning till evening. [*Fr. H.*]

During dinner, a frequent burning itching on the forehead and cheeks.

215. After dinner, hot regurgitation.

Immediately after dinner, fullness in the hypogastrium.

After meals, great lassitude.

After a meal, sensation of heat in the abdomen.

After dinner, severe palpitation and oppression of the chest, with a desire of taking a deep breath.

220. After dinner, hard distension of the abdomen, for three hours (3d d.).

Frequent eructation, without smell and taste.

Continual empty eructation, with inflation of the abdomen and stomach, during mental exertion.

Eructations, with burning in the throat.

Frequent eructation, with the taste of the ingesta.

225. Eructation after eating, with belching up of a sourish liquid which comes up into the mouth.

Hiccup after eating.

Nausea, frequently during the day.

Frequent transient fits of nausea.

Nausea in the morning, but without inclination to vomit, but rather as a premonition of swooning.

230. **Morning-sickness**, for several mornings, with inclination to vomit, while sitting and standing; but going off when lying down.

Qualmishness, with inclination to vomit. [*Stf.*]

Inclination to vomit, with running of saliva from the mouth.

Water-brash, with a flow of watery saliva from the mouth, recurring the following day at the same hour.

Constant sensation as of water rising in the œsophagus, as after eating sour things.

235 **Vomiting every morning.**

Sour vomiting, in the afternoon.

Green vomiting of acrid water and tenacious mucus, with constant nausea. [HINZE, *Hufel. Journ.*, 1815, Sept. XLI, pp. 77-79.[1]]

Vomiting of bile in the morning, after long-continued, severe retching.

Vomiting of mucus, mixed with coagulated blood.

---

[1] Effects of large doses of H. s. given for whooping cough. See also S. 644.—*Hughes.*

240. The stomach pains, while he is walking, as if it **hung loose.**

Pressure in the stomach, as if lead was lying in it.

Pressure in the stomach after a light meal.

Internal pressure in the scrobiculus cordis, every morning on awaking.

Hard pressure in the scrobiculus cordis, rising up from the abdomen and only relieved by the passage of flatus.

245. Tension across the scrobiculus cordis; he has to unbutton his clothes, and cannot bear to sit.

When blowing his nose, dull pain in the scrobiculus cordis.

The stomach distended, as if by flatulence, with ice-cold hands.

Restlessness, heaviness and sensation of acidity in the pit of the stomach during digestion.

Gnawing in the stomach, as from an acid, which also rises into the fauces.

250. **In the hepatic region, stitches,** when walking.

In the left hypochondrium, distension as from flatulence.

Painful rush of blood toward both hypochondria, at every step he takes.

Sensation as of stagnation in both hypochondria, at every step while walking.

A very disagreeable though quiet pain in the abdomen, almost as from a bruise, early on awaking, lasting for some time after getting up, with a similar headache in the forehead.

255. Pain, as from a bruise in the intestines of the hypogastrium, when walking (aft. 18 h.).

The abdomen is painfully sensitive and inflated, more while walking than when sitting (2d d.).

Pressive pain in the abdomen near to and about the hips, for fourteen days.

Severe pressure, almost lancinating, in the left side of the abdomen, when out driving.

Pressure in the abdomen below the scrobiculus cordis, while the abdomen is as hard as a stone.

260. Distended, swollen abdomen, without flatulence.

Inflated, distended abdomen.

Tension in the abdomen, all the day.

Spasmodic, pinching tension in the abdomen, several times during the day.

Cramps in the abdomen.

265. Pain, like constriction, in the abdomen before the meal.

Contractive pain in the abdomen.

Clawing in the umbilical region, from both sides of the abdomen toward the middle, sometimes rising up to the scrobiculus cordis, and causing nausea and anxious heat in the cheeks, in paroxysms; almost as if from taking cold or from the approach of the menses.

Pinching pain in the abdomen, as if from taking a cold.

In the morning, pinching in the abdomen, with a soft stool (for many mornings).

270. Colic: stitches, cutting and pinching here and there in the

abdomen, as if from flatulence, for many hours after a meal; the pain is more intense at every pulsation.

Cutting pains in the abdomen.

Cutting pain in the abdomen, without diarrhœa, for several days, toward evening.

Shooting pain in the abdomen.

Violent stitches in the left side of the abdomen, immediately below the ribs.

275. Splenetic stitches when walking.

Pain, as from excoriation in the left side of the abdomen.

Pain, as from soreness, above the umbilicus.

Pain, as from excoriation, in the hypogastrium.

Drawing pain in the abdomen.

280. Drawing pain in the epigastrium, and at the same time above the sacrum (at once).

Fermentation in the abdomen, above the navel, with eructation of hot air.

Whirling sensation above the navel.

Feeling of emptiness in the intestines.

The glands in the groin become painful, especially when touched, with a sensation as if they were swollen.

285. **Abscesses of the inguinal glands, buboes.**

Every morning, a moving about of flatus in the abdomen, with a disagreeable feeling, like a kind of colic, especially in the sides of the abdomen.

Noisy motions of the flatus in the abdomen.

Rumbling in the abdomen.

Discharge of flatus, at night.

290. Very frequent, ineffectual calls to stool, with much eructation.

Calls to stool, but the peristaltic motion of the large intestines is lacking, so as to discharge the fæces, which are not hard, and which can only be partially expelled by the exertion of the abdominal muscles.

Inactivity of the rectum; the stool is hard and insufficient, and the anus swollen.

Soft stool, which is, however, only expelled by much straining.

With much urging, difficult discharge of scanty fæces, which are not hard.

295. After much straining, a stool of hard lumps of fæces, mixed with a yellow liquid.

Frequent stools also at night; with straining, tenesmus and exhaustion, only very little is evacuated.

Diarrhœa with colic; with inclination to lie down; hot hands and cheeks.

Three diarrhœic stools, with qualmish feeling of nausea and rumbling in the abdomen.

Slight diarrhœic stools, several times a day, preceded by some pinching; then some flatus before the stool, and some more flatus afterward.

300. Diarrhœa of bloody mucus, with rumbling as if behind in the back, without pain in the abdomen.

Clay-colored stool.
Greenish stool.
Blood is passed with the stool.
Flow of blood from the rectum, with a soft stool.
305. After the stool, inflation of the abdomen.
After the stool, the nose is stopped.
After the stool, sensation of excoriation in the anus, and secretion of ichor.
The varices of the rectum protrude.
Rumbling in the rectum.
310. Crawling in the rectum, as from ascarides.
Burning at the anus.
A little lump above the anus, and a sensation of swelling there.
On the perinæum, sweat.
Weakness of the bladder; the urine only flows in a slow, perpendicular stream, and he has to wait awhile before any urine comes.
315. He never can finish urinating; some urine always seems to remain behind in the bladder.
The micturition is impeded; he has to wait awhile before the urine comes, and then it flows out slowly, for several days.
Frequent urging to urinate.
Violent urging to urinate, in the morning on awaking, and, nevertheless, difficult and slow passage of the urine.
Copious discharge of urine (aft. 4 d.).
320. Discharge of a quantity of pale urine, with pressure on the bladder.
The urine when passed is pale and clear, but becomes turbid and thick on standing, depositing a white sediment.
The urine is turbid and like whey when passed, and deposits a white sediment.
Dark-yellow urine, it scalds in passing.
Brownish-red urine.
325. Blood-red urine.
The last drops of urine are bloody.
Fatty pellicle on the urine.
Iridescent pellicle on the urine.
Acrid, scalding urine, which excoriates the inner surface of the prepuce and makes it ulcerated.
330. **The urine scalds during the emission.**
In micturition, there is a cutting pain in the female urethra.
During the emission of urine, acute, sore pain in the urethra.
The urine is sharp, and in passing, it excoriates the pudenda.
During micturition, sensation on the right scapula as if something was flowing or running inside of it.
335. Several stitches in the urethra.
The orifice of the urethra is red and inflamed.
On the penis and on the frenulum of the prepuce, itching.
Itching of the glans.
A stitch in the region of the frenulum.
340. Shooting pain in the prepuce.
Externally in the prepuce, ulcers like chancres.

Moist excoriation, with eroding, smarting pain in the fold between the thigh and the scrotum.

Itching of the scrotum.

The sexual parts are weakened, the testes relaxed and the penis of unnatural hardness.

345. Diminished sexual impulse.

The genitals are excited to seminal emission, without any amorous fancies or desire for woman.

During amorous dallying, a painful erection like excoriation and a cramp-pain in the whole penis, beginning from the bladder.

Prostatic juice passes at times with the stool.

She is very much excoriated about the pudenda and between the thighs.

350. **Flow of blood from the uterus,** almost at once, and again after ten or twelve days, after previous inflation of the abdomen.

It delays the menses by ten days and diminishes the discharge.

Before the menses, contractive headache.

During the menses, much itching on the pudenda.

* * * * * * * *

Frequent sneezing (at once).

355. Frequent sneezing, owing to itching in the nose.

Tickling in the nose, causing sneezing.

Stuffed coryza.

Coryza and much spitting of saliva.

Coryza; he has to blow his nose every moment; attended with an excessive appetite.

360. Coryza, and scraping in the throat.

Catarrhal fever, attended with internal chills and peevishness.

Frequent catarrhal fever, with heaviness in all the limbs.

Coryza, with inflammatory swelling of the nose, which pains like a boil, attended with coughing.

He blows from his nose ill-smelling mucus, even without coryza.

365. Weakness of the organs of speech and of the chest, so that she cannot speak aloud.

Tickling in the throat, and a sensation of fusty vapor, causing cough.

Scrapy, scratchy cough.

Suffocative cough, caused merely by tightness of the chest.

Deep, dry cough; from tightness of the chest when inspiring; with pain extending up into the chest at every impulse of coughing.

370. Violent fits of coughing, from time to time, threatening suffocation or vomiting.

Cough, so much aggravated by taking a deep breath that it causes him to vomit.

Cough, exciting to vomiting.

Violent, deep cough of several impulses, striking painfully against the larynx and causing retching.

An almost uninterrupted cough from an irritation in the upper part of the left side of the throat, which is worst when talking and stooping; late in the evening it always increases, and then suddenly ceases.

375. Tussiculation, at once after a meal.

The cough torments him most while walking.

Fit of coughing, as if from a cold or over-sensitiveness of the nervous system, as soon as the least member of the body becomes cool.

Morning cough, which often wakes her from sleep.

Cough, in the evening and morning.

380. She is much tormented by cough in the evening.

In the evening, impulses of dry cough.

From time to time, dry, painless, short cough.

In the evening, on going to sleep, dry cough (aft. 4 d.).

At night, from eleven to twelve o'clock, in bed, violent cough (with expectoration of mucus).

385. Cough, day and night.

Cough, with expectoration.

Cough, with expectoration of mucus, the whole day, excited by a scraping irritation in the windpipe, but especially in the throat. [*Fr. H.*]

Cough, with much expectoration, every three or four hours a violent fit; but not waking from sleep at night.

Expectoration of sourish mucus at night, almost without cough.

390. Tenacious mucus in the chest (aft. 5 d.).

Bloody expectoration from the chest, with crossness and lassitude.

Coughing of blood, after previous sensation as of a hard body in the scrobicus cordis; followed by fetid perspiration, then weakness in the head.

During coughing, obtuseness of the whole head, with throbbing in the forehead and temples.

During coughing, violent resounding throbbing in the head.

395. During coughing, stitches in the throat and headache as if everything were coming out at the forehead.

During coughing, burning in the stomach.

After the fits of coughing, sneezing.

Shortness of breath.

Frequent deep breathing as after running.

400. Pain in the chest; a pressure in the left side of the chest.

Shooting in the sternum, during respiration and walking.

Shooting pain in the side of the chest, toward the back.

Stitches in the cardiac region.

Sensation in the chest as if hot water was moving there.

405. Heat in the left side of the chest, above the heart.

Severe palpitation, with fine stitches in the heart and in the left side of the chest.

Eruption of two pimples on the outer side of the sternum, with pus in their apices and acute pain as from excoriation.

Itching on the left nipple.

Painful sensitiveness in the right half of the fleshy part of the chest, and under the right arm, on touching the chest or moving the arm.

410. A boil on the last right rib, with a stitching aching *per se* and great pain when touched.

Pain in the sacrum, frequently recurring.

In the sacrum a pain, drawing hither and thither, worst when walking. [*Fr. H.*]

Pain in the sacrum, as from fatigue, when stooping and when leaning back while sitting.

Severe pain in the sacrum, like a cutting through, during movement and at rest; so that she could neither stand, walk nor lie down.

415. Bruised pain in the sacrum, when walking (1st d.).

Bruised pain and sharp pressive pain in the sacrum and the lumbar vertebræ, but especially in the junction of the sacrum with the pelvic bones; it darts down into the lower limbs and causes a sort of limping in walking; the pain continues while sitting, standing, and lying down.

In the loins and the ossa ischii, pain as from dislocation, when sitting, and when turning the body in walking.

At night, tensive pain in the back, worst when turning the body.

Pain between the scapulæ.

420. In the morning, in bed, drawing in the whole back and in the sacrum; after rising, the whole of the back was painful, so that she could hardly move, with weariness in the limbs, aversion to eating and working, with shivering, chilliness, and adipsia.

Stitches in the back, in the left renal region.

Stitches in the left side of the back.

Stitches in the back, between the scapulæ.

Stitches in the right scapula, when blowing the nose, hawking or taking a deep breath.

425. Some violent stitches in the back.

Great weakness in the whole spine.

Shooting pains in the throat, extending into the ear, when turning the head.

Some fine stitches on the outside of the neck and behind the ears, like flea bites.

Pinching on the right side of the thyroid cartilage.

430. Bruised pain on the cervical muscles, with pain in the throat, when swallowing, as from an internal swelling.

Bruised pain in the neck, when bending the head back.

Many small, painless pimples in the nape, and on both sides of the neck. [*Fr. H.*]

The axillary glands suppurate and discharge pus.

Pain like a load on the top of the shoulder.

435. The top of the shoulder is painful, when raising the arm.

Drawing pain in the top of the shoulders.

Fine tearing in the top of the left shoulder.

Pain as of a sprain in the top of the shoulder.

In the left arm, here and there, some jerking.

440. Bruised pain in both arms.

Great fatigue of both the arms.

The arm on which he had lain is asleep, at night.

In the left upper arm, a drawing pain.

Bruised pain in the shafts of the humeri.

445. Extremely violent pains in the bend of the elbow, when stretching out the arm.

Pressive or contused pain in the olecranon process of the elbow, only on moving it, after a long walk; it went off in the open air.

Severe itching in the bend of the elbow.

In the forearms, a painful drawing in the flexor tendons.

Drawing tearing pain in the extensor muscles of the forearms and of the fingers.

450. Contused pain on a small spot on the forearm.

After midnight, pain in the interior of the forearm and over the back of the hand, aching, boring and as if excoriated, more painful when touched, less so by day.

The wrist is painful.

Sensation of heat in the palm and in the wrist.

Frequent burning sensation in the hands.

455. Heat, redness and swelling of the one hand, with intolerable pain as from a sprain, extending up into the arm, on motion.

Swelling of the right hand.

Unsteadiness in the hands, and trembling during writing.

Perspiring, cold hands.

Scaly eruption on the hands.

460. **Itching and rough, dry, grating skin on the hands.**

Continual, dull *itching in the palms.*

Small, gritty eruption on the hand and wrist, with itching.

On pressing the spread-out fingers against something, they knuckle up; the fingers are readily dislocated.

Pricks in one finger, as from needles.

465. An eroding blister on the anterior joint of the thumb, without sensation, only when pressed upon, there is a shooting pain.

Severe itching beside the nail of the left index, as if a paronychia was forming.

Tingling in the tips of the fingers.

Swelling of the fingers of both hands, with stiffness therein, when lying down.

Swelling of all the fingers, with tension on moving them.

470. The finger-joints are swollen, with gouty pains.

The nates and the posterior part of the thighs are painful, when sitting down.

A red, itching lump on the upper part of the left natis.

Two boils on one natis.

The hip-joint pains as if dislocated, when walking in the open air.

475. Excoriation in the fold between the scrotum and the thigh.

Excoriation and moisture in the fold between the scrotum and the thigh.

Profuse perspiration on the upper part between the thighs.

At night, a painful tension in the lower limbs, that prevents sleep.

Tearing pain in the thigh and leg, as from too great fatigue, also when at rest.

480. Restlessness in the lower limbs, so that she has to keep moving them, by day when at rest.

A formicating pain in the inferior extremity, which drew it quite crooked; chiefly when walking and standing.

Heaviness of the lower limbs.

Tearing in the left hip (when undressing).

Pain in the hip-joint, while walking in the open air.

485. Tearing pain in the right thigh (at once).

While sitting, tearing in the thigh, and a numb, tingling sensation in it, almost as if asleep.

Bruised pain in the anterior muscles of the thighs.

Bruised pain, transversely through the middle of the thighs.

Cramp in the muscles of the thigh and pelvis, when the thigh is drawn upward.

490. Sudden pain of exhaustion in the thigh, while walking, so that he cannot walk farther.

In the knee, cramp.

Pressive pain in the hough, on motion.

Frequently during the day, a shooting pain in the right knee.

Tearing on the outer side of the knee-joint, also when at rest, as after too great exertion and fatigue.

495. Bruised pain in the knee.

Pain in the knee as if broken.

Swelling of the knee.

Itching pimples about the knee.

Severe itching on the inner side of the knee.

500. In the leg, below the right knee, a spasmodic drawing pain, when walking.

Cramp of the calves, only when bending the kness.

Cramp-pain in all the muscles of the leg, while walking, so that he cannot walk on.

Cramp in the calves.

Restlessness in the legs, he has to keep them stretched out.

505. Restlessness in the legs at times, so that he cannot keep them still.

Tearing in the tendo Achillis, when lying in bed; and when walking, a stitch in it.

Great weariness in the legs, especially when ascending.

The left leg is asleep, in the morning in bed and heavy like lead.

Erysipelas on the leg (affected).

510. The feet are painfully sensitive in the soles, when walking on rough stones.

Sensation of pressure under the heel, when walking, as if there was a pebble lodged under it.

Cramp in the feet.

Cramp between the big toe and the heel.

Cramp in the soles of the feet and the toes.

515. Stiff feeling in the ankle-joint, with a feeling of numbness and turgidity there.

Pain in the ankle-joint, as if festering.

Tearing pain in the foot, at night.

Tearing and drawing in the soles of the feet.

Stitches on the instep.

520. Violent itching stitches on the dorsum of the foot, near the root of the toes.

In the evening, after having slept restlessly and turned over in bed, there came on the outer side of the foot on which he had lain a pain as from a knock or blow, so violent that it made him scream; the pain was only allayed by touching and stroking it with the finger, but not by motion.

Pain in the ankle-joint, as if sprained, coming in paroxysms while walking, so that he cannot continue walking for the moment.

Pain in the right ankle-joint, as if it was broken, while walking.

Cracking in the ankle-joint.

525. Formication in the soles of the feet.

Constant dull itching in the soles of the feet.

Tickling in the soles of the feet.

Hard pressure as from a little stone, on the heel, when walking.

Needle-pricking in both the heels.

530. Burning pain in the feet, especially on the dorsum of the feet, in the morning in bed.

Burning in the soles of the feet, in the morning in bed; she had to uncover them.

Drawing, burning pain in the feet up to the ankles, in the evening in bed.

Swelling of the feet about the ankles, with dyspnœa.

Coldness of the feet, by day.

535. Cold, sweaty feet.

Chilblains on the feet, which break open, with so much tenderness of these spots on healing that she cannot wear a shoe.

In the big toe, tearing, worse when walking than when standing.

Severe stitch along the big toe.

Sharp, shooting pains in the fleshy part of the right little toe.

540. Piercing stitches in the hard skin on the little toe.

Formication in the toes.

Formicating itching of the toes, for four nights.

Burning itching of the toes.

The nail of the big toe pains violently, almost like an ulcer, on slight pressure.

545. A corn that has hitherto been painless commences to have burning and shooting pains, at a slight external pressure.

Extreme sensitiveness and irritability of the nerves in various parts, *e. g.*, on the septum of the nose.

Great irritability of the nerves; every impression on body and mind excites the nervous system to a sort of internal tremor.

Drawing pain in the limbs, with paralytic sensation, especially in the thighs and legs.

Drawing pain in the shoulder-joints, the hips, and especially the knees.

550. Drawing pain in the gastric region and in the back.

Stitches in the joints, both when at rest and in motion.

The pains are worst at night.

Aggravations of the pain during the nocturnal fever, chiefly during the chill.

Sensitiveness to the open air, with chilliness and frequent nausea.

555. Even a slight wetting of the body causes painful throbbing, here and there.

When walking in the open air, trembling in the knees, with anxiety, heat in the whole body and burning of the soles of the feet.

In the forenoon, several shivers run all over him, in the open air.

Fine, stinging itching.

Constant dull itching in the sole of the feet and in the palm.

560. Burning itching on the body, chiefly in the morning on rising, with white blisters after scratching, which exude a white fluid and then soon pass away.

Eruption of pimples as large as peas, here and there on the body.

Nettle-rash, *e. g.*, on the wrist.

Cracked skin and chaps on the hands and feet.

Unwholesome, festering skin; even slight lesions fester and suppurate.

565. The part affected with an ulcer (the leg) cannot endure a pendent position.

Eroding pain in the ulcer.

An itching erosion in the ulcer.

Severe stitches in the ulcer, when laughing.

Burning and throbbing in the ulcer, at night.

570. Inflammation of the affected part.

Sour-smelling pus from the ulcer.

Bleeding of the ulcer, even when wiping it gently.

The wart is inflamed, and there are stitches in it, as if it would ulcerate.

Yellowish skin and yellow complexion.

575. An attack of jaundice; the urine is blood-red and the white of the eye yellowish.

Emaciation with chilliness in the back, redness of the cheeks, insomnia; the larynx is much affected, with hoarse, weary voice, anguish, distress, and extreme irritability as in a hectic fever.

Great heaviness in the body; he does not know what ails him.

She feels heavy in all her limbs, as if she would have a cold.

Languor and bruised feeling in all the limbs.

580. Very tired and indolent, in the morning on awaking, so that she can hardly rise from her bed.

Lassitude in the morning, after rising from bed, so that she can hardly stand upright, continuing all day, with drowsiness.

He remains long in bed in the morning, tired and slumbering.

In the morning in bed, weariness, restlessness in the legs, with stoppage of the nose.

Very tired and heavy in the body, in the morning on rising from bed, after a sound sleep.

585. Great weariness and palpitation, early on awaking.

Great lassitude in the evening, with lack of tone and palpitation.

Lassitude on walking in the open air, after a meal, with stretching in all the limbs, as if he were about to have ague; on continuing to walk, a cold sweat came over him; and in the evening in bed, a sensation of heat, so that he did not fall asleep until two A. M.

Toward evening, from a slight pain, sudden severe syncope.

Much stretching and extension of the limbs every day.

590. Frequent yawning, causing pain in the chest.

Incessant yawning, from morning till noon.

Great drowsiness toward evening, with frequent, violent, almost convulsive yawning, so that he could hardly keep from lying down.

So sleepy and tired in the evening, that he fell asleep while sitting.

Great, irresistible somnolence, in the evening; he has to lie down immediately after supper and he sleeps till morning.

595. Difficulty in going to sleep, and restless sleep.

Sleeplessness after midnight.

No sound sleep at night, only slumber.

Exuberance of ideas does not allow him to sleep after midnight.

After a lively evening's entertainment, he cannot sleep all the night.

600. In a long solid sleep, thoughts about his work kept revolving in his head, as if clouds were passing through.

For several days he was in a slumberous sleep, with constant dreaming about his daily business and many thoughts, which like clouds passed through his mind; at times he would wake up not ill-humored, give correct answers, satisfy his needs, and at once go to sleep again.

Too long and stupid a sleep, and then obtuseness of the head, as if full and stolid, with pressure in the temples, ailments as if from a spoiled stomach, eructation with the taste of the ingesta, and scraping in the throat, as if a rancid heartburn was coming.

Dreams, full of scolding.

Vexatious dreams.

605. Many dreams, at once on going to sleep, and anxiety all the night through, without awaking.

Dreams about dangerous affairs, fright and terror.

Anxious dreams, with sweat on the back on awaking.

Dreams he is vomiting pus and blood.

Anxious dreams of a conflagration; he feels as if falling, etc.

610. Dreams of escaping a danger.

Dreams that he hears shooting.

Heavy dreams, leaving behind them on awaking a state of fright.

Violent starting up in affright on going to sleep, also after a meal.

Before midnight, he sprang up out of sleep, called for help, and felt as if he could not get his breath.

615. On lying down at 10 P. M., great anxiety and restlessness in the whole body, with painful jerking of the lower limbs, which she had to keep moving for several hours; two evenings in succession.

At night, restlessness in the lower limbs, and trembling of the same.

Nocturnal nausea and vomiting.

She wakes up about midnight, with tickling in the throat, compelling her to cough and to expectorate.

He often awakes at night, with an erection and an urging to urinate.

620. At night cramp in the thigh, extending down into the foot.

In the morning in bed, cramp of the calves.

On awaking at night, though he has always been accustomed to sleep on the right side, he always finds himself lying on the back.

At night, the side on which he is lying after awhile pains him intolerably; he has to turn over.

He cannot sleep at night, for ebullition of blood.

625. At night, sleeplessness and a shaking chill for hours, so that he cannot get warm; without any subsequent heat.

Chilliness of the arms and legs, in the morning.

Chilliness; she seeks the warmth of the stove. [*Stf.*]

Chilliness, with frequent nausea and sensitiveness to the open air.

Chilliness in the open air; a disagreeable, painful sensation presses her quite down, so that she has to walk stooping forward. [*Stf.*]

630. Rigor.

Frequent shivering, extending up to the hairy scalp, where the hairs felt painful.

Rigor for an hour (aft. 10 min.).

Every evening, about six or seven o'clock, a severe chill, not followed by heat.

In the evening, at eight o'clock, severe chill, with chattering of the teeth, for a quarter of an hour, with coldness of the hands and feet, then heat with sweat, especially on the chest and forehead, with slight thirst.

635. He awakes at 2 A. M. with a febrile rigor and hot, dry skin; from time to time a shivering ague, from the nape down the back and over the chest; then some sleep, from which he awakes in a

gentle perspiration, with a pressive pain in the back, as also in and beside the hips and in the abdomen, with inclination to vomit.

In the evening, at six o'clock, fever, languor, weariness, slow pulse, chill (aft. 30 h.).

Nocturnal febrile rigor, so that he cannot get warm, not followed by heat.

During nocturnal febrile rigor, the pains present are aggravated.

Chilliness in the back, with redness of the cheeks, insomnia, while the larynx is much affected; hoarse, tired voice, anguish, apprehensiveness, extreme excitability and emaciation, as in a hectic fever.

640. Fever; now chills, now heat with photophobia.

Fever in the morning; first a bitter taste in the mouth, then after some hours a chill with thirst; and after an hour, much heat with interrupted sleep; all of this recurred twice more during the same day.

Burning fever-heat, with almost unquenchable thirst, tormenting headache, and low, delirious talk from 4 P. M. onward through the night, for three successive evenings. [HINZE, l. c.]

At night, dry heat of the body, with perspiration on the hands, which do not bear to be uncovered.

Fever, with severe, oft-repeated vomiting of green, excessively acrid water, and tenacious mucus, with constant nausea. [HINZE, l. c.[1]]

645. Perspiration frequently runs all over the body, only transiently and without heat.

He perspires very readily during every, even slight, movement.

Profuse sweat, day and night. [*Fr. H.*]

He even perspires, if he only writes a few lines. [*Fr. H.*]

At night, sweat from midnight onward, then a chill while still in bed, and after rising; every morning.

650. **Night-sweat,**

Night-sweat about midnight, especially on the back.

Night-sweat, immediately on lying down, especially on the head, so that beads of sweat stood on the face.

Night-sweat, before midnight.

Night-sweat on the whole body, while awake.

655. At night, profuse sweat, most of the night, or at least constant exhalation.

Sweat in bed, after midnight.

In the morning, profuse sweat all over the body.

In the morning, profuse, continued sweat only on the head.

Disagreeably smelling, continued exhalation of the body.

660. Sour-smelling, profuse sweat, at night.

Clammy, profuse sweat at night.

---

[1] Together with S. 237.—*Hughes.*

IODIUM. IODINE.

Iodine is obtained from various kinds of sea-wrack (*fucus*, sea-weed), by leaching the ashes, and then crystallizing the salts contained in it that can be crystallized; the residual uncrystallizable lye, consisting of iodide of sodium, is then evaporated and allowed to stand in a warm place mixed with strong sulphuric acid, in order to remove from it all muriatic acid; then manganese is added and the mass is strongly heated in a retort, whereby the iodine is separated, rising as a violet-colored vapor, which is condensed on the upper part of the retort in bluish-brown scales or leaflets. One grain of this is prepared for the homœopathic dynamization and brought up to the thirtieth potency in the manner prescribed for dry drugs at the conclusion of the first part of this work.

Even in the higher and the highest degrees of dynamization iodine is a very heroic medicine, which calls for every precaution of the good homœopathic physician; when misapplied in allopathic hands, iodine is frequently seen to cause the most fearful destruction of the body and life of patients.

Iodine has been of service especially when the following states were at the same time present:

Dizziness in the morning; throbbing in the head; excoriation of the eyes; humming before the ears; hardness of hearing; a coated tongue; mercurial salivation; bad, soapy taste; sourish eructation, with burning; *heartburn* after heavy viands; *voracious hunger;* nausea; *incarceration of flatus;* inflation of the abdomen; constipation; micturition at night; delay in the menses; cough; inveterate morning cough; difficulty in breathing; external swelling of the neck; weariness of the arms in the morning, in bed; the fingers go to sleep; curvature of the bones; dryness of the skin; night-sweats.

The abbreviations of the names of my fellow-observers are: *Gff.*, *Dr. Augustus Baron von Gersdorff; Gr.*, *Dr. Gross; Htb. u. Tr.*, *Drs. Hartlaub and Trinks*, in their *Reine Arzneimittellehre;* and *S.* (*Schreter?*).

IODIUM.

Dejection. [KUENZLI, *ueber d. Iod. Winterth.*, 1826; MAT-

In the first edition of this work (1828) Hahnemann published a list of 153 symptoms, as observed by himself from iodine. In 1829, in the second volume of their *Reine Arzneimittellehre*, Hartlaub and Trinks gave a list of 516, mainly taken from authors, but including also some symptoms from themselves and Schreter. These, with a few additions from v. Gersdorff and Gross, presumably obtained from the thirtieth dilution, constitute the present pathogenesis.—*Hughes.*

THEY, in *Gilbert's Annal.*, 1821; GAIRDNER, *Essay on the Eff. of Iod.*, etc.; RICHTER, *spec. Arzeim.-Lehre*, Vol. X.[1]]

Gloomy mood. [*S.*]

Sad, melancholy mood. [PERROT, in *med. Annal.;* V. PIERER, 1821, *Hft.* IX.[2]]

Hypochondriac mood. [GAIRDNER.]

5. Sadness. [KOLLEY, in *Hufel. Journ.*, 1824, Febr.[3]]

Very ill-humored and sensitive during the whole period of digestion, from noon till evening, with an oppressive sensation in the throat and chest, as when one is about to weep. [*Gff.*]

Oppression of the chest. [*Htb ;* GRAEFE, *Journ. f. Chir. u. Augenheilkunde*, II., 617.[4]]

Constant inclination to weeping. [PERROT.]

Now disposed to weep, then again inclined to be glad. [VOGT, *Pharmak.*, 1828.[5]]

10. Apprehensiveness after some manual work; it goes off while sitting.

Anxiety. [GAIRDNER; KUENZLI; RICHTER; GRAEFE; KOLLEY.]

Anxious oppression. [MASSALIEN, in *Rust's Magazin* XIV., p. 379.]

Great anxiety. [NEUMANN, in *Hufel. Journ.* LV., St. 1.]

Great anxiety and oppression. [GAIRDNER.]

15. Oppression, and tightness of the chest. [VOIGT.]

Anxiety and dejection; the patients generally busy themselves with the present. [GAIRDNER.]

Restless moving about; she runs about incessantly and does not get to sit down, nor does she sleep at night, so that she has to be considered as crazy [*Gr.*]

Restlessness, which keeps the body in constant activity. [KOLLEY.]

Restlessness. [GRAEFE; *Med. chir. Zeit.*, 1825, Bd. I., p. 310.[6]]

20. Aversion to sitting still.

He is afraid at every trifle, that one or another mishap may rise from it.

Discouragement. [KUENZLI.]

Discouragement and despondency, which continues also during the pains in a very depressing manner. [GAIRDNER.[7]]

Aversion to work.

25. He feels unable to do anything.

Her phlegmatic disposition has disappeared; she has become blooming, stronger and more lively. [HENNING, in *Hufel. Journ.*, Bd. LVII, St. 3, p. 90.[8]]

Peevish, cross, she is not suited by anything. [*S.*]

---

[1] To Kuenzli—Not accessible. To Matthey—"From the tincture in a goitrous subject." To Gairdner—"Observations on patients." To Richter—"General statement from authors." —*Hughes.*

[2] Not accessible.—*Hughes.*

[3] Not found at reference.—*Hughes.*

[4] To Graefe—Effects when given in scrofula.—*Hughes.*

[5] General statement from authors.—*Hughes.*

[6] Observations on patients.—*Hughes.*

[7] In the original—"Sense of sinking and faintness, which were peculiarly oppressive, and were complained of during intense pain as the thing most difficult to bear."—*Hughes.*

[8] Observation.—*Hughes.*

Inordinately great irritability to anger.

Increased sensation and irritability. [FORNEY, in *Hufel. Journ.* LII., St. 2.[1]]

30. Sensitiveness to noise.

Increased sensitiveness to external impressions. [VOIGT.]

The mind and nervous system is affected. [VOIGT; PERROT.]

Unusual excitement of the nervous system. [*Hufel. Journ.* LVII., St. 6.[2]]

Excessively merry and loquacious; she does not give any one a chance to say a word. [*Gr.*]

35. **Illusions of the sense of touch.** [GAIRDNER; KUENZLI; RICHTER.]

Delirium. [NEUMANN, l. c.]

Fixed, immovable thoughts (21st d.).

Obtuseness of the head, which renders thinking more difficult. [*Gff.*]

Obtuseness of the head, with great disinclination to serious employment. [*Gff.*]

40. Obtuseness of the head. [KOLLEY.]

Sense of obtuseness of the head, which seems to draw up the back to the nape of the head. [JOERG; *Mater. z. e. k. Heilm. Lehre*, Leipzig, 1825, Bd. I.[3]]

Obtuseness of the head, which passes over into a pressive headache (aft. 1 h.). [JOERG.]

Slightly muddled feeling in the head, with pressure in the right half of the forehead, with great hunger (aft. 1 or 2 h.). [JOERG.]

Vertigo. [RICHTER; SCHMIDT, in *Rust's Magaz.*, Bd. XVI., St. 3, p. 430.[4]]

45. Vertigo, drawing the person forward. [*S.*]

Vertigo, with lassitude, in the morning. [*S.*]

Headache. [PERROT; *Med. chir. Ztg.*]

Headache, so violent that he becomes quite frantic. [KOLLEY.]

Transient, quickly passing pain in the occiput. [JOERG.]

50. Headache in the warm air, when driving far or walking fast.

Headache in the forehead and in the upper part of the head, aggravated by every noise or talking.

Headache, as if a bandage was firmly tied around the head.

Headache in the forehead; the brain is as if bruised and extremely sensitive; the whole body, and especially the arms, are without strength, and, as it were, paralyzed; he has to lie down; attended with eructations and painful sensitiveness of the outside of the head when touched; the following day there is still obtuseness of the head and painfulness of the brain, when moved (aft. 26 d.).

Pressure on a small spot in the forehead, just above the root of the nose. [*Gff.*]

55. Pressive headache, especially in the left side toward the forehead, frequently recurring. [JOERG.]

---

[1] From tincture in a goitrous subject.—*Hughes.*

[2] The citations from *Hufeland's Journal* are all as S. 29, save where otherwise specified.—*Hughes.*

[3] Proving on several healthy persons with moderate doses.—*Hughes.*

[4] Observations on patients.—*Hughes.*

Pressure in the region of the crown, for ten minutes. [JOERG.]

Pressive headache, especially in the temples, alternately disappearing and recurring. [JOERG.]

Pressive pain in the occiput, slight while at rest, but violent when moving, and finally passing into a sensation of weary waste in the head (1st d.). [JOERG.]

Pressive headache above the eyes, toward evening. [*S.*]

60. Violent pressive pain on the lower surface of the occiput, in the afternoon, in the open air. [JOERG.]

Sharp pressive pain on the left side of the upper part of the head, above the forehead. [*Gff.*]

Drawing pressure in the left upper half of the head, extending to the temple. [*Gff.*]

Pressive and at times shooting headache. [JOERG.]

Drawing pain in the left side of the head, extending into the teeth. [*S.*]

65. Tearing, first in the left, then in the right temporal region, almost at the same time. [*Gff.*]

Tearing headache above the left eye and in the temple. [*S.*]

Pressive tearing on the right side above the forehead. [*Gff.*]

Stitches in the occiput, relieved by lying down.

Stitches in the upper part of the head (aft. 3 d.).

70. Throbbing in the forehead without pain.

Beating in the head at every motion (aft. 24 h.).

Rush of blood to the head [*Hufel. Journ.*, l. c.]

The rush of blood to the head is aggravated with those who are disposed to it. [KOLLEY.]

Rush of blood to the head, and afterward at 2 P. M. headache for half an hour, returning at 5 o'clock. [JOERG.]

75. External headache in the forehead, as if festering underneath.

Smarting, sore sensation on the right side of the occiput, above the ear, posteriorly, in the skin. [*Gff.*]

The hair falls out.

Rapid falling out of the hair. [*S.*]

Eyeache in the orbits. [*Med. chir. Ztg.*]

80. Pressure in the eyes as if there was sand in them. [*S.*]

Pressure in the eyes. [*Gff.*]

Tension above the right eye, with some inflammation of the eyes. [*S.*]

Tearing about the right eye, especially below it.

Stitches in the upper part of the left eyeball.

85. Cutting stitches in the left eye, toward the outer canthus.

Itching in the canthi.

Itching on the eyelids. [*S.*]

Redness and swelling of the eyelids, with nightly agglutination. [*S.*]

Inflammation of the eyes.

90. Watery, white swelling of the eyelids. [*Hufel. Journ.*]

Dirty yellow color of the white of the eye, traversed by injected veinlets. [*S.*]

Sensation of weariness about the eyes, as if they lay deep in, especially in the afternoon. [*Gff.*]

Lachrymation of the eyes. [*Hufel. Journ.*; KUENZLI.]
Flow of tears. [KOLLEY.]
95. Twitching in the eyes (aft. sever. h.).
Constant twitching to and fro of the lower eyelid.
Quivering of the eyelids. [KUENZLI.]
Dimness of the vision. [*Med. chir. Zeit.*]
The light seems to her weaker and more indistinct. [*S.*]
100. Objects appear to her as through a veil. [*S.*]
Obscuration of the vision. [GAIRDNER; KUENZLI; RICHTER.]
Weakness of vision. [FORNEY; SCHNEIDER; VOIGT.]
Weakened, diminished visual power. [*Hufel. Journ.*]
At times she sees objects multiplied and cannot clearly distinguish them. [*S.*]
105. Dark ringlets float down before the eyes, to the side and close to the visual axis (aft. 16 h.).
Flickering before the eyes at times. [*S.*]
She cannot do fine sewing, because the stitches flit before her eyes. [*S.*]
Sparks before the eyes. [*S.*]
Fiery, crooked rays dart down frequently obliquely to the visual direction, and also at a slight distance from the focus of the ray, round about the eye, but more in an upward direction. (aft. 24 h.).
110. Otalgia in the left ear. [*Gff.*]
Straining pain in the right ear. [*Gff.*]
Tearing pressure in the pit under the right ear and beside it on the neck. [*Gff.*]
Small, yellow scurf on the concha. [*Htb.*]
Sensitiveness of the hearing to noise (4th d.).
115. Hardness of hearing. [GAIRDNER; KUENZLI; RICHTER.]
Frequent din in the right ear, as in a mill. [*S.*]
The nose is painful in its lower part, when he blows it, without coryza. [*Gff.*]
Itching shooting, anteriorly, on the septum of the nose.
A red, burning spot on the nose, below the eye. [*S.*]
120. An itching elevation on the nose.
A small scab in the right nostril. [*S.*]
Bleeding of the nose when blowing it. [*S.*]
Profuse epistaxis. [*Htb.*]
The color of the face is changed. [KUENZLI]
125. Pale contracted face. [GAIRDNER.]
Paleness of the face. [KOLLEY; KUENZLI.]
Paleness of the face of long duration. [COINDET, in *Hufel. Journ.* LIV., A.[1]]
Pale (ghostlike?) appearance. [*Trs.*]
Yellow complexion. [*Rust's Magaz.*; NEUMANN.]
130. The yellowness of the complexion diminishes; it becomes whiter (curative action). [*Htb.*]
The face, which before was yellow, becomes brown so

[1] Symptoms of iodic saturation.—*Hughes.*

quickly, that in a few days the skin of a woman of twenty-eight looked as if it was smoked. [VOGEL.[1]]

Peculiar alteration of the features. [BAUP, in *Hufel. Jour.*[2]]

Change in the features. [*Hufel. Journ.*]

Eyes sunken. [*Trs.*]

135. **Twitching of the facial muscles.** [*Hufel. Journ.*; SCHMIDT.]

Suppurating ulcer on the left cheek, with swelling of the circumjacent glands, and a firm lump on the ulcerated spot, which was slow in dispersing; soon after, a second ulcer by the side of the first, which, however, healed more quickly. [*Htb.*]

Pressive pain in the right upper jaw. [*Gft.*]

The submaxillary glands are swollen, without pain (2d d.). [*Htb.*]

Toothache, with presive pain, now here, now there, on the right side and the left, in the molars. [*Gff.*]

140. Squeezing toothache in the right posterior molars. [*Gff.*]

Drawing pain in the teeth on the right side, toward the ear, attended with shooting pain. [*S.*]

Cutting drawing and sensation of soreness, now on the left, now on the right side, in the roots or the gums of the lower incisors. [*Gff.*]

Pain from looseness of the teeth and in the gums, while eating.

The teeth in the morning are more covered with mucus, are yellower and are more quickly dulled by weak vegetable acids. [JOERG.]

145. The gums are painful when touched.

The gums are redder. [JOERG.]

Inflammation and swelling of the gums. [*Med. chir. Ztg.*]

Bleeding of the gums. [*Gff.*]

Gumboil on the gums of a lower, hollow molar, with swelling of the cheek, extending up to below the eye.

150. In the mouth there appear, from time to time, vesicles, with swelling of the gums. [*Htb.*]

Aphthæ in the mouth, with ptyalism. [VOIGT.]

Small elevations on the inner side of the right cheek, at first only painful, with sore, pressive pain when touched; but after a few days they sting and cut like an ulcer, especially on widely opening the mouth, in eating and in reading aloud; the parts around are also inflamed. [*Gff.*]

The glands on the inner side of the cheeks are acutely painful, as if there was strong vinegar in the mouth. [*Htb.*]

Smarting and pinching on the tonsils (at once). [JOERG.]

155. Putrid smell in the mouth, even in the morning when fasting, immediately after rinsing it with clean water. [*Gff.*]

The tongue is disagreeably dry. [RICHTER.]

Coated tongue. [*Trs.;* RICHTER.]

The tongue is coated thickly, the coating being of the same color as the substances thrown up. [GAIRDNER.]

---

[1] From tincture in a goitrous subject.—*Hughes.*

[2] From tincture in a goitrous subject.—*Hughes.*

Pressure in the left half of the palate. [*Gff.*]

160. Swelling and elongation of the uvula, with much spitting.

The throat is strongly constricted. [*S.*]

Sensation of constriction in the fauces. [PERROT.]

Tormenting constriction of the throat. [*Hufel. Journ.*]

Impeding deglutition, while drinking (water), as if the œsophagus was constricted and too weak to press down the beverage.

165. Sensation of fullness in the throat (6th d.).

Pain in the œsophagus, increased by pressing on the larynx. [RICHTER.]

Pressive pain on the right side of the throat, more while not swallowing.

Tearing in the throat, above the larynx. [*Gff.*]

Shooting pain in the throat, as if it was in the larynx; also somewhat noticeable while swallowing.

170. Tickling formication in the throat, in the region of the larynx, in the morning, in bed. [*Gff.*]

Disagreeable scraping in the fauces, with frequent secretion of saliva. [JOERG.]

Quickly passing burning and scraping in the fauces. [JOERG.]

Burning and sensation of heat in the fauces. [*Med. chir. Ztg.*]

Inflammation of the fauces and ulcers therein. [PERROT.]

175. **Increased secretion of saliva,** [RICHTER; KUENZLI; VOIGT.]

Increased secretion of saliva, compelling frequent spitting, for several days. [JOERG.]

Frequently, much watery saliva in the mouth. [*Htb.*]

Very bad taste in the mouth, especially when the stomach is quite empty or quite full. [*Htb.*]

Abominable taste in the mouth. [*Htb.*]

180. **Salty taste in the mouth** (1st and 2d d.). [JOERG.]

Bitter taste in the mouth. [JOERG.]

Bitter taste in the afternoon; the sweet plums have a bitter taste to her. [*S.*]

Sourish, offensive taste in the mouth, all the day, especially while smoking. [*Htb.*]

Sweet taste on the tip of the tongue (6th d.).

185. **Thirst.** [BAUP; KUENZLI.]

Much thirst, day and night (aft. 24 h.).

Very much thirst, day and night. [JOERG.]

Unusual, increased thirst. [JOERG; NEUMANN.]

Violent thirst. [PERROT.]

190. Distressing thirst. [GAIRDNER.]

The appetite is diminished. [HENNING; RICHTER; GOEDEN, in *Hufel. Journ.*]

Diminished appetite. [HELLING and SUTTINGER, in *Rust's Magaz.* XVI., 112.[1]]

Lack of appetite. [NEUMANN.]

---

[1] From tincture in a goitrous subject.—*Hughes.*

Total lack of appetite and of sleep. [*Hufel. Journ.*]

195. **Increased appetite.** (*Trs.*; KUENZLI; BAUP; RICHTER and others.]

Continued increase of appetite. [MATTHEY; COINDET.]

Unusual hunger. [JOERG.]

Gnawing hunger (aft. 3 h.). [JOERG.]

Violent hunger. [MUHRBECK, in *Hufel. Journ.* LIV., D. 63.[1]]

200. Wild appetite. [BAUP.]

Voracity. [*Med. chir. Ztg.*]

Appetite increased even to rabid hunger. [VOIGT.]

Ravenous hunger, she cannot be satiated.

Ravenous hunger, she would like to eat again directly after a meal; she also feels much better when she has eaten to full satiety. [*S.*]

205. If he does not eat something every three or four hours, he feels anxious; but he dare not eat too much.

The whole digestion proceeds more rapidly and regularly, with normal stools. [VOIGT.]

Varying appetite, now voracious hunger, then no appetite. [VOIGT.]

Great weakness of digestion. [GOEDER; MASSALIEU; ROECHLING, in *Rust's Magaz.* XV., 137.[2]]

After dinner, feeling of weakness and general malaise. [*Gff.*]

210. **Eructation.** [*Htb*; VOIGT.]

Eructation, with the smell of medicine. [JOERG.]

Continued empty eructation, from morning till evening, as if everything partaken of changed into air.

Hiccup. [MATTHEY.]

Qualmishness in the pit of the stomach, every day; it goes off after eating; it lay heavy on the stomach.

215. **Nausea.** [GRAEFE; HENNING; PERROT.]

Nausea in the morning, at once after rising, with spasmodic pain in the stomach. [*S.*]

Inclination to vomit. [VOIGT.]

Fits of inclination to vomit, with heartburn, with a sensation as of a spoiled stomach.

Vomiting. [KUENLI; MATTHEY and others.]

220. Violent vomiting. [GAIRDNER.]

Violent, incessant vomiting. [*Trs.*]

Obstinate vomiting, which especially comes on readily after eating. [GAIRDNER.]

Incessant vomiting with diarrhœa. [GAIRDNER.]

Yellowish, salty vomiting. [*Htb.*]

225. Vomiting of bile. [*Htb.*; VOIGT.]

The secretion of bile is increased. [RICHTER.]

Increased secretion of the gastric and pancreatic juices. [RICHTER.]

Stomach troubles with constipation. [*Trs.*]

Pains in the stomach. [KUENZLI; RICHTER and others.]

---

[1] Effects when given for glandular indurations.—*Hughes.*

[2] Observations on patients.—*Hughes.*

230. Pains above the stomach. [ORFILA, *Texicol.* II.[1]]

Stomachache in the morning, going off after eructation. [*S.*]

The most violent stomachache. [KOLLEY.]

Extraordinary pain in the stomach and the bowels. [*Trs.*]

The most excruciating pain in the stomach. [GAIRDNER.]

235. Pains in the stomach, with profuse bilious evacuations. [*Trs.*]

Violent pains in the stomach and in the fauces which were tense and obstructed and did not bear touching. [PERROT.]

Pressure in the gastric region, increased every time he eats. [VOGEL, in *Rust's Magaz.*]

Fullness and inflation in the stomach, with quivering and increased warmth in the abdominal cavity, and forcing from there to the periphery of the body, as if sweat would break out. [JOERG.]

Tension in the stomach and abdomen, after previous movements there. [JOERG.]

240. Cramp-pain in the stomach. [PERROT.]

Cramps in the stomach, frequently recurring. [GAIRDNER.]

Gnawing pain in the upper part of the stomach. [GAIRDNER.]

Gnawing corroding pains in the stomach. [MATTHEY.]

Stitches in the pit of the stomach (aft. 5 d.).

245. Sharp pricking as with needles, in the upper border of the pit of the stomach. [*Gff.*]

Throbbing in the pit of the stomach. [PERROT.]

Increased warmth in the gastric region. [JOERG.]

Burning in the stomach. [LOCHER-BALBER, in *Hecker's Annal.* I., 275.[2]]

Burning in the pit of the stomach.

250. Inflammation of the stomach, in the region of the pylorus. [PERROT.]

Small, linear ulcers in the stomach, which corroded the mucous membrane, which near the pylorus was inflamed, swollen and covered with a crust of coagulated lymph; in animals. [*Htb.* and *Tr.*]

The pain in the region of the liver and the pit of the stomach is diminished (curative action). [*S.*]

Pressure in the right hypochondrium. [*Gff.*]

Pressure in the hepatic region, which also pains when touched. [*Gff.*]

255. Pressure and stitches in the hepatic region. [SUTTINGER.]

Squeezing and dull cutting in the hepatic region. [*Gff.*]

The left hypochondriacal region is hard and pains acutely when pressed upon. [*S.*]

Single impulses of sore pressure in the region of the left hypochondrium. [*Gff.*]

Sharp shooting pain in the left hypochondrium, as from incarcerated flatus. [*Gff.*]

260. Abdominal pains in the epigastrial region. [*Htb.*]

Great painfulness of the whole abdomen, as if from an inflammation of the mesenteric glands. [*Htb. u. Tr.*]

Pain in the hypogastrium, extending into the spine.

---

[1] From swallowing 20-30 centigrammes in substance.—*Hughes.*

[2] Effects on patients.—*Hughes.*

Pressive pain in the epigastrium, between the scrobiculus cordis and the navel. [*Gff.*]

Pressure in the abdomen, beside the right hip. [*Gff.*]

265. Pressure in the hypogastrium, in frequent paroxysms, chiefly when sitting, and gradually relieved by stretching; for several days in succession.

Inflation in the epigastrium, with sharp pressure here and there, as from flatulence, from dinner time, all through the period of digestion. [*Gff.*]

Swollen abdomen, very much distended; she could not lie horizontally without danger of suffocating. [NEUMANN.]

Painful tension in the abdomen, with sensation of unusual pressing. [*Hufel. Journ.*]

A drawing cramp-pain in the epigastrium, starting from the scrobiculus cordis. [*Gff.*]

270. Colic pains. [RICHTER.]

Pains in the abdomen, like colic. [*Htb.*]

Pinching and pressive pain in the abdomen.

Cutting in the umbilical region, with pappy stool. [JOERG.]

Violent cutting in the umbilical region, with call to stool. [JOERG.]

275. Drawing and pressure in the right renal region. [*Gff.*]

Burning tearing in the left side of the abdomen, near the hip. [*Gff.*]

Stitches in the side of the abdomen.

Sharp shooting pain in the left hypogastrium.

Throbbing in the abdomen. [*Rust's Magaz.*]

280. Frequent straining and pressing toward the lower opening of the pelvis, with frequent diarrhœic stools. [JOERG.]

The abdominal troubles return, especially after partaking of food. [RICHTER.]

The abdominal symptoms recur for several days, even weeks and months, on partaking of food. [*Trs.*]

Abdominal dropsy. [NEUMANN.]

In the right inguinal region, pressure. [*Gff.*]

285. The glandular swellings in the inguinal region disappear (curative action). [MARTINI, in *Rust's Magaz.* XXIII., 180.[1]]

The hernial region becomes inflamed from the (usual) truss (6th d.).

In the morning, during inspiration, there is a tangible and audible rumbling on the side of the inguinal hernia.

Obstruction of flatulence, in the left side of the abdomen.

Pressing movements in the abdomen, from the stomach to the hypogastrium, chiefly toward the os pubis, the bladder and the testes, rarely with oppression toward the chest, sometimes attended with cutting. [JOERG.]

290. Rumbling in the abdomen, frequent. [JOERG.]

Rumbling and noises in the intestines. [JOERG.]

Discharge of flatus and stool, with slight cutting in the abdomen. [KUENZLI.]

[1] Effects on patients.—*Hughes.*

Increased emission of flatus. [RICHTER.]
Emission of flatus, with a smell of rotten eggs. [JOERG.]
295. Increase of the peristaltic motion of the bowels. [KUENZLI.]
Urging to stool, without evacuation; this only results after drinking cold milk, and then it comes easy and without any effort. [*S.*]
Indolent stool. [NEUMANN.]
Difficult stool.
Constipation, sometimes of long duration. [GAIRDNER.]
300. Obstinate constipation. [*Trs.*]
Hard, knotty, dark-colored evacuation. [*Trs.*]
Irregular stool; at one time constipation, then diarrhœa. [VOIGT.]
Irregular stool; at one time constipation, then diarrhœa, with distension of the abdomen, rumbling and grumbling in it and torments from flatulence. [GOEDEN.]
At times, obstinate constipation, then again violent diarrhœa. [*Trs.*]
305. Several whitish stools during the day, softer than usual. [*S.*]
Increased evacuations. [RICHTER.]
Four times, pappy stools during the day, succeeded every time by burning in the anus. [JOERG.]
Copious papescent **evacuations,** [JOERG.]
Inclination to diarrhœas. [*Hufel. Journ.*]
310. **Diarrhœic stools.** [BAUP; KUENZLI; RICHTER.]
Diarrhœic stool. [JOERG.]
Diarrhœa, which through its long duration is very exhausting. [SUTTINGER.]
Diarrhœa, in the morning. [*Htb.*]
Violent attacks of diarrhœa, with colic. [GAIRDNER.]
315. Frequent diarrhœic stools, with pressing and straining toward the hypogastrium. [JOERG.]
Pappy stool, with cutting in the umbilical region. [JOERG.]
Violent diarrhœa of a watery, foaming, whitish mucus, with pinching about the navel, and pressure on the crown of the head. [*S.*]
Evacuations of thick mucus or of pus, while the fæces are retained, like a sort of dysentery. [*Trs.*]
Bloody, slimy, fetid, diarrhœic stools. [GAIRDNER.]
320. After the stool, in the morning, which was rather hard than soft, pressure in the hypogastrium. [*Gff.*]
Pressure in the rectum, in the evening in bed (aft. 36 h.).
Violent itching on the anus.
Violent itching on the anus, as from ascarides. [*S.*]
Small, straining stitches in the anus, when sitting. [*Htb.*]
325. Excoriation in the rectum, after a normal stool.
Frequent excoriation, itching and burning on the anus.
Burning of the anus, in the evening.
The secretion of urine is obstinately suppressed. [*Trs.*]
She passes hardly any urine, and that little is red (aft. 48 h.).
330. Scanty passage of very dark-colored urine. [NEUMANN.]
Frequent call to urinate, with little secretion. [JOERG.]

Incessant urging to urinate. [*Hufel. Journ.*]

Frequent micturition, with urging. [*S.*]

Increased secretion of urine. [RICHTER.]

335. Copious and frequent passage of light-yellow, watery urine. [JOERG.]

Increased secretion of a thickish urine, with very dark sediment. [JOERG.]

Involuntary micturition (af. 3 d.).

Dark, turbid, sometimes milky urine. [*Gff.*]

Dark urine of yellowish-green color. [JOERG.]

340. Ammoniacal smell of the urine. [JOERG.]

Urine which smarts and corrodes, when passed.

Itching erosion in the orifice of the urethra.

Keen cutting in the orifice of the urethra, when not urinating. [*Gff.*]

Pricking, as from needles, in front in the orifice of the urethra (aft. 16 d.).

345. In the penis, anteriorly, very keen drawing; it is not manifest, whether it is more in the urethra or in the glans. [*Gff.*]

Clucking tearing on the right side, close beside the penis. [*Gff.*]

Pressive pain on the right side, close to the penis. [*Gff.*]

Severe itching on the glans.

Tickling in the glans, frequently recurring. [JOERG.]

350. Violent tickling on and below the glans. [*Gff.*]

Cutting drawing in the corona glandis.

Repeated pressing and straining down toward the testes [JOERG.]

One of the testes is closely drawn up to the belly.

A painless swelling of the right testicle disperses, with violent itching and burning in it, and the breaking out of an ill-smelling sweat (curative action). [HENNING.]

355. The induration of the prostate gland is dispersed (curative action). [MARTINI.]

Excitement of the sexual organs. [KUENZLI.]

The sexual desire is startlingly increased. [*Hufel. Journ.*]

Increased sexual instinct with men. [RICHTER.]

Exaltation of the sexual instinct. [VOIGT.]

360. Erections take place slowly (5th d.)

Severe straining in the hypogastrium toward the female sexual organs. [*Hufel. Journ.*]

Labor-like spasms in the hypogastrium. [*Hufel. Journ.*]

Dropsy of the ovaries quickly disappeared (curative action?). [*Trs.*]

Induration of the uterus quickly passes into uterine cancer. [GOELIS, in *Salzb. med. chir. Ztg.*, 1821, II., 272.[1]]

365. The induration of the uterus is diminished (curative action). [KLAPPROTH, *Hufel Journ.* LVII., F. 89.[2]]

The cancerous degeneration in the neck of the uterus is

---

[1] Observation. The original is: "Scirrhus uteri quickly becomes open cancer."—*Hughes.*

[2] Observation.—*Hughes.*

diminished (curative action). HENNEMANN, in *Hufel. Journ.* LVI., B. 3.[1]]

Hysterical attacks of marriageable girls. [*Trs.*]

The menses, which were flowing, ceased. [*Gr.*]

The menses come too late by eight days, with vertigo and palpitation. [*S.*]

370. Irregular catamenia. [SUTTINGER.]

Increased menstrual flow. [FRANK, in *Rust's Magaz.* XIII., 291.[2]]

Unusually early, violent and profuse menstrual flow. [RICHTER.]

It readily causes hemorrhages from the uterus. [FORMEY, in *Hufel. Journ.*[3]]

Violent hemorrhage from the vagina. [*Hufel. Journ.*]

375. Violent hemorrhage from the vagina, for four weeks, in a plethoric woman of twenty-four years. [SCHMIDT.[4]]

A uterine hemorrhage which came with every stool, with cutting in the abdomen and pains in the sacrum and the loins, ceases (curative action). [HENNEMANN]

Before the menses, heat rises into the head, with palpitation and with tension about the neck which became thicker. [*S.*]

The premonitory symptoms of the menses disappear, and the menses set in without any trouble. [HENNING.]

During the (normal) menses, pains in the sacrum. [*S.*]

380. At the cessation of the menses, great weakness.

During the menses, great weariness. [*S.*]

The pains and derangements during the menses cease, and they proceed without any troubles. [WOLF, in *Rust's Magaz.* XIII., 292.[5]]

After the menses, palpitation. [*S.*]

The leucorrhœa ceases entirely (curative action). [KLAPPROTH.]

385. A very inveterate leucorrhœa disappears entirely (curative action). [MARTINI.]

A long-continued leucorrhœa, strongest at the time of the menses, which excoriated the thighs and corroded the linen, disappeared entirely (curative action). [GOEDEN.]

The corroding leucorrhœa becomes milder and more and more scanty (curative action). [KLAPPROTH.]

* * * * * * * *

Sneezing without coryza, with immediate and considerable protrusion of the nasal mucus. [*Gff.*]

Stoppage of the nostrils (aft. 28 h.).

390. Stuffed coryza, very frequent (chiefly in the evening); this in the open air becomes fluent with much expectoration.

Fluent coryza, with much sneezing. [*S.*]

Fluent coryza, like water.

---

1 Observation.—*Hughes.*
2 From tincture in a goitrous subject.—*Hughes.*
3 From tincture in a goitrous subject.—*Hughes.*
4 In a married woman, subject to such hemorrhages.—*Hughes.*
5 Observations on patients.—*Hughes.*

Increased secretion of mucus from the nose, for several days. [JOERG.]

Much yellow mucus from blowing his nose.

395. Increased secretion of nasal mucus. [RICHTER.]

The larynx is painful. [VOGEL.]

Pain in the throat, with expectoration of indurated mucus. [*Htb.*]

Pressure in the region of the larynx, extending to the œsophagus, as if these parts were swollen. [JOERG.]

Pressive pain, with shooting in the region of the larynx and of the sublingual glands, recurring several times in the same day. [JOERG.]

400. Pressure in the throat, forcing him to hawk up much tenacious mucus. [*Htb.*]

On pressing on the larynx, increased pain of the œsophagus. [RICHTER.]

Contraction and heat in the larynx. [*Htb.*]

Contraction and heat in the throat. [ORFILA.]

Sensation of soreness in the throat and the chest, in bed, with wheezing in the throat and drawing pain in the lungs, synchronous with the heart-beat. [*Htb.*]

405. Inflammation of the trachea. [*Trs.*]

Roughness of the windpipe, the whole day. [JOERG.]

Hoarseness. [COINDET.]

Hoarseness, in the morning. [*S.*]

Hoarseness, for more than two weeks. [*Htb.*]

410. Hoarseness in the morning, after rising, compelling him to hawk up tenacious mucus. [*Htb.*]

Hoarseness, the whole day. [JOERG.]

Deeper and quite deep voice.

Sensation, as if something lay in the larynx which he could eject by hawking, the whole day and the evening. [*Htb.*]

Intolerable crawling and tickling in the larynx, which can only be removed by hawking and coughing, with gathering of water in the mouth; in the morning, in bed. [*Gff.*]

415. Violent clearing of the throat (2d d.). [*Htb.*]

Frequent clearing of the throat, in the morning. [*Htb.*]

Increased secretion of mucus in the windpipe. [JOERG.]

More profuse secretion of the bronchial mucus. [RICHTER.]

Increased secretion of mucus in the throat, with hoarse voice. [*Gff.*]

420. The secretion of mucus extends even to the Eustachian tube, and in the throat there remains a sort of soreness. [*Htb.*]

Expectoration of mucus from the throat, in the morning after rising, with a sensation of soreness therein.

Tenacious mucus accumulates profusely in the throat, in the evening. [*Htb.*]

Expectoration of tenacious mucus from the throat, with pressure there, as if there was something lodged in the way, which he thinks he might swallow down, in the morning. [*Htb.*]

A constant inclination to a troublesome hawking up of tenacious mucus from the windpipe, with crawling and shooting in the region of the larynx, now disappears quickly and permanently (curative effect). [MARTINI.]

425. Inclination to cough. [VOGEL.]

Irritation to cough, from a severe tickling in the throat. [*S.*]

Short cough, from tickling in the throat. [*Gff.*]

Cough, with exertions, so that she comes near vomiting; after expectoration of mucus it ceases. [*S.*]

Cough, with pressure and tightness of the chest. [VOIGT.]

430. Cough in the evening.

Frequent dry cough in the evening. [JOERG.]

Dry tussiculation. [GOELIS.]

Dry cough. [MATTHEY.]

Frequent dry cough. [COINDET.]

435. Much dry cough, with tightness, pressure and burning on the chest. [JOERG.]

Frequent deep, dry cough, caused by pressure in the chest. [JOERG.]

Deep, dry cough, with shooting in the chest. [JOERG.]

Occasional excitation to cough, with tenacious expectoration. [*Htb.*]

Short cough, from a tickling in the throat, with thick, yellow expectoration, with a good appetite, but a wretched appearance.

440. Cough, with expectoration of mucus, after previous heaviness, extending from the throat into the chest, impeding the breathing. [*S.*]

Rattling of the mucus on the chest, with roughness below the sternum and heaviness of the chest. [*S.*]

Expectoration of mucus from the chest. [*Trs.*]

Mucous expectoration, sometimes mixed with blood. [SCHNEIDER.[1]]

Expectoration streaked with blood. [GOELIS.]

445. Pulmonary consumption is increased. [GUENTHER, in *Harless.*[2]]

Pulmonary consumption. [CARMINATI, in *Giern. di Fisica*, Dec., 1821.[3]]

Severe respiratory trouble. [GOELIS.[4]]

Difficult breathing. [KUENZLI.]

Difficult breathing. [MATTHEY.]

450. Short breathing (5th d.).

Tightness of the chest. [KOLLEY.]

Asthma, with pains when breathing deeply, stronger and quicker heart-beat and smaller, more frequent pulse. [JOERG.]

Asthma, and the respiration is impeded in the throat for fourteen days [*Htb.*]

Trouble in dilating the chest, during inspiration. [ORFILA.[5]]

455. Feeling when he dilates the chest, in breathing, as if he had to overcome a great obstacle. [*Htb.*]

---

1 Not traceable.—*Hughes.*

2 Not accessible.—*Hughes.*

3 Observation. The observer merely says that in three cases the emaciation and prostration was so great as to threaten a slow phthisis.—*Hughes.*

4 Not found.—*Hughes.*

5 In the original: "Breathing sufficiently free, but chest at times contracted during inspiration.—*Hughes.*

Lack of breath. [NEUMANN.]

Want of breath. [GAIRDNER.]

Suffocating catarrh. [ORFILA.[1]]

Sensation of weakness in the chest and in the region of the scrobiculus cordis. [SCHNEIDER.]

460. Pain in the chest. [MATTHEY.]

Sore pain in the chest on both sides continually during respiration and when touching it.

Pressure, somewhat deep in the right side of the chest. [*Gff.*]

Pressive pain in the right side of the chest, aggravated at every inspiration, for an hour after dinner. [JOERG.]

Pressure and tightness in the chest, as after inhaling vapors of sulphur. [JOERG.]

465. Pressure, tightness and burning in the middle and sometimes also in the sides of the chest, with dry cough. [JOERG.]

Shooting in the chest, with excitation to deep, dry cough. [JOERG.]

Sharp shooting in the middle of the right breast, only when expiring. [*Gff.*]

Sharp shooting in the lower part of the right side of the chest, near the scrobiculus cordis, when inspiring. [*Gff.*]

Rush of blood to the chest, with tendency to inflammation. [*Hufel. Journ.*]

470. Violent throbbing in the chest, and palpitation, aggravated by every muscular exertion, so that she could not stand for a minute without coming near fainting; a quiet, horizontal position gave the greatest relief. [NEUMANN.]

Palpitation. [COINDET; GAIRDNER and many others.]

Violent palpitation. [*Hufel. Journ.* and *Rust's Magaz.*]

Severe palpitation, which could be manifestly observed despite his thick clothing, and could even be heard for several steps. [NEUMANN.]

Palpitation the whole day, till he goes to sleep. [*S.*]

475. Spasmodic palpitation; she feels it down to the navel, but most severely in the scrobiculus cordis. [*S.*]

The palpitation disappears entirely (curative action). [*S.*]

Squeezing the heart together. [*S.*]

Burning, lancinating tension in the integuments of the chest.

Tearing in the integuments of the right side of the chest. [*Gff.*]

480. The female breasts enlarge, while the goitre diminishes in several females. [PERROT.]

Sometimes the breasts dwindle away. [COINDET.]

Dwindling, falling away of the breasts. [KUENZLI.]

The breasts hang down relaxed, deprived of all fat. [NEUMANN.]

Dwindling of the breasts, in two females. [*Hufel. Journ.*]

485. Dwindling away of the formerly full breasts, so that two years after the use of iodine, there was no trace of the breasts and of the lacteal glands. [*Hufel. Journ.*]

---

[1] Not found.—*Hughes.*

The glands of the female mammæ dwindle away entirely. [VOIGT.]

The desire to nurse the baby is diminished, with injurious effects.

In the coccyx and the sacrum, a pressive pain which increases and diminishes. [*Gff.*]

In the sacrum, stitches (aft. 15 d.).

490. In the back, itching above the right hip.

Cramps in the back. [*Trs.*]

Stitches in the scapulæ, when lifting something (aft. 14 d.).

Burning on the right scapula. [*Gff.*]

On the lower part of the neck, near the left shoulder, a rheumatic pinching, aggravated by touching it, seemingly relieved by an eructation, but frequently recurring afterward. [*Gff.*]

495. Rheumatic tension in the right side of the neck. [*Gff.*]

Tearing in the right side of the neck. [*Gff.*]

Tension on the outside of the neck. [*Htb. u. Tr.*]

Constriction of the throat. [*S.*]

Troublesome sensation of constriction of the neck. [PESCHIER in *Hufel. Journ.* LX., B. 97.[1]]

500. The neck becomes thicker from loud speaking. [*S.*]

The swelling of the goitre increases and becomes more painful. [GRAEFE.]

Enlargement and painful induration of the goitre. [COINDET.]

Induration of the goitre. [COINDET; PESCHIER.]

Pain and throbbing in the goitre. [GRAEFE.]

505. **Pains in the goitre.** [KUENZLI; GUENTHER, in the *Salz. med. Zeitg.*, 1822, III., 160.[2]]

Painful tension in the goitre. [BAUP.]

Constant sensation of constriction in the goitre. [*Hufel. Journ.*]

Enlargement and hardness of the goitre, during the first days, then decrease of the same. [SCHNEIDER.]

Diminution of the swelling of the neck (curative action). [*S*].

510. **Dwindling away of old and hard or doughy swellings of the thyroid glands and of large goitres** (curative effect). [COINDET; NEUMANN; GRAEFE and many others.]

Swelling of the glands on the neck and in the nape disappear permanently. (curative effect). [HENNING; MARTINI; NEUMANN.]

Redness on the neck and on the chest, as if suffused with blood. [*S.*]

Yellow spots on the neck. [*Htb.*]

Induration of the axillary glands. [ROECHLING.[3]]

515. Glandular swellings in the axillæ disappear. [HENNING; MARTINI.]

In the abnormally elevated shoulder, drawing tearing pains (2d d.).

---

[1] Observation.—*Hughes.*

[2] From local use of ointment of iodide of potassium.—*Hughes.*

[3] Instead of "induration" the original has "suppuration."—*Hughes.*

Rheumatic pains, in the left shoulder. [*Gff.*]

Severe stitches in the shoulder-joint, also at rest.

In the arm, on the outside, a pain in the bones, which wakes from sleep and keeps him from again falling asleep, aggravated by lying on it.

520. Rheumatic pains in the arms. [JOERG.]

Tearing pain in both arms, after slight manual labor.

Paralytic weariness in the arms, in the morning on awaking, in bed.

Subsultus tendinum in the arms. [*Trs.*]

Tearing in the left elbow.

525. Pressure in the bend of the left elbow.

Lancinating pain in the right wrist, when grasping or lifting anything.

Pain, as after a blow upon the metacarpal bone of the index, aggravated by touching. [*Gr.*]

Tearing in the metacarpal bone of the right index.

Heat in the hands.

530. **Trembling of the limbs.** [PERROT; GAIRDNER.]

Slight trembling of the hands. [RICHTER.]

Violent trembling of the hands, so that he could only work with them at certain hours of the day. [FORMEY.]

The hands move in zigzag fashion. [RICHTER.]

Subsultus tendinum, in the hands. [RICHTER.]

535. A round, burning, itching spot on the right hand between the thumb and the index; with two whitish vesicles upon it; it was relieved by rubbing, and went off on the third day. [*S.*]

In the finger-joints, on flexing them, a tensive pain, as if they would break; with some swelling and painfulness in pressing on them, when they are stretched out (aft. some d.).

Tearing in the posterior joint of the right thumb. [*Gff.*]

Tearing in the knuckle of the right little finger. [*Gff.*]

Tearing in the whole of the index and of the middle finger of the left hand. [*Gff.*]

540. Trembling of the fingers. [KUENZLI.]

Subsultus tendinum in the fingers. [*Trs.*]

Paronychia on the left index, from a little prick in the finger, near the nail.

In the left natis, a pressure, as if in the os ischium. [*Gff.*]

Between the left hip and the head of the femur, an intermittent sharp tearing, much aggravated by moving the joint. [*Gff.*]

545. Turgidity in the lower limbs, almost like cramp in the thighs and legs, merely in sitting, not when lying, walking or standing.

Rheumatic drawing in the whole of the left lower limb, especially in the thigh and knee, with humming in the heel, in the evening in bed; rather increased by motion. [*Gff.*]

Heaviness as of lead, in the lower limbs. [*S.*]

Swelling of the lower limbs. [COINDET.]

Swelling and trembling of the lower limbs. [KUENZLI.]

550. Œdematous swelling of the lower limbs. [NEUMANN.]

Restlessness in the lower limbs. [KUENZLI.]

Trembling of the lower limbs, which makes walking difficult, unsteady and unsafe. [KUENZLI.]

Paralysis of the lower limbs. [GOELIS.]

The thigh pains, especially at night in bed. [SCHNEIDER.]

555. Pains of a peculiar kind in the thighs. [GOELIS.[1]]

Rheumatic pain in the left thigh. [*Gff.*]

Pinching tearing in the left thigh, near to the head of the femur. [*Gff.*]

Sharp, shooting tearing in the middle of the left thigh, toward the inner side. [*Gff.*]

Twitching of the muscles of the thigh.

560. Excoriation of the female thighs, where they touch in walking.

Tearing in the left knee. [*Gff.*]

Dull tearing, on the outer side of the right hough. [*Gff.*]

A white swelling of the knee disappears (curative effect). [*Trs.*]

The leg pains on the tibia, as if festering.

565. Tearing on both sides of the leg, close above the ankles. [*Gff.*]

In the ankle-joint violent cramp, with twitchings, at night.

Cramps in the feet. [GAIRDNER.]

Pressive, spasmodic pain in the foot, from the middle toe to the ankle.

Acute, constant pain in the inner half of the right heel. [*Gff.*]

570. Single, sharp stitches in the ankles.

Heaviness of the feet, like lead. [*S.*]

Swelling of the feet, followed by their rapid emaciation and becoming thin. [*Trs.*]

Œdematous swelling of the feet. [NEUMANN.]

Subsultus tendinum of the feet. [*Trs.*; RICHTER.]

575. Sweat of the feet, so sharp that it erodes the skin.

Shooting tearing under the nail of the left big toe [*Gff.*]

The corns ache. [*Htb.*]

Erratic pains in the joints. [*Trs.*]

Rheumatic pains in the trunk, on the neck and in the arms. [JOERG.]

580. Sensation of numbness in the upper and lower extremities. [FORMEY.]

Sensation of numbness and trembling in the limbs. [VOIGT.]

Paralysis of the limbs. [GOELIS.]

Liable to catch cold, and thence inflammation of the eyes.

Shooting itching in various parts of the body.

585. Sensation as of violent flea-bites all over the body, day and night.

Itching on an old cicatrix of an ulcer (on the leg), cured many years before.

Eruption of itching pimples on the old cicatrix.

On the arms, the breast and the back, small, red, dry pimples, which at first itch. [*Htb.*]

---

[1] Preceding S. 553.—*Hughes.*

Dirty yellow color of the skin, for five or six weeks. [KOLBE, in the *Zeitschr. f. Nat. u. Heilk.* V., 1, 91.[1]]

590. Rough, dry skin. [NEUMANN.]

Induration of the glands. [ROECHLING.[2]]

The swellings of certain glands on the neck, the axillæ and the groin disappear (curative action). [MARTINI.]

It excites the glandular system, the glands of the buccal cavity, the stomach, the liver and the pancreas, and it promotes in these parts the secretion of the juices. [KUENZLI.]

Throbbing in all the arteries, at every muscular exertion. [*Rust's Magaz.*]

595. Very troublesome throbbing in all the larger arterial trunks. [NEUMANN.]

The blood is readily heated, with obtuseness of the head and subsequent headache. [VOIGT.]

The circulation is easily excited and accelerated. [VOIGT.]

Erethism of the vascular system, especially of the veins. [KUENZLI.]

Ebullitions of blood. [RICHTER.]

600. Violent ebullitions of blood. [*Hufel. Journ.*]

Disposition to hemorrhages. [*Hufel. Journ.*]

Hemorrhages. [KOLLEY.]

Hemorrhages from various organs. [VOIGT.]

Great excitement of the nervous system. [*Hufel. Journ.*]

605. Increased sensitiveness of the whole body. [*Hufel. Journ.*]

Restlessness in the limbs. [KUENZLI.]

A restless and morbid state, with a quivering motion from the gastric region toward the whole surface of the body, as if he was about to tremble or as if a general pulsation was about to break out, with a general increase of heat, seeming to come from the stomach; then a pressure in the cardiac region, a weight on the chest, with difficult breathing and acceleration of the pulse by seven or eight beats. [JOERG.]

Trembling. [COINDET; GAIRDNER.]

Trembling of the limbs. [KOLLEY; MATTHEY.]

630. Trembling of the limbs, especially of the hands. [GAIRDNER.[3]]

Trembling of the fingers and of the eyelids. [KUENZLI.]

Trembling of a peculiar kind. [GAIRDNER.]

Trembling, first of the hands, and then also of the arms, of the feet and the back, so that he can only walk tottering and unsteady, and the hand, which moves in a zigzag fashion, cannot guide anything straight to his mouth; the trembling parts can easily be held fast when at rest; general movements at the same time are painful and the circulation is accelerated, with a small, threadlike pulse. [*Trs.*]

Cramps. [KOLLEY; KUENZLI.]

635. Spasmodic movements of the limbs. [VOIGT.]

Violent cramps in the back and in the feet. [*Trs.*]

---

[1] From external applications.—*Hughes.*

[2] See note to S. 514.—*Hughes.*

[3] There is a gap here in the numbering in the original. Instead of 610, H. proceeds at once to 630.—*Trans.*

Violent cramps and convulsive twitches of the arms, the back and the legs, which are scarcely intermitted for a moment. [GAIRDNER.]

Subsultus of the tendons. [KUENZLI; NEUMANN.]

Subsultus of the tendons on the hands and the feet. [RICHTER.]

640. Subsultus tendinum on the arms, fingers and feet. [*Trs.*]

Catching at flakes. [NEUMANN.]

A sort of East Indian cholera. [*Trs.*]

Walking becomes difficult, tottering and unsteady. [RICHTER.]

Difficult, vacillating, unsteady walk from tremulousness of the limbs. [KUENZLI.]

645. Heaviness in the limbs, in the morning (8th d.).

Heaviness in the limbs. [KUENZLI.]

Heaviness in the limbs and sensation of lassitude. [KOLLEY.]

Great weariness in the afternoon, after a short walk, with a sensation of fasting, but not of hunger. [*Gff.*]

Lassitude, so that perspiration breaks out on her when she speaks.

650. **Lassitude.** [KUENZLI; NEUMANN; SCHNEIDER.]

Complete prostration of strength. [*Hufel. Journ.*]

Fatigued, cross and slow to move. [JOERG.]

Sensation of weakness. [RUDOLPH.]

Weakness of the muscles. [COINDET; KUENZLI.]

655. Long continued weakness of the muscles. [COINDET.]

Decrease of strength. [KUENZLI; COINDET.]

Loss of all strength. [COINDET; MATTHEY.]

Prostration. [BAUP; VOIGT.]

Great prostration. [SCHNEIDER; FORMEY; *Hufel. Journ.*]

660. Tendency to swoons and cramps. [VOIGT.]

Swoons. [*Hufel Journ.*]

Emaciation. [BAUP; MATTHEY; PERRAT.]

Rapid emaciation. [COINDET; VOIGT.]

Visible, manifest emaciation. [*Hufel Journ.*; SUTTINGER.]

665. **General emaciation** *of the whole body*. [CLARUS, in *Gilbert's Annal*; LOCHER-BALBER VIII., 309.[1]]

Severe emaciation. [KUENZLI.]

Extreme, sudden emaciation. [GAIRDNER.]

Severe emaciation, which may reach an extraordinarily high degree. [GAIRDNER; RICHTER.]

So severe an emaciation, that the arms and the body are almost fleshless, her breast quite flat, her calves entirely disappeared, and her thighs no thicker than her fore-arms in her days of good health. [GAIRDNER.]

670. **The greatest emaciation, till he is a mere skeleton.** [*Gr.*]

Emaciation, lasting a whole year, until he can no more be recognized, with general weakness of the muscles, attended with unusually good appetite. [LOCHER-BALBER.]

Chronic emaciation, paleness of the face, and weakness of the muscles. [COINDET]

---

[1] Observation.—*Hughes.*

Wasting away. [*Hufel. Journ.*]

Wasting away with slow fever (removed by *China*). [ZIEGER, in *Dienbach's neuest. Entdeck.* [1]]

675. Corpulence and cheerfulness return (curative effect). [MARTINI.]

Nutrition is improved (curative effect). [VOIGT.]

A girl who had been remarkably phlegmatic, loses this disposition, becomes stronger and more lively, and her muscles receive a greater mobility (after effect). [HENNING.]

Swelling and pain in the affected parts. [*Med. chir. Zeit.*]

Disappearance of a fungus articularis, which had arisen in consequence of measles (curative effect). [*Rust's Magaz.*]

680. Œdematous swelling of the whole body, which does not pass off. [ROECHLING.]

Dropsical Swellings. [FORMEY KUENZLI.]

General dropsy. [VOIGT.]

General dropsy of the skin and abdomen. [*Rust's Magaz.*]

Apoplexy. [*Rust's Magaz.*]

685. Death, with partly local and partly general inflammatory phenomena. [RICHTER.]

No desire for sleep (6th d.).

Restless sleep. [JOERG.]

Restless sleep, at night. [VOIGT.]

Restless sleep, with anxious dreams. [*S.*]

690. **Sleeplessness.** [BAUP; COINDET; FORMEY and many oth.]

Sleeplessness for eight days; she did not sleep a moment. [*Trs.*]

Sleep full of dreams. [GAIRDNER.]

Very vivid dreams, from which he would like to awake, but cannot; with sensation of fatigue after awaking. [*Gff.*]

Dreams, which he cannot recollect, during a sound sleep. [*S.*]

695. Anxious dreams. [RICHTER.]

Distressing, restless dreams. [*S.*]

Anxious dreams, about deceased persons. [*S.*]

She dreams every night; about swimming in water, walking in mud, that her daughter had tumbled into the well, etc.

At night, cold feet.

700. Coldness of the skin. [NEUMANN.]

An unusual chill frequently shakes him, even in the warm room, and he does not feel well all day. [*Htb.*]

Warmth of the skin is increased. [ORFILA; VOIGT.]

Increased animal warmth of the whole body. [RUDOLPH; RICHTER.]

Flying heat. [*S.*]

705. Fever, in which chilliness alternates with flying heat. [*Hufel. Journ.*]

Feverish states. [RICHTER; BAUP; KOLLEY and many oth.]

Fever with delirium and subsultus tendinum. [*Hufel. Journ.*]

[1] Not accessible.—*Hughes.*

Fever, with dryness and coldness of the skin, soft, quick pulse, delirium, subsultus tendinum and catching flakes. [NEUMANN.]

Quartan fever. [SUTTINGER.]

710. Pulse strong, large and full. [JOERG.]

Quick, hard pulse. [COINDET; VOIGT.]

Accelerated, increased pulse. [COINDET; MATTHEY; KUENZLI and many oth.]

Quicker pulse, accelerated by fifteen beats. [*Htb.*]

Quicker pulse, accelerated up to eighty-six beats. [ORFILA.]

715. Acclerated, full, hard pulse. [VOIGT.]

Small, threadlike, acclerated pulse. [KUENZLI; RICHTER.]

Small, hard pulse, so quick that it could hardly be counted. [GAIRDNER.]

Small, very frequent, suppressed pulse. [*Trs.*]

Soft and quicker pulse. [NEUMANN.]

720. The beats of the heart and the pulse were synchronous; the pulse was small and weak, and when she kept still, it was but little acclerated; but with every motion, it was accelerated, as also was the beat of the heart. [NEUMANN.]

Night-sweat.

Profuse night-sweat and little sleep. [JOERG.]

In the morning, she awakes in a perspiration, and feels more languid. [*Htb. u. Tr.*]

Sourish night-sweat all over, every morning, and the first hour afterward, she is very faint in her lower limbs.

KALI CARBONICUM, SALT OF TARTAR.

[Half an ounce of purified tartar, moistened with a few drops of water, is pressed together into a ball, which is rolled up into a piece of paper and allowed to dry; then it is brought to a red heat between the glowing charcoal of a grate (or of a draught furnace). It is then taken out, laid in a porcelain saucer and covered with a linen cloth; it is allowed to attract moisture from the air in a cellar, which causes the alkaline salt partially to deliquesce, and, if it is allowed to stay there a few weeks, it will deposit even the last trace of lime. A clear drop* of this preparation is then triturated three times with 100 grains of sugar of milk each time, within three hours, to the one millionth powder attenuation (Kali I); one grain of this third trituration is then raised by twenty-seven dilution vials to the decillionth dynamization (Kali X).

The carbonate of potash secured in this manner has proved itself most useful where the following morbid symptoms predominated, or at least were also present:

* This will be a salt of tartar sufficiently pure for our purposes. I would again repeat, that I have endeavored to secure the medicinal material for homœopathic use, wherever practicable, in the most simple and natural manner, and to give directions of this kind; so that every physician, wherever he may be, may secure the same substance. For this purpose, which was to me most important (and not merely to avoid every appearance of ostentation and puristic pedantry, which would in this matter have been altogether out of place), I had to avoid as far as possible all directions which would have led to difficult chemical operations, by means of costly apparatus, to secure the absolute chemical purity of the medicinal substances used.

Peevishness; *timidity;* lack of memory; *dizziness;* stolid feeling in the head; vertigo, as if rising in the stomach; headache when out driving; headache, while sneezing and coughing; morning-headache; headache with nausea; pressive pain the occiput; rush of blood to the head; hissing in the head; great tendency of the external head to catch cold; scurfy eruption of the head; dryness of the hair of the head; falling out of the hair; morning-sweat on the forehead; swelling of the eye; agglutination of the eyes in the morning; lachrymation; floating specks before the eyes; *the eye is dazzled by the light;* stitches in the ear; pains, shooting in the ears outward; weakness of the hearing, dull hearing; ulceration of the inside of the nose; dullness of olfaction; heat of the face; flying heat of the face; yellowness of the face; bloatedness of the face; drawing pain in the face; toothache, only when eating; shooting toothache; palate full of mucus; *hawking up of mucus;* sour taste in the mouth; spoiled taste; bitter taste in the mouth; rabid hunger; great liking for sugar; frequent eructation; sour eructations; nausea; anxiety, with inclination to vomit; nausea during eating; *fullness of the stomach after eating;* tension transversely across the stomach; pinching in the stomach; pressure in the liver; sprained pain in the liver when stooping; pressure in the hypogastrium when stooping; heaviness and restlessness in the abdomen; inactivity and coldness in the abdomen; labor-like colic; much flatulence; incarceration of flatus; no emission of flatus; continual emission of flatus; inactivity of the rectum; difficult evacuation of the fæces, on account of their large formation; constipation; constipation every other day; costiveness and difficult discharge of stool; mucus with the stool; anxiety before the stool; varices of the anus; *itching of the anus;* pressive pain in the rectum, before discharge of flatus; tenesmus of the bladder; frequent micturition, day and night; the sexual impulse is dormant; lack of sexual impulse; (surexcitation of the sexual instinct;) lack of erections; lack of pollutions; (too many pollutions:) swelling of the testicle; after coitus, weakness of the body, especially of the eyes; (suppression of the menses, with anasarca and ascites;) *menses too scanty; menses too early;* during the menses, an itching eruption and excoriation between the thighs; *sharpness, itching* and *erosion on and in the genitals; vaginal discharge.*

Dryness of the nose; stuffed nostrils; *stuffed coryza;* hoarseness; cough; *nocturnal cough;* expectoration of pus; *expectoration of pus when coughing;* spasm of the chest when coughing; difficult breathing; wheezing on the chest; morning-asthma; *asthma* when walking a little faster than usual; spasmodic asthma; spasm of the chest; palpitation; palpitation and orgasm of the blood in the morning on awaking; pain in the sacrum; pain in the sacrum from a fall; drawing pain from the sacrum to the middle of the back; drawing pain in the back; stiffness between the scapulæ; *stiffness of the nape;* weakness in the cervical muscles; goitre; pressure on the shoulders; the arms go to sleep; the upper arms go to sleep; weakness in the arms; lassitude of the arms, in the morning in bed; stiffness of the elbow-joint; trembling of the hands in writing; paralytic pain in the wrist; convulsive twitching of the fingers in sewing. Tearing pressure ni the thigh and leg; *nocturnal tearing in the lower limbs;* crawling shudder on the tibiæ; coldness of the feet, in the evening in bed; stiffness in the ankle-joint; swelling of the leg; burning pain in the legs and the feet; cold feet; *fetid sweat of the feet*; shooting and burning in the ball of the big toe; corns painful when touched; drawing pains in the limbs; the fingers and toes are drawn crooked; the limbs go to sleep; tendency to strains: tremulous lassitude; weakness after parturition; *readiness to take cold; lack of perspiration and inability to perspire;* anasarca and ascites; red, itching, burning, spots on the body; herpes; old warts in the face; drowsiness by day; *drowsiness early in the evening;* sleep full of fancies; anxious sleep, full of dreams; frightful dreams; twitching in sleep; tendency to shudder by day; heat in the morning in bed; great tendency to sweat while walking; *night-sweat.*

Patients suffering from ulceration of the lungs rarely get well without this antipsoric. Nitric acid is frequently homœopathically indicated after kali.

The observations marked *Gff.* are by the Royal Councilor, Baron *von Gersdorff;* those marked *Gll.* by *Dr. Goullon*, in Weimar; *Htb.*, *Dr. Hartlaub; Ng* , an anonymous contributor in Hartlaub und Trinks' *Reine Arzneimittell.*, and *Rl.*, *Dr. Rummel.*

KALI.

Great dejection, without anxiety.

Dejection (1st d.).

The mind is without tone.

Troubled mood, with disposition to weep, after bodily fatigue in the open air. [*Gff.*]

5. Sad, she feels lonesome; she seeks for company to cheer her up. [*Ng.*]

Great sadness, she has to weep without cause, in the evening. [*Htb.*]

A pathogenesis of Kali carbonicum appeared in Vol. IV. of the first edition of this work (1830), and already contained—besides Hahnemann's own—the symptoms referred to Rummel and v. Gersdorff, doubtless obtained from the 30th dil. Those of Goullon added here, presumably come from a similar source; but the main addition in the present pathogenesis is from the symptom list of Hartlaub and Nenning (chiefly the latter) in Hartlaub and Trink's *Arzneimittellehre*, Vol. III.—*Hughes.*

Lachrymose mood; she felt like dissolving in tears constantly (aft. 20 d.).

Very ill-humored; she has to weep much, because it was constantly on her mind that she had to die.

Anxious oppression, breaking out into tears (1st d.). [*Htb.*]

10. Anguish and great sadness.

Anxiety and dislike of company.

Anxiety every day.

Full of **apprehension.**

He is afraid that he might not get well.

15. **Apprehensive and anxious about her disease.**

Anxious ideas infest him in the evening.

Troubled ideas about the future.

Restlessness of the mind.

Hasty thought and action.

20. Irresolution.

Desponding and pusillanimous in a high degree.

Timidity, in the evening, in bed.

Fearful about being alone.

Great timidity.

25. Readily frightened, especially by a slight touch of the body.

She is frightened by an imaginary appearance (*e. g.*, as if a bird was flying toward the window) and she utters a loud scream.

Very peevish, in the evening, on going to sleep, and in the morning on awaking.

Cross, without cause (5th d.).

Unusual ill-humor, which is seen in his features, before he himself is aware of it. [*Gff.*]

30. Peevish mood, as if she could not do anything to suit herself. [*Ng.*]

She is always in antagonism with herself; she knows not what she wants, and feels exceedingly unhappy

Contrary disposition; he is self-willed and often does not know himself what he wishes.

Contrary mood; she demands impetuously; is not satisfied with anything; she is beside herself, and furiously angry, if everything does not go according to her wishes, and often does not herself know what she really wants.

Impatient with his children.

35. Very irritable, as after vexation.

Sensitively irritable.

Irritable mood.

Irritable, peevish mood.

Easily rendered cross.

40. Extremely cross mood (the first 11 d.).

Very peevish, she has no pleasure in anything.

He gets vexed at everything and is always cross.

Peevish, sulky mood; every trifle vexes him and every noise is disagreeable; worse at noon and in the evening.

Cross and angry thoughts, in the morning, on awaking, so that he gnashes with his teeth (aft. 4 d.).

45. Readily excited to anger. [*Gff.*]

She readily becomes violent.

Indisposed to everything and indifferent.

Indisposed to work. [*Gff.*]

Changeful mood, now good and quiet, then passionate and angry about trifles; often hopeful, often despondent.

50. Absent-minded; he finds it difficult to fix his attention on any special subject. [*Gff.*]

Lack of presence of mind; he cannot proceed right along in his business (aft. 15 h.).

He often cannot find the right word and the right expression, and makes slips in speaking.

Delirium by day and by night.

Lack of recollection, as if in the occiput, with much talking; it goes off on shutting the eyes.

55. Unconsciousness for several minutes, so violent that all his senses failed him, and he would have fallen down, if he had not held on to something (aft. 18 d.).

Sensation as if her thoughts vanished, for a few moments.

Sensation at times, as if her thoughts and her memory were gone, with whirring in the head.

Chaotic and stupid feeling in the head, in the evening. [*Rl.*]

As if intoxicated (aft. 4 d.).

60. Frequent **obtusion in the head.**

Obtuseness of the head, as after a spree, and as if the ears were stopped up, with nausea almost to vomiting (aft. 8 d.). [*Rl.*]

The head is frequently benumbed in the morning, with heaviness of the head, in the region of the eyebrows.

The whole head is benumbed, as if screwed in a vice, with shooting in the brain, in frequent intervals. [*Ng.*]

Gloomy in the head, as if he had not slept enough, in the morning, after rising, and as if overclouded, with lack of cheerfulness. [*Ng.*]

65. Weakness in the head.

Weakness in the head, just above the eyes, after walking fast (17th d.).

Vertigo, as if intoxicated, while walking, so that he staggers from one side to the other. [*Ng.*]

Vertigo, like reeling, while standing and walking; better in the open air.

Vertigo, especially after eating.

70. Vertigo, at once on rising, as if her head were too light; she has to hold on to something.

Slight fit of vertigo, as often as he rises from his chair and turns around.

Vertigo, as if there was an abyss behind him, and he was about to fall down into it, **on turning around** after looking into a mirror and after reading.

Vertigo, on turning around. [*Rl.*]

Vertigo, on quickly turning the body and **the head.**

75. **Giddy in the head, chiefly in the morning and evening.** [*Rl.*]

Very giddy, also while sitting (aft. 30 h. [*Rl.*]

Vertigo while sitting, as if tottering to and fro (before a meal.)

Vertigo while sitting, so that he dares not rise for fear of falling. [*Ng.*]

Vertigo, while writing and in the open air, everything whirls around with him. [*Ng.*]

80. Headache, relieved by sitting up in bed, worse when lying down.

Headache in the morning on awaking, for a quarter of an hour, for several mornings.

Headache in the vertex, when pressing on the head.

Cruel headache, through the eyes.

Fits of headache on one side, the right and the left with lassitude and lack of tone, almost producing nausea, in the evening. [*Gff.*]

85. Violent pain in the whole head, with throbbing and shooting in the knees, which goes off by motion; in the evening. [*Ng.*]

Pressive headache.

Pressive headache in the forehead, in the afternoon when walking, attended with peevishness (13th, 19th and 20th d.). [*Gff.*]

Pressure in the forehead, with photophobia. [*Gff.*]

Violent pressure all over the skull and down the nape; throbbing in the head and in the whole body; the pain will not bear the least touch, and is aggravated by paroxysms, with violent nausea and vomiting of bile. [*Gll.*]

90. Squeezing pressive pain in the forehead, with vomiting of mucus and acid. [*Gll.*]

Pressure and squeezing in the right temple (11th, 19th and 20th d.). [*Gff.*]

Pressure in the right temple, from morn till noon (aft. 11 d.). [*Rl.*]

Pressive headache in the left temple (6th d.). [*Gff.*]

Pressive pain in the forehead, like numbness. [*Ng.*]

95. Pressure in the forehead, in the evening on going to sleep, with qualmy nausea, as if he had spoiled his stomach; easier by resting, aggravated by walking.

Pressure above the eyes, with violent pain in the whole sinciput.

Pressive pain in the occiput, toward the nape, going off in the open air.

Violent pressive pain in the whole head, with a shivering chill over the whole body, chiefly in the forenoon. [*Htb.*]

Severe pressure in the occiput, with ebullition in the head and sensation of heaviness while standing. [*Ng.*]

100. Pressure and drawing tearing in the sinciput, extending to the eyes and the root of the nose (14th, 17th, 18th and 21st d.). [*Gff.*]

Severe pressure and drawing in the forehead, in the evening. [*Rl.*]

Pressure and burning deep in the occiput, with heaviness in the head and tendency to fall forward. [*Ng.*]

Pressive headache, from both temples toward the middle.

Pressure on top of the head, in the evening. [*Rl.*]

105. Pressure into the right side of the cranium, after rising from a stooping position. [*Ng.*]

Shooting pressure, inward into the left temple. [*Ng.*]

Boring pressing pain from without inward, above the left eye. [*Ng.*]

Pain pressing outward, in the right temple. [*Ng.*]

Severe outward pressing in the whole frontal region, while writing. [*Ng.*]

110. Severe outward pressure over the left eye, as if the brain would press forward. [*Ng.*]

Sensation in the forehead, as if it would burst her sinciput, in frequent short paroxysms. [*Ng.*]

Sensation of fullness in the head, as if the brain pressed close upon the cranium. [*Ng.*]

Heaviness in the occiput, as if it was filled with lead, the head always falls backward, with stiffness in the nape, extending to between the scapulæ.

Heaviness in the occiput, like numbness. [*Ng.*]

115. Heaviness and painfulness of the sinciput. [*Ng.*]

Severe sensation of heaviness in the left side of the head. [*Ng.*]

Squeezing pain in the whole of the upper part of the head, especially on the left side. [*Gff.*]

Squeezing pain in the left temple in paroxysms; also tearing. [*Gff.*]

Drawing in the forehead; in the forenoon and at midnight (2d, 30th d.). [*Gff.*]

120. Drawing and tearing on the vertex of the head (33d, 34th d.). [*Gff.*]

Tearing drawing in the left half of the head, above, in front of and within the temple (12th, 19th, 25th d.).

Drawing in the occiput and nape, especially on the right side, with stiffness. [*Gff.*]

Tearing in the left frontal protuberance (25th d.). [*Gff.*]

Tearing from the left temple into the articulation of the jaw, in the evening. [*Gff.*]

125. Tearing in the left and the right temples, also in the left parietal bone. [*Ng.*]

Tearing now on the right, now on the left side of the occiput, then in the forehead (1st d.). [*Ng.*]

Beating tearing on the right side of the occiput, close to the nape (16th d.). [*Gff.*]

Twitching tearing pain in the head.

Twitching in the left temple.

130. Twitching headache, the whole day.

Shooting in the temples.

Shooting in the temples, causing fright and screaming; in the right temple attended with tearing. [*Ng.*]

Stitch above the left temple and immediately afterward a stitch outward in the middle of the forehead. [*Ng.*]

Pricking in the forehead, as from needles. [*Ng.*]

135. Shooting in the sinciput.

Violent shooting in the forehead, the whole day, and at times also on the left side of the head; with violent pains in the chest, and icy coldness in the limbs.

Stitches in the forehead, in the morning.

Stitches on the upper part of the forehead and over the temples, on moving the lower jaw.

Stitches extending from the nape up into the occiput.

140. Stitches in the occiput, on treading and stooping, as if they were in the surface of the brain.

Stitch through the right side of the head, from behind forward. [*Gll.*]

Stitches through the whole head.

Dull shooting in the head (1st d.).

Beating and throbbing in the forehead, and especially in the side of the head, with frequent intermissions; also after dinner, while walking and standing. [*Ng.*]

145. Beating pain in the sinciput.

Painful throbbing in the head, when she wants to write.

Beating (throbbing) pain in the upper left side of the head; by pressing on it, the pain becomes more violent and lancinating; more external. [*Ng.*]

A burrowing throbbing in the frontal bone, above the left eye. [*Ng.*]

Ulcerative pain in the head after dinner; she had to lie down, which relieved it. [*Ng.*]

150. Rush of blood to the head, and intoxication therefrom.

Warm rising of blood to the head, with ebullition in the body, and, a few hours afterward, a slight headache (at once).

Great warmth in the head, especially on the right side of the face, frequently (5th d.). [*Ng.*]

Rising heat in the head, in the evening, before lying down; it goes off in bed. [*Ng.*]

Burning, painful sensation of heat in the head.

155. Sensation in the forehead, as if a hot body had fallen forward in it; frequently recurring when stooping and writing; it goes off on rising up. [*Ng.*]

Sensation when stooping, as if something descended from the occiput toward the forehead.

Painful feeling, as of something moveable in the head, worse on moving the head.

Constant **sensation, as if there was something detached in the head**, which turned and twisted toward the forehead.

Painful turning and twisting in the head.

160. Shaking headache.

Humming, resounding tingling in the right temple.

Crawling pain above the forehead.

Externally on the temple, an acute pressive pain.

Shooting pain externally on the head and in the nape, with a shooting swelling on the cheek, and shooting in the teeth.

165. Single tearing stitches in the left temple, extending into the zygoma.

Fine stitches, externally, on various parts of the head. [*Ng.*]

Painless, clucking, muscular twitches in the right temple. [*Gff.*]

His head was jerked several times toward the left, without loss of consciousness, after which the nape became, as it were, stiff.

Chill on the head.

170. The head readily takes cold, causing headache and toothache.

Itching of the hairy scalp.

Frequent itching of the head, chiefly on the occiput. [*Ng.*]

Itching of the skin of the scalp, with sore pain on scratching it. [*Rl.*]

Pimples on the hairy scalp.

175. Large, red pimples on the left frontal protuberance, painful when touched, and suppurating afterwards (aft. 32 d.). [*Gff.*]

Painful lump on the right side of the head, as if a furuncle was forming (aft. 6 d.). [*Rl.*]

A large, yellow, scaly spot on the upper part of the forehead.

Dryness of the hair of the head.

Falling out of the hair.

180. **Falling out of the hair of the head.** [*Htb.*]

The eyes pain, on moving them.

Pain of the left eye, when it is directed upward.

Pressure in the eyes.

Pressure on the eyelids.

185. Pressure on the eyes and in the orbits, with drowsiness, at noon (36th d.). [*Gff.*]

Pressure in the eyes, and dry pus in the eyelashes.

Pain as if the eyes were pressed inward.

The eyes pain on reading, as if pressed inward.

Pinching in the eyes.

190. Tearing in the left eye, in the morning before going to sleep. [*Gff.*]

Sharp **tearing in the** right **orbit, and in the eye at night** (30th, 31st d.). [*Gff.*]

Pressive tearing in the inside of the right eye (12th, 26th d.). [*Gff.*]

Pressive tearing in the region of the right eyebrow (26th d.).

Jerking or tearing in the eyelid, and above the right eye.

195. **Stitches in the middle of the eye.**

Stitches in the eyeball.

Stitches in the right eye (aft. 21 d.). [*Htb.*]

Stitches in the right external canthus. [*Ng.*]

Boring pain in the eyes.

200. Pain as if a boil was forming in the left eyebrow, in the evening in bed (8th. 13th d.). [*Gff.*]

Itching of the eyes.

Itching of the edge of the right eyelid.

Excoriating pain in the eye (aft. 4 d.). [*Rl.*]

Feeling of soreness in the eyelids, soon after midnight, on awaking (25th d.). [*Gff.*]

205. Smarting and transiently shooting pains in the eyes. [*Gff.*]

The boy complains of coldness in the eyelids.

Both eyes are very hot to the touch.

Burning in the eyes.

Burning in the eyelids.

210. Burning in both eyes. [*Ng.*]

Burning and smarting in both eyes. [*Ng.*]

Burning and smarting in the eyes.

Redness of the white of the eye and many distended veinlets in it.

Redness and heat in the eyes. [*Htb.*]

215. Inflammation of both eyes in the white, with burning pain (aft. 5 d.).

Inflammation of the right eyelid, with pain of the eye and inability to read by candle light.

Swelling of the right eye.

Severe swelling of the upper eyelid, toward the nose.

Swelling between the eyebrows and lids, like a little sac.

220. Swelling of the glabella between the eyebrows (21st d.).

Pimple in the left eyebrow. [*Rl.*]

Frequent excoriation of the left external canthus.

Soreness of the outer canthus, with burning pain.

Suppuration of the eyes, in the corners.

225. The eyes closed by suppuration, in the morning (aft. 16 h.).

Agglutination of the eyes by mucus, in the morning. [*Ng.*]

Lachrymation. [*Ng.*]

Lachrymation of the eyes (2d d.). [*Htb.*]

Lachrymation especially of the right eye, with smarting in a corner (27th d.). [*Gff.*]

230. Frequent lachrymation, and in the evening rays about the candle-light.

Dryness and burning of the eyes, even worse in the open air than in the room. [*Ng.*]

Sensation of dryness of the eyes (aft 2 d.).

Sensation of dryness as of sand, and overpowering sleep in the eyes.

Her eyelids close violently.

235. Difficult opening of the eyes in the morning, on awaking.

Quivering and twitching in the right eyebrow.

Staring: she can only with difficulty turn her eyes from an object, and has to fix them upon it almost against her will. [*Ng.*]

Her vision fails while writing, with small white stars before the eyes; the lower line seems to her to be above the upper one, so that she keeps writing into it. [*Ng.*]

Pain and debility of the eyes.

240. Dim-sightedness. [*Ng.*]

Obscuration of the right eye, in the morning for several minutes.

After working in water (washing) diminution of sight; she

saw only a small part of the objects; then stitches in the head above the eyes, with inclination to vomit.

Black dots and ringlets before the eyes, in reading.

Spots, gauzes and points before the eyes, when reading and when looking out doors (aft. 24 h.).

245. A small black ball floats before her eyes.

White dots seem to fall down before his face, when he looks at the snow.

Variegated colors before the eyes.

Blue and green spots before the eyes. [*Gll.*]

Yellow, shining, trembling mist before the eyes. [*Ng.*]

250. Wheels before the eyes, with yellow and white rays, while writing on paper and in the open air; they turn around and are continually enlarged. [*Ng.*]

Bright sparks before the eyes.

On coughing, sparks fly from the eyes. [*Rl.*]

Photophobia; painful sensitiveness of the eyes to daylight; the room has to be darkened.

Straining pain in the ears.

255. Straining pain in the right ear. [*Gff.*]

Straining and shooting in the ears (3d d.). [*Gff.*]

Pinching sensation in the left external ear. [*Gff.*]

Drawing pain in the one, then in the other ear (aft. 4 d.). [*Rl.*]

Tearing in the ear.

260. Tearing in the ears. [*Htb.*]

Tearing deep in the right ear, frequently renewed (1st d.). [*Ng.*]

Tearing now in the one, then in the other ear.

Tearing in the interior of the right ear. [*Gff.*]

Tearing in the right concha (24th d.). [*Gff.*]

265. Transient tearing in the left ear and around it, as if in the bone. [*Gff.*]

Tearing in the anterior border of the right ear, frequently (1st d.). [*Ng.*]

Painful tearing, extending from the left ear into the outer cartilage and at the same time in the bone above and below the right patella. [*Ng.*]

Severe tearing in and behind the ear.

Jerking behind the right ear.

270. Twitching behind and above the ear.

Stitches in both ears, in the evening, in bed.

Sharp, lancinating pain behind and above both the ears.

Sharp stitches into the left ear, startling her, in the morning. [*Ng.*]

Fine stitches out of the left ear, frequently recurring (13th d.). [*Ng.*]

275. Constant dull stitch in the left ear; it goes off by shaking the head. [*Ng.*]

Shooting and crawling in the interior of the ear, connected with a similar sensation in the stomach and in the œsophagus (30th d.). [*Gff.*]

Boring and pressive pain in the ears (1st d.).

Gnawing in the inner and outer left ear. [*Ng.*]

Ulcerative pain in the outer right ear, continuing for a long time, before midnight (3d d.). [*Ng.*]

280. Beating in the right ear, at night, only when lying on it (aft. 2 d.). [*Ng.*]

Hammering in the right ear, frequently and very disagreeably impeding the hearing.

Quivering on the left ear (aft. 10 d.).

Quivering and trembling in the right ear, on rising up after stooping. [*Ng.*]

Itching of the lobule.

285. **Violent itching in the ears** (aft. 4 d.).

Tickling in the ears. [*Gll.*]

Coldness of the ears, in the hot room (aft. 2 d.).

Heat of the lobules. [*Rl.*]

Sensation as if warmth streamed out of the left ear. [*Ng.*]

290. Redness, heat and severe itching of the external ears

Inflammation and swelling of the inner ear, with pain all around it (aft. 3 d.).

Excoriation and suppuration behind the ears, for four weeks (aft. 21 d.).

Pimples on the ears.

Running of yellow, fluid ear-wax or pus from the ear, with previous tearing therein.

295. Secretion of an ill-smelling ichor in the inner ear.

Opening of an ulcer in the ear (aft. 5 d.). [*Rl.*]

Hard swelling of the parotid gland on the articulation of the jaw, with pain when touched.

Sensation of stoppage of the ears. [*Rl.*]

One of his ears is suddenly obstructed (aft. 3 d). [*Rl.*]

300. Sudden closing of the right ear (while sitting down in the evening), and the left ear commenced to ring and to buzz, so that it shook his head somewhat.

The hearing is, as it were, dulled, in the evening (aft. 15 d.).

Diminution of the hearing in both ears, slowly increasing and decreasing (for 14 d.). [*Ng.*]

Ringing in both ears. [*Ng.*]

Loud ringing in one ear and burning in the other.

305. **Singing in the ears.** [*Gll.*]

Buzzing in the ears.

Severe **rushing sound in the ears.**

Sounds in the ears. [*Ng.*]

Detonations and raging in the ears, frequently by day. [*Ng.*]

310. **Frequent cracking in the ear.**

Cracking in the ear, during a violent expiration.

Clucking in the right ear and secretion of much soft ear-wax.

In the nose and the root of the nose, chiefly on the right side, a squeezing (23d d.). [*Gff.*]

Itching in the nose.

315. Frequent itching in the right nasal fossa. [*Ng.*]

Ulcerative pain in the right nasal fossa. [*Ng.*]
Severe burning in the nose.
Burning in the left nostril.
Burning and smarting in the upper part of the left nostril, extending into the ethmoid bone (23d d.). [*Gff.*]
320. Red, thick nose, it is, chiefly in the afternoon, both thicker and redder.
Severe swelling of the tip of the nose.
Red, hot nose, covered with many white pimples.
Pimples on the nose.
Flat, small ulcer above the left ala nasi, with pain when touched. [*Gff.*]
325. A small pimple in the left nares (aft. 5 d.). [*Rl.*]
Sore, scabby nostrils, for a long time.
Ulceration of both nostrils.
Ulcerated nostrils. [*Htb.*]
In blowing her nose, something fetid is blown out.
330. Bloody, right nostril, every morning.
Frequent epistaxis.
Epistaxis in the morning.
Acute smell.
Paleness of the face and lassitude.
335. Wretched complexion, with pale lips. [*Htb.*]
Blue rings around the eyes.
Pale, hollow-eyed face, especially in the open air, where the child looks as if frozen.
Pale face, with weary, lifeless eyes.
Heat and redness in the face, in the morning in bed.
340. Long-continued heat and redness of the face, while the feet are icy cold.
Burning red cheeks in the evening, for an hour and a half; then great paleness of the face.
Burning itching in the face.
Itching of the skin of the face, after previous quivering; he had to rub, when it burned like fire.
Severe swelling of the cheek, passing into a gum-boil, without any previous toothache.
345. Swelling on the right cheek, extending downward, with stitches and pain when touched.
Swollen cheek, with tearing and shooting.
Swollen, red cheek, with little eruptive pimples, also on the nose.
Eruptive pimples in the face.
Pimples come and go in the face.
350. Pimples in the face, continually. [*Htb.*]
Pimples in the face, with pus in their apices.
Pimples on the zygomata, with burning pain.
Painless lump on the skin, anteriorly on the cheek, below the ear. [*Gff.*]
Small, red pustule, in the middle of the forehead, going off the next morning. [*Ng.*]

355. Freckles in the face. [*Htb.*]

Dry, brittle skin on the whole face.

Pressive drawing in the muscles of the cheek, near the lower jaw. [*Gff.*]

Tearing in the left zygoma, and then on the inner side of the cheek. [*Gff.*]

Tearing in the left zygoma, only relieved by pressing on it, with a sensation as if the cheek was swollen, in the evening and through the night till next morning, so that she wept and could not sleep. [*Ng.*]

360. Tearing in the lower jaw and before the right ear. [*Ng.*]

Squeezing tearing in the right zygoma, extending to the palate. [*Gff.*]

Burning in the face, below the right eye. [*Ng.*]

Quivering in the left cheek, with fine burning stitches, with tearing extending upward into the left temple, in the evening. [*Ng.*]

Cramplike sensation in the lips.

365. Tearing in the left upper lip and in the gums; it goes off by pressing on it. [*Ng.*]

Stitch in the upper lip. [*Ng.*]

Burning on the lips. [*Htb.*]

Burning of the lower lip. [*Ng.*]

Itching about the border of the lips.

370. Eroding sore pain around the mouth on the edge of the red of the lips, very painful when touched.

Soreness of the red of the lips; in the morning on awaking they are agglutinated as if from suppuration.

Swelling of the upper lip, it cracks open in chaps, it is painful when touched and bleeds readily.

Thick, ulcerated lower lip.

Scurf on the upper lip.

375. Vesicles on the red of the lower lip, which, when touched, pain and itch.

Vesicles on the lips. [*Ng.*]

Small, pointed, itching and humid pimples on both lips and around the whole mouth.

Pimples on the lips, which smart and itch.

Painful pimple above the upper lip, near the left nostril; it pains when touched (36th d). [*Gff.*]

380. Peeling off of the lower lip (34th d) [*Gff.*]

The lips are cracked open and peel off. [*Htb.*]

The lower lip peels, cracks open and scabs off. [*Ng.*]

On the right side of the chin, a squeezing pain, near the articulation of the jaw. [*Gff.*]

Intolerable cramp in the jaws, which, as it were, contracted the throat (the fauces?) at the same time.

385. **Itching on the chin.**

The submaxillary gland pains when touched. [*Rl.*]

Swelling of the lower jaw and its glands, with looseness of the teeth.

The teeth are painfully sensitive (4th d.).

Toothache with faceache; one tooth after another became loose and sensitive, or a bone in the face became painful and seemed, like the tooth, to be all sensation; then it twitched or tore at a certain point in paroxysms.

390. Pain in the teeth, daily in the morning, on awaking. [*Htb.*]

Pain of the teeth on the left side, in the morning in bed, and the whole forenoon (2d d.). [*Ng.*]

Pain in the roots of the teeth on the left side, for several mornings after awaking, increased by eating (3d d.). [*Ng.*]

Toothache after eating, extending to the cheek-bone and ear, where there was griping and stinging.

Toothache, when partaking of any food, but not otherwise.

395. **Toothache only when eating**, a throbbing in all the teeth.

Pain in the teeth, when she takes water in her mouth. [*Htb.*]

Pain of the teeth, when he takes anything warm or cold into his mouth.

Frequent attacks of toothache as soon as he draws any cold air into his mouth; relieved by warmth. [*Ng.*]

Toothache, with subsequent swelling of the gums. [*Ng.*]

400. Toothache, like a steadily incumbent pain, as if something had got into his hollow tooth, only transiently relieved by cold water; with drawing behind the ear and on the head, finally twitches in the tooth and disappearance of the pain.

Toothache, only when eating, at noon and in the evening, often at once with the first morsel, **as if something had come into his hollow tooth,** with intolerable drawing extending to the eye and ear, only in paroxysms, with intermissions of half an hour.

Pressive toothache in the root of a posterior hollow molar, in the evening. [*Gff.*]

Drawing toothache in the evening, as soon as she gets into bed, not by day.

Drawing in the roots of the anterior teeth and in the left molars, chiefly in the evening. [*Gff.*]

405. Contractive toothache in the upper and lower rows of teeth.

Twitching and drawing in a tooth, as if it was decaying, chiefly after a meal and at night, for a long time. [*Htb.*]

Tearing toothache, during or soon after eating. [*Ng.*]

Tearing and griping in a molar and in the left zygoma, aggravated and excited by cold substances, relieved by firmly bandaging it. [*Ng.*]

Tearing in the teeth and in the lower jaw on the right side.

410. Eroding, itching, violent pain in the various teeth and in the gums, not relieved by picking the teeth.

Itching in the teeth after supper. [*Ng.*]

Itching and digging in an upper left molar, after dinner; relieved by pressing upon it. [*Ng.*]

Burrowing toothache in the left lower row, caused by picking the teeth. [*Ng.*]

Severe burrowing in an upper left molar, after dinner. [*Ng.*]

415. Boring, pressive toothache, everytime after dinner, as if something had got into the tooth.

Beating or pecking sensation in an upper right incisor, after dinner. [*Ng.*]

Throbbing and pecking in the teeth, when moving, at other times, a burning pain.

Burning, lancinating toothache, especially at night, as if a hot iron was thrust into the teeth.

Burning, shooting pain in the tooth, especially at night, with an internal chill, and swelling of the lower jaw and of the gums. (aft. 32 d.).

420. **Shooting in the teeth** and the gums, then swelling of the cheek with shooting pain (aft. 14 d.).

Severe stitches in the teeth.

Single stitches here and there in the anterior teeth, in the evening. [*Gff.*]

Single stitches in the teeth and frequent sneezing, in the morning, on awaking. [*Htb.*].

Shooting pain in the anterior teeth, with sensation of dullness at supper (32d d.). [*Gff.*]

425. A tooth is prominent and pains much in chewing.

Sensation of looseness in an upper left molar. [*Ng.*]

Looseness of all the teeth. [*Ng.*]

Bad smell from the teeth.

The gums just above the anterior incisors show a tearing pain. [*Gff.*]

430. Tickling in the gums and bleeding of the same on sucking at them with the tongue. [*Ng.*]

Redder gums.

Painful inflammation of the anterior gums.

Severe swelling of the gums above the upper molars, with swelling of the left tonsil and of the cervical glands (9th d.).

Gum-boil.

435. Ulcer on the lower gums on the right exterior side. [*Ng.*]

Soreness of the inner gums of the anterior teeth.

Fetor of the mouth, like old cheese, every morning.

Erosion of the inside of the mouth and of the tongue, as from something sharp.

Soreness of the inside of the mouth.

440. Dryness of the mouth wakes him from sleep in the morning (7th d.).

Numbness in the mouth, in the morning after awaking, as if burned. [*Ng.*]

Violent burning of the mouth, in the morning, and thirst.

Dryness in the mouth, in the morning after rising. [*Ng.*]

Dryness in the mouth, without thirst, in the evening. [*Ng.*]

445. Dry, sticky sensation in the mouth.

Sensation of dryness, and gathering of saliva in the mouth; he has to spit much.

Gathering of water in the mouth. [*Rl.*]

Continual gathering of water in the mouth. [*Ng.*]

Much saliva in the mouth, continually.

450. Much saliva runs from his mouth, even by day.

Painful blisters on all parts inside of the mouth, with burning pain.

The tongue, on awaking in the morning, is often quite dried up, and almost without sensation. [*Htb.*]

White, dry tongue in the morning, as from something acrid.

Burning of the tongue and lower lip. [*Ng.*]

455. Burning of the tip of the tongue, as if it was raw or full of blisters. [*Ng.*]

Swelling of the tongue, and many small painful vesicles on it.

Painful vesicles on the tongue and the gums.

Painful little pimple on the tip of the tongue

Soreness on the frænum linguæ.

460. Soreness of the tip of the tongue.

On the palate, itching (10th d.). [*Htb.*]

Shooting and smarting in the back part of the palate, as if from too great dryness before the breaking out of a cold, increased by deglutition, in the morning and evening (8th, 9th, 29th, 30th, 41st d.). [*Gff.*]

Sore throat, with impeded deglutition and difficult opening of the mouth.

Interference with swallowing, in the œsophagus.

465. Tendency to choke while eating.

During deglutition, pressure in the spine.

Difficult deglutition, the food descends very slowly in the œsophagus.

Sensitiveness of the œsophagus; warm food burns it; she can only eat lukewarm food.

The food does not pass down; dry and cold things she cannot swallow at all.

470. Pressure and tearing in the fauces (9th d.). [*Gff.*]

Anxious pressure in the throat.

Sensation as of a lump in the throat.

Sore throat on the left side; he feels a lump there, and stinging during empty deglutition. [*Rl.*]

Shooting pain in the fauces, as if he had a fish-bone in it, when he gets cold.

475. Elongation of the uvula, with stiffness of the nape. [*Gll.*]

Pain, as from soreness in the throat.

Pain, as from soreness, **in the throat**, in the upper part of the palate, **during empty deglutition**, and more strongly when swallowing food; but not when not swallowing.

Eroding sore throat, when swallowing.

Scrapy and scratchy in the throat (aft. 8d.).

480. Dryness in the back part of the throat. [*Rl.*]

Frequently much mucus in the throat (the first 3 d.).

Much mucus in the throat, especially in the morning. [*Htb.*]

Much mucus back in the throat, which can only be detached with much hawking. [*Ng.*]

Increased hawking of mucus (19th d.). [*Gff.*]

485. Tough mucus, back in the fauces in the morning; it can neither be swallowed down easily nor hawked up, with a constant sensation as if a plug of mucus lodged in his throat (16th d.).

Loss of the sense of taste, in the morning on awaking, but only for a short time (2d d.). [*Ng.*]

Bad taste in the mouth. [*Htb.*]

Bad taste, and much mucus in the mouth.

Disagreeable, watery taste in the mouth.

490. Disagreeable, sticky saliva in the mouth.

Bitter taste in the mouth, with nausea (1st d.). [*Ng.*]

Bitterness in the mouth.

Bitterness in the throat.

Bitter taste, in the morning.

495. Bitter-sour taste in the mouth, after breakfast.

Sour taste in the mouth, every day.

Putrid taste in the mouth.

Sweetish taste in the mouth.

Taste of blood in the morning, after awaking, for three hours. [*Ng.*]

500. Little appetite. [*Gff.*]

Little appetite, with insipidity in the mouth, but he relishes food.

Severe hunger.

Severe thirst, in the forenoon.

Thirst in the evening, before lying down. [*Ng.*]

505. Thirst, at night. [*Ng.*]

He does not relish his food, he eats without hunger.

He has a repugnance to food, especially to meat; he relishes it, indeed, when he eats it, but he cannot eat much. [*Gff.*]

He loathes rye-bread.

He loathes everything.

510. Milk does not agree with her.

Bread alone feels heavy in the stomach after eating.

Great desire for sour things.

Before and after dinner, paleness of the face and nausea, vertigo with eructation, weariness of the lower limbs and coldness of the hands and feet; but not without appetite. [*Gff.*]

While eating (fried fish), nausea even to vomiting.

515. **During a meal, he is seized with drowsiness** (aft. 2, 4 d.).

After meals, very tired and sleepy. [*Htb.*]

After meals, great drowsiness, with chill and yawning.

After meals, weariness, with throbbing in the scrobiculus cordis and headache.

During dinner, peevish, cross mood, with drawing pain in the head (30th d.). [*Gff.*]

520. After dinner, constriction of the head, like as from a hoop around it.

After meals, paleness of the face.

After eating soup, at noon and in the evening, as also after eating warm cake in the morning, pinching and restlessness in the abdomen. [*Gff.*]

After meals, especially after breakfast, pressure in the stomach as from a weight in it.

After meals, the abdomen is distended.

525. After eating but a little, there is at once fullness and violent distension of the abdomen. [*Gff.*]

After breakfast, pressive pain in the abdomen, from flatulence, only transiently relieved by the emission of flatus (14th d.). [*Gff.*]

After dinner, dull shooting in the right side of the epigastrium. [*Gff.*]

After meals, tickling urging to cough (aft. 6 d.).

After meals, a chill.

530. After eating flatulent food (vegetables), burning from the stomach up into the fauces, like heartburn.

After supper, heartburn for three hours.

After meals, sour eructations.

Frequent eructation, especially in the morning.

Ineffectual urging to eructation, and then spasmodic contraction in the stomach, in the morning and afternoon. [*Ng.*]

535. Loud eructation, with gathering of water in the mouth. [*Ng.*]

Eructation, with the taste of the ingesta.

Eructation, as from bitter-sour water. [*Ng.*]

Sour eructation, in the morning (10th d.).

Much sourish eructation, in the afternoon with inclination to vomit.

540. Acid rises from the stomach into the mouth.

Sour eructation.

Regurgitation of food and acid, after severe restlessness from the scrobiculus cordis. [*Gll.*]

Regurgitation of waters from the stomach, of this she spit out much after midnight. [*Ng.*]

Something continually tends to rise up from the stomach into the mouth (soon). [*Ng.*]

545. Heartburn.

Hiccup (at noon). [*Ng.*]

Continual hiccup before midnight. [*Ng.*]

Qualmishness all day, and much eructation at once on rising. [*Rl.*]

Qualmishness, as if he would faint.

550. **Nausea, as if she would faint,** it only went off by lying down; in the forenoon.

Nausea, as if she would faint. [*Htb.*]

Nausea, for an hour in the forenoon.

Severe nausea in the stomach, with trembling of hands and feet. [*Ng.*]

Nausea as from a spoiled or empty stomach, not passing off by eating, with frequent waterbrash. [*Ng.*]

555. Nausea with qualmishness, gathering of saliva in the mouth (and diarrhœa). [*Rl.*]

Waterbrash.

Continual loathing, as if he would vomit (soon). [*Ng.*]

Nausea, with inclination to vomit at night in bed; it goes off gradually by rising. [*Ng.*]

Very ready to vomit, especially after meals.

560. Inclination to vomit, at every internal motion, every vexation and every joy, and at every time of the day; but when she has fasted, only retching.

Retching for several evenings.

Retching in the throat, increasing for a time, then decreasing, with short breath. [*Ng.*]

Frequent vomiting, without any overloading or spoiling of the stomach; the next day she is weak, without appetite (aft. 13 d.).

Vomiting with sinking of strength, like a swoon. [*Gll.*]

565. Vomiting of food and acid, with nausea. [*Gll.*]

The child becomes glowing red in the face in the morning; it vomits up its breakfast, and then becomes pale as a corpse; after vomiting several times it recovers, but remains very languid for two days.

Frequent pain in the stomach, but seldom in the afternoon, always preceded by swashing in the abdomen, relieved by eructation and passage of flatus. [*Ng.*]

Pressure in the stomach, with rumbling, sensation of emptiness and eructation. [*Ng.*]

Frequent pressure in the stomach, in the morning, on awaking.

570. Pressure as from a stone in the stomach, in the morning, in bed, relieved by hawking. [*Ng.*]

Fits of pressure in the stomach, extending up into the chest, with want of breath even to suffocation, nausea and great exhaustion; she had to lie down, both her feet and hands trembled, relief being afforded by vomiting bitter water. [*Ng.*]

Pressure transversely across the stomach and below the hypochondria, in the evening, in bed, for half an hour.

Pressure in the scrobiculus cordis (aft. 21 d.). [*Htb.*]

Pressure in the scrobiculus cordis and the region of the lower chest, with impeded breath and rising of heat to the head, going off after one hour through eructation. [*Ng.*]

575. Pressure below the scrobiculus cordis, in the morning and the afternoon, relieved by bending the body backward and after eating.

Pressive pain in the scrobiculus cordis, compelling him to lie down.

Heaviness in the stomach.

Fullness and pressure in the gastric region.

Fullness in the pit of the stomach.

580. Feeling as if the whole gastric region was swollen. [*Ng.*]

Constant feeling in the stomach as if it was full of water. [*Ng.*]

Cramplike pains in the stomach, with pressure in the scrobiculus cordis.

Severe spasmodic pain in the stomach, almost like pressure and cutting (soon). [*Ng.*]

Violent but intermitting pains in the stomach, relieved by walking, in the morning. [*Ng.*]

585. Spasmodic contraction in the pit of the stomach and across the chest.

Violent contractive pains in the stomach, also at 1 A. M. extending to the chest and axillæ, where they become shooting pains, with choking in the throat and tightness of breath; then anxiety and brief perspiration, and eructation, which relieves; recurring in frequent paroxysms till the morning. [*Ng.*]

Painful contraction from both sides of the stomach, with sensation of fullness, relieved by vomiting clear water. [*Ng.*]

Pains as if the stomach was being screwed together, especially at night, extending into the chest and the bowels, as if they would burst the stomach, impeding the breath and speech, in paroxysms. [*Ng.*]

Constrictive pain in the stomach and toward the fauces.

590. The constrictive cramplike pains of the stomach are renewed by the least eating of (especially cold) food and drink. [*Ng.*]

The paroxysms of constrictive cramplike stomachache are frequently followed by relieving eructation, or by chills with shivering and shaking, but affecting chiefly the hands, the back and the head, with customary stools. [*Ng.*]

Drawing and cutting across the stomach, in the morning, after rising.

Cutting stomachache, toward evening. [*Ng.*]

Sensation as if the stomach was cut to pieces, with great sensitiveness of the external gastric region, in the morning [*Ng.*]

595. Painful cutting in the pit of the stomach, during and after breakfast. [*Ng.*]

Burrowing in the stomach, with painful contraction and a sensation as if everything in it was turning over, with rising of water into the mouth; it goes off through dinner, but returning afterward, with burning extending up into the throat. [*Ng.*]

Burrowing and digging in the stomach, as if it would be pierced. [*Ng.*]

Burrowing in the pit of the stomach, in the afternoon; then frequent eructation of bitter water, almost like waterbrash.

Shooting pain in the stomach, with a sensation as if everything in it would turn over, returning after dinner. [*Ng.*]

600. Shooting in the stomach, drawing up into the left axilla and later into the sacrum. [*Ng.*]

Sore pain in the pit of the stomach, both at inspiration and expiration.

Sudden blow in the stomach, passing over into eructation of air or hiccup.

Twitching on the right side, near the scrobiculus cordis (aft. sever. h.).

Throbbing in the gastric region, which pains when touched.

605. Throbbing in the scrobiculus cordis, like severe palpitation, while the scrobiculus cordis is visibly raised at every throbbing; chiefly in the morning, lasting a quarter of an hour.

Beating on the left side, near the scrobiculus cordis.

Ebullition of heat from the abdomen into the stomach, in the forenoon. [*Ng.*]

Burning in the stomach.

Burning in the stomach, after eructation, in the forenoon.

610. Sour burning, rising up from the stomach, with slight spasmodic constriction.

Sensation in the stomach, as from flatus.

Growling, rumbling and moving about in the abdomen, as from flatus, or as if diarrhœa was coming. [*Ng.*]

Great sensitiveness of the external gastric region, when touched, when eating, talking, etc. [*Ng.*]

Itching, externally on the scrobiculus cordis; it does not go off by scratching. [*Ng.*]

615. In the hypochondria, a simple pain, with growling there.

Stitches in the hypochondria and the scrobiculus cordis, taking away the breath.

Burning stitches in both costal regions frequently recurring in the afternoon (12th d.). [*Ng.*]

Pain in the liver, when walking, for several days in succession.

Pain in the liver, as if pressed sore.

620. **Pressure toward the liver,** as if starting from the right side of the chest, with throbbing in the gastric region, which is painful when touched.

It changes the pressure in the liver into a sensation of heaviness there.

Drawing pain in the liver.

Cutting pain in the right infra-costal region, with pressure in the scrobiculus cordis. [*Ng.*]

Lancinating tearing, in the right infra-costal region. [*Gff.*]

625. Shooting in the hepatic region, which feels like splenetic stitches.

Stitches under the last true rib, when taking breath (1st d.).

Stitches under the last true rib, unconnected with breathing, for four days.

Stitches between the middle ribs on the right side, when sitting (1st d.). [*Ng.*]

Dull stitches in the right side, below the ribs, in the morning. [*Gff.*]

630. Dull stitches in the hepatic and the right inguinal region. [*Gff.*]

Sharp stitches in the hepatic region. [*Gff.*]

Dull stitches frequently on a small spot of the hepatic region, with sore pain when touched (18th d.). [*Gff.*]

Pinching stitches in the hepatic region. [*Gff.*]

Shooting throbbing on a rib of the right side, opposite the scrobiculus cordis. [*Ng.*]

635. Sensation of heat in the hepatic region.

Burning pain in the hepatic region (the first days).

In the left costal region, tearing shooting, arresting the breath. [*Ng.*]

Cutting pain in the left epigastrium, coming from the lower part of the chest, where there are stitches at the same time. [*Gff.*]

Bellyache with severe pain, which at times extended even to the hip, till late at night (1st d.). [*Htb.*]

640. Bellyache, with much eructation.

Bellyache, with much eructation and spitting of saliva.

Pressure in the abdomen.

Pressive pain in the epigastrium, extending to the scrobiculus cordis, in the evening (35th d.). [*Gff.*]

Pressure in the hypogastrium (26th d.). [*Gff.*]

645. Severe pressure in the left side of the abdomen, from stooping (9th d.).

Pressive pain on a small spot in the left hypogastrium, in the evening (39th d.). [*Gff.*]

Pressive pain in the hypogastrium above the os pubis, in frequent paroxysms; it goes off by emission of flatus (1st d.). [*Ng.*]

Pressure and burrowing in the abdomen, below the navel, as from incarcerated flatus; he has to sit stooping forward, and feels worse when walking in the open air (19th d.).

Distention of the abdomen with pressive pain, sensation of fullness, lassitude and indisposition to any movement and to mental occupation. [*Gff.*]

650. Sensation of distension in the hypogastrium below the navel, going off by motion. [*Ng.*]

Abdomen much distended.

Very much inflated and distended abdomen, after the cough has disappeared on taking Kali.

Inflated abdomen. [*Gff.*]

Hard inflation of the abdomen, with painfulness of the umbilical region, when touched.

655. Inflation, pressing asunder and pinching in the abdomen, followed by a soft stool. [*Ng.*]

Bloated abdomen.

The hypogastrium, as it were, distended, and heaviness in it, when sitting and walking (aft. 3 h.).

Sensation of a heavy load in the hypogastrium, the pain is more pressive than pinching, and most intolerable when walking (aft. 3 h.).

Cramplike colic (aft. 25 d.). [*Htb.*]

660. Spasmodic contraction of the abdomen, causing a coldness.

Contractive pain in the abdomen.

Painful indrawing of the umbilical region while sitting; it goes off by moving. [*Ng.*]

Pressing out of the hypogastrium, repeatedly (aft. 10 d.).

Pinching colic in the epigastrum, in the morning (11th d.). [*Gff.*]

665. Pinching colic in the hypogastrium (30th d.). [*Gff.*]

Twitches in the hypogastrium.

Pinching below the navel during dinner, and after rising from the seat, burning in the right inguinal region, with great sensitiveness of the same, both internally and externally, and a sensation on stooping, as if something would fall out, going off gradually while at rest. [*Ng.*]

Pinching pressure in the left epigastrium as from incarcerated flatus (11th d.). [*Gff.*]

Pinching in the epigastrium, toward noon (25th d.). [*Gff.*]

670. Pinching in the abdomen, and inflation of the same.

Pinching in the abdomen in the morning in bed, after previous chill, with urging to a soft stool.

Cutting in the bowels, with severe pains; to relieve himself he has to sit bent forward, and press on the abdomen with both hands, or else recline far backward; he cannot sit up straight.

Cutting in the epigastrium as from flatus moving about, with passage of flatus while walking. [*Gff.*]

Cutting in the left epigastrium. [*Gff.*]

675. Frequent cutting in the abdomen, as if diarrhœa was imminent.

Frequent light cutting about the navel. [*Ng.*]

Cutting in the abdomen, as if everything would be torn, first deep in the hypogastrium, then higher up (1st d.).

Cutting and drawing in the abdomen, like false labor-pains (12th d.).

Tearing, at times twitching, in the right side of the abdomen or the flank, in the evening (16th, 17th d.). [*Gff.*]

680. Intermitting tearing or dull stitches in the left hypogastrium, near the hip (11th d.). [*Gff.*]

Stitches in the abdomen, in the forenoon and again in the evening.

Occasional shooting above the navel, as from flatulence.

Shooting in the right side of the abdomen, as after retaining the urine when asleep, relieved by emission of flatulence.

Shooting in the right side of the abdomen, when laughing.

685. Shooting, like fine twitches, in the right side of the abdomen.

Shooting in the left side of the abdomen, below the ribs. [*Gff.*]

Sharp stitches and shooting tearing in the left side of the abdomen, below the short ribs (8th, 9th, 17th, 24th d.). [*Gff.*]

Several violent stitches in the hypogastrium (aft. 6 h.).

Dull shooting on the right side, near the navel (19th d.). [*Gff.*]

690. Dull stitches and pressure in the left epigastrium (10th, 20th d.). [*Gff.*]

Dull stitches in the left renal region, first during expiration, afterward in close succession, going off by rubbing. [*Ng.*]

Pinching, cutting shooting deep in the left hypogastrium, as from obstructed flatus, extending to the anus and the perinæum, painfully aggravated by drawing in the belly, and but little relieved by emission of flatus (19th d.). [*Gff.*]

Sore pain in the abdomen, with pressure toward the genitals, as in the menses; and pain in the sacrum.

Pain, as from contusion, in both renal regions, long continued, in the afternoon, when sitting (1st d.). [*Ng.*]

695. Beating in the abdomen.

Burning and drawing in the abdomen.

Burning around the navel, with pinching in the abdomen, during dinner. [*Ng.*]

Sensation of cold in the abdomen, as if a cold fluid were passing through the bowels (during the menses). [*Ng.*]

Chill and swashing in the abdomen, as if it was full of water, but mostly only on the right side, in the evening. [*Ng.*]

700. The abdominal muscles are painful when touched.

Itching on the hypogastrium for several days (aft. 10 d.).

Itching about the navel. [*Gll.*]

In the right groin, pain as from something swollen. [*Rl.*]

Pain in the right inguinal region, on drawing in the abdomen (29th d.). [*Gff.*]

705. Pressure in the groin, as from a hernia.

Straining in the groins, with sensitiveness when touched (it disappears on the emission of flatus). [*Ng.*]

Painful inflation in both groins, after dinner, while sitting. [*Ng.*]

Pinching in both groins, then shooting in the anus like needle-pricks when sitting; still worse on rising; lastly it comes on when walking about and is aggravated in sitting; with tenesmus. [*Ng.*]

Drawing shooting and outward pressure in the inguinal region, as if the old cicatrix of an operation for hernia would open again. [*Ng.*]

710. Stitches in the groins and flanks, on moving or stretching. [*Ng.*]

Sudden lancinating pain in the left inguinal region, during stool, with swelling of the glands.

Intermittent, clucking, outward pressure, in the right inguinal region (27th d.). [*Gff.*]

Much trouble from flatulence (1st, 2d, 3d d.).

Colic from flatus.

715. Flatulent colic; after eructation and emission of flatus, it goes off.

Obstruction of flatus (also aft. 20 d.).

Obstruction of flatus, with bellyache.

Emission of flatus difficult and obstructed, with insufficient stool.

The flatus settles painfully on the bladder (aft. 2 d.).

720. Moving about of flatus in the abdomen with tenesmus; it goes off through emission of flatus. [*Ng.*]

Moving about in the abdomen, then cutting in the stomach, with pressure extending to the throat, both at rest and in motion. [*Ng.*]

Constant growling in the abdomen, with frequent eructation and yawning. [*Ng.*]

Cooing in the epigastrium (before dinner), as if in diarrhœa, and slight bellyache (1st d.) [*Gff.*]

Clucking in the left hypogastrium, when pressing on it.

725. Obstruction of flatus, in the beginning, then inordinately much emission of flatus.

Forcible emission of flatus, he can hardly keep it back.

Flatus emitted upward and downward, with relief. [*Ng.*]

Emission of fetid flatus. [*Gll.*]

Frequent emission of fetid flatus, at night. [*Ng.*]

730. **Much emission of flatus** (aft. 14 d.).

Ineffectual call to stool, with sensation as if the rectum was too weak to expel the fæces.

Frequent violent urging to stool, in paroxyms, but only little fæces or only some flatus is discharged. [*Ng.*]

Repeated urging to stool at night, it goes off by the emission of some flatus (aft. 3 d.). [*Ng.*]

Much urging to stool, something is passed every time.

735. Frequent call to stool, but only a little is discharged.

Frequent urging to stool; he feels as if he could not discharge all the fæces at one time (aft. 24 h.).

Insufficient evacuation; most of the fæces are retained.

Insufficient stool, after much straining. [*Gff.*]

Insufficient soft stool. [*Rl.*]

740. Tenacious stool, as if it could not be detached. [*Rl.*]

Tough, soft, dark colored evacuation. [*Gff.*]

Costiveness (aft. 3 d.).

Costiveness and painful drawing in the abdomen.

Very hard stool and restlessness in the abdomen.

745. Hard, delayed stool, at times with severe straining, or with tenesmus afterward. [*Ng.*]

Hard, scanty stool in the morning, then in the forenoon another, a soft stool (2d d.). [*Ng.*]

Very hard stool and only every other day.

Stool like sheep's dung, only discharged with pain and effort.

Three scanty stools, but else normal (1st d.). [*Ng.*]

750. Copious, brown stool. [*Gll.*]

Stools rather soft than hard, for several days (aft. 4 d.). [*Ng.*]

Soft stools with previous colic (1st d.). [*Ng.*]

Soft stool, followed by burning in anus (aft. ½ h.). [*Ng.*]

Thin stool, with pinching and restlessness in the abdomen.

755. Scanty, half-liquid stools, with bellyache and subsequent tenesmus. [*Ng.*]

Half-liquid stool in the morning, with previous abdominal pains. [*Ng.*]

Hurried call to stool, as in diarrhœa, though the evacuation was hard, with bellyache (soon after a new dose). [*Ng.*]

Diarrhœa at night, with intolerable bellyache, continuing also the following day. [*Htb.*]

Diarrhœa, in the evening. [*Htb.*]

760. Severe diarrhœa, day and night (aft. 22 d.). [*Htb.*]

Severe diarrhœa, with great lassitude (aft. 27 d.). [*Htb.*]

Diarrhœa, with pinching, deep in the abdomen, before and afterward. [*Gll.*]

Diarrhœic stool, with pinching in the abdomen before, and burning in the rectum afterward.

Severe diarrhœa, with much colic (aft. 4 d.).

765. Diarrhœic stool, with smarting pains in the anus (aft. 8 d.).

Diarrhœa without pain, with rumbling in the abdomen. [*Gll.*]

Diarrhœa for the first fourteen days, with great lassitude, lying down, lack of appetite and daily bellyache; fæces light-colored and gray.

Too liquid stools, after previous rumbling in the abdomen. [*Ng.*]

Fæces very fetid.

770. Unobserved discharge of thin stool, during emission of flatus.

Blood with the stool, for several days (aft. 4 d.).

Stools colored with blood, and then anxiety and dyspnœa.

White mucus is discharged from the anus before and during the stool.

A lumbricus is discharged with the stool. [*Ng.*]

775. Pieces of a tapeworm discharged with a solid stool. [*Ng.*]

During ordinary stool, painful straining toward the groin. [*Ng.*]

At the commencement of the stool, a severe attack of cramp in the stomach, so that she had to sit down at once; she passed urine, and while sitting, the pain increased so much that she bent double and could not speak; with nausea, regurgitation and vomiting of water, with retching; before the vomiting a shudder; during the vomiting, reeling, with shaking of hands and feet, then anxiety, and heat in the whole body; relief of the pain, deadly paleness of the face, and at last an ordinary stool (aft. ¼ h.). [*Ng.*]

With ordinary stool, colic and then a constant tenesmus, until in the afternoon another stool, a liquid one, followed (4th d.). [*Ng.*]

After the ordinary stool, renewal of the pains, in the morning (2d d.). [*Ng.*]

780. After the ordinary stool, tenesmus in the anus (1st and 4th d.). [*Ng.*]

After the stool, continual **burning in the anus**. [*Ng.*]

After the stool, shudder about the anus, for half an hour.

After a difficult, scanty stool, pressure in the abdomen. [*Gff.*]

Pain in the anus, after vomiting, as if it would burst, almost intolerable. [*Ng.*]

785. Tenesmus in the anus. [*Gff.*]

Tenesmus in the rectum and anus.

Shooting, tearing and cutting in the anus (repeated for several days). [*Gff.*]

Shooting in the rectum.

Shooting in the anus, like needle-pricks.

790. Often repeated shooting in the anus, unconnected with stool. [*Ng.*]

Itching in the anus. [*Gff.*]

Violent itching in the anus and the scrotum.

Itching in the anus after supper.

Crawling in the anus (also aft. 6 d.). [*Rl.*]

795. Violent itching and crawling in the anus, long continued, in the evening (1st d.). [*Ng.*]

Crawling and shooting in the anus, in the evening. [*Gff.*]

Stinging crawling in the anus, before every stool.

Burning in the anus, without tenesmus.

Burning in the anus, during and after the dry stool. [*Gff.*]

800. Burning in the anus, so that he could not sleep (aft 21 d.).

Burning in the rectum, after the stool.

Burning and contraction in the anus.

Burning and pinching in the anus.

Burning and pinching in the rectum, frequently (the first days).

805. Burning cutting in the anus. [*Gff.*]

Excoriation in the anus, in the evening. [*Gff.*]

Smarting sensation of excoriation on and above the anus after the (morning) stool. [*Gff.*]

Excoriation in the anus (5th d.).

Little pimples on the anus.

810. Ulcerated pimples on the anus, with shooting.

The varices of the rectum swell and protrude during a hard stool.

Protrusion of the varices, during a diarrhœic stool, with needle-pricking and burning in them, for many hours.

Large, painful varices of the anus.

The varices protrude much during urination, and emit, at first, blood, but on the following days, white mucus.

815. **The varices on the anus are thickly swollen** and there is much emission of blood from them during urination.

Much emission of blood from the swollen varices of the anus, with a normal stool.

Profuse emission of blood from the rectum, then restlessness in the blood and pulsation in the whole body.

Burning of the anus, varices, with severe pain when walking.

Inflammation of the varices of the anus (aft. 24 h.).

820. Sore pain in the varices of the anus.

Shooting in the varices of the anus.

Crawling in the varices of the anus, as from worms.

Much urging to urinate.

Urging to urinate, but it is some time before he could do so; it flowed very slowly.

825. He had to urinate frequently; but the bladder had to be pressed on a long time before the urine passed; also at night, he had to rise for it repeatedly, though he drinks but little.

She had to rise at night to urinate.

He had to rise repeatedly at night to urinate (3d, 4th d.). [*Ng.*]

She has to urinate frequently, only a little being emitted each time, but every time with a renewed subsequent urging thereto, which is almost painful (aft. 48 h.).

She has to strain during micturition, before the urine comes.

830. Scanty, pale urine (1st and 2d d.) more on 3d d. [*Ng.*]

Increase of urine, at least she has to urinate more frequently. [*Ng.*]

An unusual secretion of urine (the first days).

While busily occupied, she had to hastily pass a few drops of urine.

After micturition, a few drops follow after.

835. Passage of a few drops of urine, two or three minutes after micturition.

Turbid urine. [*Gff.*]

Greenish, pale urine, with burning during and after micturition (8th d.). [*Ng.*]

Dark yellow urine, with a cloud, an hour later, more pale urine (aft. 1 h.). [*Ng.*]

Scalding, diminished urine (at first). [*Ng.*]

840. Urine, like clayey water, with a copious sediment on standing. [*Ng.*]

Interrupted stream of urine, painless, in the afternoon (1st d.). [*Ng.*]

After micturition, emission of a milky, inodorous, flaky liquid (prostatic juice?).

Cutting in the region of the bladder.

Cutting tearing in the neck of the bladder, during micturition, increased by forcing out the urine (36th d.). [*Gff.*]

845. Tearing in the neck of the bladder, unconnected with micturition (37th d.). [*Gff.*]

Intermittent cutting in the urethra, unconnected with micturition; this becomes a tearing pain in the glans, and especially in its orifice (7th d.). [*Gff.*]

Frequent drawing and sharp tearing in the anterior part of the urethra (18th, 19th d.). [*Gff.*]

Tearing pain in the urethra.

Pinching tearing pains in the urethra (aft. 12 d.).

850. **Burning in the urethra, during micturition.**

Burning in the urethra, during micturition. [*Ng.*]

Burning in the urethra, after micturition (aft. 5 d.).

Burning smarting pain in the urethra, during and after micturition.

Burning and smarting in the orifice of the urethra and the upper part of the inner surface of the prepuce, in the morning in bed, soon after micturition (20th, 21st d.). [*Gff.*]

855. On the mons veneris, and near the genitals on the thighs, violent itching, with fine, red eruptive pimples.

On the penis, a straining sensation (aft. 24 d.).

Sharp, drawing pains through the penis (12th d.). [*Rl.*]

Tearing drawing in the penis (24th d.). [*Gff.*]

Clucking in the glans (aft. 2 d.). [*Rl.*]

860. Tearing in the glans (aft. 20 d.). [*Gff.*]

Shooting itching on the glans.

In the left testicle, a straining sensation.

Pinching in the left testicle, and in the os pubis.

Swelling of the testes and the spermatic cord, with heat perceptible externally.

865. The scrotum is painful, as if contused.

Itching of the scrotum.

Soreness of the scrotum (aft. 17 d.). [*Rl.*].

Sexual impulse much excited. [*Gff.*]

Violent sexual impulse.

870. Excited sexual instinct (aft. 24 h.).

Excites the sexual organs, with sensation of burning.

The male genitals strongly smell of semen.

Lack of sexual impulse, with undiminished morning erections.

Erections at night, without excitement of the fancy (aft. 7 d.).

875. Frequent erections (aft 13 d.). [*Ng.*]

Impetuous erections (aft. 24 h.).

Many, even painful erections, with spasmodic contraction in the spermatic cords.

No erections at all, for the first eighteen days.

Pollutions for two nights in succession (1st, 2d n.).

880. Pollutions with voluptuous dreams (the first days). [*Ng.*]

Profuse pollution with subsequent languor (aft. 23 d.). [*Ng.*]

Pollutions with great subsequent lassitude (3d, 4th, 7th n.). [*Gff.*]

The pollutions, formerly frequent, occur more rarely (aft. 14 d.).

The usual pollutions are suppressed for forty-two days.

885. Coitus without emission of semen (aft. 10 d.).

After coitus, lascivious dreams at night and pollution. [*Rl.*]

Aversion of female to coitus (the first days).

She is easily excited to coitus (aft. 29 d.).

During coitus, pinching in the vagina.

890. During coitus, sore pain in the vagina.

On the pudenda, on the left side, tearing, extending through the abdomen up into the chest.

Pinching pain in the labia.

Stitches across the pudenda.

Burning shooting on the pudenda.

895. Burning and itching on the pudenda.

Burning, smarting pimples on the pudenda.

Menses too early, by two days, immediately after a new dose (8th d.). [*Ng.*]

Menses four days too early (aft. 24 h.).

Menses five days too early, more copious and lasting longer than usual. [*Ng.*]

900. Menses six days too early. [*Htb.*]

Menses six days too early, the first day scanty, on the second more copious than usual, on the third day again scanty, ceasing entirely on the fourth day. [*Ng.*]

Menses too early by ten days, and lasting six days; during the first days, weak, but during the later days more profuse; with lassitude and drowsiness, pains in the abdomen and toothache. [*Htb.*]

The menses, which had stopped for eighty-seven days, now return again, without any other ailment than that she felt heavy in her limbs the day before (3d d.).

The suppressed menses return with a better color (5th d.).

905. Menses too late by one day, with pain in the hypogastrium. [*Ng.*]

It retards the menses (in its after-effects) by thirteen days.

The menstrual blood is very acrid, of a bad, sharp smell, and she becomes eroded from it on the thighs, which are covered with an eruption.

Before, during and after the menses, much erosion about the pudenda.

Before the appearance of the menses, on awaking from sleep in the morning, voluptuous sensations, as from coitus.

910. Before the menses, much heat, great thirst and restless nights.

A week before the menses appear, there is restlessness, as if the menses would come at once (aft. 16 d.).

Before the menses, much chilliness, trembling of the limbs and cramp-like sensations in the abdomen.

During the menses, in the morning, headache, with great heaviness. [*Ng.*]

During the menses, she feels full and sick after meals, and soon afterward she vomits.

915. When the (retarded) menses ought to have appeared, and did not come, there appeared sour eructation, swelling of the cheek, with stitches, but without any heat, and swelling of the gum.

During the menses, colic, putrid taste in the mouth, rumbling in the abdomen, great lassitude and drowsiness. [*Htb.*]

During the menses, on the second day, severe headache, from morning till evening. [*Htb.*]

During the menses, much flatus, bad taste in the mouth, and frequent eructations tasting of bile.

During the menses, cutting in the abdomen. [*Ng.*]

920. During the menses, severe pressure in the sacrum and anteriorly in the hypogastrium, as if everything was coming out at the genital organs.

During the menses, costiveness.

During the menses, pains in the sacrum, like heaviness. [*Ng.*]

During the menses, on the second day, coryza, pain in the abdomen, toothache, backache, stitches in the ears and restless sleep. [*Htb.*]

During the menses, very restless sleep, with anxious dreams.

925. During the menses, she goes to sleep again in the morning on awaking, but passes into a very disagreeable state, between sleeping and waking; she is then tormented by hearing things which distress her, though she knows she is only dreaming; but she is unable to open her eyes, and has great difficulty in tearing herself from this half-sleep.

During the menses, violent itching of the whole body.

After the menses, in the evening, coldness in the back, and

awaking after midnight with cramp and coldness in the stomach, which continues till about noon (aft. 19 d.).

A female in the fifth month of her pregnancy (after some vexation) is attacked at night with a severe hemorrhage from the vagina, with clots of coagulated blood, attended with a dull headache and a yellow complexion, but without miscarriage.

Leucorrhœa (3d d.). [*Ng.*]

930. Discharge from the vagina (the first 5 days).

Discharge, like mucus, from the vagina.

Yellowish discharge from the vagina, with itching and burning of the pudenda.

* * * * * * * *

Stuffed coryza (aft. 26 d.). [*Htb.*]

Stuffed coryza, which is loosened in the afternoon, during a walk (aft. 3 d.). [*Ng.*]

935. Stuffed coryza, with itching in the nose; she has difficulty in breathing through the nose, for several days (aft. 4 d.). [*Ng.*]

Stuffed coryza, frequently, also in the evening, in bed, with crawling in the throat (aft. 11 d.) [*Gff.*]

Severe stuffed coryza, so that he could hardly get breath.

Stuffed coryza, with much yellowish green mucus from the nose.

Stoppage of the nose.

940. Expulsion of purulent matter from the right nostril, followed by stoppage, and when blown, there arises a shooting, contractive pain, extending into the occiput. [*Gll.*]

Fluent coryza, with excessive sneezing, some thirty times a day.

Fluent coryza, almost the whole day, but especially in the evening.

Severe fluent coryza, every evening, with frequent sneezing.

Severe fluent coryza.

945. Severe fluent coryza, with much sneezing, backache and headache (aft. 10 d.).

Excessive fluent coryza (aft. 29 d.).

Coryza with bloody mucus from the nose (aft. 8 d.). [*Htb.*]

On the larynx, frequent drawing pain, with sensation of rawness.

When eating, some of the food is apt to get into the larynx, causing him to choke.

950. Rough voice.

Very rough sensation in the throat, with much sneezing.

Sore throat with cough.

Sore throat when the body is uncovered.

Very rough and hoarse in the throat, for several days. [*Htb.*]

955. Complete hoarseness and aphony (aft. 24 h.).

At first, hoarseness, then excessive fluent coryza.

Hoarseness as if something was lodged in the throat, exciting him to hawk.

It feels as if there was a plug sticking in the throat; by coughing, it is detached and the throat is cleared.

Scrapy sensation on the chest, caused by the wind.

960. Growling and slight snoring in the trachea, while respiring before the cough sets in.

Tickling in the larynx, exciting to cough, with severe hoarseness. [*Rl.*]

Crawling in the throat, exciting hawking and coughing, with sensation as if the mucus was firmly attached, in the morning and evening (12th, 22d, 29th d.). [*Gff.*]

Cough, from titillation in the throat (20th d.). [*Gff.*]

Cough, from titillation in the throat, without expectoration. [*Gll.*]

965. Scrapy, scratching cough.

Cough, which affects the chest, from tickling in the throat.

Cough, from titillation.

Cough, when playing the violin.

Severe cough, while fasting in the morning; it disappears after breakfast.

970. In the morning, hawking with expectoration.

In the morning at once at 3 o'clock, she begins to cough, and this recurs every half hour.

In the morning, much cough, with expectoration, but more yet in the evening.

Evening cough when in bed.

Every evening, severe cough, when she has lain in bed a while, for several weeks.

975. In the evening, fatiguing cough.

She has to cough every five minutes, from 9 P. M. till morning.

Nocturnal cough.

At night she is awakened by her cough.

Frequent cough before midnight, but none by day.

980. Hacking cough, with some expectoration, mostly only at night and in the morning, attended with coryza.

Frequent tussiculation, in the afternoon and the following forenoon (aft. 6 d.). [*Ng.*]

Spasmodic and irritated cough, in single strong paroxysms, even to choking, with a sore pain in the upper part of the head and great lassitude afterward.

Suffocating and retching cough, in the morning at 5 o'clock, as if from dryness in the larynx; she could not talk, for a spasm in the chest, with redness in the face and perspiration of the whole body.

Cough, which readily causes her to vomit.

985. **Cough, violent even to vomiting, in the morning.**

Fatiguing cough, so violent, that she loses her consciousness.

Dry cough, coming and going quickly.

Dry cough, almost solely by night, with shooting in the throat.

Dry cough, at night, waking from sleep, with acute pains on the chest in coughing; little coughing by day (1st d.). [*Ng.*]

990. Cough with much expectoration.

Expectoration of small, round lumps from the throat. [*Gll.*]
Cough, with expectoration of sourish taste.
Cough, with expectoration of blood-streaked mucus, three times (17th d.).
She detaches mucus in coughing, but it does not come up into the mouth, and cannot, therefore, be expectorated.
995. In coughing, rough pain in the larynx.
From coughing, shooting in the throat, with fluent coryza.
During coughing, at times shooting pain in the left breast.
In coughing, bearing scraping on the chest.
In coughing, sparks dart from the eyes.
1000. During coughing, nausea.
During coughing, pain in the varices of the anus.
During coughing, pain in the abdomen, like concussion.
Breath, very short, in the morning.
In the morning, shortness of breath.
1005. Inclination to take a deep breath.
Oppressed breathing.
Asthma, as if the chest was coated with mucus.
Asthma, with short breath, during writing (3d d.). [*Ng.*]
Oppression of the chest, with groaning, deep respiration.
1010. Oppression of the chest, with difficult, troublesome respiration, two or three times (aft. 30 d.). [*Ng.*]
Oppression of the chest, with distended abdomen.
Sensation, in the open air, as if the throat was being constricted.
Obstruction of the breath wakes him from sleep at night.
Slight rattling on the chest, at night, when lying on the back.
1015. Anguish in the chest, toward evening.
The chest is very painful, chiefly **while talking.**
Pressure on the chest, while taking breath.
Pressure, in paroxysms, anteriorly in the chest, especially on the right side, aggravated by inspiration, diminished by eructation. [*Gff.*]
Pressure in the thyroid cartilage, while coughing or when taking a deep breath (aft. 16 h.).
1020. Frequent pressure in the left side of the chest and in the cardiac region (8th d.). [*Gff.*]
Pressure in the whole of the left side of the chest. [*Gll.*]
Pressive pain in the morning on rising, on the right edge of the sternum; this is also painful when touched.
Pressure and sensation of drawing downward, in the middle of the chest. [*Ng.*]
Sharp, pressive pain behind the sternum, when breathing and in swallowing liquid food, and during eructation, for several days.
1025. Shooting pressure on the left side of the chest, when taking a deep breath.
Shooting pressure in the right side of the chest, occasionally, for several days.
Pinching pressure in the right side of the chest (26th d.). [*Gff.*]

Tension across the chest, during expiration, in walking.

Cramplike pain in the chest; it goes off by eructation. [*Ng.*]

1030. Pinching in the pectoral muscles, several times.

Pinching, obtuse shooting in the right side of the chest. [*Gff.*]

Cutting sensation in the lower part of the chest, especially on the left side; it draws down into the epigastrium, but it leaves behind a shooting pain in the left side of the chest (20th d.). [*Gff.*]

Cutting pain in the chest, in the morning, especially about the scrobiculus cordis, as from flatus accumulating there. [*Gff.*]

Cutting pain in the chest, in the evening on lying down; she did not know how to lie; worst when lying on the right side. [*Ng.*]

1035. Stitches in the sternum, in front of the right side of the chest, also during inspiration; in the evening (1st d.). [*Ng.*]

Stitches below the left breast, and at times deep up into the breast, also in the evening. [*Ng.*]

Stitches in the right side of the chest, on taking a breath.

Occasionally a stitch in the right side of the chest.

A stitch in the left side of the chest.

1040. Stitches in the left side of the chest. [*Gll.*]

Stitches in the sides, on taking breath.

Stitches in the cardiac region.

Violent stitch below the two breasts, after lifting a heavy load; later on, griping in both the epigastria, toward the front; in the afternoon. [*Ng.*]

Single cutting stitches below the right clavicle, with pain as if a thorn was lodged in it. [*Ng.*]

1045. Sudden, dull stitch in the sternum, on the eructation and the deglutition of liquid substances.

Obtuse stitches deep in the left side of the chest, under the short ribs. [*Gff.*]

Obtuse, painful stitches in the chest, below the left clavicle, only going off transiently by pressing upon it; in the evening. [*Ng.*]

Obtuse shooting, pressing and tearing below the axilla. [*Gff.*]

Burning shooting in the right side of the chest, on rising from a stooping position (aft. 1 h.). [*Ng.*]

1050. Burning shooting in the left side of the chest, when sitting; it goes off on rising (7th d.). [*Ng.*]

Boring, deep into the left side of the chest (9th d.). [*Ng.*]

Drawing pain across the chest (aft. 4 d.).

Tearing in the sternum, to the left side, above the scrobiculus cordis, in the evening. [*Gff.*]

Tearing in the left side of the chest, on the lowest short ribs. [*Gff.*]

1055. Tearing pain in the right side of the chest (9th d.). [*Gff.*]

Tearing pain in the left side of the chest (17th d.). [*Gff.*]

Pain, sore, but yet tearing, somewhat below the left axilla, aggravated and excited by strong breathing. [*Gff.*]

Sore pain in the upper part of the chest, when taking breath, when touching the parts and when she raised something heavy.

Bruised pain in the chest.

1060. Tickling in the right side of the chest (aft. 16 d.).

Clucking, like subsultus of the muscles, in the upper right side of the chest (22d d.). [*Gff.*]

Trembling or quivering, anteriorly in the chest. [*Ng.*]

The chest is affected from loud talking.

Weakness of the chest.

1065. Weakness and lassitude in the chest, from walking fast.

Painful beating in the clavicle, the shoulders, the side of the abdomen, etc. [*Ng.*]

Palpitation, frequent and violent, with oppression.

Palpitation, when he is hungry (aft. 10 d.).

Violent palpitation in the forenoon, with numbness of the head and nausea (aft. 24 h.).

1070. Frequent intermission of the heart-beats.

In or about the heart a pinching pain, as if the heart was suspended by firmly contracted bands; most noticeable during deep inspiration or coughing, but not during bodily motions (aft. several h.).

Burning in the cardiac region (aft. 2 d.).

External twitching pain on the lowest left rib.

In the breasts, tearing shooting.

1075. Itching on the fleshy part of the right side of the chest, with a fine eruption, showing only when it is rubbed.

Smarting on the chest, now here, now there, in paroxysms. [*Ng.*]

In the coccyx, violent gnawing, both at rest and in motion. [*Ng.*]

Pain in the sacrum, after standing or walking for a time.

Pain in the sacrum, only in bending backward, not while at rest.

1080. Frequent pain, just above the sacrum, when sitting. [*Gff.*]

Severe sacral pains, with labor-like pains in the abdomen and discharge from the vagina.

Pain in the sacrum, like heaviness.

Pain as from inflation in the sacrum, in the morning in bed, with a feeling as if great bubbles were accumulating in the sacral region, and with tenesmus, all of which vanishes on the emission of flatus. [*Ng.*]

Sensation in the morning, as if the sacrum was being pressed inward from both sides. [*Ng.*]

1085. Stiffness in the sacrum.

Twitching pain in the sacrum, when stooping, so that he could not raise himself up for a time.

Drawing pain in the sacrum.

Severe, constant drawing in the sacrum, alternating with throbbing there, relieved by lying down.

Throbbing in the sacrum.

1090. Severe bruised pain in the sacrum, chiefly in the morning on rising.

Violent pain in the sacrum, as if it was broken, on moving. [*Ng.*]

Itching on the lower part of the sacrum.

Tickling fatigue-pain above the sacrum.

An occasional stitch from the sacrum through the left side of the abdomen, toward the chest.

1095. Backache, paining severely.

Pressure in the back, above the right renal region, in the morning (20th d.). [*Gff.*]

Pressure in both the renal regions (7th, 8th, 15th, 19th d.). [*Gff.*]

Pressure in the left scapula.

Sharp pressure on the upper part of the back (34th d.). [*Gff.*]

1100. Drawing pressure in the scapulæ.

Drawing pressure in the back.

Tensive pressure like severe fatigue, from the right scapula, extending into the side of the back, even to the sacrum, *per se*, also early in bed, but especially while out driving. [*Gff.*]

Burning pressure in the back, worse when walking in the open air (aft. 19 d.).

Sore pressure in the right renal region (6th d.). [*Gff.*]

1105 Stiff in the back; she cannot stoop.

Stiffness and paralysis in the back and the sacrum.

Tensive pain under the left scapula, when respiring.

Several sharp, smarting pinches on the back part of the ribs, on both sides of the back.

Contractive pain in the back, while at rest after physical labor.

1110. Tearing in the right renal region (13th d.). [*Gff.*]

Tearing pain in the lumbar muscles, which arrests the breath.

Shooting and pressive tearing in the back, near the right scapula (10th, 38th d.). [*Gff.*]

Tearing in the right scapula, in the morning (4th d.). [*Gff.*]

Burning tearing on the right side, by the spine above the sacrum (18th d.). [*Gff.*]

1115. **Stitches in both renal regions** (11th, 29th d.). [*Gff.*]

Stitches on the right side of the back, extending through into the chest (25th d.). [*Gff.*]

Stitches in the right scapula, when taking breath.

Lancinating pain between the scapulæ, and oppression and anguish on the chest, almost solely while sitting, so that she has to rise and walk about.

A stitch from the apex of the left scapula into the scrobiculus cordis, while hard at work (aft. 7 d.). [*Gff.*]

1120. Obtuse shooting in the left scapula. [*Gff.*]

Pinching shooting in both scapulæ. [*Gff.*]

Sharp, tearing stitch under the right scapula. [*Gff.*]

First a pressure between the scapulæ, then from there a burning extending to the crest of the ilium equally while at rest and in motion; the burning is also felt when the hand is laid upon it.

Pulsating beating on the upper edge of the left shoulder-blade. [*Ng.*]

1125. Pain as if the flesh was detached from the bones, in the loins, when walking, but chiefly when touched.

Bruised pain in the back, while at rest, not when in motion.

Bruised pain between the shoulders and on the left shoulder; it goes off when moving. [*Ng.*]

A shooting, bruised pain in the right scapula during motion; perceptible even in the chest.

Pain as from a strain in the back.

1130. Pain as from a sprain in the left scapula.

Violently shooting pain as from a sprain in the left scapula, extending into the chest.

Itching on the back, on scratching, it changes into pain.

Pain in the nape, on bending back the head.

Violent tension in the nape, becoming more painful on moving the head. [*Ng.*]

1135. **Stiffness in the nape,** with elongation of the uvula in the throat. [*Gll.*]

Stiffness in the nape, in the morning in bed (also aft. 3 d.).

Stiffness in the nape in the morning, going off during the day; for several weeks.

Drawing pain in the neck (aft. 2 h.). [*Ng.*]

Tearing in the nape, occasionally only transient. [*Ng.*]

1140. Tearing in the right side of the nape, in the morning.

Itching little pimples in the neck, in the evening, going off after twenty-four hours. [*Ng.*]

The cervical muscles pain, on being moved.

Twitching pain on the left side of the neck (aft. 2 d.). [*Rl.*]

Pressing drawing on the right side of the neck.

1145. Tearing in the lower part of the right side of the neck (aft. 24 d.). [*Gff.*]

Rush of blood to the neck; the neck seems thicker and the cravat too narrow.

The glands on the neck are painful, as after a cold (3d d.).

Shooting in the cervical glands.

Swelling of the cervical glands (aft. 5 and 14 d.).

1150. Swelling of a cervical gland, below the chin, which is painful after taking cold.

Swelling of the cervical glands on both sides, with pain on turning the head.

Hard swelling of the cervical gland, on the corner of the lower jaw.

Tickling in the swelling of the submaxillary gland; she had to press on it with the cold hand, to ease it.

Sweat in the axillæ.

1155. The axillary gland swells and is painful when touched, as if festered (2d d.).

Swelling of the axillary gland.

Dull cutting and tearing in the right axilla (24th d.). [*Gff.*]

Tearing in the left axilla, while at rest (10th d.). [*Ng.*]

Tearing shooting in the right axilla, when raising the arm, in the morning, when writing (7th d.).

1160. Violent shooting in the left axilla. [*Ng.*]

Sensitiveness and burning in the right axilla (15th d.). [*Gff.*]

Itching in the axilla.

The top of the left shoulder aches, on violent motion of the left arm, or when it presses on anything strongly.

Pinching pressure in the right shoulder-joint, more painful when taking a breath. [*Gff.*]

1165. Severe tensive pain in the top of the left shoulder, in the morning, so that he could not raise his arm.

Tension and pressive drawing in the top of the right shoulder, with paralytic sensation in the right arm. [*Gff.*]

Drawing pain in the top of the right shoulder (17th d.). [*Gff.*]

Tearing in the top of the left shoulder, both at rest and in motion. [*Ng.*]

Tearing in the top of the right shoulder, while knitting; it goes off on motion. [*Ng.*]

1170. **Tearing in the left shoulder-joint.** [*Gff.*]

Pinching tearing, in the top of the right shoulder. [*Gff.*]

Fine shooting in the left shoulder, and then in the tendons of the left side of the neck. [*Ng.*]

Fine stitches in the top of the shoulders, both at rest and in motion. [*Ng.*]

Bruised pain under the right shoulder-joint, especially on moving or touching it.

1175. Cracking in the shoulder-joint, on moving and on raising the arm on high. [*Ng.*]

Pimples on the top of the shoulder, with violent itching and burning aftr scratching. [*Ng.*]

In the arm, severe tensive pain for eight days, so that he could not lift it up straight; but he could move it backwards on his back, lie upon it and grasp the joint without pain.

Parálytic tension and drawing in the left arm, from the top of the shoulder down into the forearm, with tendency to go to sleep, in the morning on awaking (34th d.). [*Gff.*]

Drawing pain in the left arm (aft. 21 h.).

1180. Twitching in the arm, in the evening on going to sleep. [*Ng.*]

Frequent twitching of the left arm.

Tearing in the left arm, from above down into the wrist.

Violent tearing in the whole of the left arm (7th d.). [*Ng.*]

In a cold temperature, the arms lose their warmth, become numb and almost as if asleep.

1185. Both the arms go to sleep and are benumbed in the cold; they also go to sleep after violent motion.

The arm, on which he lies at night, goes to sleep.

The arms go to sleep, in the morning in bed; they feel rigid and paralyzed with a sensation of internal pressure, and the hands are without sensation, for half an hour.

He feels paralyzed in both arms (the first days).

The arms get tired readily, when writing (aft. 3 d.).

1190. **Weakness and want of strength in both arms.**

Weakness of the arm, with swelling of the upper arms and the hands.

Itching of the arms, with little white pimples after scratching, as large as grains of millet. [*Htb.*]

On the upper left arm, quivering in the fleshy part. [*Ng.*]

Burning tension on the right upper arm, just above the elbow. [*Ng.*]

1195. Tearing in the right upper arm, above the bend of the elbow, in the evening. [*Ng.*]

Tearing in the left upper arm, occasionally extending to the top of the shoulder (11th, 16th, 20th d.). [*Gff.*]

Tearing in the upper parts of the right upper arm and in the elbow (12th and 22d d.). [*Gff.*]

Shooting tearing in the left upper arm.

Shooting in the right upper arm.

1200. **Pulsating pain in the left upper arm, at intervals.**

Subsultus of the muscles on the left upper arm (18th, 19th, 25th d.). [*Gff.*]

A pimple on the upper part of the upper arm, itching and paining. [*Gff.*]

Bruised pain in the right upper arm, especially on raising the arm. [*Rl.*]

Paralytic pain in both the upper arms, chiefly on moving them.

1205. Pain in the elbow, as if it were stiff, on stretching the right arm, after it had been bent.

Drawing and tearing in both the elbows, occasionally with a sensation of warmth in them, frequently recurring. [*Gff.*]

Tearing in the bend of both the elbows (3d, 6th and 22d d.) [*Gff.*]

Tearing stitches in the bend of the left elbow. [*Gff.*]

Severe stitches in the bend of both the elbows, in the morning in bed; going off after rising.

1210. On the fore-arm, tensive pain. [*Gff.*]

Drawing pain in the fore-arm.

Violent, short drawing, from the arm into the hand (aft. 2 d.). [*Rl.*]

Paralytic, obtusely paining, drawing from the left fore-arm into the hand. [*Rl.*]

Tearing in the upper part of both the fore-arms. [*Gff.*]

1215. Tearing in the middle of both the fore-arms. [*Gff.*]

Tearing in both the fore-arms, toward the wrist. [*Gff.*]

The hands pain in the metacarpal bones, on grasping.

Obtuse pressive pain on the dorsum of the left hand. [*Ng.*]

Drawing on the inner surface of the left wrist, aggravated by motion. [*Ng.*]

1220. Tearing in the wrists (11th and 20th d.). [*Gff.*]

Tearing in the outer process of the wrist-joint (29th d.). [*Gff.*]

Fine tearing in the left wrist-joint, extending toward the ring-finger, frequently recurring (4th d.). [*Ng.*]

Tearing in the right wrist-joint when knitting, frequently recurring. [*Ng.*]

Dull, pressive tearing in both hands, between the thumb and the index (16th, 12th and 21st d.). [*Gff.*]

1225. Violent tearing, from the dorsum of the left hand into the fingers. [*Gff.*]

Violent tearing in the dorsum of the left hand, as if in the marrow of the bones, almost intolerable. [*Ng.*]

Shooting in the left wrist-joint on motion, then also while at rest, some sharp stitches. [*Gff.*]

Cold hands.

Burning on the left hand, as from red-hot coals. [*Rl.*]

1230. **The hands go to sleep,** in the morning on awaking, with a dull headache, increasing after rising, with frequent empty eructations until toward noon. [*Htb.*]

Lack of strength in the hands.

Trembling of the hands, while writing, in the morning.

Itching on the wrist. [*Rl.*]

Violent itching of the palms, in the evening, near the fingers (1st d.). [*Gff.*]

1235. Itching above the right wrist-joint, going off by scratching. [*Ng.*]

Itching vesicles in the palm.

Red, elevated spot, shaped like a lentil above the wrist. [*Ng.*]

Rough, chapped skin on the hands. [*Htb.*]

In the fingers, drawing pain in the posterior joints.

1240. Tearing in the middle joint of the index. [*Gff.*]

Tearing under the thumb-nail. [*Gff.*]

Tearing in the phalanges and joints of several fingers. [*Gff.*]

Tearing under the finger-nails (34th d.). [*Gff.*]

Transient tearing in the fingers, and at the same time in the toes. [*Gff.*]

1245. Tearing in the left thumb. [*Ng.*]

Tearing in the joint of the left middle finger. [*Ng.*]

Tearing in the left little finger, toward the tip, passing away by motion, but frequently recurring. [*Ng.*]

Violent tearing behind the right index, extending to its tip. [*Ng.*]

Dull tearing in the ball of the thumb (9th d.). [*Gff.*]

1250. Some fine tearing pains, in the left little finger. [*Ng*]

Shooting tearing under the nail and in the tip of the index. [*Gff.*]

Drawing tearing in the tip of the little finger. [*Gff.*]

Burning tearing in the tip of the index (10th d.). [*Gff.*]

Shooting in the fingers of the right hand.

1255. Fine, painful shooting under the nail of the left middle finger. [*Ng.*]

Fine, intermitting shooting in the middle joint of the right index. [*Ng.*]

Painful shooting in the right index, as if needle and thread were passed from the posterior part toward the tip; relieved by bending the finger; renewed by stretching it. [*Ng.*]

Fine, keen shooting, as if from an ulcer, in the tips of the four fingers of the right hand. [*Ng.*]

Ulcerative pain in the posterior joint of the left thumb, in the evening. [*Ng.*]

1260. Burning pain, as from a glowing coal, on two fingers of the left hand. [*Rl.*]

Burning in the tip of the little finger. [*Gff.*]

Sore pain, in the morning, in the anterior joint of the middle finger, especially under the nail, not increased by touching it. [*Gff.*]

Crawling in the tip of the right middle finger. [*Gff.*]

The fingers open and close by jerks, in the morning in bed; then numbness, difficult motion and chilliness of the fingers.

1265. Numbness and insensibility of the right thumb, for several weeks.

The thumb goes to sleep, toward morning in bed.

The finger-tips go to sleep, chiefly in the morning.

The thumbs feel paralyzed, from knitting.

Stiffness and paralytic weakness of the right thumb and index, when writing. [*Gll.*]

1270. Little itching pimples behind the left thumb; they continue to itch after scratching. [*Ng.*]

A blister on the little finger.

An erosive blister on the left index, which, being opened, discharged for several days, not a purulent, but a watery liquid.

Around the border of the nail of the middle finger, burning pain. [*Gff.*]

Inflammation on the border of the nail of the index, like a paronychia; on pressing on it thin pus is discharged, for seven days. [*Gff.*]

1275. In the left lumbar region, tearing to and fro, while sitting, going off when in motion. [*Ng.*]

In the nates, muscular twitching.

Dull pain in the nates. [*Gff.*]

Tearing around and in the nates, near the hip-joint. [*Gff.*]

Fits of pinching tearing in the nates. [*Gff.*]

1280. Pain in the nates and thighs from sitting, as if they were festering.

Itching between the nates.

Soreness between the thighs.

In the hip-joint a pinching tearing. [*Gff.*]

Tearing pain in the left hip, from time to time.

1285. **Tearing in the hips and knees,** also when sitting.

Tearing, occasionally formicating, in the hips on their integuments (19th, 21st and 30th d.). [*Gff.*]

Twitching pain in the left hip-joint, when turning the thigh. [*Gll.*]

Fine, but very acute stinging in the left hip-joint, when standing; after sitting down there is a stitch tearing down the whole thigh, as if it were in the marrow, going off after rising from the seat. [*Ng.*]

Pain, as from a blow, in the upper part of the left hip-bone, when walking and when touched. [*Gff.*]

1290. Bruised pain of the hip-joint, with pain on moving and on sneezing.

In the lower limbs, pressure in the bones, now here, now there.

Tearing in the left thigh and in the tibia, during the menses. [*Ng.*]

Burning pain, in both the lower limbs, also at times with acute stitches.

Restlessness in the lower limbs, in the evening, she had to walk about.

1295. Restlessness in the legs, in the evening; he had to stretch them often.

Sudden great heaviness of the left thigh, so that he could only move it with difficulty; it felt paralyzed, at night in bed, and the following day when sitting. [*Ng.*]

Heaviness of the lower limbs.

Sensation of numbness in the whole of the right thigh, as if it was going to sleep, with great sensation of heaviness remaining in it, in the morning on awaking. [*Ng.*]

Sensation of numbness and great tendency to go to sleep in the whole of the right lower limb especially in the leg. [*Gff.*]

1300. **Frequent going to sleep of the lower limbs.**

The lower limb goes to sleep, while lying down.

The right limb goes to sleep and tingles.

While sitting, first one then the other lower limb goes to sleep.

Lack of strength in the lower limbs, they give way.

1305. Stiffness of the lower limb (aft. 10 d.).

In the thighs, muscular twitching. [*Gff.*]

Drawing pain in the thigh (aft. 11 d.). [*Rl.*]

Drawing pain in the left thigh, down to the knee.

Drawing pain in the thigh, when ascending, as if it would break.

1310. **Paralytic drawing in the whole thigh,** often increased to tearing, worse when standing and in the warmth of the bed, often only in the evening and at night. [*Gff.*]

Tearing on the upper and inner part of the thigh. [*Gff.*]

Tearing on the posterior part of the thigh, close to the nates, toward the genitals. [*Gff.*]

Sore pain in the middle part of the thigh, when touched.

Worn-out feeling in the thighs, as if he was fatigued by walking, many days, chiefly in the afternoon.

1315. Feeling of fatigue in both thighs, above the knees, in the evening. [*Ng.*]

Severe bruised pain, a hand's breadth above the **right** knee, as if the thigh was about to drop off, when standing; worse when sitting, and continuing afterward both in rest and in motion. [*Ng.*]

Quivering in the right thigh, on the anterior side. [*Ng.*]

Paralytic sensation of the whole thigh, with a sensation as if it would go to sleep. [*Gff.*]

Two little pimples on the left thigh.

1320. An itching spot on the thigh, near the hip; after scratching, it turns into an ulcer.

A lump above the knee, with pressive tearing pain.

On the knee, a dull pain on the side, when walking and especially when stretching the limb. [*Gff.*]

Tensive pain in the right knee, and then formication in it; only while walking, it goes off when sitting. [*Ng.*]

Stiffness in the knees (aft. two d.).

1325. Stiffness, tension and weakness in the right knee, as if tightly bandaged.

Drawing pain in the knee, when walking, extending into the thigh.

Frequent tearing in the knees. [*Gff.*]

Tearing in both knees (1st d.). [*Ng.*]

Tearing in the hough. [*Gff.*]

1330. Tearing in the knee and the knee-joint in the evening, with warmth in it. [*Gff.*]

Ripping-up pain in the knees, when walking and sitting.

Beating and throbbing in the left knee, repeated by day. [*Ng.*]

Quivering of the left knee (2d d.). [*Ng.*]

Pain as of a sprain in the knee, on rising from the seat, for several minutes.

1335. The knees go to sleep and pain, when walking fast, he could hardly bend them.

Paralytic feeling in the knee, when sitting. [*Gff.*]

Paralytic pain in the right knee, when walking (6th d.). [*Gff.*]

Itching on the knee.

Eruption in the hough.

1340. In the right leg, drawing pain down into the foot, for several days.

Paralytic drawing in the legs.

Drawing and tearing in the bones of the legs. [*Gff.*]

Tearing in the upper part of the tibia, below the knee. [*Gff.*]

Tearing in both the tibiæ, with pain in the periosteum on touching them, and tension therein when walking. [*Gff.*]

1345. Tearing in the left tibia. [*Ng.*]

Tearing in the upper part of the calf (20th d.). [*Gff.*]

Tearing in the right calf, passing inward on pressing and rubbing it, and then disappearing. [*Ng.*]

Straining sensation in the left calf, as if the tendons were too short, in standing, not in sitting. [*Ng.*]

Straining sensation in the calves, as if they were too short, on rising from the seat, by day.

1350. Cramp in the right calf (aft. 20 h.).

Shooting in the shaft of the tibia.

Quivering on the anterior surface of the left leg, when standing. [*Ng.*]

Itching on the tibia. [*Rl.*]

Violent itching on the legs, in the evening. [*Rl.*]

1355. An itching lump and three vesicles, with inflamed areola on the tibia. [*Ng.*]

Tetter on the thigh. [*Htb.*]

In the feet, tension, almost without swelling.

Pressive pain in the heel.

Pressive pain in the sole of the foot, on treading and walking.

1360. Pinching drawing in the foot, as from great weariness. [*Gff.*]

Spasmodic tearing on the ankle, with pulsation about that part, and up the tibia, extending to the knee.

Tearing about the ankles, when the feet are cold, ceasing when they get warm.

Frequent tearing in the ankle-joints. [*Gff.*]

Tearing just above the ankles (20th d.). [*Gff.*]

1365. **Tearing on the inner side of the foot and of the sole.** [*Gff.*]

Tearing in the dorsum of the foot, extending into the toes. [*Gff.*]

Tearing from the inner ankle, across to the tendo Achillis. [*Ng.*]

Drawing tearing in the feet, even into the toes. [*Gff.*]

Shooting in the left foot, inward.

1370. Shooting on the dorsum of the foot.

Stitches under the ankle.

A pain like a stitch shot into her ankle, while walking, as if the foot would break; she had to stand still.

Severe drawing and shooting, in the morning, several hours after rising, in the left ankle, when treading, paining worst in the evening, with pecking there and shooting in the heel; she dare not move her foot, she has to keep it suspended; it feels too heavy, is swollen and hot when touched at that spot.

Shooting under the heel, as from needle pricks.

1375. **Shooting in the foot.** [*Htb.*]

Violent shooting in the tendons, behind the right outer ankle, when running; going off when at rest. [*Ng.*]

Shooting and burning in the feet, after a walk. [*Htb.*]

Visible quiverings on the dorsum of the left foot, in the evening. [*Ng.*]

Formication in the soles of the feet, toward the toes.

1380. Formicating burning, in the soles of the feet, and painful sensitiveness of the same.

Heaviness and stiffness of the feet.

The feet go to sleep, after a meal. [*Htb.*]

The left foot goes to sleep, during dinner. [*Ng.*]

Cold feet, in bed.

1385. Cold feet, while the face is hot.

Sweating of the soles of the feet.

Profuse sweat on the feet, for many days. [*Htb.*]

Swelling of the feet.

Severe swelling of the feet, extending to the ankles.

1390. Swelling and redness of the soles of the feet, with burning in them, even while lying down, but much more when treading.

Severe itching about the ankle joint, in the morning in bed.

Severe itching and heat of the feet, in the evening, as if they had been frozen.

The tips of the toes pain, when walking.

Cramp in the left big toe, so that he could not stretch it, while sitting, in the evening. [*Ng.*]

1395. **Tearing in the toes** (4th, 7th, 11th and 20th d.). [*Gff.*]

Tearing in the posterior phalanx of the big toes (11th, 16th, 19th and 34th d.). [*Gff.*]

Tearing in the tips of the big toes (17th, 11th and 36th d.). [*Gff.*]

Gnawing, on the outer edge of the right big toe. [*Ng.*]

Pricking as from needles in the ball of the big toe. *Gff.*]

1400. Tickling stinging in the tips of the toes. [*Gff.*]

Fine stitches with itching in the tip of the big toe.

Pain as from a sprain in the posterior joint of the big toes, while walking, but most painful when raising them up (11th and 33d d.). [*Gff.*]

Tickling formication in the toe and sole. [*Gff.*]

Itching on the lower surface of the toes. [*Gff.*]

1405. Violent itching on the big toe, below the nail, with pain when touched. [*Gff.*]

Inflamed red (chil) blains on the toes, with pressive pain.

Chilblain on the ball of the big toe, with stinging cutting pain, red and thick.

Bluish-red chilblains on the ball of the big toe, inflamed with a cutting pain and needle pricks, especially when wearing shoes and boots.

The corns pain acutely.

1410. Stitches in the corn. [*Htb.*].

The nail of the big toe pains on the side, as if it would grow into the flesh (14th d.). [*Gff.*]

The limbs pain, in those parts on which they rest (aft. 4 d.). [*Rl.*]

The whole body is very sensitive; wherever she touched herself or moved, it pained her (3d and 4th d.). [*Ng.*]

Pressive pain in the joints of the knees, the feet and the hands, only while at rest.

1415. Pressive pain in the joints and drawing pains in the shafts of the long bones.

A sort of tension in the interior of the body, extending into the head and the eyes.

Pinching and strongly contractive sensation in the anus, in the stomach and toward the fauces.

Formication in the limbs, especially in the lower ones, when sitting, with drawing in the legs, making him restless. [*Gff.*]

Drawing pain in the whole body, now here, now there, in the nape, the scapulæ, the hands and the knees (aft. 10 d.).

1420. Drawing pain in all the limbs, with the sensation as if he had been sick for a long time, with great paleness of the face and emaciation.

Severe drawing in the abdomen, in the arms and legs, with bruised pain of the upper arms; most when resting (the first days).

Stinging in the joints and tendons.

The pains predominating in Kali are stitches. [*Gll.*]

Pain, as from festering, when pressing on any part of the body.

1425. Bruised pain of all the muscles of the body.

The parts on which she lies (arms and legs) go to sleep.

The pains come early, at 2 or 3 A. M., so that he cannot remain lying down, and they are stronger then than by day during motion.

After the cessation of the pains, at once a chill. [*Ng.*]

In the open air, she seems to feel better than in the room. [*Ng.*]

1430. The open air seems to increase the ailments, especially the feverish condtion.

On walking in the open air, drowsy with yawning.

On walking in the open air, violent tearing externally on the one side of the head.

From walking in the open air, violent headache, for several hours.

Great dislike of the open air.

1435. When walking in the open air, great readiness to take cold, and sweat at night, with restlessness and heaviness in the nape, as if from a load (4th d.).

Readiness to take cold (3d d.).

Very ready to take cold.

Very ready to take cold after being heated by exercise; he loses his appetite, has feverish shiverings, diarrhœa with colic, restless sleep, etc.

After taking cold, headache on the right side of the head and heat in the eyes.

1440. Ailments from taking cold, at every draught.

After catching cold by a draught, she feels for a moment too hot in the room, then heaviness in the limbs, tearing in the whole body, and in the head, with roaring before the ears, and general coldness, then throughout the night, a sour smelling perspiration (aft. 31 d.).

After taking a cold, there is fever in the evening; toward morning, perspiration with violent headache, and after rising, a chaotic feeling in the head.

Itching, here and there in the body, especially on the legs; on scratching, the parts are apt to bleed. [*Rl.*]

Severe itching on the abdomen and on the thighs.

1445. Itching all over the body, now here, now there, with little blotches after scratching. [*Ng.*]

Itching all over the body, in the evening, before going to sleep; it goes off in bed.

Violent itching all over the body, in the morning and evening, especially on the back, where there are small pimples (aft. 3 d.). [*Gff.*]

Severe, almost stinging itching on the whole body, at night in bed. [*Ng.*]

Itching stitches, here and there on the body.

1450. Stinging and gnawing, on the skin all over the body.

Burning itching in the face, on the back and on the head.

Burning itching in the sacrum and below the right patella. [*Ng.*]

Burning itching all over the body, in the face, on the hands, on the tibia, etc., now here, now there.

Burning on many parts of the skin, even under the axillæ, as from a **drawing plaster.** [*Gff.*]

1455. Eruptive nodules here and there on the body, also on the face. [*Rl.*]

Nettle-rash for fourteen days.

Nettle-rash, with itching so violent, that she did not know what to do, for fifteen days.

Yellow, scaly, severely itching spots all over the belly, also about the nipples; they become moist on scratching.

Tetter (on the thigh). [*Htb.*]

1460. The ulcer bleeds violently, almost without a cause.

In the cicatrix of a fontanelle, a tearing pain.

On the spot of a former ulcer (on the leg), pressure and tension.

An old wart (in the face) commences to itch.

Ebullition in the blood, and heat in the head.

1465. Ebullition in the blood, in the evening, before going to sleep, with oppression and tightness in the chest.

He feels the pulse all over the body, even in the tips of the toes.

Sensible throbbing of all the arteries. [*Gll.*]

Sensation of emptiness in the whole body, as if it was all hollow.

Heavy and languid in the whole body, as if broken on the wheel. [*Ng.*]

1470. So heavy in the limbs, that she could not set one foot before the other.

Heaviness of the body, in the morning in bed; it goes off after rising.

Heavy, especially in the feet; walking is an effort.

Indolence (aft. 2 d.).

Frequent languor and weariness (1st d.).

1475. Languor and weariness, in the evening, almost reaching nausea. [*Gff.*]

Lassitude, languor and nausea, after the afternoon nap. [*Rl.*]

Great languor in the evening. [*Ng.*]

Great weariness, in the morning on awaking, diminished on rising, but returning with increase in the afternoon. [*Htb.*]

Relaxation and lassitude of the limbs.

1480. Titillating lassitude in the limbs.

The child (of four years) wants to be continually carried.

Going up a few steps is troublesome to her; but not walking on a level.

Much talking fatigues her.

Languid, weary and bruised in the hips and lower limbs, and especially in the calves, when she walks (13th d.).

1485. Sensation of faintness every morning, as if he would swoon or have vertigo (the first 6 d.).

Threatened with syncope, as soon as he moved at all.

Fit of faintness, on returning from a short walk, so that she could reach her home with difficulty; a warm sensation in her stomach and (in winter) drops of sweat gather on her forehead, and her lower limbs tremble; after a short rest, her faintness passes off.

Attack of lassitude in the whole body, especially in the sacrum, the cervical muscles feel relaxed, the arms and legs nerveless, as if he should sink down, with a faint feeling about the heart, as from syncope (aft. sever. h.).

Attack of sudden faintness, in the evening on lying down, with aching nausea, warmth and lassitude in the pit of the stomach, and vertigo and failing of thoughts in the head; so also two fits in the morning, which leave behind them great lassitude.

1490. Attack of nausea, at once in the morning, with violent yawning, eructation, writhing about the stomach, severe heat and anguish (3d d.).

Attack of nausea and vomiting, with bruisedness of the head, drowsiness and some watery stools, with subsequent constipation.

Attack of contractive pain in the back, while at rest after physical labor; he has to lie down; then profuse sweat through the night, and in the morning a stool with mucus and blood, but painless.

Cramplike attack: A pain seized him between the shoulders like a tearing, then his nape became, as it were, stiff, and when he would move his head, it was jerked backward several times.

After the cramplike attack, eructation, giving relief, and extreme lassitude, prostration and discomfort; she could only talk quite low. [*Ng.*]

1495. Twitching in all the limbs (8th d.).

Quivering in the muscles, here and there, for several days. [*Rl.*]

Sudden tremulousness. [*Rl.*]

Violent trembling.

Tremulous in the hands and lower limbs, and easily fatigued by walking.

1500. Tremulous weariness, when walking, first in the knees, then trembling in the abdominal muscles and the arms.

Frequent yawning.

He feels as if he had not slept enough, in the morning.

Very sleepy in the morning, and waking up late.

Sleeping too long, and the head then feels chaotic, great lassitude, sensation of coryza and pressure in the eyes.

1505. In the morning, after a sound sleep, he has soon to lie down again, and after a sleep of three hours, he feels restored.

Great drowsiness by day; she goes to sleep, while sitting.

Very sleepy, with yawning in the forenoon, till noon. [*Ng.*]

Drowsiness after dinner; it goes off in the open air. [*Ng.*]

Always drowsy, in the afternoon, with yawning and wretched complexion. [*Ng.*]

1510. Great drowsiness; she felt like going to sleep at breakfast (soon). [*Ng.*]

Drowsiness in the afternoon (3d d.). [*Htb.*]

Irresistible somnolence, in the afternoon and evening.

In the evening, he gets drowsy early (aft. 10 d.). [*Rl.*]

In the evening, early drowsiness and sullen silence. [*Gff.*]

1515. Difficulty in getting to sleep, in the evening, after walking in the open air.

In the evening, he is long in getting to sleep for several days. [*Ng.*]

In the evening he cannot get to sleep before eleven or twelve o'clock, without cause.

Late in getting to sleep (the first weeks).

After mental work, he cannot fall asleep before midnight.

1520. In the evening, on going to bed at eleven, she could not get to sleep, for a stinging itching all over the body; she only slept from eleven to one o'clock. [*Ng.*]

At night in bed, he cannot fall asleep before one or two o'clock, without cause or ailment.

Insomnia at night, and if he does get to sleep, anxious dreams; in the morning, he feels dull, with hot hands.

Restless sleep (4th d.). [*Htb.*]

Very restless night; she wakes up some twenty times without any particular cause. [*Ng.*]

1525. She wakes up early, at one or two o'clock, and is too wide awake to get to sleep again.

She wakes up much earlier than usual and cannot go to sleep again.

He always awakes at four o'clock and then several times, till morning comes.

At night, after waking up, she cannot go to sleep again because of a rush of ideas.

Her night's sleep is half-awake.

1530. Only a slumbrous sleep at night.

Tendency to wake up early, without getting wide awake.

At night, after lying down, he remembers sad events, which keep him from going to sleep.

At night in bed, delirious fancies, while awake for three hours, with heat in the brain, and external heat all over the body, then some sweat, coldness of the limbs and shivering, with great timidity.

At night, she raises herself up in her bed while sleeping,

talks all manner of incoherent things with her husband, and cannot get conscious for a long time, but she knew that she was speaking with her husband.

1535. **Sleep, full of fancies and talking loud.**

Talking in sleep.

Loud talking in sleep. [*Ng.*]

Violent weeping, in a dream at night.

The child tosses about at night and cries.

1540. Sleep, full of dreams, restless. [*Gff.*]

Many dreams, with restlessness and tossing in sleep.

He falls at night from one dream into another.

He goes to sleep at once, but also begins dreaming at once.

Dreams at night, with restless sleep and frequent awaking.

1545. Dreamful sleep and frequent awaking (aft. 10 d.). [*Rl.*]

The whole sleep is full of vivid dreams, about the occurrences of the day.

Frequent voluptuous dreams (the first 14 d.).

Anxious dream, she calls for help.

Dreams about robbers (aft. 11 d.). [*Rl.*]

1550. Dreams about diseased parts of the body. [*Rl.*]

Dreams, that his approaching death is announced to him. [*Ng.*]

Anxious dream, his father was about to beat him.

Dreams, that he was tumbling down a high mountain.

Dreadful dreams disturb the sleep.

1555. Anxious dreams of threatening forms passing by her, some of which threaten to lie on her.

All manner of frightful forms before her eyes, in sleep.

Dreams of snakes, sickness and deceased persons. [*Ng.*]

Dreams of deceased persons, as if they were alive, and of quarrels with them.

Dreams of masks, ghosts and devils. [*Ng.*]

1560. **Frightened, when asleep.**

Startled, when going to sleep.

In the evening, when going to sleep, a jerk through the whole body, so that he starts up.

In the evenings after lying down, he started up, while waking in bed, with a shudder of the whole body.

In sleep, he starts up several times and trembles.

1565. In sleep, his limbs twitch and he snores.

Two nights in succession, while asleep, his whole body moved as if epilepsy was coming, with twitching in the arms and kicking with the legs, but without any rattling; after awaking, he knew nothing about it.

In the evening, after going to sleep and waking up again, she was, as it were, confused in her head, had no thoughts, knew not where she was and was then seized with a fearful anguish; then she became rational again.

At night, when lying in bed, rush of blood to the head, at times, as if he would lose his senses.

Several nights, a pressive headache, which goes off on bandaging the head.

1570. At night, gnashing of teeth, while asleep.

At night, acidity in the mouth.

At night, regurgitation of the food eaten at dinner.

At night, dryness in the mouth prevents his sleeping.

At night, an hour after going to sleep, a violent, jerking cramp in the stomach, with anguish, groaning, coldness of the tip of the nose, of the hands and feet, then vomiting of food and of an acid substance, with much eructation of air; the following night, the same, but more slight. [*Gll.*]

1575. At night, pressure and burning in the stomach. [*Gff.*]

At night, pressure below the scrobiculus cordis, with coughing.

At night, she has to spit out much mucus, often for half an hour at a time.

At night, colic for two hours, without subsequent stool, then in the morning, pain in the sacrum and chest, and in the afternoon all the limbs feel bruised.

At night, pinching in the stomach, in paroxysms, with nausea and constant eructation.

1580. At night, colic at the least movement in bed, not while at rest, a dull lancination and pressure, as if from an internal induration.

Three nights in succession, tormented by flatus.

At night, much emission of flatus.

At night, bellyache and diarrhœa.

Every night, from three to four o'clock, diarrhœa (the first week).

1585. At night, he could not get to sleep for burning on the anus.

At night, burning itching on the perinæum.

At night, sweat on the perinæum.

At night, he cannot go to sleep for itching on the scrotum.

At night, in a restless sleep, full of dreams, many erections. [*Gff.*]

1590. After midnight, violent erections, which disturb his sleep, weary him and threaten a pollution, which, however, does not occur. [*Gff.*]

In the evening, on going to sleep, constriction of the throat, so that she wakes up terrified; then stinging dryness in the throat (aft. 12 d.).

At night, an obstruction to breathing wakes him from sleep.

At night, a nightmare, with a dream as if a stone was lying on him, and as if simultaneously his throat was being constricted, while he in vain endeavors to wake up. [*Gff.*]

At night about two o'clock, she wakes up with oppression about the heart and cannot go to sleep again.

1595. At night, when she lies on the right side, she feels oppression and anguish, and she has to sit up in bed, until eructations supervene.

At night, the child is restless and anxious, cries much and reaches out for one thing and another, without accepting anything.

At night, tension in the right or the left side.

At night, stitches in the right or left side.

After midnight, violent shooting in the left side of the chest, the cardiac region and at times in the back, only to be borne while lying on the right side; intolerable, as soon as he endeavors to lie on the left side; the second night, he wakes up very early, with the most violent stitches in the chest and shortness of breath, while lying on the left side; they are intolerable only in entire rest, and go off on lying on his right side; repeated the third night while lying on his back. [*Rl.*]

1600. At night, stiffness of the nape.

At night, a throbbing pain in the upper arm awakes him.

At night, restlessness in the hands.

At night in bed, burning pains in the lower limbs.

At night on awaking, tearing and drawing with sensation of great weariness in the legs, especially in the ankle joints.

1605. **At night**, waked up twice by **cramp in the** right thigh and the **calf.**

At night in bed, on drawing up the leg, cramp in the calf and the sole of the foot.

At night, the left leg and the right arm go to sleep.

At night, restless sleep on account of pressive pain, on the side of the body on which he was lying.

At night, excessive pain in the whole body, like strokes of a hammer.

1610. In the evening in bed, such restlessness in the limbs, that she cannot find a spot on which she can rest well.

At night, severe bleeding of the ulcer.

The sleep at night is interrupted by heat in the whole body, especially on the hands, and by too vivid dreams.

In the evening in bed, very hot hands, with transient shivering and long-delayed going to sleep. [*Htb.*]

Shivering, frequent in the room, without subsequent heat. [*Ng.*]

1615. Frequent shivering, with yawning, removed by the warmth of the stove, in the forenoon (1st d.). [*Ng.*]

Shivering in the back, in the morning in bed.

Very chilly, especially after meals and toward evening.

Chill in the forenoon; in the evening hot hands.

Chilly and shivering, in the evening before lying down. [*Ng.*]

1620. Chill at every motion, also in bed (the first days). [*Ng.*]

Chill at 9 P. M., it goes off after lying down, without heat or subsequent thirst (1st d.). [*Ng.*]

Chill in the evening, in the vertex and the whole body (aft. 12 d.).

Severe chill in the evening, like fever, without thirst; for several evenings.

Chilliness, as from a coming cold.

1625. Chill of two hours, without thirst, with obtuseness of the head; on driving over a stony road.

Continual internal chill, for four days, without heat and without thirst, with icy-cold feet, obtuseness of the head, fatigue even to fainting; at the same time swelling of the lower jaw and gums, and burning toothache with stitches (aft. 32 d.).

Violent febrile rigor toward evening, for several minutes; he has to lie down; then nausea and vomiting and spasmodic pain in the chest the whole night, with short breath and much internal oppression and perspiration on the head (aft. 6 d.).

Internal chill at noon, with heat of the hands and afterward heat in the whole body, but all without thirst.

Chill and sensation of cold, in the morning in bed; then after a quarter of an hour, heat; after some hours, again a chill, but without subsequent heat.

1630. Every evening at six o'clock, at first, a febrile rigor of one hour, with thirst; then with severe fluent coryza, heat without thirst; then slight transpiration, with a sound sleep; afterward, in the morning, scrapy sensation, bad taste in the mouth; loss of appetite and the left eye closed by suppuration.

Constant chill, with severe thirst and internal heat, with hot hands and loathing of food and drink (aft. 14 d.).

First, chilliness, then heat in the face (aft. 2 d.). [*Rl.*]

Fever, after being heated to severe sweat and taking cold then in a cold bed, with burning headache, heat in the face, and severe, almost unbearable shivering of the whole body; then with a three days' sweat, so severe a stuffed coryza that he can scarcely get a breath (aft. 38 d.).

Heat, at first in the afternoon, and burning of the eyes like fever (with open windows), and immediately afterward, in the open air, a chill.

635. Dry heat on the cheeks and hands, with short breath.

Increased warmth at night, with violent pains of the zygoma. [*Ng.*]

External and internal heat, toward morning, without thirst (2d d.). [*Ng.*]

Heat in the evening in bed, without sweat afterward. [*Ng.*]

Dry heat in the evening, over the whole body. [*Ng.*[

1640. Feverish heat, every forenoon at nine and in the afternoon about five o'clock, half an hour to an hour, with deep yawning, severe thirst, headache and throbbing in the abdomen.

In the evening, chill and heat in alternation, and the following night, perspiration (3d d.).

Sweat breaks out readily by day.

Profuse sweat, while walking.

Profuse sweat, at every mental exertion, while reading, writing, etc.

1645. **Night-sweat** (the first 3 nights, aft. 2 h. and aft. 6 d.).

Night sweat (4th d.). [*Htb.*]

Morning-sweat in bed.

In the morning in bed, slight transpiration all over the body (6th d.).

During sleep, perspiration on the head, neck and trunk.

1650. Pulse slower than usual (29th d.). [*Gff.*]